Primary Care
of Women

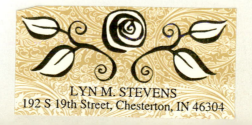

a LANGE medical book

Primary Care of Women

first edition

Edited by

Dawn P. Lemcke, MD
Section Head
Center for Women's Health
Virginia Mason Medical Center
Seattle, Washington

Julie Pattison, MD
Section of General Internal Medicine
Center for Women's Health
Virginia Mason Medical Center
Seattle, Washington

Lorna A. Marshall, MD
Section Head
Reproductive Endocrinology
Department of Obstetrics & Gynecology
Virginia Mason Medical Center
Seattle, Washington

Assistant Clinical Professor
Department of Obstetrics & Gynecology
University of Washington
School of Medicine
Seattle, Washington

Deborah S. Cowley, MD
Associate Professor
Department of Psychiatry & Behavioral Sciences
University of Washington
School of Medicine
Seattle, Washington

Medical Director
Department of Psychiatry
Harborview Medical Center
Seattle, Washington

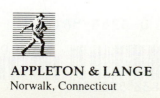

APPLETON & LANGE
Norwalk, Connecticut

Copyright © 1995 by Appleton & Lange
A Simon & Schuster Company

95 96 97 98 / 10 9 8 7 5 4 3 2 1

Prentice Hall International (UK) Limited, *London*
Prentice Hall of Australia Pty. Limited, *Sydney*
Prentice Hall of Canada, Inc., *Toronto*
Prentice Hall Hispanoamericana, S.A., *Mexico*
Prentice Hall of India Private Limited, *New Delhi*
Prentice Hall of Japan, Inc., *Tokyo*
Simon & Schuster Asia Pte. Ltd., *Singapore*
Editora Prentice Hall do Brazil Ltda., *Rio de Janeiro*
Prentice Hall, Englewood Cliffs, *New Jersey*

ISBN: 0-8385-9813-7
ISSN: 1082-1333

Acquisitions Editor: Shelley Reinhardt
Production Editor: Chris Langan
Designer: Elizabeth Schmitz
Senior Art Coordinator: Maggie Belis Darrow

PRINTED IN THE UNITED STATES OF AMERICA

ISBN 0-8385-9813-7

9 780838 598139

90000

Table of Contents

SECTION XII: GYNECOLOGIC DISORDERS

SECTION XIII: REPRODUCTIVE HEALTH ISSUES

Authors

David M. Aboulafia, MD
Section of Oncology/Hematology, Department of Internal Medicine, Virginia Mason Medical Center, Seattle, Washington.

Rosemary Agostini, MD
Clinical Assistant Professor of Orthopedics, University of Washington School of Medicine; Team Physician at Cleveland High School; Sports Medicine and Family Practice, Virginia Mason Sports Medicine Center, Seattle, Washington.

Lesley Althouse, MD, MRCP
Attending Physician, Section of General Internal Medicine, Virginia Mason Medical Center; Clinical Assistant Professor, Department of Internal Medicine, University of Washington School of Medicine, Seattle.

Tamara G. Bavendam, MD
Assistant Professor of Urology and Director of Female Urology, University of Washington Medical Center, Seattle, Washington.

James W. Benson, Jr., MD
Clinical Associate Professor, Department of Medicine, University of Washington School of Medicine; Section of Endocrinology, Virginia Mason Medical Center, Seattle, Washington.

Jane L. Becker, MD
Attending Physician, Section of General Internal Medicine, Virginia Mason Medical Center, Seattle, Washington.

Jennifer D. Bolen, MD
Clinical Faculty, Department of Psychiatry and Behavioral Sciences, University of Washington School of Medicine, Seattle, Virginia Mason Medical Center, Seattle, Washington.

James E. Bredfeldt, MD
Section of Gastroenterology, Virginia Mason Medical Center, Seattle, Washington.

Kate H. Brown, PhD
Associate Professor of Health Policy and Ethics, Center for Health Policy and Ethics, Creighton University, Omaha, Nebraska.

Dedra Buchwald, MD
Associate Professor, Department of Medicine, University of Washington School of Medicine; Director, Chronic Fatigue Clinic, Harborview Medical Center, Seattle, Washington.

Roger W. Bush, MD
Attending Physician, Section of General Internal Medicine, Virginia Mason Medical Center, Seattle, Washington.

Joanna Cain, MD
Associate Professor, Division of Gynecologic Oncology, Department of Obstetrics & Gynecology, University of Washington School of Medicine, Seattle.

Carolyn M. Clancy, MD
Director of the Division of Health Care Sciences, Agency for Health Care Policy and Research, Rockville, Maryland; Assistant Clinical Professor of Health Care Sciences, George Washington University, Washington, D.C.

Kitty Corbett, MPH, PhD
Assistant Professor, Anthropology Department and Health and Behavioral Sciences Program, University of Colorado at Denver; Adjunct Investigator, Northern California Kaiser Permanente Medical Care Program, Division of Research, Oakland, California.

Deborah S. Cowley, MD
Associate Professor, Department of Psychiatry and Behavioral Sciences, University of Washington School of Medicine, Seattle; Medical Director, Department of Psychiatry, Harborview Medical Center, Seattle, Washington.

Jennifer I. Downey, MD
Assistant Professor of Clinical Psychiatry and Consultant to the Department of Obstetrics & Gynecology, Columbia University, College of Physicians and Surgeons, New York, New York.

Mary Ann Draye, ARNP, MPH
Assistant Professor, Primary Health Care, University of Washington, School of Nursing; Fertility & Endocrine Center, University of Washington Med-

ical Center, Seattle; Family Nurse Practitioner, Seattle, Washington.

Debra S. Fetherston, MD
Attending Physician, Section of General Internal Medicine, Virginia Mason Medical Center, Seattle, Washington.

Edward F. Gibbons, MD
Attending Cardiologist and Medical Director, Critical Care Unit and Medical Director, Echocardiography Laboratory, Virginia Mason Medical Center, Seattle, Washington.

Leslie Hartley Gise, MD
Associate Clinical Professor, Department of Psychiatry and Department of Obstetrics, Gynecology, & Reproductive Sciences, Mount Sinai School of Medicine, New York, New York.

Margo C. Grady, MS
Genetic Counselor, Prenatal Diagnosis Center, Meriter Hospital, Madison, Wisconsin.

Marilyn A. Guthrie, RD
Manager of Health Promotion and Patient Education, Virginia Mason Medical Center, Seattle, Washington.

Laura J. Hart, MD
Urologist in private practice, Parma, Ohio.

Julia R. Heiman, PhD
Professor of Psychiatry and Behavioral Sciences, University of Washington School of Medicine; Director, Reproductive and Sexual Medicine Clinic, University of Washington Outpatient Psychiatry Center, Seattle, Washington.

Susan K. Hendricks, MD
Associate Professor and Director, Maternal-Fetal Medicine, University of Wisconsin Medical School.

Steven M. Juergens, MD
Assistant Clinical Professor of Psychiatry, University of Washington School of Medicine; Medical Director, Outpatient Chemical Dependency Program, Virginia Mason Medical Center, Seattle, Washington.

Robert A. Kanter, MD
Clinical Assistant Professor of Medicine, University of Washington School of Medicine, Seattle.

Raymond H. Kaufman, MD
Professor, Department of Obstetrics & Gynecology, Baylor College of Medicine, Houston, Texas.

Matthew P. Kaul, MD
Clinical Assistant Professor, Department of Reha-

bilitation, University of Washington School of Medicine, Seattle.

Michael M. Klotz, MD
Department of Obstetrics & Gynecology, Virginia Mason Medical Center, Seattle, Washington.

Irene Kuter, MD, DPhil
Assistant Professor in Medicine, Harvard Medical School, Boston, Massachusetts; Assistant Physician, Massachusetts General Hospital, Boston.

Joyce K. Lammert, MD, PhD
Clinical Instructor in Allergy & Immunology, Department of Medicine, University of Washington School of Medicine, Seattle; Section Head, Allergy & Immunology, Virginia Mason Clinic, Seattle, Washington.

Dawn P. Lemcke, MD
Section Head, Center for Women's Health, Virginia Mason Medical Center, Seattle, Washington.

Gerard S. Letterie, MD
Assistant Clinical Professor, Department Obstetrics & Gynecology, University of Washington School of Medicine, Seattle; Section of Reproductive Endocrinology, Department of Obstetrics & Gynecology, Virginia Mason Medical Center, Seattle, Washington.

Irving G. Leon, PhD
Lecturer, Departments of Psychology and Psychiatry, University of Michigan, Ann Arbor.

Patricia A. Lipscomb, MD, PhD
Clinical Associate Professor, Department of Psychiatry and Behavioral Sciences, University of Washington School of Medicine, Seattle.

Lorna A. Marshall, MD
Section Head, Reproductive Endocrinology, Department of Obstetrics & Gynecology, Virginia Mason Medical Center, Seattle, Washington; Assistant Clinical Professor, Department of Obstetrics & Gynecology, University of Washington School of Medicine, Seattle.

Charlea T. Massion, MD
Assistant Clinical Professor, Division of Family and Community Medicine, Department of Medicine, Stanford University School of Medicine, Stanford, California.

Mary Ellen Maxell, MN, RN-C, ARNP
Clinical Faculty, Department of Community Health Care Systems, School of Nursing, University of Washington, Seattle; Advanced Registered Nurse Practitioner, Center for Women's Health, Virginia Mason Medical Center, Seattle, Washington.

Jane L. Miller, MD
Assistant Professor, Department of Urology, University of Washington School of Medicine, Seattle.

Joan Ellen Miller, MD
General Internist, Department of Internal Medicine, Virginia Mason Bellevue, Bellevue, Washington.

Howard G. Muntz, MD
Section of Gynecologic Oncology, Virginia Mason Medical Center, Seattle; Clinical Assistant Professor, Department of Obstetrics & Gynecology, University of Washington School of Medicine, Seattle, Washington.

Kathleen M. Ober, PhD
Patient Care Medical Group, NAF Miramar Branch Medical Clinic, San Diego, California.

Patricia L. Paddison, MD
Psychiatrist, Center for Women's Health, Virginia Mason Medical Center, Seattle, Washington.

Laird G. Patterson, MD
Associate Clinical Professor, Department of Medicine, University of Washington School of Medicine, Seattle; Staff Physician, Virginia Mason Medical Center, Seattle, Washington.

Julie Pattison, MD
Section of General Internal Medicine, Center for Women's Health, Virginia Mason Medical Center, Seattle, Washington.

Kathy Preciado-Partida, MD
Virginia Mason Clinic, Issaquah, Washington.

Margot Putukian, MD
Assistant Professor, Departments of Orthopedics and Internal Medicine, Pennsylvania State University College of Medicine, and Team Physician, Pennsylvania State University, University Park, Pennsylvania.

Nancy L. Risser, MN, RN, CS, ANP
Clinical Assistant Professor of Nursing, University of Medicine and Dentistry of New Jersey, Newark; Pulmonary Clinical Nurse Specialist and Adult Nurse Practitioner, Department of Veterans Affairs Medical Center, Lyons, New Jersey.

Marcia E. Robbins, MSW
Psychotherapist in private practice; Adjunct Faculty, University of Washington School of Social Work, Seattle, Washington.

Romy Royce, MS, ARNP
Clinical Faculty, University of Washington, Seattle; Family Health Practitioner, Center for Women's Health, Virginia Mason Medical Center, Seattle, Washington.

Edward K. Rynearson, MD
Clinical Professor, Department of Psychiatry & Behavioral Sciences, University of Washington School of Medicine, Seattle; Virginia Mason Medical Center, Seattle, Washington.

James R. Simmons, MD
General Internist, Section of General Internal Medicine, Virginia Mason Medical Center; Associate Program Director, Internal Medicine Residency Program, Virginia Mason Medical Center, Seattle, Washington.

Beth Skrypzak, MD
Department of Obstetrics & Gynecology, Virginia Mason Medical Center, Seattle, Washington.

Paul A. Smith, MD
Attending Physician, Department of General Internal Medicine, Virginia Mason Medical Center, Seattle, Washington.

Karen C. Smith, MD
Staff Physician, Department of General Internal Medicine, Virginia Mason Medical Center, Seattle, Washington.

David E. Soper, MD
Professor, Department of Obstetrics & Gynecology and Division of Infectious Diseases, Department of Medicine, Medical College of Virginia, Richmond.

Laura R. Stone, MD
Senior Staff Physician, Department of Obstetrics & Gynecology, Alexandria Hospital, Alexandria, Virginia.

Nancy K. Sugg, MPH, MD
Assistant Professor of Medicine, University of Washington School of Medicine, Seattle; Harborview Medical Center, Seattle, Washington.

Richard C. Thirlby, MD
Clinical Assistant Professor, Department of Surgery, University of Washington School of Medicine, Seattle; Department of Surgery, Virginia Mason Medical Center, Seattle, Washington.

Catherine S. Thompson, MD
Attending Physician, Nephrology, Transplant, & Hypertension, Virginia Mason Medical Center, Seattle, Washington.

Maryann Von Eschen, MS
Genetic Counselor, Prenatal Diagnosis Center, Meriter Hospital, Madison, Wisconsin.

Edward A. Walker, MD
Assistant Professor, Departments of Psychiatry and Obstetrics & Gynecology, University of Washington School of Medicine, Seattle.

Kathe Wallace, PT
Northlake Physical Therapy, Seattle, Washington.

Faren H. Williams, MD
Assistant Clinical Professor, University of Washington School of Medicine, Seattle; Physiatrist, Virginia Mason Medical Center, Seattle, Washington.

Joseph L. Yon, MD
Clinical Professor, Section of Gynecologic Oncology, Department of Obstetrics & Gynecology, University of Washington School of Medicine, Seattle; Head, Section of Gynecologic Oncology, Virginia Mason Medical Center, Seattle, Washington.

Preface

The health care of women is generally more fragmented than that of men. This is due in part to their obstetric and gynecologic needs. It may also reflect the fact that many primary care providers feel uncomfortable dealing with some aspects of the care of women, because of unfamiliarity with or inadequate training in women's issues, particularly in gynecology and mental health. In addition, psychosocial issues, mental health issues, and lifestyle issues, all of which are important in the health of women, are time consuming and difficult to address in the context of a busy practice, leading to further referrals and fragmentation of care.

Primary Care of Women seeks to help primary care providers deal more effectively with the health care needs of women, thus delivering more integrated care. The book was originally conceived as an outgrowth of clinical work done at the Center for Women's Health at Virginia Mason Medical Center in Seattle. The Center was established in the Fall of 1988 and has experienced rapid growth both in number of providers and patient visits, with patient visits totaling 20,000 in 1993. In the Center, comprehensive care of women is provided by a team of internists, allied health professionals, obstetricians-gynecologists, psychiatrists, and social workers. This approach has been enthusiastically received by patients, provided valuable training for residents, allowed providers to learn from each other, and taught us both what we know and how much we do not know about women's unique health care needs.

Consistent with this clinical approach, *Primary Care of Women* is multidisciplinary, encompassing a variety of topics in internal medicine, obstetrics and gynecology, and mental health. Other areas covered include both more general issues such as women's access to health care, communication styles, preventative care, and cultural and racial issues as well as more specific disorders and medical conditions. The specific topics included are those which are unique to, more prevalent in, or present differently in women. It is not the intent of this text to provide in–depth discussions of specific diseases but rather a clinically useful broad overview with selected references to which the reader can turn for more details. Sections on when to refer to a specialist are included to facilitate effective referrals where indicated.

Women's health care as a distinct entity is clearly in its infancy. Increasing attention is being given to the phenomenology and treatment of illness in women and to conditions of particular concern to females, such as breast cancer, osteoporosis, eating disorders, and menopause. This heightened focus on the health care of women is reflected in the NIH Women's Health Initiative; in the burgeoning number of conferences, studies, and publications concerning women's health; and in the development of medical school and residency curricula on the health care of women. Much of the material contained in this edition will change dramatically over the next decade with the increase in research regarding women's health. For now, however, we hope this book will be of help in improving the ability of all of us to provide integrated, comprehensive, and sensitive health care to our female patients.

AUDIENCE

This book will be helpful to those providing primary care to women including internists, family physicians, obstetricians-gynecologists, allied health professionals as well as medical students and residents.

ACKNOWLEDGMENTS

The editors wish to thank the following individuals for their help in this major undertaking: The authors for their time and expertise; Dorinda Monson and Serin Posick for their talents as all around editorial assistants; Jane Lopez for the hours of word processing that she skillfully performed without complaint; Dr. Patricia Paddison for her help in the initial organization of the book; our patients from whom we learn how to be better doctors; and finally, our families and children for their patience and support.

Seattle

April 1995

Dawn P. Lemcke, MD

Julie Pattison, MD

Lorna A. Marshall, MD

Deborah S. Crowley, MD

Section I.
General Issues

Women's Access to Health Care

1

Charlea T. Massion, MD, Carolyn M. Clancy, MD, & Mary Ellen Maxell, MN, ARNP

What is "access to health care?" According to the 1993 National Academy of Sciences Institute of Medicine (IOM) report, *Access to Health Care in America,* "access is a shorthand term for a broad set of concerns that center on the degree to which individuals and groups are able to obtain needed services from the medical care system." The IOM report also describes access as "the timely use of personal health services to achieve the best possible health outcomes."

One aspect of the current national focus on health care reform is an emphasis on the importance of universal access to health services. The United States leads the world in health spending; yet, among industrialized countries, only the USA and South Africa lack national health plans that guarantee health care for all. The debate about how to provide universal access at an affordable cost has created confusion about the meaning of access. Many people equate access with insurance coverage or with the number of health providers and health facilities within a geographic area. However, having insurance or local health care services is no guarantee that people who need services will get them. Conversely, many people without insurance or who live in areas with apparent shortages of health care resources manage to receive services.

Access is affected also by attitudes toward health and health care, gender, and social and cultural factors. For example, one may consider the potential barriers to access of an indigent black teenager who is pregnant, lives in a metropolis, and lacks transportation to a prenatal clinic; of a woman who lives in rural Alabama, who is being physically abused by her husband, a prominent police official; of an elderly Vietnamese woman with a breast mass who must rely on her son-in-law as a translator and who is hesitant to describe this problem to either her son-in-law or the male physician.

Access to health care has two complementary facets: population-based strategies and personal health services. Each has important implications for national health and for an individual's ability to attain and maintain optimal health. However, population-based programs are probably more important than personal health services. For example, policies related to pollution exposure, health education, occu-

| Financial/Insurance Issues |
| Organization of Health Care |
| Provider Attitudes & Skills |
| Gaps in the Biomedical Model |
| Monitoring Access |
| Summary |

pational health, and injury control potentially can save more lives and have a greater impact on quality of life than programs to extend personal health services. However, with the tremendous amount of national resources currently devoted to personal health care, equity of access must be monitored.

Negative outcomes that can be prevented are indicators of potential problems of access to health services. Even if a particular health service is often effective, a good health outcome cannot be guaranteed. The most important consideration in access is whether people have the opportunity for a good outcome. For example, although getting regular Papanicolaou (Pap) tests does not guarantee that a woman will avoid cervical cancer, an increased incidence of advanced cervical cancer can be a national warning sign that many women have inadequate access to basic preventive services.

From 1983 to 1993, there was little evidence of progress in increasing access to personal health care services for either women or men. The IOM report states that "stagnation is the best single word to characterize our current state." Indicators of increased access, such as improvements in breast cancer screening rates, were counterbalanced by surges of infectious disease, such as tuberculosis and congenital syphilis. Most indicators of access reveal a growing division between the "haves" and "have-nots" in our society. And women, more often than men, are in the have-not sector.

Against this backdrop, this chapter reviews several factors that affect women's access to health care in our present system: financial/insurance, organization, provider attitudes and skills, and gaps in the biomedical model. The chapter also describes ways in which the monitoring of health care access can be improved and how allied health professionals can expand women's access to health care.

FINANCIAL/INSURANCE ISSUES

The current USA employer-based financing for health insurance is a historical accident that began during World War II. To avoid inflation, the War Labor Board froze wages. Trade unions proposed "hidden raises" through employer contributions for health insurance. The result was the birth of the job-linked health insurance system that dominates medical care in the USA. Today, this system functions well for fewer and fewer people; it works particularly poorly for women. The breadth of one's employee benefits reflects status and income, ie, the higher one's pay, the better the benefits.

Women use health services more frequently than men but are more likely than men to encounter financial barriers to care. Although women are more likely than men to have some insurance, they are twice as likely to be underinsured, ie, to have limited coverage with high-cost sharing, such as high copayments or high deductibles. Women have lower incomes than men and constitute a majority of the nonunionized, part-time service workers whose employers provide either no health insurance or catastrophic coverage only. Many women obtain insurance through a spouse and thus are vulnerable if the marriage dissolves or if their spouse's employer decreases or eliminates dependent coverage.

Despite recent increases of Medicaid benefits for women and children, 14 million women of childbearing age remain without any coverage, and 5 million have insurance that excludes coverage for prenatal care and delivery. Middle-aged women pay higher premiums than middle-aged men, are less likely to obtain insurance through employers, and are twice as likely to have no insurance. Analysis has demonstrated that Medicare provides better coverage for illnesses that are more common in men than for those more prevalent in women. This discrepancy occurs because acute illnesses, which are more common in elderly men (eg, lung cancer, pneumonia, prostate disorders, and myocardial infarction), generate lower out-of-pocket expenses than chronic diseases, which are more common in elderly women (eg, breast cancer, depression, hypertension, and arthritis). Coverage of prescription drugs and benefits for long-term care are excluded by Medicare. These services are of vital importance to women, who live longer and, as noted, have more chronic illnesses than men.

Ambulatory care is covered through Medicare Part B, which requires an additional premium payment. To cover costs beyond Medicare benefits and for the premiums and copayments for Part B, most elderly people have supplementary insurance. This additional coverage may be obtained through a retirement plan, by direct purchase, or if the person is eligible, through Medicaid. Because of their lower socioeconomic status and more limited retirement benefits, elderly women are more likely than men either to be solely dependent on Medicare or to have Medicaid to supplement Medicare.

Currently, 60% of persons over age 60 and 71% of those over age 85 are women. Demographic trends point to an increasing proportion of elderly women. As a result, older women constitute a disproportionate percentage of our nation's elderly, and if current gender-biased reimbursement policies continue, health care financing will diverge even further from women's needs.

Medicaid, the public insurance program, plays a critical role in ensuring access to health care for poor women, but it falls far short of providing comprehensive, uniform benefits. Within federal guidelines, states are required to provide Medicaid coverage to pregnant women who have incomes of up to 133% of the poverty level; states have the option to expand eligibility to those within 185% of this level. States also provide Medicaid coverage to single-parent families with dependent children. Medicaid covers a higher proportion of low-income women of childbearing age than any other group of adults. Because of Medicaid's income and categoric restrictions, however, only 42% of poor women are eligible.

Medicaid benefits for pregnant women are limited to treatment of pregnancy-related conditions and terminate 60 days after delivery unless a woman qualifies for welfare benefits. Thus, a medical problem such as diabetes or hypertension, detected during pregnancy, may not be followed. Medicaid reimbursement for cervical and breast cancer screening varies by state. A 1991 survey by the American College of Obstetrics and Gynecology (ACOG) revealed wide variations by state in reimbursement and in screening intervals for Pap tests and mammography.

Health care delivery for women enrolled in Medicaid is currently undergoing major changes as many states encourage or require Medicaid recipients to enroll in managed care organizations. It is too early to predict the effects of these policies on access for low-income women, because previous experience of low-income people in managed care organizations has been limited to a few pilot programs.

Women assume a disproportionate burden as caretakers for family members of all ages: the young, the sick, and the elderly. This responsibility often disrupts employment and, consequently, insurance coverage. The caretaker also may face nonfinancial obstacles to obtaining her own medical care, especially preventive services, such as lack of time, transportation, or respite care.

The current health care system in this country reflects societal inequities based on socioeconomic status and gender. Many women face prohibitive cost sharing to obtain primary care services and are at risk for developing preventable diseases or receiving inadequate care. A reformed health care system should enhance women's ability to obtain effective services without fear of unreasonable financial penalties for seeking preventive care or obtaining health advice and education.

ORGANIZATION OF HEALTH CARE

Although a woman with health insurance has financial access to care, the current way that women's health services are organized may prevent her from receiving comprehensive, coordinated primary care or from using appropriate specialized services. Historically, women's health care needs have been categorized as "reproductive" and "all other." Physicians in three specialties provide overlapping services to adult women: family physicians, internists, and gynecologists. However, gynecologists, according to an analysis of data from the National Ambulatory Medical Care Survey, were nearly twice as likely as family physicians and internists to include a pelvic examination, Pap test, and breast examination in a general medical examination. Consequently, many women, particularly during their reproductive years, may need to see more than one physician for primary care services.

Recent trends in health care financing amplify this overlap. Specifically, health maintenance organizations that require women to have primary care providers (most often family physicians or internists) now offer a "GYN benefit," which allows women, in addition to other primary care services, the opportunity to visit a gynecologist annually. Although this allowance is labeled a "benefit," it may obligate a woman to split her basic health care between two providers and possibly two locations. Also, the split may create either duplications or omissions in the coordination of basic screening tests and health education efforts.

Information from the National Health Interview Survey also reflects inadequacies in the delivery of preventive health services to women. Women who have not had a recent Pap test, breast examination, or blood pressure check are more likely to be poor, which reflects socioeconomic barriers to obtaining recommended services. Furthermore, most women who have not had recent cancer screening tests have had a recent physician contact, a fact that indicates inadequacies in access to preventive services. For example, a woman with severe asthma may have had multiple emergency visits for respiratory distress yet may never have had a mammogram, Pap test, or cholesterol check.

In the USA, many women seek health care for themselves and their families from allied health professionals (AHPs), primarily nurse practitioners, certified nurse-midwives, and physician assistants.

Since the 1925 inception of nurse-midwifery at the Kentucky Frontier Nursing Service and the start of nurse practitioner and physician assistant training programs in the mid-1960s, AHPs repeatedly have been shown to provide high-quality primary care services in a cost-effective manner in a variety of settings. AHPs are well accepted by patients and have substantially lower training and employment costs than physicians. AHPs have provided increased access to basic health services in many geographic and practice settings; in many rural and inner-city areas, they are the only providers available. In 1992 the ratio was one AHP to every twelve physicians and one to four primary care physicians. There has been no systematic effort to evaluate these ratios in relation to national health goals or decisions to fund training programs.

Despite the proven effectiveness of AHPs, major barriers to improving access to these practitioners exist. States have conflicting laws that restrict the scope of practice and prescriptive authority of AHPs. Reimbursement standards, both state and federal, are fragmented; often fees paid to AHPs are lower than fees paid to physicians for identical services. As a result, AHPs are severely hampered from achieving their potential to enhance access to primary care. These barriers could be addressed by regulatory reform through state and federal legislation.

Other barriers to AHP practice include limited acceptance by physicians, difficulties obtaining professional liability insurance, and inadequate reimbursement for preventive, screening, counseling, and educational services. When these barriers are addressed, AHPs will be able to contribute more effectively to the health care of women.

Two current developments in health care organization may affect women's access to health care in a positive way: first, the increased development of interdisciplinary women's health centers, which offer many services at a single site and which, in some models, offer more psychologic and educational services than are usually available; and second, the creation of a medical specialty in women's health, which would combine aspects of training in gynecology, psychiatry, and internal medicine with more focus on the psychologic and social aspects of women's health needs, aspects that are relatively neglected by all specialties. Several pilot residency and fellowship training programs in women's health are already underway.

Health care reform and the growth of managed care systems offer potential opportunities to address issues of reimbursement, practice patterns, liability coverage, interdisciplinary collaboration, and primary care access. Innovative models of practice with physicians, AHPs, and members of other disciplines can result in improved availability and quality of primary care services to women.

PROVIDER ATTITUDES & SKILLS

Despite adequate financial access to care, a woman may receive services based more on provider attitudes and skills than on her essential health needs. Health services researchers have reported significant disparities between women and men in the use of major diagnostic and therapeutic interventions. For example, men are consistently more likely than women to be referred for cardiac catheterization, coronary artery bypass surgery, renal dialysis, and other expensive, invasive procedures. Analysis indicates that many of these interventions are overused, ie, applied with insignificant or no effect on outcome. However, it is unclear whether men receive too many procedures, women receive too few, or both. One study suggests that women receive more appropriate cardiac services than men do. Current efforts to improve the application of technology can enhance the quality of care for both women and men and eliminate differences in utilization based solely on gender.

Another factor that can affect women's access to services is the apparent difference in the behaviors of female and male physicians. For example, a study by Lurie et al of almost 98,000 female patients enrolled in a prepaid health plan showed that women were more likely to undergo Pap tests and mammograms if they saw a female rather than a male physician, particularly if the physician was an internist or family practitioner. The screening rates were lowest for male internists and family physicians under age 38. Another study, not limited to a prepaid health plan, also showed that women whose usual source of care was a female practitioner were more likely to receive Pap tests, breast examinations, and mammograms than women whose usual source of care was a male provider.

The issue of access to abortion is another example of the effect of provider attitude and skills; it also exemplifies the complex social and political forces that affect women's access to health care. In 1977 the United States Supreme Court declared that states did not have to fund abortions through Medicaid. This decision resulted in 44 million women without financial access to abortion. Since that time, the Court also has allowed states to restrict access to abortions. State-created limitations and obstacles include waiting periods, parental consent laws, counseling and "informed consent" stipulations, and prohibition of the use of public facilities for abortion. Beyond these legal and financial restrictions is the reduced supply of physicians who are willing and trained to perform abortions. In 1992 83% of counties and nearly 25% of metropolitan areas in the USA lacked even a single abortion provider. Also, medical schools and residency programs have decreased training opportunities for first-trimester abortions. In 1991 only 13% of all obstetric/gynecologic residency programs required first-trimester abortion training, even though abortion is one of the most common surgical procedures in this field of medicine.

The content of a medical encounter is another aspect of access to health care. For example, if a woman with a vaginal infection believes she cannot discuss her psychologic and social concerns with her physician, she may not have access to appropriate services, such as contraceptive counseling and testing for sexually transmitted diseases. Studies of patient-physician communication indicate that female physicians generally conduct medical visits differently from male physicians. Although sensitive male providers certainly exist, these studies show that female physicians generally talk more, ask more questions, and engage in more positive talk and partnership building. Female physicians tend to be more informative, both medically and psychosocially. Both male and female patients talk more and appear to participate more actively in the medical dialogue when with a female physician. Positive, partnership-building communication is known to be important for facilitating life-style changes. Women's primary causes of morbidity and mortality, eg, cardiovascular disease, diabetes, and certain types of cancer, are related to life-style choices. In a partnership model, which can be created by either a female or a male physician, there is greater potential for supporting changes in unhealthy habits, such as smoking, drinking alcohol, eating high-fat foods, and maintaining a sedentary life-style.

GAPS IN THE BIOMEDICAL MODEL

At the 1993 conference "Women's Health and Primary Care," sponsored by the Center for Health Policy Research and the Department of Healthcare Sciences at George Washington University, a central question of the Women's Health Care Access Group was, "access to **what**?" The question reflected the recognition that gaps in the biomedical model have serious consequences for women. For example, domestic violence is estimated to cause more injuries to women than auto accidents, rapes, and muggings combined. Research at Yale University indicates that battering accounts for almost one of five emergency room visits for women. A 1992 study showed that, compared to a control group, abused women had triple the hospital admissions, although most of the abused women's hospital stays were for nontraumatic disorders. Physicians screen routinely for breast problems, but most do not screen routinely for domestic violence. Within the current biomedical model, women may have repeated encounters with the medical system for the treatment of problems that result directly from violence; however, if they lack services that may stop or prevent violence, they do not have effective health care access.

The health consequences of other common women's health problems, such as eating disorders or a history of sexual abuse, are currently being defined and are discussed further in Chapters 10 and 16, respectively. The health effects of these problems will not be solved by access to new drugs, surgical procedures, or machines. For example, for a woman who experiences pelvic pain as a consequence of previous sexual abuse, better access to a hysterectomy is an inappropriate solution. Extensive testing to evaluate headaches that are symptoms of an eating disorder or depression results in high bills for neurologic consultation and has little effect on outcome except to increase medical costs and, most likely, to frustrate both the patient and the provider.

The biomedical model concentrates on an individual patient treated by an individual physician or multiple physicians. However, several recent studies—of patients with breast cancer, lymphoma, and malignant melanoma, and of those recovering from heart attacks—have shown that participating in support groups not only improves people's moods and coping skills but also may help them live longer. Unfortunately, many inexpensive group interventions are not part of standard treatment but are offered as adjuncts to medical care. They are not reimbursable by insurance plans, although these interventions cost a fraction of fully covered, invasive procedures.

MONITORING ACCESS

In 1993 the IOM Committee on Monitoring Access to Personal Health Care Services reported that our system to monitor access to health care had many deficiencies. The Committee worked to define "access objectives and indicators" to assess progress toward national objectives for the personal health care system. IOM objectives that specifically relate to women are (1) promotion of successful birth outcomes and (2) early detection and diagnosis of breast and cervical cancers, assessed through rates of screening mammograms and Pap tests. For birth outcomes, the indicators of access problems include infant mortality, low birth weight, and congenital syphilis. For treatable diseases, the outcome indicators are late-stage breast and cervical cancers. The

IOM Committee suggested that these parameters can be used to improve monitoring of access to health care, similar to the use of economic indicators. The IOM report also advised the development of additional indicators to assess the impact of nonfinancial barriers to achieving optimal health outcomes, including issues of education, language, and transportation. Another indicator of access is the relation between a patient's satisfaction with her or his health care and health outcomes; however, reliable measures to assess satisfaction are still evolving.

SUMMARY

Access to health care is one of the most important social policy issues of the 1990s and has particular relevance for women. Women use health services, more frequently—and perhaps more effectively—than men do. Women tend to use primary care services more often, and they are less likely than men to receive inappropriate, expensive procedures. Health care reform should encourage more effective use of primary care services and more active collaboration of patients and practitioners to promote health rather than simply treat disease.

Current policies often pose substantial challenges to meeting women's health needs. Cost sharing that discourages use of health services, barriers to the practice of AHPs, and delivery systems that virtually mandate brief visits when a longer interaction would be more effective all pose significant threats to the development of a system more responsive to women's needs.

Eliminating financial barriers to obtaining services, the central focus of the current health care reform debate, does not guarantee an effective delivery system. When financial access is ensured, women and their providers can work together to address neglected aspects of health care, such as communication, psychosocial issues, and problems that are currently beyond the biomedical model. The challenge for all those committed to improving women's health is to ensure that increased financial access is accompanied by requisite changes in the organization and delivery of services.

REFERENCES

Bergman J: Utilization of medical care by abused women. Br Med J 1992;305:27.
Bickell NA et al: Referral patterns for coronary artery disease treatment: Gender bias or good clinical judgment? Ann Intern Med 1992;116:791.
Clancy CM: Healthcare reform: The most important women's health issue. Women's Health Forum 1994;3:1.
Clancy CM, Massion CT: American women's healthcare: A patchwork quilt with gaps. JAMA 1992;268:1918.
Collins K: Healthcare reform and women's needs: Financial access issues. Women's Health Forum 1993;2:1.
Crumholz H et al: Selection of patients for coronary angiography and coronary revascularization early after my-

ocardial infarction: Is there evidence for a gender bias? Ann Intern Med 1992;116:785.

Eckholm E (editor): Solving America's health-care crisis. The New York Times Company, 1993.

Franks P, Clancy CM: Physician gender bias in clinical decision making: Screening for cancer in primary care. Med Care 1993;31:213.

Hafner-Eaton C: Will the phoenix rise, and where should she go? The women's health agenda. Am Behav Sci 1993;36:841.

Hall J, Roter D: Examining gender-specific issues in patient/physician communication. Women's Health Primary Care [in press].

Lurie N et al: Preventive care for women: Does the sex of the physician matter? N Engl J Med 1993;329:478.

Lutz M: Women, work and preventive healthcare: An exploratory study of the efficacy of HMO membership. Women's Health 1989;15:21.

Millman M (editor): Access to health care in America. National Academy Press, 1993.

Moore Q: A survey of state Medicaid policies for coverage of screening mammography and Pap smear services. Women's Health Issues 1992;2:40.

Mullan F et al: Doctors, dollars and determination: Making physician work-force policy. Health Affairs 1993;12 (Suppl):138.

Office of Technology Assessment, U.S. Congress, HCS 37: *Nurse Practitioners, Physician Assistants, and Certified Nurse-Midwives: A Policy Analysis, 1986.*

Safriet B: Health care dollars and regulatory sense: The role of advanced practice nursing. Yale J Regul 1992;9:2.

Sofaer S, Abel E: Older women's health and financial vulnerability: Implications of the Medicare benefit structure. Women's Health 1990;16:47.

Spiegel D: Compassion is the best medicine, The New York Times, January 19, 1994.

Woolhandler S, Himmelstein D: Reverse targeting of preventive services due to lack of health insurance. JAMA 1988;259:2872.

Sociocultural Perspectives

2

Kate H. Brown, PhD, & Kitty Corbett, PhD

One of the most rewarding features of medical practice in the United States is working with patients and colleagues from a wide variety of social and cultural backgrounds. This diversity can frustrate clinicians, however, as they may feel they have not "gotten through" to their patients. Language barriers, misunderstandings, and unmet expectations can contribute to a sense of disconnection with patients and can limit clinicians' best efforts to assist patients.

The influence of gender and cultural diversity in health care is a complex issue. This chapter intends to be an orientation for medical care providers to a sociocultural perspective on women's health, illness behaviors, and communication within clinical encounters. While valuing the influence of sociocultural conditioning on individual responses, it is important to remain cautious about fitting patients into cultural categories. Patients, no less than clinicians, draw on many complex features of their lives to make sense of health and disease, giving precedence to varying combinations of these factors in specific circumstances.

DEFINITION OF SOCIOCULTURAL

A defining characteristic of human beings is the ability to create, negotiate and share meaning; anthropologists refer to these shared meanings as **culture.** Language, behavior, ideas, expectations, beliefs, and the tools used to work, eat, and play are learned through and shaped by cultural meanings shared with other group members. Culture pervades, permeates, and guides behaviors, beliefs, and artifacts. Although the influence of sociocultural framework usually remains unconscious or taken for granted as "natural," everyone is subject to these effects. Clinical encounters inevitably reflect the sociocultural influences of both patients and practitioners.

A definition of culture that refers to shared meanings goes beyond the more common use of the term, which usually refers to particular ethnic groups or nationalities. Because most people are members of many groups, they are multicultural. For instance, physicians share meanings with their medical colleagues by virtue of their intense "acculturation" in medical school, where they learned vocabularies for

| Definition of Sociocultural |
| Explanatory Models |
| Definitions of a Medical Problem |
| Causal Theories |
| Decision to Seek Health Care |
| Ethical Issues |
| Explanatory Models in Clinical Settings |
| Communication Between Clinicians & |
| Patients |
| Dynamics of Communication |
| Use of a Translator |
| Conclusion |

specific bodily functions, principles of disease processes, and culturally acceptable ways to approach and talk with patients. But physicians also carry the sociocultural messages from their parents, religious advisors, and friends about what it means to be human, sick, smart, attractive, and right or wrong and how to express these attributes in daily life. Clear communication with patients requires clinicians to appreciate their own and their patients' multiple and diverse cultural sources of information about sickness.

Patients' and clinicians' responses to illness are affected not only by culture, but also by their social position in society. Prestige, wealth, and power shape opportunities, constraints, and pressures that, in turn, are relevant to health and health care. In the USA, social class, racial classification, ethnic identity, and gender influence experience and participation in society. For example, clinicians' experiences and class identity can obscure for them the fundamentally sociologic, political, and economic nature of medical care. Practitioner-patient relationships are hierarchical. Licensed practitioners by virtue of their professional roles are gatekeepers to medication, treatment, referrals, institutions, and financing. They decide whether individual experiences of illness are legitimated as disease (whether pathophysiologic or psychological) and thus merit medical attention. They are frontline stewards of what is normative behavior in society and what is not. Providers' professional identities and their socioeconomic class, educational background, and associated values imply social distance between them and their patients. Use of the term sociocultural reminds readers that social status and culture are inextricably linked in clinical encounters with female patients.

EXPLANATORY MODELS

Although birth, sickness, suffering, and death are universal across time and cultures, anthropologists have observed that there are different patterns of response to these human experiences. The term **explanatory model** is used to describe the constellations of beliefs and behaviors people draw on when faced with these universal events. These internalized models help to make sense of an experience and guide people's actions. Although influenced by individual histories, explanatory models of health and health care are never entirely idiosyncratic responses. Explanatory models are repositories for information, biases, explanations, and assumptions that are taught and reinforced in the course of ongoing sociocultural upbringing.

Definitions of a Medical Problem

It is essential in most clinical encounters that patients and their clinicians clearly identify the issue. This seemingly straightforward task can be confounded by differing sociocultural definitions of the patients' problem. Sociomedical scientists draw on an understanding of culture in their distinction between the terms disease and illness to assist in discerning a possible source of discord between patients and clinicians. **Disease** is defined in terms of the biomedical, physiologic pathology of disorder; it is diagnosed and labeled by physicians and mentioned in scientific terms in medical texts. Disease refers to the culture of biomedicine, and its meaning is accessed most readily by members of the health care team.

The term **illness,** on the other hand, refers to a disorder as perceived by a patient involving a complex interaction of meanings, symbols, social values, and health-related behaviors in addition to biologic conditions and biomedical responses. Illness entails the personal and social acknowledgment that a person cannot fulfill her usual roles adequately, that some kind of malfunctioning is threatening the person and society, and action needs to be taken. Assessment and labeling of illness is a social process, involving a patient's reports of feelings and symptoms and other people's observations and assessments.

A clear example of the distinction between disease and illness is found in interchanges between patients and physicians about such conditions as early stages of cervical dysplasia or hypertension, both of which are observable clinically as diseases but not experienced by patients as illnesses. Less obvious disjunctures can occur when patients present symptoms consistent with their understanding of a "folk illness."

Every cultural group has identifiable folk illnesses that do not correspond in terminology, symptoms, or explanation to biomedical categories of disease. For instance, some patients with ties to traditional Mexican beliefs identify certain kinds of stomach pain as *empacho,* a folk illness attributed to a bolus of food that gets stuck on the stomach or intestinal lining. Differing sociocultural conceptions of the problematic nature of body size, teen pregnancy, and even child neglect can also be sources of misunderstanding between clinicians and patients.

A clinician may not be aware of a patient's understanding of a problem because she neglects to ask the patient or because the patient is wary about appearing unsophisticated or ignorant by disclosing such beliefs. In one such case, a physician from the USA was frustrated in her unsuccessful treatment of a patient from Laos who had chronic pelvic pain. The physician could not address the patient's needs until she understood that the woman's physical pain was exacerbated by another kind of agony: she could not bear children. Scarring from her chronic infection had caused infertility. Focusing on the disease of pelvic pain, the clinician was unaware that the illness of infertility was a major cause of the patient's distress.

Disease, responses to it, and scientific understanding of it are refracted through cultural values and social and historical contexts, as illustrated in recent work by cultural historians. Compelling evidence is found in the context of late nineteenth century American society. At the turn of the century, women's identity and roles underwent profound redefinition in response to economic and technologic changes. In an analysis of the representation of women's illnesses in fiction written between 1840 and 1940, Herndl explains the "widespread acceptance of women's innate unhealthiness" as a response by men and women to these changing role expectations for women. Herndl credits this perception as a response to a threatened status quo. Physicians, who were usually men in those days, "medicalized" women's conditions as disease and legitimated cautionary rationales against a life outside of the home or other ambitions of women that were considered abnormal. Science is never neutral, and disease categories (such as hysteria) and cures (such as prolonged bed rest—sometimes for years!) reflected social norms much more than scientific fact as understood today.

On the positive side, there may have been some secondary gain available to women through the sick role. Smith-Rosenberg suggests that women in the nineteenth century may have used the diagnosis of hysteria as an acceptable escape from familial and societal expectations of the proper woman, wife, and mother. The sick role sometimes carried grave risks and suffering for women, however. Chesler contends that the diagnosis of madness or insanity was used historically by psychiatrists, families, and communities to isolate and institutionalize rebellious women in the name of treatment.

Women's role conflicts, economic insecurity, and relative powerlessness continues to contribute to disease today. By labeling and treating certain behaviors and conditions of women as disease, the culture of the USA reinforces a medicalized response to such phenomena as pregnancy, menopause, and stress disorders. The "truth" of such a perspective is called into question by anthropologists' observations of how other societies treat these conditions. For example, Lock's findings from research on menopause in Japan present a startling contrast to women's experience of menopause in the USA. According to Lock, the interplay of physiologic state and sociocultural interpretations of aging contributes to the perception of menopause in Japan as a "nonevent," unaccompanied by the symptoms, psychologic disturbances, and prescriptions for hormonal therapies commonly associated with menopause in the USA.

Causal Theories

"Why me?" is a ubiquitous question asked by patients. Frequently, a patient's sociocultural upbringing provides a ready answer to this question, which may or may not match the explanations provided by scientific medicine. Through cultural interpretations of signs and symptoms, biologic disease can be transformed into evidence of individual moral decay or divine punishment for personal irresponsibility, as was the case in early hypotheses for the spread of the acquired immunodeficiency syndrome (AIDS). Sociocultural interpretations often are given to illnesses, birth defects, premature deaths, and other conditions and events.

The concept of "imbalance"—whether at the level of cosmic forces, temperature, stress, temperament, diet, hormones, sleep, or exercise—is a common explanation for illness. The specific nature of what is believed to be out of balance and the prescriptive recommendations vary considerably across cultures, but often when patients seek advice and treatment from healers, they want to know how to rebalance something that has gone out of kilter.

In the USA, clinical and community interventions often reflect an ongoing sociocultural controversy concerning the relative significance of the environment and of individual responsibility in causing health problems. For example, there are diseases that are seen by some people as the result of a toxic or sinister environment and by others as the fault of the patient's personality and behavior. When health practitioners make metaphoric associations of diseases with personal uncleanliness, laziness, or violations of moral codes, they reinforce mainstream cultural tendencies to define cause and prevention at the level of the individual. Control of disease is conceptualized in terms of controlling personal behaviors rather than instituting public health measures designed to control pathogens, reduce access to addictive substances, or create healthier the environments in which at-risk populations live.

Tension between values of social responsibility and in individual responsibility often remain unrecognized and unacknowledged society even as they shape clinical practice and national policies concerning health problems. For example, until recently breast cancer prevention has focused more on motivating women to have mammograms than on monitoring environmental uses of estrogenic pesticides. Similarly, concern about low birth weight has resulted in efforts to increase access to prenatal care and educate mothers about dietary and life-style changes. These programs, although important, overlook a number of societal factors that may contribute to prenatal circumstances. Such factors might include the experience of lifelong inequities, changes in the labor market, shifts in the constellations of families and responsibilities, and reductions in social service supports. Blaming the patient, implicitly or overtly, can compound the pathogenic effects of economic deprivation and insecurity and can contribute to lack of treatment or postponed treatment of preventable and life-threatening conditions for women and their families.

Nowhere are the sociocultural foundations of causal theories about disease more relevant to women's health than in the current debates about poverty and health. The epidemiologic connection between poverty and disease and reduced life expectancy rates is well documented, as is the alarming increase in the proportion of women, especially women in an ethnic minority group, and their children living in poverty in this country. As poverty rates increase for women, it should be no surprise to see a concomitant rise in women's health-related conditions: violence and abuse, pregnancy-related problems, coronary heart disease (CHD), substance abuse, and environmentally related cancers.

Outrage concerning societal inattention to these problems is tempered by mainstream USA cultural assumptions about individual responsibility for one's position in life, including poverty. In medical care, this assumption subtly informs the practice of locating patients' problems within the individual and attempting to resolve them at that level. Diseases associated with poverty may be regarded as an outcome of life-style choices and bad luck. External injustices and their consequences (eg, racism, sexism, age bias, differential exposures to environmental hazards, lack of educational opportunities) tend to be ignored or denied in clinical histories and discharge plans, not out of ill will necessarily but because of unconscious or unexamined assumptions about individual will and choice, as well as about the nature of disease.

Decision to Seek Health Care

The decision to seek help for an illness or injury is

a complicated psychologic and sociocultural process influenced by many factors. A potential patient takes into consideration the perceived seriousness of the symptom, past experience with the problem, affordability of the service in relation to other needs, and the expectation that the problem can be alleviated with attention. All these factors are subject to interpretation and weighing according to sociocultural influences. Women's perceived role demands can provide a rationale for either seeking care (eg, I owe it to my children to stay healthy) or delaying it (eg, I am too busy just now caring for my sick parents).

People are influenced by sociocultural messages about who is the most appropriate healer in a given circumstance. In consultation with significant relatives and the popular media, each person decides which is the most appropriate resource. For instance, depending on her upbringing, a patient might believe her problem is best addressed by an over-the-counter medication, a chiropractor, a spiritual healer, her mother, or a physician.

In their historical analysis of women's reproductive health care in Europe and the USA, Ehrenreich and English document the influence of cultural, political, and economic forces on how the availability and legitimacy of obstetric assistance. Even now, when licensed obstetricians are the acknowledged mainstream providers of prenatal care, it is common for pregnant women in the USA to seek help from numerous other sources. These alternative providers give pre- and postnatal dietary advice, massage, and supportive assistance. Their services sometimes are viewed as complementary to obstetricians' recommendations and interventions. Some women prefer the services and advice of these practitioners, however, because they seem more compatible with the patient's cultural expectations for care. For example, lay midwives following Mexican, African American, and Appalachian birth traditions are the first and only source of care for some pregnant women. The amalgam of "New Age" beliefs and rituals used by other lay midwives can provide valued expertise and support for some educated, middle class women living "countercultural" life-styles.

Patients often seek counsel and treatment from several providers simultaneously who practice in different traditions. It may not concern the patient that these providers do not share common theories of healing; the patient is likely to be less interested in theoretic coherence than in feeling better or giving birth to a healthy baby. Such multiple use of health care resources is not necessarily a sign of distrust of a physician's services; language compatibility, price, or kinship connections may be the primary draw to these "alternative" caregivers. Although there may be legal constraints, some medically trained obstetricians and nurse-midwives have found it advantageous to include the services of traditional birth attendants in their practices. Raphael suggests that

birth centers augment the skills of technically trained personnel with those of someone who can fulfill the role of a doula; the term **doula** refers to a birth attendant who provides the emotional and social support pre- and postpartem traditionally available from lay midwives and family members.

Researchers and clinicians have observed that patients' sociocultural background can influence how they ask for help and what they consider to be helpful. For example, Zborowski's study of patients with pain observed that those from Italian heritage were more likely than others to express their complaints verbally and request pain medication; patients with Anglo heritage tended toward stoicism; and Jewish patients, although vocal in their expression of pain, were more relieved than others by causal explanations of the pain. Expectations about pain expression are related to gender differences in some cultures. Comparing usual birth practices in Sweden, the Netherlands, the USA, and Mexico, Jordan observed quite different expectations concerning the appropriate use of pain medication during routine births for optimal birth outcomes. For example, although anesthesia is used routinely in Sweden, it is used only rarely in the Netherlands, where home birth is the norm.

Ethical Issues

Medical practitioners trained in the USA commonly assume that patients make decisions autonomously. The ethical and legal practices of "informed consent" and "advance directives" are predicated on this assumption. This method of decision-making is not practiced by all patients, however; many patients expect to make treatment decisions in consultation with others, and some expect to have little say in these decisions. Decision-making that entirely excludes the patient can appear unjust to a person raised in a culture that values the liberal traditions of autonomy. When a husband answers questions posed to his wife, who remains silent during an interview, or when a woman turns to her husband or to her elderly parents to decide on a course of treatment, a practitioner may feel frustrated or outraged. In such situations, it may be possible to find a place to talk privately with the woman, such as an examining room; it also may be helpful to remember that the woman may not wish to make decisions independently. The clinician needs to figure out whether a woman is reluctant to make a decision autonomously because she is more comfortable with joint decision-making, or whether she would prefer to decide but fears reprisals from others.

Sometimes family members ask clinicians to withhold information about diagnosis and prognosis from the patient, especially when the news might be upsetting. In companion articles, Surbone and Pellegrino reason that variation in our expectations for disclosure of information is based on different cultural understandings of patient autonomy as it relates to truth-telling. Surbone observes that "in Italian culture autonomy (autonomia) is often synonymous for isolation (isolamento) . . . [so] protecting the ill family member from painful information is seen as essential for keeping the family together and not allowing the ill member to suffer alone." Given such an interpretation, Pellegrino advises that "to thrust the truth or the decision on a patient who expects to be buffered against news of impending death is a gratuitous and harmful misinterpretation of the moral foundations for respect for autonomy." Other ethicists would consider it a form of deceitful paternalism to exclude important information from patients who need to make end-of-life decisions on their own behalf.

Explanatory Models
in Clinical Settings

Interpersonal communication between clinicians and patients, compliance with suggested regimens, and overall satisfaction and trust can be improved when physicians understand their patients' backgrounds and are ready to assist in translating between their patients' sociocultural frameworks and that of medicine. The following is a suggested strategy for working through differences in explanatory models during a clinical encounter:

- Proceed from an assumption that all persons involved share the desire both to improve the patient's health and to understand one another clearly.
- Become aware of the sociocultural foundations of one's own personal, ethnic, and possibly "medicocentric," explanatory model. A tool for self-examination follows:

  Strive for ongoing introspective inquiry that not only is personal and emotional but also is framed within a broad historical, cross-cultural, and economic perspective.

  Listen for the sociocultural nature of one's own frames of reference, conceptual maps, and explanatory schemes—the permeating influences of biomedical perspectives and of one's own ethnic, educational, family, and class-related heritage.

  While on the job, use the self as a tool for understanding, through attention to one's own irritations, other feelings, and perceptions.

  When listening to patients who are culturally different watch for unfamiliar postures, mannerisms, gestures, and vocalizations, but remain careful to suspend one's usual interpretations of these behaviors. Consider whether unfamiliar or unusual responses might be sociocultural in origin rather than assuming they have personal or clinical significance, eg, that they are signs of hostility, inattention, or psychologic disorder.

  Note subtle as well as explicit dimensions of power imbalance between providers and clients.

  Travel globally, off the beaten path, and for long periods of time.

  Read broadly, in literature and scholarship.

- Elicit the patient's explanatory model. Following is a list of questions, adapted from the work of Kleinman et al, to help physicians obtain this information:

  1. What do you think your problem is?
  2. What do you think caused it?
  3. Why do you think it started when it did?
  4. How severe is your illness? Will it have a short or a long course?
  5. What kind of treatment do you think you should receive?
  6. Who do you want involved in the decisions about your care?
  7. What are the most important results you hope to receive from this treatment?
  8. What are the chief problems your sickness has caused you?
  9. What do you fear most about your sickness?
  10. Is your financial situation an important consideration for you in deciding about medical treatment?
  11. What do your husband/family/friends think the problem is?
  12. What do your husband/family/friends think should be done about your illness?

- Openly acknowledge areas of difference and overlap in the explanatory models, explaining the basis for one's point of view.
- Tailor procedures and recommendations to fit areas of agreement between explanatory models when medically, practically, and ethically possible.

COMMUNICATION BETWEEN
CLINICIANS & PATIENTS

Dynamics of Communication

Communication between people with different sociocultural backgrounds requires more than a sensitivity to explanatory models of illness and treatment. Clinicians also must be aware of a variety of verbal and nonverbal cues that are essential to communication even when speaking with patients who speak the same language. This section reviews potential pitfalls of communication between patients and providers who do not have a common sociocultural background. Particular attention is paid to the ways that the sociocultural environment of biomedicine influences and constrains the content, direction, and flow of such interchanges.

Medical vocabulary can be problematic even between clinicians and patients who speak the same language when each is unfamiliar with the terms and metaphors used by the other to refer to an illness. For example, although the English terms hypertension, high blood pressure, and high blood seem to relate to the same condition, they may refer to different illnesses, ranging from attention-deficit disorder to a claustrophobic sensation of drowning in one's own blood. Translation from "biomedicalese" into the patient's language is a complicated endeavor, subject to misinterpretation even in the best of circumstances.

Researchers have observed that biomedical interviews, examinations, and procedures have a ritualized, hierarchical structure that can impede cross-cultural communication. Typically, practitioners direct and restrict communication so that they can carry out diagnostic and treatment activities. They control the flow of critical medical information. They initiate topics, ask the bulk of questions, and interrupt more often than patients. Practitioners signal when a consultation is over. This mode of directed questioning may present problems for some patients who share neither an explanatory model to make sense of the diagnostic reasoning shaping the questions, nor an expectation that they should be asked so many questions.

In many ways the medical encounter demonstrates the subordination of the patient's explanatory model, concerns, and autonomy to the demands of biomedical discourse. Practitioners seek to communicate their own explanatory models effectively and to receive indicators of compliance; however, in seeking information about these concerns, they unintentionally may frustrate needs and expectations of patients and their families. Although seemingly efficient, physicians who move too quickly toward a narrow diagnostic goal may miss information that is relevant either to the diagnosis or to subsequent treatment and support of the patient.

Gender also influences practitioner-patient communication; Weisman and West, in separate studies, found that female physicians tend to interrupt patients less and allow patient-initiated questions more than male physicians. According to Burgoon et al, both male and female patients seem to expect and prefer that female practitioners use "low-intensity or nonaggressive communication strategies."

A potentially transformative approach to medical care, according to Waitzkin and Britt, would involve seeking out contextual information of a broadly social or economic nature and exploring presenting problems in the context of such matters (related not merely through somatization of social distress but in relation to, for instance, societal dynamics of power relations). On the other hand, some patients may feel that such questioning is invasive and threatening to their sense of privacy about features of their lives they feel are unrelated to their medical problems.

Sociocultural differences in the presentation and timing of the key topic may contribute to miscommunication as well. To plan a medical interview, a biomedically trained practitioner typically wishes to know the patient's entire agenda at the start. It can be frustrating when a patient waits until the last minute of an office visit to mention what the clinician believes is an essential detail for framing the whole encounter. It is important to consider the possibility that this practice may reflect a cultural norm rather than denial or an irritating idiosyncrasy on the part of the patient. It is common in some cultures to introduce the key topic only after considerable preliminary talk has occurred.

Sociocultural norms also may be at odds with institutional practice with regard to greeting rituals at the beginning of the medical interview. Normative behavior of two persons who have just met one another or have met after a significant absence requires a greeting and usually at least a brief period of informal conversation before the introduction of the key topic. The expectation of most participants is that this period is a courtesy and is essential to the proper unfolding of an interpersonal encounter. This expectation is thwarted, however, when institutions attempt to eliminate such greeting time in clinician-patient meetings. Assigning less costly staff to take over greetings and history-taking has been shown to be ineffective. Despite the institutional mandate, most patients engage in greeting rituals, small talk, and an explanation of their medical history with their doctors regardless of whether they have done it all before with support staff. Aside from politeness or an attempt to establish personal contact, many patients do not trust important information to nonphysician staff or insist on repeating it to the doctor.

The potential is high for miscommunication in medical encounters also because of unshared standards about nonverbal communication. Meanings may be conveyed without words through shifts, often subtle, in posture, gesture, nonverbal utterances, and eye contact. For instance, aversion of one's gaze in many Asian cultures may be a signal of deference, not shyness or insincerity. This topic warrants extensive attention; clinicians who routinely deal with persons of different cultural backgrounds benefit from training in that group's verbal and nonverbal norms.

After years of immersion in institutional routine, providers can forget how the structural aspects of a medical care setting—architectural arrangements, accounting systems, and hierarchies of authority—shape clinical encounters. It is important for clinicians to bring to consciousness their internalized assumptions regarding medical practice so that they can communicate their intentions to patients more explicitly. For example, in the course of their daily communication with patients, physicians may need to remember that a patient does not realize that blood is drawn in the hospital's laboratory, that x-rays are taken on another floor, or that financial inquiries should be directed to an office in another building.

Use of a Translator

Most of the previous discussion has focused on the subtle dynamics of interpersonal communication between patients and physicians who share a common language. Special consideration is needed when a translator is required to facilitate even the most rudimentary communication between patients and practitioners. When using a translator, information is at risk of getting lost in both directions; however, use of specific techniques can help to prevent that loss, even if the translator is unfamiliar to the patient or unskilled in the task. Similar guidelines apply whether the translator is a professional, a friend, or a family member. The following list contains guidelines and cautions for using a translator:

Engage the patient in a brief conversation to ascertain how much of the language the patient understands before asking for a translator.

Translation is difficult to do well. Give thanks and respect when they are due.

Use only one translator at a time; if there are more than one translator available, ask the oldest person present to designate someone for the task.

If the translator is unknown to the patient and her significant others, allow time for establishment of rapport.

Ask the translator to share with the patient the instructions on how the translation will be conducted.

Arrange seating so that the patient is looking at the clinician rather than the translator.

Pause at the end of each sentence for the translator to speak, and insist that others do the same when they speak.

Speak slowly and distinctly in a normal tone of voice.

Use simple phrasing and plain vocabulary, avoiding slang, idiomatic expressions, and abstractions whether or not the translator is skilled in biomedical terminology.

Pay attention to the client's signals of comprehension, including nonverbal and verbal cues.

If possible, allow extra time for the appointment.

Ask the translator immediately after the session if there is other information such as background data that would be helpful for the clinician, patient, or family members to understand.

Write down all pertinent information to give to the patient. Include a brief explanation of the diagnosis, what it means, what should and should not be done. These notes and any additional printed materials about the condition can provide a fixed and accurate reference check in case information is lost in subsequent translations among family and friends.

CONCLUSION

Clinicians should strive to negotiate between their own explanatory models and those of the patient and her relatives or friends. Interpersonal interactions in health care settings ideally should be informed by staff's sensitization to cultural and language differences. Clinicians who routinely deal with members of a specific culturally different group should learn characteristic aspects of their heritage, dietary patterns, ethnomedical traditions, expectations regarding the sick role and providers' behavior, general value orientations, language, and communication styles.

It also is essential to recognize that such information is sensitizing but never prescriptive: individuals vary, and a person's apparent or declared sociocultural identity may correlate less with modal behaviors, beliefs, and expectations than with a recognition of shared ancestry or discrimination.

Such deep understanding of patients' cultural heritage is not always possible, of course. In addition to dealing with diverse individuals from the same sociocultural group, clinicians in the USA are likely to see patients from many different cultural groups. For instance, a practitioner who regularly and competently deals with a Mexican American population one day may find Kurdish refugees in her office waiting room and the next day be asked to treat a Jewish immigrant from Russia and a homeless white youth with multiple body piercings and tattoos.

Because vulnerability, social distance, and bureaucratic constraints will inevitably characterize many encounters between women patients and physicians, it is helpful for all involved to cultivate humility, humor, and sensitivity.

REFERENCES

Burgoon M, Birk TS, Hall JR: Compliance and satisfaction with physician-patient communication: An expectancy theory interpretation of differences. Hum Commun Res 1991;18:177.

Chesler P: *Women and Madness.* Harcourt Brace Jovanovich, 1989.

Costello C, Stone AJ (editors): *The American Woman 1994–1995: A Status Report Focus on Women and Health.* Women's Research and Education Institute, 1994.

Ehrenreich B, English D: *Witches, Midwives, and Nurses:*

A History of Women Healers. Feminist Press at City University of New York, 1973.

Facione NC: Delay versus help seeking for breast cancer symptoms: A critical review of the literature on patient and provider delay. Soc Sci Med 1993;36:1521.

Fisher S, Groce SB: Doctor-patient negotiation of cultural assumptions. Sociol Health Illn 1985;7:72.

Freeman SH: Verbal communication in medical encounters: An overview of recent work. Text 1987;7:33.

Geronimos AT: Teenage childbearing and Social and Reproductive Disadvantage: The Evolution of Complex Questions and the Demise of Simple Answers. Family Relations 1991;40(4):463.

Hahn RA, Atwood DG (editors): *Physicians of Western Medicine: Anthropological Approaches to Theory and Practice.* Reidel, 1985.

Herndl DP: *Invalid Women: Figuring Feminine Illness in American Fiction and Culture, 1840–1940.* University of North Carolina Press, 1993.

Jordan B: *Birth in Four Cultures.* 4th ed. [Revised and expanded by Davis-Floyd R.] Prospect Heights, Il: Waveland Press, 1993.

Kleinman A, Eisenberg L, Good B: Culture, illness, and care: Clinical lessons from anthropologic and cross-cultural research. Ann Intern Med 1978;88:251.

Krieger N, Rowley DL, Herman AA, Avery B, and Phillips MT: Racism, Sexism, and Social Class: Implications for Studies of Health, Disease, and Well-being. American Journal of Preventative Medicine 1993;9(6)[Supplement]:82.

Lock MM: Encounters with Aging: Mythologies of Menopause in Japan and North America. University of California Press, 1993.

Mackenzie M: The pursuit of slenderness and addiction to self-control: An anthropological interpretation of eating disorders. In: *Nutrition Update.* Weininger J, Briggs GM (editors). Wiley, 1985.

Najman J: Health and poverty: Past, present, and prospects for the future. Soc Sci Med 1993;36:157.

Pellegrino ED: Is truth telling to the patient a cultural artifact? JAMA 1992;268:1734.

Raphael D: The need for a supportive doula in an increasingly urban world. In: *Women and Health: Cross-Cultural Perspectives.* Whelehan P (editor). Bergin & Garvey, 1988.

Scheper-Hughes N: *Death Without Weeping: The Violence of Everyday Life in Brazil.* University of California Press, 1992.

Smith-Rosenberg C: *Disorderly Conduct: Visions of Gender in Victorian America.* Knopf, 1985.

Surbone, A: Letter from Italy: Truth telling to the patient. JAMA 1992;268:1661.

Trotter RT, Chavira JA: *Curanderismo: Mexican American Folk Healing.* University of Georgia Press, 1981.

Waitzkin H, Britt T: A critical theory of medical discourse: How patients and health professionals deal with social problems. Int J Health Serv 1989;19:577.

Walsh DC, Sorensen G, Leonard L: A "Society and Health" Perspective on Gender and Health: Cigarette Smoking as an Exploratory Case Study. In: Society and Health. Levine S, Walsh DC (editors). Oxford, 1995.

Weisman CS, Tietelbaum MA: Physician and the physician-patient relationship: Recent evidence and relevant questions. Soc Sci Med 1985;20:1119.

West C: Ask me no questions . . . : An analysis of queries and replies in physician-patient dialogues. Pages 75–106 in: *The Social Organization of Doctor-Patient Communication.* Fisher S, Todd AD (editors). Center for Applied Linguistics, 1983.

West C: Reconceptualizing in physician-patient relationships. Soc Sci Med 1993;36:57.

Zborowski M: *People in Pain.* Jossey-Bass, 1969.

Adolescent Medicine

3

Jane Leslie Becker, MD

The tremendous amount of growth and change that takes place during adolescence can be simultaneously exhilarating and overwhelming for a teenager, her family, and her community. The appropriate input from a health care provider can have a lasting impact on the health and well-being of a teenager. An understanding of the physical, psychological, and cognitive changes taking place increases the probability of a positive and healthy outcome, and no one is better suited to provide information and guidance than a teenager's health care provider.

The adolescent population is expected to increase from 33.8 million to 38.3 million by the year 2000. Not only is the population growing, but so are the social problems that account for an increasing proportion of the health problems in the adolescent population. Many of today's teenagers are involved in high-risk behaviors that jeopardize their health, and they are involved in these behaviors at earlier ages than ever before.

ADOLESCENT MORBIDITY & MORTALITY

The principal risks to adolescent health have changed over the past few decades and are now secondary to risky health behaviors rather than to biomedical conditions. The recently published *Guidelines for Adolescent Preventive Services* states that "changes in adolescent morbidity and mortality during the past several decades have created a health crisis for today's youth." This health crisis is caused by the social morbidities such as substance abuse, sexually transmitted diseases (STDs), adolescent pregnancy, and injury from accidents and violence. Most youths engage in some type of behavior that places their health at risk, and many engage in a multitude of high-risk behaviors simultaneously.

The four leading causes of death for adolescents, in descending order, are (1) motor vehicle accidents, (2) other accidents such as drowning and burns, (3) suicides, and (4) homicides. Accidents and violence collectively account for three-fourths of all adolescent deaths. Fifty-one percent of motor vehicle accidents involving adolescents are alcohol-related. The rate of suicide has tripled in the past 3 decades. Currently, the suicide rate is 9/100,000 for 15- to 19-

```
Adolescent Morbidity & Mortality
    Sexual Activity
    Substance Abuse
Growth & Development
    Psychological Development
    Physical Development
Office Visit
    Establishing a Patient-Physician
        Relationship
    Confidentiality
    The Interview
    Physical Examination
Screening Guidelines
Legal & Ethical Issues
```

year-olds, and 14% of these deaths are alcohol-related. There are between 50 and 200 attempts for every completed suicide. Female adolescents attempt suicide 3 times more frequently than male adolescents; however, male adolescents commit suicide 3 times more frequently than their female counterparts.

Adolescent homicide has increased at an alarming rate. From 1960 to 1987, the death rate from homicide for early adolescents (age 10–14) rose from 0.4 to 1.6/100,000; for late adolescents (age 15–19), the rate increased from 0.5 to 10/100,000; and for young adults (age 20–24), it increased from 4 to 17.8/100,000.

Sexual Activity

Sexual activity is common during adolescence and is responsible for a significant amount of adolescent morbidity. Greater than 50% of 15- to 19-year-olds have had sexual intercourse, and by twelfth grade, 55% of teenage girls and 70% of teenage boys are sexually active. Even in these dangerous times, only 27% of sexually active youths report consistent condom use, and only one-third of sexually active female adolescents regularly use a contraceptive method. Most female teenagers do not consider birth control until they have been sexually active for 6–12 months. Half of all teenage pregnancies occur in the first 6 months after the initiation of sexual intercourse, and one of ten teenagers in the United States gets pregnant every year. In the USA, there are more than one million pregnancies per year in teenagers, and most of these are in teenagers younger than 18. Pregnancy is the most common reason for teenage girls to leave school. Adolescents who are sexually active at a young age are at increased risk to have multiple partners, participate in other high-risk behaviors, and have lower educational aspirations than those who put off sexual activity until they are older.

In addition to unwanted pregnancies, these high-risk behaviors place sexually active teenagers at risk for STDs and HIV infection. It is important to note that one of six teenagers gets an STD each year, and 25% of AIDS cases involve young adults (people in their 20s) who probably got infected during adolescence, in most instances through heterosexual sex. In contrast to the USA, Western Europe and Scandinavia have a much lower rate of teenage pregnancy despite equivalent amounts of sexual activity among teenagers. Some authors attribute this difference to the nonjudgmental attitudes toward sex, easy access to contraceptive services for young people (including availability of contraceptives at low cost without the threat of parental notification), and comprehensive sex education programs that are prevalent in Western European and Scandinavian countries.

Substance Abuse

Substance abuse has reached epidemic proportions in the adolescent community. The first drug used is often nicotine. By the age of 11, one of five adolescents has smoked cigarettes, and by age 15, one of seven smokes daily. The mean age of onset for cigarette smoking is 12. Sixty percent of adults who smoke began by the time they were 14. The only population with increasing numbers of cigarette smokers is female adolescents. Besides the serious health risks posed by cigarette use itself, smoking may be the earliest sign of difficulties to come; cigarette smoking at a young age is a marker for children at increased risk for other unhealthy behaviors.

Alcohol is the most commonly abused substance among adolescents, with 39% of high school seniors reporting getting drunk within the past 2 weeks and at least 90% of high school seniors reporting some alcohol use. As many as 4.2% of high school seniors report daily use. The mean age of onset of alcohol consumption is 12.6. Alcohol-related injuries account for one of five deaths in teenagers between the ages of 15 and 20.

Marihuana, which has been shown to be the gateway to other drugs, is used daily by 9% of high school seniors. The average age of onset for marihuana use is 14.4 years. There are a multitude of other drugs that are used by teenagers with negative sequelae. Besides the dangers of the drugs themselves, poor judgment is the rule while under the influence. Adolescents who are intoxicated may engage in high-risk activities, eg, unsafe sex or riding in a motor vehicle with an intoxicated driver, that they would not engage in if they were sober.

GROWTH & DEVELOPMENT

Psychological Development

The psychological changes that occur during adolescence are dramatic; in just a few years, a teenager is transposed from childhood to adulthood. Understanding and anticipating the developmental stages enables the clinician to obtain an accurate history, address important issues, and intervene effectively.

The four major developmental tasks of adolescence are (1) gaining independence from parents, (2) acceptance of body image, (3) establishing a peer group, and (4) developing an identity (including a sexual, moral, religious, and vocational identity).

A. Early Adolescence: In early adolescence (ages 11–13 in girls), one often begins to see (1) decreased dependence on family, eg, less family activity; (2) body image concerns resulting in a preoccupation with comparing oneself to others to answer the question, "Am I normal?" (3) increased interest in the peer group (which usually involves same-sex friendships); and (4) early identity development with the first thoughts regarding future plans. Career plans at this stage are often unrealistic and may entail goals such as becoming a famous rock star. The cognitive process at this stage generally is still one of concrete operations, in which the teenager is unable to think abstractly or to hypothesize. If you ask an early adolescent, "What brought you here today?" and she answers," "The bus," you know for sure she is still in the stage of concrete operations!

B. Middle Adolescence: The four developmental tasks are exhibited at this stage (ages 14–17) by (1) an escalation of parent-child conflict as the struggle for independence increases, (2) a new comfort with the body as the teenager begins to focus on the possibility of attracting a partner, (3) increasing involvement in peer culture and sexual experimentation, and (4) identity concerns that focus on the question, "Who am I?"

An increase in risk-taking behavior is seen during middle adolescence. The teenager is separating from her family and often feels powerful both physically and psychologically. The operative mode is the "myth of immunity," wherein the teenager believes that "it won't happen to me." A concept developed by David Elkind called the "personal fable" captures the teenagers' feelings of being immortal and invulnerable. These feelings, combined with their sense of being unique, as well as the dramatic physical and psychological changes the teenager experiences often are manifested by an increase in risk taking behavior.

Cognitive development at this stage may begin to move from concrete to formal operations; the teenager gains the ability to think abstractly, appreciate time, anticipate consequences of actions, and consider her own future realistically. There may be wide individual variations here, so it is important to question teenagers carefully before making an assumption about their cognitive developmental stage.

C. Late Adolescence: During late adolescence (ages 18–21), there is (1) increasing autonomy from parents; (2) a greater comfort with the body, with puberty completed; (3) decreased importance of the peer group, with a shift in focus toward the achievement of intimacy with one person; and (4) development of practical career goals and plans. Adult cognitive processes are often evident here, as the teenager or young adult demonstrates the ability to think abstractly, hypothesize, consider probability, anticipate consequences, and appreciate time. It is important to be aware that a substantial percentage of adults never reach this cognitive level; therefore, the interview must be conducted accordingly.

Physical Development

The magnitude of physical growth and change during puberty is enormous. Growth in height during puberty accounts for 20–25% of final adult height, and pubertal weight gain accounts for 50% of an adult's ideal body weight. Although the timing of the onset of puberty and subsequent physical changes is highly variable, there is a common sequence and pattern. Chronologic age correlates poorly with biologic maturity; however, there are standards that can help assess the developmental stage of individual patients. Standard growth charts can assist in evaluating growth at puberty.

The precise trigger of the onset of puberty is not completely understood. The trigger appears to be related to decreased sensitivity of the hypothalamus and pituitary to circulating sex hormones, resulting in an increase in levels of luteinizing hormone (LH) and follicle-stimulating hormone (FSH). The gonads respond to increased levels of LH and FSH by synthesizing and secreting more estrogen, progesterone, and testosterone, which leads to the estrogen-induced LH surge that ultimately results in regular menses and ova production. Adrenal androgens promote the acquisition and maintenance of sexual hair.

Female sexual development occurs at an average age of 11.2 years, but the age of onset ranges from 9 to 13.4 years. The average length of time for completion of puberty is 4 years, with a range of 1.5–8 years. In most girls, breast budding is the first sign of puberty. Typically thelarche (breast development) is followed by pubarche (pubic hair growth), followed by the growth spurt (peak height velocity), and finally, menarche. The average age for thelarche is 10.5–11 years, with a range of from 8 to 13 years. Pubarche generally follows thelarche within 6 months to 1 year. On average, peak height velocity occurs at 12.1 years. Figure 3–1 illustrates the sequence of pubertal development.

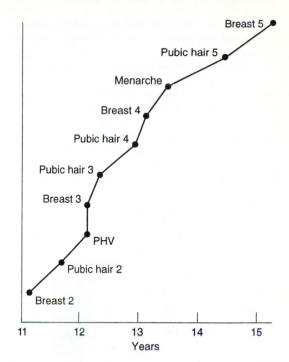

Figure 3–1. Pubertal development in female adolescents. The sequence and mean ages of pubertal events are shown. PHV = peak height velocity. (Adapted and reproduced, with permission, from Marshall WA, Tanner JM: Variations in pattern of pubertal changes in girls. Arch Dis Child 1969;44:291.)

The mean age for menarche is 12.7 years, with a range from age 9 to age 16. Menarche predictably occurs within 30 months of the onset of breast budding, generally during Tanner stage 4. (Tanner stages are explained later in this section.) Menarche always occurs after peak height velocity has been attained; growth after menarche is limited to 2–5 cm. Generally, for the first year after menarche, 50% of the cycles are anovulatory, and often the menses remain irregular for the first 6–24 months.

Besides the development of secondary sex characteristics during puberty, the ovaries, uterus, vagina, labia, and clitoris increase in size; there is an increase and alteration in body fat distribution; skeletal bone growth occurs; the sweat glands produce a characteristic odor; and the sebaceous glands increase productivity. The average growth spurt lasts approximately 24–36 months. Most often, linear bone growth is completed by 16 years of age, and height gained ranges from 5.4 to 11.2 cm. Predicting adult height can be difficult, although estimates can be made based on current height, skeletal age, and chronologic age or by using growth charts. Evaluation of abnormal height generally should be undertaken when an adolescent's height falls within the lowest 2% or highest 98% of the population. It is imperative, however, given the strong genetic component to ultimate height attainment, that the provider consider the height of the parents before beginning a complete evaluation.

In 1962, Tanner developed a sexual maturity rating scale for male and female adolescents that is used widely in clinical practice. In women, the scale is based on pubic hair and breast development. The Tanner staging system, depicted in Figures 3–2 and 3–3, divides pubertal development into five stages. Stage 1 represents the prepubescent girl, and stage 2 indicates early development. Stages 3 and 4 are intermediary stages reflecting increased maturity, and stage 5 indicates the completion of the development of secondary sex characteristics.

Variations in the timing of pubertal development may result from a number of factors, including genetic and nutritional factors and chronic medical problems. Reassurance and education about the timing of development can be comforting to concerned teenagers. Variations that are outside the standard range require evaluation. A workup for abnormal development generally is indicated if there is no breast development by age 13, menses has not occurred by age 16, or menarche occurs before 10.3 years of age.

OFFICE VISIT

Adolescents come to a medical setting for a wide variety of reasons. They may present for a routine

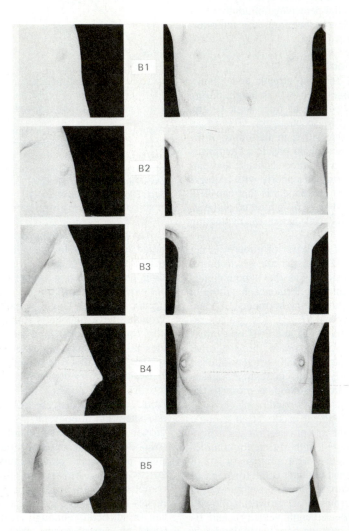

Figure 3–2. Stages of breast development, according to Marshall and Tanner. (Photographs from van Wieringen JC et al, 1971, with permission.) *Stage B1:* Preadolescent. *Stage B2:* Breast bud stage. *Stage B3:* Further enlargement of breast and areola, with no separation of their contours. *Stage B4:* Projection of areola and papilla to form a secondary mound above the level of the breast. *Stage B5:* Mature stage. (Reproduced, with permission, from Marshall WA, Tanner JM: Variations in pattern of pubertal changes in girls. Arch Dis Child 1969;44:291.) (Reproduced, with permission, from Styne DM: Puberty. In: *Basic and Clinical Endocrinology,* 4th ed. Greenspan FS, editor. Appleton & Lange, 1994.)

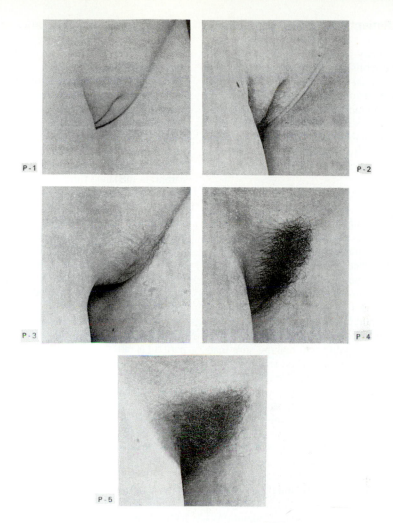

Figure 3–3. Stages of female pubic hair development, according to Marshall and Tanner. (Photographs from van Wieringen JC et al, 1971, with permission.) *Stage P1:* Preadolescent. *Stage P2:* Sparse growth of long, slightly pigmented hair, appearing chiefly along the labia. *Stage P3:* Hair is considerably darker, coarser, and curlier. The hair spreads sparsely over the junction of the pubes. *Stage P4:* Hair is now adult in type, but not in quantity. *Stage P5:* Hair is adult in quantity and type, distributed as an inverse triangle of the classic feminine pattern. Spread is to the medial surface of the thighs but not elsewhere above the base of the inverse triangle. (Reproduced, with permission, from Marshall WA, Tanner JM: Variations in pattern of pubertal changes in girls. Arch Dis Child 1969;44:291.) (Reproduced, with permission, from Styne DM: Puberty. In: *Basic and Clinical Endocrinology,* 4th ed. Greenspan FS, editor. Appleton & Lange, 1994.)

physical examination required by camp, school, an athletic team, or an employer, or one requested by their parents. Female adolescents often present for routine gynecologic care (pelvic examination, Papanicolaou smear, and contraception) and checks for STDs. Teenagers also seek care for a multitude of acute and chronic medical problems ranging from upper respiratory infections and sprained ankles to diabetes and eating disorders. Frequently an adolescent presents a noncontroversial complaint to gain access to the clinician when she has, either consciously or unconsciously, a desire to speak about something else; the true problem may be revealed if the provider takes the proper approach. Recognition of the developmental stages of adolescence and the manner in which teenagers may present to physicians can be of assistance in evaluating and treating adolescents. Behavioral changes or somatic complaints may be secondary to a variety of emotional problems; for example, abdominal pain may be the presenting complaint for school avoidance, peer group issues, fear of pregnancy, or sexual abuse.

Establishing a Patient-Physician Relationship

Although the primary goal of the visit is to screen and treat disease, establishing a relationship with the teenager is an essential first step. By taking the teenager's concerns seriously, demonstrating a genuine interest in her, and maintaining a nonjudgmental approach, it is often possible to build rapport. This approach is likely to enable the patient to discuss her health issues more readily and allow the physician to make more accurate diagnoses and provide more appropriate treatment.

Confidentiality

The chances of developing a "therapeutic alliance" improve markedly if the interview is carried out in a private setting with assurances of confidentiality. It is best to establish the principles of privacy and confidentiality early in the interview. An important aspect of a positive relationship, the assurance of confidentiality encourages the teenager to be more candid.

If both the parent and the teenager enter the office together, it is helpful to begin by reviewing the ground rules of confidentiality and making sure that everyone agrees to them. It should be stated clearly that after the initial segment of the interview, the parent will be asked to step out of the examination room. (The teenager and her parents should not be offered the choice.) The teenager then has the remainder of the interview and the examination in privacy. It is important to state specifically to the parent and teenager that, except for a disclosure by the teenager of abuse, suicidality, or homicidality, the content of what she says is confidential unless she chooses to share it. The rules of confidentiality are mandated by state law and ethical considerations. Before proceeding with the interview, it is useful to be sure that all questions regarding this policy are answered and to ascertain that everyone present agrees to the policy.

When a parent wishes to speak with the clinician alone, permission should be sought from the adolescent. Some parents feel that if they are paying the bill, they have a right to know what is discussed throughout the interview with their child. When the clinician explains the benefits derived from a confidential interview, namely, a complete and candid history, the parent generally acquiesces. Most parents have some awareness of the needs of their teenager and are grateful for the time spent by the clinician with their child. When appropriate, it is helpful to encourage the teenager to share information with her parents.

The parent and teenager should be informed of the specific situations in which the physician cannot maintain confidentiality. These situations generally are mandated by state laws and ethical considerations; they include instances in which situations where the teenager is in danger of harming herself or another, discloses sexual abuse, or is treated for a gunshot or knife wound.

The Interview

A. The Joint Interview: After reviewing the confidentiality issue, the clinician may begin by asking the teenager why she is seeking medical attention. Directing questions to the teenager rather than the parent helps empower the young person. It is important for clinicians to establish themselves as the adolescent's advocate rather than as an agent of the parent; at the same time, one must avoid an adversarial relationship with the parent. Providers should introduce themselves to the teenager first, allowing her to introduce her parent. If the clinician has previously gained knowledge of the adolescent's situation from any source, eg, a school note or phone call, it makes good sense to mention it at the beginning of the interview, thereby avoiding a difficult situation later that may compromise the provider's or the teenager's credibility.

During this limited joint interview, it is useful to include the parent in the collection of data, paying particular attention to the avoidance of personal questions, but gathering information regarding pertinent aspects of the adolescent's birth history, perinatal events, immunization history, family history, and history of allergies that the teenager may not know about. This discussion is a practical way of educating the teenager about her childhood medical history. The joint interview also can be a time to observe family dynamics and to develop a rapport with the parent. Following this brief shared interview, a feedback session may be arranged for the summation; whereby findings and recommendations can be reviewed with both the adolescent and the parent within the guidelines of confidentiality.

B. The Adolescent Interview: Teenagers often give a different reason for their visit once they are afforded privacy with the clinician. Communication may be facilitated by beginning this section of the interview with noncontroversial, open-ended questions. Data can be gathered via both verbal and nonverbal communication. It is often useful to take note of the teenager's dress and mannerisms (eg, wearing a style of clothes associated with a certain outlook—heavy metal t-shirt, pierced nose, or athletic gear). The clinician's observations may be used to open a discussion with the teenager.

The interview technique must be tailored to the developmental stage of the adolescent; for example, young teenagers may have a difficult time with open-ended questions. Establishing a rapport during this section of the interview gives the provider the opportunity to explore difficulties the teenager may be experiencing and to communicate that the provider can be a resource if difficulties of any kind develop.

1. History–The history includes questions regarding past illnesses, past surgeries, medications, allergies, and immunizations, and includes a review of systems similar to that conducted for an adult woman. In the review of systems for adolescents, particular attention should be paid to questions concerning weight changes, exercise, abdominal pains, respiratory problems, genitourinary or menstrual problems, and visual changes. To screen for an eating disorder, one may ask the teenager how she feels about her current weight, whether she has ever dieted, and if she has dieted, what her method was, eg, use of laxatives, diuretics, diet pills, or purging. The menstrual history should include onset of menarche, length of time between periods, nature of flow, cramping, intermenstrual spotting, vaginal discharge, and breast symptoms.

2. Psychosocial interview–Because the "social morbidities" (sexual behavior, substance abuse, and injury) are the most common causes of adolescent morbidity and mortality, much of the interview should focus on the psychosocial history. In adolescents, the psychosocial interview is a major portion of the history gathered. Dr. Eric Cohen at Children's Hospital in Los Angeles developed the acronym known as HEADSS to help clinicians to organize the psychosocial interview in a way that is easy to remember and conduct. HEADSS stands for Home, Education/Employment, Activities, Drugs, Sex, and Suicide/depression.

A discussion of the home is a nonthreatening way to begin the psychosocial portion of the interview. The provider might begin by asking, "Where do you live? Who lives with you?" One should not assume that an adolescent lives with one or both of her parents. Other questions related to the home include, "How do people get along at home? Have you ever run away?"

It is important to ask specific questions regarding education and employment, because teenagers usually do not volunteer information of this sort. The questions one may want to ask are, "What subject do you like the best? What subjects do you dislike? Have you ever been held back? How many schools have you attended in the last 4 years? Do you work outside of school? What goals or plans do you have for when you finish school?"

Questions concerning the adolescent's activities are next: "What do you do for fun? What are some of your friends' names (to find out if she has friends)? Do you ride a bike or in a car? Do you wear a seat belt? Do you wear a helmet when riding a bike?"

As the interview continues, the clinician asks about more sensitive topics; the next topic in the mnemonic is drugs. It often helps to ask about sensitive subjects in the third person or past tense: "Many kids use drugs; do any of your friends? What do they use? What have you used? When do you use drugs? How do you pay for them? When do you drink alcohol? Do you ever drink while driving?" Questions regarding cigarette use are appropriate during the time

questions related to drug and alcohol use are asked; cigarettes should be asked about specifically.

When discussing sexuality, it is important to be sure to ask the questions so that the teenager understands what is meant. For example, if you ask the patient if she is sexually active, she may reply, "No, not now," meaning not while she is sitting in your office or not recently (in the last week or two). Instead, the clinician might say, "Often teenagers your age choose to be sexually active. Some choose not to be. Have you ever had sex? Are you interested in males, females, or both? Have you ever had a pelvic infection? Have you ever had a pelvic examination? Have you ever been pregnant? What do you do to avoid getting pregnant? Has anyone ever touched your body when you did not want the person to?" The inquiry about which gender a teen is interested in sexually serves a number of purposes. First, the question normalizes interest in the same sex and therefore serves as an educational tool regarding other people's choices and their own. Second, it informs the teenager that if she faces this issue now or in the future, the provider can be sought out as a resource. Initially, the responses to many of these questions may be denial. As the provider and teenager develop a trusting relationship over time, however, the teenager may return to these subjects and request help.

Suicide and depression make up the final topic in the HEADSS mnemonic. Adolescents often do not "look depressed" even when they are. Useful questions include, "Do you often feel sad or mad? What do you do then? Do you often feel bored? Do you sometimes have trouble sleeping? Have you ever tried to hurt or kill yourself? Have you ever had any serious accidents? Are there guns in your home? Does anyone in your family use drugs or alcohol?"

If there are responses that cause concern, further evaluation may be required. The clinician may provide education, follow-up, or referral to an appropriate professional. It is usually best to see the adolescent again if there are concerns, even if she has been referred elsewhere, as a way of ensuring that the treatment plan is followed and as a message to the adolescent that the provider is still concerned with her care.

Physical Examination

Most adolescents are extremely sensitive and concerned about their rapidly changing body. Reassurance during the physical examination that the findings are within the normal range can alleviate many unspoken fears and concerns. Reassurance can be as simple as telling the patient how strong her heart sounds or that her lungs sound clear. Physical variations noted during the examination that could cause body image anxiety, eg, obesity, early development, or acne, should be mentioned and discussed. If the provider notices a physical problem, it is likely that the teenager has noticed it also and is concerned. Adolescents usually are grateful for the opportunity to discuss their concerns if the topics are approached sensitively. Often, education regarding the prevalence, natural history, and treatment options can relieve anxiety about a concern.

The physical examination in adolescents requires particular attention to certain areas. Because teenagers are generally self-conscious about their body, using the drapes and gown in respect for the patient's modesty is suggested.

Yearly charting of height, weight, and pubertal development (Tanner stage) is useful as a means of tracking growth. The figures can be plotted on a height velocity curve so that the physician can evaluate whether the growth spurt has begun and its pattern. Failure of a girl to reach the growth spurt by age 12 may suggest a need for further evaluation. Blood pressure should be measured, and the need for dental referral should be assessed by examination of the teeth for caries and malocclusion. Visual and auditory assessment are particularly important because deficits in these areas may be a source of embarrassment and may not be reported initially. Visual screening should be done at the initial visit and repeated every 2–3 years. Auditory testing should be done at least one time during adolescence. The thyroid should be examined for nodularity or enlargement. Examination of the skin should focus on the presence of acne or hirsutism.

Examination of the breasts allows for Tanner staging, evaluation for disparity in size, and introduction to breast self-examination (although there is controversy over the efficacy of teaching this technique to teenagers). Although breasts may begin to develop asynchronously, disparity in size often corrects itself; no consideration should be given to cosmetic surgery until pubertal development is complete. It is crucial that no one mistake the breast bud for a breast mass and biopsy it, because this error can have devastating consequences.

The orthopedic examination should focus on problems that present during puberty. This task requires an evaluation of gait to rule out slipped capital femoral epiphysis, of the tibial tubercle to rule out Osgood-Schlatter disease, and of the spine to evaluate for scoliosis. The time to detect scoliosis is during adolescence so that early treatment can be undertaken. Inspection of the external genitalia should be done yearly in every female adolescent.

For a first pelvic examination, it is worthwhile to spend some time with a model or drawing reviewing the normal female anatomy and explaining what the examination will entail. This exercise can help dispel any myths the teenager may have heard about pelvic examinations. Following this discussion with a review of the indications for a pelvic examination educates the adolescent as to what she can expect that day and on subsequent visits.

It may be helpful to acknowledge during the first pelvic examination that some girls worry about the examination being painful or embarrassing. Talking with the teenager about what she has heard about the examination and addressing those issues can be reassuring. Letting the teenager know that she is in control at all times and that the provider will stop the examination if she asks is a useful way to reframe a situation that may make the patient feel vulnerable.

A routine pelvic examination is recommended yearly beginning at age 18 in women who have never been active sexually. For teenagers who are currently active sexually, a pelvic examination is indicated every 6–12 months or with each new partner, whichever comes first. If a teenager requests a pelvic examination, one should be done, regardless of whether she meets any of the criteria. She may have a reason for this request that she is unwilling to share. If a teenager states that she thought she was to have a pelvic examination, it may be revealing to ask her why she expected one.

The routine pelvic examination in a sexually active adolescent includes a smear and screening for STDs including syphilis, gonorrhea, *Chlamydia,* and trichomoniasis, and possibly, HIV testing. In all adolescents, particular attention should be paid to inspection of the external genitalia, checking for nonambiguous genitalia, clitoral size (usually 2–4 mm wide), distribution and characteristics of pubic hair (for pubertal development), signs of mucosal estrogenization, and hymen patency. The cervix in adolescents often has ectropion, which is a red and rough area surrounding the os that represents the endocervical columnar cells extending on to the exocervix. Ectropion is of concern only if it is very large or extends onto the lateral walls of the vagina.

Aside from their role in routine health care, pelvic examinations are indicated to evaluate pelvic symptoms such as vaginal discharge, abnormal bleeding, dysmenorrhea that is not responsive to routine treatment, amenorrhea, and pelvic pain.

At the end of the visit, a summary of the findings, the diagnosis, and the recommendations is discussed with the adolescent. Following this discussion, the parent may be brought back into the room for a joint summary of the findings and treatment plan within the boundaries of confidentiality. Compliance generally is optimized if the recommendations are directed at the teenager, thereby empowering her to take on the responsibility for carrying out the plan.

SCREENING GUIDELINES

The American Medical Association recently has established recommendations known as Guidelines for Adolescent Preventive Services (GAPS). GAPS provides a framework for the organization and content of routine health care services for adolescents.

Acknowledging the impact of the social morbidities on the health of today's adolescent population, the guidelines emphasize preventive service visits, which focus on health guidance screening and prevention of physical, emotional, and behavioral conditions that are a threat to the health of adolescents. Table 3–1 depicts the major GAPS recommendations in the areas of health guidance, screening (including history, physical assessment, and laboratory tests), and immunizations for each age.

LEGAL & ETHICAL ISSUES

The legal status of adolescents can be somewhat confusing in the health care setting. The issues that come up commonly include issues of consent, confidentiality, privacy, and payment. Many of the laws are ambiguous, incomplete, or undergoing revision. Practitioners should familiarize themselves with both the federal laws and their state laws. If questions arise, appropriate legal counsel should be sought.

In most states, persons 18 years or older are legally adults and can consent to medical care. Although teenagers younger than 18 need parental consent for medical care, there are some exceptions. The exceptions generally are based on either the status of the teenager or the services required. Exceptions based on the status of the teenager involve the classifications of "mature minor" and "emancipated minor." **Mature minor** is a judicial doctrine for older teenagers who understand the risks and benefits of medical care and can give informed consent. There is no uniformity regarding the legal status of this doctrine among states. The definition of **emancipated minor** varies from state to state, but the term gener-

Table 3–1. Preventive health services by age and procedure.

Procedure	Early				Middle			Late			
	11	12	13	14	15	16	17	18	19	20	21
Health guidance											
Parenting*			•			•					
Development	•	•	•	•	•	•	•	•	•	•	•
Diet and fitness	•	•	•	•	•	•	•	•	•	•	•
Lifestyle†	•	•	•	•	•	•	•	•	•	•	•
Injury prevention	•	•	•	•	•	•	•	•	•	•	•
Screening											
History											
Eating disorders	•	•	•	•	•	•	•	•	•	•	•
Sexual activity‡	•	•	•	•	•	•	•	•	•	•	•
Alcohol and other drug use	•	•	•	•	•	•	•	•	•	•	•
Tobacco use	•	•	•	•	•	•	•	•	•	•	•
Abuse	•	•	•	•	•	•	•	•	•	•	•
School performance	•	•	•	•	•	•	•	•	•	•	•
Depression	•	•	•	•	•	•	•	•	•	•	•
Risk for suicide	•	•	•	•	•	•	•	•	•	•	•
Physical assessment											
Blood pressure	•	•	•	•	•	•	•	•	•	•	•
BMI	•	•	•	•	•	•	•	•	•	•	•
Comprehensive exam			•			•				•	
Tests											
Cholesterol			1			1				1	
TB			2			2				2	
GC, *Chlamydia,* and HPV			3			3				3	
HIV and syphilis			4			4				4	
Pap smear			5			5				5	
Immunizations											
MMR			•								
Td						•					
HBV			6			6				6	

1. Screening test performed once if family history is positive for early cardiovascular disease or hyperlipidemia.
2. Screen if positive for exposure to active TB or lives/works in high-risk situation, (eg, homeless shelter, jail, health care facility).
3. Screen at least annually if sexually active.
4. Screen if high risk for infection.
5. Screen annually if sexually active or if 18 years or older.
6. Vaccinate if high hisk for hepatitis B infection.
*A parent health-guidance visit is recommended during early and middle adolescence.
†Includes counseling regarding sexual behavior and avoidance of tobacco, alcohol, and other drugs.
‡Includes history of unintended pregnancy and STD.

ally refers to teenagers who are free from parental control, such as married teenagers, members of the armed forces, pregnant teenagers, and minors living away from home.

The second exception to the requirement for parental consent involves the particular health services involved. Every state has statutes that pertain to minors consenting to medical care for specific types of health problems. For example, emergency care can be provided without parental consent. It is recommended that the provider attempt to reach the parents and notify them of the emergency situation as soon as possible. Services for which minors who are considered otherwise capable most commonly are permitted to give their own consent are pregnancy-related care; contraception; diagnosis and treatment of STDs, HIV, and AIDS; substance abuse treatment; and outpatient mental health services. States may have age requirements or requirements for parental notification or the granting of a judicial pass. The medical record generally should document the fact that the teenager is capable of informed consent, that informed consent was obtained, and that the patient was encouraged to inform her parents but refused.

Studies show that many teenagers would not seek care for medical problems if they were not allowed to consent to their own treatment and thus assured of confidentiality. Given the tremendous numbers of pregnancies and STDs occurring in teenagers, both the adolescent and society would suffer needlessly if young people could not seek out the care required without the need for parental consent.

The issue of payment further complicates the already difficult issues of consent and confidentiality. If a teenager is seen without the consent of her parent, payment by her parent generally is not required. Even if the parent is willing to pay for care, however, an itemized bill easily can destroy the confidential nature of the encounter. Possible ways around this problem include (1) use of a nonitemized bill; (2) payment for services at the time, by the adolescent; (3) performance of the service without charge; or (4) referring the teenager for confidential services to a public health setting that will not send home a bill or charge the patient.

Particular populations of teenagers present different legal and ethical considerations. These special populations include incarcerated youth, adolescents in foster care, developmentally disabled youth, and homeless youth. When dealing with teenagers in these circumstances, it is necessary to become familiar with the appropriate state and federal laws.

REFERENCES

Cromer BA, McLean CS, Heald FP: A critical review of comprehensive health screening in adolescents. J Adolesc Health 1992;13:3S.

Elster AB, Kuznets NJ: *AMA Guidelines for Adolescent Preventive Services: Recommendations and Rationale.* Williams & Wilkins, 1994.

English A: Treating adolescents: Legal and ethical considerations. Med Clin North Am 1990;74:1097.

Epps RP, Manley MW: The clinician's role in preventing smoking initiation. Med Clin North Am 1992;76:439.

Gans JE et al: America's adolescents: How healthy are they? *AMA Profiles of Adolescent Health Series.* American Medical Association, 1990.

Goldenring J, Cohen E: Getting into adolescent heads. Contemp Pediatr 1988;5:75.

Hofmann A: *Basic adolescent gynecology: An office guide.* Stasburger V (editor). Urban & Schwarzenberg, 1990.

Klein JD et al: Access to health care for adolescents: A position paper for the Society of Adolescent Medicine. J Adolesc Health 1992;13:162.

MacKenzie RG: Approach to the adolescent in the clinical setting. Med Clin North Am 1990;74:1085.

Marshall WA, Tanner JM: Variations in pattern of pubertal changes in girls. Arch Dis Child 1969;44:291.

National Commission on the Role of the School and the Community in Improving Adolescent Health: Code Blue: Uniting for Healthier youth.

Neinstein LS: *Adolescent Health Care: A Practical Guide,* 2nd ed. Urban & Schwarzenberg, 1991.

Rickert VI, Jay SM, Gottlieb AA: Adolescent wellness: Facilitating Compliance in Social Morbidities. Med Clin North Am 1990;74:1135.

Root AW: Medical progress: Endocrinology of Puberty. J Pediatr 1973;83:1.

United States Public Health Services: *Healthy Youth 2,000: National Health Promotion and Disease Prevention Objectives for Adolescents.* American Medical Association, 1992.

Geriatric Medicine

4

Debra S. Fetherston, MD, & Lesley Althouse, MD, MRCP

The segment of the population that is elderly is expected to expand markedly as the post-World War II generation ages. It is important to provide continuous, quality health care and to promote a healthy and independent life-style for elderly women, in whom disease can lead to prolonged morbidity.

Comprehensive health care in elderly women necessitates addressing not only pathologic disease states but also important physiologic changes which occur with aging. Functional, cognitive and social status play a role in the health of the individual. As the people in the United States age over the next several decades, insuring a healthy and independent geriatric population will be vital for decreasing health care costs and the burden to the individual and society.

PRIMARY CARE

DEMOGRAPHICS

The elderly, defined as persons aged 65 years and older, currently represent 13% of the population of the United States. It is estimated that by the year 2040 this percentage will double to nearly 70 million, with more than 50 million women older than 65. Women's life expectancy currently exceeds that of men by approximately 7 years, yet women bear a higher burden of morbidity, disability, and loss of independence than men.

Comprehensive and multidimensional assessment of the elderly is critical to providing quality health care. Assessment of older women requires attention to the physical, psychosocial, and economic well-being of each patient. Loss of a spouse may lead to severe depression or financial instability. Progressive hearing impairment may lead to social isolation and thus functional decline. All these factors may influence an older woman's susceptibility to disease and disability.

Traditionally, the focus of health care in the elderly has been on the treatment of disease rather than

the promotion of health. Elderly women have been excluded from many studies because of perceived problems of hormonal changes and the comorbid conditions believed to complicate study results; therefore, knowledge regarding disease prevention and treatment in older women is seriously deficient.

IMMUNIZATIONS

There are an estimated 60,000 deaths per year from influenza and pneumococcus-related infections in the USA. An even larger number of the elderly are admitted to hospitals and extended-care facilities because of the complications of these infections. The functional reserve capacity of many organ systems in the elderly often is impaired, and a comorbid decline in the setting of acute viral or bacterial infection often is witnessed.

Influenza

Although influenza vaccine is widely available, each year an estimated 10,000 unvaccinated elderly persons die from complications of influenza. At least two influenza epidemics in this century have been responsible for more than 40,000 deaths. It is recommended that persons 65 years and older be vaccinated on a yearly basis. Health care professionals who may transmit the illness to persons at risk also should be vaccinated. Immunization provides the best immunity if given in the late fall. Immunity achieves a 65–80% efficacy in young adults, which may drop to as low as 30–40% in the frail elderly. There is a definite benefit, however, in the decrease in severity and mortality of clinical illness.

Persons exposed to an outbreak of suspected influenza A benefit from amantadine if given within 24–48 hours of the start of clinical symptoms. The dosage should be reduced to 100 mg/d in the elderly, with a further reduction if renal failure is present.

Pneumococcus

Pneumococcal infection accounts for nearly 40,000 deaths annually in the USA. Unfortunately, only 14% of persons 65 years of age and older have received the 23-valent pneumococcal vaccine. The overall effectiveness of the vaccine is estimated at approximately 50%; however, the 23 serotypes covered by the vaccine represent nearly 90% of documented pneumococcal infections in the elderly. Although pneumococcal vaccine has not been shown to affect the incidence of pneumonia, it has been shown to be effective in decreasing the rates of bacteremia and subsequent mortality. Revaccination may be considered after 6 years, especially in elderly women with illnesses that predispose them to pneumonia, such as diabetes mellitus, chronic renal failure, or congestive heart failure.

Tetanus-Diphtheria Toxoid

Approximately 100 cases of tetanus are reported to the Centers for Disease Control and Prevention (CDC) annually. Although it is not common, the disease can be fatal and often goes unrecognized by clinicians. Almost all cases of diphtheria and tetanus occur in adults who have never completed a primary immunization series. Routine immunization did not

begin until the 1940s, when military recruits and children entering school were immunized. Consequently, many elderly women never received this vaccine. It is recommended that persons who have never received a primary tetanus-diphtheria (Td) toxoid series be given the primary series of two doses 4 weeks apart of 0.5 mL Td toxoids intramuscularly, with a third dose 6 months later. A booster should be given every 10 years.

MEDICATIONS

Approximately 25% of all medications are prescribed for patients over the age of 65. It is not unusual for an older patient to be taking 6–10 medications, including over-the-counter preparations. Polypharmacy can lead to drug interactions and increases in morbidity and mortality in the elderly. Nearly 30% of hospital admissions and 50% of nursing home admissions result from iatrogenic complications from medications.

Physiologic changes that are a natural part of aging contribute to the altered pharmacokinetic parameters of many medicines. Absorption of drugs is largely intact in the elderly, although decreased gastrointestinal motility and prolonged emptying time should be taken into consideration when choosing drugs. For example, potentially ulcerogenic drugs have an increased contact time with stomach mucosa in the elderly, and unabsorbed medications may lead to a higher incidence of diarrhea. Drug distribution in the body varies significantly with age. There is a relative increase in body fat and a decrease in lean body mass. Lipophilic drugs such as barbiturates, benzodiazepines, phenothiazines, and tricyclic antidepressants distribute rapidly to fatty tissue and lead to a prolonged duration of action and risk of cumulative dose toxicity. For example, diazepam has a half-life of 24 hours in younger persons but 75 hours in older persons. Also, there is a decrease in total body water in the elderly. Hydrophilic drugs, such as digoxin, acetaminophen, and alcohol, require smaller doses because of this smaller volume of body water. Finally, plasma protein levels change with age. Serum albumin concentration declines approximately 4% each decade and may drop precipitously in the presence of concomitant disease states. Many medications that bind to albumin, such as phenytoin and warfarin, have increased free serum concentrations. This effect is most significant in drugs with a narrow therapeutic-toxicity window. In patients taking these medications, free serum concentrations rather than total drug levels should be monitored.

With increasing age, several physiologic changes result in decreases in hepatic and renal metabolism. Both hepatic and renal blood flows decrease by 40–50% with aging, with a consequent decrease in functional mass. This change has an impact on the systemic clearance of many medications.

In the liver, there is decreased activity in phase 1 metabolism, eg, the cytochrome p450 microsomal enzyme system. In the elderly, polypharmacy and drug interactions can lead to toxic drug levels for many medications. For example, cimetidine is known to inhibit the p450 system; if taken concurrently with warfarin, which also relies on this system, a toxic level of warfarin could occur. Examples of drugs that are metabolized by this system include warfarin, benzodiazepines, nonsteroidal anti-inflammatory drugs (NSAIDS), oral hypoglycemics, phenytoin, and theophylline. Clinicians should be aware that lower doses of these medications should be prescribed in the elderly to prevent potentially toxic drug levels and side effects.

The glomerular filtration rate declines approximately 10% per decade after age 40. The decrease in the number of nephrons is postulated to be secondary to progressive vascular obliteration caused by atherosclerotic changes in the afferent arteriole. Despite this physiologic decline in renal function, the serum creatinine level often remains normal, especially in elderly frail women, because of the decline in muscle mass and the tendency for this population to follow a low-protein diet. The latter problem is often multifactorial and may be related to oral problems, dysphagia, or poor hand-to-mouth coordination; it also could be the result of financial constraints. The net result is a decrease in the production of creatinine and thus the apparently stable serum level often observed. This factor has important implications for the prescription of potentially nephrotoxic medications in the elderly. Because serum creatinine is not a reliable marker of renal function, it is recommended that dosage adjustments be based on creatinine clearance, which can be calculated easily with the use of the Cockroft-Gault equation.

Men:
Creatinine clearance = (140 − age) (weight in kg)
72 × serum creatinine
Women:
Creatinine clearance = (140 − age) (weight in kg)
× 0.85 72 × serum creatinine

It is important to remember that this equation does not apply to persons with unstable or fluctuating renal function. Examples of drugs that depend highly on renal function for elimination include digoxin, diuretics, atenolol, nadolol, cimetidine, enalapril, penicillins, and cephalosporins.

Guidelines for prescribing medications in the elderly include review of the patient's drug list at each visit and use of as few medications as possible at the lowest therapeutic doses possible. The clinician must evaluate whether a medication has been helpful within the expected time frame and stop any that are

not clearly beneficial. If a patient is in decline, it is most important to review potential drug interactions and stop medications as required.

FUNCTIONAL STATUS & EXERCISE

Periodic health evaluation provides the opportunity not only for promoting health but also for detecting functional problems that may decrease the active life and independence of older patients. Functional activity is a much more powerful marker of morbidity and mortality than age alone. Accidents are the sixth leading cause of death among the elderly, with 50% of accident-related deaths caused by falls. The risk of falls increases with a decline in functional status, decrease in cognitive abilities, and use of sedatives. Although most falls do not result in serious injury, approximately 50% of elderly persons who fall develop a fear of falling, which may lead to a restriction in activity and further physical decline and social isolation. There are approximately 200,000 hip fractures per year in the USA. The loss of capacity for independent ambulation in these persons often leads to institutionalization, which may be as high as 30% in elderly women. Death is usually preceded by 8 years of functional disability and 1 year of total dependency.

Use of estrogen replacement therapy (see Chapter 21) should be encouraged strongly in elderly female patients. The benefits of improved bone strength, prevention of atrophic urologic disorders and sexual dysfunction, and possible cardiac protection are important preventive strategies in this population. It is estimated that up to 20% of elderly women past the age of 75 continue to experience hot flashes, which also are improved by estrogen therapy. If a patient has not undergone hormone replacement therapy in many years, a low dose of estrogen and, if the uterus is intact, progesterone may be tried initially to prevent untoward side effects, such as breast tenderness and fluid retention. The dose may be increased gradually to therapeutic doses if tolerated. Most elderly women prefer a noncycling regimen of hormone replacement. Recommendations regarding dosing and combination therapy are the same as in younger women.

The American College of Physicians advocates that primary care practitioners incorporate a functional assessment within their routine medical management of older patients. A variety of instruments exist to assess functional capacity. The Katz Index of Activities Scale is one of the original methods of measuring function. This scale focuses on basic activities of daily living (ADLs) such as dressing, grooming, bathing, continence, and feeding. Various measures of instrumental ADLs are employed also to evaluate ability to live independently in the community. These skills include the ability to go shopping, use a telephone, prepare food, handle personal finances, and use transportation in the community. The Get Up and Go Test and the Tinetti function-oriented evaluation of gait and balance are also excellent screening tests and can be completed in 5–10 minutes in the office setting. The patient is observed sitting and getting up from a chair, standing with eyes closed, and standing with eyes open turning the neck. While standing, the patient is given a gentle nudge on the sternum to assess balance and recovery. She is asked to walk down the hallway at her usual pace, using an aid if indicated. The patient then turns and walks back to the examination room.

Although evaluation in the office does not reproduce the home environment, it provides the best opportunity to assess ease of mobility and has been shown to be useful in improving patient outcomes. Balance and gait problems, focal neurologic difficulties, and orthostatic hypotension all may be identified early. Prompt referral for physical and occupational therapies for rehabilitative measures, adaptive devices, and strengthening may help prevent a fall or injury.

Persons who are competent in their personal and instrumental ADLs should be encouraged to exercise regularly. More than 40% of elderly persons in the USA older than 65 report a sedentary life-style. There are well-established associations between physical inactivity and many chronic disease states in older people. Obesity, glucose intolerance, hypertension, reduced high-density lipoprotein (HDL) levels, and osteoporosis all have been associated with reduced physical activity. Walking is an excellent first step in an exercise program and can improve cardiopulmonary function, improve or reverse many of the disease states previously mentioned, and improve or preserve functional capacity. Exercise programs should be individualized. Duration and intensity of exercise should be increased gradually to a goal of 20 minutes 3 times per week with an average heart rate not to exceed 60–80% of the maximal predicted heart rate for age (220 − age = maximal heart rate). Exercise not only improves overall health by decreasing cardiovascular risk but also can increase social contacts, improve cerebral functioning, and help treat insomnia and depression. Even frail elderly can benefit from an individualized program of exercise.

SMOKING & DRINKING

There are an estimated 245,000 deaths annually from coronary artery disease and a combined ischemic heart disease and stroke death rate of 500,000/yr in elderly women in the USA. Smoking is an established risk factor for stroke and ischemic vascular disease. Studies indicate that smoking cessation has benefits with regard to decreased stroke risk and vascular complications at any age, whatever the

duration or amount of cigarettes smoked. It is worthwhile to screen for alcohol abuse as a source of disease and dysfunction in elderly women. It is important to remember that substance abuse, such as alcohol abuse and smoking, may be a marker of a recent loss or depression in the elderly.

CANCER SCREENING

When considering health screening in any population, a clinician must review the benefits to the patient in light of the disease being screened for. The accuracy and acceptability of the screening test should be considered. The evidence that a preclinical diagnosis would benefit the patient more than treatment after the disease manifests itself symptomatically needs to be reviewed. Unfortunately, there are few studies that outline cancer screening strategies in elderly women, and much of the evidence available is anecdotal.

Breast Cancer

More than 50% of new breast cancers are detected in woman older than 65; the incidence in this age group is 280 cancers per 10,000 women. Obesity, nulliparity, late first pregnancy, early menarche, late menopause, atypical hyperplasia, and a high-fat diet are considered risk factors for breast cancer. A positive family history may be a significant risk factor only for women younger than age 50. Breast cancer screening with mammography and breast physical examination has been shown to decrease mortality in women older than 50. However, data regarding continued mammography past age 75 are lacking. It is suggested by some authors that annual mammography continue until age 75, with continued breast physical examinations past this age. Because a woman age 75 has an average life expectancy of 12 years, one could argue for continued mammography to age 80. The American Geriatric Society recommends mammography screening until age 85. Again, the clinician must keep in mind individual risk factors, frailty, and complicating comorbid conditions when considering screening tests. Women should be taught and encouraged to perform breast self-examination and to have annual breast examinations.

Gynecologic Cancers

Women 65 years of age and older have a greater incidence than younger women of almost all gynecologic neoplasms. Endometrial, ovarian, and vulvar carcinomas are typically much more advanced in elderly women because of fear of discovery on the part of the patient and physician neglect and attitudes of ageism. Often studies reveal higher morbidity and mortality in the elderly because of the late stage of the tumor and comorbid conditions that complicate treatment. It is recommended, therefore, that all patients over age 65 continue to have a bimanual examination annually. Departure from this recommendation may be reasonable if a patient has a decreased life expectancy, an inability to undergo treatment, or an inability or refusal to undergo the examination.

Cervical cancer has the highest USA age specific incidence and mortality rates in women older than 65. The 1988 consensus (American Cancer Society, American College of Obstetrics and Gynecology (ACOG), American Medical Association, National Cancer Institute, and other groups) recommends annual screening, but the screening interval may be lengthened if a woman has had three consecutive normal Papanicolaou (Pap) smears before age 66 and has had no new sexual partner. Other organizations, such as the US and Canadian Preventive Task Forces, have recommended that cervical cancer screening cease at age 60 on the assumption that women with normal Pap smears when younger are at negligible risk. However, 15% of women 65–75 years of age have never had adequate screening, and 38% of women over age 75 have never had a Pap smear. For women who have undergone hysterectomy and are unaware of the type of hysterectomy performed (supracervical or total), the clinician must confirm that no cervical cuff is remaining. The American College of Gynecology recommends cytologic evaluation of the vagina every 3–5 years.

MEMORY LOSS

As the population ages, there will be an increasing number of persons with cognitive impairment of sufficient severity to affect day-to-day functioning in a serious way. Not only will the longer life expectancy of women result in a higher proportion of affected women, but the burden of caring for the impaired elderly frequently falls on female members of a family. Women in their 40s, the "sandwich generation," often spend a greater number of years caring for their elderly parents or those of their partner than in raising their children to adulthood. When the condition of progressive memory loss reaches epidemic proportions in the next century, health care providers will need to counsel caregivers regarding the stress of caring for others.

INCIDENCE

Cognitive dysfunction affects 5% of the total population older than 65, with the prevalence of disease rising with age; between 40 and 50% of persons older than 85 suffer memory impairment of such severity that normal living is affected.

DEFINITIONS

The term dementia describes a symptom complex rather than a diagnosis. A **dementia syndrome** is characterized by acquired, persistent intellectual dysfunction, affecting multiple areas of neuropsychological functioning. Diagnostic criteria include (1) loss of intellectual abilities, interfering with activities of daily living at home, work, or in social situations; (2) impairments in short- and long-term memory; and (3) impaired abstract thinking, impaired judgment, or personality change. It is important to distinguish between dementia and the minor memory changes of aging alone, "age-associated memory impairment." It may require longitudinal assessment over a period of months to years to exclude progressive disease in persons with these age-associated changes. Persons with acute confusion, developing over hours to days, who are suffering from a recent onset of delirium also should be excluded.

The *Diagnostic and Statistical Manual, 4/e, (DSM-IV)* criteria indicate that the crucial difference between dementia and delirium is that confusion exists despite a normal level of consciousness in patients with a dementia; whereas, a delirium is characterized by a waxing and waning level of consciousness. There must be evidence of a specific organic factor, eg, stroke or hypothyroidism, as a cause of the symptoms to exclude a nonorganic mental disorder.

ETIOLOGY

There are more than 70 different causes for the syndrome of dementia. Alzheimer's disease (AD) is by far the most prevalent, followed by vascular disease, mixed AD and vascular disease, and the multiple other causes (Table 4–1). Some dementia syndromes may be at least partially reversible with appropriate treatment, although completely reversible dementias comprise less than 5% of all causes. Nevertheless, a comprehensive search for reversible disease in patients presenting with cognitive impairment is clearly indicated because of the high incidence of comorbidities such as depression or adverse drug effects that may affect the severity of symptoms, worsen behavioral disturbance, or contribute to disability.

In recent study of 200 consecutive patients presenting at a memory loss clinic for evaluation, it was found that more than one-half had intercurrent medical problems that influenced their condition. Primary health care providers are uniquely positioned to provide thorough assessment of all the medical, func-

Table 4–1. Differential diagnosis of dementia.

Cortical features
   Alzheimer's disease
   Pick's disease
Subcortical features
   Multiple ischemic episodes—multi-infarct dementia
   Movement disorder
      Parkinson's disease
      Huntington's disease
      Progressive supranuclear palsy
      Wilson's disease
   Affective disorder—memory loss associated with
      depression
   Normal-pressure hydrocephalus
   Chronic confusional state
      Drug reaction and toxic exposure
      Metabolic abnormality
      Endocrine disorder
      Nutritional deficiency
      Infectious disease
      Neoplasia, primary or metastatic

Adapted, with permission, from Cummings JL, Benson DF: *Dementia: A Clinical Approach.* Butterworth, 1983.

tional, and psychosocial aspects of their patients' conditions.

DEPRESSION

Although depressive symptoms are common in older persons, they may constitute a diagnostic challenge to clinicians. Depression is the disorder that is most frequently misdiagnosed as dementia. Age-associated memory impairment may be exacerbated by depression, thereby mimicking the signs of early dementia. Additionally, depression is one of the major noncognitive complications of Alzheimer's disease and may worsen the symptoms of memory loss. Because a primary goal in management of patients with dementia is to reduce excess disability, accurate diagnosis of depression and appropriate treatment are clearly important.

Elderly patients who are severely depressed usually resemble younger depressed adults and frequently give a history of previous primary, endogenous, unipolar depression or cycling bipolar disease; they present with symptoms similar to previous episodes. Older severely depressed persons usually have a markedly depressed mood, sleep disturbance (early morning awakening), reduced appetite, weight loss, anhedonia, hopelessness, and sometimes a longing for death. There may be impairment of memory and concentration, resembling the early stages of dementia. Psychotic symptoms, delusions of worthlessness, and paranoid delusions also may be present.

Many of these diagnostically useful symptoms can be found in nondepressed elderly patients too, however. For example, lack of energy may result from intercurrent disease or medication, and early morning awakening may be unrelated to disease in older patients.

A complete medical and family history generally can differentiate between depression and early dementia. A depressive illness usually is characterized by an acute, recent onset; rapid progression; and a past history of depression with clear recognition of symptoms by family members. There is vague awareness by family members of the slow onset of dementia, which has a long symptom duration and slow progression.

In some cases, formal neuropsychometric assessment may be necessary to determine the primary or secondary nature of associated depression in a cognitive disturbance. Patients with depression tend to show poor effort on tasks, may give "I don't know" answers on cognitive tests, and do not display language difficulties, agnosia, or dyspraxia. In contrast, demented patients often struggle valiantly to complete tasks, try to give some kind of answer on cognitive testing, and frequently display language disturbance and other signs of organic brain disease. If there is doubt as to the cause of the cognitive dysfunction and the patient is believed to be clinically depressed, a trial of an antidepressant drug is indicated. Selection of an antidepressant drug for use in elderly patients depends on a knowledge of the alteration in pharmacokinetics secondary to the aging process, a history of prior response to a drug, the overall health of the patient, and knowledge of the side effect profiles of the various antidepressant drugs.

The clearance of all antidepressants is delayed by aging, resulting in elimination half-lives that are an average of 2–3 times longer than in younger persons. Lower doses of such drugs as fluoxetine and trazodone, which have long half-lives, may be necessary; the dosages may be increased gradually, in keeping with the "start low, go slow" adage.

Underlying physical problems may contribute to adverse drug effects; for example, the anticholinergic side effects of the tricyclic antidepressants may worsen constipation and narrow-angle glaucoma and may exacerbate confusion in patients with Alzheimer's disease.

Cyclic antidepressants and quinidine delay electrical conduction and therefore may predispose the patient to arrhythmia and heart block. An ECG may reflect cardiotoxicity with widening of the QRS complex; a baseline ECG should be performed in all patients before a cyclic antidepressant is begun and at appropriate intervals thereafter, usually when a maintenance dosage is reached and yearly thereafter.

Desipramine and nortriptyline are recommended antidepressants in the elderly; they may be started at 10–25 mg at night and increased by 10- to 25-mg increments. Trazodone is an effective second-line drug, particularly if sleep disturbance or agitation is a problem; the starting dosage is 25–50 mg at night, with 50-mg increments. Low-dose monoamine oxidase (MAO) inhibitors have been used successfully in elderly patients who are less severely depressed, particularly when anergia and apathy are prominent symptoms. The starting dosage for phenelzine is 15 mg; it may be increased by 15-mg increments to a dosage of 60 mg/d or until maximal clinical benefit is achieved. Thereafter, an attempt can be made to taper the dosage to 15 mg/d. Fluoxetine also may be helpful when a more "energizing" antidepressant is required; the starting dosage of 5–10 mg is given in the morning. The long half-life may allow for alternate-day dosing. The use of psychostimulants, such as methylphenidate, has not been studied conclusively in the elderly, although several small trials have shown positive benefits with amotivational syndrome, apathy, and depression; the starting dosage is 2.5 mg, and the drug is taken in the morning.

As with all drugs, it is essential to provide the patient and caregivers with full information as to the nature of the drug, dosage, expected benefits and side effects, and drug and food interactions (especially with MAO inhibitors). Increases in dosage of all antidepressants should be based on the clinical response of the patient and the appearance of side effects. Response in the elderly may take longer than in younger persons, often up to 4–6 weeks, but it may occur at much lower dosages. Plasma levels may be helpful when giving a tricyclic drug. Further information on the general management of depression can be found in Chapter 13.

ALZHEIMER'S DISEASE

This tragic disorder currently affects more than 4 million persons in the USA, and it is estimated that there will be 14 million cases of AD in the USA by the year 2050. The present cost of caring for sufferers approaches $90 billion a year, more than $25 billion in nursing home care alone.

The condition of progressive, global cognitive decline was described first by the pathologist, Alois Alzheimer, in 1907, initially in patients in late middle age. At first, Alzheimer's disease referred to a presenile dementia, distinct from the mental impairment seen commonly, although by no means universally, in persons older than 65 years. Subsequently, identical pathologic changes in the brains of patients with this presenile dementia were identified in the brains of patients who had the disease in later life, and indeed the disease is rare in patients younger than 65.

Pathogenesis & Neurochemistry

The characteristic changes seen pathologically at autopsy or on brain biopsy include (1) neuritic plaques, which are spheric lesions of β-amyloid protein, surrounded by degenerating axons, found in the cerebral cortex and hippocampus and (2) neurofibrillary tangles, which are abnormal neurofibers consisting of bundles of paired helical filaments, found in the frontotemporal cortex and pyramidal cells of the hippocampus. In addition, some studies have shown that the brains of some patients with AD have lost up to 60% of cortical neurons, associated with considerable neuronal atrophy.

The pathogenesis of the principal manifestation of AD, memory loss, is attributed to the loss of neurons producing acetylcholine. Studies of postmortem brain tissue in AD patients have inconsistently shown lower concentrations of norepinephrine, dopamine, and serotonin, but the clinical relevance is unknown. Other studies have demonstrated lower levels of gamma-aminobutyric acid (GABA), vasopressin, and somatostatin; again, the clinical significance is unknown, although the findings indicate the difficulties of devising appropriate clinical drug trial strategies in the attempt to ameliorate neurotransmitter deficiencies. How the presence of the abnormal neurofibrillary tangles and neuritic plaques correlates with the neurochemical abnormalities also is unknown.

Many factors are likely to be involved in the causation and pathogenesis of Alzheimer's disease. Genetic factors have been shown to be involved in some, if not all, cases of AD. Approximately 5% of cases of AD are believed to be familial, inherited in an autosomal dominant fashion. Chromosomal studies in some of these families have demonstrated point mutations on chromosome 21. Abnormalities in chromosomes 14 and 16 have been implicated in other families, suggesting that the cause of AD is not a single genetic mutation in all cases.

It seems likely, therefore, that the pathogenesis of AD is multifactorial; it may be that exogenous factors trigger the onset of disease in those who are predisposed. Possible exogenous factors include infectious agents, toxins, head injury, and local inflammatory responses.

High concentrations of aluminum have been found in the brain tissue of patients with AD, localized in the center of the neuritic plaques. There is no convincing evidence from epidemiologic studies or from comparison with the brains of age-matched controls, however, that aluminum is causative in the development of AD; rather, it is believed that aluminum deposition may be attracted to a degenerating nervous system. Additionally, trials of metal chelators in patients with AD have shown no effect on the progression of the disease.

Head injury has been shown in epidemiologic studies to be a risk factor for development of AD; study was prompted by the observation that people who had sustained repeated head trauma such as boxers were at risk of developing dementia, termed **dementia pugilistica**. At autopsy, a greater than expected number of neuritic plaques and tangles have been found in the brains of affected persons. The mechanism by which head trauma may induce the onset of AD has yet to be elucidated.

Clinical Findings

Alzheimer's disease is a slowly progressive illness of variable duration, lasting from 5–10 years until death. Memory changes at onset can be so subtle that neither the patient nor the family may be able to give a date of onset. Frequently, there is a 2- to 3-year history of slow mental decline before the symptoms become sufficiently obvious to warrant a diagnostic evaluation, usually prompted by a family member. It is a popular misconception, however, that sufferers from AD do not realize that they are ill. On the contrary, many patients are acutely aware of their deficits, which can lead to excess morbidity in the form of depression and even mortality from suicide.

As the disease progresses, short-term memory typically is affected earlier than long-term memory, and more complex skills are lost before simpler skills learned in early life. There are no abnormal neurologic signs in the mild-to-moderate stages of the disease, a fact that has two important implications:

1. In the vast majority of cases, a presumptive diagnosis of AD can be made on the basis of the history alone if the illness has been present for more than 2 years.
2. In an illness of short duration, ie, less than 2 years, the presence of abnormal neurologic findings, including gait disturbance, should mandate an imaging study of the brain and possibly neurologic consultation.

Short-term memory lapses, eg, forgetting names, phone numbers, and appointments, are common and persistent; these are followed by more serious problems with decision making, judgment, calculation, and handling of new or more complex situations. Anxiety, depression, and social withdrawal may develop, as may anger and frustration.

As the illness progresses, other areas of brain function are affected. Language disturbances may be characterized by anomia (word-finding difficulties), echolalia (repeating words, phrases, or questions over and over), agraphia (difficulty with written communication), or alexia (loss of reading skills). Eventually, patients become aphasic and essentially mute. Mathematic ability follows a similar downhill course. Visuospatial orientation becomes impaired early in the illness; patients may get lost in their neighborhood or even in their own home and may have difficulty dressing or using household objects. Patients eventually become apraxic, ie, unable to carry out commands despite having the strength to do so.

As social skills are lost, personal hygiene may be neglected, and patients may behave inappropriately in public. Paranoid delusions are common and may result in the patient accusing others of theft, infidelity, or abuse toward family members. Hallucinations are also common; these are usually visual and may be frightening to the sufferer. Individuals may be tranquil or agitated, can be restless or lethargic, and may display different behaviors during the course of the disease. This variability in symptoms has therapeutic implications; a drug needed to assist in management for a particular behavioral disturbance may not be required for the duration of the illness.

In the later and terminal stages of the disease, patients are unable to recognize people they know, even close family members, or to recall significant life events; they become disoriented to time and place. Frequently, sufferers neglect to eat, which results in rapid weight loss. Walking becomes impaired, fecal and urinary incontinence develops, and patients ultimately become bedridden and frequently mute, requiring 24-hour custodial care. Neurologically, primitive reflexes such as grasping and rooting occur, but deep tendon reflexes are preserved, and there is no sensory loss or cerebellar ataxia. Death usually occurs from sepsis complicated by inanition; the starvation frequently is associated with dysphagia occurring late in the disease.

Alzheimer's disease is a disease of behavior as well as cognition. Behavioral problems occur with a high frequency in all dementia syndromes and greatly affect the lives of both the patient and the caregiver. Management of behavioral disturbance is discussed in the following section, "Behavioral Disturbance in Dementia."

Diagnosis

Currently, there is no single test or imaging study short of a brain biopsy that can provide a conclusive diagnosis ante mortem of Alzheimer's disease as a cause for cognitive impairment. The diagnosis of probable Alzheimer's disease rests on exclusion of other causes for cognitive decline, coupled with satisfaction of the criteria developed by the National Institute of Neurological and Communicative Disorders and Stroke–Alzheimer's Disease and Related Disorders Association (NINCDS-ADRDA) (Table 4–2). Even after these criteria are satisfied, however, the percentage of inaccurate diagnoses has been estimated, from various series, to be 15%. More refined diagnostic imaging techniques and better acceptance of formal neuropsychometric assessment should improve diagnostic accuracy.

Correct diagnosis of the cause of a dementia is of more than academic importance, even though the clinical presentation and management may be the same for all the degenerative dementias. With the advent of new and more effective drugs to enhance cognition, accurate diagnosis can prevent inappropriate treatment with potentially toxic drugs. Additionally, awareness of the fact that there are many causes

Table 4–2. Diagnostic criteria for probable Alzheimer's disease.

1. Dementia established by clinical examination and by Folstein Mini–Mental State Examination or similar tool
2. Deficits in two or more areas of cognition
3. Progressive worsening of memory and other cognitive functions
4. No disturbance of consciousness
5. Onset after age 65
6. No systemic disorder or other brain disease that could account for the findings

for a dementing illness prompts the practitioner to search for evidence of reversible disease, both neurologic and nonneurologic.

VASCULAR DEMENTIA

Vascular dementia is claimed to be the leading cause of cognitive decline in Japan and Russia and to be second only to Alzheimer's disease in Western countries. The only major cause of dementia that is preventable is multi-infarct dementia. The precise incidence is unknown, but it may approach 20–30% of all cases of dementia. There has been a resurgence of interest in the evaluation and diagnosis of vascular disease as a cause of cognitive impairment with the advent of sophisticated brain imaging techniques such as magnetic resonance imaging (MRI). According to Hachinski, MRI may be able to "delineate changes in the brain so precisely that much more can be seen than understood."

It used to be thought that mental senility was caused by slow strangulation of the brain's blood supply by gradual narrowing of the cerebral blood vessels. Fisher demonstrated, however, that cognitive impairment from blood vessel disease is caused solely by stroke. Indeed, there is a direct relationship between the extent of cerebral infarction and the presence of dementia. There is no evidence to date of a "chronic ischemic state" accounting for mental decline.

The initial definition of **multi-infarct dementia (MID)** emphasized that the vascular process is quantal, discrete, and episodic, unlike Alzheimer's disease, in which the process is chronic and continuous. Multi-infarct dementia describes a syndrome resulting from diverse causes and with multiple manifestations, depending on the number, nature, and location of strokes. Unlike Alzheimer's disease, which has a predictable pattern of progression, MID varies considerably in clinical expression and course.

In one study researchers were was able to subdivide MID patients into characteristic syndromes with particular therapeutic implications. Forty-three percent of 175 patients had multiple lacunar infarcts, usually secondary to small-vessel disease caused by hypertension. Eighteen percent of cases were thought

to be related to reduced perfusion distal to occluded or critically stenosed major arteries. Less common causes were major large strokes and multiple cortical strokes. Hypertension was the most frequent risk factor, present in 66% of cases, with other risk factors as expected for vascular disease, eg, smoking and diabetes mellitus. The type of vascular injury should be determined so that specific treatment can be given, possibly preventing further damage.

Clinical Findings & Diagnosis

The diagnosis of multi-infarct dementia requires identification of "multifocal cognitive impairment" on standardized neuropsychometric tests. The history should suggest a stepwise course with patchy residual cognitive deficits. Focal neurologic signs are present. Evidence of associated hypertension and other vascular disease may be present. Hachinski has devised an ischemic score that readily discriminates among patients with AD, MID, and mixed AD and MID (Table 4–3). General evaluation involves the determination of the presence of risk factors for vascular injury that may be amenable to treatment.

Imaging studies of the brain demonstrate whether the damage affects cortical or subcortical structures or both. Controversy exists as to the relevance of white-matter changes on MRI, because these are found frequently on imaging studies of the brains of elderly persons who are cognitively intact. Such white-matter changes are found in 40% of AD patients and in more than 80% of patients with MID. These changes are likely to be disease-related, however, in the presence of risk factors in a patient with dementia. White-matter changes in a cognitively intact patient who has risk factors for cerebrovascular disease, particularly hypertension, might place that patient in a "brain at risk" category, indicating necessity for treatment.

Other patients who fall into the brain at risk category may include smokers, diabetics, patients in

Table 4–3. Hachinski Ischemia Score.*

1. Abrupt onset (2)[†]
2. Stepwise deterioration (1)
3. Fluctuating course (2)
4. Nocturnal confusion (1)
5. Relative preservation of personality (1)
6. Depression (1)
7. Somatic complaints (1)
8. Emotional lability (1)
9. History of hypertension (1)
10. History of strokes (2)
11. Evidence of associated atherosclerosis (1)
12. Focal neurologic symptoms (2)
13. Focal neurologic signs (2)

*Reproduced, with permission, from Hachinski VC et al: Cerebral blood flow in dementia. Arch Neurol 1975;32:632.
[†]The score for each feature is given in parentheses. A score of 7 or greater suggests a vascular component to the dementia.

atrial fibrillation, and those with coronary artery disease or asymptomatic extracranial arterial disease. Patients in the predementia stages of illness, ie, those with transient ischemic attacks, subtle cognitive impairment, previous strokes, and systemic lupus erythematosus, also are likely to benefit from early intervention.

Once a dementia syndrome has developed in the presence of atherosclerotic extracranial disease, cardiac embolism, or intracranial small-vessel disease, treatment is indicated in an attempt to arrest progression and improve cognition.

Treatment

Therapeutic strategies for the brain at risk stage include smoking cessation, careful management of diabetes, dietary improvement, estrogen replacement in postmenopausal women, antihypertensive therapy (particularly with angiotensin converting enzyme (ACE) inhibitors and calcium channel blockers), lipid-lowering agents, anticoagulants (especially in the setting of chronic atrial fibrillation), and aspirin.

For patients in the predementia stage, carotid endarterectomy for significant carotid artery stenosis (70–99%), aspirin, and ticlopidine may be necessary, as well as the measures described for patients in earlier stages. These treatment measures are applicable also to the dementia stage.

There are no drugs available that unequivocally reverse the intellectual decline seen in MID. Modest improvements in a single Cognitive Capacity Screening Examination (CCSE) occurred in one study after patients underwent antihypertensive therapy. However, this study also showed that with a reduction in systolic blood pressure to below 135 mmHg, some patients experienced further cognitive decline. Any fall in cerebral blood flow may render regions of misery perfusion frankly ischemic and thereby worsen the underlying disease. The CCSE score also improved in patients who discontinued smoking and in those who underwent carotid endarterectomy. Long-term outcome of these measures is unknown.

Clinical trials of cognitive-enhancing drugs in patients with MID are particularly difficult because of the spontaneous fluctuations of the illness. Any measures of improvement should include assessment not only of performance on standardized tests but also of patient independence. At this time, the mainstay of medical treatment remains prevention. General measures for managing demented patients are discussed in the following section, "Treatment of Dementia".

OTHER DEMENTIA SYNDROMES

Dementia of Frontal Lobe Type

Although Alzheimer's disease remains the most common primary degenerative dementia, several European studies have described a second form of primary cerebral dementia that pathologically and clinically affects the frontal lobes. Some of these cases are found at autopsy to have the characteristic pathologic changes in the frontal and temporal lobes seen in Pick's disease.

Dementia of frontal lobe type (DFT) is characterized by progressive personality change and breakdown in social conduct. Affected individuals may show reduced initiative, neglect personal hygiene, become incontinent, and show bizarre or rigid behavior. Stereotypic behavior is common and may range from simple repetitive movements to ritualistic activities. Patients may be restless, disinhibited, inappropriately jocular, or apathetic with amotivational features. The most striking feature in DFT is that patients invariably lack insight into their altered character and social misconduct. Unlike the predictable memory disturbance of AD, memory disturbance is variable and idiosyncratic with concrete thinking. Neuropsychologic assessment demonstrates difficulties with tasks that require planning, abstract thought, and mental flexibility. Memory may be preserved to a greater or lesser degree. Neurologic examination is usually normal, although frontal lobe reflexes may be present. Imaging studies of the brain may show frontal or temporal lobe atrophy.

There is clearly a genetic component to DFT; almost 50% of patients have an affected first-degree relative. The incidence data suggest that between 5 and 15% of patients presenting with a dementia have DFT. Many such patients may be considered eccentric or misdiagnosed as suffering from psychotic disorders. It is likely that, with increasing sophistication in the evaluation of dementia, the true prevalence of DFT will be determined to be higher. There is no known drug therapy.

Subcortical Dementias

Some dementia syndromes are characterized by movement disorders early in the course of the disease. The most pronounced feature of the movement abnormality in subcortical dementia is psychomotor slowness, with stooped posture and abnormal gait. The patient's intellectual processes seem to be slowed along with her movements. Unlike cortical dementias such as AD or DFT, there is no dysphagia, but frequently there is difficulty with retrieving (as opposed to learning) new information and impaired processing time.

Parkinson's disease is an example of a subcortical process associated with a dementia. Other degenerative dementias of differing causes that are associated with movement disorders include **Huntington's disease, progressive supranuclear palsy,** and **Wilson's disease.** The dementia of normal-pressure hydrocephalus is thought to be a result of subcortical damage; the associated gait disturbance and urinary incontinence complete the classic triad in this disease. Multiple sclerosis and HIV-related dementia also are considered to have a basis in subcortical pathologic changes.

Potentially Reversible Dementias

In evaluating dementia, the possibility of toxic damage to the brain always must be considered. Prescription medicines not only may be the cause of cognitive decline but also may be culprits in exacerbating confusion in individuals with other causes of dementia such as AD. Many drugs have been implicated; common offenders include digoxin, propranolol, benzodiazepines, and H_2-blockers. It is worthwhile to evaluate patients' medications repeatedly in the hope of eliminating drugs that may be contributing to cognitive impairment.

Metabolic abnormalities may result in a subacute confusional state. Hyponatremia or calcium abnormalities may be relatively long-standing and may contribute to a potentially reversible dementia. Endocrine abnormalities, particularly thyroid disease, should be excluded; apathetic hyperthyroidism or occult hypothyroidism may not be apparent clinically but indicated by an abnormal level of thyroid stimulating hormone (TSH). Nutritional deficiencies, such as of vitamin B_{12} or thiamine, may cause characteristic neurologic damage. Vitamin B_{12} deficiency can result in psychologic changes without concomitant macrocytosis.

Alcohol abuse, which occurs with the same prevalence in the elderly as in younger populations, may result in thiamine deficiency caused by poor nutritional intake. Wernicke's encephalopathy and organic amnestic syndrome both are related to thiamine deficiency. Alcohol abuse may be underdiagnosed greatly in the elderly, particularly in women, because of the reluctance on the part of clinicians to question patients in depth concerning their alcohol intake. The use of a simple screening tool such as the CAGE questionnaire, discussed in Chapter 11, should be routine in the evaluation of dementia.

Infection-Related Dementia

Infectious diseases are an uncommon cause of dementia in the elderly, so that a lumbar puncture (LP) is not a mandatory investigation in the vast majority of circumstances. Neurosyphilis is seen uncommonly; an LP is required to make the diagnosis of neurosyphilis in a patient with a positive serum VDRL and dementia. Clinical response to treatment is highly variable.

Creutzfeldt-Jakob disease is an infectious, rapidly progressive dementia caused by a virus, which progresses slowly. Patients display evidence of significant cognitive decline associated with myoclonus in the later stages. EEG studies demonstrate a "burst-silence" pattern, which can be diagnostic.

Primary HIV dementia may become the most common infectious dementia and should be considered in high-risk populations.

EVALUATION OF DEMENTIA

Although the preceding review of the numerous conditions that can cause memory loss in the elderly may appear daunting, many of these conditions are associated with neurologic findings early in the course of the illness and can be diagnosed with simple blood tests.

The relative frequency of the various causes of dementia is shown in Table 4–4; the vast majority of cases of dementia presenting to a primary care provider are Alzheimer's disease or vascular disease. In evaluating a patient with memory loss, there are two key questions to answer:

1. Does the patient have more significant memory loss than expected on the basis of age alone?
2. If so, what is the cause of the memory loss?

Thorough evaluation of a patient presenting with memory loss involves a complete history and physical examination. If possible, the history should be obtained from family members (if the patient agrees) as well as the patient. An understanding of the nature, duration, progression, and severity of the deficits should be obtained; the presence of any associated behavioral issues should be noted.

A full functional assessment is mandatory to determine to what degree the patient can care for herself on a daily basis. The practitioner should be aware of the level of social support available to the patient and should assess the effect of the illness on the patient's caregivers.

The physical examination of the patient should involve a complete evaluation of any intercurrent medical problems and should allow for appropriate health screening measures as outlined earlier in this chapter.

A mental status examination is crucial, but the practitioner must recognize that sensitivity and tact are vital during the assessment. Many elderly patients with cognitive problems, particularly those with little awareness of their difficulties, believe they are being examined to determine if they are crazy and may react with anger or accuse family members

Table 4–4. Relative frequency of dementing disorders in old age.*

Disorder	Percentage
Alzheimer's disease (AD)	52
Multi-infarct dementia (MID)	17
Combination of AD and MID	14
Brain tumors and other rare neurologic conditions	7
Parkinson's disease	2
Psychiatric conditions	1
Unknown causes	7

*Reproduced, with permission, from Pieri L, Cumin R, Hinzen DH: DN&P 1989;2:248.

of conspiracy. Several visits may be necessary to build rapport to ensure as accurate and complete an evaluation as possible. A mental status examination includes assessment of the following:

1. Level of attention and alertness
2. Language skills, such as fluency, comprehension, and repetition
3. Memory, both long- and short-term
4. Calculations, writing, constructional abilities, and abstract thinking.

A great deal of information can be gleaned from a simple assessment tool that takes a few minutes to administer. There are many well-studied instruments available; frequently, such a tool is valuable in determining the anatomic location of the underlying cerebral injury, which can be useful in differential diagnosis. Table 4–5 delineates the location of various higher cognitive functions. Specific diseases demonstrate specific patterns of cognitive abnormality.

One simple tool for use in the office is the Folstein Mini-Mental Status Examination (MMSE), shown in Table 4–6, which is perhaps the most studied tool. In addition, proverb interpretation may give some insight as to a person's ability to think abstractly. These instruments do not by themselves make a diagnosis of dementia; they are screening tools for the evaluation of cognitive dysfunction and determination of which patients require more comprehensive evaluation with neuropsychometric testing.

For example, normal elderly persons have a mean score of 27.6 on the Folstein MMSE, but the sensitivity of the test depends on the underlying educational level of the patient. A highly educated but impaired person may achieve a normal test result; such individuals may fall into a gray area, in which the history is suggestive but the preliminary office evaluation does not detect gross deficits. Neuropsychometric evaluation may provide additional information and thus assist with diagnosis. Such evaluations also may help distinguish between dementia and stroke-related

Table 4–6. The Folstein Mini–Mental State Examination.*

Function	Task	No. Points
Orientation	Patient asked, "What is the (year) (season) (date) (day) (month)?"	5
	"Where are we (state) (county) (town) (hospital) (floor)?"	5
Registration	Patient asked to name three objects with 1 sec to say each. Patient asked to repeat all three. (One point for each correct answer. Count and record number of trials.)	3
Attention and calculation	Patient asked to begin with 100 and count backward by 7 (stop after 5 answers), or to spell *world* backward.	5
Recall	Patient asked for the names of the three objects repeated earlier.	3
Language	Patient shown a pencil and a watch and asked to name them.	2
	Patient asked to repeat, "No if's, and's, or but's."	1
	Patient given a three-stage command: "Take a piece of paper in your right hand, fold it in half, and place it on the floor."	3
	Patient asked to read and obey the following written command: "Close your eyes."	1
	Patient asked to write a sentence.	1
	Patient asked to copy a design (intersecting pentagons).	1
Total score possible		30

*Reproduced, with permission, from Folstein MF, Folstein SE, McHugh PR: "Mini-Mental State" a practical method for grading the cognitive state of patients for the clinician. J Psychiatr Res 1975;12:189.

Table 4–5. Location of higher integrative functions.*

Location	Assessment
Frontal lobes	Points finger each time examiner makes fist; makes fist each time examiner points
Temporal lobes	Dominant: standard aphasia testing Nondominant: interprets affect
Parietal lobes	Dominant: names fingers, knows left and right, reads Nondominant: constructs copy of matchstick figure
Occipital lobes	Matches colors and objects

*Reproduced, with permission, from Shuttleworth EC: Memory function and the clinical differentiation of dementing disorders. J Am Geriatr Soc 1982;30:365.

disease, in which the deficits are patchy, and may assist in excluding depression.

The physical examination should include a neurologic assessment. Specific attention should be paid to evaluation of gait, which may suggest the presence of a subcortical dementia or normal-pressure hydrocephalus. The finding of any other neurologic abnormalities should prompt ongoing evaluation to exclude conditions other than Alzheimer's disease.

Laboratory evaluation is usually straightforward; most metabolic causes of dementia can be excluded by a complete blood count (CBC); a chemistry panel; thyroid function studies, especially TSH; vitamin B_{12} and folate levels; and a test for syphilis. Special clinical circumstances may prompt other tests such as an erythrocyte sedimentation rate (ESR) for vasculitis or an HIV antibody test in a high-risk individual.

Imaging studies of the brain have been used in an

attempt to diagnose AD and to exclude other conditions that might coexist. Computed tomography (CT) of the brain shows various abnormalities cross-sectionally in the lateral ventricles, sulci, and temporal lobes. Some studies have shown that CT analysis of the temporal lobe can discriminate AD patients from controls with an accuracy of 94%. In most circumstances, the CT scan is most useful to exclude other intracerebral diseases such as stroke, tumor, or hematoma.

If a patient has had evidence of a dementia for longer than 2 years and the neurologic examination is normal, the diagnostic yield is low; the scan is likely to show atrophy only. Longitudinal assessment of the degree of atrophy may have a higher degree of diagnostic accuracy with respect to the severity of disease.

MRI may be most useful in discriminating between AD and vascular dementia. MRI findings that support the diagnosis of AD include ventricular enlargement and widening of the subarachnoid spaces at the temporal regions of the brain, both of which correlate with disease severity.

Positron emission tomography (PET) can assess the rates of glucose utilization, oxygen consumption, and regional cerebral blood flow, thereby providing a functional rather than merely morphologic assessment of the brain. Some PET changes correlate with cognitive impairment; for example, decreased activity in the left hemisphere is associated with speech impairment. In general, PET scanning is limited to research centers.

Single photon emission computed tomography (SPECT) is less expensive and clinically more available than PET. As in PET, a variety of cerebrally active isotopes can be used to delineate areas of less active uptake. The presence of bilateral temporoparietal defects without other defects is indicative of a high probability of AD. Unilateral deficits are not predictive of AD, as their frequency is similar in patients with vascular or Parkinson's dementia.

Patients in the early stages of AD may have normal SPECT scans because of the low sensitivity of the test. Nevertheless, a suggestive SPECT scan, together with the clinical impression, especially if temporoparietal dysfunction is present on neuropsychometric assessment, may increase diagnostic accuracy greatly in the absence of a definitive test.

TREATMENT OF DEMENTIA

General Principles

The management of dementia in the home and in the long-term-care setting is a problem that is expected to grow as the population ages, with a disproportionate burden of care falling on female caregivers, including spouses, sisters, daughters, and female nurses.

Longitudinal studies suggest that survival time of patients who are suffering from dementia is increasing. A recent study demonstrated that the 50% survival rate from onset of disease was 8.1 years in AD, 6.7 years in MID, and 6.2 years in mixed disease. According to another study in a nursing home setting, demented individuals were cared for at home by family members for an average of 4.7 years before admission to the nursing home, with an average survival time in the nursing home of 2.5 years. Survival was decreased in patients in both studies when significant behavioral disturbance was present. Providers should establish close relationships with primary caregivers in a supportive and educational role.

General Health Maintenance

As dementia progresses, sufferers may experience problems with eating, grooming, and personal hygiene and may have difficulty exercising regularly. Proper nutrition is vital; weight loss is a common problem in dementia. Patients may forget to eat or how to prepare food or may develop cravings, particularly for sweet foods. Provision of food supplements and monitoring of appropriate textures may be indicated. Early discussion should take place with the patient, if she is able to participate, and with the family regarding provision of artificial feeding devices in the event of irreversible dysphagia.

The establishment of clear daily routines for exercise, grooming, meals, and toileting can minimize greatly the confusion and disorientation of daily life. Clothing should be simple and easy to change. If incontinence develops, a search should be made for reversible causes such as infections, drugs, or fecal impaction before assuming the cause to be related to cognitive decline.

As the patient with AD loses cognitive function, loss of muscular control, abnormal posture, and rigidity increase the risk of falling. Medications that potentiate hypotension and dizziness also may increase the risk. An uncluttered house, handrails, adequate lighting, and secure carpets are common sense approaches to decreasing the risk of falls.

The caregiver and clinician should assess driving skills; one recent study demonstrated a relationship between lower scores on the Mini-Mental Status Examination and difficulty with driving. Warning signs for the caregivers that the patient should discontinue driving include a growing tendency to get lost and extremely slow driving, indicating that memory and reaction time are declining. If the patient will not give up driving voluntarily, the caregiver may have to intervene by taking away the car keys or with other measures. Financial management problems may come to light when patients forget to pay bills, cannot balance a checkbook, spend irresponsibly, or make false accusations of stolen money. Caregivers may have to set up joint accounts or even apply for guardianship of the estate. Clinicians can provide caregivers with names of some of the excellent manuals available to assist in caregiver education.

Behavioral Disturbance in Dementia

Although Alzheimer's disease is a disorder of both cognition and behavior, the scientific and clinical establishment has concentrated on the evaluation and treatment of the cognitive decline rather than on the clinical management of the behavioral problems. There are few controlled clinical trials of the pharmacologic and nonpharmacologic strategies for improving behaviors.

Behavioral problems are estimated in a variety of studies to affect between 70 and 90% of patients with AD; they include agitation, aggression, depression, difficulties with personal hygiene and care, wandering, and screaming. The most common problem according to a recent outpatient study was restlessness. The frequency of most behavioral problems and the average total number of problems per patient increased with the level of cognitive impairment as measured by the Folstein MMSE. Behavioral problems often are reported by families to be their major source of stress and may be the main reason that patients are admitted to institutions. Wandering, particularly at night; incontinence; and physical violence are the three highest predictors of institutionalization.

Before beginning any form of treatment, whether with drugs or nonpharmacologic means, the behavioral disorder needs to be assessed. A useful way of cataloging behaviors is by assessment of the amenability of the disorder to specific treatments. Most behavioral disorders in the geriatric population are not treatable with psychotherapeutic medication and could be classed as nonpsychiatric behaviors. Dysfunctional behaviors of this type include aimless wandering, incoherent verbalizing, screaming or yelling, repetitive movements, hypersexuality, hoarding, spitting, inappropriate undressing, eating inedible objects, hiding things, physical self-abuse, inappropriate urination or defecation, constant commenting or questioning, and physically disruptive activity such as dumping food on the floor.

In contrast, there is a small group of behaviors that may respond to pharmacologic treatment; these might be termed psychiatric behaviors and include anxiety, depression, delusions and hallucinations, insomnia, and psychomotor hyperactivity and extreme aggression, which could include punching, slapping, kicking, biting, or scratching.

Evaluation of the cause of a behavior should involve assessment of the medical context by eliminating the iatrogenic causes of discomfort or agitation, eg, poorly timed diuretics, and treating painful conditions that the patient may not be able to describe, eg, arthritis, constipation, or dental problems.

The environmental approach to managing behavioral difficulties includes recognition of the need for a safe space for patients to wander in; the attempt to avoid restraints; matching staff to patients appropriately, eg, providing aides of the same sex for personal care; and maintaining a familiar, predictable, and nonthreatening environment.

The psychiatric approach includes recognition of specific behavioral reactions to mental illness, eg, an agitated response to a frightening hallucination, and in recognizing that an acute confusional state may represent a superimposed delirium secondary to a new and potentially treatable medical problem.

Treatment of Behavioral Disturbance

A. Nonpharmacologic Treatment: Treatment goals in the care of persons with dementia are to maximize participation in life through interaction and autonomy, to promote physical and emotional comfort, to maximize safety, and to maintain dignity and human contact.

Studies at the University of Washington have indicated the value of attempting to analyze behavior to improve management. This approach uses the ABC analog, which states that problem behavior occurs in three stages:

1. The *a*ntecedent or triggering event; what happens to instigate the behavior
2. The *b*ehavior itself
3. The *c*onsequence of the behavior.

An example of the use of this method of analysis involves an AD patient who becomes restless or agitated when her daughter is trying to prepare dinner. The antecedent event is the fact that the patient is left alone and feels isolated from family life. The problem behavior is the restless pacing that ensues. The consequence is the sense of frustration or annoyance that the caregiver feels at the patient's agitation or seeming dependence. The best approach to this type of problem is not to administer a drug to calm the patient as evening approaches but to attempt to increase her sense of self-worth and autonomy and her feeling of participation in family life by giving her a small task. Clearly, the management of demented patients in the home relies heavily on the commitment of the caregiver (see the section following, "Caregiver Issues").

B. Pharmacologic Treatment: Psychotherapeutic medications should be used judiciously in elderly patients, particularly in the setting of dementia, in which cerebral functioning already is compromised. Nonpharmacologic means of treatment should be tried first in all cases and should continue throughout all medication trials. Decisions should be made on the bases of safety and efficacy. Side effects of a drug must be acceptable for the patient under treatment. The decision to use a drug should take into account the patient's age, medical condition, and other drugs being taken. An appropriate starting dosage and dosage range must be determined. Efficacy involves identifying a specific "target behavior" to be treated, determining how to demonstrate that a drug is effective in treating that behavior, and deciding on a timeframe that allows demonstration of efficacy.

The most commonly used psychotherapeutic drugs to treat behavioral disorders can be classified into six groups as follows:

1. Antianxiety agents
2. Neuroleptics
3. Carbamazepine
4. Beta-blockers
5. Lithium
6. Miscellaneous drugs: trazodone, buspirone, L-deprenyl, valproic acid, and the selective serotonin reuptake inhibitors (SSRIs)

Many of the drugs in the preceding list have demonstrated beneficial effects in limited trials and situations, and many have been used only on the basis of clinical experience over time. There is a paucity of reliable clinical research on the use of psychotherapeutic medications in general in the demented elderly population.

1. Antianxiety drugs–These drugs are most useful for the short-term treatment of the target behaviors insomnia and "fidgety" restlessness. The class of drug most useful in the elderly is that of the benzodiazepines, especially those with short half-lives and no active metabolites, such as lorazepam (which is the only benzodiazepine that is well absorbed intramuscularly), oxazepam, or alprazolam. Doses should be low to start and should be tapered gradually to avoid rebound anxiety or insomnia. Lorazepam is also useful for patients who need sedation; for example, it may be given 1 hour before a medical or dental examination at a dose of 0.5 mg intramuscularly.

Benzodiazepines can precipitate rage reactions or increased agitation in an unpredictable fashion in some patients (the paradoxic response) and may exacerbate confusion.

2. Neuroleptics–These drugs are currently the mainstay of pharmacologic treatment for the severe agitation, paranoia, hallucinations, and other psychotic-type symptoms that can complicate dementia. These drugs should not be used indiscriminately for the long-term treatment of aggression because of the high potential for serious side effects, particularly tardive dyskinesia and akithisia. As with all psychoactive drugs, target behaviors should be identified and the drug closely monitored for efficacy and side effects.

Any neuroleptic may be effective for aggressive behavior; the choice should depend on the unique side effect profile of the drug. Low dosages should be used, especially if the drug is given on a daily basis; for example, haloperidol at a dosage of 0.25 mg twice daily may be effective in controlling assaultive behavior in a frail elderly patient.

There are few data to suggest the benefits of one neuroleptic over another, and few studies have attempted rigorously to compare neuroleptic drugs with other classes of drugs in the treatment of psychotic behavior. The paucity of data on the usefulness of neuroleptics is ironic given the fact that they are the most commonly used drugs in the management of patients with AD. At one time or another, almost every patient receives at least one psychoactive agent.

3. Carbamazepine–Several studies have shown that carbamazepine may be effective in patients with dementia with the target behaviors of combativeness, agitation, rage, and mood lability. The drug is particularly useful in patients with abnormal EEG findings in the temporal lobes; however, it also has been found to be helpful in patients who have violent outbursts but normal EEGs, suggesting that the beneficial effect may not be the result of the anticonvulsant effect. Clinical improvement can occur at levels below or in the low therapeutic range for seizure disorders. Side effects are sedation, drowsiness, skin rash, and ataxia. Bone-marrow suppression remains the most life-threatening complication. Because of the toxicity of the drug, carbamazepine should be used only after other drugs have failed.

4. Beta-blockers–Beta-adrenergic blocking medications have been used commonly in patients with organic cerebral dysfunction with a variety of diagnoses since the late 1970s. These drugs have been shown to be efficacious in controlling aggressive behavior, particularly in patients with dementia, schizophrenia, and mental retardation. Propranolol and pindolol are lipid-soluble, thereby crossing the blood-brain barrier; however, response of the target behavior of impulsive rage outbursts may be delayed in onset and may require relatively high doses. The adverse effect profile, particularly the risk of provoking bronchospasm or congestive heart failure or aggravating peripheral vascular disease, precludes use in most elderly individuals.

5. Lithium–There are few data in the literature concerning the use of lithium in the demented elderly, although it has been reported on anecdotally in patients with manic-type behavior. The drug may work best in combination with other medications such as neuroleptics or benzodiazepines. When used to treat aggression, lithium may be efficacious at doses lower than those needed to treat bipolar disease. Thus, serum levels of 0.3–0.6 meq/L may be therapeutic. As with all the psychotherapeutic drugs discussed, the clinical data are insufficient to permit recommendation of the drug except in infrequent circumstances when other approaches have failed.

6. Miscellaneous drugs—

a. Trazodone—This drug has been used in several small uncontrolled trials in patients with agitation, with generally positive results. It is a useful drug in elderly demented patients with insomnia or depression because of the low side effect profile. Sedation and edema are commonly reported side effects; otherwise, the drug is well tolerated. Clinical response to trazodone may be delayed.

b. Buspirone—There are few clinical data available as to the efficacy of this well-tolerated drug in the management of anxiety or agitation in the demented elderly.

c. L-deprenyl—This drug is an irreversible inhibitor of MAO type B that has been shown to slow the course of early Parkinson's disease. A recent study of the cognitive and behavioral effects of L-deprenyl in patients with AD showed no measurable impact on cognitive function and little on behavior over a 15-month period; it did not appear to slow the progression of the disease.

d. Serotonergic drugs—Potentiation of serotonergic transmission recently has been investigated in the treatment of the behavioral and cognitive symptoms of dementia. The finding that postmortem cortical tissue concentrations of serotonin are reduced in AD prompted these studies, as did the observation that behavioral symptoms can be altered substantially by antidepressants.

Pharmacotherapy for Dementia

In most circumstances, there are no drug treatments that reverse, cure, or otherwise attenuate the clinical course of a dementia syndrome. When a definite metabolic or biochemical abnormality can be identified, treatment may result in the restoration or normalization of cognitive function to a variable degree.

Treatment of vascular dementia depends on prevention by modification of risk factors as outlined previously. The movement disorder of Parkinson's disease may be improved by modification of dopaminergic transmission in the brain, but such treatment does not affect the associated memory disturbance.

The present strategy for treatment of Alzheimer's disease focuses on replacement of deficient acetylcholine. As discussed earlier in this chapter, the major biochemical abnormality in AD appears to be a relative deficiency of acetylcholine in specific areas of the brain. One approach has been the use of acetylcholine esterase inhibitors in the hope that acetylcholine levels in the brain will be enhanced if biochemical breakdown is attenuated and that such enhancement will improve cognitive function.

One such drug, tacrine (tetrahydroaminocridine or THA), currently is approved by the United States Food and Drug Administration (FDA) for treatment of Alzheimer's disease. A recent 30-week randomized, double-blind, placebo-controlled trial studied the efficacy and safety of high-dose tacrine. Outcome measures included clinical cognitive assessment. Tacrine was shown to produce statistically significant, dose-related improvement in most patients on objective, performance-based tests; clinician and caregiver evaluations; and measures of quality of life. The drug was generally well tolerated. Major adverse reactions, related to the cholinergic activity of the drug, were gastrointestinal, chiefly nausea and diarrhea. Fifty percent of treated individuals experienced asymptomatic elevations of liver transaminases, which were readily reversible on discontinuation of the drug. No cases of irreversible liver disease have occurred as a consequences of tacrine administration. Patients usually can be rechallenged successfully with the drug once the transaminases have returned to normal. The dose-response efficacy of tacrine continues up to 160 mg/d, and the beneficial effect has persisted for longer than 30 weeks.

CAREGIVER ISSUES

Although a diagnosis of Alzheimer's disease can be difficult to accept, it may come as a relief to caregivers to understand the nature of the problems they are facing. Caregivers face an enormous burden, emotionally, physically, socially, and financially.

The primary health care provider for the patient has the additional responsibility to assist the caregiver by providing education and support. Monitoring the responses of the caregiver to the burdens of caring for a sufferer from AD can be vital in attempting to avoid the serious problem of "caregiver burnout."

People who care for an AD patient frequently are fatigued from caring for the person all day, not getting adequate sleep, and living with constant stress, which may lower resistance to illness. Caregivers also may suffer from emotional reactions such as anger, guilt, embarrassment, helplessness, depression, grief, and isolation. Warning signs of caregiver burnout include weight loss from inadequate nutrition or depression, dependence on drugs or alcohol, verbal or physical abuse of the patient, and even suicidal isolation.

To prevent caregiver burnout, it is important to encourage the caregiver to take time out to enjoy hobbies or vacations. Respite care on an hourly, daily, or even weekly basis provides the caregiver with necessary free time. Counseling or joining a support group can be helpful. Two organizations that can assist families in caring for an AD patient are the Alzheimer's Disease Education and Referral Center (ADEAR) and the Alzheimer's Disease and Related Disorders Association (ADRDA), both of which have national and local chapters.

REFERENCES

Alessi C: Managing the behavioral problems of dementia in the home. Clin Geriatr Med 1991;7:787.

American Geriatrics Society: Screening for cervical carcinoma in the elderly. J Am Geriatr Soc 1989;37:885.

Applegate W, Blass J, Williams TF: Instruments for the functional assessment of older patients. N Engl J Med 1990;322:1207.

Christman K et al: Chemotherapy of metastatic breast cancer in the elderly. JAMA 1992;268:57.

Cooper JK: Drug treatment of Alzheimer's disease. Arch Intern Med 1991;151:245.

Diagnostic and Statistical Manual of Mental Disorders, 4/e (DSM-IV). American Psychiatric Association, 1994.

Desforges J: Gait disorders in the elderly. N Engl J Med 1990;322:1441.

Eddy DM: Screening for cervical cancer. Ann Intern Med 1990;113:214.

Fisher CM: Dementia in cerebral vascular disease. In: *Cerebral vascular disease, sixth conference.* Siekert R, Whisnant J (editors). Grune & Stratton, 1968.

Folstein MF, Folstein SE, McHugh PR: "Mini-mental state": A practical method for grading the cognitive status of patients for the clinician. J Psychiatr Res 1975;12:189.

Gallo JJ, Reichel W, Andersen L: *Handbook of Geriatric Assessment.* Aspen, 1988.

Gardner P, Schaffner W: Immunization of adults. N Engl J Med 1993;328:1252.

Giacobini E: Pharmacotherapy of Alzheimer's disease: New drugs and novel strategies. Prog Brain Res 1993;98:447.

Guralnik JM, FitzSimmons SC: Aging in America: A demographic perspective. Cardiovasc Clin 1986;4:75.

Hachinski VC: Preventable senility: A call for action against the vascular dementias. Lancet 1992;340:645.

Hachinski VC et al: Cerebral blood flow in dementia. Arch Neurol 1975;32:632.

Kawachi I et al: Smoking cessation and decreased risk of stroke in women. JAMA 1993;269:232.

Kenny DE, Oettinger EN: *The Family Care Book,* 2nd ed. CAREsource Program Development, 1991.

Knapp MJ et al: A 30-week randomized controlled trial of high-dose tacrine in patients with Alzheimer's disease. JAMA 1994;271:985.

Lamy P: The elderly and drug interactions. J Am Geriatr Soc 1886;34:586.

Larson EB et al: Diagnostic tests in the evaluation of dementia: A prospective study of 200 elderly outpatients. Arch Intern Med 1986;146:1917.

Mace NL, Rabins PV: *The 36-Hour Day.* Johns Hopkins University Press, 1991.

Maletta G: Treatment of behavioral symptomatology of Alzheimer's disease, with emphasis on aggression: Current clinical approaches. Int Psychogeriatr 1992;4:117.

Mandelblatt J et al: Breast cancer screening for elderly women with and without comorbid conditions. Ann Intern Med 1992;116:722.

Montamat P, Cusack B, Vestal R: Management of drug therapy in the elderly. N Engl J Med 1989;321:303.

Mor V et al: Risk of functional decline among well elders. J Clin Epidemiol 1989;42:895.

Neary D: Dementia of frontal lobe type. J Am Geriatr Soc 1990;38:71.

Ouslander J: Drug therapy in the elderly. Ann Intern Med 1981;95:711.

Prevention and Control of Influenza: Recommendations of the Immunization Practice Advisory Committee. MMWR 1992;41(RR-9).

Schneider LS, Sobin P: Non-neuroleptic treatment of behavioral symptoms and agitation in Alzheimer's disease and other dementia. Psychopharmacol Bull 1992;28:71.

Shapiro ED et al: The protective efficacy of polyvalent pneumococcal polysaccharide vaccine. N Engl J Med 1991;325:1453.

Sloan R: Principles of drug therapy in geriatric patients. Am Fam Physician 1992;45:2709.

Stern GM: New drug interventions in Alzheimer's disease. Curr Opin Neurol Neurosurg 1992;5:100.

Teri L et al: Management of behavior disturbance in Alzheimer disease: Current knowledge and future directions. Alzheimer Dis Assoc 1991;6:77.

Tinetti M: Performance-oriented assessment of mobility problems in elderly patients. J Am Geriatr Soc 1986;34:199.

Tinetti M, Ginter S: Identifying mobility dysfunctions in elderly patients. JAMA 1988;259:1190.

US Senate Special Committee on Aging America: *Trends and Projections,* 1987–1988.

Wenger N: Coronary heart disease in women: A new problem. Hosp Pract 1992;59.

Whalley LJ: Drug treatments of dementia. Br J Psychiatry 1989;155:595.

Williams WW et al: Immunization policies and vaccine coverage among adults: The risk for missed opportunities. Ann Intern Med. 1988;108:616.

5

Health Care for Lesbians

Jennifer I. Downey, MD

Lesbians are a significant, yet invisible, minority. Many women whose primary erotic attractions and relationships are with other women, nevertheless, do not openly adopt a lesbian social role. Between 3 and 5% of women in the United States identify themselves as a lesbian.

DISCLOSURE OF SEXUAL ORIENTATION

Although lesbian patients have the option of "coming out" to their health care providers, disclosing their sexual orientation is fraught with potential hazards. A number of studies suggest that health practitioners (like people in the general population) often have false beliefs about homosexuality. A lesbian patient who discloses her sexual orientation risks rude treatment, inadequate medical care, or breach of confidentiality. She may even be denied treatment. As a result of these risks, a substantial number of lesbians may decide not to give complete information about their medical histories or avoid seeking health care altogether.

In an effort to avoid discrimination, lesbians may turn to alternative sources of treatment such as chiropractors, nutritional counselors, and other holistic health practitioners. Lesbians also tend to avoid routine screening procedures such as Papanicolaou tests and breast examinations significantly more often than heterosexual women.

In order for health care providers to be able to respond to the unique medical and social needs of lesbian patients, an awareness of attitudes prevalent in society that may affect care is essential. **Homophobia** (the irrational fear, dislike, or hatred of homosexual people) is extremely prevalent. Until recently, much medical literature suggested that homosexuality was caused by childhood psychopathology, and sexual orientation toward a same-sex partner was considered worthy of a psychiatric diagnosis. This situation lasted until 1980, when the American Psychiatric Association removed homosexuality from the *Diagnostic and Statistical Manual.*

Another attitude that affects clinicians' approach to patients is **heterosexism,** which is the belief that heterosexuality is superior and should be encouraged. Several decades ago, the mental health community

---

Disclosure of Sexual Orientation
Health Issues Specific to Lesbians
    Definition
    Gynecologic Care
    Assisted Reproduction
Mental Health
Practical Strategies in Delivering Health Care

---

often recommended that homosexual individuals who aspired to psychologic health undergo treatment to "convert" them to heterosexual orientation. "Conversion" therapy has been found to be unsuccessful for the vast majority of homosexual people, and it is rarely undertaken today. Sexual orientation is considered to have a complex etiology with a biological component, at least in many people.

Homophobia and heterosexism have no valid scientific basis. Because providers were raised in a society pervaded by these prejudices, it is inevitable that clinicians—even gay and lesbian ones—are affected by them to a variable extent. Therefore, practitioners need to be as aware as possible of potential negative biases.

HEALTH ISSUES SPECIFIC TO LESBIANS

Definition

Most authorities define a **lesbian** as a woman whose erotic fantasies and experiences are predominantly about and with other women for a specified period of time (ie, over the previous year). Although the components of fantasy and erotic experience are crucial, two other components are also important (1) identifying oneself as a lesbian and (2) identifying oneself to others as a lesbian. "Coming out" to oneself is a matter of self-knowledge and self-naming, while "coming out" to others affects the person's social role. Many combinations of these four components are possible. For instance, a woman may have predominantly same-sex fantasies and privately believe she is a lesbian although she has never had a sexual encounter with a female partner; she may even maintain her social role as a wife in a traditional marriage. Another woman—perhaps a college student—could have sexual fantasies about men and women in equal amounts, have about equal amounts of erotic experience with both, and think of herself as heterosexual. A woman with the same types of fantasy and experience but with strong affiliations to feminist groups on campus might identify herself as a lesbian. Yet, a sex researcher would describe the experience of these two women as bisexual.

Hence, it is important to realize that individuals label themselves as lesbian, bisexual, or straight depending not only on their behavior but also the meaning they place on their behavior. Johnson et al found 77% of self-labeled lesbians have had coitus with men; whereas Robertson and Schachter reported a figure of 89%. Many of these women, however, identify themselves as lesbian, not bisexual. Because coitus with men increases exposure to a variety of gynecologic ailments, the provider needs to clarify the meaning of the terms the patient uses regarding sexual orientation.

Gynecologic Care

Many studies have addressed the issue of sexually transmitted diseases in lesbians; however, no studies found any gynecologic problems unique to or more frequent among lesbians than among bisexual women. In fact, some diseases (eg, cystitis, syphilis, gonorrhea, and chlamydial infections) occur less frequently in women who have been sexually active with women only.

HIV infection is a special instance of this factor. As of November 1990 the Centers for Disease Control and Prevention reported that almost all lesbian AIDS cases in the USA have been related to injecting drug use, and that only two instances of female-to-female sexual transmission of HIV have been reported. This finding does not imply that safe-sex practices between women should not be observed; they should. On the other hand, it is vital for practitioners to realize that lesbians do not share the elevated risk of HIV infection that homosexual men experience. This elevated risk is not because of sexual orientation per se, but to particular sexual practices of homosexual men and not of homosexual women, specifically, the tendency for gay men to have more sexual partners and to engage in anal penetration.

Lesbians require routine gynecological care because some disorders—even infectious ones—occur in women who have never had heterosexual intercourse. These infections include *Candida albicans, Trichomonas vaginalis,* and nonspecific vaginitis (*Gardnerella vaginalis*). Genital herpes also is found in women who have never experienced intercourse because oral-genital transmission of virus can occur, and both herpes simplex virus (HSV) and human papilloma virus (HPV) have been reported. Abnormal cervical cytologic findings have been reported in a high proportion of lesbian patients at several clin-

ics. Other conditions such as endometriosis, endometrial cancer, and breast disease would be expected to occur at the same rate as in heterosexual women with comparable parity.

Johnson et al have suggested that screening for cervical cancer among lesbians and bisexual women should be carried out in accordance with standard clinical practice, with the frequency based on the individual's risk factors and not on the basis of sexual orientation. Similarly, these authors have suggested that screening for sexually transmitted diseases should be individualized and that routine treatment of female partners for vaginal infections should not be done unless the partner has a demonstrated infection. It should be kept in mind that the patient's current sexual orientation does not mean she has not had sexual contact with men or that she has no need of routine care.

Assisted Reproduction

Another aspect of medical care important to lesbians involves efforts to achieve parenthood. Because so many lesbians have a history of sexual relationships with men, it has always been the case that lesbians have been mothers. It was only in the 1980s that large numbers of lesbian couples began to request their clinicians' help to enable them to become pregnant, usually via artificial insemination by donor (AID).

Clinicians have disagreed about the ethics of using AID to help unmarried women to become pregnant—regardless of their sexual orientation. The American Fertility Society's 1993 *Guidelines for Gamete Donation* lists as one indication for therapeutic donor insemination that the patient is a single female. It generally is agreed that a health care practitioner who believes that it is not acceptable to assist unmarried women by using this intervention should not be required to do so, but that he or she should refer the patient to a practitioner who would be able to honor her request if she is adequately prepared emotionally, socially, and economically to take on the responsibility of raising a child.

Some practitioners will experience concern about purposefully creating families in which no father will have a role. A single woman contemplating a pregnancy by AID—whether heterosexual or lesbian—might be asked what plans she has made to provide her child with male figures. Often lesbians have excellent relationships with male friends or family members who are able to act as support persons. A number of studies in the 1980s compared children of lesbians to children of divorced heterosexual women and found insignificant differences in gender role behavior, behavior problems, and social relationships with peers. Because the children studied had not reached adulthood, long-term outcome on such variables as sexual orientation and mental health is unknown. However, there were no indications that the children growing up in lesbian families were developing any differently than children growing up in the traditional nuclear family. Although it is sometimes believed that children of homosexual parents have an increased likelihood of growing up to be homosexual themselves, preliminary data do not support this assumption.

Studies of lesbian mothers who conceived with the help of AID have shown that, similar to other mothers of planned babies, they were highly motivated to obtain medical care and give their babies a good start in life.

A common stereotype of lesbians has been that they are uninterested in families, children, or motherhood. Although individuals can be found who fit a stereotype such as this one, the notion clearly is not true for lesbians in general. For instance, when Johnson et al queried 1921 self-described lesbians and 424 self-described bisexual women, 58.8% of the lesbians and 60.6% of the bisexuals said they had considered having a child. Concerning the different options by which one can achieve parenthood, 61% of the lesbians had considered AID, 62% adoption, 37% intercourse with a cooperative man, and 15% intercourse with an unsuspecting man. Of the bisexual women 38% had considered AID, 53% adoption, 65% intercourse with a cooperative man, and 22% intercourse with an unsuspecting man. Given numbers like these, it seems likely that biologic parenthood will be sought by larger numbers of lesbians as time goes on and that help from medical practitioners will be requested.

Lesbian patients have noted that they appreciate an attitude of respect in practitioners that avoids assumptions about heterosexuality, relationship status, and method of conception. If a lesbian is pursuing pregnancy with her partner she should be offered the opportunity to have the partner present for medical treatments, childbirth classes, and the delivery.

Because legal and custody implications vary from state to state and community to community, a clinician should never document sexual orientation in a chart without informed consent. The partner who is not the biologic parent usually does not have any legal claim on the child (adoption is available to couples who are not married only in a few states), and may tend to feel excluded from the pregnancy and birth as a result; therefore, the practitioner needs to be particularly sensitive to the feelings of this woman.

MENTAL HEALTH

Because women are more frequent users than men of mental health services, as well as general medical services, lesbians are likely to seek some kind of psychologic counseling. Several large population-based studies comparing heterosexual with homosexual women have found few differences in psychopathology. Bell and Weinberg reported higher rates of loneliness and depression in homosexual than in heterosexual women. Also, a higher rate of attempted suicide among lesbians has been reported (ie, 25% in white homosexual women versus 10% in white heterosexual women). Saghir and Robins found that more homosexual than heterosexual women have a problem with alcohol abuse, a finding that has been substantiated by a number of other investigators. The reasons for these differences are not clear, although important factors that should be considered are the stress of being a member of a stigmatized minority and the importance of the gay bar as one of the few places to meet other lesbians.

Issues that commonly cause a lesbian to seek psychologic help include internalized homophobia (feelings of shame and disappointment about being lesbian) and difficulties with coming out to family, friends, or colleagues. Other issues include relationship problems, depression, and substance abuse. In addition, many women, especially younger ones, may have feelings of confusion about whether they are predominantly heterosexual or homosexual. Sexual problems—especially regarding whether a coupled relationship is to remain exclusive and regarding differences in level of sexual interest—also may lead to consultation.

Primary care clinicians can be most helpful to lesbians who have complaints in the emotional and psychiatric spheres by facilitating communication and education between the patient and her concerned family members or partner. Psychiatric emergencies include suicidal or homicidal ideation, psychosis, severe self-destructive behavior, and battery. Patients with problems such as these should be referred to a psychiatric professional immediately, and a concerned member of the patient's network should be informed so that he or she can stay with the patient and ensure that the contact with the mental health practitioner is made. Less urgent situations warrant referral if the distress persists over several weeks and does not respond to education and support or if the condition appears to require expertise that the primary practitioner does not have, for example, the use of certain psychotropic medications or sex therapy.

It is helpful for clinicians to be informed concerning which psychiatric facilities, including treatment centers for substance abuse, in their geographic area are particularly sensitive to female clients and nontraditional family structures. When referring to private practitioners in the community, discretion and previous screening are advised. It is not helpful to refer a lesbian patient to a practitioner who still believes that homosexual orientation is not consistent with mental health. Treatment by such a person can result in damaged self-esteem and worsening of symptoms as well as failure to address the patient's clinical problems. It is equally unhelpful to refer a confused adolescent or young adult who is unclear about her sexual orientation to a therapist who is so fixed in a gay-affirmative stance that he or she will reassure the patient about being gay without exploring the meaning and extent of the confusion. Some young people who are not homosexual acquire the conviction that they are gay as a way of explaining to themselves global psychopathologic impairments. Such individuals need treatment by professionals skilled in treating severe neurotic difficulties and character problems, not education and reassurance.

If the primary care clinician lacks skills in psychologic evaluation and the problem is complex, the best approach often is to refer the patient, couple, or family for evaluation by the most sophisticated and well-trained practitioner available. Some patients do not need extended treatment. Patients who do require treatment can be referred by the evaluating clinician. Thus, referral can be viewed as a two-step procedure: first, evaluation; second, treatment (if needed). This approach avoids the problem of trying to make an appropriate referral for treatment when the referring practitioner has neither the time nor the training to perform an adequate psychologic evaluation.

PRACTICAL STRATEGIES IN DELIVERING HEALTH CARE

A number of studies of lesbians' satisfaction with practitioners have yielded suggestions from patients about to deliver health care more sensitively. In general, women have asked that clinicians not assume that everyone is heterosexual. Thus, when the medical history is taken, it is helpful if the practitioner allows for clarification rather than implying that a certain answer is expected. Instead of asking, "Are you married?", the clinician can inquire, "Are you involved in an intimate relationship (or with a life partner)?" or "Whom do you live with?" Instead of asking, "Are you sexually active?" or "What kind of contraception do you use?" the practitioner may ask, "Are you sexually active—with men, women, or both?" "Do you have need of contraception?"

Lesbians are keenly attuned to cues as to the open-mindedness of a provider. They take note of the health questionnaires they are given and the literature that is available in the waiting room. It is not necessary for every patient to disclose her sexual orientation; however, if the clinician believes it is important to know the patient's sexual orientation (eg, in gynecologic interactions or in mental health treatment), he or she may preface the inquiry with an explanation of why the information would be helpful. In addition, the matter of confidentiality can be discussed; many lesbians are willing to disclose their sexual orientation when reassured that it will not be revealed in the chart. When a patient does not want her lesbian identity documented, the clinician may consider using a

coded entry in the chart to remind him or her about the patient's sexual orientation while preventing breaches of confidentiality. Some women simply need more time to develop a trusting relationship with a physician before they are willing to discuss a matter as sensitive as sexual orientation.

Clinicians can build rapport with lesbian patients in other ways as well. For instance, they can offer to include partners in medical discussions and ensure access for the partner to the delivery room or intensive care unit. They can make sure that all next-of-kin policies and discussions of advance directives include the possibility of a lesbian partner, help their patients get up-to-date information about topics of medical interest to lesbians such as safe sex and substance abuse, and refer patients for appropriate counseling about such issues as parenting, coming out, battery, and hate crimes.

The sexual orientation of the practitioner can become an issue. Some clinicians and health care consumers have advocated that health care providers for lesbians ideally should be lesbians. The rationale for this argument is that in a homophobic culture, episodes of bias against lesbians in the health care setting would be reduced if not eliminated. The particular danger of recommending that minority groups be treated by members of the same group is that this practice may lead to **peripheralization** (the exclusion from the society mainstream of both patients and clinicians). Thus, except in special instances, it is suggested that the provider need not be lesbian or gay as long as she or he is sensitive to and informed about the issues affecting the patient.

The sexual orientation of the health professional may become an issue with individual patients in another respect. Some lesbians who have been traumatized by negligence or abuse in the health care setting may seek to reassure themselves in future interactions by asking to know the sexual orientation of the practitioner. Although revealing this information is a matter of clinical judgment and personal style, the clinician's willingness to be frank about his or her sexual orientation often is helpful.

In an article discussing the care of gay and lesbian adolescents Ramafedi and Blum wrote eloquently about the duties of the clinician:

> The care of gay and lesbian adolescents is an important issue that unfortunately rests less heavily in scientific fact than in the personal discretion of the provider. Pediatricians are strongly urged to consider carefully how their own attitudes impact on their care of families, to promote discussion of the issues within their communities, to support and to participate in research in the area of adolescent sexuality, and to provide education and care to all children and adolescents, regardless of sexual preference.

This statement applies also to clinicians who treat lesbian patients of all ages. It is a reminder that clinicians must act as community leaders as well as physicians, support research as well as treatment, and

perhaps most of all, consider carefully the impact of personal attitudes on the patients.

REFERENCES

American Fertility Society: *Guidelines for Gamete Donation: 1993.* American Fertility Society, 1993.

Bancroft J: Commentary: Biological contributions to sexual orientation. In: *Homosexuality/Heterosexuality: Concepts of Sexual Orientation.* McWhirter DP, Sanders SA, Reinisch JM (editors). Oxford, 1990.

Bell AP, Weinberg MS: *Homosexualities: A Study of Diversity among Men and Women.* Simon & Schuster, 1978.

Chu SY et al: Epidemiology of reported cases of AIDS in lesbians, United States 1980–1989. Am J Public Health 1990;80:1380.

Edwards A, Thin RN: Sexually transmitted diseases in lesbians. Int J STD AIDS 1990;1:178.

Friedman RC: *Male Homosexuality: A Contemporary Psychoanalytic Perspective.* Yale University Press, 1988.

Friedman RC, Downey J: Neurobiology and sexual orientation: Current relationships. J Neuropsychiatry 1993; 5:131.

Janus SS, Janus CL: *The Janus Report on Sexual Behavior.* Wiley, 1993.

Johnson SR, Palermo JL: Gynecologic care for the lesbian. Clin Obstet Gynecol 1984;27:724.

Johnson SR, Smith EM, Guenther SM: Comparison of gynecologic health care problems between lesbians and bisexual women: A survey of 2345 women. J Reprod Med 1987a;32:805.

Johnson SR, Smith EM, Guenther SM: Parenting desires among bisexual women and lesbians. J Reprod Med 1987b;32:1987.

Kinsey AC et al: *Sexual Behavior in the Human Female.* Saunders, 1953.

Ramafedi G, Blum R: Working with gay and lesbian adolescents. Pediatr Ann 1986;15:773.

Robertson P, Schachter J: Failure to identify venereal disease in a lesbian population. *Sexually Transmitted Diseases.* 1981;8:75.

Saghir MT, Robins E: *Male and Female Homosexuality: A Comprehensive Investigation.* Williams & Wilkins, 1973.

Ethical Issues

6

Lorna A. Marshall, MD, & Joanna Cain, MD

Ethics is the formal study of moral behavior in which moral obligations are analyzed in terms of recognized values and principles of society. Ethics becomes important in health care when personal determinations about what is right and wrong become inadequate to reach resolution of conflicting values. A logical and disciplined approach to a complex ethical problem becomes necessary. A full discussion of the various theories and processes of ethics that can be used in clinical decision making is beyond the scope of this chapter. Four basic ethical principles frequently are used in approaching clinical situations:

1. Autonomy–the respect for self-determination of the patient.
2. Beneficence–the duty to do what is good for the patient.
3. Nonmaleficence–the duty to avoid harming the patient.
4. Justice–the right of the patient to be treated fairly and to a fair allocation of society's resources.

Ethical issues that are specific to women often involve choices regarding reproduction, including choices that involve obligations to the fetus. However, ethical issues can be identified in all stages of a woman's life.

CHILDHOOD

Parents are the recognized surrogate decision makers for their children. If the parents disagree about health care decisions, or if the health care provider believes that the parents are not acting in the best interest of the child, conflict may occur. Such disagreement sometimes arises in cases of young women who have been victims of abuse or rape. One or both parents may refuse to give permission for health care, perhaps because of the involvement of a family member, perhaps for idiosyncratic reasons. The health care provider must consider whether the parent is acting in the best interest of the child; if it is believed that the parent is not acting in the child's interest, the court may be asked to appoint a guardian. Choices such as these are not made in a vacuum but

Childhood
Adolescence
Pregnancy
Abortion
Reproductive Technologies
Other Ethical Issues of Adult Women
Elderly Women & End-of-Life Issues

with consideration for all the facts of the case. The potential harm to children of causing a rift between their parents can be a compelling reason against proceeding further.

ADOLESCENCE

The identification of a surrogate decision maker for adolescents becomes especially difficult when decisions about contraceptive care and abortion are called for. It is important for health care providers to know the laws in their state regarding parental notification or consent. Most states allow minors to give consent for treatment of sexually transmitted diseases. Most states also allow pregnant minors to give consent for procedures on themselves and usually on their offspring. However, the majority of states require parental consent or notification before a provider can perform an abortion on a minor, although many states do not enforce these laws.

In some cases, laws requiring parental permission may conflict with the health care provider's assessment of what is best for the patient. Identification of who is the patient—the adolescent or her parents—becomes problematic. Furthermore, the broader social interests, eg, protecting other members of society from sexually transmitted diseases, must be considered in formulating ethical solutions.

PREGNANCY

In obstetrics, the health care provider has the interests of two patients in view; these interests are interrelated and sometimes conflicting. In the past, obstetricians clearly identified the mother as the patient.

The well-being of the fetus was of course important, but the well-being of the mother generally was considered to be the primary concern. In recent years, there have been changes in our perception of the fetus as a patient. For example, fetuses now can undergo surgery and other treatments for disorders in utero. The definition of the fetus as a patient is changing gradually. More than ever, the obstetrician must balance maternal health and maternal autonomy with the needs of the fetus.

The mother generally has been considered the surrogate decision maker for the fetus, because decisions that affect the fetus almost always directly affect her. Usually, women are willing to accept considerable risk to themselves for the good of the fetus. When treatment that may be beneficial to the fetus is refused by the mother, the obstetrician is faced with competing interests. To override the patient's wishes may be in the best interest of the fetus but also violates the patient's autonomy and right to refuse care. Recently, husbands or other, unrelated third parties have attempted to make decisions concerning the fetus, despite disagreement with the wishes of the mother.

Rarely, a court has ordered a cesarean section to be performed on a pregnant woman, indicating that in rare circumstances concerns of the fetus may be as important as or more important than the interests of the mother. However, such choices may not be in the long-term interest of society if they discourage women from seeking care because of fear of loss of autonomy. Because of the complexity of these decisions for individuals as well as society, involvement of the courts is discouraged by many major groups.

Mandatory screening for HIV infection in pregnant women is being considered in some jurisdictions and provides an example of a possible conflict between the interest of the mother and that of the fetus. If the mother is HIV-positive, therapy is now available prenatally that may benefit the health of the fetus. However, the identification of an HIV-positive woman in a nonconfidential screening may have significant economic and social consequences for the woman, such as social discrimination and denial of insurance coverage or employment.

Decisions concerning specific pregnant women may have unexpected far-reaching implications for other women. For example, in states in which drug abuse in pregnancy is being considered for inclusion in criminal codes, pregnant women who are drug abusers could be jailed to protect the fetus. As a consequence, other pregnant women who abuse drugs may become reluctant to seek prenatal care or admit drug use to their provider for fear of criminal prosecution. Their fetuses would be unintended victims of these legal interventions and potentially more harmed than if the mother continued abusing drugs but received prenatal care.

Finally, judgments about futility of treatment and withholding and withdrawing care need to be made even in the field of obstetrics, in which the outcome involves fetal health or survival. Subjecting the mother to the risks of cesarean section may not be appropriate when fetal distress occurs at 22 weeks of gestation or when the result will be an anomalous infant who has no chance of survival; the situation may be different at 26 weeks, when the infant may survive. Informed consent is a difficult issue when the outcome is uncertain; it is especially difficult for a woman who is first presented with the complex consequences of accepting or withholding treatment after she has initiated labor.

ABORTION

Few topics in health care have received as much attention from society as the issue of abortion. The 1973 Supreme Court decision in *Roe v Wade* upheld the right of a woman to terminate her pregnancy until the time of fetal viability and thereafter when necessary to protect her own life or health. In 1992, the Supreme Court reaffirmed the decision in *Roe v. Wade*. Considerable conflict still exists in the United States regarding this issue. Although the legal right to an abortion is ensured, abortions often are not publicly financed. Respect for women's wishes for health care becomes biased, therefore, on socioeconomic grounds. The issue of financing abortions as part of just health care reform has become a major source of conflict.

In general, the main ethical issue regarding abortion is the conflict between respect for a woman's autonomy and society's interest in the fetus. Central to the issue is the definition of life and whether or not to differentiate among the fertilized egg, preembryo, embryo, fetus, and newborn infant in that definition. In one point of view, a fetus whose survival is contingent on using the woman's body could be assigned fewer rights than one who is able to survive independently. Whether and by what vehicle society should be involved in topics about which there is such strong moral disagreement are important questions.

The potential use of prenatal diagnostic methods to determine the gender of a fetus, followed by abortion for gender selection, raises a myriad of ethical issues. Whereas in this country gender selection is rare, it is common in India and some other countries. If abortion for gender selection were to become prevalent, questions such as the following would be raised: Can the potential for serious societal harm justifiably lead to restriction of the choices available to parents? Is autonomy with regard to reproductive matters an absolute right?

REPRODUCTIVE TECHNOLOGIES

The advances and greater availability of the reproductive technologies have raised new ethical issues. Again, defining the beginning of life is central to an approach to this topic. It is argued by some that the preembryo, which is multicellular but not differentiated, deserves special respect, but not the full rights of an individual.

The increased use of egg donation for older women and those with premature ovarian failure also has raised new ethical issues. The egg donor must undergo the risks of ovarian stimulation and egg retrieval with no benefits except for minimal monetary compensation. Because the monetary compensation is more attractive to less affluent than more affluent women, egg donors are more likely to have lower socioeconomic status. Because medical insurance usually does not cover ovum donation in this country, egg recipients usually have higher socioeconomic status. Thus, the potential exists for socioeconomic inequity between donor and recipient. This situation is markedly different from that of other types of transplants, such as kidney, in which organs are allocated on the basis of greatest and most immediate need.

OTHER ETHICAL ISSUES OF ADULT WOMEN

Although most ethical issues specific to adult women involve reproduction, there are some that do not; some aspects of informed consent and surrogate decision making apply specifically to women.

In general, women consider themselves to be less powerful in society than men. When they are ill and in a hospital setting, they feel even less powerful. The task of consenting to treatment may be given to the "more powerful" person, with the patient incompletely informed. The health care provider must take pains to ensure that the patient is truly informed and that she feels she has the freedom to consent to or refuse care without coercion.

All patients should be encouraged to appoint a durable power of attorney for health care. When such an appointment has not been made, each state has a hierarchy for surrogate decision making. In some circumstances, such as regarding lesbian couples, states may not recognize the person most able to make surrogate decisions unless a durable power of attorney has been appointed. Patients should be encouraged to express their feelings about withdrawal and withholding of support to both her health care provider and her durable power of attorney or surrogate decision maker. It is the physician's responsibility to be sure that the surrogate does not make a decision that would be in conflict with the patient's previously stated wishes. Preparation of advance directive documents should be encouraged strongly; all institutions accepting Medicare payments are required to ask about the existence of these documents.

ELDERLY WOMEN & END-OF-LIFE ISSUES

Advance directives and other end-of-life issues become even more important when the patient is elderly. Because women are likely to outlive their spouse, arrangements for a durable power of attorney for health care other than the spouse need to be made.

An additional problem with the elderly is the determination of a patient's competence and her ability to make choices. When treatment is refused by the patient and competence is questioned, the provider may have to decide whether to follow the desires of the patient or of her surrogate.

Because of limited economic resources, health care reform at the federal and state levels may have a dramatic impact on elderly women. For example, age-based rationing of expensive treatments such as kidney transplants has been discussed as a means to limit health care expenditure. Because women's life expectancy is greater than men's, such rationing may be unfairly applied to women who may otherwise have many years to live. Guidelines or mandates about the termination of care for chronically or terminally ill patients also would affect women disproportionately, for the same reason.

REFERENCES

Annas GJ: The supreme court, privacy, and abortion. N Engl J Med 1989;321:1200.

Appelbaum PS, Grisso T: Assessing patients' capacities to consent to treatment. N Engl J Med 1988;319:1635.

Council on Ethical and Judicial Affairs, American Medical Association: Mandatory parental consent to abortion. JAMA 1993;26:82.

Dunstan GR: The moral status of the human embryo: A tradition recalled. J Med Ethics 1984;1:38.

Ethics Committee of the American Fertility Society: Ethical considerations of assisted reproductive technologies. Fertil Steril 1994;62(Suppl 1).

Jonsen AR, Siegler M, Winslade WJ: *Clinical Ethics: A Practical Approach to Ethical Decisions in Clinical Medicine,* 3rd ed. McGraw-Hill, 1992.

McCullough LB, Chervenak FA: *Ethics in Obstetrics and Gynecology.* Oxford University Press, 1994.

Section II.
Preventive Health Care

7

Preventive Services

Paul A. Smith, MD

Because clinicians often see women with medical problems that could have been avoided, it is easy for them to appreciate the importance of disease prevention. They also see patients with advanced stages of disease that may be difficult or impossible to treat successfully and for which the outcome would have been more favorable had the condition been recognized and treated earlier. The benefit from the application of preventive services can be seen readily in the worldwide eradication of smallpox, the prevention of poliomyelitis epidemics in the United States, and the marked reduction in deaths from cervical cancer.

Despite their benefits, however, preventive services should be selected with great care. Because all people are potential recipients of preventive services, the financial costs may be enormous. In choosing interventions for healthy women, one must be certain that the benefit will be greater than the harm done. Randomized prospective studies provide the most reliable of evidence to support a recommendation of a preventive intervention. This type of study has shown that the use of mammography to detect breast cancer in women older than 50 results in decreased mortality. Benefit can only be strongly suggested from well-done case-controlled studies such as decreased mortality from colon cancer through the use of sigmoidoscopy.

For other interventions there may be insufficient data on clinical efficacy, such as with self-examination of the breast. There are many examples of screening tests or preventive treatments that looked promising on a theoretic basis but when studied in randomized trials were shown to have no benefit. Examples are routine chest radiographs to detect lung cancer in cigarette smokers and medical therapy for hyperlipidemia in young, healthy people without other risk factors for cardiovascular disease.

The Canadian Task Force (CTF) on the Periodic Health Examination (1979; 1987), the United States Preventive Services Task Force (USPSTF), and the American College of Physicians (ACP) (Eddy, 1991) have evaluated preventive services with exhaustive critical reviews, using explicit criteria to grade the evidence and link it with the strength of each recommendation. Review articles by Hayward et al and Sox have summarized these findings; these reports

> Types of Preventive Services
>   Periodic Health Assessment
>   Screening
>   Counseling
>   Chemoprophylaxis & Immunizations
> Cardiovascular Disease
>   Smoking
>   Hypertension
>   Hypercholesterolemia
>   Exercise
>   Chemoprophylaxis
> Cancer
>   Breast Cancer
>   Cervical Cancer
>   Ovarian Cancer
>   Endometrial Uterine Cancer
>   Colorectal Cancer
>   Lung Cancer
> Counseling to Prevent Disease & Injury

form the basis of this discussion. Selected recommendations are summarized in Table 7–1: the emphasis is on services for which the evidence is strongest or for which controversy exists.

Other published recommendations come from medical specialty societies, national governmental agencies such as the National Cholesterol Education Program, professional and scientific societies such as the American Cancer Society, and individual experts; often there is no a clear consensus among reports.

TYPES OF PREVENTIVE SERVICES

Preventive services include screening for disease with physical examination, history taking, and testing; counseling about health behaviors; and providing immunizations and chemoprophylaxis. A critical review of the screening physical examination by Oboler and LaForce has left little to be recommended universally, with the exception of blood pressure measurement and breast examination. Some of the most effective interventions are recommendations that affect health practices such as smoking, physical activity, diet, alcohol and drug use, and recommen-

Table 7–1. Prevention and screening recommendations for women.

Intervention	Health Condition	Target Group	Recommendation
Physical Exam **Blood Pressure**	CHD, cerebrovascular disease, renal disease		
Routine		18 year+	Every 1–2 years and every visit for other reasons
High risk		18 year+, diastolic BP is 85–90 mmHg, 1 or more CHD risk factors present	Every year
Clinician Breast Examination	Breast cancer		
Routine		40 year+	Every year
High risk		18 year+ (ACP), 35 year+ (CTF, USPSTF), history of premenopausal breast cancer in a first-degree family member	Every year
Laboratory Testing **Mammography**	Breast cancer		
Routine		50–75 year+	Every year (ACP, CTF) Every 1–2 years (USPSTF)
High risk		35–40 year, history of premenopausal breast cancer in a first-degree family member, other risk factors (ACP)	Every year (ACP, CTF, USPSTF)
Papanicolau Smear	Cervical cancer		
Routine		18 year+, no other risk factors (see text)	Every 1–3 years
		65 year+, low risk and regular negative screening throughout past 10 years	Discontinue
High risk		18 year+ or onset of intercourse, presence of risk factors	Every year
Sigmoidoscopy	Colorectal cancer		
Routine		50 year+ (ACP)	Every 3–5 years (ACP), no recommendation (CTF, USPSTF)
High risk		40 year+ (CTF), 50 year+ (USPSTF), hx one first-degree family member with colon cancer or personal hx of endometrial, ovarian, or breast cancer	Every 3–5 year (CTF, USPSTF)
FOBT	Colorectal cancer		
Routine		50 year+ (ACP)	Every year (ACP), no recommendation (CTF, USPSTF)
High risk		Same as sigmoidoscopy	Every year (CTF, USPSTF)
Colonoscopy	Colorectal cancer		
Very high risk		More than 1 first-degree family member with colon cancer (especially if < 40 years old at diagnosis); familial polyposis coli; personal hx colon cancer, ulcerative colitis > 10 years or adenomatous polyps	Every 3–5 years (ACP, CTF, USPSTF)
Nonfasting Cholesterol	CHD		
Routine		18 year+ (ACP, USPSTF)	Every 5 years, not recommended (CTF)
High risk		18 year+, 1 or more CHD risk factors	More frequently (ACP, USPSTF) individual clinical judgement (CTF)
Counseling **Tobacco Use**	Cardiovascular disease, some cancers, lung disease	All women (ACP, CTF, USPSTF)	Actively counsel smokers to quit, primary prevention messages to adolescents
Alcohol Use	Accidents, suicide, homicide, hypertension, heart and liver disease, etc.		
Routine		All women	Counsel alcohol moderation, abstention when driving and during pregnancy
High risk		Problem drinkers	Case finding strategy

(continued)

Table 7–1. Prevention and screening recommendations for women. (continued)

Intervention	Health Condition	Target Group	Recommendation
Dietary Fat, Sodium, Fiber	CHD, hypertension	18 year+ (ACP, USPSTF), no comment (CTF)	Advise diet to maintain desirable weight, total fat < 30% of calories, saturated fat < 10% of calories, cholesterol < 300 mg/d, high fiber foods, limit salt
Calcium Intake	Osteoporosis	18 year+ (USPSTF, CTF)	Counsel to maintain adequate calcium intake by natural diet and supplements
Exercise	CHD, osteoporosis, other	18 year+ (USPSTF), 40 year+ (CTF)	Educate about the role of exercise in disease prevention (USPSTF), teach effect of immobility on bone mass (CTF)
Injury Prevention Seat Belt Use	Motor vehicle accidents	All women	Advise seat belt use (ACP, CTF, USPSTF)
Sexual Behavior	Unwanted pregnancy, sexually transmitted diseases	All women	Advise contraceptives (CTF, USPSTF), barrier methods and safe sexual practices to prevent STD (USPSTF)

dations for accidental injury prevention. Conventional clinical activities such as diagnostic testing may be less important than counseling and patient education in some instances.

There has been increasing recognition of the importance of selectivity in ordering screening tests and providing preventive services. Knowledge of the conditions for which the patient is at greatest risk is essential. This determination requires consideration of the patient's past medical history, age, sex, family history, and personal health habits. Individual risk assessment with appropriate selection of services should reduce the risk of adverse consequences of screening.

Periodic Health Assessment

The evaluation of asymptomatic people has changed from the traditional complete history and physical examination. The periodic health examination focuses on history-taking to assess individual risk (eg, smoking, family history of colon or breast cancer, use of seat belts), directed physical examination, and counseling. Barriers to accomplishment of these measures include lack of payment to providers for screening visits and other preventive services, uncertainty over which services are recommended, and lack of time or training on the part of clinicians to enable counseling or assessment of risk. Because most Americans see a physician at least once a year, these episodic visits can also be used as opportunities to provide preventive services.

Screening

Screening is performed to detect disease before symptoms are evident. Tests that are useful in the diagnosis of symptomatic patients or in following patients with established disease may be of no value in screening, eg, use of CA-125 for monitoring of ovarian cancer. Whether or not a screening method leads to improved outcome depends on the characteristics of the disease, the screening test, and the patient population. The disease must cause significant morbidity and mortality. The natural history should include an asymptomatic period in which the diagnosis can be made, and the results of early treatment must be superior to those obtained after symptoms appear. The test must be sensitive and specific, with reasonable cost and patient acceptance. The condition must be prevalent enough in the population to justify screening. The patient must have sufficient life expectancy to warrant intervention and be willing to undergo the screening and potential treatment.

Counseling

Counseling interventions are those in which patients are given information and advice regarding personal behaviors to reduce the risk of illness and injury. For an intervention to be considered effective, it must be shown that clinicians can influence the personal behavior through counseling and that behavior change may improve outcome. A good example is cigarette smoking cessation.

Chemoprophylaxis & Immunizations

Chemoprophylaxis refers to the use of drugs by healthy people as primary preventive measures to decrease the risk of disease, eg, aspirin to prevent vascular disease, or hormone replacement therapy to prevent heart disease and osteoporosis. Use of chemoprophylaxis requires demonstration of reduction in morbidity or mortality from the disease in question without other adverse effects, as well as the ability of patients to comply.

Immunizations are given to prevent viral and bacterial illness. Risk assessment is required to guide individual recommendations (see Chapter 8).

CARDIOVASCULAR DISEASE

Cardiovascular disease is the leading cause of death in American women, accounting for more than 359,000 deaths from coronary heart disease (CHD) and 87,000 deaths from stroke in 1990, according to Boring et al. Thirty-five percent of all deaths among women are caused by CHD, and 50% of all people who die from CHD are women. Although women have CHD as frequently as men do, disease generally develops 6–10 years later. The most effective strategy for disease reduction is primary prevention through risk factor modification. The modifiable risk factors are cigarette smoking, hypertension, hypercholesterolemia, and physical inactivity.

Smoking
There is a consensus among the three panels mentioned previously (CTF, USPSTF, and ACP) that all patients who smoke should be counseled during every clinical encounter to stop. Currently 29% of adult American women smoke, and smoking rates are rising faster in adolescent women than in any other group. Brief office interventions have been shown to be effective in reducing smoking rates (see in Chapter 9). There is much evidence that risk of myocardial infarction is reduced by smoking cessation in both women and well as men. Benefit from stopping smoking is realized almost immediately, and by 5–10 years, the ex-smoker's risk approximates that of people who have never smoked.

Hypertension
The USPSTF, CTF, and ACP all recommend blood-pressure measurement at every clinical encounter and at least every 2 years in normotensive persons, yearly if diastolic pressure is 85–90 mmHg. The diagnosis of hypertension (systolic blood pressure greater than 140 mmHg, diastolic blood pressure greater than 90 mmHg) should not be made on the basis of one reading; it should be based on three separate visits with at least two measurements at each visit. The benefit from early detection and medical treatment of hypertension, with reduction in cardiovascular events and mortality, is well established by randomized controlled trials in men. The greater the severity of blood-pressure elevation, the greater the clinical improvement with treatment. A greater than

40% reduction in age-adjusted stroke mortality in women observed since 1972 has been attributed largely to early detection and treatment of hypertension, according to the Joint National Committee on Detection, Evaluation, and Treatment of High Blood Pressure. Once hypertension has been established, patients should be counseled on sodium reduction, weight reduction if appropriate, exercise, and reduction of other cardiovascular risk factors. Drug therapy should be advised in accordance with recently published guidelines of the aforementioned committee.

Hypercholesterolemia
Hypercholesterolemia is associated with accelerated atherosclerosis and CHD in a continuous, graded fashion over most of the range of cholesterol values. This association appears to be less strong in women than in men, although the Framingham data, as reported by Lerner and Kannel, indicate it may be more important in elderly than in young women. Controversy exists over who benefits from screening. The USPSTF, the ACP, and the National Cholesterol Education Program (NCEP) recommend periodic screening in all adults, whereas the CTF (1993) recommends case finding in middle-aged men only. Screening generally is done by nonfasting total cholesterol measurement. However, the NCEP guidelines recommend measurement of both nonfasting total and high-density lipoprotein (HDL) cholesterol as the initial screen. Although a high level of low-density lipoprotein (LDL) does increase CHD risk, a low HDL level may be a more important risk factor in women.

Primary prevention of CHD by diet or drug therapy to lower blood cholesterol has been shown to benefit middle-aged men with high blood cholesterol levels but no clinical disease (especially those with other risk factors for CHD); however, information on primary prevention in women is limited. Of the two trials with significant numbers of women (one drug trial reported by Dorr et al using colestipol, and one dietary intervention trial reported by Frantz et al), neither showed a mortality benefit from intervention. One angiographic study of secondary prevention in patients with known CHD and hypercholesterolemia included significant numbers of women who were treated with drug therapy. Reduction in LDL cholesterol and regression of coronary artery stenosis were shown, according to Kane et al.

Screening followed by primary prevention is not without risk. Smith et al reported increased mortality from causes other than CHD in treated groups compared with those given placebo in trials using medical therapy: those with low risk of CHD had increased mortality from all causes.

Women chosen for hypercholesterolemia screening should belong to a group in which the benefit of treatment is known to outweigh the risks. These groups include women with known CHD or peripheral vascular disease and women at high risk because of age and multiple risk factors, eg, diabetes mellitus, smoking, hypertension, family history of premature CHD.

Although there is insufficient evidence for or against a general recommendation to lower dietary saturated fat, and cholesterol to decrease mortality from CHD in women, there is no evident risk and much potential benefit. Premenopausal women and those at low risk of CHD may be served best by such dietary advice, by encouragement to exercise, and by thoughtful, selective screening.

Exercise

Regular physical activity is associated with decreased cardiovascular risk in men and is recommended by the USPSTF for all adults. This recommendation assumes a similar benefit to women and does not address the fact that the effectiveness of counseling to change exercise behavior is unproved.

Chemoprophylaxis

Prevention of CHD with hormone replacement therapy in selected women is recommended by the ACP (see Chapter 21).

Routine use of aspirin in the primary prevention of CHD events and stroke in women is not recommended by the CTF (1991). Large trials in women are lacking. Trials in middle-aged men have failed to show a clear benefit in all- cause mortality. A reduced rate of nonfatal myocardial infarction needs to be balanced against potential adverse effects such as hemorrhage and stroke. Women with known coronary artery disease may benefit from aspirin in secondary prevention, and the decision to prescribe it should be made on an individual basis.

CANCER

Breast Cancer

Breast cancer is the second most common cause of cancer death in women in the United States, surpassed only by lung cancer; it accounted for an estimated 46,000 deaths and 182,000 new cases in 1994, according to Boring et al. Lifetime risk of the development of breast cancer is estimated to be 11%. Because tumors detected at an early stage have a favorable prognosis with treatment, screening is an attractive option.

A. Mammography: Several randomized trials have shown a clear reduction in breast cancer mortality in women older than 50 who have received regular screening mammograms. All three panels previously mentioned recommend annual or biannual screening in this age group. The optimal frequency of screening has not been established. The Health Insurance Plan of Greater New York (HIP) performed the first controlled trial to demonstrate the benefit of annual mammograms. Subsequent trials have demonstrated a similar mortality benefit using mammograms at a frequency of every 2–3 years. The age at which the benefit of screening is lost has not been established, and the decision to screen should be individualized based on comorbidity. The USPSTF recommends stopping at age 75; the American Geriatrics Society recommends cessation at age 85.

The most controversial issue in screening for breast cancer is whether to screen women at average risk between the ages of 40 and 49, a practice that has become common in the United States. The HIP study included women between the ages of 40 and 64. The initial analysis of the data showed a mortality benefit only in women aged 50 and older. Analysis after 18 years of follow-up showed a small benefit in the younger group, although the numbers were insufficient to reach statistical significance. None of the subsequent trials were able to show benefit in women younger than 50, although there were insufficient numbers in the individual trials to rule out a possible benefit. The Canadian National Breast Screening Study (CNBSS), designed specifically to answer this question, failed to show a decrease in mortality in younger women receiving clinical breast examination plus routine mammograms compared to those receiving the usual care, according to Miller et al (1992a). Although there was no mortality benefit, a large number of women had cancers detected at an early stage, with possible increased chance of cure. The CNBSS has been criticized for its relatively short follow-up period of 7 years and poor-quality mammograms.

A recent analysis of pooled data from five randomized Swedish trials, reported by Nystrom et al, confirmed the benefit in women older than 50, with benefit seen as early as 3 years into the follow-up period; however, this analysis failed to show significant benefit in women younger than 50. In these studies a small benefit may be caused by detection of cancer in women in their early 50s who entered the study in their 40s. Overall, there is no convincing evidence that routine mammography in women under age 50 is of benefit.

Although there are no large studies of screening with mammography in high-risk groups, the recommendation is to screen women at greatest risk with annual examinations beginning at age 35 or 40, including those with a first-degree family member who had premenopausal breast cancer and women with a personal history of breast cancer.

B. Breast Examination: An annual clinical breast examination is recommended beginning at age 40. There are no randomized trials comparing screening with examination alone to no screening. In the nonrandomized Breast Cancer Detection Project and the controlled HIP study, which combined mammography with breast examination, it is clear that the two interventions are complementary. In these studies, 50–67% of the value of screening was from the physical examination. The CNBSS confirmed the benefit of clinical examination, according to Miller et al (1992b).

C. Breast Self-Examination: Breast self-examination is relatively insensitive, especially in older women, who are at higher risk. No evidence is available from randomized trials to support breast self-examination. Retrospective studies have suggested that women who practice breast self-examination are more likely to present with early-stage tumors, but this finding may be biased by an increased tendency to seek medical attention in the group that regularly practices self-examination. None of the three panels makes specific recommendations for this practice.

D. Genetic Testing: A genetic test for the uncommon familial premenopausal breast cancer gene may become available in the next few years. As with other potential genetic tests (those for hereditary ovarian and hereditary colon cancer), this test should not be applied to the general population, and its use will need to be coupled with genetic analysis and counseling.

Cervical Cancer

Cervical cancer is a common gynecologic malignant disease in the United States; Boring et al report more than 15,000 new cases annually and more than 4600 deaths estimated to occur in 1994. Since the practice of routine Papanicolaou testing has become widespread, mortality from cervical cancer has decreased by 70% in this country. Observational studies have documented similar results in Canada and several European countries; Eddy reports marked reduction in cervical cancer death rates temporally related to adoption of routine Pap smears. Randomized trials have not been performed; because of the strength of the evidence to date, they will not be done for ethical reasons.

There is consensus that all women should be screened beginning at the time of first intercourse or at age 18; more than 60% of women in the United States experience intercourse by the age of 18. Screening should occur every 1–3 years, with the frequency dependent on individual risk. Women who are at higher risk should receive annual Pap tests; risk factors include three or more lifetime partners, intercourse before age 21, evidence of human papilloma virus on previous Pap smears, prior cervical cancer or dysplasia, history of cigarette smoking, and low socioeconomic status. With so many women in one or more of these categories, it may be easier for clinicians to perform annual Pap smears unless there is low risk. In women at low risk, testing every 3 years gives 96% of the benefit of annual testing, according to Eddy. It has been recommended that women at low risk who have three consecutive negative Pap smears may, at the clinician's discretion,

have longer intervals between Pap smears. It is not clear when Pap testing should be concluded. If a women is at low risk, and has had regular screening with consistently normal smears up to the age of 65–70, additional screening may not be necessary. Even if Pap smears are not deemed necessary, inspection of the genital tract to detect other pelvic malignant disease and gynecologic problems should continue.

Women who have not had intercourse are at very low risk for cervical cancer, and some authorities recommend no screening. Women with prior hysterectomy for a benign condition, adequate histologic evidence that the cervix has been removed, and no previous abnormal Pap smears require no further screening for cervical cancer. Women who have had vaginal or cervical neoplasia at hysterectomy and those with prior endometrial cancer are at higher risk for developing vaginal neoplasia and need continued screening with vaginal smears. Women with human immunodeficiency virus (HIV) infection are at high risk for invasive neoplasia, and Pap testing every 6 months is recommended. Women who have had in utero diethylstilbestrol (DES) exposure require annual Pap smears but no other special screening.

Ovarian Cancer

Ovarian cancer is the leading cause of gynecologic cancer death and the fourth leading cause of all female cancer deaths in the USA; Boring et al estimated 24,000 new cases and 13,600 deaths in 1994. For those at average risk, lifetime occurrence is 1.2%. Risk is increased with first- or second-degree family members with ovarian cancer, and it is decreased with oral contraception use, parity, and breast-feeding. A rare form of hereditary ovarian cancer carries a lifetime risk of up to 50% and is suggested by multiple family members in two to four generations with early-onset ovarian cancer.

Routine screening is not recommended. Bimanual pelvic examination, serum CA-125 testing, and transvaginal ultrasonography all lack sufficient sensitivity to detect cancers early enough to alter prognosis. Routine screening with CA-125 or ultrasonography in women older than 50 would result in more than 30 false-positive tests for each ovarian cancer detected, with women testing falsely positive undergoing undue stress and invasive testing, including laparotomy. Women from families who have the rare hereditary ovarian cancer syndrome should be referred to a gynecologic oncologist. For further discussion of ovarian cancer, see Chapter 50.

Endometrial Uterine Cancer

Routine screening for endometrial cancer is not recommended. Women should be counseled to report all abnormal uterine bleeding, and those with such findings should be evaluated by endometrial sampling or other diagnostic testing. For a discussion of the evaluation of postmenopausal bleeding, see Chapter 21.

Colorectal Cancer

Cancer of the colon and rectum is the third most common cause of cancer death among American women, with 70,000 new cases and 28,000 deaths estimated for 1994, according to Boring et al. At the time of diagnosis, more than half of the colorectal cancers are at an advanced stage. Surgical treatment is far more effective at an earlier stage. Because it is thought that most colorectal cancers arise from polyps, screening strategies to identify localized cancers and find polyps for removal may decrease mortality. These methods include fecal occult blood testing (FOBT) and sigmoidoscopy. There has been no consensus on whether or how to screen people of average risk for colorectal cancer because, until recently, there have been no studies showing a mortality benefit.

Special screening has been recommended for those at high risk; risk factors include colorectal cancer in a first-degree family member; familial polyposis coli; personal history of endometrial, ovarian, or breast cancer; ulcerative colitis; and prior colon cancer.

A. Fecal Occult Blood Testing: The ACP recommends annual fecal occult blood testing (FOBT) after age 50. The USPSTF and the CTF found insufficient evidence for or against FOBT to make a recommendation. Of the five large randomized controlled trials of FOBT, one group, Mandel et al, recently published its final results. This study compared FOBT using six guaiac-impregnated rehydrated slides performed every year, every 2 years, or not at all. There were equal numbers of men and women in all three groups. After 13 years of follow-up study, a 33% reduction in mortality from colorectal cancer was found in the screened group compared with the unscreened control group. No difference in mortality was observed between the annually and the biannually screened groups. With the use of rehydrated slides, the number of false-positive results was greatly increased. In this study, the positivity rate of each screening was nearly 10%, with a positive predictive value for cancer of only 2.2%. All patients with positive results were referred for further study, usually colonoscopy; it has been estimated that one-half to one-third of the screening benefit may have been caused by chance selection for colonoscopy. The sensitivity of FOBT for colorectal cancer is poor, at about 30%. Given the modest mortality benefit, poor positive predictive value, and low sensitivity, FOBT is a less than ideal method for screening.

B. Sigmoidoscopy: There are no randomized trials of sigmoidoscopy, although a well-designed case-controlled study by Selby et al offers strong evidence for reduced mortality from colorectal cancer by screening with rigid sigmoidoscopy. This study found that patients who died from cancers of the rectum and distal colon (within the view of the 20-cm rigid scope) were much less likely than matched controls to have had a screening sigmoidoscopy in the previous 10 years. Although bias could have accounted for the difference, the investigators performed a powerful test for hidden bias: they studied patients who died from cancers above the reach of the sigmoidoscope and found no difference in the number of screening sigmoidoscopic examinations between this group and controls, suggesting a true efficacy of screening rather than unmeasured selection factors. The estimated mortality reduction from distal tumors was 59%. The mortality benefit for screening 10 years previously was as strong as that for screening within 2 years. Because approximately half of the currently diagnosed colorectal cancers are within the view of the longer, 60-cm flexible sigmoidoscope, the authors estimated an overall colorectal cancer mortality reduction of 30% with screening by this method. The ACP recommends screening every 3–5 years for those at average risk; the USPSTF and the CTF have not recommended screening, although new guidelines may be forthcoming soon from these groups.

C. Colonoscopy: All three panels recommend screening with colonoscopy for those at very high risk for colorectal cancer. Although the indications and timing of screening vary somewhat among the groups, all recommend colonoscopy for those with a first-degree family member with colorectal cancer, with screening to begin at age 40. Screening as early as age 18 is recommended for those with ulcerative colitis of 10 years duration, personal history of colon cancer or adenomatous polyps, or familial polyposis syndromes. The ACP recommends a frequency of every 3–5 years and that an air contrast barium enema may be substituted for colonoscopy.

Lung Cancer

Lung cancer is the leading cause of cancer death in women in the United States, with an estimated 72,000 new cases and 59,000 deaths in 1994, according to Boring et al. Screening by any means is ineffective. Seventy-nine percent of lung cancers in women are attributed to cigarette smoking. Primary prevention by promoting smoking cessation is the most effective clinical intervention. All women who smoke should be advised of the cancer risk and be counseled to stop.

COUNSELING TO PREVENT DISEASE & INJURY

All the panels previously mentioned recommend encouragement of the use of seat belts to prevent automobile injury and death. Also recommended is counseling on the use of motorcycle helmets, home fire safety precautions, and the danger of firearms.

There is consensus to advise smoking cessation for all smokers, and for counseling to prevent tobacco use in nonsmokers. All persons should be advised to limit their use of alcohol, stop alcohol consumption during pregnancy, and avoid driving after any alcohol use. Clinicians should use a case-finding strategy to identify problem drinkers (see Chapter 11); they should educate patients about the dangers of illicit drugs and counsel against their use.

The USPSTF recommends safe sexual practices to reduce the risk of sexually transmitted disease, and counseling to prevent unwanted pregnancy.

Functional and cognitive assessment of the elderly is recommended and is discussed in Chapter 4.

Dietary counseling is discussed in Chapter 9. In addition, the USPSTF recommends that women and adolescent girls be counseled on adequate calcium and iron intake and that they receive specific guidelines for intake during pregnancy.

REFERENCES

Ahlquist DA et al: Accuracy of fecal occult blood screening for colorectal neoplasia. JAMA 1993;269:1262.

American Cancer Society: *Summary of Current Guidelines for the Cancer Related Checkup: Recommendations.* American Cancer Society, 1988.

American College of Physicians: Guidelines for counseling postmenopausal women about preventive hormone therapy. Ann Intern Med 1992;117:1038.

Baker LH. Breast Cancer Detection Demonstration Project: Five year summary report. CA 1982;32:194.

Boring CC et al: Cancer statistics, 1994. CA 1994;44:7.

Canadian Task Force on the Periodic Health Examination: Can Med Assoc J 1979;121:1193.

Canadian Task Force on the Periodic Health Examination: The periodic health examination. 2. 1987 update. Can Med Assoc J 1988;138:618.

Canadian Task Force on the Periodic Health Examination: Periodic health examination, 1991 update. 6. Acetylsalicylic acid and the primary prevention of cardiovascular disease. Can Med Assoc J 1991;145:1091.

Canadian Task Force on the Periodic Health Examination: Periodic health examination, 1993 update. 2. Lowering the total cholesterol level to prevent coronary heart disease. Can Med Assoc J 1993;148:521.

Carlson KJ, Skates SJ, Singer DE: Screening for ovarian cancer. Ann Intern Med 1994;121:124.

Dorr AE et al: Colestipol hydrochloride in hypercholesterolemic patients: Effect on serum cholesterol and mortality. J Chronic Dis 1978;31:5.

Eddy DM (editor): *Common Screening Tests.* American College of Physicians, 1991.

Eddy DM: Screening for breast cancer. Ann Intern Med 1989;111:389.

Eddy DM: Screening for cervical cancer. Ann Intern Med 1990;113:214.

Frantz ID et al: Test of effect of lipid lowering by diet on cardiovascular risk. The Minnesota Coronary Study. Atherosclerosis 1989;9:129.

Hayward RSA et al: Preventive care guidelines: 1991. Ann Intern Med 1991;114:758.

Hulley SB et al: Should we be measuring blood cholesterol levels in young adults? JAMA 1993;269:1416.

Joint National Committee on Detection, Evaluation, and Treatment of High Blood Pressure: The fifth report of the Joint National Committee on Detection, Evaluation, and Treatment of High Blood Pressure. Arch Intern Med 1993;153:154.

Kane J et al: Regression of coronary atherosclerosis during treatment of familial hypercholesterolemia with combined drug regimens. JAMA 1990;264:3007.

Lerner D, Kannel W: Patterns of coronary heart disease morbidity and mortality in the sexes: A 26 year follow-up of the Framingham population. Am Heart J 1986;111:383.

Mandel JS et al: Reducing mortality from colorectal cancer by screening for fecal occult blood. N Engl J Med 1993;328:1365.

Miller AB et al: Canadian National Breast Screening Study. 1. Breast cancer detection and death rates among women aged 40 to 49 years. Can Med Assoc J 1992;147:1459.

Miller AB et al: Canadian National Breast Screening Study. 2. Breast cancer detection and death rates among women aged 50 to 59 years. Can Med Assoc J 1992;147:1477.

National Cholesterol Education Program: NCEP Adult Treatment Panel II Report. JAMA 1993;269:3015.

Nystrom L et al: Breast cancer screening with mammography: Overview of Swedish randomised trials. Lancet 1993;341:973.

Oboler SK, LaForce FM: The periodic physical examination in asymptomatic adults. Ann Intern Med 1989;110:214.

Preventive Services Task Force: *Guide to Clinical Preventive Services: Report of the United States Preventive Services Task Force.* Baltimore: Williams & Wilkins, 1989.

Selby JV et al: A case-control study of screening sigmoidoscopy and mortality from colorectal cancer. N Engl J Med 992;326:653.

Smith GD, Song F, Sheldon TA: Cholesterol lowering and mortality: The importance of considering initial level of risk. Br Med J 1993;306:1367.

Sox HC Jr: Preventive health services in adults. N Engl J Med 1994;330:1589.

8

Immunizations

Karen C. Smith, MD

Immunization guidelines in the United States are well-standardized by the Advisory Committee on Immunization Practices (ACIP), and little controversy exists regarding their implementation. The general recommendations are presented here along with recent updates in practices. Special considerations that apply to women who are pregnant or may become so in the near future are also discussed.

THE CHALLENGE OF UNIVERSAL IMMUNIZATION

The most challenging issue facing health care providers is how to provide universal coverage effectively. It is incumbent on primary care specialists to review their patients' immunization needs periodically, to update services as appropriate, and to provide documentation in the patients' charts of services rendered. In a 1988 study, the estimate of the rate of appropriate tetanus vaccinations from surveys of physicians' practice patterns and chart audits revealed only 12–24% compliance. Influenza vaccines in patients 65 years or older were given and documented in 12–68% of the charts.

In many primary care practices, compliance with guidelines is hampered by the lack of a consistent review process with patients, inadequate time to discuss the rationale for making the recommendations, and absence of a referenced chart documenting when immunizations are updated. It is strongly suggested that practitioners scrutinize their practice styles for efficiency of providing universal coverage to their patients. In addition to the aforementioned areas in which improvement may be made, the use of patient-held minirecords has been suggested as a means to increase patients' awareness of their need for receiving immunizations on schedule. Using these minirecords has shown an increasing compliance with children's immunizations. Providing printed guidelines concerning anticipated immunization requirements by age during routine office visits may also be helpful.

The Challenge of Universal Immunization
Diphtheria & Tetanus
Influenza
Pneumococcus
Hepatitis B
Rubella
Measles
Mumps
Polio
Vaccinations in Pregnancy
Special Needs of Travelers

DIPHTHERIA & TETANUS

A diphtheria-tetanus (dT) combined vaccine may be updated every 10 years in adults. It appears that people over the age of 55, and especially over age 65, are frequently at risk for tetanus infections in the USA. Reasons for this statistic include the lack of primary immunization in some elderly patients and waning immunity to tetanus in people who have been immunized in the past. A careful history should be obtained regarding any past tetanus vaccines. If doubt exists as to the last booster date, the patient may be vaccinated without concern for significant side effects even if the previous vaccine was given within 10 years. The schedule for primary immunization includes three injections given (1) at time zero, (2) 4 weeks or longer after the first injection, and (3) 6–12 months after the second dose. Local side effects such as itching or swelling at the injection site are common, but major side effects are extremely rare. An alternative strategy was recently advised by the Task Force on Adult Immunization (comprised of representative from American College of Physicians, Infectious Diseases Society of America, and Centers for Disease Control and Prevention). If a completed pediatrics series of primary immunization and an adolescent or adult booster can be documented, a single booster at age 50 provides life-long protection. This new recommendation does not alter management of the injured patient. In the setting of a minor wound, a dT booster should be administered unless there is documentation of a booster within the last ten years. When immunization status is doubtful or remote and a patient presents with a large, dirty wound, tetanus immune globulin should be given simultaneously with a dT booster.

Diphtheria is becoming more prevalent in poor urban populations in the USA and is seen increasingly in third-world populations abroad. The vaccine is conjugated with tetanus so that compliance with the tetanus guidelines ensures immunity to diphtheria. The dT combination is preferred over a tetanus booster alone because of the continued need to protect patients from both diseases. Pregnancy is not a contraindication to use of the dT vaccine.

INFLUENZA

Influenza control is markedly improved by immunizing people who are at high risk for complications of infection and of low-risk people who may be exposed to people at risk. Those who should be immunized because of higher risk are people over age 65 and younger patients with the following medical conditions: chronic cardiovascular or lung disease, kidney failure, liver disease, HIV infection, cancer, and diabetes. In addition, others who qualify are residents of chronic-care facilities, organ transplant recipients, and alcoholics. Low-risk people who should consider immunization are health care workers and others caring for high-risk patients, anyone with a high risk of exposure, and anyone who chooses prophylaxis to avoid potential loss of work time. Parents of children at risk for complications from influenza infection should consider immunization. The only contraindication is a history of anaphylaxis to eggs or other components of the vaccine. In high-risk people with a significant risk of allergic reaction to the vaccine, desensitization may be considered. Adults with acute febrile illnesses should wait until resolution of the acute infection before receiving the vaccine, but concurrent minor illnesses do not necessitate a delay in immunization.

Side effects are relatively uncommon. The most frequently reported symptom is soreness at the injection site, which lasts approximately 48 hours. Rarely, systemic reactions of fever, malaise, and myalgia appear 6–12 hours after injection and last 1–2 days. These symptoms occur most commonly in people who never have been exposed previously to any influenza virus or vaccine. A delayed-type local allergic reaction is induced occasionally by thimerosal, which is included in the vaccine. Finally, it should be noted that reports of Guillain-Barré sequelae related to the influenza vaccine have not increased since the 1976–1977 "swine flu" season. Influenza vaccine may be given concurrently at different sites with any one of the following vaccines: pneumococcal, measles-mumps-rubella (MMR), oral polio, *Hemophilus influenza,* Group B (HIB), dT, and pertussis.

Use of amantadine should be considered in spe-

cific instances. The agent is both prophylactic and therapeutic in treating influenza A but not B. It may be given concurrently with the flu vaccine in patients exposed to influenza A and should be continued for 2 weeks after immunization. It also may be administered to patients who probably have acute influenza A infection; it is most valuable when started within 48 hours of the onset of symptoms. Finally, amantadine may be useful in patients who are at high risk throughout the flu season if the influenza vaccine is definitely contraindicated (see preceding discussion). This drug is especially appropriate in people who may be exposed to large numbers of others, eg, a nursing home resident. Recommended dosages of amantadine are 100 mg daily for prophylaxis and 100 mg twice daily for treatment. The higher dosage should be reduced at times in elderly patients or in those with impaired renal function. It should be noted that a significant number of drug-related neurologic reactions have been reported. Its use is recommended only when potential benefits clearly outweight anticipated complications.

Pregnancy is not a contraindication to influenza immunization in women who meet any of the aforementioned criteria. The vaccine also is considered safe in lactating women. Amantadine is classified in pregnancy category C; it should be used, therefore, only when the benefits are felt clearly to outweigh the potential complications of infection.

PNEUMOCOCCUS

There is general agreement that pneumococcal vaccine should be given once at age 65 for additional protection against otherwise life-threatening pneumococcal illness, which is common in this age group. Certain adults should receive the pneumonoccocal vaccine before age 65. This group is composed of people with the following medical illnesses: chronic cardiac or pulmonary disease, sickle cell anemia, any lymphoma or hematologic malignant condition, asplenia, diabetes mellitus, alcoholism, chronic liver disease including cirrhosis, multiple myeloma, chronic renal disease (especially with the need for dialysis or with nephrotic syndrome), and other conditions associated with immunodeficiency, including HIV infection. People living in facilities where there is a greater risk of exposure also should be immunized. This vaccine may be given concurrently with influenza vaccine but in a different injection site. It is not usual practice to give boosters of the vaccine because of the frequency of side effects associated with reimmunization. However, the Task Force on Adult Immunizations has recently recommended a second pneumococcal vaccine after age 65, especially for people immunized at an earlier age because of risk factors. A minimum of 6 years should elapse between immunizations.

Pregnancy is not a contraindication to use the pneumococcal vaccine in women who should be immunized based on the aforementioned criteria.

HEPATITIS B

As of 1991, the Centers for Disease Control and Prevention (CDC) estimated a lifetime risk of 5% of contracting hepatitis B in the USA. Completion of a series of the hepatitis B vaccine is 85–90% effective in preventing clinical hepatitis and viral infection. If the vaccine recipient develops measurable hepatitis B surface antibody, protection from infection appears to be 100%. Hepatitis B vaccine currently is recommended only in adults at higher than average risk of exposure to the virus. Health professionals and others (eg, police officers) likely to have an occupational exposure to blood products are advised to receive the vaccine series. Others who appear to be at higher risk of infection because of exposure include patients undergoing dialysis, those who have hemophilia or for other reasons receive blood products regularly, some residents of chronic-care facilities, injection drug users, household contacts of hepatitis B carriers, sexually active persons with multiple partners, Alaskan Eskimos, Pacific Islanders, and homosexual and bisexual men. People in these categories should receive hepatitis B vaccine if they have negative serologic test results for hepatitis B surface antibody or antigen. In some circumstances it is advisable to offer concurrent initiation of hepatitis B vaccine with passive immunization, or hepatitis B immune globulin (HBIG). These instances include (1) a needle or splash exposure with fluids contaminated with or at high risk of containing hepatitis B and (2) sexual contact with a person suspected of having acute hepatitis B. The recommended schedule for immunization is (1) time 0, (2) 1 month later, and (3) 6–12 months later. If there is a delay in obtaining the second booster, it should be administered as soon as possible, and the third dose should be given no sooner than 2 months following the second dose. Completion of the immunization series confers 80–95% protection against clinical hepatitis and chronic hepatitis. When the recipient is known to have developed a hepatitis B surface antibody response to serologic testing, immunity is thought to be 100%.

Postvaccination assessment of immunity may be advisable in recipients older than 30 years because seroconversion rates may be lower in older individuals. Those recipients who are at greatest risk of exposure through daily activities or life-style (eg, patients undergoing dialysis and staff at dialysis units) or whose immunity response is likely to be low (eg, those taking immunosuppressive medications or who have immunosuppressive diseases) should consider testing for immunity within 6 months of completing the series. If antibody levels are below 10 mIU/mL, one or more boosters should be considered.

Side effects are limited to minor reactions. Between three and twenty-nine percent of vaccinees have local pain. Between one and six percent have a fever above 37.7 °C and associated constitutional symptoms. Questions have been raised about a low incidence of associated Guillain-Barré syndrome, but this relationship appears to be doubtful.

Pregnant women considered at high risk of exposure to hepatitis B should be immunized. It is widely accepted that hepatitis B surface antigen testing is included in standard prenatal laboratory screenings.

RUBELLA

Adults born after 1956 should receive one vaccine containing measles (rubeola), mumps, and rubella (MMR) unless there is evidence from medical records indicating prior infection, immunization after age 12 months, or serologic documentation of immunity. Many adults born in the early 1960s or later have received this immunization, but documentation should be confirmed when possible, or serologic testing may be considered. Inadvertent repeat immunization is not likely to be harmful if immunization status cannot be determined easily. The rubella vaccine currently administered is believed to give lifelong immunity; therefore, boosters are unnecessary.

Rubella antibody testing usually is included in prenatal laboratory evaluations and often is available to practitioners caring for women with children. Furthermore, a woman lacking evidence of immunity to rubella during her pregnancy should be immunized immediately after delivery. Documentation of this immunization should be obtained.

Side effects to rubella vaccine include rash, lymphadenopathy, and arthralgias or frank arthritis. Adult women appear to be more susceptible than others to these complications.

Rubella vaccine is contraindicated during pregnancy. It is a live-virus vaccine, and there is concern that a low incidence of congenital rubella syndrome (CRS) may result from vaccinating women in the first trimester of pregnancy. There are no substantial data, however, linking inadvertent vaccine administration during pregnancy to fetal abnormalities. Theoretic concerns about the possibility of CRS lead to the aforementioned recommendation but are not grounds for pregnancy termination. Women should be counseled to avoid pregnancy for 3 months after receiving the vaccine.

MEASLES

Adults born after 1956 should receive one MMR vaccine unless there is evidence of prior infection,

Table 8–1. Immunization recommendations.

Immunization	Recommendations	Recommendations During Pregnancy
Diphtheria/tetanus	Complete primary series; booster every 10 years*	Not contraindicated
Influenza	Annually starting age 65 and in others who meet criteria*	If otherwise indicated
Pneumococcal	Once at age 65 or older; once in younger women who meet criteria*	If otherwise indicated
Hepatitis B	High-risk women*	If otherwise indicated
Measles, mumps, rubella	Once if born after 1956	Contraindicated; pregnancy should be avoided for 3 months after receiving
Rubella	*	Contraindicated
Measles (Rubeola)	*	Contraindicated

*See text for additional information.

immunization after age 12 months, or serologic conversion. Because immunity after measles vaccine has been noted to wane, adults born after 1956 who have an increased risk of exposure to measles should receive a booster. This vaccine may be administered as attenuated measles virus or as a second MMR. Those who are thought to be at increased risk of exposure are students, health care workers, and travelers to areas where measles is prevalent.

Adverse reactions to the vaccine have been reduced since a new, attenuated virus has been used beginning in 1979. Between 5 and 15% of patients have a fever lasting up to 48 hours and beginning 5–12 days after immunization. Mild rash may accompany the fever. Up to 50% of people who received the killed virus vaccine that was used between 1963 and 1968 have a mild reaction when reimmunized with the current, live-virus vaccine.

Pregnancy is a contraindication to vaccination and the same precautions apply as for the rubella vaccine. Specifically, women should be counseled to avoid pregnancy during the 3 months following immunization.

MUMPS

The mumps vaccine is considered to confer lifelong immunity and is included in the MMR vaccine. Adverse reactions to this vaccine are rare. Pregnancy is a contraindication to mumps vaccination.

POLIO

Rare indications exist to give live polio vaccine to adults. Inactivated polio vaccine (IPV) may be con-

sidered in certain circumstances, largely when risk of reexposure is high or a state of partial immunization is present. It also may be used as a booster in patients who are immunocompromised, especially if there is an increased risk of exposure through travel or from household or occupational contacts.

VACCINATIONS IN PREGNANCY

Use of the aforementioned vaccines in the setting of pregnancy or potential pregnancy is discussed in most of the preceding recommendations. Table 8–1 contains a summary of the standard immunizations discussed in this chapter and includes advice related to pregnancy. These recommendations are in agreement with those of the American College of Obstetrics and Gynecology.

SPECIAL NEEDS OF TRAVELERS

Special considerations govern decisions to advise additional immunizations for international travelers. Many large institutions include travel advisory consultants or clinics. Many community health departments counsel travelers regarding up-to-date recommendations specific to the destination. For additional information, practitioners may wish to contact the CDC Travel Reference Service at (404) 332-4559 or request written material from International Traveler, Superintendent of Documents, U.S. Government Printing Office, Washington, DC 20402.

REFERENCES

Briggs GG et al: *Drugs in Pregnancy and Lactation: A Reference Guide to Fetal and Neonatal Risk,* 3rd ed. Williams & Wilkins, 1990.

Centers for Disease Control and Prevention: Prevention and control of influenza: Recommendations of the Advisory Committee on Immunization Practices (ACIP). MMWR 1993;42(No.RR-6):1.

Cunningham FG et al: *Williams Obstetrics,* 19th ed. Appleton & Lange, 1993.

Dickey LL: Promoting preventive care with patient-held minirecords: A review. Patient Educ Couns 1993;20:37.

Guide for Adult Immunization, 3rd ed. American College of Physicians, 1994.

Hayward RSA et al: Preventive Care Guidelines: 1991. Ann Intern Med 1991;114:758.

Kottke TE et al: Making "time" for preventive services. Mayo Clin Proc 1993;68:785.

Lewis CE: Disease prevention and health promotion practices of primary care physicians in the United States. Am J Prev Med 1988;4(Suppl):9.

Payne T et al: Development and validation of an immunization tracking system in a large health maintenance organization. Am J Prev Med 1993;9:96.

Shulman ST et al: Principles of immunization. In: *Biologic and Clinical Basis of Infectious Diseases,* 4th ed. Shulman ST et al (editors). Saunders, 1992.

Task Force on Adult Immunization: Adult Immunizations 1994. Ann Intern Med 1994;121(No. 7):540.

Tetanus—United States, 1987 and 1988. MMWR 1990; 39(No.3):37.

U.S. Preventive Services Task Force: *Guide to Preventive Services.* Williams & Wilkins, 1989.

Update on adult immunization: Recommendation of the Immunization Practices Advisory Committee. MMWR 1991;40(No. RR-12):Table 7.

Health Promotion

Marilyn A. Guthrie, RD, Nancy L. Risser MN, RN, CS, ANP, & Kathleen M. Ober, FNP, PhD

9

Life style and health habits influence most major chronic conditions that affect women, including heart disease, breast cancer, obesity, and osteoporosis. Nutrition and weight management, smoking cessation, exercise, and stress management strategies remain the mainstays of a health-promoting life style. In addition, these practices form the foundation for the management of the aforementioned and other chronic conditions. For example, many women find relief from the symptoms of premenstrual syndrome and menopause by making changes in their diet or by increasing their level of physical activity.

NUTRITION

Historical Perspective

Nutrition plays a critical role both by optimizing health and well-being and by reducing the risk of chronic disease. Even if there exists a propensity toward a certain condition, a balanced and adequate diet can prevent or attenuate the associated symptoms or risk factors.

Over the past half century, eating patterns in the United States have changed dramatically largely because of changes in women's role in society and the workplace. As women have entered the workforce in significant numbers, greater emphasis has been placed on convenience foods, fast foods, and dining out. Consumption of refined sugars, sodium, animal fat, and protein has increased, and intake of fresh fruits and vegetables and whole grains has decreased. Current eating patterns and recommended levels of intake are reflected in Table 9–1.

Screening

Many women are at high risk of nutritional deficits, excesses, and imbalances that may affect their health and well-being negatively. The goal of nutrition screening is to identify women at risk before their health has deteriorated to the point that they develop acute or chronic disease or complications of disease and require medication or hospitalization. Brief, simple questions in the following areas as part of the patient assessment and history taking can single out women who need attention to issues of diet and nutrition.

Nutrition
  Historical Perspective
  Screening
  Calories & Obesity
  Fat, Heart Disease, & Cancer
  Fiber & the Antioxidant Nutrients
  Calcium & Osteoporosis
  Alcohol
  Caffeine
  Dietary Recommendations
  Issues of Pregnancy & Nutrition
  Psychosocial Issues
Smoking Cessation
  Risks of Smoking
  Incidence
  Benefits of Cessation
  Strategies for Cessation
  Practical Clinical Approaches
  Prevention in Adolescents
  Issues of Pregnancy & Smoking
  Follow-up & Relapse Prevention
Exercise
  Benefits
  Screening
  General Recommendations
  Motivational Factors
  Issues of Pregnancy & Exercise

A. Body Weight: Changes in body weight and composition reflect dietary intake and serve as general indicators of nutritional and overall health. Body mass index (BMI) is a weight:height ratio that is strongly correlated with body fat; BMI is calculated by dividing body weight (kg) by height squared (m^2). An increase or decrease in weight of more than 10 pounds in the past 6 months could indicate imminent or present disease. Even when the weight change is associated with an emotional cause, eg, depression, the health consequences can be significant. Women who are obese (BMI greater than 27 or weighing 120% or more of their desirable body weight) are at increased risk for a number of related conditions, eg, hypertension, diabetes, and osteoarthritis. Women who are underweight (BMI less than 24) are at increased risk for illness and poor nutritional status.

Table 9–1. Current and recommended intake of nutrients and alcohol.

Nutrient	Current Dietary Intake	Recommended Intake
Fat	40–45% of total calories	25–30% of total calories
Protein	15–18% of total calories	15–18% of total calories
Carbohydrate	30–35% of total calories	55–60% of total calories
Fiber	15 g/d	25–30 g/d
Salt	10 g/d	5 g/d
Alcohol	200 kcal/d	5% of total calories

B. Eating Habits: A woman may appear to be the appropriate weight and look well, but if she restricts her food intake, the risk for specific diseases increases. Unfortunately, assessing dietary intake can be difficult because of impaired recall. Restrictions in diet, poor appetite, difficulty eating or swallowing, and overeating are clues to possible nutritional deficiencies or malnutrition.

C. Clinical Features: Many signs found on physical examination are likely to be associated with poor nutritional status. Problems with the mouth, teeth, or gums; history of bone pain or fractures; and skin changes may be indicators of nutritional inadequacies. Obesity, hypertension, and lipid abnormalities may indicate poor or imbalanced dietary intake. Some of the women who are identified to be at nutritional risk may benefit from seeing a registered dietitian to ensure adequate intake or for dietary modification to accommodate specific conditions, such as hypercholesterolemia, hypertension, or obesity.

D. Functional Status: Any decline in self-care or home management activities should be regarded as a possible risk factor for and an indicator of poor eating habits. Particular attention should be paid to changes in functional status of instrumental activities of daily living (IADLs) that relate to the likelihood of the patient obtaining, preparing, and eating the foods that make up an adequate diet. Patients who do not have sufficient resources to purchase nutritional foods should be referred to a social service worker who can identify community resources.

Calories & Obesity

Weight management is a key to improving health and quality of life for women and offers great potential to prevent costly disease. Obesity increases a woman's risk for at least five of the leading causes of death: heart disease, stroke, diabetes, atherosclerosis, and some types of cancer.

Caloric needs change throughout a woman's life cycle. During adolescence, the energy needs increase to accommodate the additional growth that occurs. The caloric needs of adult women stabilize, except during pregnancy and lactation, when the consump-

tion of additional calories is necessary. After the age of 30, the metabolism and corresponding caloric requirement gradually decrease. Without a concomitant adjustment in eating patterns at this time, weight management becomes a concern. Weight gain peaks in both sexes between the ages of 35 and 44 years, after which it tends to decline in men but continues to increase in women. Between the ages of 25 and 54, women's average weight gain is more than one-third above that of men.

In adjusting intake for weight loss, one must limit calories sufficiently to produce a caloric deficit while providing adequate energy to meet basal needs and avoid a "starvation effect" with subsequent lowering of metabolic rate. Diets that provide less than 800 kcal/d can result in significant initial weight losses but with major regains of weight within 2 years following treatment. Questions have been raised regarding potential deleterious effects of the weight cycling that occurs with repeated attempts at low-calorie dieting.

Eating frequency and dietary composition are relatively new areas of study with regard to gender differences, effect on energy balance, and potential effects on overall health. It seems reasonable that total energy load; the proportions of protein, fat, and carbohydrate; and the frequency with which meals are eaten could influence overall metabolism. Compared with a traditional three-meal diet, a nibbling or grazing type of eating pattern has been shown to reduce serum total cholesterol, low-density lipoprotein (LDL) cholesterol, apolipoprotein B, and serum insulin. Evidence also suggests that significant favorable differences in total body energy and body composition could be elicited by a high-carbohydrate diet compared with a high-fat diet.

Fat, Heart Disease, & Cancer

Heart disease is the major cause of death among women, and nutrition plays an integral role in its causation and management. Several major coronary heart disease risk factors, such as elevated blood lipids, excess body weight, and hypertension, are responsive to nutritional intervention. In addition, women respond more positively than men to dietary changes for risk reduction.

Although epidemiologic studies give conflicting results, there may be a causal relationship between dietary fat and the development of breast cancer. Women, particularly those with other risk factors for breast cancer, are well advised to consume a low-fat diet to promote health and lessen the likelihood of development of breast cancer.

A high intake of fat, particularly saturated fat, can lead to elevated levels of serum cholesterol. Use of unsaturated fatty acids, especially when substituted for saturated fatty acids, can lower the levels of total cholesterol and LDL cholesterol. Consumption of a diet low in total fat and high in carbohydrate, particularly complex carbohydrate, is an important factor in the primary prevention of heart disease and possibly cancer as well. In addition to its role in prevention of chronic disease, this type of diet can be helpful in weight management and health promotion, because a greater proportion of calories come from fiber-and nutrient-rich foods, which tend to be low in calories.

Fiber & the Antioxidant Nutrients

Fiber, both soluble and insoluble, plays an important role in health maintenance in several ways. Some types of fiber (primarily soluble) can help lower cholesterol levels, whereas other types of fiber can help regulate blood glucose levels. The role of fiber (primarily insoluble) in regulation of bowel activity is well known; it also plays a role in maintaining the integrity of the intestinal tract lining and possibly in reducing the risk of colon cancer. Perhaps less appreciated is the contribution of fiber to weight management owing to the adsorption of water and subsequent expansion as the fiber-containing food enters the digestive tract. This factor may be particularly important for women, who face a greater challenge than men do in maintaining a healthy weight.

Increasing one's intake of fruits and vegetables is important for health maintenance; information is growing concerning the potential benefit of these foods in lowering the risk for heart disease, cancer, and other conditions. These foods, especially those that are dark green, deep orange, or yellow and those belonging to the cabbage family (cruciferous vegetables), contain specific substances that are be beneficial to health, including antioxidant nutrients, vitamins C and E, and beta-carotene. Antioxidant nutrients may be important in ameliorating the aging process and tissue damage that occurs during oxidative processes as a result of free radical formation. There is no evidence to indicate benefit from consuming megadoses of such nutrients in supplement form; the emphasis should be on food sources of these nutrients.

Calcium & Osteoporosis

Nutrition plays a key role in reducing the risk of osteoporosis, which leads to more than 1.5 million bone fractures each year. Of the 25 million people in the USA with this disease, most are women.

Dietary calcium exerts its greatest effect on bone-mineral density during two phases of life: (1) the bone building years of childhood and adolescence and (2) the elderly years. Studies show that adequate dietary calcium intake throughout the adolescent period is critical for the attainment of optimal bone mineral density and thus reduce the risk of future osteoporosis. It is prudent, therefore, to recommend a high calcium intake during this critical period. Between 1200 and 1500 mg of calcium is suggested for female adolescents. To avoid depletion of the skeletal bone tissue during the elderly years, pre-

menopausal women should consume 1000 mg/d of calcium, and elderly women not taking estrogen should consume 1500 mg/d. In addition, these adult women may need vitamin D supplementation to enhance calcium absorption if sun exposure is limited.

Dietary sources of calcium include milk and other dairy products, canned fish, tofu, and dark green leafy vegetables. Dairy products contain the added benefit of lactose and, in milk, vitamin D, which increase the rate of calcium absorption. Because only a few calcium-fortified foods are available currently, supplements constitute a major source of calcium for many women. A form of supplemental calcium often recommended is calcium carbonate; however, this form can lead to constipation and abdominal distention. In addition, large doses can bind and limit absorption of the dietary iron. Divided doses of calcium lactate or calcium citrate are advised. Because calcium lactate is only 13% elemental calcium, the number or size of pills must be increased in comparison with calcium carbonate, which contains 40% elemental calcium.

Alcohol

There is no clear evidence that moderate alcohol consumption causes any long-term deleterious health effects. In fact, moderate alcohol consumption is related positively to HDL cholesterol levels in both women and men. There are many potential harmful effects, however, of excess use. In addition to increasing the risk of liver disease, some cancers (particularly of the head and neck region), cardiomyopathy, and pancreatitis, excess alcohol consumption may increase the likelihood of migraine headaches and depression and act as a trigger for hot flashes during menopause. Heavy alcohol consumption increases the risk for osteoporosis and fractures in older women in several ways. Excess alcohol intake interferes with the bone remodeling process and prevents bone cells from building new bone; it also increases the loss of calcium in the urine. Women who consume alcohol in large amounts also typically eat less calcium-rich foods and exercise less.

Although alcohol is not harmful in moderate amounts, it represents a source of empty calories that contributes to the overall energy intake without concomitant nutrients. For women concerned about weight management, it is important that alcohol not compromise the nutritional composition of the diet.

Caffeine

Contrary to popular belief, extensive research on caffeine has not linked moderate caffeine consumption to any health risks, including cancer, cardiovascular disease, or teratogenesis. The effects of caffeine differ greatly, however, depending on level and acuteness of intake and the development of tolerance.

Because caffeine imposes pharmacologic actions, excesses can be toxic. The symptoms related to acute or chronic high caffeine intake include anxiety, restlessness, tremulousness, irritability, dry mouth, restless leg syndrome, myalgia, palpitations, arrhythmias, mood and sleep disturbances, gastrointestinal disturbances, and exacerbation of symptoms of premenstrual syndrome.

Menopausal women report an increase in hot flashes when they drink caffeinated beverages and find that decreasing their level of intake can offer considerable relief from this symptom. Any link between caffeine and the development of benign breast disease in women remains unclear. Caffeine appears to stimulate breast pain before menses in some women. When women with benign breast disease give up caffeine, the discomfort often regresses remarkably within 4–6 months.

Because it is so widely used, caffeine is one of the most thoroughly investigated ingredients in the food supply. After being studied carefully for decades, the preponderance of scientific evidence demonstrates that caffeine is safe when consumed in moderation.

Dietary Recommendations

Even if there exists a propensity toward a medical condition, a balanced and adequate diet can prevent or attenuate the symptoms or risk conditions associated with that disease. A well-balanced diet comprises the following key components:

A. A Wide Variety of Foods: Women often fail to consume a wide variety of foods because of concerns about fat and calories. They tend to be narrower in their food choices than men, sometimes eliminating a key group of foods and, therefore, the corresponding nutrients. Consuming a wide variety of foods ensures that the nutritional needs are met, with minimal risk of overconsumption of empty calories.

B. A Healthy Weight: Recommendations for weight management include a moderate reduction in caloric intake (no more than 500–1000 kcal) with a concurrent increase in aerobic exercise.

C. Moderate Intake of Fat and Cholesterol: The current recommendation is to consume no more than 30% of the total calories as fat calories, with less than 10% from saturated fat. A practical approach is to determine the woman's energy needs on the basis of her age, height, and weight; compute the fat allowance in grams; and budget fat intake throughout the day.

D. Adequate Intake of Fiber: Carbohydrates, primarily complex carbohydrates such as whole grains, pastas, cereals, and fruits and vegetables, should provide more than 55% of the energy intake for the day. A high carbohydrate intake contributes to the recommended fiber intake of 25–30 g/d, because most of the dietary fiber is found in complex carbohydrates. This level can be achieved by consuming the recommended number of servings of grains,

fruits, and vegetables shown in the Food Guide Pyramid (Fig 9–1).

E. Adequate Intake of Calcium: Although food is the ideal vehicle for obtaining calcium, a person's diet, if devoid of dairy products, contains only approximately 300 mg of calcium per day. Therefore, regular intake of dairy products or calcium-fortified orange juice needs to be a part of the daily diet.

F. Moderate Intake of Alcohol and Caffeine: A rule of thumb for alcohol intake is not to exceed 1–2 ounces of alcohol per day, which represents one mixed drink, 4–6 ounces of wine, or 12 ounces of beer. This level of intake is considered an upper daily limit for moderation, not a daily average.

Depending on individual tolerance for caffeine, moderate amounts of caffeine-containing foods and beverages do not pose a health risk for most women.

G. Supplementation as Needed: Depending on the overall profile of the diet and the woman's individual needs, vitamin or mineral supplementation, or both, may offer some benefit. For example, women, particularly in their later years, require calcium in greater amounts than typically can be provided solely by dietary sources. At the time of menopause or at age 50, women would be well advised to take a calcium supplement in combination with vitamin D to enhance calcium absorption.

Women following strict weight-control diets or who have restricted their caloric intake because of poor appetite, pain, illness, substance abuse, or emotional problems typically do not eat enough to get all the necessary nutrients; such women should consider a multi-vitamin supplement.

Issues of Pregnancy & Nutrition

Women who are considering pregnancy should be aware of the potential deleterious effects of alcohol on the fetus. Although it is unclear at what level these effects occur, it may be prudent to advise women considering conception to limit alcohol intake to low amounts. Such women also should consider folate supplementation to reduce the risk of neural tube defects in the fetus.

A woman's primary nutritional concern during pregnancy is for adequate energy to support the accelerated growth of the fetus. During pregnancy, the woman's caloric needs increase by at least 300 kcal above nonpregnant needs. Because there is a concomitant increase in the requirements for most other nutrients, a prenatal vitamin-mineral supplement may be recommended.

Because caffeine crosses the placenta and enters the fetal circulation, it affects the fetus. The use of caffeine during pregnancy appears to stimulate the fetal heart. Possible effects of excessive caffeine use on the fetus include skeletal abnormalities, a decrease in intrauterine growth, and a low birth weight. Pregnant women are advised to avoid caffeine-containing foods and beverages.

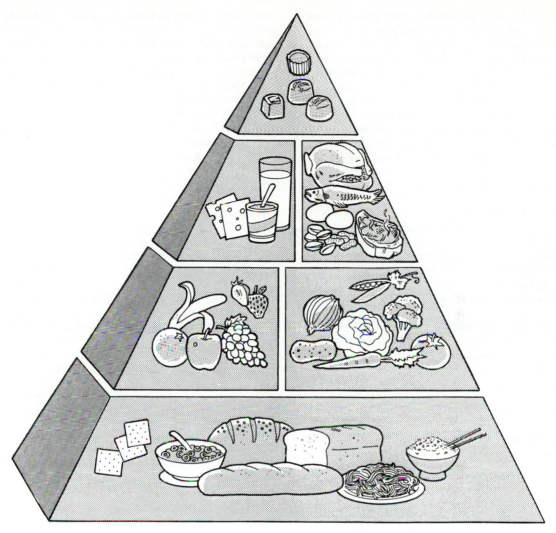

MAJOR FOOD GROUP	RECOMMENDED DAILY AMOUNTS	FATS and SUGARS (relative amounts)
Fats, oils, and sweets	Use sparingly	▼▼▼▼▼▼▼▼▼▼▼▼▼▼▼▼ ▼▼▼▼▼▼▼▼▼▼▼▼▼▼ ●●●●●●●●●●●
Milk, yogurt, and cheese	2–3 servings	▼▼▼▼ ●●●●●●●●
Meat, poultry, fish, dry beans, eggs, and nuts	2–3 servings	●●●●●●●●●●
Fruits	2–4 servings	▼▼▼▼▼
Vegetables	3–5 servings	●●●●●
Bread, cereal, rice, and pasta	6–11 servings	▼▼▼▼▼▼▼▼ ●●●●●●●●

▼ Sugars (added)

● Fat (naturally occurring and added)

Figure 9–1. The food guide pryamid.

There has been much debate concerning the safety of consuming aspartame during pregnancy. On the basis of current research, there is no reason to suggest that aspartame in moderate amounts poses a significant health risk to pregnant women or their babies. On the other hand, milk, fruit juice, and water are better beverage choices for mothers-to-be, and pregnancy is not a time to use diet foods.

Because nausea, vomiting, and heartburn are common symptoms during pregnancy, adjustment of the size and frequency of meals is recommended. Eating smaller, more frequent meals and avoiding spicy, fried foods may help relieve some of the discomfort.

Psychosocial Issues

It is important to keep in mind that food provides more than nutrition. Eating satisfies physiologic, emotional, social, and psychologic needs. There are no "good foods" or "bad foods," only unhealthy eating patterns. It is the role of health professionals to help women define the appropriate role of eating in meeting their needs and, if indicated, to refer women to other professionals and resources to help them manage their eating habits. Clinicians can challenge the norms, messages, and role models that are presented in media and advertising that create unhealthy and unrealistic expectations in young women about body image and eating habits (see Chapter 10).

SMOKING CESSATION

Risks of Smoking

Cigarette smoking remains the chief preventable cause of death and illness in the United States, responsible for one-sixth of all deaths. In women younger than 50 years of age, two-thirds of myocardial infarctions can be attributed to smoking. Smoking is associated with the negative pregnancy outcomes of low birth weight, preterm delivery, abruptio placentae, placenta previa, and antepartum hemorrhage. Smokers have an increased risk of spontaneously aborting a chromosomally normal fetus, with an odds ratio of 1.2–1.8 compared with nonsmokers. Ectopic pregnancy and tubal infertility also occur more frequently among smokers, possibly related to the increased risk for pelvic inflammatory disease.

Incidence

The prevalence of smoking in women did not exceed 25% until World War II, when it was still one-half that of men. Smoking prevalence in men has dropped by almost half, from 52% in 1965 to 28% in 1991, whereas that of women fell by one-third from 34% to 23.5%, leaving 22 million women in the USA who continue to smoke. From 1990 to 1991, the prevalence of smoking continued to decline in most population subsections but increased among blacks and women. Recruitment of new smokers continues,

with women having a greater prevalence of smoking than men among adolescents and young adults. Among women 20–24 years of age with less than a high school education, there was a 10% increase in smoking prevalence from 1974 to 1985; at the same time, there was a small decline for women with a high school education.

Gender, race, and educational differences also exist for success in quitting. Women are less successful in cessation attempts than men, and blacks are less likely to quit than whites. Smokers who are unemployed or unmarried, who have low incomes, or who have less than a high school education also are less likely to quit. Depression occurs twice as often among those with a history of nicotine dependence compared with people who have never smoked and has been linked to increased smoking initiation and to failure in efforts at smoking cessation.

Benefits of Cessation

All patients, including the elderly, receive substantial and immediate health benefits from stopping smoking. For example, carboxyhemoglobin levels normalize within days of quitting. Smoking cessation reduces the risk for lung, esophageal, head and neck, bladder, and other cancers; coronary heart disease; stroke; and chronic lung disease. Because coronary artery disease develops in women at a later age than men, there is greater opportunity for primary prevention by smoking cessation. Within 2–3 years after quitting, women's relative risk of coronary heart disease returns to that of nonsmokers. A woman who stops smoking before the onset of disease experiences a 24% reduction in the mortality risk from all causes within 2 years of quitting.

Strategies for Cessation

Even with brief interactions, clinicians can influence their patients to stop smoking. Because 70% of adults in the USA see a physician at least annually, a small increase in the percentage of smokers who quit would justify the effort involved. Girls and adolescent women average four physician contacts a year, creating millions of opportunities for prevention or cessation counseling annually.

Effective interventions require the use of multiple methods to motivate and assist behavioral change, involve both physicians and nonphysicians in individualized efforts, and provide the messages on multiple occasions over the longest possible time period. A successful approach includes use of cues to intervene, eg, chart stickers; advising every smoker to quit at each visit; setting a quit date; prescribing nicotine replacement therapy; providing self-help materials; and providing follow-up contact.

Clinicians who refer smokers to other resources for help need to recognize that different methods work for different people. Most smokers are interested in quitting on their own, using self-help guides or books. Work-site group programs may be especially helpful to women smokers, who seem to benefit more than men from social support during the quitting process. Most methods, including hypnosis; group programs; and repeated, serious self-help quitting attempts, result in similar long-term success rates. Initial dramatic smoking reductions are followed by relapse. On the average, only 30–40% of smokers remain abstinent after 3–6 months, and only 10–20% are successful after a year. Multicomponent programs that allow smokers to select individualized strategies seem the most promising. They apply social learning principles to skills training and emphasize maintenance as well as initial cessation. Because the long-term success rate in most public service and research programs has been 20–30% consistently, claims of more impressive results should be viewed with skepticism; careful long-term evaluation data often are not available.

Practical Clinical Approaches

The following are minimal interventions that clinicians can use:

1. Ask every patient about smoking habits during each visit.
2. Deliver a clear, firm, unequivocal message to quit to each smoker, regardless of age or health status.
3. Inform each smoker of the health benefits of quitting, personalizing reasons for cessation.
4. Try to obtain an agreement from the patient to quit smoking.
5. Monitor progress at follow-up visits.

A counseling approach along with other methods helps the smoker to develop a plan for cessation and is associated with higher cessation rates than simply telling the patient to stop smoking. When feasible, the clinician should add the following steps:

1. Assure the patient that he or she can quit.
2. Discuss the smoker's personal reasons for quitting and previous attempts. Portray quitting as an evolving process; successful quitting usually occurs only after several unsuccessful attempts.
3. Motivate cessation by linking abnormalities such as wheezes, cough, abnormal results on spirometry, or other symptoms to smoking. Convince the patient that smoking may injure others such as family members.
4. Address weight-control concerns if fear of gaining weight appears to motivate continued smoking. Suggest a food diary to evaluate caloric intake and an exercise program.
5. Provide assistance in the development of alternative behaviors for reward, relaxation, and coping with stress.
6. Secure a commitment to a specific quit date within 3 weeks and give the patient an appointment to return on that date. Record the agreement on a signed prescription form and in the chart. Emphasize the importance of total abstinence after a quit attempt.
7. Provide self-help materials, such as the American Lung Association's "Freedom From Smoking" manuals.
8. Provide a list of local resources for referral, and refer smokers to formal "quit-smoking" treatment.
9. Emphasize the relative importance of strategies for behavioral change (Table 9–2) compared with nicotine replacement products alone to learn relapse-prevention skills for long-term abstinence.
10. Offer nicotine replacement therapy to smokers who demonstrate symptoms of nicotine addiction (smoke their first cigarette within half an hour of awakening, smoke more than one pack of cigarettes daily, or report significant withdrawal symptoms during previous quit attempts) (Table 9–3). Use of nicotine replacement therapy doubles the abstinence rates compared with placebo; the highest success rates are achieved when it is combined with intensive behavioral therapy. Remind smokers that the nicotine ther-

Table 9–2. Behavioral strategies for smoking cessation.

Strategy	Method
Aversive techniques	Before quitting, associate smoking with negative consequences (eg, rapid smoking, rubber band snap to wrist for urge).
Self-monitoring	Log time, and circumstances of each cigarette; identify smoking triggers.
Contingency reinforcement	Plan daily and long-term rewards for steps toward quitting.
Stimulus control	Disrupt usual routine; reduce or eliminate trigger situations (eg, coffee, alcohol, time spent with smokers).
Response substitution	Substitute something else for smoking in trigger situation (eg, gum, deep breathing, or candy); increase positive habits (eg, exercise, time spent with nonsmoking friends).
Enhance personal commitment to quit	List benefits of quitting; announce quitting plans to friends; sign contract that specifies quit date.
Enlist social support	Quit with a friend; join a group program.
Manage anxiety	Learn meditation and relaxation techniques.
Coping-response training/cognitive rehearsal	Practice ways to turn down cigarette offers; have plans for frequent trigger situations; rehearse response for anticipated barriers; use imagery and picture self a nonsmoker.

Table 9–3. Nicotine withdrawal symptoms.

Craving for tobacco
Headaches
Insomnia
Altered bowel habits
Mood changes, irritability, anxiety
Craving for sweets
Difficulty concentrating
Change in appetite

apy costs little more than the cigarettes it replaces (Table 9–4).

Prevention in Adolescents

During adolescence, attempts to quit smoking decline with age. The earlier the experimenting teenager can be counseled, the better the chance of cessation. The most successful prevention programs for adolescents have been school-based ones that employ peer leaders to provide psychosocial interventions that include refusal skill training and contingency management. At office visits, clinicians can provide information on peer smoking prevalence because adolescents often overestimate peer smoking.

Issues of Pregnancy & Smoking

Although 20–40% of women who smoke at the beginning of pregnancy quit, 20–25% of pregnant women continue to smoke. Smoking cessation before pregnancy or during the first trimester leads to infant outcomes similar to those for nonsmokers. Quitting at this time can be an opportunity for a permanent change in life-style that can reduce the risk of smok-

ing-related chronic disease later in life. Because of the risks of nicotine use during pregnancy, it is important to offer intensive behavioral therapies for smoking cessation to women who are attempting to conceive and those who are pregnant. For pregnant women who cannot stop smoking with behavioral therapies alone, Benowitz (1991) concludes that nicotine replacement therapy is likely to present less risk to the fetus than cigarette smoking, particularly in heavy smokers.

Follow-up & Relapse Prevention

Relapse after initial success is the greatest problem facing smokers who want to quit. Smoking status during the first 2 weeks of nicotine replacement therapy is highly correlated with long-term success. In addition to the follow-up visit on the quit date, additional appointments or telephone contacts within the first 2 weeks are important. Smoking status and relief of withdrawal symptoms should be assessed.

For the person who almost has achieved abstinence and still is motivated to stop, more intensive pharmacotherapy or referral to a formal cessation program may be considered. If smoking continues near or at baseline levels, or the patient reports feeling defeated, pharmacotherapy can be stopped and the smoker allowed to regroup. At a future office visit, a new quit date may be set possibly with plans to use a more intensive intervention. Prevention of relapse requires continued use of skills learned during the quitting process. Often, smokers who relapse blame themselves rather than attributing the slip to external causes. A relapse should not be viewed as a

Table 9–4. Nicotine replacement therapy.

Product	Dose	Directions	Cost
Nicotine polacrilex chewing gum (nicorette)	2 mg (one piece) q 20–30 min PRN for urges; max 30/24 hrs; use enough gum (avg one piece of gum/2 cigaretts); use for 3–6 mo.	Do not smoke and chew gum. Chew gum slowly so it is absorbed through buccal mucosa and not swallowed. To maintain proper pH, use no liquids while chewing gum. Provides nicotine on demand. Side effects include jaw pain, hiccups, nausea, and oral ulcers.	$35–40 for a box of 96 pieces
Transdermal nicotine delivery system (Habitrol, Nicoderm, Nicotrol, ProStep)	Use high-dose patch for 4–8 wks. If smoker weighs < 100 lb, smokes < $\frac{1}{2}$ pack/day, or has cardiovascular disease, begin with lower dose. Taper dosage over 4–8 wk.	Do not smoke and use patch. Remove patch after 16–24 hr. Apply new patch to different area of intact skin on upper body. May bathe and exercise. About $\frac{1}{2}$ of users experience skin irritation. Other side effects include nausea, headaches, lightheadedness, insomnia, and nightmares. Provides constant blood levels but higher possibility of overdose.	$45–55 for a box of 14 patches

failure. Most smokers need more than one quit attempt to learn what is necessary for their ultimate success. The clinician should continue to repeat a clear, consistent, personalized nonsmoking message.

Clinicians should provide positive reinforcement to those who have quit and continue to emphasize the benefits of quitting. These patients can be helped to recognize high-risk situations for relapse and to develop coping behaviors. Relapses after the first week often are associated with negative emotional states (eg, work, family crisis, other stress), smoking triggers (eg, alcohol, coffee), and social situations (eg, parties, presence of other smokers).

Weight should be monitored, and behavioral strategies offered early in an attempt to limit total calories. Although weight gain after the cessation of smoking may be prevented by nicotine replacement therapy and possibly by serotoninergic drugs such as D-fenfluramine, weight often increases when drug therapy is discontinued. Behavior modification strategies must be the foundation of long-term weight control.

Before reducing or stopping nicotine replacement therapy for smokers who have quit, the clinician should assess for persistent withdrawal symptoms. Some people need continued high doses or longer term patch therapy to maintain cessation.

EXERCISE

Benefits

In recent years, the recognition of possible associations between a sedentary life-style and disease states has led to the widespread acceptance that regular physical exercise can contribute to improved health. Research has demonstrated that regular exercise is effective not only in the prevention of coronary heart disease but also in the management of chronic conditions such as diabetes, hypertension, arthritis, osteoporosis, obesity, and chronic respiratory disorders. Increased information is available pertaining to positive changes in the cardiorespiratory capacity, body composition, rate of bone loss, and coronary heart disease risk factors in women resulting from participation in regular aerobic exercise.

According to Bovens et al, persons with higher levels of physical fitness or physical activity have better coronary risk profiles, based on amount of body fat, blood pressure, and smoking habits, than persons who are less fit or active. Because the incidence of cardiovascular disease in postmenopausal women is three times greater than in premenopausal women, it seems reasonable to encourage and facilitate physical activity at an early age. Although the findings of studies of physical inactivity and cancer are inconsistent, Sternfeld suggests that activity may provide a protective effect with some types of cancer (eg, colon cancer).

Women engaged in regular exercise have reported psychologic benefits such as improved self-esteem and body image; elevated mood; and reduced anxiety, stress, and depression. Attainment of cardiovascular fitness can be achieved at any age and in a variety of ways. Regular exercise alone, however, is not adequate to attain optimal health and reduce the risk of disease. Exercise should be considered an integral part of a total health program.

Screening

Although exercise is considered safe for most people, some form of health and fitness screening is desirable before recommending life-style modifications such as an exercise program. The purposes of the health and fitness screening are (1) to detect the presence of disease; (2) to provide information on the presence of risk factors for coronary disease (see Chapter 32); (3) to assess health behaviors, personal fitness goals, perceived benefits, preferences for types of activities, the need for barriers or support, and potential financial constraints; and (4) to design a safe exercise program.

Age, sex, health status, and coronary artery disease risk factors determine the nature and extent of the health and fitness screening. The screening may vary from a short interview or self-administered medical history questionnaire, such as the Physical Activity Readiness Questionnaire (PAR-Q), to a comprehensive medical evaluation that may include exercise-tolerance testing and laboratory tests. The PAR-Q has undergone several revisions to increase the specificity for detecting contraindications to exercise and reduce the number of unnecessary referrals. The advantages of this preparticipation questionnaire are its (1) ease of administration and cost-effectiveness; (2) ability to identify persons with coronary risk who need a medical evaluation before embarking on a vigorous exercise program; (3) ability to identify medications that may affect cardiorespiratory or metabolic responses to exercise and thus safety; (4) ability to identify persons with special needs, eg, pregnancy; and (5) ability to identify apparently healthy women over age 65 who warrant a medical evaluation before initiating a moderate or vigorous exercise program (Table 9–5).

The American College of Sports Medicine (ACSM) provides guidelines for the identification of persons at high risk who require medical clearance and a diagnostic exercise test before initiating an exercise program. A high-risk person is defined as one who has two or more cardiac risk factors whether or not there are symptoms or disease. The ACSM recommends conducting an exercise-tolerance test (1) to assess cardiopulmonary fitness; (2) to aid in the diagnosis of coronary heart disease (CHD) in asymptomatic or symptomatic persons; and (3) to assess the safety of vigorous exercise before an exercise program is begun.

Table 9–5. Physical activity readiness questionnaire, revised version.

1. Has a doctor ever said you have a heart condition and recommended only medically supervised physical activity?
2. Do you have chest pain brought on by physical activity?
3. Have you developed chest pain within the past month?
4. Do you tend to lose consciousness or fall over as a result of dizziness?
5. Do you have a bone or joint problem that could be aggravated by the proposed physical activity?
6. Has a doctor ever recommended medication for your blood pressure or heart?
7. Are you aware, through your own experience or a doctor's advice, of any other physical reason against your exercising without medical supervision?

According to the ACSM guidelines (Table 9–6), "women under age 50 who are asymptomatic, apparently healthy, with fewer than two CAD risk factors do not require medical evaluation by a practitioner prior to starting on a program of vigorous exercise training (Harris et al, 1993)." Moreover, it is unnecessary for asymptomatic, apparently healthy women, regardless of age or coronary risk profile, to undergo a medical evaluation before starting a moderate exercise training program. The criteria for vigorous and moderate exercise training are greater than 60% maximal oxygen consumption and 40–60% maximal oxygen consumption, respectively.

Although these guidelines suggest that medical evaluation is often unnecessary, the practitioner plays an important role as counselor. The counselor role includes education on general exercise principles and injury prevention, modification of a training program after an injury, and enhancement of an exercise program for currently active women based on their needs and goals.

General Recommendations

General recommendations can be made for healthy, low-risk women who are interested in beginning an exercise program. Although a person may exercise on a regular basis, the conditioning effect may be suboptimal secondary to either lack of knowledge or improper application of basic principles of exercise. The achievement of a healthier lifestyle can be accomplished by teaching the patient the key components of a balanced program: cardiorespiratory endurance, muscular strength, muscular endurance, body composition, and flexibility. Because physical fitness can be measured more objectively than the other factors, it is appropriate to note the ACSM definitions of each of these components:

1. **Cardiorespiratory endurance,** or **aerobic capacity,** is the sustained ability of the heart, lungs, and circulatory system to transport oxygen to working muscles, where it is used, and remove waste products. Cardiorespiratory endurance is enhanced through aerobic exercise, which allows more oxygen to be delivered to the working muscles.
2. **Muscular strength** is the force a muscle produces in one maximal effort.
3. **Muscular endurance** is the ability of a muscle to perform a series of forceful contractions for a prolonged period of time.
4. **Body composition** refers to two components of total body weight, lean body mass and total body fat.
5. **Flexibility** is the capacity to use muscles and joints freely throughout full range of motion.

Optimal levels of cardiorespiratory fitness and body fat can be attained by following established

Table 9–6. Guidelines for exercise testing and participation in women.*

	Apparently Healthy		Higher Risk[1]		
	Younger (≤ 50 ys)	Older	No Symptoms	Symptoms	With Disease[2]
Medical examination and diagnostic test recommended prior to:					
Moderate exercise[3]	No[4]	No	No	Yes	Yes
Vigorous exercise[5]	No	Yes[6]	Yes	Yes	Yes
Physician supervision recommended during exercise test:					
Submaximal testing	No	No	No	Yes	Yes
Maximal testing	No	Yes	Yes	Yes	Yes

*Reproduced, with permission, from American College of Sports Medicine.
[1]Persons with two or more cardiac risk factors or symptoms.
[2]Persons with known cardiac, pulmonary, or metabolic disease.
[3]Moderate exercise (exercise intensity 40–60% VO_2 max); exercise intensity well within the individual's current capacity and can be sustained comfortably for a prolonged period, ie, 60 min; slow progression and generally noncompetitive.
[4]The no responses in this table mean that an item is not necessary, not that the item should not be done.
[5]Vigorous exercise (exercise intensity greater than 60% VO_2 max); exercise intense enough to represent a substantial challenge and ordinarily would result in fatigue within 20 min.
[6]A yes response means that an item is recommended.

guidelines from the ACSM for mode of activity, intensity, duration, and frequency. Proper manipulation of these major exercise variables on a consistent basis gently disrupts homeostasis initiating adaptation to or improvement in functional capacity. In addition, the exercise principles of overload, specificity, and rate of progression must be addressed relative to the patient's fitness goals. The **overload principle** refers to the introduction of stimuli that trigger body adaptations. The **principle of specificity** states that the body's adaptations to exercise training generally are specific to the muscle groups that have been trained. The rate of progression is dictated by the person's improvement in functional capacity, health status, age, needs, and goals.

A. Mode of Activity: Development of the cardiovascular system requires aerobic exercise consisting of continuous movement using large muscle groups for a specified length of time. Activity selection should be based on personal preferences, finances, and physical limitations. The aerobic component could include activities such as walking, jogging, swimming, water aerobics, cross-country skiing, aerobic dancing, circuit training, hiking, and stair climbing. Swimming, cycling, and walking are the activities of choice for persons who are overweight or have joint problems.

B. Intensity: Cardiovascular endurance (functional capacity) improves when the muscle works at 50–85% of maximal oxygen consumption or 65–90% of maximal heart rate (MHR). The ACSM suggests a training level of 60–80% of MHR. Maximal heart rate can be obtained by either the Karvonen formula or a maximal exercise test. Although the maximal exercise-tolerance test is a direct method and therefore more accurate in determining maximal heart rate, it is costly and unnecessary for persons at low risk.

For the low-risk population, the Karvonen formula can estimate the intensity needed to overload sufficiently the cardiovascular, respiratory, and vascular systems. The heart rate method of prescribing exercise intensity is based on the assumption that heart rate is a linear function of exercise intensity. This method is based on the fact that the percentage of maximal heart rate is related to the percentage of maximal oxygen consumption. Several methods were developed by Karvonen and colleagues. In the simplest method, MHR is computed by subtracting the person's age from 220. The next step determines the lower and upper ranges of the training zone by taking 65 and 90% of MHR, respectively. This method is easy to teach and low in cost. The disadvantage is that, in some cases, the target heart rate may not be a true indication of the person's exercise effort.

The application of this method for apparently healthy women must be based on their level of fitness. Recommendations for appropriate exercise intensity are as follows for low, average, and advanced

fitness levels: 60–70% MHR, 70–80% MHR, and 80–90% MHR, respectively.

The Rate of Perceived Exertion (RPE) scale provides a subjective form of evaluation used to monitor exercise intensity or level of difficulty. Borg developed the scale to approximate the range from resting to maximal heart rates, ie, 60–200 beats per minute. A modified version of this scale ranges from 0 (no exertion) to 10 (approaching exhaustion) (Table 9–7). The training zone ranges from 4 to 7, ie, from somewhat strong to very strong. The RPE scale is a useful tool to help regulate and monitor intensity of exercise. In addition, it is an alternative method for use with patients who take medications that may affect the heart rate.

C. Frequency: Ideally, a person should engage in aerobic exercise 3–5 times per week. Current evidence indicates that three training sessions per week performed on nonconsecutive days will maintain cardiovascular endurance. For sedentary persons, this strategy can minimize the risk of soreness and injury and increase exercise adherence. Once adaptation is accomplished, the number of sessions per week can be increased to perpetuate the training effect or response.

D. Duration: Existing evidence concerning the duration of exercise leads to the recommendation that a person perform 20–60 minutes of continuous aerobic activity. The duration of an exercise session should be inversely related to the intensity of the activity. Generally, lower intensity activity of longer duration is recommended for unfit adults because of the potential hazards and compliance problems associated with high-intensity activity.

Each exercise session must include a warm-up and a cooldown period in addition to the training or conditioning phase. Warm-up should consist of a minimum of 5 minutes of low-level activity to increase body temperature and blood flow. Metabolism increases, and nutrients are transported to muscles. The performance of lower intensity exercises with the pri-

Table 9–7. Rate of Perceived Exertion (RPE) Scale.*

Rating	Amount of Exertion
0	No exertion at all
0.5	Extremely weak
1	Very weak
2	Weak
3	Moderate
4	Somewhat strong
5	Strong
6	
7	Very strong
8	
9	
10	Extremely strong; maximal

*Reproduced, with permission, from Borg GV: Med Sci Sports Exerc 1982;14:377.

mary muscle groups to be used during the cardiorespiratory endurance phase prepares the joints, muscles, and connective tissues for more vigorous exercise. Gentle stretching increases flexibility and resilience of tissues in preparation for higher intensity exercise. The intensity of exercise is increased gradually to achieve the target heart rate zone for 20–60 minutes based on intensity and level of fitness.

Cooldown is the gradual reduction in exercise intensity at the end of the training phase. Slowly lowering the intensity helps promote venous return to the heart, thus minimizing problems associated with inadequate blood flow to the brain (vasovagal response). This phase can be accomplished by performing the same movements at a slower pace for a minimum of 5 minutes. Completion of the cooldown phase with gentle stretches can prevent extreme muscle soreness and promote improvements in flexibility with a reduced risk of injury.

Motivational Factors

Successful initiation of and adherence to an exercise program can be achieved when the patient is able to make appropriate decisions and adopt health behaviors that are satisfying and comfortable. The practitioner must be cognizant of each patient's unique needs and goals and be prepared with strategies and techniques to facilitate the adoption of activities and enhance adherence.

The practitioner can enhance exercise adherence by understanding and applying appropriate strategies. Initially, rapport must be developed between the practitioner and patient. A positive factor influencing a patient's satisfaction and adherence is her perception of the genuine interest and caring of the practitioner.

The practitioner must be able to stimulate the patient to participate in planning the exercise program by explaining the benefits of exercise for her health and fitness status. Once the decision is made to begin an exercise program, the practitioner can use a behavioral technique called contracting to increase the level of commitment. **Contracting** involves an agreement between the practitioner and patient specifying the desired goal, steps to attain the goal, sources of support or positive reinforcement, measurement of progress, potential barriers, and rewards or incentive strategies.

When planning an exercise program, a number of factors must be considered to enhance adherence. It is important to develop a program that fits the woman's schedule, income, and life-style. The exercise setting may be a health club, park or recreational facility, or home. The focus of the personal exercise program must be on setting attainable goals for weight loss, stamina, strength, speed, and muscular development. If the woman's goal is weight control, for example, cardiorespiratory, or aerobic, exercise would be the most effective form.

The clinician may suggest that the patient select several enjoyable activities to avoid boredom and recommend varying these activities from season to season. The program's progression must be slow, methodical, and safe. For some women, it may be appropriate initially to recommend that they incorporate exercise into their leisure or daily activities. A patient with a low level of fitness may start by going out dancing, playing tennis, walking or riding her bicycle to do errands, or parking far from the mall entrance when shopping to improve her fitness level before progressing to a more moderate exercise regimen. Patients should be reminded that improvement takes time and involves a lifetime commitment.

Issues of Pregnancy & Exercise

The emphasis on health promotion and disease prevention by engaging in positive health behaviors such as exercise and adequate nutritional intake has increased the number of women continuing to exercise during prenatal and postpartum periods. Although pregnancy results in specific physiologic and anatomic changes, most women can exercise with a minimum of risk to themselves or the fetus, in the absence of obstetric or medical complications. Women with certain other medical or obstetric conditions, including chronic hypertension or active thyroid, cardiac, vascular, or pulmonary disease, require careful evaluation to determine whether an exercise program is appropriate.

The primary concern of the medical provider is to ensure maximal safety of mother and fetus while maintaining the highest level of fitness. The American College of Obstetrics and Gynecology (ACOG) established guidelines to assist health and fitness professionals in the safe prescription of exercise. The medical provider must (1) understand the modifications of specific exercise regimens that are necessary because of physiologic changes during pregnancy (Tables 9–8 and 9–9); (2) assess the patient's needs and physical abilities; (3) know the contraindications for exercise (Tables 9–10); and (4) recognize potential risks for continued exercise.

Recently, the ACOG guidelines were revised in the following areas: exercise recommendations for women with a history of regular exercise before pregnancy and for sedentary, pregnant women wanting to start an exercise program; monitoring of exercise intensity; and maintenance of maternal core temperature.

Generally, women participating in regular, noncompetitive exercise before pregnancy may continue the same program and modify it according to their training response. Studies have indicated that women typically decrease intensity and duration with the progression of pregnancy and associated changes. Sedentary pregnant women should obtain medical clearance and begin with low-intensity, low-impact, or non-weight-bearing exercise and increase the in-

Table 9–8. Exercise guidelines for pregnancy and the postpartum period.

There are no data in humans to indicate that pregnant women should limit exercise intensity and lower target heart rates because of potential adverse effects. For women who do not have any additional risk factors for adverse maternal or perinatal outcomes, the following recommendations may be made:

1. During pregnancy, women can continue to exercise and derive health benefit even from mild to moderate exercise routines. Regular exercise (at least three times per week) is preferable to intermittent activity.
2. Women should avoid exercise in the supine position after the first trimester. Such a position is associated with decreased cardiac output in most pregnant women; because the remaining cardiac output will be preferentially distributed away from splanchnic beds (including the uterus) during vigorous exercise, such regimens are best avoided during pregnancy. Prolonged periods of motionless standing should also be avoided.
3. Women should be aware of the decreased oxygen available for aerobic exercise during pregnancy. They should be encouraged to modify the intensity of their exercise according to maternal symptoms. Pregnant women should stop exercising when fatigued and not exercise to exhaustion. Weight–bearing exercises may under some circumstances be continued at intensities similar to those prior to pregnancy throughout pregnancy. Non–weight–bearing exercises, such as cycling or swimming, will minimize the risk of injury and facilitate the continuation of exercise during pregnancy.
4. Morphologic changes in pregnancy should serve as a relative contraindication to types of exercise in which loss of balance could be detrimental to maternal or fetal well being, especially in the third trimester. Further, any type of exercise involving the potential for even mild abdominal trauma should be avoided.
5. Pregnancy requires an additional 300kcal/d in order to maintain metabolic homeostasis. Thus, women who exercise during pregnancy should be particularly careful to ensure an adequate diet.
6. Pregnant women who exercise in the first trimester should augment heat dissipation by ensuring adequate hydration, appropriate clothing and optimal environmental surroundings during exercise.
7. Many of the physiologic and morphologic changes of pregnancy persist four to six weeks postpartum. Thus, pre–pregnancy exercise routines should be resumed gradually based upon a woman's physical capability.

Reproduced, with permission, from American College of Obstetricians and Gynecologists: *Exercise During Pregnancy and the Postpartum Period.* Technical Bulletin No. 189, 1994.

Table 9–9. Physiologic and anatomic changes during pregnancy.*

Cardiovascular
  Increased blood volume
  Increased cardiac output
  Increased resting heart rate
  Decreased systemic vascular resistance
  Decreased cardiac output with supine position and motionless stance
Respiratory
  Increased minute ventilation
  Increased arterial oxygen tension
  Increased oxygen uptake
  Increased baseline oxygen consumption
Mechanical
  Shift in center of gravity
  Increased joint laxity
Thermoregulatory
  Increased basal metabolic rate
  Increased heat production
Metabolic
  Extra 300 kcal/d needed if inactive

*Modified and reproduced, with permission, from Special Medical Reports, *American Family Physician,* 1994;49:1258.

ture below 38 °C also was deleted from the guidelines. In the past, there was concern that core temperatures elevated above 38 °C were capable of inducing neural-tube defects. According to McMurray et al, however, thermoregulatory studies of pregnant women exercising within normal limits have not demonstrated an increase in neural-tube or other birth defects.

Generally, low-risk, physically fit women deliver infants of normal birth weight for gestational age. Conditions that may affect fetal growth adversely are strenuous physical work, nutritional stress, and prolonged standing. An association has been found between lower birth weight infants and performance of strenuous work or exercise by the mother during pregnancy.

The type of exercise recommended depends on the patient's needs and health status during pregnancy. Examples of exercise considered safe during pregnancy are walking, swimming, water aerobics, low-impact aerobic dancing, bicycling, golf, and cross-country skiing.

The adaptation to exercise by the woman and fetus depends on the person's past exercise history, current

tensity gradually. Inclusion of exercise can lead to improved maternal health with minimal risk to fetal outcome.

Previously, the ACOG recommended limiting training heart rates to 140 beats per minute. However, recent studies have reported that heart rates greater than 140 beats per minute did not increase the potential for adverse maternal or perinatal effects. Moreover, an increase of the maternal resting heart rate of 15–20 beats per minute rendered the training heart rate formula ineffective. Therefore, the ACOG advocates the use of RPE to monitor intensity.

The issue of maintaining maternal core tempera-

Table 9–10. Absolute contraindications to exercise in pregnancy.*

Pregnancy–induced hypertension
Preterm rupture of membranes
Preterm labor during the prior or current pregnancy or both
Incompetent cervix/cerclage
Persistent second– or third–trimester bleeding
Intrauterine growth retardation

*Modified and reproduced, with permission, from Special Medical Reports, *American Family Physician,* 1994;49:1258.

exercise habits, pregnancy status, and physical limitations. Potential exercise benefits include a lesser weight gain, improved tolerance of labor pain, faster return to prepregnancy weight and fitness level, better regulation of blood glucose levels, and improved general sense of well-being.

REFERENCES

Alameda County Low Birth Weight Study Group: Cigarette smoking and the risk of low birth weight: A comparison in black and white women. Epidemiology 1990;1:201.

American Academy of Family Physicians: *Nutrition Interventions Manual for Professionals.* American Academy of Family Physicians, American Dietetic Association, National Council on Aging, 1992.

American College of Obstetrics and Gynecology: *Exercise During Pregnancy and the Postpartum Period.* Technical Bulletin No. 189, 1994.

Bak AA, Grobee DE: Caffeine, blood pressure and serum lipids. Am J Clin Nutr 1991;53:971.

Benowitz NL: Nicotine replacement therapy during pregnancy. JAMA 1991;266:3174.

Benowitz NL: Pharmacologic aspects of cigarette smoking and nicotine addiction. N Engl J Med 1988;319:1318.

Borg GV: Psychophysical bases of perceived exertion. Med Sci Sports Exerc 1982;14:377.

Bovens AM et al: Physical activity, fitness, and selected risk factors for CHD in active men and women. Med Sci Sports Exerc 1993;25:572.

Breslau N et al: Nicotine dependence and major depression: New evidence from a prospective investigation. Arch Gen Psychiatry 1993;50:31.

Caralis DG et al: Smoking is a risk factor for coronary spasm in young women. Circulation 1992;85:905.

Centers for Disease Control and Prevention: Cigarette smoking among adults—United States, 1991. MMWR 1993;42:230.

Fentem PH: Exercise in prevention of disease. Br Med Bull 1992;48:631.

Flay BR et al: Smoking: Epidemiology, cessation, and prevention. Chest 1992;102:277S.

Foreyt JP, Goodrick K: Weight management without dieting. Nutr Today 1993;28(2):4.

Gilpin EA et al: Physician advice to quit smoking: Results from the 1990 California tobacco survey. J Gen Intern Med 1993;8:549.

Glassman AH et al: Smoking, smoking cessation, and major depression. JAMA 1990;264:1546.

Hankin JH: Role of nutrition in women's health: Diet and breast cancer. J Am Diet Assoc 1993;93:994.

Harris M, Stead L: *ACSM's Resource Manual for Guidelines for Exercise Testing and Prescription,* 2/e. Lea & Febiger, 1993.

Hatch MC et al: Maternal exercise during pregnancy, physical fitness, and fetal growth. Am J Epidemiol 1993;137:1105.

Hurt RD et al: Nicotine patch therapy for smoking cessation combined with physician advice and nurse follow-up: One-year outcome and percentage of nicotine replacement. JAMA 1994;271:595.

Kaufman NJ: Smoking and young women: The physician's role in stopping an equal opportunity killer. JAMA 1994;271:629.

Kawachi I et al: Smoking cessation in relation to total mortality rates in women: A prospective cohort study. Ann Intern Med 1993;119:992.

Kenford SL et al: Predicting smoking cessation: Who will quit with and without the nicotine patch? JAMA 1994;271:589.

Kottke TE et al: Attributes of successful smoking cessation interventions in medical practice: A meta-analysis of 39 controlled trials. JAMA 1988;259:2883.

Kris-Etherton PM, Krummel D: Role of nutrition in the prevention and treatment of coronary heart disease in women. J Am Diet Assoc 1993;93:987.

Leviton A: Caffeine consumption and the risk of reproductive hazards. J Reprod Med 1988;33:175.

Marlatt GA, Gordon JR: *Relapse Prevention Maintenance Strategies in the Treatment of Addictive Behaviors.* Guilford, 1985.

McMurray RG et al: Recent advances in understanding maternal and fetal responses to exercise. Med Sci Sports Exerc 1993;25:1305.

Munro JF et al: Appraisal of the clinical value of serotoninergic drugs. Am J Clin Nutr 1992;55:189S.

Ockene JK et al: Increasing the efficacy of physician-delivered smoking intervention: A randomized clinical trial. J Gen Intern Med 1991;6:1.

Rodin J: Weight change following smoking cessation: The role of food intake and exercise. Addict Behav 1987;12:303.

Rosenberg L et al: Decline in the risk of myocardial infarction among women who stop smoking. N Engl J Med 1990;322:213.

Scholes D et al: Current cigarette smoking and risk of acute pelvic inflammatory disease. Am J Public Health 1992;82:1352.

Silagy C et al: Meta-analysis on efficacy of nicotine replacement therapies in smoking cessation. Lancet 1994;343:139.

Spring B et al: Post–smoking cessation weight gain: Preventive intervention with D-Fenfluramine. Pharmacol Biochem Behav 1990;36:431.

St Jeor ST: The role of weight management in the health of women. J Am Diet Assoc 1993;93:1007.

Sternfeld B: Cancer and the protective effect of physical activity: The epidemiological evidence. Med Sci Sports Exerc 1992;24:1195.

US Department of Health and Human Services: *The Health Consequences of Smoking for Women: A Report of the Surgeon General.* Department of Health and Human Services, Public Health Service, Publication No. 0-326-003, 1980.

Wardlaw GM: Putting osteoporosis in perspective. J Am Diet Assoc 1993;93:1000.

Section III.
Psychiatric and Behavioral Disorders

Disordered Eating

10

Patricia A. Lipscomb, MD, PhD, & Rosemary Agostini, MD

Disordered eating is a concern to many women and a serious health problem to some. It can take the form of anorexia nervosa, bulimia nervosa, or a nonspecific version such as emotion-based overeating.

Eating disorders appear to arise from a combination of sociocultural, physiologic, and psychologic factors. Sociocultural factors include societal pressures on women to be physically attractive, with the current Western ideal of feminine beauty at a standard that is thinner than is medically healthy. Misguided attempts to achieve an unrealistic weight can contribute to the development of eating disorders, both by direct physiologic effects (caloric deprivation producing a physiologic predisposition to binge) and by psychologic issues (an erosion of self-esteem related to the inability to measure up to an unrealistic ideal). Even in the absence of vigorous attempts to lose weight, unrealistic ideals of thinness can interfere with women's acceptance of their feminine shapes. To the extent that this ideal interferes with self-esteem, negative emotions (eg, dejection, anxiety, or resentment) can result. Vulnerable persons may use the temporarily soothing effects of pathologic eating to try to regulate these feelings. No matter how strong environmental pressures are, however, eating disorders do not develop in the absence of individual psychopathology. Therefore, effective treatments must address more than just the problematic eating behavior.

ANOREXIA NERVOSA

Essentials of Diagnosis

- Refusal to maintain minimal normal weight for age and height (weight less than 85% of recommended level)
- Morbid fear of becoming fat
- Disturbance of body image
- Absence of menstrual periods for at least three consecutive cycles

Incidence

The prevalence of anorexia nervosa is estimated to be approximately 0.3% of the female population from age 18 to 35. It occurs in men at a rate that is approximately 5–10% of that in women and is more prevalent among homosexual than heterosexual men. It is more common among whites than nonwhites and among middle- to upper-income groups than other economic groups.

Pathogenesis

Family psychopathology is typical and presumably contributes to the expression of the illness. Disturbances in the family may include enmeshment among members, particularly patient and mother; low tolerance for affective expression, such as anger, which is labeled as negative; poor communication in general; and lack of empathy by the parents for the children's emotional experience.

A precise mechanism for the development of the

disorder cannot be described. However, the development of symptoms appears to represent a form of passive rebellion against the parents. Before the development of overt symptoms of an eating disorder, patients were often "model children" whose excellent behavior was taken for granted by the parents. Patients typically felt confined and controlled by their parents' expectations regarding behavior and achievement. In addition, there is often inadequate psychologic differentiation between the patient and her mother, so that the two of them are joined in an ambivalent and mutually dependent dyad. The refusal to maintain body weight may represent a desperate attempt by the girl to seize control from the parents, especially the mother, in an area of her life that she truly can control, ie, what she eats. Ambivalence about adult roles, including sexual ones, also may play a part, as evidenced by the fact that extreme weight loss results in a body shape resembling that of a prepubertal girl and in loss of reproductive functioning.

Anorectic patients, although typically bright in many respects, often lack age-appropriate abstracting ability. They often think and behave quite illogically. They typically displace their various other problems onto an overconcern about weight and body shape, as if maintaining an emaciated shape will magically mean that everything else in life is fine.

Signs & Symptoms

The cardinal sign is excessive thinness. This condition may be accompanied by hyperactivity, even when the girl appears too frail to maintain a high level of activity. There may be ritualization of eating behavior, including hoarding of food and compulsions about weighing, measuring, and counting, eg, counting the number of Cheerios eaten for breakfast.

Anorectic patients generally deny that they have a problem, and insist they are too fat even when they are frankly cachectic. Most patients are intensely preoccupied with food. Despite the fact that the word **anorexia** means absence of appetite, these patients are hungry most of the time.

Clinical Findings & Diagnosis

Laboratory findings are as follows:

- Prepubertal levels of follicle-stimulating hormone and luteinizing hormone
- Diminished response to gonadotropin-releasing hormone
- Postmenopausal (low) levels of estrogen
- Absence or reversal of normal circadian rhythm of plasma cortisol
- Reduction of metabolic clearance rate of cortisol
- Incomplete suppression of adrenocorticotropin and cortisol by dexamethasone.

The principal indicator of anorexia nervosa is refusal to maintain a minimally normal body weight. Guidelines such as the various versions of the Metropolitan Life Insurance weight tables are used to determine normal weight levels.

Girls and women with anorexia nervosa are intensely fearful of weight gain and body fat and typically do not feel reassured even by ongoing weight loss. Instead they continue to feel fat even when emaciated. This disturbance of body image often reaches delusional proportions.

The amenorrhea of anorexia nervosa is a consequence of low estrogen levels (due to decreased pituitary secretion of FSH and LH) and typically follows weight loss but may precede it in some individuals. Menarche can be delayed if anorexia nervosa is already present.

Some anorectic patients alternate periods of severe restriction of their caloric intake with periods of binge eating followed by purging. These bulimic anorectic patients appear to represent a distinct subtype, and they may have more in common with patients who have bulimia nervosa than with purely restrictive anorectic patients.

Individuals with anorexia nervosa are unlikely to seek treatment on their own and are typically brought to a clinician by family members concerned about their extreme weight loss.

Complications

Complications include electrolyte imbalance (metabolic alkalosis and hypokalemia), cardiovascular disturbances (bradycardia, tachycardia, hypotension, congestive cardiac failure, various ECG changes, ventricular arrhythmias, and sudden death), renal abnormalities (decreased glomerular filtration rate, increased blood urea nitrogen, and pitting edema), hematologic problems (pancytopenia and reduced serum complement levels), skeletal abnormalities (osteoporosis and associated pathologic fractures), endocrine abnormalities (amenorrhea and hypogonadism), metabolic abnormalities (low basal metabolic rate, hypercholesterolemia, altered glucose metabolism, impaired temperature regulation), and dermatologic abnormalities (lanugo, scaly skin, and hypercarotenemia). When self-induced vomiting is present, the gastrointestinal and dental complications of bulimia nervosa (see following section, "Bulimia Nervosa") may occur also.

Treatment

The first goal of treatment is restoration of normal body weight, followed by the an establishment of healthy eating patterns. Treatment of the underlying psychologic problems (including low self-esteem, disturbed interpersonal relationships, erroneous beliefs about weight, ineffective affect regulation, and intrapsychic conflict) is required to reduce the chance of relapse.

A. Hospitalization: Hospitalization is indicated when weight has dropped below 85% of ideal body weight and continues to fall. Severe electrolyte imbalance also mandates hospitalization, even if weight has not reached a critically low point.

The inpatient treatment team determines a target weight (generally a range rather than a single figure) that will support normal menstrual cycles and reverse bone demineralization. There is a trend toward using body mass index, ie, weight (kg)/ [height (m)]^2, rather than weight alone, and toward taking into account the patient's age.

Typically, a behavior modification program is set up in which the patient's adherence to daily weight and behavior goals leads to previously agreed-on results, including positive reinforcers (eg, increased privileges) and negative reinforcers (eg, withholding of privileges). Discussions about food generally are held only with the dietitian to avoid engaging the whole team in struggles about food. Patients are encouraged to gain weight only at the recommended rate and not any faster. Forced feeding via nasogastric tube is a last resort reserved for life-threatening situations. The goal is for the patient to assume responsibility for a rational pattern of eating rather than for the staff to impose its program on the patient.

B. Psychotherapy:

1. Individual therapy–Forms of individual psychotherapy for anorexia nervosa include cognitive restructuring (especially with respect to beliefs about food and attractiveness), interpersonal therapy, and psychodynamic approaches that emphasize an understanding of the psychologic conflicts underlying the problem behavior. When significant character disorders are present, psychoanalysis or psychoanalytic psychotherapy provides the best chance of lasting results.

2. Family therapy–Patients with anorexia nervosa tend to be younger than patients with other eating disorders. The younger the patient, the more likely she is to benefit from therapy that addresses pathologic dynamics within the family, on whom she is still emotionally dependent. Without family therapy, the patient may not be able to sustain gains made in individual therapy because of the pressure exerted by the family system to retain its status quo.

Family therapy helps the members of the family understand that the anorectic patient bears symptoms on behalf of the whole family system, whose pathologic condition exceeds the patient's problem behavior. The dynamics of the family tend to perpetuate the eating disorder and must be identified and addressed.

Another way of stating this dynamic is that the patient's symptoms serve some purpose in the family system. In order for the patient to recover successfully in her family setting, the family must figure out how to solve the problems that will be unmasked if the patient relinquishes her symptoms. An example

would be a family in which parents are alienated from each other but their common focus on their daughter's illness keeps them from divorcing.

3. Group therapy–Group therapy for patients with anorexia nervosa may be most useful in nonacute stages of treatment to provide ongoing support over a period of years and to help the patient maintain therapeutic gains made earlier in a more intensive treatment setting. At any stage of treatment, group therapy offers one distinct advantage over other forms of treatment: the opportunity for group members to confront each other about the ways in which they try to fool themselves and their clinicians as well as the problematic ways in which they interact with peers.

C. Medication: There are few data concerning the usefulness of medications in treating anorexia nervosa and no double-blind placebo-controlled studies. If major depression is present, indications for antidepressant medication are the usual ones (severe and pervasive mood disturbance accompanied by several vegetative symptoms such as insomnia and extreme fatigue). Patients with anorexia nervosa may be more susceptible to orthostatic hypotension as a side effect of some antidepressants. Because cardiac arrhythmias are a complication of anorexia nervosa, the least cardiotoxic antidepressants should be favored.

Prognosis

In studies of hospitalized or tertiary referral populations followed for at least 4 years after onset of illness, approximately 44% of the patients had their weight restored to within 15% of the recommended level and attained regular menstruation, about 24% did not come within 15% of the recommended level and continued with absent or sporadic menstruation, and about 28% had an intermediate outcome. Fewer than 5% died. Poorer outcomes are correlated with vomiting, previous treatment failures, family dysfunction, being married, and lower initial weight. The mortality rate (generally from cardiac arrest or suicide) approached 20% among patients followed for more than 20 years. The mortality rate from suicide alone is estimated to be between 2 and 5%, underscoring the necessity of psychotherapy.

After inpatient treatment, approximately two-thirds of patients have continued difficulties with eating behavior and psychologic problems.

Referral to a Specialist

Because of the possibility of grave complications, every patient with anorexia nervosa should be referred to a specialist in eating disorders and should be followed closely by the primary care physician.

Issues of Pregnancy & Anorexia Nervosa

Anorectic women may have great difficulty conceiving because of prolonged anovulation. Low prepregnancy weight and poor nutritional status during pregnancy both are associated with low birth weight. If a pregnant anorectic patient purges through vomiting or diuretic/laxative abuse, electrolyte imbalance may put the fetus in further jeopardy. Anorexia nervosa is associated with increased rates of stillbirth and preterm birth.

Psychiatric Comorbidity

Depression is extremely common in patients with anorexia nervosa, with a lifetime prevalence reported at 60% as long as 10 years after treatment for the eating disorder.

Anorexia nervosa also may be related to obsessive-compulsive disorder, based on symptom overlap, family history, neuroendocrine abnormalities, and responses to psychopharmacology.

Anorectic patients often have significant personality disorders. At least one-half of these patients meet the criteria for borderline personality disorder. Avoidant features are also common.

Controversies & Unresolved Issues

Patients who meet the diagnostic criteria for anorexia nervosa form a heterogeneous group with respect to weight-control practices. An area of current research involves refining the typology of the various presentations of the illness. One question concerns whether different behaviors, eg, purely restrictive behavior versus binge/purge behavior, correspond to different underlying psychopathology.

BULIMIA NERVOSA

Essentials of Diagnosis

- Uncontrolled binge eating averaging at least twice weekly for at least 3 months.
- Recurrent inappropriate compensatory behavior to prevent weight gain, such as self-induced vomiting, laxatives or diuretics, strict dieting or fasting, or vigorous exercise, averaging at least twice weekly for at least 3 months.
- Overconcern with weight and body shape.

Incidence

Current point prevalence rates are estimated at about 1%. (Earlier studies, based on the looser diagnostic criteria of the American Psychiatric Association's *Diagnostic and Statistical Manual,* 2/e, yielded much higher prevalence rates, up to 19%.) Women make up approximately 90–95% of those afflicted. Most bulimics are young, white, and middle- or upper-class.

Pathogenesis

Pathologic family systems probably contribute sig-

nificantly to the development of bulimia nervosa. There is often overt conflict within the family and an emphasis on achievement that may be even greater than that seen in the families of nonbulimic anorectic patients. The pressure to achieve may be implicitly contradicted by a mandate to be passive, dependent, and unassertive.

The onset of symptoms tends to be later in bulimia nervosa than in anorexia nervosa. The mean age of onset of binge eating is approximately 18 years, with self-induced vomiting beginning about 1 year later. The onset of symptoms often follows a significant loss, such as separation from family in the course of going away to school or a romantic rejection. The overconsumption of food may be undertaken initially in an attempt at soothing oneself when overcome with negative emotion. Also, the onset of binge eating frequently occurs after a protracted period of severe caloric restriction.

Such stringent dieting produces a physiologically based predisposition to binge-eat when the self-imposed restriction is lifted. A disturbance of serotonin neurotransmission may operate as an additional physiologic factor. Because the normal consequence of overconsumption is, of course, weight gain, the girl may try to control weight gain by additional stringent dieting. This behavior sets up a cycle of alternating fasting (or near-fasting) and binge eating. Often girls first learn of vomiting as a means of controlling caloric intake from a friend. They may copy the behavior initially on a trial basis but later become reliant on the practice to avoid weight gain after the binge eating that has become habitual.

Signs & Symptoms

There are usually few if any outward signs to alert the clinician. Body weight is usually normal, although premorbid obesity is common. Erosion of dental enamel from stomach acid is common. A few bulimic women have visible calluses on the dorsal aspects of their hands (Russell's sign, caused by teeth abrading the skin), as well as fresh abrasions and scarring. Some patients have obvious parotid hypertrophy.

Clinical Findings & Diagnosis

Bulimia nervosa is characterized by regular binge eating and inappropriate compensatory behaviors to prevent weight gain. Overeating is considered binge eating when the individual consumes in a discrete time period, (eg, 2 hours or less) an amount of food that is definitely more than most persons would eat in a similar length of time and other similar circumstances.

The food consumed during binges varies according to the individual's tastes and to what is available, but sweet, high calorie foods are generally favored, as well as foods that require little or no preparation (eg, chips that can be eaten from the bag.)

Binges are often precipitated by negative feelings, life stress, or extreme hunger by dieting. The individual usually conducts the binge in private, consuming the food rapidly, and continuing even after uncomfortably full. Most persons with bulimia nervosa induce vomiting after binge eating. Feelings of shame and disgust often follow the binge, with or without the self-induced vomiting.

Laboratory findings are generally nonspecific, although the serum amylase level may be elevated and the result of a dexamethasone suppression test may be abnormal. Diagnosis is made through history, which is extremely difficult because most bulimic patients are secretive about their binging out of a sense of shame. Questioning about abnormal eating and weight-control practices should be matter-of-fact and nonjudgmental and should persist as long as the physician suspects an eating disorder. For example, a physician might say, "Some young women are extremely concerned about their appearance and weight and do things like throwing up after eating to try to avoid the calories. Is that something that you ever do?" A patient may deny the problem initially but later acknowledge it and accept help.

Complications

Complications include electrolyte imbalance (metabolic alkalosis and hypokalemia), gastrointestinal problems (constipation, esophagitis, gastritis, and perforations of the esophagus or stomach [Mallory-Weiss tears]), cardiovascular disturbances (orthostatic hypotension and potentially lethal arrhythmias), dental problems (increased caries and upper incisor erosions), and endocrine disturbances leading to irregular menses or amenorrhea.

Treatment

A. Hospitalization: Bulimia nervosa usually does not require inpatient treatment. Hospitalization should be considered when the binge eating and purging occupy so much of a patient's time that normal work and socialization are impossible. Although hospitalization is required to treat suicidality and life-threatening electrolyte imbalance, treatment is directed at stabilizing the patient in the face of these complications rather than at the underlying eating disorder.

B. Psychotherapy:

1. Individual psychotherapy—Cognitive-behavioral therapy has received the most systematic study and appears to bring about in most patients substantial change in eating and weight-control practices and in the attitudes that contribute to the disordered behaviors. This approach includes (1) modification of attitudes with respect to body shape and its relation to self-worth; (2) education in nutrition and rational weight regulation (eg, many bulimic patients do not know that severe caloric restriction predisposes to binge eating); (3) identification of precipi-

tants of binge eating (primarily through record-keeping); (4) increasing "damage-control" skills (getting back on track after a binge); (5) increasing the repertoire of maneuvers for dealing with intensely unpleasant affective states (which often act as precipitants of binge eating); (6) increasing problem-solving skills in general (for some patients, binge eating becomes an all-purpose approach for dealing with problem situations); (7) increasing social contacts.

One especially promising behavioral approach known as exposure with response prevention combines having the patient consume food in the treatment setting with preventing the usual pathologic response (vomiting). For some patients, the binge eating occurs only when vomiting can be guaranteed, so learning to resist the urge to vomit translates into stopping binge eating.

Lasting behavioral change is more likely to occur in patients who receive long-term individual psychotherapy or psychoanalysis, in which intrapsychic and interpersonal issues can be addressed more definitively than is possible in therapeutic approaches that focus primarily on behavior change. Individual therapy often includes work on developmental issues, conflict with respect to sexual and aggressive drives, affect regulation, and gender-role expectations.

2. Group therapy—In group therapy for bulimia nervosa, psychoeducational approaches plus the cognitive-behavioral methods described previously are the most widely used techniques. In the group format, there is also the opportunity to observe and modify disturbed interpersonal interactions in a setting that approximates interactions with friends and family more closely than does individual therapy.

3. Family therapy—It is unusual for bulimic patients to undergo family therapy except for adolescents still living with their families of origin. Family therapy also may have some usefulness in younger adult patients who are not emotionally emancipated from their parents. The basic strategy is the same as in anorexia nervosa, ie, to identify the ways in which the family system perpetuates and maintains the symptoms of the patient and to work at breaking the cycle.

C. Medication: Several antidepressants have been shown in double-blind placebo-controlled studies to reduce bulimic symptoms significantly better than placebo. Depressed and nondepressed bulimic patients appear to respond equally well to the "antibinge" effects of antidepressants. This finding suggests that the drugs may exert direct central effects on the neurotransmitter systems that regulate appetite and eating behavior. Fluoxetine hydrochloride has shown the best results published to date. Dosages of up to 60 mg/d often are required, which is 3 times the usual antidepressant dosage. Other antidepressant medications, including desipramine and nortriptyline, appear to be effective in the normal antidepressant dosage range. Monoamine oxidase inhibitors also appear to be effective in producing short-term reduction of bulimic symptoms, but the decision to prescribe a medication that requires stringent dietary restrictions must be considered carefully in patients who have serious problems with impulse control concerning oral intake.

Although antidepressants appear to be effective in bringing about short-term behavior change in some patients, relapses are common following cessation of medication. Medication should be tried for 5–8 months initially; if relapse occurs, a longer trial is indicated, and maintenance treatment with antidepressant medication should be considered. Outcome data for long-term treatment of bulimia nervosa with antidepressants are not available. Approximately one-half of the patients studied do not have a therapeutic response to the drugs in the first place. Psychotherapy is therefore the mainstay of treatment of bulimia nervosa.

Prognosis

With adequate treatment, the prognosis is good for bringing the problem behavior under control. Approximately 70% of patients completing treatment programs consisting of psychotherapy, medication, or both, report considerable improvement. Poorer outcomes are associated with more severe initial symptoms requiring hospitalization and with alcohol abuse. In one treatment group examined 3 years after treatment ended, only approximately 27% of the patients were binge eating and purging less than once a month, 33% were binge eating and purging daily, and 40% had an intermediate outcome. The prognosis for untreated bulimia nervosa is unknown.

Referral to a Specialist

Most bulimic women benefit from referral to a skilled therapist who is experienced in treating eating disorders. The primary care physician remains a vital part of the treatment team but usually lacks the specialized training required for specific treatment of eating disorders. Suicidal ideation mandates referral to a psychiatrist or psychologist.

Issues of Pregnancy & Bulimia

Menstrual disturbances are common and may interfere with the ability to conceive. Purging is potentially deadly to the fetus because of the severe electrolyte imbalance that can occur. Low birth weight and low 5-minute Apgar scores have been associated with bulimia nervosa; also associated are increased rates of stillbirth, breech delivery, and cleft palate.

Psychiatric Comorbidity

No single psychologic profile applies to all cases, but common characteristics include chronically lowered mood, recurrent anxiety, poor tolerance for frustration, feelings of alienation, difficulty expressing negative feelings such as anger, impulsive behavior, substance abuse (alcohol and drugs), and other behavioral disturbances (such as shopping sprees and theft).

Almost all bulimic patients have a history of major depression, and at any given time, about one-half are depressed. Suicidal ideation is common and requires careful assessment.

Personality disorder is common, with more than one-half of bulimic patients meeting criteria for borderline personality disorder.

Controversies & Unresolved Issues

There are limited data comparing the outcomes of various treatments for bulimia. Current outcome measures that focus narrowly on binge/purge behavior may not discriminate well among treatments that aim to bring about change at a deeper level. For example, an adolescent might gain adequate behavioral control and stop having symptoms of an eating disorder while retaining the underlying conflicts that caused the behavior in the first place. Such a patient might grow up to interact pathologically with her own daughter in such a way that facilitates the development of an eating disorder rather than helping the daughter deal with similar conflicts.

An area of controversy concerns the threshold at which inpatient treatment is necessary for bulimic patients and when outpatient therapy is adequate. A model that categorized bulimia nervosa as an impulse-control disorder related to alcohol abuse might dictate that at least the early stages of treatment should be attempted only in an inpatient setting, where access to the abused substance (food) can be controlled. On the other hand, the cost of even a short hospitalization can buy a great deal of outpatient therapy, which is needed after hospitalization anyway.

COMPULSIVE OVEREATING

Compulsive overeating is not a diagnostic category but a term applied to various forms of pathologic eating in which overconsumption of food is driven by emotions. In some instances, it may represent a nonpurging form of bulimia. It also may precede the development of bulimia, although this situation is uncommon. Many overeaters do not binge but "graze," ie, overconsume food over the course of the day, sometimes with the overeating concentrated toward the end of the day. The prevalence of pathologic overeating is not known, but one can assume that it plays a part in most cases of obesity, and approximately 25% of the US population is at least 20% heavier than ideal body weight (see Chapter 18). The overeating referred to in this category does not necessarily involve the consumption of massive quantities of food, as in bulimia, but rather the chronic consumption of more calories than necessary to maintain ideal body weight.

Patients may be helped through psychotherapy to work out the psychologic issues that cause the problem behavior. When obesity has already resulted, the added weight is generally refractory to treatment. Although diets may be successful in the short term, patients typically regain the weight lost. A sensible eating plan coupled with appropriate exercise is the most rational approach. Many patients find support groups helpful for increasing self-esteem and for exchanging useful strategies for avoiding overeating.

THE FEMALE ATHLETE TRIAD: DISORDERED EATING, AMENORRHEA, & OSTEOPOROSIS

The Female Athlete Triad is a term coined by Dr. Kim Yeager in 1992 to describe the interrelatedness of disordered eating, amenorrhea, and premature osteoporosis in athletes.

Although exercise and sports generally have great health benefits for both women and men, young female athletes may be at increased risk of development of this triad of disorders; the emphasis in sports on body weight may lead to eating disorders and to amenorrhea, with the resultant low estrogen level, which may result in premature osteoporosis.

Athletes may display a spectrum of disordered eating which includes restriction of calories and overexercising to burn calories. Even though these young women do not meet all the *DSM-IV* criteria for eating disorders, they are at increased risk for development of serious endocrine, skeletal, and psychiatric disorders. The prevalence of disordered eating in female athletes has been reported to be 15–62%.

Amenorrhea is defined as the "absence of menstrual bleeding." Women who have **primary amenorrhea** have not had a menstrual period by the age of 16; **secondary amenorrhea** is the absence of menstrual periods in a women who has had established menstrual cycles. It is essential that young women, including athletes, be evaluated appropriately for all causes of amenorrhea. There has been much confusion in the literature in terms of the prevalence because different authors have used different numbers of missed menstrual cycles in the definition of amenorrhea. Endocrinologists define amenorrhea as three missed menstrual cycles, clinicians define it as six missed cycles, and bone researchers use the criterion of less than two cycles in 1 year. It is appropriate for clinicians to begin an evaluation when an athlete has missed 3–6 menstrual cycles.

Oligomenorrhea, a menstrual cycle length of 35–90 days, also has medical consequences. The prevalence of oligomenorrhea in athletes ranges from 3.5 to 66%.

Osteoporosis is defined as premature bone loss or inadequate bone formation, resulting in low bone mass, microarchitectural deterioration, and increased skeletal fragility, resulting an increased risk of fracture. The prevalence of osteoporosis in athletes is unknown, but it is clear that the progress can be rapid, and bone loss may not be completely reversible. It is much more severe in amenorrheic athletes who have moderate-to-severe eating disorders.

All female athletes are at risk for the female athlete triad. Characteristics that increase an athlete's risk for development of one or more components of the triad include (1) a pressure to excel at her sport at all costs; (2) achievement or maintenance of a body weight or level of body fat that is not appropriate for her, especially during her normal growth period; (3) participating in an "appearance" or endurance sport, eg, gymnastics, diving, or track and field; (4) harmful training techniques; (5) inadequate nutrition or failure to meet energy needs for the sport or amount of exercise; (6) excessive pressure to perform and please the coach or the parents; (7) social isolation; (8) a specific psychologic profile, ie, the propensity to do whatever is necessary to win, even risking one's health, well-being, and life; and (9) a sport-athlete mismatch, eg, a large-framed girl trying to meet the expectations of a petite gymnast.

Primary care physicians caring for female athletes should support these patients to be the best they can be, focusing on performance rather than weight or appearance. They must recognize that amenorrhea is not a normal consequence of exercise and training but a sign that something is wrong and that it must be evaluated appropriately. The long-term consequences of amenorrhea and its hypoestrogenic state in young women are only beginning to become known. It is known, however, that estrogen levels in most amenorrheic women drop to postmenopausal levels and that there can be rapid loss of bone, which may be irreversible. Amenorrheic athletes are at increased risk for stress fractures and other musculoskeletal injuries. There is great concern about possible future consequences of premature osteoporotic fractures as these women grow older.

Physicians must include questions about amenorrhea, oligomenorrhea, and disordered eating in their preparticipation physical examinations. It is important to ask questions about menstrual cycles and disordered eating of any young person with stress fractures and overuse injuries, especially if healing is not taking place.

Amenorrheic athletes who have been evaluated fully for other causes of amenorrhea should be encouraged to increase their energy intake until they resume normal menstrual function; for those who do not, hormone replacement should be considered to help maintain bone and prevent further bone loss and other potential consequences of hypoestrogenemia. In short, physicians can help athletes to reach their full potential while protecting them from the short-

and long-term endocrine, skeletal, and psychiatric complications of disordered eating, amenorrhea, and osteoporosis.

REFERENCES

Abbott DW, Mitchell JE: Antidepressants vs. psychotherapy in the treatment of bulimia nervosa. Psychopharmacol Bull 1993;29:115.

American Psychiatric Association: *Practice Guidelines for Eating Disorders.* American Psychiatric Association, 1993.

Franko, DL, Walton, BE: Pregnancy and eating disorders: A review and clinical implications. International Journal of Eat Disord 1993;13:41.

Gwirtsman HE: Bulimic disorders: Pharmacotherapeutic and biologic studies. Psychopharmacol Bull 1993;29:109.

Kennedy SH, Garfinkel P: Advances in diagnosis and treatment of anorexia nervosa and bulimia nervosa. Can J Psychiatry 1992;37:309.

Nattiv A et al: The female athlete triad. In: *Medical and Orthopedic Issues of Active and Athletic Women.* Agostini R (editor). Hanley & Beyus Inc., 1994.

Nattiv A et al: The female athlete triad: The interrelatedness of disordered eating, amenorrhea, and osteoporosis. (Agostini R, guest editor). Clin Sports Med 1994;13:1.

Sharp CW, Freeman CPL: The medical complications of anorexia nervosa. Br J Psychiatry 1993;162:452.

Skonich AA: Medical news and perspective: The female athlete triad, risk for women. JAMA 1993;270:8.

Yeager KK et al: Commentary: The female athlete triad: Disordered eating, amenorrhea, and osteoporosis. Med Sci Sports Exerc 1993;25:775.

Chemical Dependency

11

Steven M. Juergens, MD

DEFINITIONS & DIAGNOSTIC CRITERIA

Addiction in women is a major public health issue. Physicians need to be skilled in the prevention, recognition, and treatment of addictive disorders. Addiction, also termed **chemical dependence** or **psychoactive substance dependence,** has been defined as a chronic, progressive disease characterized by continuous or periodic uncontrolled use of and preoccupation with a psychoactive substance and continued use despite related social, physical, emotional, and legal consequences. It is potentially fatal. **Denial** (a range of psychologic maneuvers designed to reduce awareness of the fact that alcohol or drug use is a cause of the person's problems) is an integral part of the disease and an obstacle to recovery.

The diagnostic criteria for psychoactive substance dependence in the *Diagnostic and Statistical Manual of Mental Disorders (DSM-IV)* provide a framework from which to make the diagnoses of abuse and dependence (Table 11–1). Tolerance and withdrawal may be part of but are not essential to the diagnosis of addiction. There are 10 classes of psychoactive substances:

1. Alcohol
2. Amphetamines or similar-acting sympathomimetics
3. Cannabis
4. Cocaine
5. Hallucinogens
6. Nicotine
7. Inhalants
8. Opioids
9. Phencyclidine (PCP) or similar-acting arylcyclohexamines
10. Sedatives, hypnotics, and anxiolytics.

The symptoms of addiction are the same across the categories but may be more or less salient depending on the class.

EPIDEMIOLOGY

Recent estimates are that 8.2% of women have a lifetime history of alcohol dependence, with 3.7%

continuing to be dependent in the last 12 months. There is a 5.9% lifetime prevalence of drug dependence (not including nicotine) with 1.9% dependent in the last 12 months. Overall, women have a lifetime prevalence of 17.9% of any substance abuse or dependence and a 6.6% 12-month prevalence, about one-half that of men, who have a 35.4% lifetime and 16.1% 12-month prevalence. The highest prevalence is in the 25- to 34-year-old age group, and it appears addiction problems have increased in younger cohorts.

GENDER DIFFERENCES IN SUBSTANCE ABUSE

On the whole, women drink less than men, and alcoholic women drink less than alcoholic men. More women than men abstain at any age. Women are less likely than men to drink daily, to drink continuously, or to engage in binges, but their drinking is more often solitary. Women begin drinking later than men do, and their pattern of alcohol abuse begins at a later age. They appear for treatment at about the same age, however, revealing a "telescoping" of the course of their addiction. Women are more likely to date onset of their drinking problems to stressful events. They are much more likely than men to stay with an alcoholic partner but are more likely to be divorced when they enter addiction treatment. In seeking treatment, women are more likely to be motivated by health and family problems, whereas men more often enter

Table 11–1. *DSM-IV* criteria for substance abuse and dependence.*

Abuse

A. A maladaptive pattern of substance use leading to clinically significant impairment or distress, as manifested by one (or more) of the following, occurring at any time during the same 12-month period:

1. Recurrent substance use resulting in a failure to fulfill major role obligations at work, school, or home (eg, repeated absences or poor work performance related to substance use; substance-related absences, suspensions, or expulsions from school; neglect of children or household).
2. Recurrent substance use in situations in which it is physically hazardous (eg, driving an automobile or operating a machine when impaired by substance use).
3. Recurrent substance-related legal problems (eg, arrests for substance-related disorderly conduct).
4. Recurrent substance use despite having persistent or recurrent social or interpersonal problems caused or exacerbated by the effects of the substance (eg, arguments with spouse about consequences of intoxication, physical fights).

B. The symptoms have never met the criteria for substance dependence for this class of substance.

Dependence

A maladaptive pattern of substance use, leading to clinically significant impairment or distress, as manifested by 3 (or more) of the following occurring at any time in the same 12-month period:

1. Tolerance.
2. Withdrawal.
3. The substance is often taken in larger amounts or over a longer period than was intended.
4. There is a persistent desire or unsuccessful efforts to cut down on or control substance use.
5. A great deal of time is spent in activities necessary to obtain the substance (eg, visiting multiple doctors or driving long distances), use the substance (eg, chain-smoking), or recover from its effects.
6. Important social, occupational, or recreational activities are given up or reduced because of substance use.
7. The substance use is continued despite knowledge of having had a persistent or recurrent physical or psychologic problem that is likely to have been caused or exacerbated by the substance (eg, current cocaine use despite recognition of cocaine-induced depression, or continued drinking despite recognition that an ulcer was made worse by alcohol consumption).

Specify if:
With physiologic dependence: evidence of tolerance or withdrawal.
Without physiologic dependence: no evidence of tolerance or withdrawal.

*Reproduced, with permission, from American Psychiatric Association: *Diagnostic and Statistical Manual of Mental Disorders,* 4th ed. American Psychiatric Association, 1994.

treatment because of job and legal problems. Women abuse prescription drugs more than men do and use them with alcohol; however, they use illicit drugs to a much lesser extent than men do, except for cocaine and amphetamines, which often are used for weight loss. Women experience greater societal stigmas for their addiction, which is a factor in keeping their problem hidden.

Addicted women in treatment are likely to have lower self-esteem and report more psychiatric symptoms than men. Female problem drinkers are more likely to seek care for alcoholism in health care settings that are not specifically set up for alcoholism, eg, mental health, emergency, and primary care settings, and to report greater alcohol-related symptom severity. Depression and anxiety may be addressed, but addiction is ignored in these settings. Women have a higher incidence of anxiety and depression with addiction than men. In women, addiction also is associated with character pathology, anorexia and bulimia nervosa, dissociative disorders, posttraumatic stress disorder, and sexual abuse.

Role deprivation (a lack or loss of role of wife, mother, or worker) appears to increase the use of alcohol by reducing self-esteem, feelings of self-worth, and contact with role partners who could provide feedback about excessive drinking. However, divorce or separation in women who are problem drinkers leads to fewer problems with alcohol, perhaps because the marriage was dysfunctional (ie, an "alcoholic marriage").

GENETIC VULNERABILITY

Women appear to have a genetic vulnerability to alcoholism at least as great as that of men. It is estimated that at least one-half the liability to alcoholism is a result of genetic factors, a figure that is higher than for coronary artery disease, stroke, peptic ulcer disease, or major depression.

EVALUATION

Screening

It is important to recognize that addiction is a chronic, progressive, potentially fatal illness that affects the quality of life of patients and those around them in a profoundly negative way. Women may present to their physician with psychologic or somatic complaints when addiction is the main, although undetected, issue. It is important, therefore, to include effective systematic screening procedures in clinical practice to facilitate diagnosis and referral of women with alcohol and drug problems. Inquiry should be in a routine, nonjudgmental manner, and evasiveness and defensiveness should be noted. Screening for chemical dependency is best done using historical information that focuses on adverse consequences (eg, family or marital problems, blackouts) rather than relying on laboratory testing. Further inquiry should be made regarding alcohol use, however, if there is an elevation in levels of (1) mean corpuscular volume (MCV), (2) liver function tests, such as serum gamma-glutamyl transpeptidase (SGGT; a particularly sensitive test), serum glutamic-oxaloacetic transaminase (SGOT), serum glutamic-pyruvic transaminase (SGPT), and lactic dehydrogenase (LDH), (3) uric acid, (4) high-density lipoprotein (HDL) cholesterol, (5) triglycerides, or (6) amylase. Positive tests for hepatitis B and HIV and the presence of bacteremia may indicate present or past injecting drug use (IDU). Urine and blood screenings for drugs and alcohol are valuable but limited by the length of time tests remain positive after drug use. Physical signs of addiction include changes in vital signs, agitation or somnolence, miosis or mydriasis, needle marks or scars, unexplained trauma, enlarged liver, alcohol on breath, and acne rosacea. Physicians screening for alcoholism should ask patients for specific information in a matter-of-fact manner. People may be evasive when asked about their alcohol and drug use (eg, saying "not much" or "only on weekends"); the clinician should not accept such vague answers but attempt to define quantity and consequences.

There are more than 100 addiction screening questionnaires in use; although most were developed for use with men, there is no strong evidence suggesting that they are less sensitive for women. Two of the most frequently used, are the Short Michigan Alcoholism Screening Test (Table 11–2) and the CAGE Questionnaire (Table 11–3). These tests are recommended for standard office practice. Patients also should be screened for drug abuse. Patients should be asked about recent or past use of marihuana, cocaine, amphetamines, benzodiazepines, narcotics, and other illicit drugs. The Drug Abuse Screening Test (DAST) is a 28-item test that can be given easily in office practice. Both the screening test questions and *DSM-IV* give guidelines for pursuing a fuller history of drug and alcohol addiction. Investigating the ways that addiction has affected a person's life (eg, arrest for driving while intoxicated, objections from friends or family, school or work difficulties, history of treatment for addiction) gives a fuller appreciation of the extent and context of the patient's addiction.

Further Evaluation

If a diagnosis of a substance dependence is made or suspected, the physician needs to discuss the diagnosis with the patient and negotiate further evaluation or treatment. These issues are best discussed in the context of a supportive relationship with the patient. Information is presented in a nonjudgmental, empathic, and optimistic manner; the clinician lists the specific components in the history, physical examination, and laboratory evaluation that are related to problems with alcohol or drugs. In the discussion, it should be emphasized that chemical dependency is a treatable disease and the patient is not at fault for having it but that there is a responsibility to accept treatment.

Because most physicians rarely treat substance

Table 11–2. Short Michigan Alcoholism Screening Test (SMAST).*

1. Do you feel you are a normal drinker? *(No)*†
2. Does your spouse, a parent, or other close relative ever worry or complain about your drinking? *(Yes)*
3. Do you ever feel guilty about your drinking? *(Yes)*
4. Do friends or relatives think you are a normal drinker? *(No)*
5. Are you able to stop drinking when you want to? *(No)*
6. Have you ever attended a meeting of Alcoholics Anonymous? *(Yes)*
7. Has drinking ever created problems between you and your spouse, a parent, or other close relative? *(Yes)*
8. Have you ever gotten into trouble at work because of your drinking? *(Yes)*
9. Have you ever neglected your obligations, your family, or your work for 2 or more days in a row because you were drinking? *(Yes)*
10. Have you ever gone to anyone for help about your drinking? *(Yes)*
11. Have you ever been in a hospital because of drinking? *(Yes)*
12. Have you ever been arrested for drunken driving, driving while intoxicated, or driving under the influence of alcoholic beverages? *(Yes)*
13. Have you ever been arrested, even for a few hours, because of other drunken behavior? *(Yes)*

*Reproduced, with permission, from Selzer ML, Vinokur A, van Rooijen L: A self-administered Short Michigan Alcoholism Screening Test (SMAST). J Stud Alcohol 1975; 36:117.
†Answers suggestive of alcoholism are shown in parentheses after each question. Three or more indicate a diagnosis of alcoholism; two indicate the possibility of alcoholism; one or less indicates that alcoholism is unlikely.

abuse themselves but facilitate referrals to treatment resources, it is important for them to become familiar and comfortable with treatment options for chemically dependent women. Going to an open Alcoholics Anonymous (AA) meeting, visiting a reputable treatment center, and getting to know a professional counselor in the field are concrete ways to carry out this task. The patient may deny that drugs or alcohol is a problem. It is helpful to involve the closest family members to get their input and

Table 11–3. CAGE Screening Test for Alcoholism.*

Have you ever felt the need to	**C**ut down on drinking?
Have you ever felt	**A**nnoyed by criticism of your drinking?
Have you ever felt	**G**uilty about your drinking?
Have you ever taken a morning	**E**ye opener?

INTERPRETATION: Two "yes" answers are considered a positive screen. One "yes" answer should raise a suspicion of alcohol abuse.

*Modified and reproduced, with permission, from Mayfield D et al: The CAGE questionnaire: Validation of a new alcoholism screening instrument. Am J Psychiatry 1974; 131:1121.

support for treatment. The physician may refer the family to an addiction counselor who does **interventions** in which family, friends, and other important people in an addicted person's life (eg, employer) are brought together by the therapist for a surprise confrontation of the addicted person. These people talk about the negative consequences of the patient's addiction in an objective yet caring manner so that the patient will agree to enter treatment.

Other strategies for motivating patients to assess their alcoholism include contracting with the patient for a 3-week period during which use of alcohol is limited (eg, the patient agrees to take no more and no less than 1 oz of liquor or the equivalent per day); if the patient fails to keep to this agreement, the clinician suggests that the patient is unable to control her use, indicating a problem with alcohol. The physician asks the patient to go to a few AA meetings or asks her to see a counselor for a second opinion.

Long-term follow-up is essential for anyone who is suspected of being addicted. If the patient is in denial initially, continuing discussion and concern may allow her to accept treatment later. After the patient has been treated, continued monitoring of her abstinence from alcohol and addicting drugs is important because relapse is common. If an addicted patient states that she has returned to "controlled" use of alcohol or drugs, the physician should be concerned; the popular saying "once an addict, always an addict" usually holds true.

Addiction is a chronic illness, and controlled use is often transient. The physician should discuss with the patient the fact that relapse to addiction is frequent in chemically dependent women who are not abstinent. An important concept for the clinician to appreciate is **cross-addiction.** If a patient had a primary problem with one drug (eg, cocaine) and becomes abstinent but begins to use another drug (eg, alcohol or benzodiazepines), she is at higher risk for subsequent relapse to the initial drug or for developing problems with the new substance. Thus, abstinence from all addicting substances is important.

EFFECTS ON PREGNANCY & THE NEWBORN

Children of chemically dependent women are profoundly affected. Fetal alcohol syndrome (FAS) and fetal alcoholic effects (FAE) are among the leading causes of mental retardation in the Western world. The incidence of FAS is between 1 and 3 of 1000 births; rates are as high as one of one-hundred births in some Eskimo villages.

The minimal criteria for FAS include (1) prenatal or postnatal growth retardation (weight, length, or head circumference below the 10th percentile); (2) central nervous system involvement (signs of neurologic abnormality, developmental delay, or intellec-

tual deficit); and (3) characteristic facial dysmorphology with at least 2 of the following signs: (a) microcephaly; (b) microphthalmia or short palpebral fissures, or both; and (c) poorly developed philtrum, thin upper lip, or flattening of the maxillary area. Children with FAE appear to have a continuum of effects ranging from subtle cognitive-behavioral dysfunction to severe morphologic abnormalities. Because there is no safe amount of alcohol a woman can consume in pregnancy, abstinence is recommended; however, a reduction in heavy drinking in pregnancy is associated with improved neonatal outcomes compared with continued heavy drinking. Over the long term, the craniofacial abnormalities of FAS diminish and weight normalizes, but microcephaly and short stature remain. Mental retardation remains, as do maladaptive behaviors such as poor judgment, distractibility, and difficulty perceiving social cues, which cause serious lifelong psychosocial and adjustment problems.

An estimated 9–11% of women have used an illicit drug in their pregnancy; the exposure to such drugs in pregnancy results in significant impairments. Infants exposed to narcotics in utero have serious interactive difficulties with problems engaging and being consoled by a caretaker, are more tremulous and irritable than other babies, and have unpredictable emotional responses. These factors interrupt the maternal-infant bonding. Lower birth weight and smaller head circumference are noted in infants whose mothers use narcotics. Neonatal growth catches up by 12 months of age, with the exception of smaller head circumference, which is reported to be predictive of poor developmental outcome. The outcome for children whose mothers take part in methadone maintenance therapy during pregnancy is better than for those whose mothers use heroin.

Treatment of the neonatal narcotic abstinence syndrome in infants (high-pitched cry, sweating, tremulousness, excoriation of the extremities, and gastrointestinal upset) should be largely supportive. Pharmacologic therapy with paregoric, diazepam, or phenobarbital is used if withdrawal is severe and other causes of symptoms are ruled out.

Cocaine use in pregnancy is associated with abruptio placentae, placenta previa, stillbirth, and prematurity. There is an increase in congenital abnormalities including neural tube defects, genitourinary malformations, ileal atresia, and cardiac abnormalities. Use of cocaine or marihuana in pregnancy is related to intrauterine growth retardation. Babies exposed to cocaine have a high degree of irritability and tremulousness. Cessation of cocaine use does reduce the risk of maternal and neonatal complications. Long-term effects are under study.

Addiction uniformly affects a mother's ability to parent effectively. Abandonment, neglect, abuse, physical and cognitive deficits, decreased interpersonal skills, and emotional difficulty and lability occur more frequently in children with addicted parents than in others.

MEDICAL COMPLICATIONS

There are some health consequences of addiction specific to women. Women have higher blood alcohol levels and become more intoxicated than men when given the same amount of alcohol, even when their size is taken into consideration. This finding may be because (1) the lower body water content among women leads to a smaller volume of distribution and higher blood alcohol concentration; (2) there is diminished activity of alcohol dehydrogenase (the primary enzyme in the metabolism of alcohol) in the stomach of women; or (3) fluctuation of gonadal hormone levels in the menstrual cycle may affect the rate of alcohol metabolism, although findings are inconsistent.

Women show an increased susceptibility to alcoholic liver disease, including fatty liver, hepatitis, and cirrhosis, with a shorter duration of heavy drinking and a lower level of daily drinking compared with men. Based on the risk of developing alcoholic liver disease, heavy drinking for women is defined as one and one-half or more drinks per day (one drink equals $1\frac{1}{2}$ oz—one shot—of liquor, 12 oz of beer, or 5 oz of wine) compared with 4 or more drinks per day for men.

Compared with nondrinkers, moderate drinkers have an increased risk of breast cancer. Heavy alcohol consumption is a risk factor for osteoporosis. Women who drink heavily may have increased susceptibility to neuropsychologic impairment in a shorter length of time than men.

There is an association between hypertension and alcohol intake in women after shorter periods of heavy drinking than in men. In both men and women, 1–2 alcoholic drinks per day produces an elevation of HDL cholesterol, which may protect against cardiovascular disease. However, this level is at the threshold of dangerous drinking for women and cannot be recommended. Women who drink heavily have a much higher mortality rate than men from most major alcohol-related causes of death, natural and unnatural.

Less information is available regarding the differential effects of other drugs in women compared with men. Menstrual disorders (eg, painful menses, heavy flow, premenstrual discomfort, and cycle irregularity or absence) have been associated with multiple drugs and alcohol. Addicted women run the risk of exposure to sexually transmitted diseases because of impaired judgment. If there is injecting drug use, there is risk of hepatitis B and C, HIV infection, and bacteremias with the attendant complications of these infections.

TREATMENT

The general principles of alcohol and drug treatment are identical. Indeed, many women in addiction treatment are polydrug- and alcohol-dependent. Most programs are group-oriented with some individual sessions with a counselor, and family is included in some sessions. The patient initially is detoxified, and abstinence from addicting drugs is stressed. Treatment includes educational sessions regarding various aspects of addiction and therapy sessions that center on "here and now" issues, eg, adjustment to life without chemicals, breakdown of denial, and stresses on family, friends, and job. Alcoholics Anonymous and other self-help programs such as Women in Sobriety are introduced, and attendance is encouraged or required. Programs may be outpatient or inpatient with a fixed or variable length of stay. Inpatient treatment is more intensive, eliminates drug access, and may offer more medical and psychiatric services; however, it is more disruptive, more expensive, carries a greater stigma, and may be artificially safe, postponing critical learning tasks.

There has been no clear advantage demonstrated in outcome in women treated in same-sex versus coed programs, although the woman's preference should be honored if possible. Treatment services that may be particularly important for women are assertiveness training, special help for victims of sexual and physical abuse, issues of parenting, self-esteem, and childcare, and provision of positive female role models in recovery.

Detoxification

A. Alcohol: Alcohol withdrawal includes a highly variable group of symptoms. These symptoms range from those that are relatively mild, such as sweating, hypertension, tachycardia, and anxiety, to more serious problems of delirium tremens and convulsions. Withdrawal can be accomplished on an outpatient basis unless there are significant medical, psychiatric, or social complications. Adjunctive pharmacologic therapy for alcohol withdrawal should be considered for patient comfort and to prevent seizures and delirium. More severe withdrawal requiring higher doses of medication and closer monitoring is best accomplished with inpatient detoxification.

Benzodiazepines are the most common treatment for alcohol withdrawal. A regimen may include 25–50 mg of chlordiazepoxide; 1–2 mg of lorazepam; or 5–10 mg diazepam, taken 4 times daily for 1 or 2 days, followed by oral tapering by 20%/d for outpatient withdrawal, with daily visits to the physician to assess symptoms. The patient should stay with someone who will monitor her condition and, if difficulties arise, call a physician. The patient should not drive a motor vehicle. Lorazepam has a shorter half-life than the other two drugs, can be given intramuscularly, and does not accumulate if there is significant liver disease. Thiamine, 100 mg twice daily, and multivitamins should be given as well. Beta-adrenergic blockers (atenolol and propranolol), alpha-adrenergic agonists (clonidine), and carbamazepine may have a role but are more experimental.

To help a patient establish a long-term pattern of sobriety, disulfiram may be a useful adjunct. Disulfiram inhibits aldehydehydrogenase, which leads to increased levels of acetaldehyde in the metabolism of alcohol. The result is the toxic reaction of nausea, vomiting, tachycardia, flushing, dyspnea, and headache if alcohol is ingested. The usual dosage is 250 mg daily; if an aversive agent is appropriate, the drug can be begun 48–72 hours after cessation of alcohol ingestion.

B. Sedative and Hypnotic Drugs: Benzodiazepine and barbiturate withdrawal should be approached pharmacologically. Even a low dose of a benzodiazepine for months requires some detoxification because there is a risk of delirium or seizures with sudden discontinuation. Conservative detoxification is a slow process that takes weeks (eg, 10% every 3–7 days). For patients taking shorter-acting benzodiazepines such as alprazolam, it may be advantageous to switch to a longer-acting agent such as clonazepam for withdrawal because withdrawal symptoms are less severe with longer-acting benzodiazepines. In the presence of (1) significant difficulty with withdrawal, (2) an unclear history, (3) high-dose abuse, (4) inadequate social support, or (5) medical or psychiatric complications, inpatient detoxification in a facility with experienced personnel is recommended.

C. Opiates: Detoxification in patients with opiate dependence is accomplished by gradual reduction of the opiate dose over several days or weeks. One approach is to use a long-acting opioid such as methadone in equivalent doses and reduce it over a 14-day period. Clonidine, an alpha-agonist that suppresses hyperactivity in the locus coeruleus, is effective in suppressing autonomic signs and symptoms of withdrawal but is less effective in decreasing subjective discomfort.

Naltrexone is an opioid-receptor antagonist used after opioid detoxification to prevent the euphoric effects of opiates. Dosage is 100–150 mg 3 times weekly. There are high dropout rates related to motivation and opioid craving that limit use to patients who have family support, psychotherapeutic support, and a source of external limits on behavior.

Methadone maintenance, primarily indicated for "hard-core" addicts, is an attempt to interrupt an addict's life-style by decreasing criminality, promoting stability and employment, and reducing IV drug abuse and thus risk of HIV infection. It is a valuable and underused treatment of indeterminate length. Some patients have been able to interrupt their addictive life-style and become gradually detoxified.

D. Cocaine, Cannabis, Hallucinogens, and Inhalants: General supportive measures are usually adequate for treatment of patients withdrawing from these substances; there are no clear-cut detoxification regimens.

REFERENCES

American Psychiatric Association: *Diagnostic and Statistical Manual of Mental Disorders,* 4th ed. American Psychiatric Association, 1994.
Blume S: Women and addiction. In: *Comprehensive Handbook of Drug and Alcohol Addiction.* Miller NS (editor). Marcel Dekker, 1991.
Chasnoff I: Drug and alcohol effects on pregnancy and the newborn. In: *Comprehensive Handbook of Drug and Alcohol Addiction.* Miller NS (editor). Marcel Dekker, 1991.
Closser MH, Blow FC: Special populations: Women, ethnic minorities and the elderly. Psychiatr Clin North Am 1993;16:199.
Cyr MG, Moulton AW: The physician's role in prevention, detection and treatment of alcohol abuse in women. Psychiatr Ann 1993;23(8):454.
Cyr MG, Moulton AW: Substance abuse in women. Obstet Gynecol Clin North Am 1990;17:905.
Davis SK: Chemical dependency in women: A description of its effects and outcome on adequate parenting. J Subst Abuse Treat 1990;7:225.
Frances RJ, Franklin JE: Treatment approaches to alcoholism and other psychoactive substance use disorders. In: *Concise Guide to Treatment of Alcoholism and Addictions.* Frances RJ, Franklin JE (editors). American Psychiatric Press, 1989.
Kendler KS et al: A population-based twin study of alcoholism in women. JAMA 1992;268:1877.
Kessler RC et al: Lifetime and 12-month prevalence of DSM-III-R psychiatric disorders in the United States: Results from the National Comorbidity Study. Arch Gen Psychiatry 1994;51:8.
Klatsky AL, Armstrong MA, Friedman GD: Alcohol and mortality. Ann Intern Med 1992;117:646.
Skinner HA: The Drug Abuse Screening Test. Addict Behav 1982;7:363.
Streissgath AP et al: Fetal alcohol syndrome in adolescents and adults. JAMA 1991;265:1961.
Weisner C, Schmidt L: Gender disparities in treatment for alcohol problems. JAMA 1992;268:1872.
Wilsnaek SC et al: Predicting onset and chronicity of women's problem drinking: A five-year longitudinal analysis. Am J Public Health 1991;81:305.

Anxiety and Panic Disorder

12

Deborah S. Cowley, MD

Anxiety is a common experience that serves as an adaptive response to danger or threat. In anxiety disorders, however, anxiety occurs without clear cause or out of proportion to the magnitude of external events. Such "pathologic" anxiety is distressing and debilitating and interferes with normal functioning.

Anxiety disorders affect at least 5–10% of the general population. Many forms of anxiety, particularly panic disorder and agoraphobia, are significantly more prevalent in women than in men. Because they occur during the childbearing years, important questions are raised regarding their course and management during pregnancy and lactation. Most patients with anxiety disorders are seen and treated in primary care rather than psychiatric settings. Thus, skill in recognition and management of anxiety disorders is important for primary care providers.

Incidence & Risk Factors

Anxiety disorders have lifetime prevalence rates in the general population of 1.5–3.5% for panic disorder, with or without agoraphobia; 5% for generalized anxiety disorder; 2.5% for obsessive-compulsive disorder; and 2% for social phobia. Rates of posttraumatic stress disorder (PTSD) vary considerably (1–14% lifetime) depending on the population sampled. Specific phobias occur in approximately 10% of the general population. Approximately 5–10% of patients presenting to both primary care and subspecialty medical clinics have clinically significant anxiety disorders.

Although anxiety disorders can begin at any stage of life, they are most likely to develop in childhood, adolescence, or young adulthood. The peak age of onset of panic disorder is between the late teens and mid-30s. Generalized anxiety disorder (GAD) usually begins in childhood or adolescence. The peak period of onset of obsessive-compulsive disorder (OCD) is in childhood or adolescence in male patients, but in the 20s in women. The onset of social phobia is typically in childhood or the teens, childhood, often following a history of shyness or specific humiliating experiences.

The reasons for the greater prevalence of anxiety disorders in women than in men are unclear but may include hormonal factors, sexual differences in the structure and neurochemistry of the regions of the

Incidence & Risk Factors
Characteristics
Complications & Associated Conditions
Diagnosis
Treatment
Prognosis
Referral to a Specialist
Issues of Pregnancy, Lactation,
& Menstruation
Controversies & Unresolved Issues

brain that mediate anxiety, and the types of life stressors and feelings of powerlessness experienced by women. Women are 2–3 times more likely than men to develop panic disorder, twice as likely to have GAD, 2–3 times as likely to suffer from specific phobias, and more likely to report significant social phobia. Obsessive-compulsive disorder occurs at about the same rate in men and women.

Panic disorder is familial and probably inherited; the risk of developing the disorder increases to 17% in first-degree relatives of affected people. Precipitants of initial panic attacks include life stress and exposure to stimulant drugs, such as cocaine, amphetamines, and caffeine.

Obsessive-compulsive disorder has a genetic component and has been linked to altered serotonin function in the brain. This disorder may result from disturbances in a neural circuit involving the frontal cortex, thalamus, and basal ganglia. Symptoms of OCD may develop in patients with disorders of the basal ganglia such as Sydenham's chorea, Tourette's syndrome, and other movement and tic disorders.

Social phobia is transmitted in families, may be inherited, and often begins as marked shyness in childhood. Posttraumatic stress disorder depends on exposure to an unusual and extreme stressor. However, the risk of PTSD increases with greater intensity and duration of the stressor and is higher in people with fewer social supports and those who have preexisting psychiatric disorders.

Characteristics

During the past 15 years, several distinct anxiety disorders have been described. These conditions differ in clinical presentation, cause, and treatment. Most patients presenting to primary care providers with anxiety symptoms have situational anxiety or an adjustment disorder with anxious mood, in which clinically significant anxiety occurs in the context of ongoing life stress. More chronic anxiety disorders include panic disorder, phobic disorders (agoraphobia, social phobia, specific phobias), generalized anxiety disorder, obsessive-compulsive disorder, and posttraumatic stress disorder. The American Psychiatric Association's *Diagnostic and Statistical Manual, 4/e (DSM-IV)* lists diagnostic criteria for these disorders, which are summarized briefly in the following paragraphs.

Panic disorder is characterized by recurrent, unexpected attacks of intense fear, associated with four of the following thirteen symptoms:

1. Palpitations/accelerated heart rate
2. Sweating
3. Trembling or shaking
4. Shortness of breath
5. Choking
6. Chest pain
7. Nausea or abdominal distress
8. Dizziness
9. Feelings of unreality (derealization) or detachment from oneself (depersonalization)
10. Fear of losing control or going crazy
11. Fear of dying
12. Numbness or tingling
13. Chills or hot flushes.

At least one panic attack must lead to a month or more of worry about having another attack (anticipatory anxiety), anxiety about the possible consequences or meaning of the attack, or a significant change in behavior as a result of the attack.

Generalized anxiety disorder is characterized by chronic (6 months or more), excessive worry that is difficult to control, causes significant functional impairment, and is accompanied by three of the following six symptoms: restlessness or the feeling of being "on edge"; fatigability; trouble concentrating, or experiencing the mind as "going blank"; irritability; muscle tension; and sleep disturbance.

In **obsessive-compulsive disorder,** persistent irrational thoughts or images (obsessions) or repetitive behaviors that the patient feels driven to perform to reduce anxiety (compulsions) significantly interfere with her life. Examples of compulsive rituals include handwashing, checking, counting, or arranging objects in a rigid order.

Posttraumatic stress disorder follows a traumatic, life-threatening event and is marked by a reexperiencing of the trauma in dreams, intrusive memories, or flashbacks; avoidance of situations associated with the trauma; emotional numbing; and increased arousal in the form of an exaggerated startle response, temper outbursts, and insomnia. Posttraumatic stress disorder has been described and studied primarily in male combat veterans. In women, PTSD may follow rape or sexual abuse, other traumatic events, and accidents.

In **phobic disorders,** particular situations or objects are feared and avoided. Specific phobias are common and include fear of heights, spiders, the dark, and so on. In **social phobia,** the patient fears being judged, being the center of attention, or standing out in a situation such as public speaking, meeting new people, or eating or writing in front of other people. **Agoraphobia** refers to numerous fears of situations or settings in which escape would be difficult without embarrassment (eg, crowds, tunnels, bridges, movie theaters, checkout lines at grocery stores). Agoraphobia often accompanies panic disorder, but it may occur alone.

Complications & Associated Conditions

Panic disorder usually is accompanied by fear of having another panic attack (anticipatory anxiety) and often leads to phobic avoidance or agoraphobia. Two-thirds of patients with panic disorder have a lifetime history of depression, and one-third have coexisting depression and panic disorder. The latter group has been shown to have lower treatment response rates than patients with panic disorder alone. Panic disorder also has been linked with an increased rate of suicide attempts.

Depression commonly coexists with OCD, PTSD, and social phobia. Most anxiety disorders are associated with an increased rate of alcohol and sedative abuse and dependence. Abuse of these drugs may alleviate anxiety symptoms temporarily and represent a form of "self-medication"; however, repeated use and withdrawal may provoke more anxiety. OCD may be associated with neurologic conditions, Tourette's syndrome, and other movement or tic disorders.

Diagnosis

Most patients with anxiety disorders do not seek psychiatric help but present to primary care providers, often quite preoccupied with the physical symptoms of their disorder and convinced that they have a dangerous or even life-threatening medical problem. This focus on somatic symptoms can divert attention from the underlying anxiety disorder and result in costly and invasive medical workups with negative findings.

There are several rating forms available to assess anxiety symptoms. These include the Hamilton Rating Scale for Anxiety and the Yale-Brown Obsessive-Compulsive Scale. Although these rating forms can be helpful in evaluating treatment, a few diagnostic questions are more helpful in diagnosing an anxiety disorder.

For example, for panic disorder, the patient can be asked, "Have you ever had an attack when you suddenly felt frightened or anxious?" If the answer is yes, the patient should be asked whether this ever has happened for no apparent reason, or "out of the blue." Some people may not admit to feeling frightened but report instead sudden attacks of racing heart, shortness of breath, or dizziness. For OCD, screening might include questions such as, "Is there anything that you have to do over and over again and you can't resist doing it, like washing your hands again and again or checking something several times to make sure you've done it right?" Patients can be asked a general question about phobias such as, "Is there anything you fear so much that you always avoid it, like animals, heights, crowds, closed spaces, driving, public speaking, or being the center of attention?" To screen for PTSD, the patient can be asked whether she has experienced a traumatic or life-threatening event that still affects her. In screening for anxiety disorders, it is important to assess how much the symptoms impair the patient's function and interfere with her life.

The psychiatric differential diagnosis of anxiety disorders includes agitated depression, mania, and psychotic disorders. Anxiety symptoms also may result from medical illnesses or substance abuse or withdrawal. Some of the conditions to include in the medical differential diagnosis are listed in Table 12–1. Most of the conditions listed in Table 12–1, however, are uncommon causes of significant anxiety symptoms. In the presence of a clear-cut, typical history of an anxiety disorder in a young and apparently healthy woman, the medical work-up need not be exhaustive; it should be designed to rule out only the conditions strongly suggested by the patients history and physical examination. In older patients and those not responding to initial treatment for the anxiety disorder, a more extensive medical workup is indicated.

Several medical conditions warrant special mention. Mitral valve prolapse often occurs together with panic attacks, especially in women. This usually benign medical condition most often requires no specific treatment and does not change the approach to diagnosis or treatment of panic attacks. Irritable bowel syndrome also commonly coexists with anxiety disorders and may respond well to treatment of anxiety, especially with tricyclic antidepressants. Chest pain can be a symptom of panic attacks and may lead to invasive, expensive cardiac workups.

The most common and most frequently overlooked conditions causing anxiety symptoms are substance abuse and depression. Alcohol or sedative withdrawal, caffeine, marihuana, and stimulants such as cocaine and amphetamines often provoke anxiety or panic symptoms, but the patient may not spontaneously report drug or alcohol use. Many depressed people complain primarily of anxiety, and their de-

Table 12–1. Medical differential diagnosis of anxiety.

System or Agent	Disorder or Drug
Cardiac	Arrhythmias
	Coronary artery disease
	Congestive heart failure
Respiratory	Hyperventilation
	Asthma
	Pulmonary embolus
	Chronic obstructive pulmonary disease
Endocrine	Cushing's syndrome
	Hyperparathyroidism
	Hyper- or hypothyroidism
	Hypoglycemia
	Menopausal symptoms
	Pheochromocytoma
	Carcinoid
	Insulinoma
Neurologic	Temporal lobe epilepsy
	True vertigo
	Tic disorders (obsessive-compulsive disorder)
	Tumor
	Akathisia
Medication or drugs	Alcohol withdrawal
	Caffeinism
	Sedative withdrawal
	Cocaine
	Amphetamines
	Marihuana
	Steroids
	Sympathomimetics
	Theophylline
Other	Electrolyte disturbance
	Collagen vascular disease

pressive symptoms may be missed. Because major depression frequently coexists with anxiety, all anxious patients should be asked about symptoms of depression. Screening for depression and for substance abuse is described in Chapters 13 and 11, respectively.

Treatment

A. General Measures: Patients with anxiety disorders usually are quite relieved to be given a diagnosis and be told that they have a treatable condition. Many of these patients believe they are "going crazy" or suffering from a life-threatening disorder. Providing information about their anxiety disorder is extremely helpful. A small number continue to insist that they have a "medical" disorder or that there is something wrong with them that the doctors have been unable to diagnose. Such patients may benefit from an empathic approach in which the provider does not attempt to argue or convince them otherwise but instead sympathizes with the difficulty of their position, discusses anxiety disorders using a medical model (eg, emphasizing the increased adrenalin), and explains that psychologic factors such as life stressors can exacerbate any condition, including theirs, and thus deserve attention.

In addition to education, general measures helpful for people with anxiety disorders include avoidance of caffeine, alcohol, and illicit drugs; adequate sleep; exercise; and when possible, avoidance of life stressors such as moving to a new home or major changes in routine. In initiating treatment, the provider needs to be reassuring, optimistic, and available to answer questions and take telephone calls.

B. Pharmacotherapy: Effective medication is available for panic disorder, OCD, GAD, and social phobia. Medications provide useful adjuncts in the treatment of PTSD. Specific phobias, on the other hand, should be treated with psychotherapy (see the following section) and do not respond to pharmacotherapy.

The best studied medications for panic disorder are the tricyclic antidepressants, primarily imipramine; however, it now appears that most antidepressants are effective. Exceptions are bupropion and trazodone. The selective serotonin reuptake inhibitors (SSRIs), fluoxetine, sertraline, and paroxetine, have not been well studied for panic disorder, but they appear to be helpful and to have few side effects. Although monoamine oxidase (MAO) inhibitors may be the most effective antipanic medications, they usually are not considered the first-line treatment because they require a tyramine-free diet and carry the risk of hypertensive crisis. A full list and discussion of antidepressants and their side effects is given in Chapter 13.

There are several important points to keep in mind when prescribing antidepressants for panic and anxiety disorders. First, many anxious patients are exquisitely sensitive to and phobic of medication side effects. Thus, these drugs should be started at very low doses, eg, 10 mg imipramine or 2 mg fluoxetine syrup daily. Second, anxious patients often develop increased anxiety or "overstimulation" in the first week or two of antidepressant treatment. They should be warned that this effect might occur and reassured that it will pass. If necessary, benzodiazepines can be prescribed initially to help reduce anxiety. Although small dosages of antidepressants are necessary at first, patients with panic disorder usually require full antidepressant dosages for therapeutic efficacy and thus need to have their dosages steadily increased, as rapidly as they can tolerate, to the usual antidepressant level. Finally, antidepressants may take up to 10–12 weeks to reach their full effect in anxiety disorders, as opposed to 4–6 weeks in depression. In general, success rates for antidepressant treatment of panic disorder are approximately 70–80%, with a placebo response rate of about 30%.

Specific types of antidepressant medications are helpful in other anxiety disorders. The treatment of choice for social phobia is an MAO inhibitor, although the SSRIs appear to be effective also and produce fewer side effects. Beta-blockers such as atenolol, 50–100 mg/d, may be helpful prescribed regularly or as needed in circumscribed social phobias such as fears of performance or public speaking. Sedating antidepressants may be beneficial in GAD.

The treatment of choice for OCD is prescription of one of the serotonergic antidepressants: clomipramine, 150–300 mg/d; fluoxetine, 20–40 mg/d; sertraline, 50–200 mg/d; or paroxetine, 20–50 mg/d. A moderate-to-marked therapeutic response occurs in 40–60% of patients given one of these medications; the response can take up to 12 weeks and is rare with placebo. If one of these agents is ineffective, another may work for the patient. Although all four agents are effective, clomipramine has more anticholinergic side effects.

In patients with PTSD, antidepressants may be helpful in treating depression, panic attacks, and intrusive symptoms. SSRIS may alleviate emotional numbing and avoidance.

Traditionally, people presenting with anxiety symptoms have been treated with anxiolytics, primarily benzodiazepines. Benzodiazepines are indeed quite effective for generalized anxiety disorder and situational anxiety symptoms. Alprazolam (Xanax), 2–6 mg/d; clonazepam (Klonopin), 1–3 mg/d; lorazepam (Ativan), 3–8 mg/d; and diazepam (Valium), 20–60 mg/d, all have been shown to be effective in panic disorder, with alprazolam being comparable in efficacy to imipramine but with a much more rapid onset of action. The starting dosage for panic disorder is 0.25–0.5 mg alprazolam (or an equivalent dosage of another benzodiazepine) (Table 12–2) 3 times daily.

Benzodiazepines are also useful as treatment adjuncts in OCD and social phobia, although the high rate of alcohol abuse and dependence in patients with social phobia dictates caution in prescribing these medications in this group. Patients with other anxiety disorders usually require lower doses of benzodiazepines than do patients with panic disorder.

The advantages of benzodiazepines include a rapid onset of action, efficacy when used as needed, and a low rate of adverse effects, especially cardiac side effects. The greatest disadvantage is the development of tolerance (need for a higher dose to achieve a therapeutic effect or loss of anxiolytic effects altogether) and dependence. Anxious patients without a history of substance abuse are unlikely to abuse benzodiazepines; however, they may develop tolerance and withdrawal symptoms with attempted discontinuation, especially with higher doses and longer duration of treatment. Other side effects of benzodiazepines include memory loss for recently acquired information (anterograde amnesia), sedation, impaired driving ability, and incoordination. The patient should be advised not to drive if she feels sleepy while taking the medication.

The primary indications for use of benzodiazepines in anxiety disorders are (1) disabling symp-

Table 12–2. Pharmacokinetics of benzodiazepines commonly prescribed for anxiety disorders.

Generic Name (Trade Name)	Dosage Equivalent (mg)	Onset of Action	Elimination Half-Life (hours)*	Hepatic Metabolism
Alprazolam (Xanax)	1.0	Intermediate	6–20	Oxidation
Chlordiazepoxide (Librium)	20.0–25.0	Intermediate	5–100	Oxidation
Clonazepam (Klonopin)	0.5	Intermediate	18–50	Oxidation, nitroreduction
Clorazepate (Tranxene)	15.0	Fast	30–100	Oxidation
Diazepam (Valium)	10.0	Fast	30–100	Oxidation
Lorazepam (Ativan)	1.5–2.0	Intermediate	10–20	Conjugation
Oxazepam (Serax)	30.0	Slow	5–21	Conjugation

*Elimination half-lives include those of all active metabolites.

toms, with significantly impaired function at school, at work, or in caring for children and (2) inability to tolerate other medication or to benefit from psychotherapeutic treatments. Benzodiazepines should be avoided in people with a history of alcohol or substance abuse themselves or a family history of alcoholism in a first-degree relative.

The pharmacokinetic properties of the benzodiazepines commonly used for anxiety disorders are given in Table 12–2. Compounds with a more rapid onset of action are more suitable for use "as needed." Elimination half-lives increase with age and liver disease. The risk of side effects of benzodiazepines increases with age; hip fractures are significantly more frequent in elderly people taking benzodiazepines with a long than with a short half-life. This is a particularly important consideration in elderly women with osteoporosis. Benzodiazepines that are metabolized by conjugation, have no active metabolites, and have relatively short half-lives, such as oxazepam and lorazepam, are preferable in elderly or medically ill patients.

Buspirone (BuSpar), a non-habit-forming and nonsedating medication, is now available for treatment of generalized anxiety. Buspirone takes 2–3 weeks at dosages of 30–60 mg/d for full effect. Its most common side effects include dizziness, gastrointestinal upset, and headaches. No tolerance or withdrawal symptoms have been reported with this medication. Its benign side effect profile makes buspirone the current treatment of choice for GAD.

C. Psychotherapy: The mainstay of treatment for phobic disorders (agoraphobia, specific phobias) is behavior therapy, in which the patient confronts the feared situation either in her imagination, with the therapist, or on her own (exposure therapy), often using relaxation or other techniques to become less and less fearful of it (desensitization). Behavior therapy is also quite effective in OCD, for which it consists of a combination of exposure and response prevention, eg, preventing the patient from washing her hands if she fears dirt and contamination.

Recently, a specific form of cognitive-behavioral therapy has been developed for panic disorder and generalized anxiety disorder. In this therapy, the patient identifies and confronts distorted thoughts (eg, "If I have a panic attack, I will have a heart attack and die") and learns specific techniques to deal with and tolerate anxiety symptoms. Cognitive-behavioral therapy has a high success rate (80–90%), takes about 12–20 sessions, and gives the patient a valuable feeling of mastery of her disorder. Although this therapy usually is done best with the help of a trained therapist, patient manuals such as one by Barlow and Craskee are available. Cognitive-behavioral therapy is being developed presently for social phobia.

Posttraumatic stress disorder usually requires more intensive psychotherapeutic approaches, including both group and individual treatment. Specific forms of psychotherapy for PTSD are reviewed by Solomon et al and include desensitization, flooding, and stress inoculation therapy. The general goal is to allow the patient to confront or recall the trauma and integrate the event into their life while reducing intrusive memories, flashbacks, and hyperarousal. Patients can be gradually desensitized to stimuli or situations that remind them of the traumatic event, either in their imagination, by talking about the event, or by confronting real life situations that arouse painful memories or flashbacks. Sudden, overwhelming exposure to feared situations, or flooding can be a very effective treatment but may exacerbate comorbid depression, substance abuse, panic attacks, or suicidal ideation and so should be used with caution. Stress inoculation therapy emphasizes identifying stress reactions, rehearsing coping skills, and applying these skill in feared situations. All of these approaches are best carried out by a therapist with expertise in treating PTSD.

The optimal treatment for most anxiety disorders usually is a combination of medication and psychotherapy. Some people prefer to avoid medication or cannot tolerate side effects and so may choose psychotherapy alone, whereas others prefer a medical model and do not wish to spend the time required for psychotherapy. The success of treatment can be monitored using rating scales and diaries; many of the treatments for anxiety disorders take weeks to work, and identifying small gains in the first few weeks of treatment can be encouraging.

Prognosis

Surprisingly little is known about the long-term prognosis of anxiety disorders. In general, they tend to have a chronic, fluctuating, waxing and waning course with exacerbations during periods of life stress. Naturalistic studies of patients with panic disorder treated in anxiety clinics show improvement in about 40–50%, worsening or continued symptoms in 15–30%, and discontinuation of symptoms in approximately 30%. The prognosis for anxiety disorders is worse in those with comorbid depression, substance abuse, or personality disorders.

Referral to a Specialist

Anxiety disorders often can be treated successfully in the primary care setting with a combination of reassurance, education, medication, problem-solving to assist in dealing with life stressors, and encouragement of the patient to confront feared situations. Referral to a psychiatrist, psychologist, or other mental health provider is indicated in the following situations:

1. **Diagnostic uncertainty**–If the presenting complaints are confusing, complicated, or atypical, a psychiatric evaluation may be helpful to clarify the diagnosis and the appropriate approach to treatment.
2. **Treatment failure**–When the first-line treatments outlined in this chapter do not help, other diagnoses should be reconsidered. Evaluation by a specialist is helpful to obtain suggestions of alternative treatments or to initiate a specific psychotherapeutic or medication treatment program.
3. **Comorbidity, severe illness, or suicidality**–Patients with comorbid depression, substance abuse, or personality disorders or who are very ill or are suicidal are more difficult to treat and should be referred to a specialist. Acutely suicidal patients should be referred for emergent consultation or hospitalization.

Issues of Pregnancy, Lactation, & Menstruation

Many women with anxiety disorders note that their symptoms worsen premenstrually, even in the absence of premenstrual syndrome. The course of these disorders during pregnancy is quite variable. Symptoms of OCD often begin or worsen during pregnancy, whereas panic attacks may subside. These conditions usually have their onset during the childbearing years, however, so that a large number of women develop anxiety disorders or continue to be symptomatic during pregnancy and lactation.

It is clearly preferable to plan a pregnancy during an asymptomatic period, discontinue medication, and use psychotherapeutic approaches as needed during the pregnancy. It is important to taper benzodiazepines slowly to avoid uncomfortable withdrawal symptoms or seizures. In the case of an unplanned pregnancy or severe symptoms, it may be necessary to make difficult choices concerning treatment, taking into account both the safety of the fetus and the mental health of the mother. These decisions should be made, when possible, with the full, informed collaboration of the woman and, if appropriate, with the participation of her partner.

Medications should be avoided whenever possible during pregnancy but especially in the first trimester. A recent study by Pastuszak et al of women taking tricyclic antidepressants or fluoxetine during the first trimester revealed no increased rate of fetal malformations or adverse pregnancy outcome in comparison with women using nonteratogenic medications. However, the rate of miscarriages was significantly higher (13.5% for fluoxetine, 12.2% for tricyclics, and 6.8% for nonteratogens). MAO inhibitors have been associated with congenital anomalies and should be avoided.

First- and second-trimester exposure to benzodiazepines has been associated with an increased risk of cleft lip and palate and cardiocirculatory defects, although these findings have not been replicated in more recent, large studies and may be attributable, at least in part, to concurrent heavy smoking. Both tricyclics and benzodiazepines given close to term may provoke a neonatal withdrawal syndrome. Animal studies suggest that prenatal exposure to antidepressants and benzodiazepines may result in behavioral differences in offspring, although this finding has not been observed in humans.

Concerns about medication use in pregnancy must be weighed against evidence that maternal anxiety can affect the fetus adversely. In primates, anxiety leads to placental vasoconstriction and fetal hypoxia; in humans, there has been one case report of a spontaneous abortion during a panic attack. Given the paucity of knowledge and lack of clear clinical guidelines, it may be helpful to obtain psychiatric consultation, gather information from the company manufacturing the drug to be prescribed and a local teratogen information service, and keep in close contact with the patient's obstetrician.

Tricyclics, fluoxetine, and benzodiazepines all

cross into breast milk. Benzodiazepines are contraindicated during lactation because they may cause lethargy, jaundice, and poor feeding in the infant. The effects of antidepressants on the infant are less well known. Clearly, the most conservative approach is to avoid combining lactation and medication. If medication is to be prescribed during nursing, however, the baby's pediatrician and the American Academy of Pediatrics guidelines regarding use of medication during lactation should be consulted.

Controversies & Unresolved Issues

The pathophysiology of anxiety disorders remains incompletely understood. Although genetic factors have been implicated in panic disorder, OCD, and social phobia, the specific genetic differences inherited in these conditions have not been identified. In panic disorder, underlying mechanisms are still un-

clear despite numerous studies. This disorder may involve altered function of the locus coeruleus, the major brain region regulating central noradrenergic tone; increased sensitivity to carbon dioxide and other signals of suffocation or anoxia; or changes in brain handling of lactate. The development of frequent panic attacks and agoraphobia may be linked to childhood separation anxiety and to a cognitive style characterized by increased sensitivity to cues related to threat, danger, or physical symptoms.

The optimal length of treatment of anxiety disorders is also undetermined but probably depends on the duration of the disorder, with illness of longer duration requiring longer treatment. In a study of imipramine in the treatment of panic disorder, Mavissakalian and Perel demonstrated that most people can cut their dosage in half after 6 months but that discontinuation of medication at this point results in high relapse rates.

REFERENCES

American Psychiatric Association: *Diagnostic and Statistical Manual of Mental Disorders,* 4th ed. American Psychiatric Association, 1994.

Barlow DH: *Anxiety and Its Disorders.* Guilford Press, 1988.

Barlow DH, Craske MG: *Mastery of Your Anxiety and Panic.* Graywind Publications, 1989.

Cowley DS, Roy-Byrne PP: Panic disorder during pregnancy. J Psychosom Obstet Gynecol 1989;10:193.

Goodman WK et al: The Yale-Brown Obsessive-Compulsive Scale (Y-BOCS). Part I. Development, use, and reliability. Arch Gen Psychiatry 1989;46:1006.

Greist JH: An integrated approach to treatment of obsessive-compulsive disorder. J Clin Psychiatry 1992;53:4 (Suppl):38.

Hamilton M: The assessment of anxiety states by rating. Br J Med Psychol 1959;32:50.

Katon W et al: Chest pain: Relationship of psychiatric illness to coronary arteriographic results. Am J Med 1988;84:1.

Mavissakalian M, Perel JM: Clinical experiments in maintenance and discontinuation of imipramine therapy in panic disorder with agoraphobia. Arch Gen Psychiatry 1992;49:318.

Nezirogly F, Anemone R, Yaryura-Tobias JA: Onset of obsessive-compulsive disorder in pregnancy. Am J Psychiatry 1992;149:947.

Pastuszak A et al: Pregnancy outcome following first-trimester exposure to fluoxetine (Prozac). JAMA 1993; 269:2246.

Roy-Byrne PP et al: Psychopharmacological treatment of panic, generalized anxiety disorder, and social phobia. Psychiatr Clin North Am 1993;16:719.

Solomon SD, Gerrity ET, Muff AM: Efficacy of treatments for posttraumatic stress disorder: An empirical review. JAMA 1992;268:633.

13

Mood Disorders

Jennifer D. Bolen, MD, & Marcia Robbins, MSW

Numerous population and cross-cultural studies have shown that depression, mood disturbances, mood cycling, and loss reactions have a higher prevalence in women than in men. This gender difference begins to emerge in early adolescence.

Continuing research into mood disorders highlights the fact that these disturbances are complex and have multifactorial causes. There are unique biopsychosocial factors that predispose women to these reactions, such as hormonal changes, reproductive losses, poverty, cultural influences, and abuse. A clinician, determining treatment for a woman suffering from disordered mood must rely on an integrated model that includes all the factors that may influence the patient's mood status.

Prevalence of, risk factors for, and biopsychosocial influences on mood disorders are reviewed in this chapter, especially as they pertain to women. The most commonly seen diagnoses from the American Psychiatric Association's (APA) *Diagnostic and Statistical Manual, 4/e (DSM-IV)* are outlined to provide a review of presenting signs and symptoms and to help with differential diagnosis. The major emphasis of the chapter is on the evaluation and treatment recommendations, including history gathering, clinical workup, treatment methods, and risks of nontreatment.

Epidemiology

Epidemiologic studies demonstrate repeatedly that 13–20% of people in any community sample exhibit depressive symptoms. Other studies show 1-year prevalence rates for major depression in the range of 2.6–6.2%. Lifetime prevalence for male and female patients combined is 14% (9–26%) in women; 5–12% in men), and the female-to-male ratio is 2–3:1. The highest rates of major depression occur in patients who are between 18 and 44 years old, with the highest occurrence between 25 and 34 years.

Thirty percent of depressions in women start in association with a reproductive event such as menarche, menses, pregnancy, childbirth, infertility, menopause, or oral contraceptive exposure. Additionally, women predominate with respect to unipolar depression, seasonal depression, and rapid-cycling mood disorders.

Epidemiology
A Biopsychosocial Model
Risk Factors
Clinical Findings & Diagnosis
Evaluation
Treatment
Issues of Pregnancy & Treatment for Depression
Age-Related Aspects of Depression
Referral to a Specialist
Summary

A Biopsychosocial Model

A biopsychosocial model currently is used to attempt to understand the causes of mood disorders. Biologic factors include heredity, age, physical illness, circadian cycles, and endocrine physiology. Psychological factors include personality features that may predispose to mood disturbance. Some personality traits found more often in women are correlated with vulnerability to depression; these include passive, avoidant, dependent, and learned helplessness features. Social factors particularly prevalent in the lives of women include poverty, abuse, gender discrimination, caretaking burdens, and low social status. Factors such as culture and ethnicity impact differently on men and women. All of the above influences are hypothesized to affect people on a biochemical level, causing dysregulation of basic neurophysiology at the cellular level of the brain, leading to mood disturbance.

Serotonin, norepinephrine, dopamine, and the endorphins are four of the chemoreceptor systems believed to be important in mood regulation. Additional neuroreceptors are being studied. Both estrogen and progesterone have effects on these receptor systems and are hypothesized to be significant in female-specific disturbances such as premenstrual syndrome (PMS) and perimenopausal complaints. The additional dysfunction in the hypothalamic-pituitary-adrenal axis seen in depression currently is being studied. Mood disorders also may be associated with thyroid dysfunction, particularly hypothyroidism.

Risk Factors

A. Hormonal Fluctuations: Hormonal fluctuations are known to interact with neurotransmitters, the neuroendocrine axis, and circadian systems. Girls begin to outnumber boys in rates of depression at the time of menarche. A significant percentage of women report mood or somatic changes premenstrually. Between 30 and 50% of women report depressive symptoms as a side effect of oral contraceptives; this factor accounts for approximately 40% of discontinuations of these agents. Pregnancy generally is associated with the lowest rates of psychiatric disorders, whereas the postpartum time period is associated with the highest rates of depression. Menopause—more accurately, perimenopause—has not been associated clearly with an increased risk for major mood disorders but is certainly a time for increased complaints of insomnia, irritability, lability, concentration and memory problems, and fatigue. Infertility and reproductive losses have a negative impact on mood in many women. Reproductive hormonal manipulation to enhance fertility or treat perimenopausal irregular bleeding sometimes disrupts mood homeostasis.

B. Genetic Factors: The effects of genetic factors on mood are well documented. A major study by Kendler conducted on female twin pairs showed a substantial influence from genetics on the 1-year prevalence for major depression. Another study of first-degree relatives of depressed and normal subjects showed a doubling of risk for depression in the relatives of affected compared to nonaffected individuals. In this study by Weissman et al, the female relatives of depressed subjects had a 1:3 chance of a depressive episode, and the male relatives had a 1:6 chance.

C. Sleep Disturbance: A sleep disturbance may contribute to the risk of major depression. Sleep studies show that female patients have higher total sleep requirements than male patients and yet often are relatively sleep-deprived. Insomnia often precedes the onset of depression; perimenopausal women, in particular, may have disrupted sleep because of vasomotor symptoms at night; or postpartum women may have disrupted sleep related to infant feeding.

D. Psychologic Factors: Cognitive and personality styles, as discussed previously, may affect mood. Family and culture-bound traditions regarding female roles emphasize responsibility toward family over self, dependency, compliance, self-sacrifice, and physical beauty, rather than assertiveness, self-direction, physical expression in work and play, and independent creativity.

E. Social Factors: Women and children comprise 75% of the population of the United States living in poverty. Although marriage decreases the risk of depression in men, married women are more likely to be depressed than their single counterparts. An unhappy marriage is a major risk factor for depression in women, whose depression rates are 3 times higher than those of their spouses. The number of children in the home has a positive correlation with rates of depression. Domestic violence and history of prior or current victimization also afflict women more commonly than men and are major risk factors for depression. Dysfunctional work environments, in which low status, poor pay, and sexual harassment are factors, contribute toward an increased risk for dysphoric and depressed mood. Bereavement in women triggered by reproductive losses, death of a child, divorce, or widowhood can precipitate a depressive episode.

F. Predisposing Psychiatric and Medical Illnesses: Examples of the many illnesses associated with mood disorders include anxiety disorders, substance abuse, eating disorders, posttraumatic stress disorder, sleep disorders, hypothyroidism, and hyperthyroidism. Autoimmune illness is more prevalent in women than in men, and the resultant pain symptoms and steroid exposure are added risk factors for depression and mood instability. Also, stroke and dementia often are accompanied by depression.

G. History of Depression: Current data support a high risk for recurrent depression in patients over the life cycle. A prospective study by the National Institutes of Mental Health of 555 patients with unipolar depression shows a relapse rate following recovery of the index episode of up to 61% at the 5-year mark.

H. Medications: Among the agents that may cause mood disturbances are prednisone, beta-blockers, and antihypertensives. A careful evaluation of any patient's mood would include a review of current and recent medication exposure.

Clinical Findings & Diagnosis

The most common depression diagnoses in primary care settings are major depressive episode, adjustment disorder with depressed mood, and dysthymic disorder. The criteria for these and most of the other, less common forms of depression described in the following sections are taken directly from the *DSM-IV*. For all of these diagnoses, the symptoms must not be caused by substance use or an organic condition.

A. Major Depressive Episode: The *DSM-IV* criteria for a major depressive disorder require that "five (or more) of the following symptoms have been present during the same 2-week period and represent a change from previous functioning; at least one of the symptoms is either (1) depressed mood or (2) loss of interest or pleasure."

The additional symptoms referred to in the APA criteria include (3) weight loss or gain, (4) insomnia or hypersomnia, (5) psychomotor agitation or retardation, (6) fatigue or low energy, (7) feelings of worthlessness or excessive guilt, (8) diminished ability to think or concentrate, and (9) recurrent thoughts of death, suicidal ideation, or suicide attempt. Beck Depression Inventory scores are usually in the range of the upper teens to greater than 20 on a scale of 0–63. (The Beck Depression Inventory, a self-administered multiple-choice questionnaire that takes minutes to complete, is a well-established and easily understood clinical tool that indicates both presence of depression and degree of severity.)

B. Adjustment Disorder With Depressed Mood: This condition is defined as the development of symptoms, either emotional or behavioral, in response to an identifiable stressor (or stressors) that has occurred in the preceding 3 months; and the patient experiences a drop in mood and other symptoms common to depression but does not fulfill criteria for major depression. The reaction (1) causes impairment in social or occupational functioning and distress in excess of what would be expected from exposure to the stressor, and (2) is of a significant level and has not lasted longer than 6 months. Once the stressor has been eliminated, the symptoms do not last for longer than another 6 months.

C. Dysthymic Disorder: A patient who is chronically depressed for at least 2 years and has at least two of the following symptoms is diagnosed as having dysthymic disorder: (1) changes in appetite, (2) insomnia or hypersomnia, (3) low energy or fatigue, (4) diminished self-esteem, (5) poor concentration or difficulty with decision-making, and (6) feelings of hopelessness. Scores on the Beck Depression Inventory usually are elevated but not in the range seen for major depression. During the 2-year period, the person has never been free from the symptoms for more than 2 months at a time. No major depressive episode has been present during the first 2 years of the disturbance. The symptoms cause clinical distress or impairment in social or occupational functioning.

D. Seasonal Depression: Known also as seasonal affective disorder (SAD), seasonal depression requires identification of a regular temporal relationship between the onset of mood episodes and a particular time of the year, eg, regular occurrence of a depressive episode in the fall or winter. The change from depression to euthymia or hypomania also occurs at a characteristic time of the year, eg, depression disappears in the spring. In the previous 2 years, two depressive episodes must have occurred following the same seasonal pattern, and no nonseasonal depressions may have occurred outside the pattern. Seasonal depressive episodes must outnumber the nonseasonal episodes that have occurred over the patient's lifetime. This disorder is more common in female than male patients and often presents with striking hypersomnia, lethargy, weight gain, and dysthymia.

E. Rapid-Cycling Bipolar Disorder: Rapid-cycling bipolar disorder is a disturbance of mood meeting criteria for major depression at times and for mania or hypomania at other times. These cycles must occur at least 4 times annually, and the episodes must meet the criteria for a major depressive, manic, mixed, or hypomanic episode. This disorder is much more common in female than male patients.

F. Bipolar Disorder: Bipolar disorder has several separate criteria sets depending on the subtype as defined in *DSM-IV*. This disorder refers to an individual suffering from a mood disturbance that includes cycles of elevated mood states. **Mania** is defined as a period of elevated mood with at least 3 of the following symptoms present: (1) sense of grandiosity, (2) decrease in the need for sleep, (3) increase in talkativeness, (4) thought racing, (5) distracted or agitated easily, (6) buying sprees, (7) sexual indiscretion.

G. Cyclothymia Disorder: Criteria for this disorder include at least a 2 year history of cyclic mood disturbance with elevation of mood and depression of mood. Neither of these mood states fulfills criteria for major depression or mania. The person has not been without symptoms for more than 2 months during the 2 year period.

H. Postpartum Depression: Postpartum depression occurs in 10–20% of women who give birth; it may have a delayed onset of from 6 weeks to 3–4 months after delivery and a course of from 6 months to 1 year. *DSM-IV* criteria require onset within 4 weeks of delivery and may include manic or mixed episodes as well as episodes of major depression.

Puerperal psychosis occurs after approximately 1 in 1000 deliveries. A prior episode carries a risk of a repeat episode of 1:3.

I. Premenstrual Dysphoric Disorder: Also known as premenstrual syndrome (PMS), premenstrual dysphoric disorder is a constellation of symptoms that often includes a disturbance in mood confined to the premenstrual phase. A period of at least 2 weeks of each cycle is not affected. Diagnosis is made most accurately with prospective daily calendar ratings (see Chapter 44).

Evaluation

Up to 75% of patients with identified depressions are treated in the primary care setting, although many cases go unrecognized and untreated. Depression can be missed easily if other presenting complaints such as somatic symptoms are emphasized, if the depression is masked, or if the patient is not asked specific questions about depressive symptoms. Unfortunately, inquiry into the patient's mental health in the medical setting can be perceived as a lack of validation on the part of the provider of the patient's presenting complaints. Providers need to attend to the patient's presenting problems seriously, as well as to offer educational information regarding the importance of additional inquiry concerning mental health. If depression is identified coincident with the patient's presenting illness or routine well care, timely evaluation of the mood problem is indicated assuming the patient is willing. If additional evaluation by a mental health specialist is indicated, further education may be necessary for the reluctant patient.

Brochures that define depression and mood disturbance are available for placement in waiting areas; these materials inform patients of the contemporary understandings of depressive illness, ie, that it is not a weakness, that often it does not abate without treatment, that lack of treatment has ramifications in terms of quality of life and risks of suicide and substance abuse, and that treatment is successful when well-established clinical guidelines are followed.

Women who have depression often present in medical settings with conditions such as fatigue, pain, or headache. If depression is suspected, a screening tool such as the Beck Depression Inventory can be used during the visit. The inventory also can direct a clinician to critical problem areas such as suicidality, sleep disturbance, and weight change, although it cannot substitute for the provider's careful history.

In brief visits there may not be time to attend to more than the primary presenting problem; if a mood disorder is suspected, the patient should be asked to come back as soon as possible for additional evaluation and history.

A thorough past and current medical and mental health history, including psychosocial aspects, is the standard for evaluation. Included also are a history of recent stressors, medication exposure, prior treatment efforts, past or current abuse, and depression in other family members; most important are the patient's mind-set concerning her mental health and the provider's impression of her psychologic status.

The history must include attention to hormonal status, cyclic mood changes, pregnancy or prepregnancy status, any physical condition that can aggravate or cause depression, medication (over-the-counter and prescribed), and substance exposure. Inquiries are made concerning job and family satisfaction, recent loss or trauma, and recent major stressors. Evaluation of suicidal or homicidal ideation, self-harm impulses, and parenting safety are priorities in history gathering.

Studies show that the strongest predictors for major depression are recent stressful life events, a positive family history, a prior episode, and the presence of other psychiatric disorders. A positive history in these areas warrants further evaluation of depression and predepression symptoms. The discovery of predepression symptoms such as sleep disturbance, mild anhedonia, and beginning loss of motivation might prompt preventive measures to attempt to circumvent the development of a more chronic and refractory depression subtype. The recommendation of increased exercise, stress reduction and relaxation training might prevent a major depressive episode. With a positive history one might intervene earlier with medications and\or therapy. Certainly, monitoring a patient under these circumstances is warranted.

Additional evaluation of a patient with a mood disorder generally includes a physical examination; a test of thyroid function, especially in women older than 50; additional laboratory studies if indicated; and an ECG if the patient is elderly or has a history of cardiac disturbance. A patient with perimenopausal and depression symptoms might benefit from obtaining a measure of follicle-stimulating hormone (FSH) or estradiol.

Psychologic testing is not routine in the workup of patients with mood disorder; however, it is indicated if the differential includes the possibility of dementia or unusual memory and cognitive problems beyond those typical to depressed patients. Many perimenopausal and geriatric patients complain of memory difficulties, and the extent of the evaluation depends on the provider's clinical intuition regarding the presence of organic factors.

Treatment

Dysfunction in terms of parenting, work, interpersonal relationships, marriage, and general quality of life is high for depressed people. Suicide rates of depressed people range from 10% to 15%. Susceptibility to other illnesses may be increased. Poor self-care and high-risk health behaviors such as smoking, overeating, lack of exercise, and alcohol abuse are additional problems associated with depression. It is hoped that identifying depressed patients and initiating treatment will minimize the morbidity of untreated depression.

Excellent studies have been done proving the efficacy of treatment for mood disorders; rates of response to treatment are reported to be in the range of 60–80%. Studies of mild-to-moderate depression have shown equal effectiveness of antidepressant pharmacotherapy and cognitive/behavioral or interpersonal psychotherapy. Antidepressant medications are indicated strongly for severe depressions. A combination of antidepressants and weekly psychotherapy is often the initial treatment of choice.

Patients who have been in psychotherapy in the past andare presenting with an acute or chronic depression may opt for pharmacotherapy only. Patients in whom depression is refractory or recurrent often benefit from supportive psychotherapy because medications may take longer to be effective in subsequent episodes, and the interim suffering is often great. Feelings of hopelessness and the possibility of suicide must be monitored in more refractory and treatment-resistant patients.

In addition to initiating one of the treatments outlined in the following sections, it is helpful for the clinician to provide educational material for the patient. An excellent book for patients to read is *Depression and Its Treatment* by Griest and Jefferson.

A. Psychotherapy: Psychotherapy alone may be recommended in adolescents with depression, patients with mild and situational mood disturbances, and women who are strongly opposed to taking medication. Pregnant patients and those planning a pregnancy are good candidates for psychotherapy alone. The initial response to psychotherapy may be somewhat slower than to medication, a fact best explained to the patient when weighing the pros and cons of the options for treatment.

Psychotherapy is practiced by a diverse group of providers with a variety of academic degrees and training; the most common practitioners are therapists with an masters degree, psychologists with a PhD degree, and psychiatrists with an MD degree. Referrals should be made to known therapists with excellent reputations, good training, and a track record of reasonable outcomes. Attempting to provide a good match between therapist and patient is beneficial. Most states have licensing boards for mental health practitioners and have on record any disciplinary actions related to licensed professionals. Boundary violations such as sexual abuse are not uncommon in the therapy profession and can be highly damaging to patients. Referrals should be made with caution and the patients told to trust their instincts regarding therapists. It is helpful to inform patients that they have several options and to encourage them to recontact the primary provider if an initial referral does not work well.

"Side effects" of psychotherapy need to be considered. In some instances, increased insight may precipitate life changes, with subsequent increase in stressors, eg, a patient who leaves a miserable marriage and undergoes a change in financial status, a major relocation, or a reduction in contact with her children. Therapy also may be the setting in which child abuse experiences that have been "tucked away" for years are brought into conscious awareness, with the attendant psychologic pain.

B. Pharmacotherapy:

1. Antidepressants–Pharmacotherapy is indicated in cases of severe depression, of milder but chronic depression that has not responded to an adequate trial of psychotherapy, and of depression with anxiety and multiple vegetative symptoms. At times medications are tried because a depressed patient is unwilling or unable to seek psychotherapy. Numerous other factors may contribute to the decision to prescribe antidepressants, such as a history of severe pain, fibromyalgia, long-standing fatigue, or severe PMS.

When a provider decides to recommend a medication trial to a patient, the first action is inform the patient of pros, cons, and alternative options of pharmacotherapy. It is helpful to stress that the initial prescription is a trial of medication and that if the benefits outweigh the side effects, the trial will become longer term treatment.

Choosing an initial agent depends on the provider and the patient. Providers should prescribe agents with which they are familiar and that they use frequently; patients often can participate in the selection when given adequate information about the side-effect profiles common to these agents.

It is important to inform patients that all antidepressants studied demonstrate equal efficacy in the treatment of depression; greater than 70% of depressed patients respond with mood improvement. The tricyclic antidepressants (TCAs), which have stood the test of time (up to 4 decades), are often a good choice for patients with pain syndromes or headaches. They are generally inexpensive and provide latitude in terms of flexibility of dosage. Data on long-term exposure to these older agents are abundant. The downside of these drugs is their side-effect profile (Table 13–1) and high lethality in overdose. The selective serotonin reuptake inhibitors (SSRIs), which are newer medications, have a minimal side-effect profile, are much safer in overdose, but are expensive. Antidepressant effects are not immediate with either kind of drug therapy but often take from 10 days to 6 weeks to appear.

Studies and experience show that side effects of all antidepressants are most common in the initial and early phases of treatment. One study of patients taking antidepressants found minimal complaints of side effects at the 6-month point. Dry mouth and constipation tend to be persistent side effects with the TCAs. Women are especially prone to weight gain with the TCAs. Active and athletic women often complain of decreased tolerance for aerobic exercise when taking a TCA. A tendency toward lighter sleep, which may persist in patients taking an SSRI, can be treated with low dosages of trazodone at bedtime, in addition to the primary daytime agent. Gastrointestinal complaints of patients taking SSRIs tend to be early-phase side effects and rarely persist beyond 3–5 weeks.

Patients should be warned that antidepressants can augment the effects of ethyl alcohol. In general, taking antidepressants is a contraindication to alcohol use because of the negative interactions between alcohol and antidepressants, such as the depressive effects of alcohol on the central nervous system, and the negative effects of alcohol on sleep quality. Table 13–2 compares the advantages and side effects of TCAs with those of SSRIs.

Bupropion, neither a TCA nor an SSRI, has the following advantages: minimal side effects, no sexual side effects, efficacy in SAD, a tendency toward activation rather than sedation, and no weight gain. Its drawbacks include the necessity to take it 3 times daily, lowering of seizure threshholds, minimal anxiolytic effects, and lightening of the sleep cycle (bedtime dosage should be avoided).

Trazodone is an antidepressant that usually causes sedation; its use as a primary antidepressant is lim-

Table 13–1. Side-effect profiles of antidepressant medications.*

| | Side Effect† | | | | | | |
| | Central Nervous System | | | Cardiovascular | | Other | |
Drug	Anticholin-ergic‡	Drowsiness	Insomnia/ Agitation	Orthostatic-Hypotension	Cardiac Arrhythmia	Gastroin-testinal Distress	Weight Gain (Over 6 kg)
Amitriptyline	4+	4+	0	4+	3+	0	4+
Desipramine	1+	1+	1+	2+	2+	0	1+
Doxepin	3+	4+	0	2+	2+	0	3+
Imipramine	3+	3+	1+	4+	3+	1+	3+
Nortriptyline	1+	1+	0	2+	2+	0	1+
Protriptyline	2+	1+	1+	2+	2+	0	0
Trimipramine	1+	4+	0	2+	2+	0	3+
Amoxapine	2+	2+	2+	2+	3+	0	1+
Maprotiline	2+	4+	0	0	1+	0	2+
Trazodone	0	4+	0	1+	1+	1+	1+
Bupropion	0	0	2+	0	1+	1+	0
Fluoxetine	0	0	2+	0	0	3+	0
Paroxetine	0	0	2+	0	0	3+	0
Sertraline	0	0	2+	0	0	3+	0
Monoamine Oxidase Inhibitors (MAOIs)	1	1+	2+	2+	0	1+	2+

*Reproduced from Depression Guideline Panel: *Depression in Primary Care: Detection, Diagnosis, and Treatment. Quick Reference Guide for Clinicians.* (Clinical Practice Guideline No. 5, AHCPR Publication No. 93-0552.) Department of Health and Human Services, Public Health Service, Agency for Health Care Policy and Research, 1993.
†0 = absent or rare.
1+
2+ = in between.
3+
4+ = relatively common.
‡Dry mouth, blurred vision, urinary hesitancy, constipation.

ited, therefore, because of difficulty achieving a therapeutic dose. It also can cause heart block and priapism on rare occasions and has less of an antipanic effect than other agents. It is an inexpensive agent useful at bedtime to promote stage 4 sleep and may be used with more activating agents, such as SSRIs and bupropion.

Venlafaxine is a newly marketed antidepressant with both SSRI and norepinephrine reuptake inhibition activity. It is sometimes effective for patients in whom treatment with TCAs or SSRIs has failed to help. The common side effects of this agent are similar to those seen with the SSRIs (see Table 13–1).

Monoamine oxidase inhibitors (MAOIs) can be

Table 13–2. Comparison of tricyclic antidepressants (TCAs) with selective serotonin reuptake inhibitors (SSRIs).

	TCAs	SSRIs
Advantages	Effective Dosage flexibility Variety of types available Long-term data available Inexpensive Better with pain conditions	Effective Single daily dose Three types available Newer than TCAs Expensive Better with obsessive-compulsive disorder
Disadvantages	Dry mouth Constipation Heart block Tachycardia Postural changes in blood pressure Weight gain Sedation in some types of depression Anorgasmia Lethal in overdose	Occasional loose stools, flatulence Can trigger premature ventricular contractions in some patients Rare reports of bradycardia Weight loss Lightens sleep cycle Anorgasmia Much safer than TCAs in overdose Gastrointestinal side effects Jitteriness Akathisia

used in patients who have a history of a positive response to these agents or in whom TCAs and SSRIs have failed to help. They are believed to be safer than other agents in bipolar depression because there is less risk for the induction of mania. The significant drawbacks of MAOIs include hypertensive crisis if combined with tyramine-containing foods or sympathomimetic drugs, dietary restrictions, weight gain, drug interactions, postural hypotension, and the necessity for a washout period of approximately 2 weeks between stopping one of these drugs and beginning another type of antidepressant. The serotonin syndrome is a risk factor for patients exposed to SSRIs and MAOIs in a close temporal relationship. This syndrome of autonomic instability can be life-threatening.

2. Mood stabilizers–Mood stabilizers are prescribed for patients with bipolar disorder, rapid cycling, and refractory and recurrent unipolar depression. Medications in this category include lithium, carbamazepine, and valproic acid. They all require close monitoring of the patient and lab screening of drug levels and specific blood tests (such as CBC, LFT, or TSH depending on the agent during treatment. Because lithium can cause hypothyroidism, levels of thyroid-stimulating hormone (TSH) should be monitored during exposure. Often combinations of two of these three agents are prescribed in patients with rapid-cycling bipolar or unipolar disorders or patients with refractory mania.

3. Augmentation–The term augmentation applies to the addition of a second agent to a patient's regimen when the primary agent has provided a partial response, or when a mild relapse has occurred and the clinician does not want to increase the dosage of the primary agent. The augmenting agent boosts the positive treatment effect of the primary agent. Common augmentation agents include lithium in low dosage (300–900 mg/d); thyroid medication, such as sodium liothyronine (Cytomel) (25–50 µg/d); buspirone; trazodone; TCAs; and SSRIs.

4. Dosage guidelines–Table 13–3 presents the

Table 13–3. Pharmacology of antidepressant medications.*

Drug	Therapeutic Dosage Range (mg/d)	Average (Range) of Elimination Half-Lives (h)[†]	Potentially Fatal Drug Interactions
Tricyclics			
Amitriptyline (Elavil, Endep)	75–300	24 (16–46)	Antiarrhythmics, monoamine oxidase inhibitors (MAOIs)
Clomipramine (Anafranil)	75–300	24 (20–40)	Antiarrhythmics, MAOIs
Desipramine (Norpramin, Pertofrane)	75–300	18 (12–50)	Antiarrhythmics, MAOIs
Doxepin (Adapin, Sinequan)	75–300	17 (10–47)	Antiarrhythmics, MAOIs
Imipramine (Janimine, Tofranil)	75–300	22 (12–34)	Antiarrhythmics, MAOIs
Nortriptyline (Aventyl, Pamelor)	40–200	26 (18–88)	Antiarrhythmics, MAOIs
Protriptyline (Vivactil)	20–60	76 (54–124)	Antiarrhythmics, MAOIs
Trimipramine (Surmontil)	75–300	12 (8–30)	Antiarrhythmics, MAOIs
Heterocyclics			
Amoxapine (Asendin)	100–600	10 (8–14)	MAOIs
Bupropion (Wellbutrin)	225–450	14 (8–24)	MAOIs (possibly)
Maprotiline (Ludiomil)	100–225	43 (27–58)	MAOIs
Trazodone (Desyrel)	150–600	8 (4–14)	—
Selective Serotonin Reuptake Inhibitors (SSRIs)			
Fluoxetine (Prozac)	10–40	168 (72–360)[‡]	MAOIs
Paroxetine (Paxil)	20–50	24 (3–65)	MAOIs[§]
Sertraline (Zoloft)	50–150	24 (10–30)	MAOIs[§]
Monoamine Oxidase Inhibitors (MAOIs)[∥]			For all three MAOIs: Vasoconstrictors,[¶] decongestants,[¶] meperidine, and possibly other narcotics
Isocarboxazid (Marplan)	30–50	Unknown	
Phenelzine (Nardil)	45–90	2 (1.5–4.0)	
Tranylcypromine (Parnate)	20–60	2 (1.5–3.0)	

*Reproduced from *Depression Guideline Panel: Depression in Primary Care: Detection, Diagnosis and Treatment. Quick Reference Guide for Clinicians.* (Clinical Practice Guideline No. 5, AHCPR Publication No. 93-0552.) Department of Health and Human Services, Agency for Health Care Policy and Research, 1993.
[†]Half-lives are affected by age, sex, race, concurrent medications, and length of drug exposure.
[‡]Includes both fluoxetine and norfluoxetine.
[§]By extrapolation from fluoxetine data.
[∥]MAO inhibition lasts longer (7 days) than drug half-life.
[¶]Including pseudoephedrine, phenylephrine, phenylpropanolamine, epinephrine, norepinephrine, and others.

standard dosage ranges for antidepressants. In patients with high anxiety or panic, SSRIs should be started at low dosages (2–5 mg fluoxetine, 25 mg sertraline, 10 mg paroxetine); short-acting benzodiazepines should be prescribed as needed in the early phase to treat adrenergic side effects, which generally clear in 2–3 weeks. If the patient's sleep pattern is a significant presenting problem or deteriorates, trazodone or an alternative agent may be added at bedtime. The bedtime agent can be discontinued after a few weeks to months, although some patients continue to need it for the duration of treatment.

Elderly patients should be started on antidepressant therapy with low dosages, eg, nortriptyline 10 mg, fluoxetine 2–5 mg. All patients must be monitored carefully for side effects and drug interactions.

5. Trial and treatment time guidelines–An adequate trial of an antidepressant is 3–4 weeks for TCAs or 6 weeks for SSRIs. For patients who respond initially and relapse partially during their treatment, one can increase the dosage within the drug's therapeutic range. The side-effect profile and recommended dosage guidelines often dictate the drug's upper dosage limit. Blood levels of the drugs are called for infrequently because of lack of availability or reliability; it is best to leave it to a psychiatric consultant to order these tests.

Medications are started at low dosages and increased during the first 1–2 weeks depending on tolerance. It is best to see patients again within 7–14 days of initiating medication to evaluate mood, anxiety, sleep, functional status, side effects, and suicidal ideation. If a patient is feeling better and having minimal side effects, one can adjust the dosage at this first return visit and see the patient again in 2–6 weeks. If the patient is doing well and a therapeutic dosage has been determined with reasonable certainty, subsequent visits can be scheduled for every 2–4 months. Frequency of visits in the first 3 months of antidepressant therapy depend in part on side effects, clinical response, and confidence in the dosage adjustment. Patients should be told to call or schedule an appointment if their mood falters and cycles down over a period of several days or if associated symptoms of depression reemerge, such as sleep disturbance or panic. At the 9-month point for patients with first-onset, single-episode depression, one can begin to educate the patient about tapering off medications. Tapering may start after 9–12 months of therapy and is best done over a period of several weeks with monitoring. If symptoms of depression return, medication can be restarted or increased to the level that was most effective or brought full remission.

C. Refractory and Recurrent Illness: Refractoriness is most common in patients with complex psychiatric conditions, such as those with depression and anxiety or with major depression superimposed on chronic dysthymia, dissociative disorder, posttrau-

matic stress disorder, or personality disorder. Patients who responded in the past but relapsed after drug discontinuation and failed to respond again after retreatment are another example of refractory patients. Patients with refractory illness are best referred for psychiatric consultation because they may require multiple medications, electroconvulsive therapy, or mood stabilizers. These patients also need increased support for living with a chronic illness.

Even in the best of circumstances, relapse rates for major depression are as follows: 50% after one episode, 70% after two, and 90% after three. Longer periods of medication maintenance currently are being recommended for patients with recurrent depression, and the guidelines for duration of treatment are being determined.

D. Additional Therapies: Electroconvulsive therapy (ECT) is helpful in some conditions such as rapid-cycling mixed mania and dysphoria, psychotic depression, and refractory depression. The side effects include short-term memory impairment, stigma, and often, rapid relapse after treatment stops even when medications have been restarted.

Phototherapy is indicated if a patient has SAD alone or in combination with major depression, dysthymic disorder, or both. Two types available include a phototherapy panel and the dawn simulator. The former has been studied more extensively than the latter but requires sitting near the light panel daily for 30–60 minutes. Headache is a possible side effect. A family history of retinal eye disease is an indication for ophthalmologic consultation before panel exposure. The dawn simulator turns light on gradually in the bedroom, simulating a spring dawn. Outdoor midday exposure to natural light for 1 hour also has been shown to have benefit.

Other therapies include support groups, group psychotherapy, day treatment, exercise, movement therapies, and acupuncture, their effectiveness is variable. Vitamin B_6 may be tried in patients with oral-contraceptive-related mild depression; a dosage of 25–50 mg twice daily is recommended. Stimulants are tried sometimes in elderly patients. Sleep deprivation is another intervention that has demonstrated some effectiveness.

Issues of Pregnancy & Treatment for Depression

All women of childbearing age must be considered at risk for pregnancy. It is important to ask these patients about pregnancy plans or prevention before initiating pharmacotherapy. If the patient is planning a pregnancy, the safest treatments are psychotherapy, support, phototherapy if indicated, and exercise. A review of risks of psychiatric medications during pregnancy was published recently by Miller. Tricyclics and fluoxetine have not been associated with increased risks of malformations, but neonates exposed in utero to TCAs have some risk for withdrawal symptoms at birth. Longer term behavioral teratogenicity has not been studied and is a concern until further research addresses this issue. A study by Pastuszak showed increased risk of first-trimester miscarriage in women taking TCAs or fluoxetine.

Age-Related Aspects of Depression

A. Adolescence: Adolescents often experience moodiness that seems related to their stage of development. For severely distressed patients, referral to psychotherapy is often advisable in lieu of medication treatment because adolescents have many psychosocial issues to be unraveled and appreciated, which may require a considerable amount of time. The effectiveness of medication is less well studied and demonstrated in this age group, and these patients are often sensitive to the side effects. Adolescents also present challenges in the areas of compliance and impulsivity.

For adolescents who continue to be depressed after a course of psychotherapy, a trial of medication is indicated. The provider should keep in mind cardiac sensitivity (ie, sinus tachycardias, postural sensitivity) to TCAs and check the patient's pulse rate and postural blood pressure. SSRIs are much safer than other drugs if taken in overdose, and they are better tolerated in athletic girls. Because antidepressants are rapidly metabolized in adolescents and children, they require the same weight-adjusted doses used for adults. Split-dose regimens sometimes sustain a more even blood level in adolescents, related to the more rapid biodegradation of these agents in this age group.

B. Mid-Life: For women in their 20s, 30s, and 40s, pregnancy and prepregnancy issues must be assessed in terms of treatment options. These women are in the age group most commonly treated for depression and often experience a number of the reproductive factors believed to be important in depression onset eg, delivery, hormonal changes associated with birth and lactation, miscarriage, oral contraceptive exposure, perimenopausal changes, and PMS. Additional factors to be considered include death of aging parents, caretaking burdens, work stress, divorce, financial stressors, and at times, the onset of conditions related to aging such as breast cancer or autoimmune illnesses. This age group is better informed than older generations in terms of treatment for depression and is an optimal group for both psychotherapy and pharmacotherapy.

C. Later Life: Older women with depression are a particularly challenging group to treat. They are often medically complex and may be taking many medications. Some older women are recently widowed, and bereavement symptoms may confuse their diagnosis. Members of this generation has been less open about mental health, and may feel more stigmatized than younger people do today if a psychiatric diagnosis is applied to themselves or a family member. In this age group, compromised physical health, memory impairment, high-risk for falling, and sensitivity to the side effects of antidepressants are important aspects of clinical treatment. Supportive psychotherapy, social services, and personal support are important treatment interventions. Medication trials should be started with low dosages that are raised gradually; the provider should not hesitate to check blood levels and should watch for drug interactions with other medications being taken.

Referral to a Specialist

Referral of the patient to a psychiatrist depends on the clinician's level of comfort with differential diagnosis of mood disorders, ability to distinguish affective illness from primary anxiety disorders, and confidence in working with the pharmacotherapy of mood disorders; another factor is the patient's willingness to see a consultant.

Patients with the following characteristics should be referred: (1) those considered at high risk of suicide, homicide, or self-abusive behavior; (2) patients with a history of past or current psychosis, dissociation, rapid cycling, refractory symptoms, mania, eating disorder, severe personality disorder, or active substance abuse; (3) noncompliant patients; (4) those highly sensitive to side effects of medication; (5) patients with partial or no response to two adequate medication trials; (6) those who relapse or experience breakthrough during treatment; and (7) those with complex medical conditions.

Referral for psychotherapy is common in the primary care setting. Phototherapy, electroconvulsive therapy, day treatment, inpatient treatment, and psychologic testing are less frequent referral requests. When a psychiatrist is consulted, he or she may take over the treatment of the patient, initiate treatment and refer the patient back to the primary care provider for continuation, or make recommendations to the primary provider, who initiates or tailors the treatment.

Summary

Mood disorders in women across the lifespan are common and multifactorial in origin. Early intervention rests on detection of these disorders and appreciation of related health issues: such as perimenopausual symptoms, sleep difficulties, hypothyroidism, anemia, and the range of psychosocial effects noted in the text of this chapter. The busy provider in today's health environment is under pressure to see more patients on a daily basis which makes detection and treatment of mood disorders in patients at times a challenge. A cooperative approach in the health care setting utilizing teamwork between physicians, nurses, and support staff and including consultative back-up from mental health providers will provide more optimal detection and quality treatment of mood disordered patients. Newly released guidelines for depression treatment from the Ameri-can Psychiatric Association and the U.S. Department of Health and Human Services are evident of strong support for detection, diagnosis, and treatment.

REFERENCES

American Psychiatric Association: *Diagnostic and Statistical Manual of Mental Disorders,* 4th ed. American Psychiatric Association, 1994.

American Psychiatric Association: Practice guidelines for major depressive disorder in adults. Am J Psychiatry 1993;150:1-51.

Angold A, Worthman CW: Puberty onset of gender differences in rates of depression: A developmental, epidemiologic and neuroendocrine perspective. J Affective Disorders 1993;29:145.

Angst J: Epidemiology of depression. Psychopharmacology 1992;106:71.

Beck AT et al: An inventory for measuring depression. Arch Gen Psychiatry 1961;4:561.

Blazer D et al: Depressive symptoms and depressive diagnoses in a community population. Arch Gen Psychiatry 1988;45:1078.

Bromberger JT, Costello EJ: Epidemiology of depression for clinicians. Soc Work 1992;37:120.

Depression Guideline Panel: *Depression in Primary Care.* Vol 1. *Diagnosis and Detection.* (Clinical Practice Guideline No. 5, AHCPR Publication No. 93-0550.) US Department of Health and Human Services, Public Health Service, Agency for Health Care Policy and Research, 1993.

Depression Guideline Panel: *Depression in Primary Care.* Vol 2. *Treatment of Major Depression.* (Clinical Practice Guideline No. 5, AHCPR Publication No. 93-0551.) US Department of Health and Human Services, Public Health Service, Agency for Health Care Policy and Research, 1993.

Depression Guideline Panel: Depression in Primary Care: Detection, Diagnosis and Treatment. *Quick Reference Guide for Clinicians.* (Clinical Practice Guideline No. 5, AHCPR Publication No. 93-0552.) Department of Health and Human Services, Public Health Service, Agency for Health Care Policy and Research, 1993.

Griest J, Jefferson J: *Depression and Its Treatment,* 2nd ed. American Psychiatric Press, 1993.

Jatlow PI: Psychotropic drug disposition during development. In: *Psychiatric Pharmacosciences of Children and Adolescents.* Popper C (editor). American Psychiatric Press, 1987.

Kendler KS et al: The prediction of major depression in women: Toward an integrated etiologic model. Am J Psychiatry 1993;150:1139.

Miller LJ: Psychiatric medication during pregnancy: Understanding and minimizing risks. Psychiatr Ann 1994;24:69.

Narrow WE et al: Use of services by persons with mental and addictive disorders: Findings from the National Institute of Mental Health epidemiological catchment area program. Arch Gen Psychiatry 1993;50:95.

Parry BL: Reproductive-related depressions in women: Phenomena of hormonal kindling? In: *Postpartum Psychiatric Illness.* Hamilton JA, Harberger PN (editors). University of Pennsylvania Press, 1992.

Pastuszak A et al: Pregnancy outcome following first-trimester exposure to fluoxetine (Prozac). JAMA 1993;269:2246.

Schmidt PJ, Rubinow DR: Menopause-related affective disorders: A justification for further study. Am J Psychiatry 1991;148:844.

Weissman MM: Advances in psychiatric epidemiology: Rates and risks for major depression. Am J Public Health 1987;77:445.

Weissman MM, Kidd KK, Prusoff BA: Variability in rates of affective disorders in relatives of depressed and normal probands. Arch Gen Psychiatry 1982;39:1397.

Weissman MM et al: Affective disorders in five United States communities. Psychol Med 1988;18:141.

Weissman MM et al: Sex differences in rates of depression: Cross-national perspectives. J Affective Disorders 1993;29:77.

Bereavement

Edward K. Rynearson, MD

The presumption that pathologic responses to death occur in coherent form, duration, and incidence is based on early reports of cases in treatment rather than reliable measurement and comparison. Freud's brilliant speculation that mourning (normal bereavement) and melancholia (pathologic grief) were separate but related was transformed into an a priori principle by subsequent theoreticians. This fruitful model was so compelling that clinical facts were strained to make them fit. The belief in the model led to a number of clinical axioms:

> The world is despised with mourning—the self is despised with grief.
> Mourning is inevitable and necessary and resolves in months.
> Mourning follows a sequence of discrete stages.
> Grief is a denial or aberrant fixation of mourning.
> Catharsis and active mourning promise recovery.

These clinical suppositions of the nature of grief were excessively simple; they were misleading, not because they were wrong, but because they were not entirely right. Several authors have reviewed the empirical work available to verify these presumptions about grief, and in all cases, the data cannot support them. The danger of such empirical refutation, however, is that the concepts, which have usefulness and relevance, will be discarded entirely.

To study so subjective and diverse a referent as pathologic grief requires, first, a tentative approach that is tolerant of multiple hypotheses, and second, a softening of the demand of empirical validation until the development of precise and specific measurement tools. Until then, it is advisable to remain skeptical when presented with certainties about the nature of pathologic grief and its treatment.

THE RISK OF GENDER

A review of clinical studies of grief demonstrates that a disproportionate number of women present for psychotherapy (3–4 times the frequency of men). The increased risk in women to develop unrecovered grief is consistent with recent epidemiologic surveys that demonstrate the high risk among women in the

---

The Risk of Gender
A Preliminary Typology of Pathologic Grief
    Dependent (Chronic) Grief Syndrome
    Unexpected Loss (Distorted) Grief
        Syndrome
    Conflicted (Delayed) Grief Syndrome
Therapeutic Implications
    Death & Symbology
    Psychotherapy
    Comorbidity & Medications
    Psychiatric Consultation
    Nonrecovery

---

general population for affective disorders, anxiety disorders, and somatization disorders.

The explanation for the apparent vulnerability of women remains obscure. To overemphasize the biologic and neuropsychologic uniqueness of women denies the uniqueness of their emotional attachments, of their primary role as caregivers, and of their economic calamity and role dysjunction when their spouse dies—all of which alone or in combination might be overwhelming. It would be misleading to deny the significance of any of the biopsychosocial variables that differentiate women's responses to grief from men's. Perhaps seeking help for intense grief responses is a more adaptive response than the prototypical male behavior of persistent stoicism and resistance of support. Clarification of these possibly gender-related responses to loss must await further, controlled research.

A PRELIMINARY TYPOLOGY OF PATHOLOGIC GRIEF

The development of a precise diagnostic classification of pathologic grief has been stymied by the vagueness and diversity of grief responses. In an effort to bring order, researchers have used several divergent research strategies:

1. Comparison of "abnormal" responses of grief with "normative" responses of bereavement.

2. Comparison of grief responses with categories of affective and anxiety disorders from the American Psychiatric Association's *Diagnostic and Statistical Manual (DSM-IV)*. (Although *DSM-IV* disorders offer some degree of reliability and a descriptive similarity to grief responses, there is no assurance that they are homologous entities.)
3. Enrollment of bereaved people in long-term prospective studies so that the emergence of dysfunctional responses can be monitored as they develop.

The long-term, prospective research strategy offers a more rigorous and systematic approach than the others while illuminating responses that are specific for nonrecovery. Because grief is measured in years instead of weeks or months, the slow, painstaking prospective study of the bereaved is required to delineate and monitor a typology of nonrecovery. Only a few researchers have committed themselves to such an arduous inquiry. Preliminary findings from prospective research suggest three distinct descriptive syndromes of intense, prolonged, and dysfunctional grief. Unfortunately, the studies lack standardized measures, which limits the predictive power and cross-validation of the data. The clinical usefulness of this typology lies in its linkage of descriptive syndromes of nonrecovery with premorbid phenomena within the individual and the relationship with the deceased as well as with the independent effects of specific forms of dying. The linkage sharpens the clinician's capacity to predict course and outcome as well as to shape strategies for intervention. The detailed description of this typology is contained in the authoritative works of Parkes and of Raphael, who cite their own data and review other longitudinal studies. Although their descriptions of the three pathologic syndromes of nonrecovery are nearly identical, the two researchers have labeled them differently. Raphael's label of each syndrome is shown parenthetically in Table 14–1.

Data are sufficient to suggest that dependent (chronic) grief is the most common of the three syndromes and conflicted (delayed) is the rarest. It must be emphasized that the three syndromes may be present in combination and that the interactive effects have not been clarified.

Dependent (Chronic) Grief Syndrome

Dependence here refers to a relationship of relative nondifferentiation, in which one's image is contingent on the availability of another person. Such dependence demands continuing interchange as a requisite in maintaining an image of self as whole and acceptable. The death of the person depended on initiates a pathogenic shift in the self-image toward the state of being weak, uncaring, and incompetent. Those pathologic self-images are potent and compelling organizers of perception and independently affect the thoughts, feelings, and behavior of the pathologic grief syndrome.

Unexpected Loss (Distorted) Grief Syndrome

The explanatory model for this syndrome proposes that the mode and onset of the dying itself has pathogenic effects. In assuming that focus, the model does not disregard the pathogenicity of premorbid ambivalence or dependency, but it cites the specific effects of sudden and unnatural dying.

A dysfunctional syndrome that reflects the incomplete and fragmentary resolution of grief is the **posttraumatic stress syndrome (PTSD)** of hyperreactivity (startle reactions, explosive outbursts of anger) and recurrent intrusive recollections of the dying (flashbacks, nightmares) alternating with a compensatory psychic numbing, constriction of affect and social functioning, and loss of a sense of control over one's destiny. Posttraumatic stress phenomena, identified as stages of shock or numbness by other authors, are observed commonly in the initial adjustment to death from any cause. However, these phenomena are intensely preoccupying and enduring following unexpected loss.

When unexpected loss is associated with an unnatural cause, such as accident, suicide, or homicide, the bereaved is further traumatized by the obligatory involvement in the investigation and media coverage of the death. With accidental and homicidal dying, there may be a continuing participation in the trial and punishment of a dying that bears the social stigma of transgression. Violence, violation, and volition are elements of unnatural dying that catalyze a prolonged traumatic bereavement. Preliminary studies of persons bereaved by unnatural dying have suggested specific syndromal effects associated with those "three Vs": violence associated with posttraumatic stress, violation with victimization, and volition with compulsive inquiry to establish blame and punish the perpetrator.

Table 14–1. Pathologic syndromes of nonrecovery.

1. **Dependent (chronic) grief syndrome:** Links clinging or over-reliant attachment to responses of immediate pining and chronic grief.
2. **Unexpected loss (distorted) grief syndrome:** Links unexpected loss to responses of immediate disbelief, avoidance, and anxiety, leading to chronic anxious withdrawal.
3. **Conflicted (delayed) grief syndrome:** Links conflicted ambivalent attachment to minimal immediate responses of anxiety and pining.

Conflicted (Delayed) Grief Syndrome

The conflicted (delayed) grief syndrome follows the death of an ambivalently valued figure in a situation in which ambivalence cannot be psychologically tolerated. The model suggests that these patients are unable to tolerate the unexpressed anger they have harbored toward the deceased. When intense anger for the lost figure is felt, it is directed at the self. Freud originally identified that dynamic as the basis of depression, in which the self is viewed as bad and worthless, in contrast to mourning, in which the external world seems impoverished. Although this model is limited as an explanatory principle for conflicted (delayed) grief syndrome, the unconscious denial of ambivalence might be operative when the grief appears after an inordinate delay.

THERAPEUTIC IMPLICATIONS

Death & Symbology

The way to become a part of the grief experience with the patient is through mutual exploring of the death. Death is not a generic event; it is the form and context of dying, rather than death itself, that gives meaning and structure to the grief experience.

Understanding the patient's concept of death may point to a personal symbology that has provided meaning and coherence. The meaningless, disintegrating impact of death distorts one's continuing efforts to anticipate the future with hope and purpose. Although most authors cite the issue of figuring out the "meaning of the death" as a final task that follows emotional adjustment and acceptance, it may be of paramount concern to a patient whose grief is fresh. Because the "hopeless and purposeless" distortion of the future may be operative from the outset of treatment, and because its presence presumably impedes recovery by its pessimism regarding engagement (including engagement with a therapist in therapy), establishment of sustaining and generative symbology is important throughout therapy. Focusing on activities that provide a basis for meaning, (eg, family, work, altruism, and religion), as well as deflecting the patient's nihilistic view of self into a search for meaning in the surrounding world, may enable the patient to divert her thoughts from the indeterminateness of death.

Psychotherapy

There are few controlled studies of the psychotherapy of unrecovered grief. Studies limited to support groups and short-term (15–20 sessions) individual psychotherapy demonstrate a measurable effectiveness during the first year of treatment. Patients undergoing treatment show a significant increase in their rate of recovery, but untreated patients show the same frequency of recovery after 2 years. Both treated and untreated patients demonstrate the same frequency of nonrecovery (15–30%).

It now appears that forms of intervention that are appropriate for one type of pathologic grief syndrome may be useless or even harmful in another. Presumably, abreactive strategies are appropriate for conflicted grief syndrome, cognitive and behavioral strategies for dependent grief syndrome, and techniques to modify posttraumatic stress for unexpected loss syndrome. The strategies are not mutually exclusive; a balanced combination that matches the changing percepts of the patient is clinically indicated. The exclusive use of a single therapeutic model would fail if misapplied, not from therapeutic resistance, but from therapeutic incongruity.

Comorbidity & Medications

Affective and anxiety disorders include many of the signs and symptoms of pathologic grief. Nearly one-half of patients with uncomplicated bereavement meet diagnostic criteria for depressive disorder during the first year of bereavement, and one-third meet criteria for an anxiety disorder as well. Those affective and anxiety responses begin to subside after 4–6 months of bereavement without treatment, but a sizable minority of persons (20%) remain depressed or anxious for many years.

Withholding medication from patients who present with refractory affective and anxiety disorders would border on clinical negligence, yet no study of the effectiveness of antidepressant and antianxiety drugs in patients with pathologic grief has been undertaken. Clinicians have not been discouraged from the use of medications in grieving patients, even though the practice has no empirical basis. The judicious use of medication in combination with psychotherapy seems a reasonable alternative, particularly in cases of refractory or intense and dysfunctional affective and anxiety disorders, for which there is abundant evidence of their effectiveness. Knowing that the patient and members of the extended family have a history of effective use of pharmacotherapy may alert the clinician to the inclusion of medication during the early phase of treatment.

Psychiatric Consultation

Referral to a psychiatrist should not be delayed by the promise of spontaneous recovery. Recent studies have documented that patients who show a particularly intense and dysfunctional response within the first 3–6 months of grieving are at high risk for nonrecovery. Patients who are unable to function at home or at work because of their despondency or who become preoccupied with suicide at any point during their recovery should be encouraged to seek psychiatric consultation.

Nonrecovery

Careful studies of patients treated for pathologic

grief invariably report that 15–30% are nonresponders. Grief-stricken patients should not be demoralized further by the offer of a therapy that promises short-term recovery or a narrow model that insists on one of several underlying causes. Because failed recovery is common to every prospective outcome study of pathologic grief, clinicians must be prepared to recognize and acknowledge therapeutic limitations rather than anticipate short-term recovery.

There is no known strategy or combination of strategies that ensures recovery, and patients should be reassured that failed recovery is not tantamount to personal failure. For purposes of ongoing support, clinicians need to maintain an optimism about the future, including an image of self-stability, that does not require "recovery" of what has been lost. Accommodating to this distressing subjective state requires steadfast courage and commitment. Perhaps all that can be offered is an empathic reassurance that both the clinician and the patient are doing their best.

REFERENCES

Bergen L: *Death and Dying: Theory, Research, Practice.* William C. Brown, 1979.

Freud S: Mourning and melancholia. In: *Complete Psychological Works of Sigmund Freud* (standard edition). Vol 14. Hogarth Press, 1957.

Horowitz MJ et al: Pathologic grief and the activation of self-image. Am J Psychiatry 1980;137:1157.

Jacobs SC: Attachment theory and multiple dimensions of grief. Omega 1987–1988;18:41.

Jacobs S: *Pathologic Grief: Maladaption to Loss.* American Psychiatric Press, 1993.

Kessler RC et al: Lifetime and 12-month prevalence of DSM-III-R psychiatric disorders in the United States: Results from the National Comorbidity Survey. Arch Gen Psychiatry 1994;51:8.

Parkes CM, Weiss RS: *Recovery from Bereavement.* Basic Books, 1983.

Raphael B: *The Anatomy of Bereavement.* Basic Books, 1983.

Rynearson EK: Psychologic adjustment to unnatural dying. In: *Biopsychosocial Aspects of Bereavement.* Zissok S (editor). American Psychiatric Press, 1987.

Rynearson EK: Psychotherapy of pathologic grief: Revision and limitations. Psychiatr Clin North Am 1987; 10:487.

Wortman CB, Silver RC: Coping with irrevocable loss. In: *Cataclysms, Crises, and Catastrophes: Psychology in Action.* VandenBos CR, Bryant BK (editors). American Psychological Association, 1987.

Wortman CB, Silver RC: The myths of coping with loss. J Consult Clin Psychol 1989;57:349.

Zisook S: Measuring symptoms of grief and bereavement. Am J Psychiatry 1982;139:1590.

Zisook S, Schuchter SR: Depression through the first year after the death of a spouse. Am J Psychiatry 1991; 148:1346.

15

Domestic Violence

Nancy Sugg, MD, MPH

Throughout any woman's life span, she will be at risk for violence from partners and family members. If she is abused, she will be confronted by a society that may blame her for the actions of her abusers. Although the law no longer sanctions domestic violence, the attitude that the beating of wives or partners is not truly criminal still prevails in the American culture.

INCIDENCE

Adolescent Women

Adolescence is a time of transition between living with family and living independently. It is a time of separating from the dependent relationship with family and forming new relationships with intimate partners. Unfortunately, for many young women, it is also a time of experiencing physical violence at the hands of family members, intimate partners, or both. Because adolescence is a period when behavior patterns and role models are formulated, violence experienced during this time may affect a woman's future significantly.

Rates of abuse of adolescents are difficult to find. Straus and Gelles' nationwide study of families found that 91 of 1000 adolescents between the ages of 15 and 17 were victims of severe or very severe assaults by their parents. McLeer and Anwar found that 42% of patients presenting to an emergency room with injuries related to domestic violence were between the ages of 18 and 20. Although studies vary regarding the relative rates of physical violence committed against female and male adolescents, young women clearly are more often the victims of sexual abuse. The health consequences for adolescents are less often injury from the abuse and more likely to be risky behaviors. Included in the destructive behaviors associated with abuse are chemical dependency, suicidal ideation or attempts, and running away from home.

Violence in intimate relationships is also a risk for teenage women. One study found that 9% of high school juniors and seniors, the majority of whom were female (65%), had been recipients of violence from a dating partner. More alarming is the effect violence had on the relationship: 23% felt the violence

| Incidence |
| Adolescent Women |
| Adult Women |
| Pregnant Women |
| Elderly Women |
| Clinical Findings |
| Chronic Pain |
| Somatic Complaints |
| Injury |
| Alcohol Abuse |
| Psychiatric Illness |
| Evaluation |
| Intervention |
| Referral |
| Follow-up |
| Documentation |

improved the relationship, 35% felt it did not change the relationship, and only 23% ended the relationship as a result of the violence. Jealousy and alcohol use were said to be common causes of the violence, and 35% of the adolescents interpreted the violence as an act of love.

Adult Women

Domestic violence often occurs in the privacy of the home and does not come to the attention of the medical or the criminal justice system. Because of this lack of reporting, reliable statistics on the annual incidence of domestic violence are unavailable. The best estimate of domestic violence in the general adult population comes from a study done in 1975 by Straus and Gelles. A nationwide, random sample of married and cohabitating couples were given an 18-item survey that described tactics that could be used to resolve conflicts. The tactics included physical violence, (eg, slapping), and severe violence (eg, beating up or using a knife or gun). The study revealed that 3–4% of both men and women had experienced at least one episode of severe violence in the year of the study. When extrapolated to the general population, this figure represents 1.8 million women per year who are subjected to severe violence. When couples experience severe violence, it is often not an

112

isolated event. In this study, of the women who experienced severe violence, 47% had three or more episodes per year.

One problem with the aforementioned study is that it did not include women who were in relationships but not cohabitating or women who were separated or divorced. The period of separation and divorce can be one of the most dangerous times for women in abusive relationships. When these groups are taken into account, it is estimated that 3–4 million women per year are victims of severe violence by their intimate partners.

Recently, researchers have begun to study the prevalence of domestic violence in primary care settings. Studies from areas as geographically diverse as Southern California, North Dakota, and the Midwest have found prevalence rates of 14–28%. Battering may present to medical providers more often as stress-related illnesses or somatic complaints than as broken bones or lacerations. Because of this fact, primary care providers are in a key position to intervene in cases of intentional violence.

Pregnant Women

Pregnancy is often thought to be a time of joyful expectation and closer commitment for a couple. For many women, however, it is a time of increased physical violence and fear. During this period, physical violence affects not only the health of the mother but also the health and safety of the unborn child.

McFarlane studied the frequency and severity of abuse in black, Hispanic, and non-Hispanic white pregnant women who attended public prenatal clinics. When all women were grouped together, it was found that 17% reported physical abuse during pregnancy. The abuse tended to be recurrent, with 60% experiencing two or more episodes of physical violence. White women experienced not only the most episodes of abuse, but also the most severe episodes of abuse. According to McFarlane's study, women who were abused were twice as likely to enter prenatal care in the third trimester as women who were not abused. Many women reported being denied access to transportation by their abusers, as well as being denied the use of vitamins or antibiotics that were prescribed during pregnancy.

Little research has been done on the pregnancy outcomes for battered women. One study looked at the incidence of low birth weight (< 2500 gm) babies born to battered and nonbattered women. After controlling for other factors associated with low birth weight, researchers found that battered women had a fourfold increase in low-birth-weight deliveries. The exact cause of the low-birth-weight deliveries is unknown, but Newberger offers several hypotheses, including blunt trauma to the abdomen; exacerbation of existing medical conditions such as diabetes, hypertension, or asthma; an increase in unsafe health habits such as smoking or alcohol use because of the psychologic stress of battering.

The sharp increase in numbers of teenage pregnancies is well known. Pregnancies in teenagers are already considered high-risk pregnancies, and battering only adds to the likelihood of a poor outcome. Nearly one-third of McFarlane's study group were teenagers. The pregnant teenagers had a higher rate of abuse during pregnancy (27.3%) than adult women (15.7%). They differed from older pregnant women in that they often identified multiple perpetrators. They were at risk for abuse not only from their boyfriend but also from their family members.

It is imperative that all pregnant women be screened for physical violence during prenatal visits throughout the pregnancy. Furthermore, any pregnant woman who presents with an injury needs to be asked if the injury was inflicted intentionally.

Elderly Women

Estimates of the rate of abuse of elderly women are difficult to obtain because of the hesitancy of victims to report the abuse and the problems of defining abuse. The best prevalence data come from a study done in Boston by Pillemor, reported by Benton and Marshall, in which 3.2% of elderly adults were found to have experienced physical abuse, psychologic abuse, or neglect. In 86% of cases of abuse of elderly women, the abuser is a relative, and 40% of the time, the relative is a spouse.

Although no single definition of abuse exists, most are similar to that of the American Medical Association Elderly Abuse Reporting Act; included in the definition are physical and psychologic injury; sexual abuse; and withholding of food, clothing, and medical care. However, other definitions have gone beyond physical and psychologic injury and included areas such as financial exploitation, isolation, and neglect.

Psychologic abuse of the elderly includes threats, humiliation, harassment, and isolation from friends and family. The mental health consequences of depression, anxiety, and insomnia are similar to those experienced by adult women.

Neglect includes failure to provide clean clothing and bedding; provision of inadequate food, water, or shelter; improper administration of medication; poor personal care. Some of the elements of neglect may fall more precisely under Fulmer and O'Malley's definition of "inadequate care of the elderly." The neglect may not be intentional; rather the neglect results from the caregiver's lack of education regarding the proper care of a dependent elderly person.

Exploitation of the elderly usually involves inappropriate use of financial resources. Elderly patients may give a relative or caregiver power of attorney only to find that their finances have been drained. Caregivers or relatives may move into the elderly woman's home and deny her control of her home or finances through threats or manipulation.

CLINICAL FINDINGS

Any woman, regardless of socioeconomic class, level of education, professional status, ethnic or religious group, age, or race, has the potential to be a battered woman. There is no "classic" battered woman; therefore, screening for abuse in all patients is essential. However, there are symptoms and signs that should compel the medical provider to ask direct questions regarding violence.

Chronic Pain

Chronic pain, such as headache, abdominal pain, or pelvic pain, may be a signal of ongoing abuse. Domino found that most patients with chronic headache referred to a pain clinic for evaluation had a history of physical or sexual abuse. Drossman found that of women referred to a gastroenterologic practice for workup of abdominal pain, 36% admitted to experiencing physical or sexual abuse as an adult. Patients with the diagnosis of functional bowel disorder had a higher risk of physical abuse than those who had organic bowel disorders, with an odds ratio of 11:39. Similarly, Rapkin found a significant percentage of women with chronic pelvic pain without pelvic pathology who had a history of physical abuse as an adult. Clearly, patients with chronic pain have high rates of clinic attendance and often receive exhaustive and expensive workups seeking an organic explanation for their pain. It is extremely important that questions about a history of abuse, both physical and sexual, be part of any evaluation for chronic pain.

Somatic Complaints

Somatic complaints also may be a sign of battering. Ratner found that women who were physically abused scored significantly higher on the somatic complaint subscale of the General Health Questionnaire. Patients may present with vague symptoms for which an organic source cannot be found even after an exhaustive workup. The patients may be labeled as **hypochondriacal** or **hysterical,** thereby obscuring the underlying problem of abuse.

Injury

Multiple injuries in the central region of the body should raise a strong suspicion of abuse. Injuries to the head, breast, abdomen, back, and genitalia are common. Injuries to the head include facial hematomas, nasal and mandibular fractures, and ruptured tympanic membranes. A study by Zachariades found violence inflicted by a male partner to be the third leading cause of facial injuries for women. Other red flags of intentional injury are old injuries and bruises

in various stages of healing, burns in unusual places, and human bites. Any injuries that do not match the explanation given by the patient certainly need further investigation.

Marital rape is a common form of physical violence in abusive relationships. Russel found that 40% of battered women experienced marital rape. Campbell and Alford found that forced vaginal intercourse accounted for the majority of marital rape incidents but that anal intercourse, being hit, kicked, or burned during sex, and insertion of objects into the anus and vagina also were described frequently by abused women. The women studied associated these acts with urinary tract infections, vaginal and anal bleeding, urinary incontinence, unwanted pregnancies, and sexually transmitted diseases. Because rape may not result in obvious injuries and because women may be embarrassed to describe marital rape, it often is not revealed unless the medical provider asks direct questions about abuse.

Alcohol Abuse

Battered women are at higher risk than others for alcohol abuse. One study found that 16.3% of battered women are alcohol-dependent compared with 2.4% of nonbattered women. Stark found that battered women had rates of alcoholism similar to nonbattered women before the first episode of battering. After battering began, however, the rates of alcoholism rose to fivefold. For many women, the use of alcohol may be a means of calming the anxiety and numbing the pain of abuse.

Conversely, Miller compared women who were in treatment for alcohol addiction with women randomly selected from households and found that alcoholic women have endured a significantly greater amount of violence. It is clear that alcoholic women need to be screened for violence and that battered women need to be screened for alcoholism. Both issues need to be addressed to provide optimal treatment.

Unfortunately, the use of alcohol by battered women may have a negative influence on the way that their victimization is perceived. When Kurz studied physicians who were treating domestic violence victims in an emergency room, he found that in 40% of the cases, the physicians did not respond to the battering. When physicians were asked their perception of the patient treated, they often cited the use of alcohol as their reason for not pursuing the battering issues. Alcohol was considered a discrediting trait that made a woman less of a "true victim." This perception clearly decreases a battered woman's access to appropriate treatment.

Psychiatric Illness

As can be expected, repeated physical violence has a major effect on women's mental health. Anxiety is a common symptom of battered women, and many women are placed on low-dose antidepressant or anxiolytic medication without the physician knowing about the underlying problem. Patients with psychiatric diagnoses are rarely screened for battering. Jacobsen found that 81% of inpatient psychiatric patients had a history of physical or sexual assault. However, therapists rarely ask about assault, and Jacobson found that only 9% of the assaults were recorded in the medical charts.

Depression is an extremely common sequela of domestic violence. Cascardi found that wives who were physically assaulted scored significantly higher on the Beck Depression Inventory than wives from discordant marriages without violence. This higher level of depression may be responsible in part for the higher rates of suicide among battered women. One study found that of women who presented to an emergency room as the result of a suicide attempt, 28.6% were battered women. Another study by Stark found that one of four battered women had attempted suicide at least once. It is crucial that all patients being treated for depression or for attempted suicide be screened for domestic violence.

EVALUATION

One of the first steps in asking about abuse is to provide an environment that encourages women to reveal the abuse. Hanging posters on the subject of domestic violence in the waiting room or having brochures available in the women's bathroom conveys a willingness to attend to the issue. If health history forms are available, a question about physical violence or threat of violence is important; abused women will know that the health provider is concerned about the issue, and nonabused women will understand that it is a standard question asked of all women. Although health surveys are useful in collecting information, the patient also should also be asked verbally about abuse. One study found that 7.3% of women were identified as abused after completing a self-report health history, whereas the same questions asked verbally revealed a prevalence of 29.3%.

Creating a safe environment for the discussion of abuse is also critical. At some point in the interview, the patient must be spoken with alone. The presence of a partner, parent, or caregiver who refuses to leave should raise suspicion of abuse. It is sometimes difficult to compel an overly protective partner to leave the room. Asking the partner to fill out forms, or sending the patient to the bathroom for a urine sample and having a female nurse or physician follow her in are techniques that have been used. It is also important to make sure that children, if there are any, are in a safe place. Ideally, the children could be invited to play in a supervised playroom. If this is not available, a social worker, nurse, or staff member could entertain the children in an area separate from the waiting room. Caution must be used in offering to entertain the children to avoid arousing the suspicion of the abuser. Fear that the partner may take the children will constrain the patient from revealing abuse.

The patient must be reassured that all the information she relays will be kept confidential and will not be shared with the abuser. The issue of confidentiality is especially important if the practitioner or physician also provides health care to the batterer. However, confidentiality cannot be maintained if a child or elderly person is at risk of or is being abused. If a report to the appropriate state protective department needs to be filed, it is essential that the patient be made aware of the pending report and that issues of safety be discussed.

When asking about physical violence, the best approach is a direct question aimed at specific behavior. Initially, asking general questions about how things are going at home or with the partner is reasonable, but at some point a direct question needs to be asked.

The physician should avoid using phrases such as **abused, battered woman,** or **domestic violence,** because these terms may mean different things to different women. It often is helpful to begin the questioning by pointing out the health risks of violence or by stating that many women find themselves in violent situations. Another approach is to ask how conflicts are resolved between the woman and her partner and if hitting ever is used by either partner. These openings should lead into direct questions about being hit, hurt, or threatened at home.

Methods of asking pregnant women about abuse have been well studied by McFarlane, who developed three simple screening questions that were found to be effective in identifying abused patients:

1. Within the past year, have you been hit, slapped, kicked, or otherwise physically hurt by someone?
2. Since you have been pregnant, have you been hit, slapped, kicked, or otherwise physically hurt by someone?
3. Within the past year, has anyone forced you to have sexual activity?

McFarlane's study found significantly higher levels of abuse than had been reported previously in the literature. Two reasons for this increase were cited by the author: first, that the patients were verbally questioned about abuse by their primary provider, and second, that the questions were asked in each trimester.

The physical examination is of paramount importance in looking for evidence of physical abuse and neglect in elderly women. The skin is often the most revealing organ because it can provide information on hydration, hygiene, nutrition, and physical abuse. Evidence of neglect may be found in poorly cared for decubiti or burns from prolonged exposure to urine or feces. Evidence of restraints around the wrist or waist should be noted. The genital and rectal areas need to be examined for signs of sexually transmitted diseases and trauma.

Many forms of abuse of elderly women cannot be identified by a physical examination, however. Rather, the medical provider needs to ask questions of both the patient and the caregiver to discover potential abuse. Patients need to be assessed concerning their daily activities such as cooking, eating, bathing, dressing, and walking, as well as regarding issues such as incontinence and ability to use a bathroom. This assessment gives the provider an idea of the types of stress a caregiver encounters and a sense of whether basic needs are being met appropriately. It is important to obtain information regarding who lives in the home, whether drugs or alcohol are abused by household members, what financial arrangement exists, and whether the elderly patient has social support other than that of the caregiver.

Many elderly patients do not provide information about abuse out of fear of retaliation or fear that if the caregiver leaves they will be forced to move into a nursing home. However, some elderly patients do not provide the information because they do not recognize neglect or financial exploitation as abuse. Again, it is important to ask direct questions about being hit or hurt, as well as questions regarding the use of restraints, being locked in a room, verbal intimidation, and failure to be fed, cleaned, or given medication in a timely and appropriate manner.

INTERVENTION

Once a patient reveals abuse, it is important for the provider to communicate to the patient that the problem is serious and that he or she is concerned about the issue. There are multiple ways of approaching the problem, such as stressing to the patient that she does not deserve to be beaten, addressing the fact that assault is a criminal act and that the patient has the right to be safe in her own home, or focusing on the health consequences of ongoing abuse. One of the most devastating responses a health care provider can make is lack of any response. If the provider does not address the issue, the woman's sense of hopelessness and isolation is intensified.

Assessing safety is the next critical step. The primary issue is whether it is safe for the patient to return home that day; the provider should ask her that question directly. If she wishes to return home, she needs to begin making a safety plan in case the violence starts again. A detailed plan does not need to be completed in the office or clinic, but the patient needs to be encouraged to think about safety. The pa-

tient should plan escape routes from each room in the house. She should think about how she will access money and transportation if she needs to leave suddenly. She should think about where she could go in an emergency, such as the home of a friend or relative, and possibly leave clothing there for future needs. She should have important documents, such as children's birth certificates, health insurance cards, bank books, and credit cards, and her prescription medication easily accessible.

If the patient does not feel it is safe to return home, a safe place must be located. The place may be the home of friends or relatives or may be a shelter whose location is confidential. The safety plan does not stop here, however, because the period of separation and divorce can be one of the most dangerous for an abused woman. She may need a protection order or a restraining order, and it is important to find out whether she knows how to obtain these documents.

Campbell studied risk factors for domestic violence ending in homicide. Although it is not always possible to ask about each danger sign, it is crucial to be aware of factors that may increase the risk of a lethal outcome. The following situations were found to be associated with risk of homicide:

1. Increase in frequency or severity of violence in the last year.
2. Presence of firearms in the home.
3. Sexual abuse.
4. Abuse of drugs or alcohol by the batterer.
5. Violent episodes outside the home perpetrated by the abuser.
6. Threats to kill the woman by the abuser (or she believes he is capable of killing).
7. Attempts by the abuser to control all aspects of the woman's life.
8. Violent jealousy expressed by the abuser.
9. Battering during pregnancy.

Referral

It is important for health care providers to investigate the resources available in their community. If one has personal contact with a staff member at the local shelter, there is someone to turn to with questions. Keeping an up-to-date list of resources saves time and prevents frustration.

Before an abused woman leaves the office, she should know how to contact the police and the local shelter in an emergency. Some areas have city- or statewide hotlines that can give the patient the telephone numbers she needs for her area. Brochures are handy, but they may be dangerous if they are found by the batterer. It may be prudent to have the woman memorize the most important numbers or hide them in a safe place.

Teenage women are at a disadvantage when it comes to accessing social services. Because most teenagers are under the age of majority, representatives of social service organizations are not as likely to get involved without parental consent. Child protective services are geared to respond to abuse of young children and often do not expend great effort in protecting adolescents from abuse. Because of their age, female adolescents often are denied access to shelters for battered women; legally, they cannot file assault charges unless they are emancipated adults. This state of affairs often leaves abused adolescent women without advocacy or resources. Caught in limbo between childhood and adulthood, adolescent women are at risk for battering from multiple sources and lack appropriate avenues for help. Helping the adolescent find someone to confide in, such as a school guidance counsellor, minister, or counsellor at a local teen center, may be the most valuable action that can be taken. However, for some teenagers, the health care provider may be the safest advocate, and subsequent visits will need to be scheduled to talk about issues such as safety, defining limits in relationships, and building self-esteem.

Elderly women may have difficulty finding shelters that can address their specific needs, especially if they are physically or mentally impaired. Many women may remain in abusive situations or relationships because they fear that nursing home placement is their only alternative.

Follow-up

Ending a battering relationship is a process. For some women the process may take one day; for others it may take 10 years; and for still others, the relationship may never end. There are a variety of reasons that women remain in an abusive situation. One of the most compelling is the real threat of death if she leaves. It is important for the provider to respect the serious dilemmas that many women face in leaving an abusive relationship, including fear, economic insecurity, religious convictions, and family pressures.

Health care providers need to follow the course of a battering relationship as they would follow any health problem. Domestic violence should be listed on the problem list and the situation reassessed at subsequent visits. Continued support for the woman is crucial.

Documentation

Proper documentation in the medical chart is crucial for any criminal or civil proceedings that may follow for the patient. It is also important as a means of verifying that the medical provider has acted responsibly in intervening in a situation of domestic violence.

For an acute assault, the date, time, and place of the incident need to be recorded. The most important aspect to record, however, is the name of the alleged assailant and the relationship to the patient. Terms such as "boyfriend" and "cousin" are not specific enough. Recording the relationship is necessary also because violence by an intimate partner or caretaker has a higher probability of being repeated than violence inflicted by a stranger. The mechanism of injury should be described and all visible signs of injury should be documented. Any evidence of old injuries should be documented also. Finally, one should document the fact that safety was assessed and information on appropriate resources was given.

REFERENCES

Appleton W: The battered wife syndrome. Ann Emerg Med 1980;9:84.

Bayatpour M et al: Physical and sexual abuse as predictors of substance use and suicide among pregnant teenagers. J Adolesc Health 1992;13:128.

Benton D, Marshall M: Elder abuse. Clin Geriatr Med 1991;7:831.

Bullock L, McFarlane J: The birth-weight/battering connection. Am J Nurs (Sept) 1989;89:1153.

Campbell J: Risk of homicide with battered women. Adv Nurs Sci 1986;8(4):36.

Campbell J, Alford P: The dark consequences of marital rape. Am J Nurs 1989;89:946.

Cascardi M: Marital aggression: Impact, injury, and health correlates for husbands and wives. Arch Intern Med 1992;152:1178.

Council on Scientific Affairs: Elder abuse and neglect. JAMA 1987;57:966.

Council on Scientific Affairs, American Medical Association: Adolescents as victims of family violence. JAMA 1993;270:1850.

Domino J: Prior physical and sexual abuse in women with chronic headache: Clinical correlates. Headache 1987;27:310.

Drossman D: Sexual and physical abuse in women with functional or organic gastrointestinal disorder. Ann Intern Med 1990;113:828.

Farber E, Falkner M: Violence in families of adolescent runaways. Child Abuse Negl 1984;8:295.

Gin N: Prevalence of domestic violence among patients in three ambulatory care internal medicine clinics. J Gen Intern Med 1991;9:317.

Goldberg W, Tomlanovich M: Domestic violence in the emergency department. JAMA 1984;251:3259.

Hamberger L: Prevalence of domestic violence in community practice and rate of physician inquiry. Fam Med 1992;24:283.

Hilberman E: Overview: The "wife-beaters" wife reconsidered. Am J Psychiatry 1980;137:1336.

Jacobson A: The failure of routine assessment to detect histories of assault experienced by psychiatric patients. Hosp Community Psychiatry 1987;384:386.

Jacobson A et al: Assault experiences of 100 psychiatric inpatients: Evidence of the need for routine inquiry. Am J Psychiatry 1987;144:908.

Kurz D: Emergency department responses to battered women: Resistance to medicalization. Soc Probl 1987; 34:69.

Lachs L: Recognizing elder abuse and neglect. Clin Geriatr Med 1993;9:665.

McFarlane J: Abuse during pregnancy: The horror and the hope. AWHONNS 1993;4:350.

McFarlane J: Assessing for abuse: Self-report versus nurse interview. Public Health Nurs 1991;8:245.

McFarlane J et al: Assessing for abuse during pregnancy. JAMA 1992;267:3176.

McLeer S, Anwar R: A study of battered women presenting in an emergency department. Am J Publ Health 1989;79:65.

Miller B et al: Spousal violence among alcoholic women as compared to a random household sample of women. J Stud Alcohol 1989;50:533.

Moon A, Williams O: Perceptions of elder abuse and help-seeking patterns among African-American, Caucasian American, and Korean-American elderly women. Gerontologist 1993;33:386.

Newberger EH et al: Abuse of pregnant women and adverse birth outcomes. JAMA 1992;267:2370.

Parker B: Abuse of adolescents: What can we learn from pregnant teenagers? AWHONNS 1993;4:363.

Rapkin A et al: History of physical and sexual abuse in women with chronic pelvic pain. Obstet Gynecol 1990;76:92.

Rath D: Rates of domestic violence against adult women by male partners. J Am Board Fam Pract 1989;2:227.

Ratner R: The incidence of wife abuse and mental health status in abused wives in Edmonton, Alberta. Can J Public Health 1993;8:246.

Richards J: Battering in a population of adolescent females. J Am Acad Nurse Pract 1991;3(4):180.

Roscoe B, Callahan J: Adolescents' self-report of violence in families and dating relations. Adolescence 1985; XX(79):545.

Rosenberg M et al: Interpersonal violence: Homicide and spouse abuse. In: *Public Health and Preventive Medicine,* 12th ed. Last JM (editor). Appleton-Century-Crofts, 1986.

Russel D: *Rape in Marriage.* Indiana University Press, 1990.

Stark E, Flitcraft A, Frazier W: Medicine and patriarchal violence: The social construction of a "private" event. Int J Health Serv 1979;9:461.

Stark E et al: *Wife Abuse in the Medical Setting.* Monograph 7. Washington, DC, Office of Domestic Violence, 1981.

Straus M, Gelles R: *Behind Closed Doors: A Survey of Family Violence in America.* Doubleday, 1980.

Straus M, Gelles R: *Physical Violence in the American Family.* Transaction Publishers, 1990.

US Department of Health and Human Services: *Study Findings: Study of National Incidence and Prevalence of Child Abuse and Neglect.* US Department of Health and Human Services, 1988.

Washington State Medical Association: *Elder Abuse: Guidelines for Intervention by Physicians and Other Service Providers.* Washington State Medical Association, 1985.

Zachariades N: Facial trauma in women resulting from violence by men. J Oral Maxillofac Surg 1990;48:1250.

Sexual Abuse

16

Patricia L. Paddison, MD, & Jennifer D. Bolen, MD

The prevalence of long-term effects on health of childhood sexual abuse in women finally is being recognized. Clinicians who finished training 10 years ago had little exposure to or training in the effects of childhood sexual abuse. Health care providers have begun to be aware of the connections among health, health-related behaviors, and abuse, and the demand for training in these areas is on the rise.

In a rural Midwestern area, women who had been sexually abused as children sought medical care 3–5 times as frequently as nonabused women. Headaches, exacerbations of asthma, and abdominal distress were the most common presenting symptoms, according to a study by Cunningham et al. Lechner et al queried 523 patients in a family practice clinic via questionnaire and found that sexual abuse victims reported problems in the respiratory, gastrointestinal, and neurologic areas 2–3 times more frequently than the nonabused group. Only 5.1% of the abused group had disclosed this information to a physician. In a random review of nonpsychotic adult patients presenting to a psychiatric emergency room, only 6% of the charts noted a history of childhood sexual abuse, according to Briere and Zaida. However, when physicians were asked to query their next 50 patients verbally about abuse, 70% of patients reported sexual contact before the age of 17 initiated by someone 5 or more years older. This study demonstrates the importance of asking all patients about a history of sexual abuse, because many patients fail to disclose the information spontaneously.

Sexual abuse can be defined as any act with sexual overtones perpetrated by a needed or trusted adult, whom a child is unable to refuse because of age, lack of knowledge, or the context of the relationship. The perpetrator is usually 5 or more years older than the child, a factor that differentiates abuse from consensual exploration. **Major** sexual abuse involves genital touching or oral, anal, or vaginal intercourse. **Minor** sexual abuse involves clothed molestation or exhibitionism. Major sexual abuse, particularly abuse that has gone on for years, is more damaging than minor abuse and causes more numerous and profound sequelae.

INCIDENCE

Nonclinical population studies of the prevalence of childhood sexual abuse indicate that between 12 and 40% of adult women have experienced sexual abuse before the age of 17. A national survey by Timnick conducted among 2000 adults revealed that 27% of the women had been sexually abused. Russell surveyed a random sample of 933 women in San Francisco and discovered that 38% had been sexually abused before age 18. Seventy-eight percent of those who reported sexual abuse experiences in childhood felt that these experiences were associated with long-term effects. Wyatt found no differences in the rate of sexual abuse among ethnic groups in a study of 248 women in Los Angeles; no differences were found among women of different economic status either, according to Wyatt and Peters. Although this chapter addresses the concerns of women, it should be noted that 7–10% of men have been sexually abused in childhood.

Girls are more likely to be victimized within the family than by an outsider, most often by a male relative. The occurrence of major sexual abuse and the length of abuse have been correlated with particularly long-lasting sequelae, according to Briere. The clinical presentation often is complicated further by other potentially damaging experiences such as physical and psychologic abuse, parental psychopathology, parental neglect, alcoholism, and severe family dysfunction. These and other factors combine with the child's innate personality style, developmental stage, and resiliency to influence the long-term effects of the abuse.

There are few studies of the impact of abuse on function involving children from nonclinical settings. Our understanding is based principally on generalizations from what is observed in children in clinical settings. A nonclinical population study by Hibbard et al, looking at abuse histories and health-related feelings and behaviors in 712 middle school children, found a significant correlation between a history of sexual abuse and the occurrence of substance abuse, laxative abuse, and suicidal behavior during the middle school years.

SCREENING

Clinicians should inquire routinely of all patients at the initial interview about adverse sexual experiences. How and when to obtain these histories are matters of clinical judgment. Generally, an appropriate time to ask about abuse is when taking the past medical history after inquiring about menses and pregnancy. The clinician may ask questions such as: "Has anyone ever touched you against your will in childhood or adulthood? Have you had any adverse sexual experiences?" If a patient says yes, the physician should ask, "How old were you when it started, and how old when it stopped? Was it oral sex, anal sex, or intercourse? What made it stop? Who and how old was the abuser?" Framing the initial question in two ways, ie, using the words **against your will** and **adverse experiences** allows the patient to define the abuse in her own way. Specifically naming the types of abuse is an attempt to take away the shame patients have in describing the acts. Knowing the duration of abuse and whether the perpetrator lived in the home helps the clinician to evaluate how damaging the abuse was. Inquiring about what made the abuse stop gives the clinician information about what the patient experienced and the degree of family dysfunction. Increased durations of abuse and penetration are associated with poorer outcomes. Children rarely disclose sexual abuse. If a child does disclose such information and the mother or primary caretaker is supportive, the outcome is usually more positive than otherwise.

Although clinicians may fear that raising the subject of abuse may cause decompensation on the part of the patient, ignoring the subject only contributes to continued isolation and possible development of psychopathology. The patient needs to understand the value of determining the effects of sexual abuse, namely, the complex interplay of childhood experiences with adult health and body experiences. The clinician can express concern that retraumatization during the examination be minimized and problem-solve with the patient to reduce that risk, eg, by talking and keeping eye contact. It is appropriate at this time to ask the patient if she feels she has worked through the effects of the abuse; if the abuse appears to be unresolved, one may refer the patient to a mental health professional experienced in abuse. When to refer to a mental health professional is discussed in greater detail later in this chapter.

CLINICAL FINDINGS

Medical complications that may be associated with sexual abuse include chronic pelvic pain, premenstrual syndrome (PMS), somatization disorder, pain syndromes, pseudoseizures, headaches, asthma, and gastrointestinal (GI) complaints (Table 16–1). Chronic pelvic pain with normal laparoscopic findings has been associated with a history of sexual abuse. Forty percent of women presenting to a PMS clinic reported a history of sexual abuse, according to Paddison et al. Multiple bodily complaints were common in women with somatoform disorders and a history of sexual abuse according to a study by Loewenstein performed in a primary care setting. Barsky et al compared hypochondriacal with non-hypochondriacal outpatients in a general medical clinic and found that the hypochondriacal patients had significantly more traumatic sexual contacts as well as more instances of physical violence and major parental upheaval in childhood. Clinicians have noted that cancer patients with a history of sexual abuse may be more problematic in their pain management. Patients referred to a GI clinic who had a history of abuse (sexual and physical) reported more medical symptoms and were more frequent users of health care services than nonabused patients, according to Drossman et al.

Psychiatric complications that may be associated with sexual abuse include substance abuse, depression or suicide, eating disorders, sexual disorders, borderline personality disorder, anxiety disorders (posttraumatic stress disorder [PTSD]), and dissociative disorders (multiple personality disorder [MPD]) (Table 16–2).

Many women in the early stages of recovery from sexual abuse engage in self-destructive behaviors including substance abuse, involvement in abusive relationships, promiscuity, and self-cutting; self-cutting is considered self-mutilation rather than a suicide attempt. High rates of sexual abuse are seen in women in substance abuse treatment programs, and even higher rates are found in the resistant or treatment-unresponsive groups.

One model of the way that childhood trauma predisposes individuals to numerous medical and psychiatric complications uses the concept of inescapable stress. In animal models, as reported by

Table 16–1. Medical complications of sexual abuse.

Chronic pelvic pain
Premenstrual syndrome
Somatization disorder
Hypochondriases
Pseudoseizures
Headaches
Asthma
Gastrointestinal complaints

Table 16–2. Psychiatric complications of sexual abuse.

Substance abuse
Depression
Suicide
Sexual disorders
Eating disorders
Borderline personality disorder
Anxiety disorders (eg, PTSD)*
Dissociative disorders (eg, MPD)†

*PTSD = posttraumatic stress disorder.
†MPD = multiple personality disorder.

van der Kolk, this concept involves inescapable shock, and the effects of exposure include (1) deficits in learning to escape novel adverse situations, (2) decreased motivation for learning new contingencies, (3) chronic subjective distress, and (4) increased tumor genesis and immunosuppression. The "learned helplessness syndrome" that follows is caused by lack of control. In humans this syndrome is related to depression and PTSD. van der Kolk notes that outcome is also influenced by the severity of the stressor, genetic predisposition, developmental phase, presence of a social support system, prior traumatization, and preexisting personality. Thus, abuse survivors may be at risk for medical and psychiatric sequelae such as depression, revictimization, and stress-related illnesses.

When faced with repeated trauma, the victim commonly uses the defense mechanisms of dissociation, repression, and denial. Each mechanism is an appropriate way to cope with present trauma when no other modes of coping are available. Continuing to use these defense mechanisms in adulthood, however, long after the original trauma has occurred, may be maladaptive. Many trauma survivors, including war veterans, use dissociation; they may say, "It's happening to someone else," or describe being "in the wallpaper" while the abuse was taking place. Repression involves pushing the memories into the unconscious mind. Denial manifests itself as minimization of the abuse experiences (or history); the patient claims they are unimportant. Using these defense mechanisms in adulthood may predispose the woman to manage current stress by somatizing anxiety. Thus, a woman may present to her practitioner with nonspecific somatic complaints, such as PMS, abdominal pain, or headaches, when the real issue is marital discord or work problems.

If clinicians view their patients with a history of abuse in the context of the inescapable stress concept and the defense mechanisms of dissociation, repression, and denial, they may understand better their patients' underlying psychopathology and ultimately be more helpful (see the following section, Treatment).

TREATMENT

Clinicians should be aware that abuse survivors are usually quite anxious at their first visit and, as a result, may appear disorganized and forgetful. The pelvic examination can be difficult for these patients. It may help to delay the pelvic examination until the next visit if the patient is particularly anxious. These patients may call back for instruction on medications or procedures that were discussed during the office visit; anxiety often causes them to "space out" or dissociate through part of the interview or examination. Therefore, written instructions can be helpful.

After determining that a patient has suffered sexual abuse, the clinician should inquire whether the patient feels that further work on or help with the abuse would be useful at this time. Every primary care clinician should have the names of at least two experienced clinicians who work in the area of sexual abuse so that a referral may be made when needed. When it is ascertained that the presenting physical complaints are not the result of an underlying illness, the clinician may want to use the concept of bodily memories as a way to help engage the patient to consider psychotherapy: the clinician may want to state that it is fortunate that no cause of the symptoms has been found, that some of the symptoms may be due to the body "remembering" or "holding onto" the abuse, and that therapy can be helpful. Physical therapy involving pelvic floor exercises, biofeedback, or other types of movement therapy for chronic pelvic pain with no underlying pathology also are quite helpful. Here, too, the referral should be made to someone experienced in the area of sexual abuse. Patients usually accept the information that the body retains the tension of abuse, which causes pain, and that learning how to relax the pelvic floor may lessen the pain. Asking the patient to try a different approach before proceeding with invasive diagnostic procedures is usually appreciated. Reassuring the patient that she is to return for a follow-up visit at a later date helps her to feel listened to and not dismissed.

One also should refer a patient to a mental health provider if she is experiencing severe symptoms, eg, posttraumatic sequelae, severe panic attacks, sleep disturbance, depression, self-mutilation, or involvement in abusive relationships. The difficult-to-manage patient who is noncompliant with the treatment of serious medical problems also should be referred.

An in-depth mental health evaluation can help determine treatment recommendations. Often a combination of individual psychotherapy, pharmacotherapy, and possibly, group therapy is advised. Antidepressant medication often is the most helpful type of pharmacotherapy because these drugs target mood, panic, and the "positive" symptoms of PTSD (autonomic hyperarousal, hypervigilance, nightmares, and flashbacks). The selective serotonin reuptake inhibitors (SSRI) such as paroxetine (Paxil), sertraline (Zoloft), and fluoxetine (Prozac) are effective and easy to use. Although the literature primarily deals with tricyclic antidepressants and monoamine oxidase (MAO) inhibitors, one study suggests that fluoxetine is helpful for PTSD. Clinically, the medications seem to be equally effective. Sometimes the addition of low-dose trazodone (Desyrel) in the 25 to 50 mg range helps with the nightmares and sleep disturbances. One should avoid prescribing habit-forming agents such as the benzodiazepines, although they are helpful in treating the acute reactivation of memories on a short-term basis (less than 3 weeks). These drugs may be helpful for someone whose symptoms have caused extreme impairment. Neuroleptics should be avoided. For a more comprehensive review, one may refer to Saporta's work.

The patient should be an active participant in treatment planning, although there are situations in which the survivor is so disabled that participation in the planning of the initial phase of treatment is minimal. At other times, patients may have their own, fixed agenda for treatment. These agendas are sometimes helpful and always illuminating, and they should be listened to before decisions are made; however, the caregiver needs to stay within his or her domain of ethical, sensible, and well-founded treatment. If in doubt, one may consult with an experienced colleague.

Establishing good health care as an adult is a symbol of taking control of and responsibility for one's life. Treatment and recovery, when possible, enable a patient to go from feeling like a victim to feeling like a survivor and ideally to becoming someone who thrives in life. The health care provider plays an integral part in the development of a new relationship between the survivor and her body and between the survivor and her support network.

SPECIAL ISSUES OF PREGNANCY

Because pregnancy is a time of change and refocusing, many women begin to retrieve memories of abuse during pregnancy or delivery. They may have negative feelings toward a particular sex of their baby. Some women state that a male child reminds them of the abuse, that they fear the child will grow up to be an abuser, and thus that they prefer a female child. Other women fear a female child will be subjected to abuse and prefer a male child. What is important is that the clinician explore the woman's feelings about her baby and refer her for mental health treatment when conflict is present. Some women fear touching their baby's genitals and changing diapers. They fear their touch may be abusive or that memories of their own abuse may surface at this time. Some mothers become overly protective of their children in fear that the children may be abused. Clearly,

these issues relate to unresolved childhood sexual abuse, and treatment with a skilled therapist is indicated.

Another important issue surrounding pregnancy in abuse survivors has to do with the relationship of the survivor to her health care provider. The patient may distort the relationship due to her experiences with authority figures in the past; the distortion may be toward either a heightened positive or an increased negative perception. Clinicians should be cautious and maintain professional boundaries to avoid these distortions. This issue is discussed further in the next section.

CONTROVERSIES & UNRESOLVED ISSUES

Many patients who file malpractice claims against physicians or therapists for sexual contact have been sexually abused in childhood. Kluft's review of the psychiatric literature and his discussion of this occurrence as related to the vulnerability to revictimization is helpful. Many women who were sexually abused in childhood have problems recognizing a sexual/personal boundary violation and do not recognize dangerous situations. Too often they blame themselves and fail to take appropriate measures either to end the abuse or to seek treatment for the consequences.

The fact that the true prevalence of sexual abuse has been debated may account for the discrepancies (12–40%) previously reported. Factors related to the accuracy of data include the use of surveys of both major and minor sexual abuse at the same time. Another factor has to do with the shame involved in reporting sexual abuse. Researchers who use same-sex interviewers and preface the data collection with remarks such as, "This information may be helpful in preventing abuse of others," report higher rates of abuse. Face-to-face interviewing as opposed to telephone surveying also results in higher rates of reported abuse. Because of these issues regarding the prevalence of sexual abuse, it is difficult to determine the true significance of the clinical conditions associated with sexual abuse.

Another controversy involves the accuracy of memories. Some professionals have disputed claims of childhood sexual abuse, stating that the patients were susceptible to suggestions made by unskilled therapists or while under hypnosis. The current questions under study include the veracity and the malleability of memory. In a study of the verification of sexual abuse memories, Herman and Schatzow reported that outside information was obtained in 74% of cases and statements indicating a strong likelihood of occurrence were obtained in 9%. A recent study involving interviews with 129 women who had been seen as children 17 years earlier in a city hospital with well documented histories of sexual victimization showed that 38% had no recall of the reported abuse. Women who could not recall the abuse in this study tended to be a younger age at the time of the abuse and were abused by someone they knew well. Lack of recall for the abuse in childhood does not mean that the abuse did not occur and this study supports that it may be common. False reporting may be more common in legal battles over child custody than in therapy settings because of the possibility of using the accusation as a way to secure custody.

Many survivors experience few clear memories, although they may have body memories. A recent review by van der Kolk of trauma and memory formulates that these memories, also known as somatic memories, are a somatosensory level of organizing prior trauma effects in the memory function of the brain. These include physical sensations and visual images that persist and activate long after the original trauma and seem impervious to change. Examples of these body memories include a certain sexual position activating a fight or flight response during routine sex, seeing a perpetrator's face in place of their partner's face during sex, and having the smell of alcohol on their partner's breath may activate flashbacks (if the perpetrator was an alcohol abuser). Although retrieval and accuracy of memory warrant further study, it is a fact that most patients continue to be reluctant to disclose their abuse and therefore are unrecognized and undertreated.

The impact of multiple types of trauma is an issue that remains unresolved by researchers. Frequently, researchers do not recognize that patients who have had numerous types of abuse are more pathologic in their clinical presentation than patients with only one type of abuse, eg, patients who have had sexual abuse only versus those who have had sexual abuse and also experienced physical or emotional abuse or domestic violence. Focusing on only one type of abuse in a study may yield faulty data. Researchers also may fail to distinguish between major and minor sexual abuse and fail to account for the duration of abuse, eg, a one time occurrence versus sexual abuse lasting 6 years.

REFERENCES

Barsky AJ et al: Histories of childhood trauma in adult hypochondriacal patients. Am J Psychiatry 1994;151:397.

Bolen JB: The impact of sexual abuse on women's health. Psych Ann 1993;23:446.

Briere J: The long-term clinical correlates of childhood sexual victimization. Ann NY Acad Sci 1988b;528:327.

Briere J: *Therapy for Adults Molested as Children: Beyond Survival.* Springer, 1989.

Briere J, Zaida LY: Sexual abuse histories and sequelae in female psychiatric emergency room patients. Am J Psychiatry 1989;146:1602.

Cunningham J. Pearce T, Pearce P: Childhood sexual abuse and medical complaints in adult women. J Interpersonal Violence 1988;3:131.

Drossman DA et al: Sexual and physical abuse in women with functional or organic gastrointestinal disorders. Ann Intern Med 1990;113:828.

Herman JL, Schatzow E: Recovery and verification of memories of childhood sexual trauma. Psychoanal Psychol 1987;4:1.

Hibbard MD et al: Abuse, feelings, and health behaviors in a student population. Am J Dis Child 1988;142:326.

Kluft RP: Incest and subsequent revictimization: The case of therapist-patient sexual exploitation, with a description of the sitting duck syndrome. In: *Incest-Related Syndromes of Adult Psychopathology.* Kluft RP (editor). American Psychiatric Press, 1990.

Lechner ME et al: Self-reported medical problems of adult female survivors of childhood sexual abuse. J Fam Pract 1993;36:633.

Loewenstein RJ: Somatoform disorders in victims of incest and child abuse. In: *Incest-Related Syndromes of Adult Psychopathology.* Kluft RP (editor). American Psychiatric Press, 1990.

Paddison PL et al: Sexual abuse and premenstrual syndrome: Comparison between a lower and higher socioeconomic group. Psychosomatics 1990;31:265.

Root MPP: Treatment failures: The role of sexual victimization in women's addictive behavior. Am J Orthopsychiatry 1989;59:542.

Russell DEH: *The Secret Trauma: Incest in the Lives of Girls and Women.* Basic Books, 1986.

Saporta JA: The role of medications in treating adult survivors of childhood trauma. In: *Treatment of Adult Survivors of Incest.* Paddison PL (editor). American Psychiatric Press, 1993.

Springs FE, Friedrich WN: Health risk behaviors and medical sequelae of childhood sexual abuse. Mayo Clin Proc 1992;67:527.

Timnick L: 22% in survey were child abuse victims. Los Angeles Times, 1985;8:25.

van der Kolk BA: *Psychological Trauma.* American Psychiatric Press, 1987.

van der Kolk BA: The body keeps the score: Memory and the evolving psychobiology of posttraumatic stress. Harvard Review of Psychiatry 1994;1:253.

Walker D et al: Relationship of chronic pelvic pain to psychiatric diagnoses and childhood sexual abuse. Am J Psychiatry 1988;145:75.

Williams LM: Recall of childhood trauma: A prospective study of women's memories of child sexual abuse. J Consult Clin Psychol [in press].

Wyatt GE: The sexual abuse of Afro-American and white American women in childhood. Child Abuse Negl 1985;9:507.

Wyatt GE, Peters SD: Methodologic considerations in research on the prevalence of child sexual abuse. Child Abuse Negl 1986;10:241.

17

Evaluating Sexual Dysfunctions

Julia R. Heiman, PhD

Sexual dysfunctions are disorders that impair or prevent participation in sexual activity. Many women experience a sexual dysfunction but either do not choose to view it as a problem or are unwilling to volunteer the information to a primary care physician. The reasons for the latter usually include some combination of the woman's discomfort, her perception of discomfort in her health care provider, or the fact that her physician inadequately questions her on this topic. This stalemate has continued for many generations, assisted by broader cultural resistance to the idea that sex can be a problem or to the acknowledgment that women's sexuality is important. Women's sexuality has been seen as incidental in comparison to diseases and conditions that are life-threatening or severely compromising of general functioning. On the other hand, male erectile problems have been the subject of extensive research on pathogenesis and medical interventions.

The prevalence of sexual dysfunction is not known precisely, and epidemiologic studies that include sexual dysfunction are rare, especially in women. There have been studies showing that satisfaction with one's marriage does not presume adequate sexual functioning or satisfaction. Frank et al found that 63 of 100 women who considered themselves happily married reported dysfunctions including lack of sexual arousal and orgasm. Other data suggest sexual dysfunctions are common. For example, according to a study by Rosen et al of 329 women between 18 and 79 years old sampled from a gynecologic clinic, orgasm difficulties were reported by 58% and painful intercourse by 29%.

DIAGNOSIS & TREATMENT

Diagnosing sexual dysfunctions in women is a straightforward task. Table 17–1 shows the categories of the American Psychiatric Association's *Diagnostic and Statistical Manual, 4/e (DSM-IV)* used as a guide for clinical assessment. There are six major categories that, when modified by the variables lifelong/not lifelong and generalized/situational, provide a thorough description of the extent of the sexual problem. It is important to ask about each basic category, even if the patient states only one, and to

Diagnosis & Treatment
  Desire Disorders
  Sexual Arousal Disorders
  Orgasmic Disorders
  Sexual Pain Disorders
  Other Sexual Complaints
Screening
Referral to a Specialist
Controversies & Unresolved Issues

identify which dysfunction occurred first. For example, a pain disorder preceded by an arousal disorder (lack of lubrication) suggests a different treatment from a pain disorder that preceded an arousal disorder. In addition, the symptoms must be accompanied by marked distress or interpersonal difficulty to qualify as a disorder in the *DSM-IV*.

Desire Disorders
A. Hypoactive Sexual Desire Disorder:
1. Diagnosis–When a woman reports a desire disorder, it is important to clarify whether she is simply uninterested in sex but able to respond sexually or she is aversive to sex. Hypoactive sexual desire disorder is a common complaint; 30–50% of patients (mostly women) in sex therapy clinics report the condition.

There are two major problems with this diagnosis: (1) there are no norms for sexual desire across ages and (2) the reasons for the development and maintenance of the complaint are variable and imprecise, suggesting it is a heterogeneous diagnosis. Certainly, physical factors can play a role (Table 17–2); in particular, general health, depression, hormonal status, and use of recreational drugs and medications should be reviewed. Psychological and interpersonal factors are as likely if not more likely to play a role. Sudden events such as job loss or family trauma and cumulative factors such as the psychologic response to aging (an especially sensitive issue in women because of the stricter cultural norms for women's attractiveness), life milestones such as children leaving home, or ongoing relationship distress commonly have an impact on sexual desire.

Table 17–1. Female sexual dysfunctions.*

Sexual desire disorders
  Hypoactive sexual desire disorder: Persistent absence or deficiency of sexual feelings and desire for sexual activity. Take into account factors that affect sexual functioning such as age, sex, life context. Rule out other psychiatric disorders such as major depression.
  Sexual aversion disorder: Persistent or recurrent aversion to and avoidance of genital contact with a sexual partner. Rule out other psychiatric disorders such as major depression or obsessive-compulsive disorder.
Sexual arousal disorder
  1. Partial or total lack of physical response as indicated by lack of lubrication and vasocongestion of genitals, or
  2. Persistent lack of a subjective sense of sexual excitement and pleasure during sex. (This criterion is omitted from *DSM-IV*, but it is important for clarification.)
Inhibited female orgasm
  Persistent delay or absence of orgasm. Lack of coital orgasm is usually considered a normal variation of female sexual response if the woman is able to experience orgasm with a partner using other, noncoital methods.
Sexual pain disorders
  Dyspareunia: Recurrent genital pain before, during, or after intercourse. Rule out vaginismus and lack of lubrication.
  Vaginismus: Recurrent involuntary spasm of the outer third of the vagina interfering with or preventing coitus. Rule out physical disorder or other psychiatric disorder (rare).
Sexual dysfunctions not otherwise specified
  Examples: Anesthesia with arousal and orgasm; too-rapid orgasm; genital pain during noncoital activities; lack of pleasure during sex.
Sexual satisfaction
  A woman may be satisfied despite the preceding symptoms, but the partner may be dissatisfied. The problem may be a difference in desire rather than hypoactivity of one partner.

*Using modified *DSM-IV* classification with expansion (Schover et al, 1982). For all diagnoses, specify psychogenic, biogenic, or both; lifelong or not lifelong; generalized or situational.

2. Treatment–Appropriate treatment depends on the outcome of the assessment of the patient's health and psychosocial issues. Generalized and lifelong low sexual desire suggests the need for a screening for endocrine disorders, illness, and long-term medication use. Depression is a possible diagnosis in women with low sexual desire. The use of testosterone has been shown to increase desire but is viewed cautiously as a long-term intervention because of its potential cardiovascular side effects. Kaplan and Owett recommended that low doses of testosterone be used in women with clear androgen deficiencies, such as those produced by bilateral oophorectomy or chemotherapy, because the therapy provides replacement for low androgen levels. These authors do not state recommended dosage levels, however, except to note that 15 mg of testosterone enanthate in aqueous solution (bimonthly injections) restored libido and orgasmic response, with no signs of virilization, in one patient. Other chemical treatments such as yohimbine, antidepressants, and dopamine agonists all appear to carry more of a placebo than a true effect on low desire, although there may be a subgroup that is as yet undescribed for whom these interventions are effective.

The patient also may benefit from information conveyed by the physician. For example, a woman can be informed that there are no current norms for sexual desire at different ages. On the other hand, sexual desire is not expected to go from 2–3 times per week to zero times per week between the ages of 20 and 40 unless something is wrong. Desire and behavioral frequencies (the latter more dependent on the availability of a partner) remain quite stable in women, decreasing generally with age or in the context of a long-term relationship in most couples, regardless of sexual orientation. There are no data on the percentage of couples who stop having sex while maintaining a good relationship; this occurrence may be more common in lesbian couples.

If there is no medical disorder, individual or couples therapy can be recommended. A controlled treatment study has not been published, and differential effectiveness of treatment is likely but unknown; however, the clinical literature provides an estimate of the effectiveness of treatments. Hypoactive sexual desire is one of the more difficult sexual disorders to treat with psychotherapy. One study showed a success rate below 50%. Treatment duration varies but is often 15–45 sessions. Better treatment outcomes are associated with the absence of a global and lifelong desire disorder and with strong commitment to a relationship.

B. Sexual Aversion Disorder:
1. Diagnosis–A much rarer desire disorder, sexual aversion disorder usually is accompanied by low sexual desire and occasionally by vaginismus or dyspareunia. Women with this disorder may have a history of sexual or physical abuse or may have extensive negative, unexpressed feelings about their relationships. Physical factors rarely are involved, although there may be concomitant significant anxiety or obsessive compulsive symptoms that may respond to specific treatment.

2. Treatment–Psychologic intervention, combining individual and couples therapy, can be useful. Therapy typically includes cognitive-behavioral techniques, desensitization, and working through of past issues of abuse. Couples work often focuses on conflict areas, emotional differences, and issues of control. Specific aversions of phobic dimensions, such as aversion to semen, can be difficult to remove and may need to be diminished somewhat and then worked around (eg, avoiding manual stimulation to orgasm). In occasional cases, a significant level of anxiety augments rather modest aversion symptoms, and a course of anxiolytics can be helpful. However,

Table 17–2. Summary of factors and treatment approaches for female sexual dysfunction.*

Physical Factors†	Treatment Action
1. Illness/disease	
Diabetes, neurologic disorder, pelvic inflammatory disease, endometriosis	Treat illness; inform of its sexual effects; refer if adjustment to illness remains a problem.
Depression, anxiety, panic	Refer for consultation concerning medication or psychotherapy, or both.
2. Endocrine status	
Menstrual disorders including anovulatory cycles, thyroid conditions, elevated prolactin	Endocrine workup; consider nonhormonal treatment; with hormonal and other medication, consider sexual side effects and inform patient.
Menopausal	Discuss alteration of hormonal status; consider topical lubricants. For patient information, have list of reference books on menopause available; discuss sexual consequences.
3. Medications	
Antidepressants, neuroleptics, diuretics, hormones, other vasoactive substances	Change medication or reduce dosage if appropriate. Note drug interactions (eg, antidepressants and hormones).
4. Recreational drugs	
Alcohol, nicotine, cocaine, cannabis	If heavy use, refer to treatment; if moderate use, ask if patient can stop for 3 months or dramatically reduce. If not able to do latter, refer for substance abuse treatment or more extensive evaluation.
5. Surgeries	
Abdominal repairs, hysterectomy	Careful physical examination and review of records. If over one year since surgery and no physical signs of problems, refer for consultation.
6. Genitourinary pain	
Interstitial cystitis	Alleviate symptoms of recurrent pain. If no improvement, refer for specialized or psychologic treatment of pain.

Psychological Factors	Treatment Action
1. Acute or chronic stress	
Symptoms of fatigue, poor motivation, sleep disturbance, distractibility, poor coping style	Rule out depression; acknowledge degree of stress; refer for evaluation.
2. Gender identity	Refer for consultation.
3. Sex role satisfaction	Give information and book list; refer for counseling.
4. Sexual knowledge	Give information; refer.
5. Sexual attitudes and values (including religious)	Give information; refer for psychological or religious counseling.
6. Negative body image	
Negative history, aging, illness, surgery, trauma, body weight	Give book list; refer for therapy.

Interactional Factors	Treatment Action
1. History of physical, sexual, or emotional abuse (as a child or adult)	Consider books; refer for therapy.
2. Prior relationships	
Patterns of attachment (chaotic, stressed, clinging) and sex (always poor, decreasing, stopped suddenly)	Consider broader interpersonal issues that may benefit from treatment.
3. Current relationship	
Partner's health, satisfaction, commitment	Give information about impact of relationship on sex; offer to speak with partner; refer.
4. Sexual preferences	
One partner focused on one sexual position or pattern	Recommend discussion with partner; if refused or no effect, refer.

*The examples given here are not inclusive. See text for more details.
†Although listed separately, physical, psychologic, and interactional factors overlap and interact with each other.

it is probably wise to have a clinician experienced in sexual and anxiety disorders give a second opinion before trying an antianxiety medication. Although no outcome statistics are available for these disorders, the duration and success of therapy are estimated to be similar to those of hypoactive sexual desire.

Sexual Arousal Disorders

A. Diagnosis: These disorders are uncommon in women unless there are concomitant menopausal, dyspareunia, or anorgasmic symptoms. Women who report lack of lubrication are most likely to be menopausal or perimenopausal. It should be noted that physical and subjective sexual arousal are not necessarily correlated in women; however, a continual lack of lubrication may lead to discomfort in sex, which will then impair subjective arousal. Also, women's partners sometimes interpret lack of lubrication to mean lack of interest, which can result in a distressed sexual relationship.

B. Treatment: Reviewing possible physical causes for this complaint is the first step. The recommendation of topical lubricants such as K-Y Jelly, Astroglide or estrogenic compounds depends on the woman's physical condition and her risk factors for estrogen therapy. If the woman has another, concurrent sexual dysfunction that preceded her sexual arousal problem, such as lack of orgasm or genital pain, that condition should be addressed first and the woman referred for therapy. The effectiveness of treatment for sexual arousal disorder is essentially unknown because the condition is so rarely treated in the absence of pain or orgasmic dysfunction. A discussion of both of these disorders follows.

Orgasmic Disorders

A. Diagnosis: These disorders are common sexual complaints, with approximately 10% of women reporting global, lifelong lack of orgasm and at least 50% reporting situational and intermittent orgasmic problems. Until recently, it has been rare for an orgasmic problem to have a physical basis, although it is important to review surgeries, use of recreational drugs and alcohol, and medications carefully. With the advent and frequent prescription of serotonin-reuptake inhibitor antidepressants, reports of medication-induced anorgasmia have become more frequent. Orgasm delay also can occur with other medications, including the monoamine oxidase (MAO) inhibitor antidepressants.

Psychological and interpersonal factors frequently contribute to lack of orgasm, including early family history messages about sex as shameful, a view of the parents as untrustworthy or abandoning, unpleasant earlier sexual experiences, and ineffective current sexual techniques of both partners. Male partners of nonorgasmic women often are quite distressed by and feel responsible for the woman's orgasm problem. Although the partner can be helpful by providing physical and emotional attention, taking primary responsibility for a woman's orgasm is counterproductive and can contribute to a continuing lack of orgasm, because the female partner is likely to feel pressured to perform. The woman often feels inhibited and embarrassed about this problem, which makes her less likely to disclose it to a primary care provider than if she had a sexual pain problem.

B. Treatment: It is rare that primary (lifelong, generalized) orgasmic disorder has a physical basis. There is evidence that it can be treated effectively by masturbation or traditional sex therapy techniques or both. Individual, group, and couples therapy have been shown to be effective. Books are available dealing with body image, relaxation, self-observation, tolerance of sexual arousal tension, acceptance of sexual feelings, and sensual touching that may be used alone or with a partner. Lack of progress using

any of the techniques described in the books should be evaluated by a brief counseling consultation. Therapy is usually effective in the 88–90% range for becoming orgasmic during masturbation and in the 75% range for experiencing orgasm in partner activities. Therapy usually takes 15–20 sessions, unless there are issues in the woman's history such as sexual assault or other interpersonal trauma or serious conflicts. Situational or intermittent problems with orgasm are more likely to be related to relationship problems and require additional therapy.

Sexual Pain Disorders

A. Dyspareunia:

1. Diagnosis–Of the sexual pain disorders, dyspareunia—recurrent genital pain before, during, or after intercourse—is the most variable in presentation. Its diagnosis requires a careful physical examination to identify the type of pain and possibly its physical basis, which may be injury, endometriosis, scarring, or unusual skin sensitivity. Pain of a diffuse and long-term nature is more difficult to treat, and the clinician should keep in mind the possibility of referral during the assessment to evaluate potential psychologic factors that could be addressed simultaneously. Psychologic factors include development issues such as guilt and shame surrounding sex, traumatic sexual events such as rape or even painful sex from consensual experiences, and relationship distress such as unresolved conflicts and anger.

2. Treatment–Dyspareunia may be related to organic factors, not all of which can be treated. For example, pain sensitivity may remain after scar tissue is removed. Nevertheless, referral to a psychotherapist could help because behavioral patterns and emotions, eg, fear or tension, may be maintaining the pain. Letting the patient know when no more can be done about the pain on a physical level is important. In addition, it is useful for the patient to discuss with her partner the need to rely on noncoital sexual expression. Low doses of antidepressants may provide temporary help for dyspareunia but are best considered reluctantly, only after consultation with a specialist in sexual disorders, because of the likelihood of the medications affecting desire or orgasmic response. Referral to a specialist also may help in managing the pain by finding ways for the patient to control her focus and relax.

B. Vaginismus:

1. Diagnosis–Recurrent involuntary spasm of the outer third of the vagina interfering with intercourse, vaginismus often is accompanied by much embarrassment on the part of the patient and frustration for the couple. Vaginismus is less common than dyspareunia, but both are infrequent and together account for about 10% of sexual complaints. A primary care provider is likely to see patients with this disorder when symptoms have existed for some time and either relationship distress or desire for pregnancy is prominent. Again, a careful physical examination is important, as is questioning about the initial conditions under which symptoms appeared. Once established, the vaginismus response is enduring and usually requires both a mechanical and a psychologic approach to treatment. Psychologic factors typically include past and present strong sexual inhibition; less commonly include sexual trauma (rape or incest); and frequently involve unexpressed negative feelings toward a sexual partner or other important male figures. Phobia about sexual response or intercourse also may be part of the clinical picture. Finally, in vaginismus, as in dyspareunia, a repeated experience with pain can establish a pain-tension-pain cycle that maintains itself independently of overt psychologic factors.

2. Treatment–The usual recommendation is a dilation procedure, using a series of graduated dilators coupled with relaxation. Gradual involvement of the partner includes his use of dilators or fingers, gradual insertion of his penis, and reliance on the woman's guidance to control the pace and duration of the sexual activity. For severely phobic women, additional techniques and systematic desensitization may be necessary. Although clinicians 20 years ago reported rapid and easy success with vaginismus (10–14 sessions), more recently they report more demanding problems; perhaps patients with milder problems are being treated through self-help methods. There is a book available on this topic by Valins that has been reported to be a useful resource.

Other Sexual Complaints

Lack of sensation in the genital area may be an issue for women who have experienced neurologic disease or injury; the potential for recovery from the underlying illness determines whether the problem can improve or the patient needs to accommodate to the problem. Lack of feeling without physical findings suggests the need for a referral for evaluation to help identify and manage psychologic factors. A patient with noncoital genital pain, like those with other pain disorders, needs careful evaluation for possible physical sensitivity or injury. Early psychologic referral is recommended unless symptoms remit quickly, given the propensity for pain to result in behavioral patterns that may maintain it. When sexual dissatisfaction is based on different levels of sexual desire between the patient and her partner, but both are within the limits of typical variation (eg, 2–3 times a week; one time a month), it may be helpful to let the patient know the usual variations in desire. If differences in desire are well outside the usual range (several times a day; less than once in 6 months), referral for therapy may be offered.

SCREENING

Office screening formats usually include some combination of symptom checklists and interviews. Brief questions about sexual functioning can be included in the general screening. (Research suggests that patients are more likely to answer questions than to initiate sexual information.) Two possible questions are as follows:

1. Are you currently experiencing any sexual concerns or problems? (If an interview format is used, the clinician may consider probing for information about problems of desire, arousal, orgasm, or pain.)
2. (If the patient has answered yes to the previous question.) Does the problem bother you enough that you want to do something about it?

The first question allows the person to raise a wide variety of issues, including contraception, sexual abuse, and safe sex. In fact, separate questions about these issues can be asked in the same period of time. The second question helps the clinician to evaluate whether the person expresses enough distress to want to pursue help. If she does not, the information is useful in determining whether the symptoms are related to another problem such as depression, genital injury or sensitivity, endocrine problems, or medication-related disorders, or whether they fit into a broader disease pattern such as that of diabetes or a neurologic disorder.

It is important for the clinician not to assume that a patient is heterosexual until this fact has been made clear by the patient. Some sexual complaints, such as vaginismus, are clearly less common in lesbian women; others are just as common. For example, lack of lubrication can be a bothersome issue regardless of sexual orientation.

REFERRAL TO A SPECIALIST

Primary care practitioners cannot be expected to provide all the treatment options available for sexual disorders. In some cases, even the diagnostic workup may benefit from a specialist's consultation to avoid inefficient referral or unnecessary treatment. Conditions under which a referral should be considered include the following:

1. The physician is uncertain of the diagnosis. If the problem appears to be long-term yet situational, and possibly contributed to by a myriad of physical, psychologic, and interpersonal factors, an early referral may prevent dissatisfaction and save both money and time for the patient.
2. The factors surrounding the sexual problem appear to be in an area in which the primary care

provider has limited expertise. Common areas include psychological and interpersonal factors as well as the nonphysical consequences of illness or normal physiologic processes. For example, some women have a mixture of psychological reactions to menopause and the events surrounding it, as do their partners. The psychologic reactions can be even more extensive in response to a disease like multiple sclerosis; the complaint of loss of sexual functioning may be a patient's "flag" for fears of a number of interpersonal losses. Lack of specialized training and knowledge in the area of sexuality may be an issue, particularly regarding the factors that determine a good sex life, predictors of relationship endurance and happiness, and sexual values and attitudes. Well-intentioned advice to "have a glass of wine to relax before sex" or "take a vacation" has been offered in the past by primary care providers. For an ongoing sexual problem, the patient may benefit more from a brief consultation with a therapist.

3. The symptoms are intense or severe. A 35-year-old woman who has never been able to have intercourse because of vaginismus is best referred to a specialist in sexual problems after a careful history and physical examination. Similarly, a patient who reports extensive distress or serious relationship problems associated with a sexual dysfunction may benefit most by rapid referral to a specialist in sexuality or relationships.

Whether referring for a second opinion, an evaluation, or treatment, several factors can increase the likelihood of success. One should know the ability of the clinician referred to and have confidence that he or she will do a thorough job. It is useful to keep a short list of names of specialists in the areas of sexuality, psychiatry, psychology, relationship distress, and endocrinology. One should ask for verbal or written feedback from the referral agent; written reports take longer and bear a cost to patients. It is possible, however, that the patient may refuse to give permission for information exchange, especially in the case of a referral for psychotherapy or management of psychiatric medication. Also important are the manner and message used in presenting the referral to the patient. One should explain briefly the reason for the referral; if referring to a nonmedical specialist, one might state that both normal and problematic functioning are established to be result from an interaction of the mind and the body. If referring to a psychiatrist, psychologist, social worker, or nurse, one should specify the referral agent's area of expertise, eg, sexuality, pain disorders, diagnosis, medication interactions. The recommendation of a therapist for recovery from rape, sexual abuse, or physical abuse might be accompanied by the statement that some people find that therapy speeds the recovery process. In the case of a referral to a marital or relationship therapist, it may be worthwhile to mention that distressed relationships take a toll on individual family members' health (increased clinic visits have been reported), work efficiency, and general functioning. Perhaps the most important message the patient needs to hear is that a referral will increase the likelihood that the problem will be dealt with quickly and thoroughly, with less cost to health and quality of life.

CONTROVERSIES & UNRESOLVED ISSUES

Sexual problems can be a source of distress, causing pain and discomfort; can result from a disease such as diabetes; and can have a ripple effect on other areas of a woman's life. Examples of effects in other areas of life are the avoidance of forming enduring relationships, the avoidance of having children although they are desired, ongoing relationship distress or dissolution, or discontinuance of a sexuality impairing medication prescribed for a serious medical condition. A woman may feel that a sexual complaint is not only embarrassing but insignificant. It is the responsibility of the health care provider to include sexual disorders in the realm of health care. Unfortunately, little attention traditionally is given in medical and professional training programs concerning how to appropriately ask about sexual complaints, the treatment of sexual complaints, and the connections between sexual complaints and other areas of a woman's life.

Just as hormone replacement therapy (HRT) remains controversial, so does prescription of hormonal agents to deal with vaginal lubrication (estrogens) and sexual desire (androgens). Although androgens have been found to increase sexual desire in surgically menopausal women, the long-term effects of the use of these drugs has not been evaluated. One must recognize and weigh the possible effects of androgens and HRT on each patient. Even when data on large samples of women become available, the decision to treat will continue to involve weighing risks and benefits.

Also unresolved is the issue of how to manage patients who insist on a medical treatment when a less invasive, nonmedical treatment is recommended. One example is a woman who requests yohimbine instead of psychotherapy for low sex drive. Given the modest effectiveness of yohimbine and the uncertain effectiveness of psychotherapy for her disorder, a trial of yohimbine may seem appropriate. If she later requests treatment with testosterone, however, the primary care provider should look at her current testosterone levels, be familiar with her medical profile, making sure the woman understands the risks and benefits of both drug treatment and psychotherapy. Sexual disorders are caught in the ever-expanding web of concern and controversy regarding provider and patient roles in making informed treatment decisions.

REFERENCES

American Psychiatric Association: *Diagnostic and Statistical Manual of Mental Disorders,* 4th ed. American Psychiatric Association, 1994.

Blumstein P, Schwartz P: *American Couples.* Morrow, 1983.

Burman B, Margolin G: Analysis of the association between marital relationships and health problems. Psychol Bull 1992;112:39.

Frank E, Anderson A, Rubinstein D: Frequency of sexual dysfunction in "normal" couples. N Engl J Med 1978;199:11.

Heiman J, LoPiccolo J: *Becoming Orgasmic: A Sexual and Personal Growth Program for Women,* 2nd ed. Prentice Hall, 1988.

Kaplan HS, Owen T: The female androgen deficiency syndrome. J Sex Marital Ther 1993;19:3.

Kilmann PR et al: Perspectives of sex therapy outcome: A survey of AASECT providers. J Sex Marital Ther 1986;12:116.

Levine SB: Intrapsychic and individual aspects of sexual desire. In: *Sexual Desire Disorders.* Leiblum SR, Rosen RC (editors). Guilford, 1988.

Rosen RC, Leiblum SR: Assessment and treatment of desire disorders. In: *Principles and Practices of Sex Therapy.* Leiblum SR, Rosen (editors). Guilford, 1989.

Rosen RC, Leiblum SR (editors): *Erectile Disorders: Assessment and Treatment.* Guilford, 1992.

Rosen RC et al: Prevalence of sexual dysfunction in women: Results of a survey study of 329 women in an outpatient gynecological clinic. J Sex Marital Ther 1993;19:171.

Schover L et al: A multiaxial problem-oriented system for the sexual defenses: An alternative to DSM III. Arch Gen Psychiatry 1982;39:614.

Segraves RT: Drugs and desire. In: *Sexual Desire Disorders.* Leiblum SR, Rosen RC (editors). Guilford, 1988.

Sherwin B, Gelfand M, Brender W: Androgen enhances sexual motivation in females: A prospective, cross-over study of sex steroid administration in the surgical menopause. Psychosom Med 1985;47:339.

Valins L: *When a Woman's Body Says No to Sex: Understanding and Overcoming Vaginismus.* Penguin, 1992.

Verhulst J, Heiman J: A systems perspective on sexual desire. In: *Perspectives on Sexual Desire.* Leiblum SR, Rosen RC (editors). Guilford, 1988.

Section IV.
Metabolic & Endocrine Disorders

Obesity

18

Robert A. Kanter, MD

Essentials of Diagnosis
- Twenty percent or more above ideal body weight.

Incidence & Risk Factors

Obesity has become a major public health problem in the United States and in other economically developed countries. In 1994, the latest National Health and Nutrition Examination Survey (1988–1991) found that 35% of women in the USA 20 years of age or older were 20% or more above their ideal body weight. The prevalence of obesity has doubled in the USA since 1900. Obesity has a higher prevalence in minority and lower socioeconomic status populations. Its prevalence increases with age, especially in women. When multiple risk factors coincide, as in black women aged 45–75, the prevalence rates are up to 60%.

Morbidity & Mortality

Obesity is associated with significant excess morbidity and mortality. An NIH Consensus Conference reported that at 160% of ideal weight, obese people have twice the death rate of nonobese people, and at 200% of ideal weight, the death rate is 3 times as high. Other smaller studies report up to 8-fold increases in death rate. Mortality is caused primarily by increased rates of cardiovascular disease. Increases in diabetes, hypertension, gallbladder disease, arthritis, and cancer also contribute to excess morbidity and mortality. Obese women experience increased rates of cancer of the gallbladder, uterus, ovaries, and breast.

The distribution of the excess fat mass (upper body versus lower body) and the total fat mass are independent determinants of risk (see the section, "Evaluation"). Although fat deposited in the upper body, particularly in the intra-abdominal cavity, carries a greater risk of hypertension, diabetes, cardiovascular disease, and breast cancer, excess fat in a lower body distribution (on the buttocks and thighs), as is most common in women, also is associated with increased rates of these illnesses. The Nurse's Health Study followed 115,000 women prospectively for 8 years and found that even mild degrees of obesity were associated with increased rates of cardiovascular disease. After the data were adjusted for age and smoking status, women 130% or more above ideal

Essentials of Diagnosis
Incidence & Risk Factors
Morbidity & Mortality
Etiology
Evaluation
Treatment
Issues of Pregnancy & Obesity
Psychosocial Concerns

weight had 3.3 times greater risk of cardiovascular disease than women at ideal body weight.

Etiology

A. Historical Perspective: The prevailing theory of the cause of obesity has undergone marked shifts in the last 40 years. In the 1950s, psychoanalysts postulated that obesity was caused by a basic personality problem and that the patient was acting out unconscious conflicts. Later, behavior therapists wrote that obesity was a learned disorder caused by conditioning. Published accounts of successful short-term behavioral treatments led to the widespread use of such therapy in commercial and hospital-based programs.

In the 1970s and 1980s, animal studies showed that weight is regulated by a complex interaction of neural, hormonal, and metabolic factors, and led to the development of a set-point theory. Genetic studies in humans showed that obesity often clustered in families, which reinforced the idea of a predetermined weight that the body would attempt to keep.

The problem with all of these theories is that they assume obesity is a single disease with a single cause. Obesity is a heterogeneous condition, however, with many contributing factors. It is no longer believed that body weight is regulated to one precise point but that it varies over a range, affected by a complex interaction of genetic and environmental influences.

B. Genetic Influences: In the late 1980s, twin studies established conclusively that the regulation of body weight has a significant genetic component. Unfortunately, these studies were carried out primarily in lean people and the results do not necessarily apply to the obese. When the data were examined more carefully, it was found that the concordance rates for obesity were much lower in the heavier than the leaner twin pairs (36% versus 60%, respectively). It was concluded that genetics plays a much greater role in the weight of lean than of obese people. Bouchard examined more than 1700 relatives in 409 families in Quebec and estimated that the regulation of body fat had a genetic component of 25%, whereas 30% was culturally transmitted and 45% was nontransmissible.

Practitioners should explain to overweight patients that their weight is not genetically "cast in stone." People inherit only a tendency toward obesity, and this tendency can be modulated by diet and exercise. Evidence of this gene-environment interaction is provided by migration studies comparing genetically similar populations. Japanese-American men living in Hawaii and California are 2–3 times more likely to become obese than Japanese men living in Japan.

Genetic factors appear to influence the resting metabolic rate (RMR), which is the energy expended to sustain the body's vital functions when at rest. RMR accounts for 60–75% of the total calories burned each day, and its level appears to be influenced greatly by heredity. Longitudinal studies have shown that subjects with low metabolic rates are more likely to gain weight than those with normal or high rates. The RMR can vary by as much as 1000 kcal/d in obese women of similar age, weight, and height. Thus, some obese people are more energy-efficient than others, and a low RMR is a risk factor for obesity.

C. Environmental Influences: One of the best studies to demonstrate the interaction of environmental and genetic influences on body weight was the Iowa Adoption Study of Price et al. The authors compared the adult weights of children adopted at birth with the weights of their biologic and adopted parents. The weights of the adoptees as adults more closely resembled their biologic parents' weights, demonstrating a clear genetic component. The biologic parents' weights explained only 50% of the variance in the adoptees' adult weights, however. The other 50% was explained by environmental factors.

Children adopted into rural families weighed more as adults than children adopted into urban families. In addition, those adopted into stressful families also weighed more as adults. Stressful families were defined as families with premature death or divorce of an adopted parent or the presence of alcoholism or emotional illness in an adopted parent. Thus, both environmental and genetic factors were found to influence body weight. The rural-urban effect has been confirmed by studies in Denmark, and recently, additional studies of the association of psychosocial stress and obesity have appeared.

Felitti (1991) and Springs and Friedrich reported the association of a history of sexual abuse and obe-

sity in general medical patients. McGann reported an association of parental alcoholism and obesity. In a case-controlled study of patients seeking treatment for obesity, Felitti (1993) found increased rates of early parental loss; parental alcoholism; and personal history of depression, anxiety, substance abuse, and current marital dysfunction in obese patients compared with never-obese controls. Most recently, Lissau and Sorensen found that parental neglect during childhood increased the risk of adult obesity.

D. Interaction of Genetic and Environmental Factors: It has been accepted for a long time that the classic eating disorders, bulimia nervosa and anorexia nervosa, are complex biopsychosocial phenomena. The results of the more recent research on obesity lead to the conclusion that obesity also is caused by a complex interaction of biologic, psychological, and social factors.

For example, not all children of alcoholics or all incest survivors are obese. These stress factors by themselves are not sufficient to cause obesity. In those who have inherited a "thrifty metabolism," however, these stress factors might interfere with the ability to compensate for that slow metabolism. Not all obese people are survivors of early trauma or children of dysfunctional families. Some may have counterproductive life-styles, eg, two jobs and no time for themselves, work in the food-service industry, or sedentary hobbies. Failure to address these psychosocial factors may contribute to high relapse rates. The encouraging fact is that these psychosocial stress factors are all treatable.

E. Eating Styles: Early studies concluded that there was no difference in eating style or level of caloric intake between obese and nonobese people. More recent studies challenge this view. The doubly-labeled water technique now allows accurate estimation of the 24-hour energy expenditure in nonhospitalized people. Both obese and nonobese people underestimate their caloric intake as recorded in diet diaries. In obese people, the underestimation ranges from 30 to 50% and is significantly greater than that seen in nonobese people.

Furthermore, 25–45% of obese patients seeking weight-loss treatment in university- and hospital-based programs report problems with binge eating. These patients report eating large amounts of food in a short period of time and that they feel out of control of their eating during the episodes. Obese binge eaters generally do not attempt to compensate for their overeating by purging, which distinguishes this disorder from bulimia nervosa.

In two multisite field trials of newly proposed diagnostic criteria for binge-eating disorder (BED), the prevalence of binge eating in nonpatient community samples was low, about 2.5%. In the nonpatient obese population, the prevalence was 5–10%. Among patients seeking weight-loss treatment, the rates were much higher. Binge eating was reported by 16% of participants in a commercial weight-loss program, by 30% in hospital-based programs, and by 71% in Overeaters Anonymous, a self-help group for "compulsive overeaters."

Several studies have shown that binge eating is associated with greater degrees of obesity. In many people, binge eating without purging of calories is a major cause of weight gain. Others, however, become obese, attempt to lose weight by dieting, and start binge eating in response to severe caloric deprivation. In the multisite field trials, 49% of those with BED reported that their binge eating started before they began dieting for weight loss, and 37% reported that they began dieting before beginning binge eating. The remainder of the respondents believed that the two behaviors began at the same time.

Other studies of adults have confirmed that binge eating more commonly precedes dieting. This important finding has not been appreciated by those in the "antidiet" movement, who counsel the overweight not to diet because it may lead to an eating disorder. A careful history of which came first, binge eating or dieting, is critical in planning treatment for obese women who binge.

Initial treatment studies employing standard behavioral methods showed that binge eaters dropped out of treatment and regained weight sooner than nonbinge eaters. More recent studies using more comprehensive multidisciplinary treatment protocols showed no difference in initial weight loss or weight loss sustained at 1 year between binge eaters and non-binge eaters.

F. Physical Activity: Obese adults are less physically active than nonobese adults, and many treatment studies have concluded that increased physical activity is a critical ingredient in long-term weight management. However, these findings alone do not prove that obesity is caused by inactivity. It is clear that in some cases obesity causes inactivity. Many relapsing dieters have been observed to maintain their exercise programs until the added weight makes vigorous exercise uncomfortable. In these people, weight gain leads to inactivity, which perpetuates the weight gain; the inactivity does not cause the obesity.

Evaluation

A. Classification by Weight: For the purpose of helping patients select among treatments, a simple three-level classification of obesity has proved useful. The three levels are defined by the percentage overweight* according to standard tables of height and weight: mild 20–40%, moderate 41–100%, and

*The benchmark weight being the midpoint of the recommended weight range at a specified height for people of medium build from the 1983 Metropolitan Life Insurance Company Table.

Table 18–1. Classification of obesity in women by degree of severity.

Class	Percentage Overweight*	Body Mass Index (BMI)	Prevalence Among Obese (%)
Mild	20–40	25–30	90
Moderate	41–100	30.1–35	9.5
Severe	> 100	> 35	0.5

*Midpoint of recommended weight range for medium build at specific height, from 1983 Metropolitan Life Insurance Company tables as benchmark.

severe over 100% (Table 18–1). The corresponding BMIs are 25–30, 30.1–35, and over 35, respectively. The threshold for obesity of 20% overweight or a BMI of 25 (27 for men) was recommended by a National Institutes of Health Consensus Conference, which determined that risk to health begins when the body mass exceeds this level, and weight loss becomes medically indicated. A weight that is 40% above ideal weight (BMI above 30) corresponds to an inflection upward in the mortality curve and represents a level at which medical intervention becomes strongly indicated. At 100% above ideal weight, the risks to health may be great enough to warrant consideration of surgical intervention.

Percentage overweight is a concept easily understood by patients and practitioners. From a practical standpoint, it is the weight criterion used most often by insurance companies to determine which weight-management service (none, medical, or surgical) the company will authorize for reimbursement. Percentage overweight, however, is subject to arbitrary changes in the tables defining ideal weight.

The body mass index (BMI), or weight in kilograms/height in meters^2, has gained favor in research. It does not depend on complicated tables; it corrects the degree of fatness by height and allows more accurate comparisons between people of different heights. The disadvantage of using BMI is that most patients and physicians are not familiar with BMI units. This makes it difficult for them to appreciate the significance of the value and to use the measure in clinical work.

B. Pattern of Regional Fat Distribution: The distribution of excess fat mass is a risk factor independent of the total fat mass or degree of overweight. Because fat deposited in the upper half of the body carries greater risk of morbidity and mortality, body fat distribution should be measured in each patient.

From a clinical standpoint, the ratio of the circumferences of the waist and hips (waist:hip ratio [WHR]) is a simple, objective method for estimating the pattern of regional fat distribution. A WHR equal to or greater than 0.8 in women is considered a degree of upper body fat distribution sufficient to increase risk and thus to warrant recommendation of weight reduction.

C. Medical Evaluation: The following conditions are contraindications for aggressive weight-loss therapy:

Malignant arrhythmias
Unstable angina
Acute myocardial infarction or cerebrovascular accident
Active peptic ulcer, thrombophlebitis, or gout
Lactation or pregnancy
Protein-wasting diseases, eg, lupus, Cushing's syndrome
Major system failure, eg, hepatic or renal failure
Drug-induced protein wasting, eg, antineoplastic agents, steroids equivalent to or greater than 20 mg/d prednisone
Symptomatic cholelithiasis
Active bulimia nervosa
Active substance abuse

Other conditions mandate caution in managing weight loss; these include the following:

History of peptic ulcer, thrombophlebitis, or gout
History of cholelithiasis (without cholecystectomy)
History of eating disorder
Prepubertal age
History of suicide attempt
Chronic drug therapy, eg, insulin, oral hypoglycemics, lithium, nonsteroidal anti-inflammatory drugs, diuretics, antihypertensives, antiangina agents

1. History–In addition to a routine medical history, it is important to look for any condition that might be contributing to obesity, such as Cushing's disease, insulinoma, hypothyroidism, polycystic ovarian syndrome, or ovarian failure. The first two conditions can be treated surgically. The last three may cause mild obesity alone or may combine with other factors to cause major obesity. They can be treated medically, and their treatment enhances other treatments of obesity. Several rare syndromes associated with obesity—Prader-Willi, Laurence-Moon-Biedl, and Fröhlich's syndromes and hyperostosis frontalis—are beyond the scope of this chapter.

It is important to document medical conditions that will be improved by weight loss, because this information may help motivate the patient to follow through with treatment. Such conditions include hypertension, diabetes mellitus, hyperlipidemia, sleep apnea, loud snoring, arthritis of weight-bearing joints, low back pain, reflux esophagitis, angina, intermittent claudication, congestive heart failure, chronic obstructive pulmonary disease, peripheral edema, and intertriginous dermatitis. Sleep apnea deserves special attention because it is common in moderate and severe obesity and often is unrecognized. Major symptoms include morning headache, daytime hypersomnolence, restless sleep, nightmares, nocturnal awakening with dyspnea, and dramatically loud snoring. Family members may be able to confirm apneic episodes. A history suspicious for sleep apnea should prompt a referral to a sleep center, because treatment will enhance the patient's ability to follow any weight-management program.

It is important to identify any conditions that might be aggravated by weight loss so that they can be monitored carefully and treatment adjusted if necessary. These conditions include renal or hepatic failure, history of cholelithiasis, peptic ulcer, thrombophlebitis, and gout. Similar monitoring is necessary if the patient is being treated with diuretics, antihypertensives, antiangina drugs, antineoplastic agents, insulin, oral hypoglycemics, steroids, or nonsteroidal anti-inflammatory drugs (NSAIDs).

Contraction of the blood volume and the catabolic stress of aggressive weight loss can worsen renal or hepatic failure. Dehydration can increase the risk of a recurrence in patients with a history of thrombophlebitis. Patients with a history of these conditions should attempt only conservative regimens that produce weight losses of $\frac{1}{2}$–1 pound/wk.

Patients with past peptic ulcer disease should be treated prophylactically with H_2-blockers, because hypocaloric diets often lead to increased acid production. A history of gout warrants prescription of low-dose allopurinol and monitoring of serum uric acid, which often rises with dieting. Patients who require NSAIDs or steroids should be treated prophylactically with misoprostol to protect the gastrointestinal tract. Dosages of diuretic, antihypertensive, antianginal, and oral hypoglycemic agents and of insulin may have to be reduced as weight is lost.

A history of symptomatic cholelithiasis warrants ultrasonography of the gallbladder and pretreatment laparoscopic cholecystectomy or concurrent ursodiol therapy if stones are found. Weight loss increases the lithogenicity of bile and can precipitate acute cholecystitis in patients with asymptomatic stones. Ursodiol corrects the increased lithogenicity of bile during weight loss.

Recent myocardial infarction or stroke, or peptic ulcer (within 3 months), current thrombophlebitis, unstable angina, major arrhythmias, lactation, and pregnancy are absolute contraindications to aggressive weight loss (greater than $\frac{1}{2}$ lb/wk).

The menstrual and reproductive history are important, also. Many obese women have oligo- or amenorrhea and are infertile. Because weight loss often restores regular cycles and fertility, a reliable method of birth control is necessary during weight loss. Diaphragms may become loose with weight loss; the fit must be checked for each 20 pounds of weight loss.

A thorough weight history should be obtained, including onset of obesity, weight changes over the years, lifetime maximum weight, events associated with rapid weight gain or loss, and effects of pregnancy on weight. Prior attempts at weight loss should be documented, including the type of program; duration of treatment; amount of weight loss; length of time weight loss was sustained; and use of anorectic drugs, very-low-calorie diets, or obesity surgery. Patients should be asked to identify any special problems or risk factors that perpetuate obesity or cause weight regain.

Because patients may be reluctant to volunteer information on emotional or social factors, special attention should be given to these areas. Specific questions about substance abuse, unusual eating patterns, and history of physical or sexual abuse should be asked in person, because patients often decline to answer the same questions on a self-report questionnaire or review of systems form.

A thorough family history is important. The heights and weights of immediate family members should be obtained, as well as any history of complications of obesity; eating disorders; substance abuse; emotional illness; or loss of parental contact through premature death, divorce, or disability.

2. Physical examination–A complete physical examination is necessary, with particular attention to the systems affected by obesity. Evidence of diabetes; hypertension; thrombophlebitis; or gallbladder, heart, or acid peptic disease should be sought. The upper airways should be checked for narrowing, especially if symptoms of sleep apnea are present. Skin breakdown in intertriginous areas, peripheral edema, and venous stasis changes are all more common in obese people. Conditions that might interfere with treatment or exercise should be investigated, including foot ulcers, arthritis, and deformity of the spine, legs, or feet.

3. Laboratory tests–Recommended laboratory tests include (1) complete blood cell count (CBC); (2) fasting chemistry panel, including electrolytes, glucose, renal and liver function studies (including a measure of gamma-glutamyltransferase [GGT] to screen for alcohol abuse), and uric acid; (3) lipid profile including total cholesterol, high-density lipoprotein (HDL), low-density lipoprotein (LDL), and triglycerides; (4) thyroid panel including free thyroxine index and thyroid-stimulating hormone (TSH); and (5) urinalysis.

If hypertriglyceridemia, major obesity (more than 50 pounds above ideal weight), or a family history of diabetes is present, a formal 2-hour oral glucose tolerance test and glycohemoglobin level should be obtained. An overnight dexamethasone suppression test should be ordered only if the clinical picture strongly suggests Cushing's syndrome.

If there is a history of biliary colic or stones, or if right-upper-quadrant tenderness is noted on physical examination, an abdominal ultrasonographic examination should be obtained to assess biliary pathology.

D. Psychological Evaluation: An in-depth psychological evaluation is beyond the expertise of most primary care practitioners. It is more effective for the practitioner to do a brief screening and, if necessary, suggest an appropriate referral to a specialist.

It is important to obtain information about diet readiness, relative behavioral contraindications to weight-loss treatment, and psychosocial stress factors. For patients who are ready to lose weight, who have no behavioral contraindications or significant psychosocial stress factors, referral can be made to a registered dietitian or a low-intensity program such as the ones described in the following section, "Treatment." Patients who have behavioral contraindications or significant psychosocial stress are best referred to a professional multidisciplinary weight-management program or to an individual therapist so that more in-depth assessment can be made and more intensive therapy employed.

1. Diet readiness–A patient should be encouraged to consider whether the time is right to lose weight. Is her job (or her partner's job) stable? Does she have the time to devote to weight management? Are her family members in reasonable physical and emotional health? Will family and friends be supportive? Is it realistic for her to become more physically active?

One effective way to stimulate patients to consider their state of readiness is to suggest reading on the subject. Many self-help books on weight loss have excellent chapters on diet readiness. They often include brief self-administered questionnaires that let the patient draw her own conclusions. The section "Are you ready"? in *Thin for Life* by Fletcher is a good example. Other helpful chapters can be found in *The Truth About Addiction and Recovery* by Peele and Brodsky and *The Weight Maintenance Survival Guide* by Brownell and Rodin.

2. Behavioral contraindications to weight loss–Bulimia nervosa is characterized by uncontrolled binge eating, with subsequent purging (induced vomiting or laxative abuse). It is likely to interfere with any attempt at weight loss without the support of a therapist or multidisciplinary team well versed in eating disorders. Patients with active bulimia or who have recovered from bulimia should attempt to lose weight only with conservative balanced deficit diets of 1200–1500 kcals/d and with the support of an eating-disorder therapist (see Chapter 10). Binge eating without purging, which is present in 25–50% of obese patients who seek professional help to lose weight, also is treated best in a professional multidisciplinary weight-management program or by an individual therapist with an interest in eating disorders.

Depression can be a contributing cause of weight gain and an impediment to successful participation in a weight-management program. Up to 26% of patients who seek professional help to lose weight meet the criteria outlined in the *Diagnostic and Statistical*

Manual, 3/e Revised *(DSM-III-R)* for a current affective disorder (7.4% major depression; 16.7% dysthymia, ie, mild depression; and 1.9% bipolar illness). The Beck Depression Inventory is a simple, one-page questionnaire that can be used by primary care practitioners to screen for depression. Patients who score in the severely depressed range (Beck score higher than 29) should be referred for treatment of the depression first and pursue weight loss at a later time, when the depression has lifted. If it is clear that the weight problem is a major cause of the depression, participation in a weight-loss program with a professional behavioral component can lead to rapid improvement in mood. Patients with moderate degrees of depression (Beck score 20–29) should be referred to a multi-disciplinary program in which antidepressants can be prescribed and professional counseling can be offered or to a therapist for individual psychological counseling that can take place while the patient participates in a structured weight-loss program. If the patient reports a history of diet-induced depression, she should be referred for therapy before she begins any weight-management program and should continue with therapy concurrent with any attempt to lose weight. For such patients, slow, steady weight loss with a conventional 1200–1500 calorie diet may be preferable to rapid weight loss using a formula diet.

Patients experiencing an acute psychiatric disorder, such as anxiety or psychosis, should not attempt weight loss until the condition is treated. The distress of the psychiatric condition will interfere with program compliance, and the deprivation of dieting may exacerbate the emotional disorder. Close collaboration between the patient's mental health professional and the providers of the weight-management program should continue throughout weight-loss treatment.

Current or past substance abuse is about twice as common in women who seek professional help for weight loss as in women in the general population. Weight-loss treatment is inappropriate for patients with active substance-abuse problems, including abuse of alcohol, barbiturates, cocaine, and marihuana. Patients should be referred for treatment of the substance-abuse disorder before they are encouraged to devote attention to their weight. It is likely that many of the issues that underlie the substance-abuse disorder also play a role in their use of food. Any skills or insights gained in substance-abuse recovery may prove helpful in the patient's weight-management efforts.

Tobacco use is not a contraindication to weight-loss treatment. Patients should be advised, however, not to try to stop smoking and lose weight at the same time. The emotional and physiologic changes caused by smoking cessation are likely to interfere with adherence to a weight-management program.

Patients should be advised to stop smoking several months before or after losing weight.

Because many women cite weight gain as one of the major reasons they restart smoking, it may be preferable for some women to lose weight before they stop smoking. The skills gained in a weight-loss program may help the patient to limit weight gain after she has stopped smoking. Patients should be informed, however, that smoking usually places one at far greater health risk than does obesity.

Patients experiencing marked stress from marital or occupational problems, illness, death of a loved one, or other major life events may not be good candidates for weight loss. A recent study has shown that the more adverse life events experienced at the time a weight-loss program is started, the more likely the patient is to drop out before completing treatment. Patients have difficulty fully embracing a weight-reduction program if their concentration and energies are focused on a life crisis. On the other hand, if a patient insists she can meet the demands of a weight-management program, that decision should be supported. Some patients report that weight is the one area of their life that they can control when the rest of their life seems beyond control.

Some psychosocial stress factors are not of crisis proportions but are long-standing issues. These "roadblock issues" drain sufficient energy from the patient that she does not have the personal resources to be successful at weight management. Two of the most common issues are parental alcoholism and past physical or sexual abuse. A simple screening questionnaire has been developed to elicit a history of these and other psychosocial stress factors (see Appendix A: Roadblock Questionnaire). These stress factors impair a patient's ability to develop the "empowered" state of mind that is necessary for successful long-term weight management.

If the patient endorses the presence of roadblock issues, one should refer her for either appropriate counseling concurrent with attempts at weight loss or treatment at a comprehensive program that can address both psychosocial issues and weight-management skills.

Treatment

A. Treatment Philosophy: A discussion of weight management in a book on women's health must address the issue of whether it is reasonable to try to change one's body weight at all. The "antidiet" movement has argued against dieting because of high relapse rates and, in women, because dieting can be a symbol of yielding to the pressure of male stereotypes that emphasize the cultural definition of beauty at the expense of developing other talents. Antidiet advocates note that studies indicate that body shape has a large genetic component that cannot be changed at will. Furthermore, they state that attempts to alter one's shape by repeated dieting can lead to increased weight variability, which may be associated with adverse health outcomes.

Professional literature and the lay press have paid much attention to a few observational studies noting a possible adverse health effect of weight variability (yo-yo dieting). Some of these studies have suggested that remaining overweight may be preferable to repeated attempts at weight loss. A recent national task force, however, reported that the evidence was inconclusive. Studies have not differentiated between intentional and unintentional weight loss and were not designed to determine the effects in obese as opposed to nonobese people. Thus, the above arguments are applicable to average weight people, but not for obese people. The antidiet movement will make a positive contribution if it discourages dieting and dissatisfaction with the body in people of normal weight and the seeking of unrealistically low weights in overweight people.

On the other hand, society will not be well served if overweight people are convinced that diets are ineffective in the obese, that dieting is a greater risk to health than staying heavy, and that excess weight is an unimportant health risk. The fact remains that people who are more than 20% above ideal body weight, as defined by the 1983 Metropolitan Life Insurance Tables for desirable weights, are at increased risk for excess morbidity and mortality.

B. Treatment Goals: Several lines of evidence support the efforts of obese patients to achieve lower weights. Long-term (4–5 year) follow-up studies of patients undergoing obesity surgery show that weight loss greatly reduces mortality rates, even though few patients reach ideal body weight.

Studies of nonsurgical weight loss also have shown that it is not necessary to attain an ideal body weight to achieve significant health benefits. As little as a 10% loss of body weight (20–30 pounds) can normalize blood pressure in obese patients who are hypertensive. Modest losses of 10–20 pounds can significantly improve diabetes control in adult obese patients with type II diabetes. Cholesterol and triglyceride levels also can improve with similar losses. Even if some of the weight is regained, these health benefits may persist for up to 2 additional years.

It may be effective to encourage patients to set short-term goals for moderate weight loss. Maintaining the health benefits that accompany moderate weight loss can be a central goal of treatment, even if more weight is to be lost later. The aim is to help the patient to feel successful and enhance her self-esteem despite the fact that she has not attained her ideal weight. Brownell and Rodin have proposed a set of questions (Table 18–2) to help guide patients in selecting reasonable weight-loss goals.

Reliable data on short-term weight loss and maintenance of weight loss are available for only a small percentage of obesity treatment programs. The best-

Table 18–2. Questions to ask for setting a reasonable weight goal.*

1. Is there a history of excess weight in your parents or grandparents?
2. What is the lowest weight you have maintained as an adult for at least 1 year?
3. What is the largest size of clothes that you feel comfortable in, at the point you say "I look pretty good considering where I have been?" At what weight would you wear these clothes?
4. Think of a friend or family member (of your age and body frame) who looks "normal" to you. How much does that person weigh?
5. At what weight do you believe you can live with the required changes in eating and exercise?

*These questions represent clinical impressions and are based in part on criteria proposed by Brownell KD, Rodin J: The Weight Maintenance Survival Guide. American Health Publishing, 1990. Research-based criteria have not been established.

documented programs are university-based research programs employing behavioral therapy, very-low-calorie diets, pharmacotherapy, or surgery. These programs serve relatively few people. On the other hand, self-help groups, commercial programs, and popular diet books reach millions of people, but almost nothing has been published about their efficacy.

From reviews of the published literature, Bennett concluded that the greater the structure and the intensity of treatment, the greater the weight loss. Conventional 1200-calorie diets combined with behavioral therapy result in an average of 18–20 pounds lost in 20 weeks. Two-thirds of this loss is maintained over the next year. Patients treated more intensively under medical supervision, using very-low-calorie diets (420–800 calories) and behavioral therapy, lose 45–55 pounds in 12–16 weeks and maintain one-half to two-thirds of this loss in the following year. Programs using very-low-calorie diets and behavior therapy that provide opportunities for long-term treatment achieve better long-term results. Average weight losses of up to 48 pounds (72% of initial weight loss) have been sustained at 5-year follow-up examinations.

About 50% of severely obese patients who are treated surgically maintain a 50% or greater reduction in excess weight 5 years after surgery. This figure corresponds to sustained weight losses of 50–100 pounds. Surgery requires lifelong postoperative care to avoid vitamin and mineral deficiencies. Noncompliance with the postoperative diet can lead to vomiting after gastroplasty and diarrhea and dumping syndrome after gastrointestinal bypass. Weight may be regained from maladaptive eating and patients may demand surgical reversal after either procedure. Combining surgery with psychological counseling and other recovery interventions may improve long-term weight loss by enhancing postoperative dietary compliance.

Unfortunately, the surgical procedures that produce the greatest weight loss (partial gastrointestinal bypasses) have the greatest long-term complication rates. Vitamin and mineral deficiencies and anemia are more common (15–30%) in patients who have a gastric bypass than in those who have only a gastroplasty. Partial gastrointestinal bypass can cause diarrhea, "dumping" (a syndrome of weakness, palpitations, and diaphoresis), and intolerance of dairy products. In addition, serious liver disease, kidney stones, and arthritis can occur if too much of the small intestine is bypassed.

The tendency of obese patients to underestimate their caloric intake explains in part why more highly structured programs using formula diets or prepackaged foods produce better weight losses than conventional diets. Patients are more likely to consume the prescribed number of calories if they do not have to determine their own portions.

Regular exercise (both aerobic and resistance types) enhances the results of any program of calorie restriction. Exercise not only expends calories, but also prevents the loss of lean tissue. Because lean tissue mass is the major determinant of metabolic rate, regular exercise keeps the metabolic rate from falling as is usually the case when only calorie restriction is employed. The patient's energy expenditure is greater, therefore, even when she is at rest. Greater overall energy expenditure accelerates fat loss and makes maintenance of weight loss easier.

In many studies, regular exercise has been shown to be one of the strongest predictors of long-term weight loss. Perhaps more important than the number of calories burned, exercise may be more helpful as a stress reducer. Furthermore, someone who makes the time to engage in regular exercise is demonstrating evidence of a more "empowered" life style. Thus, regular exercise may be a marker of an important attitude change that is essential for long-term success.

Considering all the available treatment approaches for obesity, the greater the intensity of treatment, the greater the weight loss and the greater the expense.

C. Provider's Role:
1. Understanding the disease—To be an effective primary care provider for an obese woman, it is important for the practitioner to understand the disease of obesity. It is a complex biopsychosocial condition that usually needs multicomponent treatment. The patient often has low self-esteem and poor interpersonal relationships. Depression, "codependency," and family dysfunction are common comorbidities. Personal growth and general problem-solving skills may be as important as diet and exercise.

Obesity is a chronic disease like hypertension or atherosclerosis that requires long-term treatment and thus long-term supportive, nonjudgmental relationships with practitioners. Relapse often is part of the recovery process; therefore, multiple treatment cycles are likely to be needed. Because the patient has to feel comfortable enough to return to her primary care provider to seek support for the next cycle of treatment, it is important for the practitioner not to make weight loss the basis of the relationship with the patient. If weight loss is the only basis for acceptance, the patient will not return to the provider.

The primary care practitioner's message should be: "I am happy to be your physician no matter what your weight. My job is to monitor and treat any complications of obesity. I will support any efforts you make to control your weight." Thus, no matter what the outcome of the weight-loss attempt, the patient still has a physician.

2. Recognizing one's attitude—It is important for practitioners to recognize their own emotional responses to their patients' attempts to lose weight. The practitioner may feel frustration and even anger. At such times, the practitioner is vulnerable to criticizing the obese patient for "not trying hard enough" or "not really wanting to change." Such statements are far more likely to diminish the patient's self-esteem than to bring about any behavior change. Practitioners should realize that patients feel the same, or greater, frustration and anger in response to their perceived failure.

Clinicians must resist being cast in the prosecutor's role and strive to be supportive. Patients may be so accustomed to receiving criticism from family and other professionals that they try to elicit it by discussing their lapses in great detail until the criticism they believe they deserve is meted out. Additional strategies for supporting patients' weight-loss efforts are detailed in Appendix B, Weight-Management Primer for Primary Care Practitioners.

D. Initial Treatment: No single approach can be used with all patients; each program is effective for some people. The challenge is to match each patient with the program that best suits her needs. A useful three-step approach to this process has been proposed by Brownell and Wadden and is outlined in Figure 18–1. First, the patient is classified by degree of obesity. Patients at increasing levels of obesity are at greater health risk and therefore warrant more intensive treatment. At each level of obesity, a range of options is available.

The second decision imposes a stepped-care approach to the treatments considered appropriate for each level of obesity. Thus, the least expensive and least dangerous approach should be used first. Nonresponders are advanced to the next (more intensive) step, and so on. Last, the patient's personal characteristics are used to select the specific treatment program and ancillary support services that best meet her needs.

As an example, one should consider a woman 50% above her ideal weight. She is classified at level 3, suggesting programs in steps 2, 3, or 4. If the patient

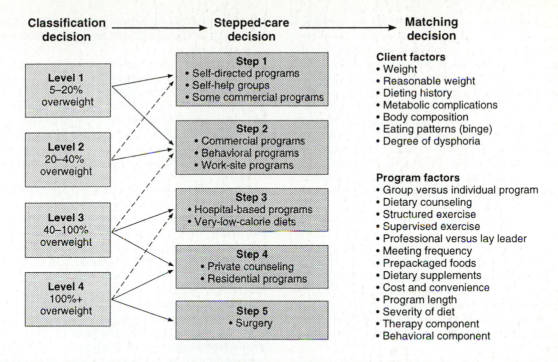

Figure 18–1. A conceptual scheme showing the three-stage process of selecting a treatment. The first step, the classification decision, divides patients according to percentage overweight into four levels. These levels dictate which of the five steps is reasonable in the second stage, the stepped-care decision. The least intensive, costly, and risky approach should be used. The third stage, the matching decision, is used to make the final selection of a program and is based on a combination of client and program variables. The dashed lines with arrows between the classification and stepped-care stages show the lowest level of treatment that may be beneficial, but more intensive treatment is usually necessary for people at the specified weight level. (Reproduced, with permission, from Brownell KD, Wadden TA: Etiology and treatment of obesity: Understanding a serious prevalent and refractory disorder. J Consult Clin Psychol 1992;60:511.)

previously has tried programs in step 2 without much success, a step 3 program is the least expensive place to start. The patient should assess the types of hospital- or clinic-based programs that exist in her community and choose the one best suited for her situation. If exercise is a difficult area for her, one of the institutions with a strong, perhaps supervised, exercise component would be a good match. On the other hand, if the patient reports problems with binge eating or a history of sexual abuse, seeking individual counseling as an adjunct to a group weight-loss program might provide the best chance for long-term success.

E. Maintenance of Weight Loss: No matter what form of treatment is employed to lose weight, there is a tendency to return to the baseline weight after a period of time. Thus, the maintenance of weight loss remains the greatest challenge. Researchers have identified several methods for enhancing maintenance of weight loss: taking part in an extended treatment program, participating in a regular exercise routine, and learning coping skills (problem-solving skills directed at eating behavior and general life issues).

The results of studies of patients successful at long-term weight loss have been published by Colvin and Olson, Kirschenbaum, and Fletcher. Although a variety of approaches were used to achieve the initial loss, all the successful patients appeared to share particular qualities, which are best described as a sense of personal empowerment (see Table 18–3). Successful patients realized that they alone were responsible for making their programs work. They gave up blaming others when things did not work out as well as expected. Assertiveness was required to set limits with family and associates in the workplace so that private time was available: time to exercise, plan low-fat meals, or just relax. Successful patients resolved to deal with problems directly and not to use food to cope with unpleasant feelings. They were able to acknowledge small changes as partial victories and were persistent in spite of many lapses and relapses. Successful patients who came from abusive or addictive families sought out recovery programs, making use of either twelve-step groups or traditional psychotherapy.

After reviewing the characteristics displayed by patients who are successful at long-term weight reduction, it becomes clear why long-term treatment is necessary. The qualities described can take years to develop. They are not "quick fixes" or simplistic formulas but sophisticated life skills that require much experimentation and refinement. One can appreciate also why so many patients who seek obesity treatment (at least 50%) come from dysfunctional families. These empowerment traits are qualities that children of dysfunctional families do not learn; they learn instead the characteristics that currently are termed **codependent.** Table 18–3 demonstrates that empowerment and codependency are mirror images.

Rather than displaying ownership and personal responsibility, typical dieters are focused on external factors, blaming others and events out of their control.

Rather than being assertive, these dieters are passive and have great difficulty setting limits and boundaries. Participating in regular exercise and following a low fat diet takes extra time and effort. Adult children of dysfunctional families (ACDFs) have difficulty taking that time without feeling guilty. They are too busy taking care of everyone else.

Rather than displaying food awareness and "mindful eating," patients seeking treatment often binge-eat to numb feelings and escape self-awareness. In the extreme, abuse survivors who learned to dissociate to cope with earlier traumas dissociate when eating. Rather than being in touch with their feelings, a hallmark of dysfunctional family members is being out of touch with their own feelings and focused on everyone else's feelings.

Recovery requires self-awareness, reaching out for support, and persisting for the long haul. Instead of having patience with the process of recovery, accepting small wins, and gaining confidence, these dieters display rigid perfectionism. That is to say, these dieters will set an unrealistic goal; if they do not accomplish this goal they will only see the negative and abandon the effort instead of taking credit for the partial accomplishment.

Rather than self-awareness, ACDFs display magical thinking: "The next fad diet or new diet pill will fix the problem," "Once I get to my goal weight, life will be perfect," "Thin people have no problems."

Table 18–3. Empowerment compared to codependency.

Empowerment	Codependency
1. Ownership	1. Externality
2. Assertiveness, self-protection	2. Passivity, poor boundaries
3. Exercise	3. No time for self
4. Low-fat diet, mindful eating	4. Binge eating, dissociation
5. In touch with feelings	5. Out of touch with feelings
6. Accept small changes	6. Perfectionism
7. Recovery work	7. Isolation, shame, guilt, magical thinking

Isolation is the operating principal for ACDFs. They are too full of shame and guilt to easily connect with others for support.

From the previous discussion, it is obvious that developing the skills necessary for long-term weight management takes time, perhaps 3–5 years or more. The journey from co-dependency to empowerment is not a short one. Because at least 50% of patients who seek professional help to lose weight were raised in dysfunctional families, it is easy to appreciate why long-term treatment is so vital for many obese patients.

It is important, however, to emphasize to patients that although nonempowerment takes a long time to correct, it is a learned behavior pattern that can be **unlearned.** It is not a genetic trait. This should be conveyed to the patient as a hopeful message. People do recover from nonempowerment, if they take a holistic approach by looking at both what and why they are overeating.

In summary, practitioners must recognize that the major forces behind nonempowered behavior are shame, guilt, and fear of abandonment. Physicians should support their patients' efforts to resolve these feelings through both (1) weight management and (2) personal growth and recovery interventions. Recovery work restores the patient's self esteem and self efficacy, which allows the patient to have the resilience to persist for the long-term.

This clinical formulation is supported by two lines of research that demonstrate that (1) childhood sexual abuse, parental alcoholism or emotional illness, and parental neglect are risk factors for adult obesity; and (2) success at long-term weight loss is associated with regular exercise, directly confronting problems, seeking social support and not eating in response to emotional stress.

Issues of Pregnancy & Obesity

A. Risks to Obese Women and Offspring: The risks of maternal and fetal complications are increased in pregnancies of obese women. The mother is at greater risk for preeclampsia, diabetes, acute chorioamnionitis, obstructive labor, and cesarean section. Babies of obese pregnancies have an increased incidence of macrosomia and of neural tube, great vessel, ventral wall, and other intestinal malformations. Because of these risks, it is best to counsel obese women to lose weight before becoming pregnant.

B. Recommendations for Weight Gain: It is well established that both maternal prepregnancy BMI and weight gain during pregnancy affect fetal growth. Overweight women and those who gain a large amount of weight during pregnancy have a greater incidence of macrosomia. The impact of maternal weight gain during pregnancy is less, however, as the mother's prepregnancy weight increases (Fig 18–2).

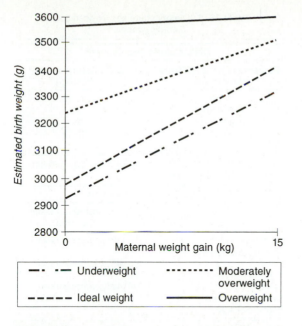

Figure 18–2. Birth weight of liveborn infants at term by prepregnancy body mass and weight gain adjusted for maternal age, race, parity, socioeconomic status, cigarette consumption, and gestational age (n= 2964). (Reproduced, with permission, from Abrams, BF, Laros RK: Prepregnancy weight, weight gain, and birth weight. Am J Obstet Gynecol 1986;154:503.)

Based on this information, the Institute of Medicine has recommended different amounts of weight gain depending on the woman's prepregnancy weight for height (Table 18–4). Unfortunately, there are not enough data to establish exactly how much weight obese women (BMI greater than 30, or weight greater than 135% of ideal body weight) should gain. The Institute of Medicine recommends individual dietary assessment and counseling for obese pregnant women and a weight gain of at least 15 pounds, which is the total estimated weight of the products of

Table 18–4. Weight gain recommendations for pregnancy.*

Body Mass Index (BMI)†	Recommended Gain
Low (BMI < 19.8 or < 90% ideal body weight (IBW))‡	12.5–18 kg (28–40 lb)
Normal (BMI 19.8–26.0 or 90–120% IBW)	11.5–16 kg (25–35 lb)
High (BMI 26.0–29.0 or 120–135% IBW)	7–11.5 kg (15–25 lb)
Obese (BMI > 29.0 or > 135% IBW)	6+ kg (15+ lb)

*Reproduced, with permission, from National Academy of Sciences: *Nutrition During Pregnancy.* National Academy Press, 1990.
†Body mass index = (weight in kg/height in m²) or (weight in lb/height in in.²) × 700.
‡Ideal body weight, based on 1959 Metropolitan Life Insurance Company standards.

conception. The report recognizes, however, that obese women can have healthy offspring with smaller weight gains.

C.   Obesity and Diabetes in Pregnancy: Because obesity is associated with increased risks to the mother and fetus, it is tempting to recommend calorie restriction in obese pregnant women, especially in those with gestational or type II diabetes mellitus. This recommendation is controversial because of concern raised about the risks of inducing ketosis. Two studies, one in 1969 and another in 1977, reported that ketonuria during pregnancy was associated with impaired neuropsychological development of the offspring. These reports resulted in warnings to avoid calorie restriction in any pregnancy. Later studies raised serious questions about the methods employed and whether chorioamnionitis caused both the ketonuria and the intellectual impairment. Coetzee reported that pregnant outpatients who were obese, had diabetes, and followed 1000-calorie diets always had serum acetoacetate levels below 1 mmol/L even though urine acetone was 2+ on reagent strips. These serum levels were considered nontoxic. Furthermore, the birth weights of these offspring were normal, and no adverse neonatal events occurred. More recently, Magee et al demonstrated that on a metabolic ward, a diet of 1200 kcal/d raised serum ketone levels and therefore advised against this level of intake. Other well-controlled studies, using less restrictive diets of 1500–1800 kcal/d, have shown improved glycemic control without ketonuria or marked ketonemia.

In the largest study to address this issue, Rizzo et al studied 223 pregnant women (women with type I diabetes, women with gestational diabetes, and normals) and their offspring. Scores on IQ tests of offspring were correlated inversely with third-trimester levels of beta-hydroxybutyrate and free fatty acids. It is interesting to note, however, that the women with elevations of these metabolites had poorly controlled type I diabetes and were not women on calorie-restricted diets. The authors questioned whether there is a difference between the effect of starvation ketosis and of the ketosis associated with poorly controlled diabetes. They noted that ketosis developed in 10–20% of normal pregnancies after an overnight fast and indeed may protect the fetus from starvation. Although the ideal caloric level for obese pregnant women (diabetic or nondiabetic) has not been established conclusively, the best recommendation at the current time is to limit the diet to 1500–1800 kcal/d so that the total weight gain for the pregnancy is limited to 15 pounds or less.

The addition of a low-impact aerobic exercise program (20 minutes, 3 times a week) can improve glycemic control additionally without harm to the fetus when added to intense dietary therapy. Because glucose intolerance is greatest after the morning meal, exercise may be most effective if performed after breakfast.

Diets with lower carbohydrate content (40% carbohydrate, 40% fat, 20% protein) may be more effective in controlling blood sugars than typical, 60% carbohydrate diets, especially if the carbohydrate content of breakfast is reduced compared to that of lunch and dinner (Table 18–5). If fasting or postprandial blood sugars become elevated despite diet and exercise, insulin treatment becomes necessary.

Postpartum counseling is important for obese women who had gestational diabetes whether they required insulin or only dietary treatment during pregnancy. If they remain overweight after delivery, their chance of developing overt type II diabetes is 60% over the next 20 years. If they maintain an ideal weight, the risk is reduced to less than 25%. Also, the risk of development of gestational diabetes with subsequent pregnancies is reduced if the patient can achieve a body weight closer to ideal before the next pregnancy. These considerations argue strongly for encouraging patients to devote time and energy to managing their weight once the pregnancy is over.

Psychosocial Concerns

Obese people in our society are subject to widespread prejudice and discrimination. Children as young as 6 years, when asked to describe silhouettes of obese children, use negative words such as "lazy, dirty, stupid, cheats, ugly, lies." As adults, obese people encounter discrimination in college admissions, work promotions, and personal relationships. These findings led Stunkard and Wadden to suggest that the psychological perils of obesity may exceed its medical complications.

Obese binge eaters have increased levels of psychopathology compared with the nonbingeing obese. Increased rates of depression, panic disorder, drug and alcohol abuse, impaired work and social functioning, past physical and sexual abuse, and borderline and avoidant personality disorders have been found. In addition, obese binge eaters report alcohol abuse more frequently in parents and significant others. The relationship between psychopathology and binge eating is likely a complex one. Increased levels of psychological distress may lead to binge eating, but is also has been shown in treatment studies that depression and other psychological symptoms are reduced when binge eating declines.

Table 18–5. Dietary strategies for gestational diabetic women.*

Daily Caloric Requirement	
Percentage of Ideal Body Weight (IBW)	Daily Caloric Intake[†] (kcal/kg)
< 80	35–40
80–120	30
120–150	24
> 150	12–15

These calories are divided into three meals and four snacks composed of 40% high–fiber carbohydrates, 20% protein, 40% fat (polyunsaturated).

Daily Caloric Distribution	
Meal	Percentage of Daily Calories
Breakfast	10 (33% carbohydrate)
Midmorning snack	5
Lunch	30 (45% carbohydrate)
Afternoon snack	10
Dinner	30 (40% carbohydrate)
Midevening snack	5
Bedtime snack	10

*Adapted, with permission, from Mulford MI et al: Alternative therapies for the management of gestational diabetes. Clin Perinatol 1993;20:619.
[†]Based on present pregnant weight.

REFERENCES

Abrams B: Maternal nutrition. In: *Maternal-Fetal Medicine: Principles and Practice,* 3rd ed. Creasy RK and Resnick R (editors). Saunders, 1994.

Bennett GA: Behavior therapy for obesity: A quantitative review of the effects of selected treatment characteristics on outcome. Behavior Therapy 1986;17:554.

Bouchard C: Genetic factors in obesity. Med Clin North Am 1989;73:67.

Brownell KD: Whether obesity should be treated. Health Psychol 1993;12:339.

Brownell KD, Rodin J: *The Weight Maintenance Survival Guide.* American Health Publishing, 1990.

Brownell KD, Wadden T: Etiology and treatment of obesity: Understanding a serious prevalent and refractory disorder. J Consult Clin Psychol 1992;60:505.

Coetzee EJ, Jackson WPU, Berman PA: Ketonuria in preg-
nancy—with special reference to calorie restricted food intake in obese diabetics. Diabetes 1980;29:177.

Colvin RH, Olson SC: *Keeping it Off.* Gilliland, 1989.

Felitti VJ: Childhood sexual abuse, depression, and family dysfunction in adult obese patients: A case control study. South Med J 1993;86:732.

Felitti VJ: Long-term medical consequences of incest, rape and molestation. South Med J 1991;84:328.

Fletcher AM: *Thin for Life.* Chapters Publishing, 1994.

Kanter RA, Williams BE: Effect of pre-treatment binge eating on long-term weight loss. Obesity Res 1993;1(Suppl 2):115S.

Kanter RA, Williams BE: Personal and parental alcohol abuse, and victimization in obese binge eaters and nonbingeing obese. Addict Behav 1992;17:439.

Kanter RA, Williams BE: Post-treatment contact affects

long-term weight loss. Obesity Res 1993;1(Suppl 2):116S.

Kayman S. Bruvold W, Stern JS: Maintenance and relapse after weight loss in women: behavioral aspects. Am J Clin Nutr 1990;52:800.

Kirschenbaum DS: *Weight Loss Through Persistence: Making Science Work for You.* New Harbinger, 1994.

Kuczmarski RT et al: Increasing prevalence of overweight among U.S. adults: The National Health and Nutrition Examination Surveys, 1960–1991. JAMA 1994;272:205.

Lissau I, Sorensen TIA: Parental neglect during childhood and increased risk of obesity in young adulthood. Lancet 1994;343:324.

Magee MS, Knopp RH, Benedetti TJ: Metabolic effects of 1200-kcal diet in obese pregnant women with gestational diabetes. Diabetes 1990;39:234.

McGann PK: Self-reported illnesses in family members of alcoholics. Fam Med 1990;22:103.

Metropolitan Height and Weight Tables. Stat Bull Metropol Life Ins Co 1984;64:2.

Moore TR: *Diabetes in Pregnancy.* In: *Maternal-Fetal Medicine: Principles and Practice,* 3rd ed. Creasy RK, Resnick R (editors). Saunders, 1994.

Mulford MI, Jovanovic-Peterson L, Peterson CM: Alternative therapies for the management of gestational diabetes. Clin Perinatol 1993;20:619.

National Institutes of Health Consensus Development Panel on the Health Implications of Obesity: Ann Int Med 1985;103 (6 pt 2):1059.

National Task Force on the Prevention and Treatment of Obesity: Weight cycling. JAMA 1994;272:1196.

Peele S, Brodsky A: *The truth about addiction and recovery.* Simon & Schuster, 1991.

Price RA et al: Genetic contributions to human fatness: An adoption study. Am J Psychiatry 1987;144:1003.

Pronk NP, Wing RR: Physical activity and long-term maintenance of weight loss. Obesity Res 1994;2:587.

Rizzo T et al: Correlations between antepartum maternal metabolism and intelligence of offspring. N Engl J Med 1991;325:911.

Springs FE, Friedrich WN: Health risk behaviors and medical sequelae of childhood sexual abuse. Mayo Clin Proc 1992;67:527.

Stunkard AJ, Wadden TA: Psychologic aspects of severe obesity. Am J Clin Nutr 1992;55(Suppl):524S.

Wadden TA, VanIlallie TB (editors): *Treatment of the Seriously Obese Patient.* Guilford Press, 1992.

Waller DK et al: Are obese women at higher risk for producing malformed offspring? Am J Obstet Gynecol 1994;170:541.

19

Hirsutism

Lorna A. Marshall, MD

Essentials of Diagnosis

- Polycystic ovarian syndrome is most common diagnosis when hirsutism and oligomenorrhea are present.
- Idiopathic hirsutism–no identifiable ovarian or adrenal androgen overproduction.
- Adult onset congenital adrenal hyperplasia is much less common than idiopathic hirsutism.
- Adrenal and ovarian tumors are rare but need to be excluded.

Essentials of Diagnosis
Incidence & Risk Factors
Clinical Findings & Diagnosis
Treatment
Prognosis
Referral to a Specialist
Issues of Pregnancy & Hirsutism
Psychosocial Concerns
Controversies

Incidence & Risk Factors

Hirsutism is the presence of excess body hair in women; it is usually an androgen-dependent process. Close to one-third of women between the ages of 15 and 44 have hair growth on the upper lip, lower abdomen, or breasts. In addition, 6–9% have hair growth on the chin and sides of the face.

Polycystic ovarian syndrome (PCOS), defined as chronic anovulation with hyperandrogenism, is common, although its estimated prevalence depends on how it is diagnosed. Up to 90% of women who present with hirsutism and have irregular menses have PCOS.

Adult-onset congenital adrenal hyperplasia has a higher incidence in Ashkenazi Jews, Hispanics, and those of central European ancestry, and a lower incidence in those of Northern European ancestry.

Idiopathic hirsutism, with no identifiable adrenal or ovarian androgen excess is common in women of Mediterranean ancestry.

Because the concentration of hair follicles per unit area is greater in Caucasians than Asians, Asian women can have very elevated ovarian or adrenal androgen levels with only mild hirsutism.

Clinical Findings & Diagnosis

The evaluation of a hirsute woman should document the severity of hirsutism and exclude any serious underlying disorders. When treatment is desired, an attempt should be made to determine whether the patient has ovarian or adrenal androgen overproduction, or if the hirsutism results from an abnormality of peripheral androgen metabolism. The causes of androgen-dependent hirsutism are as follows:

Polycystic ovarian syndrome
Congenital adrenal hyperplasia
Ovarian tumors
Adrenal tumors
Cushing's syndrome
Idiopathic hirsutism
Exogenous drugs
Acromegaly
Hyperandrogenism insulin resistance–acanthosis nigricans (HAIR-AN) syndrome
Ectopic ACTH-secreting tumors

A. History: A menstrual history should be taken. Most women with polycystic ovarian syndrome have oligomenorrhea, although primary or secondary amenorrhea can occur when the androgen excess is severe. Women with idiopathic hirsutism or adult-onset congenital adrenal hyperplasia usually have regular menses. The elevated androgen levels present in patients with adrenal or ovarian tumors or hyperthecosis often result in amenorrhea. A careful history of medications should be obtained to exclude androgen containing preparations.

Any methods that were used to control hirsutism should be documented. Frequency of shaving, waxing, plucking, or electrolysis treatments should be recorded so that the effectiveness of therapy can be quantified.

B. Symptoms: For most hirsute women, symptoms begin at the time of menarche and worsen gradually with age. Rapidly progressive hirsutism or hirsutism that is noted first before menarche raises the possibility of an androgen-dependent tumor or Cushing's syndrome. Use of oral contraceptives may delay the onset or arrest the progression of hirsutism. A woman may first complain of hirsutism in her mid-30s after she has stopped taking oral contraceptives. Weight gain may worsen the endocrinologic profile and the signs of hyperandrogenism in polycystic ovarian syndrome. Acne is another sign of hyperandrogenism, and its history should be elicited.

Significant scalp hair loss, deepening of the voice, increased muscle mass, and clitoromegaly are considered signs of virilization. They usually are associated with higher androgen levels, although some scalp hair loss and slight changes in pitch can be seen with milder androgen excess. Before signs of virilization appear in a woman with an androgen-producing tumor, decrease in breast size and change in body contour to a more masculine habitus often are noted.

C. **Physical examination:** The type, amount, and distribution of the excess hair growth should be documented carefully. **Hypertrichosis** is a generalized increase in hair throughout the body, is present in both men and women, and does not warrant an investigation. Hirsutism is central in distribution, following the midline of the body. Coarse, terminal hairs suggest androgen excess, whereas finer, less pigmented, and slower growing vellus hairs do not.

Examination may be difficult if the patient has used mechanical methods frequently to control the hair growth. Correlation between history of hair growth and examination results should be ascertained carefully. Several scoring systems are available for quantifying the severity of hirsutism; they may not be useful in the clinical management of this disorder, however. Instead, careful documentation is made of hair growth on the upper lip, chin, breast and midsternal area, midline upper abdomen, lower abdomen and escutcheon, upper arm, inner thigh, upper back, and lower back. Sometimes, photographs are useful for documenting the findings of the baseline examination and for monitoring treatment.

Acanthosis nigricans refers to velvety, verrucous, hyperpigmented skin changes, usually at the nape of the neck, at the axilla, and underneath the breasts. Its presence suggests the severe androgen excess associated with hyperthecosis, which may be a severe form of polycystic ovarian syndrome.

A pelvic examination should be performed for all women who present with hirsutism. Varying degrees of clitoral enlargement are seen in hirsute women. In general, the glans should be less than 7–8 mm in diameter. A glans size greater than 1 cm in diameter suggests virilization. Most androgen-producing ovarian tumors are too small to be palpated on examination. However, some larger nonsecreting ovarian tumors are associated with hyperplasia of the surrounding stroma and subsequent hirsutism.

Other signs of virilization, such as general body habitus signs or temporal balding, should be noted. Sometimes previous pictures of the patient are sometimes useful for comparison.

Central obesity, hypertension, pigmented striae, proximal muscle weakness, facial plethora, and increased dorsocervical and supraclavicular fat suggest Cushing's syndrome.

D. **Laboratory Tests and Imaging Techniques:** It has been argued that a hormonal evaluation is not necessary if hirsutism is mild or moderate and has been slowly progressive since puberty. An androgen-producing tumor would be unlikely, and treatment to suppress ovarian androgen production, and possibly an antiandrogen, can be offered.

If hirsutism is severe, recent in onset, or rapidly progressive, an evaluation should be initiated. The two key tests for exclusion of androgen-producing tumors are measures of testosterone and dehydroepiandrosterone sulfate (DHAS).

Testosterone is the best marker for ovarian androgen secretion. In nonhirsute women, approximately two-thirds of circulating testosterone can be considered ovarian-derived, either from direct secretion or from peripheral conversion of androgen precursors. In hirsute women with ovarian androgen overproduction, an even higher percentage of testosterone is ovarian-derived. If the testosterone level is greater than 200 ng/dL, an androgen-producing tumor, usually ovarian, is likely to be present and a referral should be initiated. Some women with hyperthecosis but no ovarian tumors have testosterone levels that are close to 200 ng/dL. On the other hand, some postmenopausal women with testosterone producing tumors may have testosterone levels slightly less than 200 ng/dL. If the testosterone level is greater than 100 ng/dL and a tumor is strongly suspected in a woman of this age group, the evaluation to locate a tumor should continue.

DHAS is almost exclusively an adrenal product. Although it is not an androgenic steroid, it is a marker of androgenic steroid production by the adrenal gland. When DHAS levels are greater than 700 μg/dL, an adrenal tumor should be suspected. DHAS measurement is not a suitable screening tool for adult-onset adrenal hyperplasia.

If Cushing's syndrome is suspected from the history and clinical findings, a dexamethasone suppression test should be done. One milligram of dexamethasone is given at bedtime; the 8:00 AM cortisol level should be less than 6 μg/dL to exclude Cushing's syndrome.

Selective use of 17-hydroxyprogesterone (17OH-P) is appropriate as a screening method for the most common type of adult-onset congenital adrenal hyperplasia, 21-hydroxylase deficiency. Its use should be considered in patients who are members of ethnic groups that are at high risk for this disorder. The test also should be performed in young women with severe hirsutism, especially if their menstrual periods are normal. Identification of this attenuated form of adrenal hyperplasia allows the provider to offer the appropriate treatment options. If the 17OH-P level is less than 3 ng/dL, 21-hydroxylase deficiency is unlikely. If it is greater than 8 ng/dL, the diagnosis is likely and a referral should be initiated. If the level is between 3 and 8 ng/dL, an ACTH-stimulation test should be performed.

The response of 17OH-P to administration of ACTH is believed to differentiate women with attenuated adrenal hyperplasia from those who have a slightly elevated baseline 17OH-P caused by another process, such as PCOS. The interpretation of this test is sometimes difficult, and referral to a medical or reproductive endocrinologist to determine the protocol and interpret the results is useful.

There is usually little reason to subcategorize further various functional androgen excess conditions. Free testosterone, sex-hormone-binding globulin, and androstenedione levels generally are not useful in the differential diagnosis or treatment recommendations and add expense to the evaluation. Prolactin and gonadotropin levels should be measured when appropriate as part of an evaluation for oligomenorrhea or amenorrhea.

Suppression tests with oral contraceptives or dexamethasone or stimulation tests with human chorionic gonadotropin (HCG) have been used in the past to identify the location of an androgen-producing tumor. However, the results have correlated poorly with more accurate methods such as catheterization. Occasionally, administration of dexamethasone is used to help distinguish between an adrenal tumor and adrenal hyperplasia when the DHAS level is greater than 700 μg/dL.

The term HAIR-AN syndrome has been applied to cases of severe hirsutism associated with insulin resistance, acanthosis nigricans, and usually oligomenorrhea or amenorrhea. This syndrome is thought by some to be the extreme of polycystic ovarian syndrome, with findings of hyperthecosis (large clusters of luteinized cells in the ovarian stroma). Initially it was thought that the hyperandrogenism caused the hyperinsulinism, but more recent evidence suggests that the converse may be true. Lesser degrees of insulin resistance are associated with polycystic ovarian syndrome.

Women with polycystic ovarian syndrome have been shown to have lifelong increased risk for unfavorable lipoprotein profile, heart disease, diabetes, and endometrial cancer. Screening for lipoprotein abnormalities should be part of the evaluation. Pelvic ultrasonography is not recommended as a screening test for hirsutism. Polycystic ovarian syndrome is a clinical diagnosis, confirmed by laboratory tests. Its diagnosis does not depend on the ultrasonographic appearance of the ovaries, although enlarged ovaries with multiple tiny cysts in the cortex have been described in association with PCOS. A wide spectrum of sonographic appearances of the ovary in PCOS has been described. When the testosterone level is greater than 200 ng/dL, ultrasonography, preferably transvaginal, is recommended to exclude a tumor. However, few investigators have reported on transvaginal scanning as a screen for ovarian androgen-producing tumors. These tumors are small, often 1–2 cm in size, and sometimes cannot be detected clearly with any imaging technique. For the adrenal gland, computed tomography and magnetic resonance imaging are the best tests to localize a tumor.

When a tumor cannot be detected but suspicion remains high, selective catheterization of the ovarian and adrenal vessels can be useful in localizing the tumor. Adrenal tumors occasionally produce testosterone, so that both ovarian and adrenal veins need to be catheterized when testosterone levels are elevated.

Treatment

Mechanical treatments are effective by themselves for mild hirsutism and can be used in conjunction with medical therapy for more severe hirsutism. Bleaching is most successful with vellus hair growth, but frequent use can result in skin irritation. Plucking is painful but can be useful for mild hirsutism in localized areas. Plucking has not been shown to decrease or increase the rate of hair growth. For larger areas, shaving commonly is used, but it carries a stigma when stubble is apparent. Depilatories and waxing also are used for larger areas but can cause significant skin irritation. Electrolysis is not really permanent, although it is often advertised to be. It can be expensive and time-consuming and may eventually cause skin thickening.

Most women without tumors should be treated with oral contraceptive pills (OCPs) with or without an antiandrogen (Table 19–1). Estrogen opposes the effect of androgen on the hair follicle, resulting in a reduced rate of hair growth and finer, less pigmented hair. In addition, OCPs suppress pituitary secretion of luteinizing hormone (LH), which drives ovarian testosterone production. Gonadotropin-releasing hormone agonists plus estrogens and progestins are also useful but are much more expensive and should be used only in selected cases.

Most monophasic OCPs are appropriate for the

Table 19–1. Medical treatments of hirsutism.

Mechanism	Medication
Ovarian suppression	Oral contraceptive pills
	Gonadotropin-releasing hormone analogs
Adrenal suppression	Glucocorticoids
Antiandrogens	Spironolactone
	Cyproterone acetate
	Flutamide
Combination therapy	Antiandrogens
	Oral contraceptive pills

treatment of hirsutism. Preparations with ethynodiol diacetate have not been shown to be more effective than those with ethinyl estradiol. No more than 30–35 µg of ethinyl estradiol is necessary. The 19-nortestosterone derivatives such as levonorgestrel should be avoided because of their greater androgenic activity. The best progestins to prescribe are norethindrone and the newer, less androgenic progestins (desogestrel, norgestimate, and gestodene).

The addition of glucocorticoids, even for women with late-onset congenital adrenal hyperplasia, usually has little benefit. In general, OCPs are preferred over corticosteroids because of the better safety margin. If dexamethasone is given, the dosage should be low (0.25–0.5 mg), and cortisone levels should be monitored to exclude adrenal suppression. Adjustments in dosage should be made if the 8 AM cortisol level is less than 2 µg/dL.

Spironolactone is the only antiandrogen available in this country for which efficacy and safety have been established clearly. Cimetidine is a weak antiandrogen and not clinically useful. Cyproterone acetate is used widely in Europe but not available in the United States. Flutamide is being studied currently as a treatment for hirsutism.

Because spironolactone competitively inhibits the androgen receptor, it should be effective for the treatment of hirsutism of all causes, if a tumor has been excluded. It also may inhibit biosynthesis of ovarian and adrenal androgens. Spironolactone is most effective when given in doses of 100–200 mg/d. An undesirable side effect is abnormal bleeding; the addition of OCPs corrects the abnormal bleeding and augments the treatment of hirsutism. Because hyperkalemia is a theoretic risk of treatment, potassium levels should be monitored at follow-up visits.

Currently the combination of OCPs and spironolactone is the most practical and effective therapy in most circumstances. Usually the OCPs are started first, and blood pressure is monitored before therapy with spironolactone is initiated.

When the effectiveness of any medical therapy is to be monitored, the 3-month growth cycle of hair should be considered. Any interruption in androgen-mediated growth cannot be seen until the next cycle of growth. The patient should be advised that 3–6 months of treatment may be required before any improvement is seen. It is also important to advise the patient that excess hair will not fall out and needs to be removed by mechanical means after about 6 months of medical therapy. The goal of therapy is to arrest or attenuate the growth of new hair.

Prognosis

For most women with moderate or severe hirsutism, the disorder is a long-standing problem that may improve somewhat with medical and mechanical therapies but may never go away completely. Younger women request medical treatment more of-

ten and adhere to the prescribed treatment to a greater degree than do older women, who often choose to accept less complete control of their symptoms. Women who respond well to oral contraceptives can use them for the duration of their reproductive years, and this can be a quite satisfactory long-term treatment option.

Women who have severe hirsutism and virilization from an androgen-producing tumor have rapid improvement in some but not all of their symptoms after removal of the tumor. For example, a deepened voice is never restored to normal.

Women with polycystic ovarian syndrome are at increased risk for a variety of other disorders. Thirty percent of young women with endometrial cancer have polycystic ovarian syndrome. In addition, these women are at increased risk for cardiovascular disease and diabetes.

Referral to a Specialist

Both medical endocrinologists and reproductive endocrinologists can care for patients who have complicated forms of hirsutism. Referral should be considered if androgen levels are in the tumor range, if ACTH testing is required, or if initial attempts at treatment are unsuccessful. Referral to a general surgeon should be made if an adrenal tumor is identified. If an ovarian tumor is suspected, the patient should be referred to a reproductive endocrinologist or gynecologist for removal. Androgen-producing ovarian tumors are rarely malignant, and consultation with a gynecologic oncologist usually is not needed.

Issues of Pregnancy & Hirsutism

Many of the disorders associated with hirsutism result in oligomenorrhea or amenorrhea. Such patients usually require ovulation induction to conceive. In women with high levels of androgens, ovulation induction is often difficult, requiring high doses of clomiphene or human menopausal gonadotropins. In some cases, electrocautery of the ovarian cortex is necessary in combination with ovulation-inducing agents. These women are also at higher risk for complications of ovulation induction, including ovarian hyperstimulation and multiple pregnancies.

Increased rates of spontaneous pregnancy loss have been associated with elevated LH levels, such as those seen in polycystic ovarian syndrome.

The effect of pregnancy on the progression of hirsutism is variable. Mechanical methods are the only treatments recommended during pregnancy. The effect of spironolactone on the developing fetus is unknown.

Couples in which one partner has attenuated congenital adrenal hyperplasia should undergo genetic counseling, preferably before conception. Classic congenital adrenal hyperplasia is one of the most common autosomal recessive disorders. In some cases, the carrier state may present as attenuated or adult onset congenital adrenal hyperplasia.

Psychosocial Concerns

A patient's reaction to hirsutism depends on her racial and cultural background, her perception of body image, and the severity of her symptoms. Most women in whom the onset of hirsutism occurs after puberty do not show any changes in gender identification. Compared with nonhirsute women, hirsute women tend to have greater body weight, more mood disturbances, fewer sexual partners, more body image problems, and more somatic complaints.

The effect of excessive androgens on behavior in women is not known; studies on this topic have contradictory findings. Some studies have shown that high androgen levels correlate with greater sexual interest, especially with regard to masturbation. Antiandrogens given for the treatment of hirsutism may diminish this effect. This potentially undesirable side effect should be considered when counseling hirsute women about treatment options for hirsutism.

Controversies

Controversy surrounds both the diagnosis and the management of patients with androgen excess. The diagnosis of "idiopathic hirsutism" has been questioned recently. Most women with normal ovarian and adrenal androgen levels are believed to have a disorder of peripheral androgen production. Specifically, they are thought to convert testosterone to dihydrotestosterone, the androgen active at the hair follicle, more quickly than normal women do. There may be a small subset of women who have an abnormality in the hair cycle; if so, these patients can be described more accurately as having idiopathic hirsutism.

A good marker of peripheral androgen activity is 3α-androstanediol glucuronide (3α-diolG). An elevated level suggests a defect in peripheral androgen metabolism only if DHAS and testosterone levels are normal. When this marker should be measured, if at all, is currently controversial.

The diagnosis of attenuated forms of congenital adrenal hyperplasia remains controversial. When to perform and how to interpret ACTH-stimulation tests is debated.

Polycystic ovarian syndrome remains one of the least understood disorders in the field of endocrinology; as currently defined, it may encompass a large number of disorders. Finally, when to treat hirsutism with corticosteroids is quite controversial. Any risks of long-term therapy may not be justified by the benefits achieved. Currently it is believed that the treatment should be reserved for young women with severe hirsutism, in whom an attenuated form of congenital adrenal hyperplasia has been diagnosed clearly.

REFERENCES

Dunaif A et al (editor): *Polycystic Ovary Syndrome*. Blackwell Scientific Publications, 1992.

Lobo RA: Androgen excess in women: The enigma of the hirsute female. In: *Controversies in Reproductive Endocrinology and Infertility*. Soules MR (editor). Elsevier, 1989.

Pittaway DE (editor): Hyperandrogenism. Infertil Reprod Med Clin North Am 1991;2:455.

Sawaya ME, Hordinsky MK: The antiandrogens: When and how they should be used. Dermatol Clin 1993;11:65.

Schriock EA, Schriock ED: Treatment of hirsutism. Clin Obstet Gynecol. 1991;34:852.

Speroff L, Glass RH, Kase NG: Hirsutism. In: *Clinical Gynecologic Endocrinology and Infertility,* 5th ed. Williams & Wilkins, 1994.

Thyroid Disorders

20

James W. Benson, Jr, MD

Thyroid disorders are more common in women than men. Graves' disease favors women by a ratio of 10:1, and thyroid nodules are 3 times as common in women. Postpartum autoimmune thyroiditis and struma ovarii are of course unique to female patients.

PHYSIOLOGY

To appreciate the changes in circulating thyroid hormone concentrations in thyroidal and nonthyroidal disease, it is necessary to understand normal thyroid physiology, including synthesis, protein binding, and peripheral metabolism.

Synthesis

Inorganic iodide is transported actively into the thyroid gland for use in synthesis of thyroid hormone, which involves three steps (Fig 20–1): (1) Organification occurs when iodide is bound to tyrosine residues attached to the large intrathyroidal protein thyroglobulin, (2) Iodotyrosines are coupled to form triiodothyronine (T3) and thyroxine (T4), and (3) Proteolysis frees T4 and T3 from thyroglobulin for release into the circulation. Both iodide uptake and thyroid hormone synthesis are stimulated by thyrotropin, or thyroid-stimulating hormone (TSH), secreted by the pituitary gland. Circulating thyroid hormones exert negative feedback on TSH, which is under the control of hypothalamic thyrotropin-releasing hormone (TRH) (Fig 20–2).

Protein Binding

More than 99% of thyroid hormone in the bloodstream is bound to thyroxine-binding globulin (TBG), albumin, and prealbumin. Only unbound, "free" T4 and T3 are biologically active. Processes that increase TBG transiently decrease the levels of free T4 and T3, because hormone attaches to open binding sites. Rapid equilibration occurs, however, as the low level of free thyroid hormone decreases its own disposal rate by autoregulation, reaching a new steady state with normal levels of free T4 and T3.

Peripheral Metabolism

The peripheral metabolism of T4 is critical for hormone action and is affected significantly by non-

thyroidal factors, especially during acute illness. Thyroxine is degraded by removal of iodine (deiodination) (Fig 20–3). Removal of an iodine from the outer ring by 5′-deiodinase to form T3 accounts for 50% of the metabolic fate of T4. Of circulating T3, 80% is produced by deiodination of T4 and 20% by direct thyroidal secretion. Biologic activity of T3 is at least twice that of T4, although the plasma concentration is only 1/50 that of T4. Because T4 is converted intracellularly to T3, it is unclear whether T4 is just a prehormone for T3 or has independent bio-

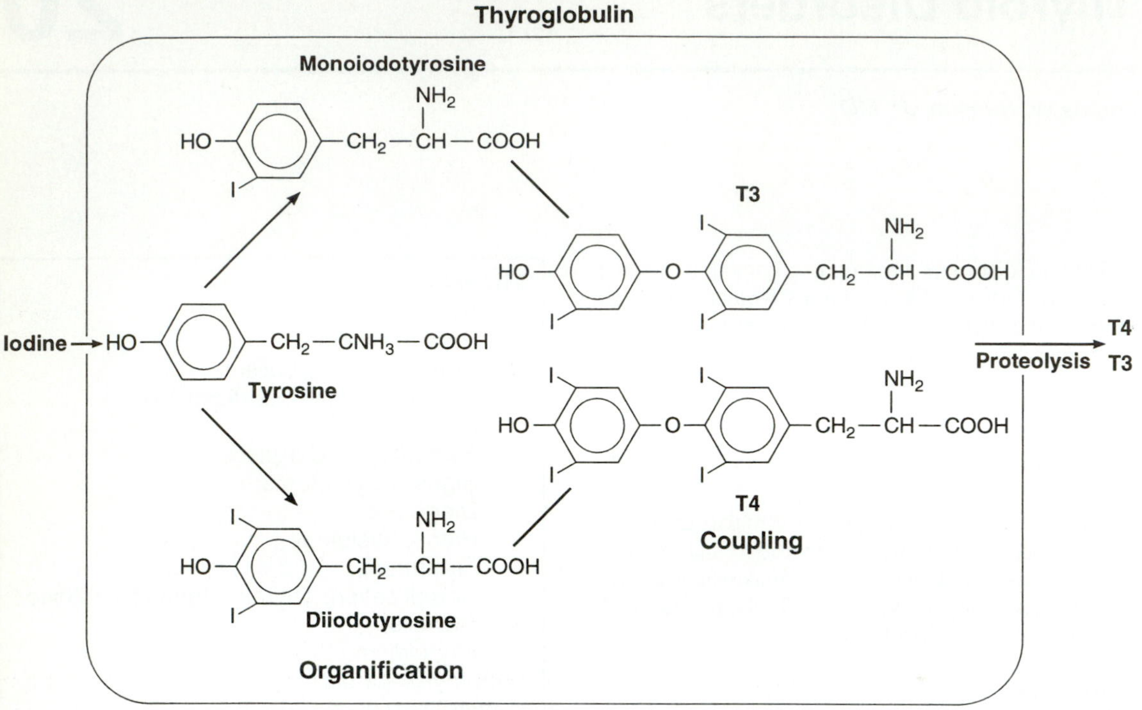

Thyroglobulin

Monoiodotyrosine

NH_2

HO—⬡—CH_2—CH—COOH

Iodine →HO—⬡—CH_2—CNH_3—COOH

Tyrosine

T3

NH_2

HO—⬡—O—⬡—CH_2—CH—COOH

NH_2

HO—⬡—O—⬡—CH_2—CH—COOH

T4

Coupling

NH_2

HO—⬡—CH_2—CH—COOH

Diiodotyrosine

Organification

$\xrightarrow{\text{Proteolysis}}$ T4 / T3

Figure 20–1. Thyroid hormone synthesis.

logic potency. The other 50% of T4 is deiodinated at the inner ring by 5-deiodinase to form reverse T3 (rT3), which is biologically inactive.

HYPERTHYROXINEMIA (Increased T4)

An elevated T4 is not uncommon, and the differential diagnosis for it is large. Table 20–1 outlines the possible causes of this condition. It may occur with thyrotoxicosis or euthyroidism.

THYROTOXICOSIS

Essentials of Diagnosis
- Tachycardia
- Tremor
- Hyperkinesis
- Weight loss
- Nervousness

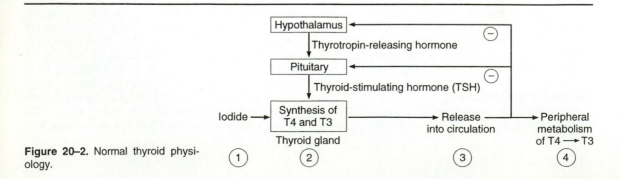

Figure 20–2. Normal thyroid physiology.

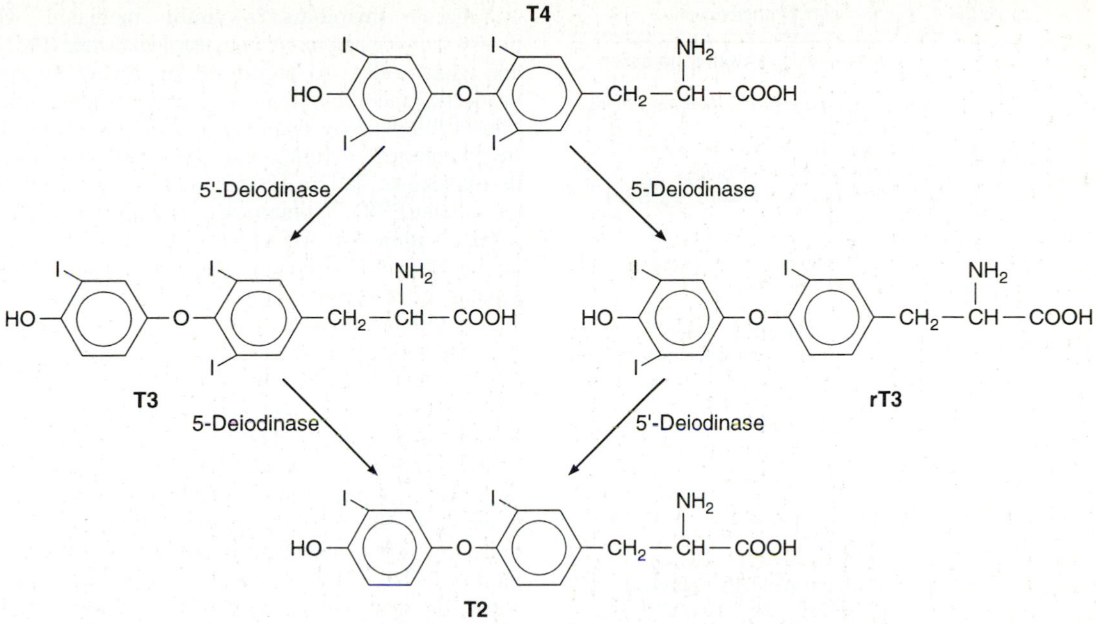

Figure 20–3. Peripheral metabolism of T4.

Signs & Symptoms

The first step in evaluating the patient is to identify clinical thyrotoxicosis. Thyrotoxic patients under the age of 60 years usually manifest all the signs and symptoms of hyperthyroidism. In the elderly, only weight loss, tachycardia (especially atrial fibrillation), or failure to thrive may be present. Detection during pregnancy may be particularly difficult because findings of hypermetabolism (except for weight loss) are consistent with pregnancy itself. The signs of thyrotoxicosis are as follows: (1) tachycardia, (2) tremor, (3) skin changes, (4) hyperkinesis, (5) lid lag, (6) muscle weakness, and (7) systolic hypertension (wide pulse pressure).

Patients may present with a variety of possible symptoms: weight loss, palpitations, heat intolerance, shakiness, hyperdefecation, insomnia, nervousness, polydipsia, oligo- or amenorrhea, or easy fatigability.

Diagnosis

Almost all patients with thyrotoxicosis have an elevated free thyroxine index (FTI). Confirmation requires a suppressed level of TSH (except in the rare conditions of TSH overproduction). In most cases, the TSH is less than 0.1 mIU/L. A normal TSH rules out the diagnosis. If the FTI is normal but clinical suspicion is high, a T3 level should be obtained; "T3 toxicosis" may occur, particularly in toxic nodules, or recurrent Graves' disease after radioactive iodine therapy. Other laboratory abnormalities include mild hypercalcemia, elevated aspartate aminotransferase (AST) and alkaline phosphatase, low cholesterol, and mild neutropenia.

Pathophysiology

The mechanism of thyrotoxicosis can be classified as either thyroid overproduction or "other." The critical test in differentiating between these two categories is the 4-hour radioactive iodine uptake (RAIU), which is nearly always high (occasionally normal) in patients with overproduction and suppressed in those with all other causes of thyrotoxicosis. Although the RAIU is mandatory to obtain, a thyroid scan is unnecessary except in defining a single toxic nodule or struma ovarii (which would require pelvic scanning).

Graves' disease, the most common cause of thyrotoxicosis, is an autoimmune disorder mediated by thyroid-stimulating immunoglobulin (TSI) usually presenting in patients between 20 and 50 years of age. Graves' orbitopathy can be detected in most patients using sensitive testing, but clinically significant disease characterized by exophthalmos, congestive findings of conjunctival injection and chemosis, periorbital edema, and paresis of extraocular muscles occurs in only 50% of patients. In most patients in whom eye disease develops, clinical findings occur within 6 months before or after the onset of thyrotoxicosis. The severity of orbitopathy is unrelated to the level of thyroid hormone and probably is mediated by a related but different immune phenomenon. Lid lag alone is not an indicator of Graves' orbitopathy

Table 20–1. Causes of hyperthyroxinemia.

Suppressed RAIU	I. Clinical thyrotoxicosis with suppressed TSH
	A. Increased release from damaged thyroid gland
	  1. Subacute thyroiditis
	  2. Autoimmune thyroiditis
	B. Amiodarone and iodides, eg, SSKI
	C. Factitious
	D. Struma ovarii

Increased RAIU	E. Overproduction by thyroid gland
	  1. Graves' disease
	  2. Toxic nodule
	  3. Toxic multinodular goiter
	II. Clinical thyrotoxicosis (with pathologic increase in TSH)
	A. Hydatidaform mole and choriocarcinoma
	B. Thyrotropin-producing pituitary tumor

III. Clinical euthyroidism
A. Normal TSH
1. Increased TBG
a. Pregnancy
b. Hereditary TBG excess
c. Acute intermittent porphyria
d. Hepatitis and primary biliary cirrhosis
e. Drugs
i. Estrogens and oral contraceptives
ii. Methadone
iii. Heparin
iv. Perphenazine
v. 5-fluorouracil
2. Familial dysalbuminemia
3. Peripheral conversion defect
B. Low TSH: first trimester of pregnancy
C. High TSH
1. Acute psychiatric illness
2. Thyroid-resistance syndrome

because it is mediated by sympathomimetic activity, which is increased in all forms of thyrotoxicosis. Decreased visual acuity from optic nerve compression is a rare complication. Patients with clinically apparent orbitopathy should be referred to an ophthalmologist for baseline measurement of exophthalmos and visual acuity. Any patient complaining of progressive exophthalmos, decreased visual acuity, or diplopia should be reassessed by an ophthalmologist.

The cause of toxic nodule and toxic multinodular goiter is unknown, but these conditions do not appear to be autoimmune in nature and are not associated with eye disease or other autoimmune diseases. Hydatidiform mole and choriocarcinoma both can produce human chorionic gonadotropin (HCG), which is homologous to TSH. Occasionally enough HCG is produced to cause clinical thyrotoxicosis. This unusual cause of hyperthyroidism should be considered if there is anything to suggest retained products of conception. Thyrotropin-producing pituitary tumors causing thyroxicosis are rare, and patients in whom such a tumor is suspected should be referred to an endocrinologist.

Subacute thyroiditis is virally mediated, with biopsy showing polymorphonuclear leukocytes (PMNs) and giant cells. A prodrome of fever, myalgia, headache, and occasionally upper respiratory infection is followed by exquisite tenderness of the diffusely enlarged thyroid gland, signs and symptoms of thyrotoxicosis, and an elevated erythrocyte sedimentation rate (ESR). Spontaneous resolution occurs uniformly within 4–6 weeks, usually with a transient period of hypothyroidism. Permanent thyroid dysfunction or recurrence is rare.

Autoimmune (painless) thyroiditis is an indolent disorder; biopsy shows lymphocytic infiltration. The thyroid gland is diffusely enlarged and nontender. The ESR is normal, and antithyroid antibodies are detected in 50% of patients.

The mechanism by which thyrotoxicosis occurs in both forms of thyroiditis is leakage of stored hormone from the inflamed gland. Although autoimmune thyroiditis may occur in anyone, the most common setting is within 6 months postpartum. In fact, about 5% of women develop this condition after delivery with spontaneous remission occurring within 3–6 months. Spontaneous remission usually includes a period of transient hypothyroidism; however, permanent hypothyroidism may develop in 20% of patients. Women with postpartum depression should be screened for painless thyroiditis, particularly the hypothyroid phase. Because there is also an increased incidence of Graves' disease during the postpartum period, diagnostic separation of these two entities is important and may be difficult in a woman who is breast-feeding. RAIU is contraindicated because radioactive iodine is excreted in breast milk for up to 1 week after oral administration to the mother. Ideally, breast-feeding would be terminated to permit RAIU and definitive treatment. If cessation of breast feeding is not an acceptable option, measurement of TSI is appropriate, although false-negative findings may occur. If the test for TSI is positive, medical treatment of Graves' disease should be initiated.

Struma ovarii (benign or malignant ovarian dermoid containing thyroid tissue) is a rare cause of thyrotoxicosis. Suspicion is raised if RAIU is suppressed, no thyroid tissue is palpable, and spontaneous resolution does not occur, or if a pelvic mass is palpable. Factitious thyrotoxicosis must be considered if RAIU is suppressed, particularly among medical personnel. Iatrogenic exogenous thyroid hormone excess historically has been a frequent cause of elevated T4, but with titration of dose using sensitive assays for TSH, this cause is becoming less common. Finally, a unique form of thyrotoxicosis in which overproduction of thyroid hormone occurs but RAIU is decreased because of dilution by nonradioactive iodine can be precipitated by iodine-rich medications such as amiodarone and saturated solution of potassium iodide (SSKI).

Treatment

Because thyroiditis (whether painful or silent) resolves spontaneously, treatment is warranted only for symptomatic patients, ie, beta-blockers for heart rate in excess of 100 beats/min or severe tremor. The usual starting dose of atenolol is 25–50 mg daily, with increases as needed to keep the heart rate below 100 beats/min. Because iodine uptake is impaired and synthetic processes damaged, treatment with either radioactive iodine or thionamides would be unsuccessful. Beta-blockers are relatively contraindicated during breast-feeding because they are concentrated in breast milk, which may lead to bradycardia in the infant.

Analgesic treatment initially should consist of acetaminophen, nonsteroidal anti-inflammatory agents, or salicylates. Although salicylates are probably the most effective medication, there is some risk of displacing thyroid hormone from TBG, thereby worsening the thyrotoxic state. Salicylates should be avoided in severely thyrotoxic patients. High-dose steroids (prednisone, 30–40 mg/d) should be reserved for patients with severe pain unresponsive to the previously mentioned measures because the recurrence rate may be as high as 20% following cessation of therapy.

For treatment of Graves' disease, there are three standard options in addition to use of beta-blockers. In the USA, ablation with I-131 is the most frequently recommended method. Treatment with a single oral dose of 6–12 mCi has a 95% cure rate at 6 months. The major side effect is permanent hypothyroidism, which develops in 60% of patients by 1 year and 90% by 10 years. There is no evidence of an increased incidence of cancer or abnormalities of reproduction. Radioactive iodine is contraindicated in pregnancy and breast-feeding. It is not used commonly in children or adolescents, although there are few data to suggest toxicity in this age group. In elderly or severely thyrotoxic patients, pretreatment with a thionamide may be appropriate for 6–8 weeks to reduce the risk of radiation thyroiditis causing an unacceptable rise in circulating thyroid hormone levels.

The second option is treatment with thionamides (propylthiouracil, 100 mg orally 3 times daily, or methimazole, 30 mg orally daily), which interfere with thyroid hormone synthesis. Thionamides can modulate cellular immunity in vitro, although a similar effect in clinical disease is unclear. Propylthiouracil also decreases peripheral conversion of T4 to T3. A euthyroid state is reached in about 4–12 weeks, after which titration of the dosage downward is necessary at a rate of 30% every 2–4 months. Treatment is continued for 1 year. After discontinuation of treatment, remission persists in only 40% of patients by 5 years. Most recurrences appear within the first 6 months after therapy is stopped. Remission is unlikely if TSI, TSH, or T3 is abnormal. Although standard practice is to treat with ablative therapy (I-131 or surgery) if thyrotoxicosis recurs after 1 year of thionamide treatment, there is some evidence, particularly in children, that the remission rate continues to increase with longer duration of therapy; the rate may be as high as 70% after 5 years of treatment.

Radioactive iodine is preferred over medical treatment for Graves' disease because of predictability of rapid cure and lack of side effects. Rash or arthralgias occur in about 1–5% of patients who take thionamides, and 0.5% suffer transient life-threatening agranulocytosis. Patients should be advised to obtain a WBC count with differential if any fever or sore throat develops. Periodic WBC counts are not recommended because both thyrotoxicosis and treatment with thionamides can cause mild neutropenia.

The third treatment option, thyroidectomy, is reserved for patients in the second trimester of pregnancy who are unable to tolerate propylthiouracil (methimazole is contraindicated because of scalp defects in the fetus) and patients in whom treatment with the other two approaches has failed.

Thyrotoxicosis during pregnancy constitutes a high-risk pregnancy; treatment should be managed by an endocrinologist or perinatologist. Fetal demise is increased in patients with untreated hyper- or hypothyroidism. Because thionamides cross the placenta easily but thyroid hormones do not, a maternal plasma concentration of T4 must be maintained in the high-normal range. The baby is at risk for neonatal goiter, which may compromise delivery, and transient neonatal thyrotoxicosis, because TSI crosses the placenta. Both complications may occur even if the mother is euthyroid if the presence of TSI persists. Both the pediatrician and the obstetrician must be aware of the diagnosis. Patients should not become pregnant until their thyrotoxicosis has remitted or been treated definitively. Propylthiouracil is the treatment of choice if the mother does not wish to terminate breast-feeding to receive radioactive iodine, although hypothyroidism and goiter may occur in the infant.

The oral cholecystographic agents sodium ipodate and iopanoic acid are structurally similar to T4 and consequently interfere with deiodination of T4 to the more biologically active triiodothyronine. T3 decreases rapidly, reaching normal values within a few days. Because these are iodinated compounds, they also inhibit release of hormone stored in the thyroid gland, thereby decreasing T4 as well. The usual dosage of sodium ipodate is 500 mg orally twice daily. Because it is not approved by the US Food and Drug Administration (FDA) for this treatment, use of sodium ipodate is restricted to severe cases that are life-threatening and cases in which thionamides cannot be used. As occurs with any iodinated compound, the diluting effect on thyroidal radioactive iodine uptake makes definitive treatment with I-131 impossible for up to several weeks after treatment is stopped.

Except as a temporizing measure, thionamides are not appropriate for treatment of toxic uni- or multi-del-nodular goiters because remission is unlikely. Definitive therapy with radioactive iodine is recommended. Surgery is an acceptable option, but pretreatment with thionamides to achieve euthyroidism is recommended to decrease the risk of thyroid storm precipitated by surgical manipulation of the toxic gland.

Complication: Thyroid Storm (Thyrotoxic Crisis)

The acute, life-threatening worsening of thyrotoxicosis called thyroid storm is fortunately rare. Manifestations include fever, tachycardia, vomiting, diarrhea, abnormal liver function tests, and altered mental status (usually agitation but occasionally apathy or coma). High-output congestive heart failure and tachyarrhythmias may require treatment.

The mechanism of thyroid storm—a medical emergency—is unclear. In some cases, direct injury to the thyroid gland, from either surgical manipulation or I-131 therapy may release stored thyroid hormone. Most cases are associated with nonthyroidal conditions, however, such as infection, other surgery, or trauma. Circulating total T4 and T3 do not correlate with the severity of disease and in fact are no higher in thyroid storm than in typical thyrotoxicosis. Free thyroid hormone levels are higher in thyroid storm, perhaps because an inhibitor of binding to TBG is released during acute illness, thus displacing thyroid hormone into the unbound, biologically active state.

Immediate treatment of thyroid storm must be initiated in the hospital. Because there are no definitive tests to confirm thyrotoxic crisis, clinicians should treat as such if the diagnosis is suspected. Treatment includes inhibition of thyroidal hormone synthesis and release, blockade of peripheral conversion and

action, and supportive measures (Table 20–2). All therapies should be initiated simultaneously except that propylthiouracil must be given before iodide or ipodate to prevent enrichment of intrathyroidal iodine stores and continued production of thyroid hormone. For temperature control, salicylates should be avoided because they inhibit binding to TBG and thus may increase free hormone levels. Steroids traditionally have been used because patients may have unsuspected autoimmune adrenal insufficiency. If congestive heart failure (CHF) is present, beta-blockade may be highly effective in decreasing the high-output state, but it should be administered in an intensive care unit with hemodynamic monitoring because sympathetic blockade may worsen CHF, particularly in patients with underlying cardiac disease. Treatment of the underlying illness is critical to survival.

EUTHYROIDISM

Particularly in the inpatient setting, elevation of T4 without clinical thyrotoxicosis is common, usually caused by increased TBG levels or decreased conversion to T3. In contrast to the situation in thyrotoxicosis, TSH is not suppressed. The conditions and medications associated with increased TBG and consequent high T4 are accompanied by a low resin-T3-uptake (RT3U) and a normal FTI. In familial dysalbuminemia, an aberrant albumin is produced with an unusually strong affinity for T4 (but not T3). The pattern of blood tests is unique—high T4, normal RT3U, normal T3, and normal TSH.

As described previously, T4 is metabolized peripherally by deiodination. In various conditions, 5'-deiodinase is inactivated, causing circulating T3 to fall, frequently below normal, with a reciprocal increase in reverse T3 (rT3) (Fig 20–4). Inhibition of 5'-deiodinase may be caused by acute illness, starvation, and medications such as amiodarone, oral cholecystographic agents, propylthiouracil, steroids,

Table 20–2. Treatment of thyroid storm.

Medication	Inhibitory Site
Propylthiouracil, 300 mg po q6h (give before iodide or ipodate)	Synthesis and deiodination
SSKI, 10 drops in water po tid or sodium iodide 1 g IV over 24 h	Release
Sodium ipodate (Oragrafin), 500 mg po bid	Deiodinase
Atenolol 50 mg po q6h prn or propanolol 1 mg IV prn	Sympathomimetic and deiodinase
Supportive measures: IV hydration Acetaminophen/cooling blanket Hydrocortisone, 100 mg IV q8h Digoxin for congestive heart failure	

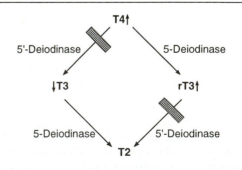

Figure 20–4. Peripheral thyroid hormone metabolism in acute illness.

and beta-blockers. In 10% of patients, T4 increases to above the normal level, because of both decreased peripheral metabolism and increased TSH responding to low T3 levels. Because there is no binding abnormality, the FTI parallels the level of T4, and these patients are truly hyperthyroxinemic. Confirmation of this condition is made by demonstrating a normal or minimally elevated TSH level. The level of T3 is low, although it is not always measured. No treatment is required. A low T3 during acute illness is meaningless, unless T4 is also low and TSH is elevated. Amiodarone and oral cholecystographic agents are structurally similar to T4 and compete for 5'-deiodinase. Although the mechanism is uncertain in acute illness, free fatty acids released during acute physiologic stress may inhibit this reaction.

A small subset of clinically euthyroid patients without a conversion defect have mild elevations of TSH. As many as 20% of acutely hospitalized patients with a spectrum of psychiatric illnesses are hyperthyroxinemic. Because the T3 level is normal and the TSH level is normal or mildly elevated, central pituitary stimulation is the presumed mechanism. Such patients are not clinically thyrotoxic, and laboratory test results return to normal within 1–3 weeks.

Peripheral thyroid hormone resistance is a rare condition, probably caused by an intracellular defect in pituitary and peripheral tissues. Despite high levels of T4 and T3, patients are clinically normal or mildly hypothyroid with increased TSH. A pituitary tumor must be ruled out. No treatment is available or necessary.

Table 20–3. Causes of hypothyroxinemia.

I. Hypothyroidism
  A. Primary (thyroidal failure)—increased TSH
     1. Post-ablative (I-131 or surgery)
     2. Thyroiditis
        a. Transient (recovery phase in subacute or autoimmune thyroiditis)
        b. Permanent (autoimmune including Hashimoto's)
     3. External radiation
     4. Congenital dyshormonogenesis
     5. Medications
        a. Amiodarone
        b. Lithium
        c. Iodides (eg, SSKI)
        d. Thionamides (propylthiouracil and methimazole)
  B. Secondary (pituitary or hypothalamic failure)—low TSH
     1. Tumor (primary or metastatic)
     2. Infiltrative (sarcoidosis, hemachromatosis, histiocytosis, lymphoma)
     3. Inflammation (hypophysitis)
     4. Ablation (surgery or radiation therapy)
     5. Medications
        a. Dopamine
        b. Steroids
II. Euthyroidism—normal TSH
  A. Decreased binding to TBG
     1. "Euthyroid sick" syndrome
     2. Hereditary decreased TBG
     3. Nephrotic syndrome
     4. Chronic renal failure
     5. Cirrhosis
     6. Medications
        a. Androgens
        b. Steroids
        c. Salicylates
        d. L-asparaginase
  B. Altered intracellular metabolism
     1. Phenytoin
     2. Carbemazapine

HYPOTHYROXINEMIA

The multiple causes of hypothyroxinemia are given in Table 20–3.

HYPOTHYROIDISM

Signs & Symptoms

The signs and symptoms of hypothyroidism can be nonspecific and subtle. Common signs include (1) bradycardia, (2) hypothermia, (3) hypokinesis, (4) skin changes (skin may be doughy, dry, and cold), (5) hoarseness, (6) pericardial effusion, (7) delayed relaxation phase of deep tendon reflexes, and (8) diastolic hypertension. A variety of symptoms may manifest: fatigue, cold intolerance, failure to lose weight or modest weight gain, constipation, muscle cramps, weakness, or menorrhagia.

The signs and symptoms are reversible with thyroid hormone replacement therapy, including hyper-

tension. The laboratory abnormalities, which include combined hyperlipidemia (increased triglycerides and low-density lipoprotein cholesterol), macrocytic anemia, elevated liver function levels, high creatine phosphokinase (CPK), and hyponatremia, also resolve with correction of thyroid hormone deficiency. The possibility of hypothyroidism should be considered in any patient with hyperlipidemia. Measurement of TSH is mandatory to confirm primary hypothyroidism. If T4 is unequivocally low and there is no other reason for an inappropriately low TSH, eg, euthyroid sick syndrome, evaluation for pituitary disease is indicated. When total T4 is low because of decreased binding to TBG, the RT3U is appropriately increased (except in euthyroid sick syndrome) yielding normal FTI and TSH.

EUTHYROID SICK SYNDROME
(Low T4, Low T3)

As many as 70% of critically ill patients have T4 levels below normal; often the levels are undetectable. On the basis of their normal TSH and return of T4 to normal with resolution of the intercurrent illness, these patients are euthyroid. The low T4 level is caused by interference with binding to TBG. The inhibitor remains speculative, but the same fatty acid purported to inactivate 5′-deiodinase during acute stress has been implicated, as have immunoglobulins. Careful measurement of unbound T4 by equilibrium dialysis shows a normal or minimally depressed result, confirming euthyroidism. Unfortunately, the FTI is often deceptively low because the interfering substance also inhibits binding to the resin in the RT3U. If the TSH level is not immediately available or it is below normal, the single most important piece of data is a recent normal T4, because even discontinuation of replacement therapy should decrease the plasma concentration by only 50% in the course of 1 week. Thyroid hormone replacement is unnecessary because the patient is euthyroid.

The euthyroid sick syndrome has prognostic implications: the lower the FTI, the higher the mortality rate, probably as a reflection of the severity of the underlying illness. The FTI will improve concurrently with improvement in the acute illness. Mild secondary hypothyroidsm also may be present in acute illness because TSH is normal or mildly decreased despite a free T4 level slightly lower than normal. The response of TSH to TRH is blunted in the presence of high-dose steroids (either exogenous or endogenous) and dopamine infusion. From a teleologic perspective, this response may be appropriate (as is the shift to biologically inactive reverse T3,) because the body is already in a catabolic state. Only if TSH is undetectable or there is other reason to suspect pituitary insufficiency should an additional workup be initiated. A transient increase in TSH to above normal usually is seen during the recovery phase either because of transient decrease in free T4 caused by increased binding to TBG as the inhibitor is removed or because of recovery from mild secondary hypothyroidism. In both acute and recovery phases, serial measurements of FTI and TSH every 3–7 days are appropriate.

Treatment

In symptomatic hypothyroidism with low FTI and high TSH, the decision to treat is straightforward. In patients with subclinical hypothyroidism, however, with normal FTI and a mild elevation of TSH to less than 10 mIU/L, the decision is more difficult. There is disagreement concerning whether these patients are normal, recovering from painless thyroiditis, or in the process of developing frank hypothyroidism. Studies have shown that frank hypothyroidism develops at a rate of 5% per year in patients with antithyroid antibodies and not at all in patients without antibodies. When patients with subclinical hypothyroidism are treated with replacement thyroid hormone, no changes in body weight or lipids are ob-

served, but improvement in some cardiac parameters and subjective symptoms has been reported. This condition is recognized in about 8% of men and 15% of women over the age of 60. Replacement therapy should be started if one of the following exists:

1. Positive antimicrosomal or antithyroglobulin antibodies
2. Goiter
3. TSH above 10 mIU/L
4. Development of low FTI
5. Strong clinical suspicion of symptomatic hypothyroidism (bradycardia, delayed deep tendon reflexes, unexplained fatigue, or weight gain)

In the absence of these indications, observation with repeat TSH every 6 months is adequate.

Replacement of thyroid hormone should be with synthetic L-thyroxine, which has a plasma half-life of 7 days; this treatment avoids the swings in plasma concentration encountered with T3 (sodium liothyronine [Cytomel]) or with desiccated thyroid, which contains T3 in the amount of 15%.

Because peripheral conversion of T4 accounts for 80% of circulating T3, it is unnecessary to prescribe additional T3. If for some reason a T3-containing preparation is used (usually because of patient preference), plasma T4 measurement will be lower than expected. If the patient is allowed nothing by mouth for more than 1 week, L-thyroxine may be given intramuscularly (intravenously is preferrable) in equivalent dosages because oral absorption is at least 80%. Oral absorption may be impaired by malabsorption syndrome or by ingestion of ferrous sulfate, cholestyramine, sucralfate, or aluminum hydroxide. Generic preparations should be avoided because problems of bioavailability have been reported.

In the past, most patients have received too much hormone, as determined by suppressed TSH, although they have not been symptomatic. Overreplacement may have particular implications for women because decreased bone mineral density has been demonstrated in such patients with attendant increased risk of symptomatic osteoporosis. The level of TSH should be maintained within the normal range, which requires approximately 1.6 µg/kg/d. L-thyroxine needs to be given only once daily. Patients without coronary artery disease may be started immediately on full replacement dosage. Adjustment of the dosage to normalize TSH should be made no sooner than 8 weeks after initiation of therapy. Once TSH is in the normal range, a change in dosage is rarely needed, and periodic measurement of TSH is not necessary. Increases in circulating thyroid hormone levels increase myocardial oxygen demand, thereby increasing risk of angina pectoris or myocardial infarction in patients with coronary artery disease. In such patients, treatment should be started with 0.025–0.050 mg/d and increased by 0.025–0.05

mg every 4–8 weeks if tolerated. Antianginal medications may need to be initiated or increased.

For patients requiring surgery, preoperative treatment of hypothyroidism is preferable but not mandatory. Increased sensitivity to anesthetics and narcotics, decreased ability to excrete a water load with consequent risk of hyponatremia, and decreased inotropic and chronotropic myocardial function are reasons to delay elective surgery such as laminectomy or cholecystectomy. Fortunately, however, there are good data showing that most patients with undiagnosed hypothyroidism undergoing major nonelective surgery such as coronary artery bypass grafting do well, with minimally increased morbidity and no increased mortality. Emergent and semiemergent surgery should proceed without rapid replacement therapy but with careful perioperative monitoring.

Complication: Myxedema Coma

Profound hypothyroidism, usually in the setting of intercurrent illness such as sepsis, congestive heart failure (CHF), or cerebrovascular accident (CVA), may lead to myxedema coma. The clinical findings can include hypercapnea caused by decreased ventilatory drive, hypothermia, bradycardia, CHF, and hyponatremia. Supportive measures include adequate ventilation, body warming, water restriction, treatment of CHF, and administration of steroids in case autoimmune adrenal disease coexists. Adequate thyroid hormone replacement should be administered immediately, although the dosage is controversial. Because T3 is not available commercially for intravenous administration, L-thyroxine, 500 µg intravenously, is recommended, followed by 100 µg daily thereafter.

Because in acute illness there is almost always inhibition of 5'-deiodinase, it is reasonable (but unproved) to provide T3 orally also, if possible, at a rate of about 10 µg every 8 hours. There is an increased risk of acute myocardial infarction or arrhythmia during rapid replacement therapy.

THYROID NODULE

Incidence & Risk Factors

About 5% of the population over the age of 40 years have a palpable thyroid nodule; however, at autopsy half the population have at least one nodule. Exposure to face or neck irradiation in childhood increases the risk of palpable abnormality to 30%, with peak incidence at age 30. Most nodules, even those appearing after exposure to irradiation, are benign; only 5% of nodules are malignant. In irradiated patients, 30% are malignant. The benign lesions include cysts, colloid nodules, and cellular follicular adenomas.

Screening

Patients with a history of face or neck irradiation in childhood for thymus enlargement, tonsil and adenoid hypertrophy, acne, or cancer should have annual neck palpation for at least 30 years after exposure. A patient with a family history of medullary carcinoma of the thyroid requires annual examination; members of families with multiple endocrine neoplasia syndrome II (hyperparathyroidism, pheochromocytoma, and medullary carcinoma of the thyroid) should be screened annually with a provocative test of calcitonin secretion such as pentagastrin or calcium infusion. Ultrasonography is not an appropriate screening method because of the high incidence of abnormality (50%) with no discrimination between benign and malignant lesions.

Signs & Symptoms

Thyroid nodules are usually palpable if they are larger than 1 cm in diameter. They are usually round, smooth, and nontender. Physical examination and history rarely can distinguish between benign and malignant lesions. Even rock-hard nodules may represent benign thyroiditis. Sudden onset of painful, tender nodule usually represents hemorrhage into a preexisting solid or cystic nodule. Rapid growth, particularly in an irregular, hard nodule, suggests anaplastic carcinoma. Presence of cervical nodes must raise concern about malignant disease. Size is not a good discriminator.

Diagnosis

First, euthyroidism should be confirmed by determining the level of TSH. If hypo- or hyperthyroidism is detected, attention should be directed to diagnosis and treatment of the metabolic abnormality. Separation of benign from malignant lesions has been enhanced and simplified by fine-needle aspiration biopsy, which is safe and inexpensive. Adequacy of specimen and accuracy of cytologic interpretation depend on experience; patients should be referred to a center specializing in this procedure—one in which at least 30 biopsies are performed yearly. About 70% of biopsies are read as benign; the false-negative rate is 1–5%. A malignant cytologic classification is the result in 5% of biopsies, with a false-positive rate of 0–5%. A suspicious classification is given in 10–15% of biopsies, of which 25% are cancer. Approximately 10–15% of biopsies are indeterminate because of an inadequate number of cells, usually in the setting of hemorrhage.

Fine-needle aspiration biopsy should be the first step in diagnosis. Ultrasonography cannot discriminate between benign and malignant nodules. Because most nodules are "cold" (nodules that do not take up radionuclide) on radionuclide scan, ultrasonography is not helpful as an initial procedure. If cytologic findings are suspicious, however, a "hot" nodule (ie, a nodule that takes up more radionuclide than the rest of the thyroid, which is suppressed) is rarely cancerous. Cancer can be expected in about 30% of patients undergoing surgery if the diagnostic approach charted in Figure 20–5 is employed.

Treatment

Malignant lesions and suspicious lesions that are not hot on scan should be removed by an experienced surgeon. Near-total thyroidectomy is indicated for clearly malignant nodules, most of which are papillary carcinoma. The extent of surgery for suspicious nodules remains controversial. The differential diagnosis between follicular carcinoma and adenoma may be equally difficult to confirm at frozen section. If there is considerable doubt, at least a subtotal thyroidectomy should be undertaken.

If cancer is confirmed, referral to an endocrinologist is appropriate. Papillary carcinoma, which represents 70% of malignant lesions, has an excellent prognosis, with no decrease in life expectancy if (1) the patient is under 40 years of age, (2) the lesion is less than 3 cm in diameter, and (3) there is no vascular or capsular invasion. Lymph-node invasion is common and unrelated to mortality rate. Follicular carcinoma accounts for 20% of malignant lesions and is more aggressive, with a 10-year mortality rate of 30%; most of the mortality is the result of local recurrence. Treatment in both types of differentiated carcinomas includes adequate surgical removal, suppressive doses of L-thyroxine (enough to suppress TSH to below normal), and usually, ablation of residual normal and malignant thyroid tissue with I-131. Anaplastic carcinoma is unresponsive to any treatment and uniformly fatal. Medullary carcinoma and lymphoma are intermediate in responsiveness to therapy.

Treatment of benign nodules remains controversial. Although suppression with L-thyroxine is standard procedure in some centers, many institutions do not recommend it routinely for three reasons: (1) controlled studies of up to 3 years show no difference in likelihood of shrinkage or enlargement between patients who undergo thyroid suppression and those who do not; (2) administration of suppressive doses of L-thyroxine may have adverse consequences, including atrial fibrillation and decreased bone mineral density; and (3) there is no evidence that suppression prevents malignancy. Suppression of remaining thyroid tissue following removal of benign nodule is equally uncertain; however, in patients who were exposed previously to face or neck irradiation, the incidence of recurrent nodule decreases from 30% to 7% with suppression. Annual palpation of the benign nodule or remaining gland after surgery is recommended; if progressive enlargement or recurrence is found, biopsy should be repeated.

THYROID FUNCTION DURING PREGNANCY

Early Pregnancy

Thyroid function changes in a predictable manner during the first trimester of pregnancy. Coincident with rising HCG levels, FTI increases and TSH decreases, consistent with the thyroid-stimulating activity of HCG. These alterations peak at 6–12 weeks and return to normal by 20 weeks. Even when FTI or TSH is beyond the normal range, clinical thyrotoxicosis is not observed. Treatment is not necessary for this normal physiologic phenomenon. In fact, understanding of this condition is critical for prevention of unnecessary intervention. Close follow-up is equally

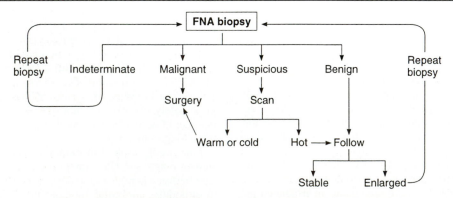

Figure 20–5. Evaluation of thyroid nodule. (FNA–fine-needle aspiration.)

important, however, because Graves' disease can present during pregnancy and must be aggressively managed. If the patient is symptomatic or thyroid function fails to normalize by 20 weeks, the level of TSI should be obtained and treatment with propylthiouracil initiated.

The relationship of this physiologic phenomenon to hyperemesis gravidarum remains controversial. Although up to 50% of women with hyperemesis gravidarum have an elevated FTI, they are not clinically thyrotoxic, and conversely, most pregnant patients with high FTI do not have hyperemesis gravidarum. Because FTI elevation is self-limited, treatment with propylthiouracil should be avoided if possible.

Late Pregnancy

Throughout pregnancy, TBG levels increase progressively under the influence of increasing circulating estrogen levels. Consequently, T4 levels increase progressively to above normal limits by the third trimester, with an expected decrease in RT3U. Although equilibration does occur, T4 does not increase as much as would be expected from the increase in TBG. Consequently, there is a modest decrease in FTI and increase in TSH, with both remaining within the normal range. In 50% of patients receiving thyroid replacement therapy for hypothyroidism who are unable to respond to TSH stimulation, frankly elevated TSH can be documented. Therefore, a TSH level should be obtained at the twenty-fifth week of gestation in patients receiving replacement therapy.

The dosage of thyroid replacement should be increased to normalize TSH, although the significance of these mild abnormalities late in pregnancy is unclear. Finally, the thyroid gland enlarges by about 20% as detected by ultrasonography during pregnancy. In the iodine-sufficient United States, however, there is no increase in incidence of clinical goiter during pregnancy.

MEDICATIONS THAT ALTER THYROID FUNCTION TESTS

Many commonly prescribed medications have an effect on thyroid function tests either by altering binding to proteins or by changing thyroid metabolism. These medications are classified here according to mechanism of action and in Table 20–4 by changes in thyroid function tests.

A. Increased TBG
   1. Estrogens (including oral contraceptives)
   2. Methadone
   3. Heparin
   4. Perphenazine
   5. 5-Fluorouracil (5-FU)

Table 20–4. Medications affecting thyroid function.

Medication	T4	Resin-T3-Uptake	Free Thyroxine Index	T3	Thyrotropin	Mechanism
Dopamine	D*	D	D	D	D	Pituitary suppression
Steroids	D,N,I	D,N,I	D,N,I	D,N	D,N,I	Pituitary suppression; deiodinase block
Methimazole	D	D	D	D	I	Decreased synthesis
Propylthiouracil	D	D	D	D	I	Decreased synthesis, deiodinase block
Inorganic iodides and amiodarone	D	D	D	D	I	Synthetic defect
	I	I	I	I	D	Block release Iodine repletion
Amiodarone	N,I	N,I	N,I	D	N,I	Deiodinase block
Ipodate	N,I	N,I	N,I	D	N,I	Deiodinase block
Beta-blockers	N,I	N,I	N,I	D	N,I	Deiodinase block
Lithium	D	D	D	D	I	Block release
Estrogens Methadone Heparin 5-fluorouracil Perphenazine	I	D	N	I	N	Increased thyroxine-binding globulin
Androgens Steriods L-asparaginase Salicylates	D	I	N	D	N	Decreased thyroxine-binding globulin
Phenytoin Carbamazepine	D	D	D	N	N	Decreased intracellular metabolism

*D = decreased; N = normal; I = increased.

B. Decreased TBG or binding to TBG
   1. Androgens
   2. Steroids
   3. Salicylates
   4. L-asparaginase
C. Increased synthesis of thyroid hormone
   1. Amiodarone
   2. Inorganic iodide, eg, SSKI
D. Decreased synthesis of thyroid hormone
   1. Thionamides (propylthiouracil and methimazole)
   2. Inorganic iodides, eg, SSKI, in patients with intrinsic defect in thyroid hormone synthesis such as Hashimoto's thyroiditis
   3. Amiodarone (same mechanism as SSKI)
E. Decreased release of stored thyroid hormone
   1. Inorganic iodide, eg, SSKI
   2. Amiodarone
   3. Lithium carbonate
F. Decreased peripheral conversion of T4 to T3
   1. Sodium ipodate or iopanoic acid
   2. Propylthiouracil (not methimazole)
   3. Steroids
   4. Amiodarone
   5. Beta-blockers
G. Altered intracellular metabolism of thyroid hormone
   1. Phenytoin
   2. Carbamazepine
H. Decreased TSH secretion
   1. Steroids
   2. Dopamine

A few medications require special comment. Inorganic iodides act at multiple steps in thyroid hormone physiology. They uniformly interfere with diagnostic radioactive iodine uptake by competition for uptake into the thyroid gland. They may precipitate reversible myxedema in patients with damaged synthetic processes but paradoxically may cause thyrotoxicosis in iodine-deficient patients with autoimmune thyroid disease. Finally, they inhibit release of thyroid hormone from the gland, leading to hypothyroidism and goiter. The class III antiarrhythmic agent amiodarone, because of structural similarity to the thyronines and its iodine content, has many, often clinically important, effects on thyroid hormone synthesis and action. Depending on the baseline status of the thyroid gland, amiodarone may cause either hypo- or hyperthyroidism, both of which are reversible. In addition, amiodarone is a potent inhibitor of 5'-deiodinase.

The mechanism of action of antiseizure medications on thyroid hormone metabolism is obscure, but it appears to involve increased intracellular disposal accounting for decreased circulating hormone levels but normal TSH and euthyroid clinical status. A low FTI may occur as often as 20% of the time. No treatment is indicated, but if there is any other reason to suspect pituitary dysfunction, further evaluation should be undertaken.

GLOSSARY OF THYROID FUNCTION TESTS

T4–total thyroxine concentration, of which 99.9% is inactive, bound to plasma proteins.
RT3U–resin-T3-uptake, which is an indirect reciprocal measurement of T4 binding to TBG; ie, if TBG increases, RT3U decreases.
FTI–free thyroxine index, which is an indirect calculation of biologically active, unbound thyroxine.

$$FTI = \frac{\text{patient's T4} \times \text{patient's RT3U}}{\text{laboratory mean normal RT3U}}$$

The normal range for FTI is the same as for T4.
Free T4–an indirect measurement of unbound thyroxine performed by equilibrium dialysis, which is more sensitive and accurate but much more difficult to perform than a test for T4.
T3–total T3, of which 99% is bound to protein.
TSH–thyrotropin (thyroid-stimulating hormone), which is secreted by the pituitary gland and controls thyroid function. Most laboratories now use sensitive assays capable of measuring 0.1 mIU/L (second generation) or 0.01 mIU/L (third generation). Discussion in this chapter refers to the second-generation assays.
RAIU–radioactive iodine uptake, which is the percentage of an oral dose of I-123 or I-131 taken up by the thyroid gland in 4 or 24 hours.
Thyroid scan–nuclear imaging with I-123 or ^{99}Tc to show functional anatomy of the thyroid gland.

REFERENCES

Burrow GN: Thyroid function and hyperfunction during gestation. Endocr Rev 1993;14:194.
Gharib H: Fine-needle aspiration biopsy of the thyroid: An appraisal. Ann Intern Med 1993;118:282.

Ingbar SH, Braverman LE (editors): *Werner's The Thyroid.* Lippincott, 1986.
Roti E et al: The use and misuse of thyroid hormone. Endocr Rev 1993;14:401.

Menopause & Hormone Replacement Therapy

21

Dawn P. Lemcke, MD, Lorna A. Marshall, MD, & Julie Pattison, MD

Although menopause results in similar hormonal changes in most women, the experience of each woman depends on variables such as her age, cultural background, health, type of menopause (spontaneous or surgical), desire for more children, and contact (or lack thereof) with her medical practitioner. In the United States, many women view menopause as a signal of major change in their lives, either positive change, such as freedom from the need for contraception, or negative change, such as experiencing mood swings or feeling "old." In some Asian cultures, women reach menopause without much notice at all and rarely seek medical help or hormonal treatment for symptoms. One woman might be sad that her reproductive years are over. Another may be happy to find her migraine headaches have resolved. Women undergoing surgical menopause may experience vasomotor symptoms and osteoporosis more abruptly than women with spontaneous menopause.

The postmenopausal years may be as variable as menopause is, depending on development of the diseases associated with menopausal hormonal changes at menopause and the decision of whether or not to undergo hormone replacement therapy (HRT). Although some practitioners consider menopause primarily a hormone-deficient state necessitating HRT, the experiences and needs of patients are much more variable and complex than that description indicates.

PHYSIOLOGY

Menopause, by definition, is the last menstrual period. The perimenopause refers to the years surrounding menopause, in which ovarian function begins to change. Number of eggs diminish, and the ovaries become more resistant to the action of follicle-stimulating hormone (FSH). The ovaries start to produce decreasing quantities of estrogen, progesterone, and androgen. Loss of the negative feedback from ovarian estrogen production causes increased secretion of FSH and luteinizing hormone (LH). There is also declining secretion of the ovarian glycoprotein inhibin, which selectively inhibits FSH.

The eventual result is sustained elevation of FSH, which may be a sign that menopause is near.

Vasomotor symptoms may start at this point. The exact cause of these symptoms is not known, although several mechanisms have been postulated. The symptoms occur in only 75% of women and usually last between 2 and 5 years; they last much longer and may be lifelong in a few women. Menstrual cycles may be anovulatory, resulting in missed menses or irregular bleeding. With declining estrogen levels, women may experience insomnia, problems with concentration, minor short-term memory loss, and irritability. Eventually, ovarian estrogen and progesterone production ceases, but ovarian testosterone production drops by only 30%; it accounts for 40% of postmenopausal testosterone production, with the rest produced by the adrenal gland. Androgens from both sources are aromatized in some peripheral tissues, especially fat cells, into the weak estrogen, estrone; therefore, obese women may have higher postmenopausal endogenous estrogen levels and fewer estrogen-deficiency symptoms.

CLINICAL FINDINGS & DIAGNOSIS

The diagnosis of menopause is made when amenorrhea occurs or when FSH is elevated to a level greater than 30 mIU/mL. Menopause is probably present when the FSH is near this level in a woman with the typical clinical picture. FSH can be used only to make the diagnosis of menopause, not to monitor estrogen replacement, because even high doses of estrogen inhibit FSH only partially (inhibin also inhibits FSH).

The average age of menopause is 51 years. Premature menopause, occurs before age 40. A woman who has had a hysterectomy without an oophorectomy may have no vasomotor symptoms. Such women should be evaluated for signs of estrogen deficiency at their yearly gynecologic examinations and should have an FSH level checked yearly when they near the age of menopause.

If hormone replacement is not elected, urogenital atrophy may occur within 2–3 years. The vagina and urethra are estrogen-sensitive tissues, and estrogen deficiency causes atrophy of both. Age-related vaginal changes not affected by estrogen also occur. Through both processes, the vaginal mucosa atrophies, causing problems with lubrication and dyspareunia. Urethral atrophy causes dysuria, urgency, and urge (but not stress) incontinence. Urethral strictures also may occur.

Accelerated bone loss occurs in the perimenopausal years and in the first 2–3 years after menopause. Depending on the bone mass when entering menopause and the propensity toward menopausal bone loss, osteoporosis may result. Symptoms of osteoporosis, such as fractures and chronic bone pain, do not appear until 10 or more years after menopause. Although other medical diseases cause osteoporosis, estrogen-related menopausal bone loss accounts for the vast majority of cases (see Chapter 22).

Premenopausal cardiovascular protection from estrogen is lost after menopause. Adverse lipid changes occur. Although coronary artery disease (CAD) generally develops 6–10 years later in women than men, by the time women reach their 70s–80s, their death rate from CAD is equivalent to that in men.

Controversy exists regarding association of psychologic symptoms with the biologic changes caused by menopause. Few studies are available to sort out the multiple potential causes of mood depression in some women perimenopausally. There is evidence that many women experience a significant deterioration in mood during menopause. Most likely more important than estrogen deficiency are a woman's psychologic make-up, cultural background, intercurrent stresses, and changing role in her family.

Currently, there is little knowledge concerning the effects of menopause on sexuality. Studies generally have been small and sometimes have included women who were not yet menopausal. Definitions of sexuality have varied, and few data correlating symptoms to hormonal levels are available. It has been difficult to isolate the effect of ovarian failure from the effect of other factors that influence sexuality, such as the changing body image and stressful life events. The studies that are available show decreases in sexual activity and thoughts and in vaginal lubrication in postmenopausal women. Dyspareunia has been shown to be associated significantly with loss of sexual desire. In one study, previous sexual problems were reported to be exacerbated at menopause.

HORMONE REPLACEMENT THERAPY

Most of the data available to assess the benefits and risks of HRT are from retrospective studies primarily of estrogen alone, usually in higher doses than are used today. These cohort and case-control studies are helpful but introduce biases, such as selection, detection, and observational bias. For instance, women who take menopausal hormones have been found to be more highly educated, thinner, more affluent, and more compliant with other beneficial preventive health practices than women who do not; therefore, the beneficial effects of HRT may be related partially to healthier life-styles. Additionally, either patients or their practitioners may have selected to use or not use HRT based on a perception of intrinsically greater HRT benefit (woman with coronary disease) or HRT risk (strong family history of breast cancer). Alternatively, women may undergo more frequent or target-organ-specific medical evaluations because they are undergoing HRT, perhaps causing earlier or more frequent detection of diseases proposed to be related to hormones. Data from the large, prospective Women's Health Initiative, which includes a hormone replacement therapy trial, are not expected to be available until approximately the year 2006. Therefore, decisions regarding use of HRT currently must be based on the data available.

Benefits

The benefit from HRT has been associated mostly with prevention or improvement in coronary heart disease, osteoporosis, urogenital atrophy, and overall mortality.

A. Cardiovascular Disease: Coronary heart disease (CHD) is the leading cause of death of women in the USA. The average postmenopausal woman has a 46% lifetime probability of developing and a 31% probability of dying from CHD. Because CHD is so common and deadly, any benefit of HRT would outweigh a small increase in risks from HRT in most women. Multiple retrospective studies using estrogen alone have shown a protective effect of exogenous oral estrogen (primarily conjugated equine estrogen) in postmenopausal women, although many of the studies were small and the duration of therapy short. Most studies showed a relative risk of 0.55–0.65 for development of CHD and of 0.5–0.63 for death from CHD. Two independent meta-analyses of published data found that estrogen users had approximately a 50% lower risk of CHD than nonusers, with the data adjusted for cardiac risk factors. The Framingham study is the only prospective cohort study that found a statistically significant increase in cardiovascular risk among women taking estrogen. However, a reanalysis of the data that excluded chest pain as an end point, which correlates poorly in women with angiographic evidence of CAD, found a beneficial effect of estrogen on ischemic heart disease in women under the age of 60. Although observational bias may play some role in these 40–50% risk reductions, it is unlikely to explain the consistency and magnitude of risk reduction. In addition to these studies of fatal and nonfatal myocardial infarction (MI), several studies of angiographically defined CAD have shown a lower (60–70%) incidence of significant coronary artery stenosis in women taking estrogen.

A few studies of combined therapy with estrogen and progestin are available, but most studies were small, were inconclusive, or produced inconsistent results. In a large, prospective, Swedish cohort study, women who used combined therapy at some time had a 50% risk reduction in MI, a reduction that is at least as large as that of women taking estrogen alone. In a small population-based case-control study by the Group Health Cooperative, the risk reduction for current users of combined therapy was the same as that for current users of estrogen alone (0.68 and 0.69, respectively).

Current use of estrogen seems to confer more benefit than former use of estrogen. The large, prospective Nurses' Health Study found that current estrogen use was associated with a relative risk of major CAD of 0.56 and that former use was associated with a relative risk of 0.83, after adjustment for cardiac risk factors.

In addition to the evidence of cardiac benefits, there is also some evidence that combined therapy may decrease the risk for stroke. A recent large case-control study in England showed that the incidence of stroke was lower in women undergoing combined therapy than in controls, although only 16% of patients who took hormones took them for a mean of 15 months. In contrast, the Nurses' Health Study did not show a similar reduction in stroke risk with estrogen replacement. There is some evidence that HRT may reduce the risk of subarachnoid hemorrhage in women who have smoked at some time.

There is no evidence that venous thromboembolic disease is increased in women undergoing estrogen replacement therapy (ERT). All too often, ERT is discontinued inappropriately in postmenopausal women in whom deep venous thromboses develop.

The mechanism of the cardiovascular benefit of estrogen is probably multifactorial. It is likely that the most studied benefit has been the effect on serum lipoproteins. Oral estrogen therapy alone reduces serum low-density lipoprotein (LDL) cholesterol by 10–15% and increases high-density lipoprotein (HDL) cholesterol by 20–30%, especially the HDL_2 subfraction; both of these are considered desirable effects. It also increases the level of triglyceride minimally, which is not believed to be a significant adverse effect. Transdermal and parenteral estrogen have only insignificant effects on lipids. The addition of progestins to estrogen replacement has an adverse lipid effect, such that the beneficial effects of estrogen of decreasing LDL and increasing HDL are lessened. The degree of effect depends on the progestin androgenicity, dosage, and regimen. However, a recent large population-based cross-sectional analysis showed that the addition of cyclic progestin (usually medroxyprogesterone acetate) to estrogen therapy (mainly conjugated equine estrogen) was associated in current users with improvement in HDL, LDL, other lipoproteins, fibrinogen, antithrombin III, and fasting serum glucose and insulin. Women undergoing combined therapy showed even more improvement than women taking estrogen alone, who showed more improvement than untreated women.

In addition to the beneficial effects on lipoprotein, HRT may have beneficial effects on coagulation and fibrinolysis. There is also evidence that estrogen may act locally on the endothelial wall to slow the incorporation of oxidized LDL and other atherogenic lipoproteins into the intima. Estrogen also may inhibit tonic arterial vasoconstriction, an effect that may be reversed by progestins. Hypertension appears to remain unchanged or to improve slightly with ERT. Therefore, hormones may exert their effect both through short-term metabolic, vasoactive, and coagulation effects and through long-term synthetic effects.

B. Osteoporosis: Osteoporosis and increased risk for fracture most frequently result from estrogen deficiency. A postmenopausal woman has a 15% probability of development of a hip fracture. ERT inhibits bone resorption and increases intestinal absorption of calcium, preventing bone loss and even minimally increasing bone density. Combination therapy with estrogen and progestin is of no less benefit to bone density than estrogen alone. Numerous studies have shown that estrogen replacement protects against the development of osteoporotic fractures in the hips and vertebrae. No studies are available yet of the effect of combined therapy on fractures, but it is believed that the effect is similar to that of estrogen alone. There is some evidence that estrogen also may decrease fractures by improving coordination and thus preventing falls.

The greatest impact of HRT on bone occurs when the therapy is begun early in menopause. If begun within the first few years after menopause, there appears to be a long-lasting protective effect. If HRT is discontinued at any point, bone loss returns to the former, accelerated early postmenopausal rate. Hormone replacement may be started in older women who develop osteoporosis, but significant reduction in fracture risk does not occur until after 7 years of HRT. The daily dosage of conjugated estrogen required to prevent bone loss is 0.625 mg. A decreasing fracture risk correlates with longer durations of therapy. A more in-depth discussion of this topic is available in Chapter 22.

C. Vasomotor Symptoms: Hot flashes occur in approximately 75% of menopausal women, but only a minority of women seek medical treatment for them. The symptom varies widely in severity and may cause secondary insomnia. Estrogen replacement can alleviate these symptoms within a few days to 1 month. Progestins are the second most effective hormone to treat these symptoms.

D. Urogenital Atrophy and Sexual Dysfunction: Systemic or local ERT is effective in preventing or reversing the urogenital changes caused by estrogen deficiency. Whether or not hormones improve sexuality is controversial. As mentioned previously, research on sexuality is scant and difficult to perform. In addition to a possible hormonal contribution, several factors that may be involved in sexual dysfunction should be considered, including psychosocial factors, hypothyroidism, hyperprolactinemia, and other medical problems in the patient or sexual partner.

The improvement in vaginal fluid and blood flow induced by estrogen has been shown to decrease dyspareunia. Estrogen relieves vasomotor symptoms and related sleep disturbances and, in this manner, improves quality of life. These benefits of estrogen may improve sexual dysfunction indirectly. Of the studies available, some show improvement in libido with estrogen, but others show no effect. No detrimental effect on sexuality has been shown for estrogen. Progestins have not been well studied for their effects on sexuality, but in replacement doses they may be potential second-line agents because of their effect on vasomotor symptoms.

Androgens—more specifically, testosterone—have been even more difficult to study because the ovary and the adrenal gland continue to produce them after menopause. Only limited data are obtained from single testosterone measurements because the levels fluctuate. Oophorectomized women often have participated in studies without differentiation from women who enter menopause naturally. One study of testosterone with estrogen replacement showed a 13% incidence of adverse virilizing side effects such as increased facial hair, acne, and hoarseness. Because androgens have a negative effect on lipids, most authorities believe they are not a good choice for long-term therapy and should be reserved for

short-term use in women with refractory sexual dysfunction.

E. Neuropsychologic Symptoms: There are few studies of the effects of HRT on psychologic symptoms. Estrogen has been shown to improve overall quality of life, and a few studies have shown improvement in psychologic symptoms with estrogen, although the benefits are not major. The addition of a progestin to the replacement regimen caused adverse mental health symptoms in one study. There is some evidence that estrogen replacement may improve cognition.

F. Mortality: Several studies have shown an improvement in overall mortality in women taking estrogen alone, primarily secondary to the cardiovascular benefit. No studies are available of the effect of combined therapy. Life expectancy in women undergoing ERT is increased on average only 2 years; the major effect of hormone replacement is not on mortality but on decreased morbidity and improved quality of life.

Risks

Many of the studies of the potential carcinogenicity of menopausal ERT were based on early use of relatively high doses of unopposed estrogens. Few studies have been performed of the newer replacement regimens with lower estrogen doses with or without progestins.

A. Endometrial Cancer: Several case-control studies of the risk of endometrial cancer in menopausal women using unopposed estrogen compared with nonusers have shown an increased risk: the risk is 2–6 times higher in women who have used unopposed estrogen at any time and 7–12 times higher in long-term users. Cyclic use of estrogen alone (eg, 25 days of the month) was not enough of a change to lower the risk. The risk is increased after only 3 years of unopposed estrogen use and persists for longer than 10 years after the estrogen has been discontinued. The risk of endometrial cancer also increases with the estrogen dose, although there is no level of unopposed replacement below which added risk does not occur. At the time of diagnosis, endometrial cancer in women who have used estrogen is generally of a lower grade pathologically and at an earlier stage with better survival potential than endometrial cancer in nonusers. Whether or not to use HRT in women with a personal history of endometrial cancer is discussed later in this chapter.

The addition of a progestin in sufficient dosage and for sufficient duration to the estrogen therapy significantly reduces the risk of development of endometrial cancer, possibly to a lower level than in women who use no hormones at all.

B. Breast Cancer: The risk of breast cancer to women using HRT remains controversial. Only observational studies are available, and many are small and have failed to control for important variables such as premenopausal hormone use, estrogen dosage, and family history of breast cancer. The primary end point has been discovery of breast cancer, which may lead to bias if earlier detection occurs because of closer surveillance of women taking hormones.

An early, small meta-analysis concluded that there was no increase in the risk of breast cancer with noncontraceptive estrogen use. Since that time, two larger meta-analyses of the risk of ERT have been performed. The authors of one study concluded that treatment of menopausal women with 0.625 mg/d of conjugated estrogen does not increase the risk of breast cancer. The other study's authors concluded that risk was increased significantly only after 15 years of ERT. Because women with family or personal histories of breast cancer were excluded from the studies, no conclusions could be made concerning these subgroups. Whether or not to use HRT in women with a personal history of breast cancer is discussed later in this chapter. Few studies have been performed with combined therapy.

Women in whom breast cancer develops while they are taking estrogen seem to have a better survival rate than women who are nonusers, suggesting either earlier detection through closer surveillance or a less aggressive tumor type.

Overall, the risk for development of breast cancer in an average postmenopausal woman who is not undergoing HRT is 10%, with a 3% chance of dying from the disease. If there is no or only minimal increased risk of development of breast cancer secondary to HRT, the probable significant cardiovascular benefits would far outweigh any adverse effects of hormones in most women. Clearly, more research is needed.

C. Other Conditions: Although the incidence of migraine headaches usually decreases with age, they may improve or worsen with menopause. Estrogen replacement may exacerbate migraine headaches in some women. Regimens to diminish this effect are discussed later in this chapter.

There may be a slight increase in incidence of gallbladder disease in women undergoing ERT.

Endometriosis reactivation can occur with ERT, but combined therapy or progestin therapy alone for 6 months before estrogen is added may prevent reactivation and pain.

Prescribing Hormone Replacement Therapy

- All postmenopausal and perimenopausal women should be counseled concerning HRT.
- HRT alleviates vasomotor symptoms, prevents and treats genitourinary atrophy, prevents osteoporosis, and may play a key role in preventing cardiovascular events.
- Risks including that of endometrial cancer can be managed by using appropriate HRT regimens and

surveillance. The impact of HRT on the risk of breast cancer remains controversial; mammograms at appropriate age-determined intervals are recommended.

A. Indications: Most menopausal women are candidates for hormone replacement therapy. In particular, hormone replacement therapy should be considered for the following women:

- All menopausal or perimenopausal women with symptoms of estrogen deficiency, including vasomotor symptoms (hot flushes, night sweats) and genitourinary atrophy.
- Women with or at risk for osteoporosis, particularly women with premature ovarian failure or who have undergone oophorectomy before age 50.
- Postmenopausal women with or at risk for CHD.

Many physicians use a selective approach to HRT, recommending it only to symptomatic women, or asymptomatic women who are at high risk for osteoporosis and have decreased bone-mineral density documented by densitometry. This approach has been shown to be cost-effective and to decrease overall morbidity secondary to estrogen use. Because HRT may have other benefits, however, such as decreasing the risk of both primary and secondary cardiovascular events, improving overall sense of well-being, and decreasing mortality, many physicians suggest a less selective approach to starting HRT.

B. Contraindications: Absolute contraindications to HRT include the following:

- Undiagnosed vaginal bleeding
- Acute vascular thrombosis (eg, deep venous thrombosis, stroke, or transient ischemic attack)
- Undiagnosed breast mass
- A personal history of breast cancer or other estrogen-dependent tumors including endometrial carcinoma.

The last-mentioned contraindication continues to be a source of great controversy, with few objective data to draw conclusions from. HRT does not appear to present a risk for women who have had noninvasive stage I endometrial cancer treated with hysterectomy. On the basis of a small, nonrandomized study of patients with stage I endometrial cancer, it was reported that women who received estrogens had fewer recurrences. Most clinicians would recommend HRT to these women. The American College of Obstetrics and Gynecology (ACOG) has issued a committee opinion regarding this issue stating that in "women with a history of endometrial cancer, estrogens could be used for the same indications as for any other women except that the selection of appropriate candidates should be based on prognostic indicators and the risk the patient is willing to assume."

For women with a personal history of breast cancer, the appropriate recommendation regarding HRT is particularly unclear. Such a history is considered by most clinicians to be an absolute contraindication to HRT based on the biologic evidence that estrogen can stimulate the growth of breast cancer cells. Despite the biologic evidence, there are no randomized, prospective studies that support HRT as a risk for reactivating or causing recurrence of breast cancer. It seems appropriate, therefore, for the patient and her physician to weigh the patient's individual risks and benefits before making a decision regarding the appropriateness of HRT. It appears that short-term treatment (1–2 yr) to address severe vasomotor symptoms may not have adverse effects. Many women with premenopausal breast cancer who have undergone chemotherapy have premature ovarian failure and significant symptoms of estrogen deficiency. In addition, they are at high risk for osteoporosis. In these women, careful evaluation for osteoporosis should be undertaken and discussions of treatment initiated. Again, the individual risks and benefits should be discussed with the patient and a joint decision made regarding the appropriateness of estrogen.

A relative contraindication to estrogen therapy is impaired liver function, a condition that should not deter the use of estrogen but may call for a transdermal rather than an oral route of delivery. This change in delivery is recommended because liver failure markedly affects the first-pass liver effect on the concentrations of estrogen in the serum.

A history of venous thromboembolic disease (VTE) should not be considered a contraindication to HRT. Presence of this condition may be another reason to change the route of delivery from oral to transdermal. Administration of oral estrogen promotes hepatic synthesis of coagulation factors that may promote VTE, whereas the transdermal route does not have the same effect. This situation is in contrast to that of a prior history of VTE and use of oral contraceptive agents. Oral contraceptives contain supraphysiologic doses of estrogen and therefore may promote VTE.

Migraine headaches, which are common in women, are not either an absolute or a relative contraindication to HRT, but the route and regimen are important factors in avoiding exacerbation of headaches. If a woman has recurrence or exacerbation of her headaches with HRT, the following strategies can be tried to alleviate the headaches: Initially, a lowering of the estrogen dosage may be tried, with attention paid to the minimal effective dose to prevent osteoporosis. Changing from a cyclic to a continuous regimen prevents the fluctuations in estrogen and progestins that may initiate migraine headaches. In addition, changing from conjugated estrogen to 17-beta-estradiol or changing from oral to transdermal administration also may help in the management of headaches.

Available Hormones

Once the physician and patient have agreed on hormone replacement therapy, deciding on the appropriate hormones and regimen can be a challenge. Each provider should become familiar with one or two HRT regimens to be given initially to most patients. Adjustments can be made after the first 3–6 months of HRT administration.

A. Estrogens: Oral estrogen preparations are the most commonly used preparations, with the largest amount of supporting clinical data and experience. Oral administration of estrogen leads to high concentrations of estrogen within the liver, which leads to hepatic synthesis of coagulation factors and apolipoproteins. This effect may be problematic if hypercoagulability occurs or beneficial if there is an improvement in lipid profiles.

Conjugated equine estrogens (Premarin) are a combination of estrone, equilin, and in small amounts, 17-alpha-estradiol and 17-alpha-dihydroequilenin. The minimal dosage necessary to treat or prevent osteoporosis is 0.625 mg/d. This dosage is usually effective for treatment of vasomotor symptoms, but some women require higher dosages (1.25–2.5 mg/d). Although these dosages may be safe in the short term, long-term need for higher doses of conjugated estrogen should prompt the clinician to search for other causes for the symptoms or consider a change in the delivery system of estrogen. The dosage necessary for a cardioprotective effect also appears to be 0.625 mg/d.

Estradiol is used commonly in Europe; because serum levels of estradiol can be measured, one can evaluate women who have ongoing vasomotor symptoms despite a reasonable dosage of oral medication. Oral 17-beta-estradiol is available in the USA in a micronized form as Estrace. The minimal dosage approved for the prevention of osteoporosis is 0.5 mg, if intake of calcium is 1500 mg. However, 1 mg is closer to the bioequivalent of 0.625 mg conjugated estrogens. One milligram of 17-beta-estradiol is usually effective for amelioration of vasomotor symptoms and may represent the cardioprotective dosage also, although this has not been studied.

The hormone, 17-β-estradiol, is also available in a transdermal delivery system. The advantage of this delivery system is that it avoids the first-pass effect of the liver, which may avoid an increase in coagulability in patients who have had VTE. Transdermal delivery also may be an advantage in smokers; according to one study, smokers do not gain the benefit of decreased fracture risk from oral estrogen. Because the transdermal delivery system offers continuous delivery of the drug, there is a well-balanced therapeutic effect. The minimal dose is 0.05 mg twice weekly for prevention of osteoporosis, which is equivalent to 0.625 mg of conjugated estrogen. The major disadvantage of the transdermal system is that it may not offer the same initial beneficial effects on lipoproteins as the oral preparations. Recent data suggest, however, that the same benefit eventually is achieved with long-term administration. Whether or not transdermal preparations offer the same cardio-protective effect as oral preparations is not known. Other minor inconveniences include local allergic skin reactions to the adhesive, and in active women, difficulty keeping the patch in place.

There are few data on the bioavailability of vaginal preparations of estrogens. They are well absorbed through the vaginal mucosa, but whether the levels are consistently high enough for protection from cardiac disease and osteoporosis is unclear. It is known that vaginal preparations are helpful in the treatment of women with urogenital atrophy. For women with severe symptoms, they can be used on a short-term basis while an oral preparation is being initiated to provide more rapid relief of symptoms. They might be appropriate also in low doses for women who wish to treat genitourinary atrophy but do not wish therapy for other risk factors. Continual use of vaginal estrogens in women who have a uterus mandates the addition of a progestin.

B. Progestins: The most commonly used progestin in the USA is medroxyprogesterone (MPA). MPA is favored over norethindrone and norgestrel, because MPA has less androgenic activity and therefore less negative impact on the lipid profile. There are now available a newer class of progestins, 19-nortestosterone derivatives that have negligible androgenic effects. These agents—desogestrel, norgestimate, and gestodene—are currently available only in oral contraceptive agents; they are available separately in Europe, however, and are being studied as a component of postmenopausal HRT. All these agents are synthetic progestins; unaltered oral progesterone is poorly absorbed. Some pharmacies prepare micronized oral progesterone, which can be considered in patients who have many side effects with the synthetic preparations. Although it is absorbed well because of the micronization process, its duration of action is short, suggesting that twice- or thrice-daily dosing is probably necessary, which may present a compliance issue. Two hundred milligrams of micronized progesterone is probably equivalent to 2.5 mg of MPA.

C. Androgens: Recently, there has been an increase in interest in androgen administration as part of HRT. In the past, testosterone was used widely in parenteral preparations for postmenopausal HRT. The recognition that androgens adversely affect the lipid profile and may be implicated in coronary heart disease resulted in a marked decrease in use. Studies of the effects of lower doses of testosterone or oral methyltestosterone have suggested that sexual motivation and interest may be restored with minimal or no changes in the lipid profile. Some clinicians now recommend routine use of estrogen/androgen therapy when libido is decreased or when menopausal symptoms are not relieved by increased dosages of estrogen. It is important for clinicians and patients to recognize that there are no long-term data concerning the effect of androgens or estrogen/androgen preparations on the risk of coronary heart or other diseases.

Androgen therapy is indicated rarely in women who have undergone a spontaneous menopause. Usually, careful adjustments in the estrogen/progestin combination can alleviate symptoms. The addition of androgens may be useful occasionally, in young women who have undergone surgical menopause and continue to complain of malaise and diminished libido. The lowest possible dosage (1.25 mg methyltestosterone) should be used initially and adjustments made if necessary. Estrogen/androgen preparations are more widely available than androgens alone. Androgens should be continued only if they clearly alleviate symptoms.

Available Regimens

A. Estrogen Only: When determining the best estrogen regimen for a patient, the physician must consider, in addition to patient preference and willingness to comply, other medical problems such as hyperlipidemia, whether the patient smokes, and any difficulties she has had with progestins. The menopausal patient who has had a hysterectomy is started most easily on HRT, because she can be placed on daily estrogen in any form without the addition of a progestin. Daily estrogen most closely approximates the physiologic state. A "time-off" period from estrogen is not required; in fact, it may cause a return of the patient's vasomotor symptoms. The menopausal patient with an intact uterus represents a greater challenge for HRT. Most such patients should have the addition of a progestational agent. If a woman with an intact uterus cannot take progestins because of intolerance, unacceptable bleeding, or return of headaches, she may be a candidate for unopposed estrogens. These women require yearly endometrial surveillance, and many need to discontinue treatment because of endometrial abnormalities.

B. Combination Estrogen and Progestin: Postmenopausal women with an intact uterus should take estrogen opposed with a progestational agent to decrease the risk of endometrial hyperplasia and subsequent endometrial cancer. Progestins may be added in a varying number of days per month. As the number of days of progestin therapy increases, the risk of endometrial hyperplasia decreases (Fig 21–1). The duration of progestin therapy correlates better than the daily dosage with a decreased occurrence of endometrial hyperplasia.

The progestin component should be used in the minimal dosage necessary to prevent hyperplasia so

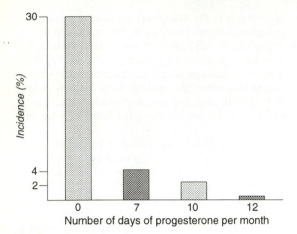

Figure 21–1. Endometrial hyperplasia in women receiving estrogen therapy. The number of days/mo that progesterone is taken is correlated with the occurrence of endometrial hyperplasia.

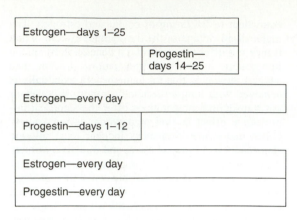

Figure 21–2. Estrogen/progestin prescribing schedules.

that unwanted side effects are avoided, including elevated lipids, bloating, irritability, and worsening depression.

The ideal estrogen/progestin combination relieves symptoms of menopause, prevents osteoporosis, prevents endometrial cancer, has a favorable effect on the lipid profile, and avoids vaginal bleeding and other undesirable side effects. Two regimens of combination therapy may meet these criteria, cyclic and continuous combined therapy.

1. Cyclic estrogen/progestin therapy–Cyclic estrogen/progestin therapy combines any form of estrogen in a minimal dosage along with a progestin, generally MPA, in a dosage of 5–10 mg/d for 10–13 consecutive days per month. Figure 21–2 presents two common variations of this regimen. The authors recommend the cyclic regimen using daily estrogen with the progestin administered on days 1–12 of the month. One of the advantages of this regimen is that vasomotor symptoms may be less with no break from estrogen administration. This regimen also tends to result in lighter withdrawal bleeding than in the regimens in which estrogen and progestin are stopped at the same time.

These cyclic regimens have specific advantages: predictable withdrawal bleeding, ease of monitoring, and reduced dysfunctional uterine bleeding in the perimenopausal period. This regimen is most successful with and appropriate for women in the perimenopausal years who continue to have occasional menses. The patient on a cyclic regimen experiences ongoing withdrawal bleeding that is usually lighter and briefer than her menstrual bleeding was and without other menstrual symptoms. Many women find this situation acceptable. Withdrawal bleeding on the cyclic regimen rarely continues past age 65.

Cyclic regimens allow for the screening of endometrial pathologic conditions based on the onset of withdrawal bleeding. In programs with 12–14 days of progestin administration, withdrawal bleeding before day 10 for three cycles is associated with an unfavorable pathologic state of the endometrium. In regimens with 10 days of progestin administration, any bleeding before the end of progestin administration for three cycles should be investigated.

2. Continuous combined estrogen/progestin therapy–Continuous combined HRT is an option for patients who find the idea of ongoing vaginal bleeding a deterrent to HRT (see Fig 21–2). This regimen consists of any of the forms of estrogen taken daily in a minimal dosage, combined with daily progestin, usually medroxyprogesterone in a dosage of 2.5–5.0 mg/d. The continuous combined regimen has several advantages. It eliminates cyclic withdrawal bleeding and can produce amenorrhea while effectively relieving menopausal symptoms. A daily progestin dosage has not been shown to have consistent adverse side effects on the lipid profile and appears to protect against endometrial hyperplasia. However, clinical experience with this protocol is short in duration. The few studies of long-term administration have reported cases of endometrial cancer, a fact that should be kept in mind when decisions about endometrial surveillance are made. During the first year of this regimen, 50–80% of women experience irregular uterine bleeding, a disadvantage that may discourage the patient from taking hormones. Patients who are informed of this possibility are more likely to continue therapy until achieving amenorrhea. This regimen may be most appropriate for women who are a few years past their last spontaneous menses, because they are likely to have less irregular uterine bleeding. On this regimen, bleeding that continues for longer than 6 months should be evaluated.

Fine-Tuning the Regimen

Although HRT has many beneficial aspects, many women have side effects. To help with compliance and continuation of HRT, a follow-up visit 2–3 months after initiation of therapy is appropriate. At this visit, a discussion of side effects and bleeding patterns can take place, and minor dosage adjustments can be made.

If the patient continues to experience vasomotor symptoms, it is appropriate to consider increasing the dosage of estrogen for 3–6 months. After this time, a gradual taper to the lowest dosage can be tried. Some patients experience better relief of their symptoms with twice-a-day dosing of an oral preparation. If these strategies are not effective, a trial of a transdermal delivery system can be helpful. Measurement of serum estradiol levels, for patients taking estradiol preparations, may reassure the patient with continued symptoms that absorption of the medication is occurring. If none of these strategies is helpful, it may be appropriate to consider androgens, particularly in patients who have had surgical menopause.

If a patient reports persistent symptoms of urogenital atrophy at the 3-month follow-up visit, addition of a vaginal estrogen preparation may be helpful.

Many patients, particularly older women, complain of breast pain in the initial months of therapy. Reassurance that this symptom is usually short-lived often is the best course of action, but in many women, a change to the transdermal system or a temporary lowering of the estrogen dosage may be appropriate.

Symptoms of bloating or irritability usually are associated with the progestin component of the regimen. The lowest dose of progestin appropriate for the patient's regimen always should be used, and a change to continuous therapy to allow a lower progestin dosage may be considered if these symptoms are disabling to the patient.

An important fact to remember when following patients undergoing HRT is that the clinical signs and symptoms, not the laboratory FSH level, are the most appropriate guides in monitoring estrogen dosage. The FSH level is appropriate for diagnosing menopause, but is inadequate to monitor estrogen replacement. In some women, supraphysiologic dosages of estrogen never lower the FSH to normal.

Duration of Therapy

The decision of how long to continue a patient on HRT depends on the indications and reasons for beginning HRT initially. If the therapy is being given only to alleviate vasomotor symptoms 2–5 years is an appropriate length of time. If symptoms recur after discontinuation of therapy, HRT may be reinstituted for an additional 2–5 years. Some women may require lifetime therapy to alleviate menopausal symptoms.

If HRT was started to prevent or treat osteoporosis or to decrease the risk of cardiovascular events, therapy ideally should be lifelong. For prevention of osteoporosis, it is important to begin HRT as soon after menopause as possible, preferably within 3 years of a natural menopause and 6–12 months of a surgical menopause, which are the periods of rapid bone loss. Because bone loss in women may plateau significantly at age 70, it may be possible to discontinue HRT between the ages of 70 and 75 and still decrease the risk of fracture.

There are no definitive data concerning the duration of HRT necessary to achieve the cardioprotective effect. According to the studies to date, current users of estrogen alone are afforded maximal protection. This finding translates logically to the need for lifelong therapy for ongoing benefit. There are few studies that have demonstrated an equivalent cardioprotective effect for the combined estrogen/progestin regimens. Future results of trials may resolve this issue.

If HRT is begun to improve a patient's sense of well-being, lifelong therapy might be appropriate.

Alternatives to Estrogen

ERT may be absolutely contraindicated or a patient may decide that the risks outweigh the benefits for her. There are alternatives to estrogen that may help to ameliorate symptoms but do not abolish these symptoms as estrogen does.

For vasomotor symptoms, progestins are probably the best alternative; they have been shown in double-blind, placebo-controlled studies to decrease vasomotor symptoms, but not abolish them. Regimens include MPA, 20 mg/d; megestrol, 40 mg/d; and depo-MPA, 50–150 mg/1–3 mo.

Clonidine, an alpha-adrenergic agonist, has been used also, but its efficacy usually is limited because the doses required often lead to hypotension. Methyldopa has met with limited success. A new steroidal preparation, tibolone, has been introduced in Europe for treatment of vasomotor symptoms. It is a weak estrogen, androgen, and progestin combination without adverse effects on the endometrium. Nonpharmacologic methods to relieve vasomotor symptoms are being investigated. These include deep breathing exercises, and relaxation techniques monitored with biofeedback equipment.

For symptoms related to urogenital atrophy, a woman who elects not to use oral estrogen therapy may consider low-dose intravaginal estrogen. Lubricants such as Replens or Astroglide may be helpful to prevent dyspareunia.

Follow-up Care

As discussed previously, follow-up of patients beginning HRT increases compliance and reduces start-up problems. If therapy is going well, the patient should visit her physician annually for age-appropriate health screening.

POSTMENOPAUSAL BLEEDING

In the past it was axiomatic that any uterine bleeding in a postmenopausal woman required a diagnosis. After a careful history and examination were performed to exclude other sources of bleeding such as urinary, vaginal, or rectal, an evaluation of the endometrium was performed. This axiom still applies to postmenopausal women who are not undergoing HRT, but the management of postmenopausal bleeding in women undergoing HRT is more complex.

Women using combined estrogen/progestin regimens are expected to have uterine bleeding. The challenge of the clinician is to determine when the bleeding represents significant endometrial or uterine pathologic states, and when it can be managed expectantly or with an adjustment in HRT dosage or regimen. Endometrial biopsies add to the cost of HRT, and repeated biopsies are poorly tolerated by most women. Primary care clinicians should learn the technique of endometrial biopsy but only with the clear understanding of when to biopsy and how to manage the results. A discussion of the technique of endometrial biopsy may be found in Chapter 47.

Data are increasing that suggest that transvaginal ultrasonography can be substituted for endometrial biopsies in selected circumstances, thus avoiding the pain and expense of sampling. Other diagnostic tests such as hysteroscopy should be performed when abnormal bleeding continues in a patient with normal biopsies. Hysteroscopy should be performed by a skilled endoscopist; often this is done in an outpatient setting.

Indications for Endometrial Biopsy

There are no clear, published guidelines for when endometrial sampling is indicated. The authors recommend the following guidelines established on the basis of experience and a review of the literature:

1. Postmenopausal women who are not undergoing HRT–A biopsy should be performed for any episode of bleeding. For repeated episodes in patients with previously normal biopsies, a referral for dilation and curettage (D&C), hysteroscopy, or both, should be made.
2. Women in whom HRT has not yet been initiated–A biopsy is not recommended if the woman is amenorrheic or has been having consistent cyclic bleeding, because these women have a very low incidence of endometrial abnormalities. A biopsy is recommended for women with acyclic bleeding before HRT is initiated.
3. Women undergoing ERT only, with a uterus–A biopsy should be performed yearly. Ultrasonography usually cannot be substituted because of the thick endometrial lining in these women. A

baseline biopsy before starting HRT should be considered.
4. Women using combined regimens with cyclic progestin–A biopsy should be performed when bleeding is acyclic or lasts 10 days or longer. If bleeding is cyclic but begins before the tenth day of progestin administration, one should increase the dosage or duration of progestin or both before performing a biopsy. If bleeding early in the course of progestin administration persists in spite of these manipulations, a biopsy should be performed.
5. Women using continuous estrogen/continuous progestin regimens–The incidence of acyclic bleeding is high in the first 3–4 mo, and such bleeding usually does not represent a pathologic condition of the endometrium Sampling is indicated when bleeding is unusually heavy and persistent in the start-up months. If acyclic bleeding continues for 6 months after HRT is initiated, a biopsy is indicated, although transvaginal ultrasonography sometimes can be substituted. Long-term data are scant at this time but suggest that endometrial evaluation must be performed when bleeding occurs after amenorrhea has been established in these regimens.
6. Women using innovative regimens–When providers choose to use alternative therapies that are not well studied, usually because of poor tolerance of progestins, the endometrium should be evaluated liberally. For example, if cyclic progestins are given every 2–3 mo, a biopsy or transvaginal ultrasonography should be performed yearly to assess the patient's response to the regimen.

Managing Biopsy Results

Appropriate interpretation of endometrial biopsy results is important in the management of postmenopausal bleeding. Women with endometrial cancer or adenomatous hyperplasia with or without atypia should be referred to a gynecologist or gynecologic oncologist for management. When simple or cystic hyperplasia or proliferative endometrium is present, the dosage or duration of progestin administration should be increased. A repeat biopsy should be performed after 4–6 months when hyperplasia is present but is not necessary for proliferative endometrium if the bleeding abnormality is corrected. Findings of secretory, nonproliferative, or atrophic endometrium are reassuring. The description "insufficient for diagnosis" is reassuring only if the clinician is certain that the endometrial cavity was entered and an adequate sample was obtained. Otherwise, repeat sampling is indicated. Alternatively, transvaginal ultrasonography can be performed to document an atrophic endometrium.

When transvaginal ultrasonography is performed, both endometrial layers should be measured at the widest part of the endometrium. An endometrial thickness of 5 mm or less is associated with a very low risk of a significant pathologic condition, although endometrial cancer has been documented in rare instances when the thickness was 5 mm. An endometrial biopsy is indicated in postmenopausal women when the endometrial thickness is 6 mm or greater.

COUNSELING & EDUCATION

Counseling peri- and postmenopausal women concerning menopause and hormone replacement therapy is becoming increasingly difficult. Available information, and sometimes misinformation, has increased dramatically in the past few years. The physician is not the only source or even the primary source of information. Thus, the clinician must consider the biases of the patient when planning a counseling session.

Menopause should be considered by the health care provider and the patient as a time to reevaluate a womans health, life-style, and other factors that may have an impact on her risk of disease. Whether or not HRT is to be prescribed should be viewed as only one portion of a perimenopausal counseling session. Because the issues concerning HRT are complex, however, they often require the bulk of the interview time. It is useful to begin to discuss these issues when the woman reaches her 40s so that decision-making will be easier at the time of menopause.

Multiple studies have shown that when women are informed and involved in the decision-making process concerning HRT, they are much more compliant in taking their hormones. The role of the clinician in this area is to facilitate decision-making—clearly not to make a decision for the patient. The symptoms a woman is experiencing should be reviewed, and she should be informed concerning which ones are related to estrogen deficiency. Her risk status for breast cancer, osteoporosis, and cardiovascular disease should be reviewed. The risks and benefits of HRT should be summarized, and the value of each of these to the patient should be discussed. For example, a woman whose mother died of a hip fracture will assign a high value to the prevention of osteoporosis by HRT. Finally, the physician should help the patient make a decision, and then help her feel comfortable with the decision that has been made.

If a woman chooses to undergo HRT, she should be informed fully about the expected risks and side effects. She should recognize that standard regimens are used at first and that adjustments can be made if undesirable side effects occur. A return visit after 3 months of HRT is often useful to address the patient's concerns and make minor changes in an attempt to increase long-term satisfaction with HRT.

In addition to counseling regarding HRT, the increased calcium needs that occur with menopause should be reviewed (see Chapter 22). If a woman elects not to use HRT or it is contraindicated, she should be advised of recommendations for timing and frequency of bone-mineral density testing to screen for osteoporosis (see Chapter 22). Because ovulation occasionally occurs in the year after menopause, women should be advised to continue to use some form of contraception for this period of time. Low-dose oral contraceptives, tubal ligation, vasectomy, an intrauterine device, and barrier contraceptives are all good choices for some patients (see Chapter 51).

The provider can employ a variety of tools besides a prolonged counseling session to facilitate decision-making. Pamphlets are available from a variety of sources, or the patient can be referred to one of the more informative and accurate books available for laypersons. Group sessions in a classroom format may be used to show a videotape, provide additional written and didactic information, and allow an interchange of information among perimenopausal women. Carefully constructed videotapes, or perhaps interactive video, may allow greater efficiency in providing counseling.

CURRENT CONTROVERSIES

Interest in menopause and HRT has grown considerably during the past 10 years. The conception and funding of the Women's Health Initiative provide one example of the commitment of the medical community to this area of womens health care. Many controversies exist in this area, however, and will continue to exist for many years, such as who should take HRT, what regimens are optimal, for how long therapy should be given, and what is the impact on breast cancer risk, heart disease risk, and life expectancy.

Formal, quantitative, and individualized risk-benefit analyses such as that proposed by the American College of Physicians may become a tool to help physicians counsel perimenopausal women. Counseling will continue to be based on less than optimal long-term studies, however.

Data on the drug tamoxifen, an estrogen antagonist for breast tissue, suggest that it may have the same effects as other oral estrogens on the prevention of bone loss, stimulation of endometrial lining, and changes in lipid profile. It does not prevent genitourinary atrophy, however, and it may even worsen vasomotor symptoms. Estrogens with combined agonist and antagonist effects may increase the options for safe administration of HRT to postmenopausal women.

There are even fewer long-term data regarding progestins than estrogens, and concerns continue about the possible impact of progestins on risk for cardiovascular disease and patient compliance with acceptability of HRT regimens containing progestins. Few clinicians are comfortable routinely administering estrogen alone to women with a uterus because of the four- to eightfold increased risk of endometrial cancer. Recent studies suggest that less frequent administration of progestins, eg, every 3 months, may provide adequate endometrial protection in most women and increase compliance. Local routes of progestin administration such as intravaginal or by intrauterine device also are being studied as a means to provide endometrial protection with minimal systemic effects.

REFERENCES

American College of Obstetrics and Gynecologists, Committee on Gynecologic Practice:*Estrogen Replacement Therapy and Endometrial Cancer.* ACOG Committee Opinion No. 80. American College of Obstetricians and Gynecologists, 1990.

American College of Physicians: Guidelines for counseling postmenopausal women about preventative hormone therapy. Ann Intern Med 1992;117:1038.

Barrett-Connor E, Bush TL: Estrogen and coronary heart disease in women. JAMA 1991;265:1861.

Belchetz PE: Hormonal treatment of postmenopausal women. N Engl J Med 1994;330:1062.

Creasman WT: Estrogen replacement therapy: Is previously treated cancer a contraindication? Obstet Gynecol 1991;77:308.

Falkeborn et al: The risk of acute myocardial infarction after oestrogen and oestrogen-progestogen replacement. Br J Obstet Gynecol 1992;99:821.

Ferguson KJ, Hoegh C, Johnson S: Estrogen replacement therapy: A survey of women's knowledge and attitudes. Arch Intern Med 1989;149:133.

Gassman A, Santoro N: The influence of menopausal hormonal changes on sexuality: Current knowledge and recommendations for practice. Menopause 1994;1:91.

Goldstein et al: Endometrial assessment by vaginal ultrasonography before endometrial sampling in patients with postmenopausal bleeding. Am J Obstet Gynecol 1990;163:119.

Grady D et al: Hormone therapy to prevent disease and prolong life in postmenopausal women. Ann Intern Med 1992;117:1016.

Karlsson B et al: Endovaginal scanning of the endometrium compared to cytology and histology in women with postmenopausal bleeding. Gynecol Oncol 1993;50:173.

Laufer LR et al: Effect of clonidine on hot flushes in postmenopausal women. Obstet Gynecol 1987;156:428.

Leather AT, Savvas M, Studd JWW: Endometrial histology and bleeding patterns after 8 years of continuous combined estrogen and progestogen therapy in postmenopausal women. Obstet Gynecol 1991;78:1008.

McClure RD, Marshall L: Endocrinologic sexual dysfunction. In: *Sexual Dysfunction: A Neuro-Medical Approach.* Singer C, Weiner JW (editors). Futura Publishing, 1994.

Padwick ML, Pryse-Davies J, Whitehead MI: A simple method of determining the optimal dosage of progestin in postmenopausal women receiving estrogens. N Engl J Med 1986;315:930.

Paganini-Hill A, Ross RK, Henderson BE: Postmenopausal oestrogen treatment and stroke: A prospective study. Br Med J 1988;297:519.

Petitti DB: Estrogen use in women who have survived breast cancer. Womens Health Forum 1993;2:1.

Psaty BM et al: The risk of myocardial infarction associated with the combined use of estrogens and progestins in postmenopausal women. Arch Intern Med 1994;154:1333.

Schiff I et al: Oral medroxyprogesterone in the treatment of postmenopausal symptoms. JAMA 1980;244:1443.

Silberstein SD, Merriam GR: Estrogens, progestins, and headache. Neurology 1991;41:786.

Stampfer et al: Postmenopausal estrogen therapy and cardiovascular disease: Ten year follow-up from the nurses' health study. N Engl J Med 1991;325:756.

Stampfer MJ, Coldlitz GA: Estrogen replacement therapy and cardiovascular disease: A quantitative assessment of the epidemiologic evidence. Prev Med 1991;20:47.

Steinberg et al: A meta-analysis of the effect of estrogen replacement therapy on the risk of breast cancer. JAMA 1991;265:1985.

Sullivan et al: Estrogen replacement and coronary artery disease. Effect on survival in postmenapausal women. Arch Int Med 1990;150:2557.

Summary of the Second Report of the National Cholesterol Education Program (NCEP) Expert Panel on Detection, Evaluation, and Treatment of High Blood Cholesterol in Adults (Adult Treatment Panel II). JAMA 1993;269:3015.

Thompson SG, Meade TW, Greenberg G: The use of hormonal replacement therapy and the risk of stroke and myocardial infarction in women. J Epidemiol Community Health 1989;43:173.

Wood H, Wang-Cheng R, Nattinger A: Postmenopausal hormone replacement: Are two hormones better than one? J Gen Intern Med 1993;8:451.

Osteoporosis

22

Dawn P. Lemcke, MD

Osteoporosis, defined as bone mass 2.5 standard deviations below the mean of a young, normal person, is a major cause of morbidity and mortality, particularly in postmenopausal women. A decline of bone mass by 1 standard deviation is by definition **osteopenia,** which increases the relative risk of fracture by 50–100%. At present, prevention is clearly the most effective way to decrease this morbidity and mortality. The current mainstays of prevention are estrogen replacement therapy, calcium and vitamin D supplementation, and appropriate exercise. Treatments for established osteoporosis continue to be in a state of flux as new agents are evaluated.

Essentials of Diagnosis
Pathophysiology
Incidence
Risk Factors
Secondary Causes
Screening
Clinical Findings & Diagnosis
Prevention & Treatment
Referral to a Specialist
Controversies & Unresolved Issues

Essentials of Diagnosis

- Low bone mass
- Microarchitectural deterioration of bone tissue
- Bone fragility
- Presence of fractures

Pathophysiology

Bone mass in women peaks shortly after puberty, at the end of the growth period (approximately age 17), although small gains in bone mass may be achieved up to age 30. This period is followed by progressive loss of bone mass. Women differ from men in their pattern of bone loss in that women not only have a slow, protracted phase, which is also present in men, but also have an accelerated phase that occurs in the postmenopausal period. It is this accelerated phase in menopause that is believed to account for up to 40% of loss of bone mass. The accelerated phase may last for 5–10 years and generally ceases by age 70 (Fig 22–1).

The slow phase of bone loss is due to decreased bone formation. There is continued activity of osteoclasts, but osteoblasts fail to recreate bone, leading to a decrease in bone mass. In the accelerated phase of osteoporosis, there is a marked increase in osteoclastic activity, with continued osteoblastic activity, which cannot maintain the same rate of activity as osteoclasts. A major contributor to the accelerated phase of bone loss in menopausal women is the loss of intrinsic estrogen. The primary effect of estrogen on bone is to decrease bone turnover by decreasing osteoclastic activity. Other factors that contribute to osteoporosis are decreased absorption of calcium

from the gastrointestinal tract, which occurs with aging; elevated parathyroid hormone (PTH) levels caused by decreased serum calcium levels; and decreased vitamin D levels, which occur with aging. The risk of fracture, particularly in the elderly, is affected by the type of fall and use of protective devices. Although it may not be possible to change the aging process, the pathophysiology of osteoporosis gives clues concerning the prevention and treatment of this disease.

Incidence

Osteoporosis represents a major public health problem in the United States, affecting 15–20 million persons per year, most of whom are postmenopausal women. The disease accounts for 1.3 million fractures per year. The major manifestations of osteoporosis are proximal hip fractures accounting for 250,000 fractures per year, distal forearm and Colles' fractures representing another 250,000 fractures per year, and vertebral fractures in the amount of 500,000 fractures per year. In 1986 dollars, these fractures cost approximately $10 billion. Conservative estimates, taking into account the aging of the population and increase in incidence of osteoporotic fractures, place the cost of these fractures in the year 2020 at $62 billion. It is estimated that 15% of white women will fracture a hip in their lifetime, with a mortality rate between 5 and 20% in the year following the fracture related to complications. For many women, a fracture means the loss of independent living and a marked change in the quality of life, factors that add to the impact of the disease.

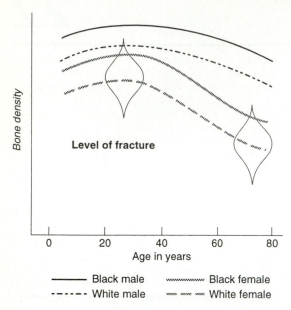

Figure 22–1. Effect of sex and race on peak bone mass. Individual values about regression lines (for white women this is given by a top-shaped figure). This figure illustrates the rapid perimenopausal bone loss, but also that low bone density at young ages predisposes to fractures in later life. (Reproduced, with permission, from Riggs BL: Osteoporosis. In: *Textbook of Endocrinology*, 2nd ed. DeGroot LJ et al [editors]. Saunders, 1989. Reproduced, with permission, from Riggs BL, Melton LJ: The prevention and treatment of osteoporosis. N Engl J Med 1992;327:620.)

Table 22–1. Risk factors for osteoporosis.

Nonmodifiable
  Female sex
  Age over 65 years
  Slight build
  Family history of osteoporosis
  White or Asian race
  Premature menopause
  Surgical menopause
  History of atraumatic fracture
  Loss of 1 in or more in height
Modifiable
  Estrogen deficiency
  Sedentary life-style
  Low calcium intake
  Failure to achieve peak bone mass
  Weight below normal
  High alcohol consumption
  Cigarette smoking

Risk Factors

Although there are known risk factors for osteoporosis, risk factor assessment in individual patients may miss up to 30% of women who are at highest risk for fracture. Risk factor assessment is important, however, it should not be the sole method by which preventive measures or treatment are offered to patients.

Definitive risk factors for osteoporosis are shown in Table 22-1. Of these factors, the most important are menopausal status or estrogen deficiency, calcium deficiency, inactivity, and failure to achieve peak bone mass in adolescence.

Recommendations for calcium intake have been somewhat controversial, but it is clear that failure to achieve peak bone mass in adolescence can be related directly to calcium intake (Fig 22–2). The attainment of peak bone mass helps later in the prevention of osteoporosis. After menopause, appropriate calcium intake along with other measures also can help in the prevention of osteoporosis.

Physical inactivity markedly reduces bone mass secondary to the loss of mechanical loading on bone, which acts to increase bone mass. Athletes have somewhat greater bone mass, unless they are suffering from the female athlete triad; this triad consists of the interrelated medical disorders of disordered eating, amenorrhea, and osteoporosis (see Chapter 10).

Alcohol intake in women also may increase risk of osteoporosis because alcohol impairs bone remodeling. Alcoholic women are at higher risk of fractures from falls that are associated with lower bone mass. It has been shown that taking one or more drinks per day increases risk of hip fracture in women by 15–40% over their lifetime.

Smoking represents a risk factor for decreased bone mass and thus a preventable cause of osteoporosis. A recent study comparing female twins who were discordant for smoking revealed that those who smoked one pack of cigarettes a day throughout their

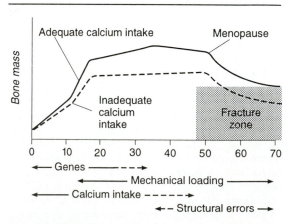

Figure 22–2. Major determinants of bone mass at various ages. (Reproduced, with permission, from Heaney R: Nutritional factors in bone health. In: *Osteoporosis: Etiology, Diagnosis, and Management.* Riggs BL, Melton LJ III [editors]. Raven Press, 1988.)

adult life had an average decrease in bone density of 5–10% compared with their nonsmoking twins. This decrease is in the range that effectively increases the risk of fracture. Female patients of all ages who smoke should be urged to discontinue smoking; physicians should be attentive to opportunities for early intervention concerning possible osteoporosis in these patients.

Amenorrhea, usually caused by a decreased level of estrogen, is a clear risk factor for osteoporosis. Important causes of amenorrhea are natural or surgical menopause, anorexia nervosa, and prolactinoma. Other important types include hypothalamic amenorrhea and exercise-induced amenorrhea. Drugs, including luteinizing hormone releasing hormone (LH-RH) agonists and antiestrogens, also provoke anovulation. A careful history including menstrual and exercise history should help the physician to decide which women need further testing. Early intervention in amenorrheic women is important, although a study reported that anorectic women who achieved 80% of recommended weight and took estrogen and calcium supplementation did not fare any better in bone mass preservation than those who had no intervention.

Other modifiable risk factors for osteoporosis include excess dietary consumption of caffeine, phosphorus, and protein, all of which increase urinary excretion of calcium.

Secondary Causes

In a patient who has documented osteoporosis, a careful history and physical examination and several laboratory tests should be performed to rule out secondary causes of osteoporosis. These factors, listed in Table 22–2, may be identified in 20% of women with vertebral fractures. The most common causes of secondary osteoporosis are endocrinopathies. Other causes that should be considered are malignant tumors, (particularly multiple myeloma), renal insufficiency, and liver disease.

In searching for secondary causes, the history should include a drug and alcohol history and a menstrual history. Standard laboratory tests should include a chemistry battery, complete blood count, creatinine level, and urinary calcium test. Additional laboratory tests that may be performed if indicated from the preceding evaluation are tests for PTH, thyroid-stimulating hormone (TSH), serum protein electrophoresis (SPEP), urine protein electrophoresis (UPEP), 25-OH-vitamin D, prolactin, and urinary calcium. The level of urinary calcium excretion in a woman with documented osteoporosis may help in determining not only the cause of the osteoporosis but also the effective therapy. Normal urinary calcium excretion in women is 100–250 mg/d. Factors that increase calcium excretion include high calcium intake, renal calcium leak, high level of bone resorption, and furosemide therapy. Decreased levels of calcium excretion may be secondary to vitamin D deficiency, small-bowel disease, low calcium intake, and thiazide therapy.

Medications as secondary causes for osteoporosis deserve special mention. Glucocorticoid therapy represents a significant risk for osteoporosis. Although the true incidence of glucocorticoid-induced osteoporosis is not known, current data suggest the incidence to be 30–50%. Doses of prednisone of 7.5 mg or greater appear to cause significant loss of trabecular bone in most patients. Lesser doses do not appear to have a significant effect in premenopausal women, but postmenopausal women lose bone when taking lower doses. The mechanism of glucocorticoid-induced osteoporosis is both systemic and skeletal. The systemic effects include a decrease in calcium absorption and increase in renal excretion of calcium, decrease in gonadal hormone secretion, and muscle wasting. The skeletal effects of glucocorticoids that lead to osteoporosis are an inhibition of osteoblastic activity, increased sensitivity to PTH and 1,25-[OH]2D3, and possibly, stimulation of osteoclasts.

Thyroid hormone replacement, used commonly by many women, may present a risk for osteoporosis if the patient is "overreplaced," thus suppressing the TSH level. It is recommended, therefore, that the new, supersensitive TSH measurements be used to follow women undergoing thyroid replacement to maintain their hormone levels in the normal range to prevent bone loss.

Prolonged use of heparin and anticonvulsants also may accelerate bone loss in women and increase the risk for osteoporosis.

Although it may not be possible to avoid the use of the forementioned medications, special attention should be given to other interventions that may offset the effects of the medications. These interventions might include ensuring appropriate calcium intake,

Table 22–2. Secondary causes of osteoporosis.

Endocrinopathies
  Hypogonadism
  Hyperthyroidism
  Hyperparathyroidism
  Cushing's syndrome
  Hyperprolactinemia
  Acromegaly
Gastrointestinal diseases
  Malabsorption syndromes
  Chronic obstructive jaundice
  Primary biliary cirrhosis
  Subtotal gastrectomy
Drugs
  Anticonvulsants
  Chronic use of heparin
  Overreplacement with thyroid hormone
  Glucocorticoids

recommending exercise, and treating estrogen deficiency or documented osteoporosis at an early stage.

A brief mention of the effect of the injectable contraceptive depot medroxyprogesterone acetate (DMPA) on bone mass and osteoporosis is appropriate given the recent widespread use of this form of contraception in young women. Many women who take DMPA become amenorrheic. It has been noted that levels of estradiol and estrone are slightly decreased in women who take this drug, approximating the early- to mid-follicular range. A small study performed in New Zealand found that women using DMPA for at least 5 years had bone-mineral densities that ranged between those of age-matched nonusers and postmenopausal women. The researchers found no clinical evidence for osteoporosis and found that the effects were reversed with discontinuation of the DMPA. This study has been criticized by some because the measure of bone mass was not corrected for other variables, particularly smoking. A prospective, randomized trial is needed to evaluate the effects more closely. In the meantime, DMPA remains an acceptable alternative for young women and should not cause great concern for severe effects on bone mass.

Screening

Bone mass can be measured accurately in a number of ways. It is clear from many studies that the bone mass measure is correlated with risk for subsequent fracture at all sites. The following currently available methods for measuring bone density allow documentation of osteoporosis and prediction of fracture risk:

1. Single-photon absorptiometry–This method is limited to peripheral sites and cannot be used to measure spine and hip density. It is well tolerated by patients, with short scan times of 10–20 minutes and a cost of $35–125. It is relatively accurate and precise and may be most helpful in hyperparathyroidism, in which peripheral cortical bone is reduced more than trabecular bone.
2. Dual-photon absorptiometry–This method measures spine and hip density. From a patient standpoint, it is more cumbersome than single-photon absorptiometry, with scan times of up to 60 minutes. It is slightly more costly than single-photon absorptiometry.
3. Dual-energy x-ray absorptiometry (DEXA)–This method largely has replaced the other types of absorptiometry and currently represents the best method of determining bone density. It is rapid, with scan times of 10 minutes, costs approximately $100, and is precise. An excellent test for following patients over time, it can measure density at any site; most commonly, the hip and spine are evaluated.
4. Quantitative computed tomography (QCT)–An accurate method of determining bone density, its use is limited because of its cost ($100–400) and radiation exposure, which makes it unsuitable for following patients.

To date, none of the major health organizations (eg, American College of Physicians and United States Preventative Services Task Force) recommend routine screening for bone density, and there are no clear guidelines regarding intervals of screening and subsequent treatment. If a mass screening strategy were employed, according to one study, the percentage of women receiving estrogen therapy would increase and lifetime risk of hip fracture would decrease. The cost-effectiveness of such a strategy has not been determined. At present, most authorities recommend a selective screening approach to osteoporosis. The indications for bone mass measurement as recommended by the National Osteoporosis Foundation are as follows:

1. Estrogen-deficient women, to make decisions regarding estrogen replacement.
2. Patients with vertebral abnormalities or radiographic evidence for osteopenia, to diagnose spinal osteoporosis to make decisions regarding diagnostic evaluations and therapy. Radiographic osteopenia does not always represent osteoporosis, and no further evaluation should be pursued if bone density is normal.
3. Patients receiving glucocorticoid therapy, to diagnose low bone mass so that therapy can be adjusted, if other effective therapies are available and appropriate for the patient.
4. Patients with primary hyperparathyroidism, to diagnose low bone mass to determine risk for severe skeletal disease and possible candidacy for early surgical intervention.

Besides the possibility of a mass screening that included menopausal women potential indications for bone density measurement include the following:

1. Therapy for osteoporosis–Bone mass would be monitored to assess therapeutic efficacy. DEXA scanning is the most appropriate for this indication because of its precision. Unfortunately, there are no protocols for monitoring therapy in this way.
2. To identify "fast losers" of bone–Such patients would benefit from aggressive therapy.
3. Patients at high risk for osteoporosis–Evaluation would be done for patients undergoing anticonvulsant therapy and thyroid replacement therapy and those with amenorrhea, anorexia nervosa, alcoholism, multiple atraumatic fractures, or breast cancer.

Besides the recommendations for who should be screened, there are also recommendations for who should not be screened. If the decision to treat or alter treatment will not be affected by the results of bone density testing, it is not appropriate to measure bone mass. For example, some menopausal women plan to undergo hormone replacement therapy regardless of the results of bone mass screening.

Deciding when to measure bone mass is also important. There is no clear consensus on this issue. Most authors recommend an initial measurement in the perimenopausal period for women in whom treatment decisions might be altered. There is controversy concerning when or if further determinations are necessary. In a patient undergoing glucocorticoid therapy, bone density measurements every 6 months for the first 2 years of therapy might be reasonable.

The National Osteoporosis Foundation has made helpful recommendations regarding the decision to treat after screening. An amenorrheic patient with a bone mass density that is 1 standard deviation below "young normal" should be considered strongly for estrogen therapy. Women whose bone mass is 1 standard deviation above young normal are protected against osteoporosis and have a low risk of fracture. This group may benefit from reassessment in 5 years

to ensure that there has been no change in bone mass. Women with intermediate values should have their bone mass measured again in 2–3 years to look for further bone loss and to guide treatment decisions (Fig 22–3). Besides the methods previously discussed, techniques that are being evaluated for use in measuring bone density include ultrasonography, osteography, magnetic resonance imaging, and use of chemical markers of bone turnover.

Clinical Findings & Diagnosis

Most often osteoporosis is a silent disease without signs and symptoms until fractures occur. Some of the manifestations of the disease are loss of height, spinal deformity (especially kyphosis), and fractures, which may lead to pain. Although osteomalacia may present with diffuse bone pain, osteoporosis does not, unless the patient has suffered a fracture. If a patient with known osteoporosis without fractures experiences back pain, the pain is usually caused by other factors such as nerve compression, facet joint arthropathy, degenerative disk disease, or muscle dysfunction. Diagnosis of osteoporosis is made on the basis of a finding of decreased bone density by one of the methods described in the preceding section, "Screening".

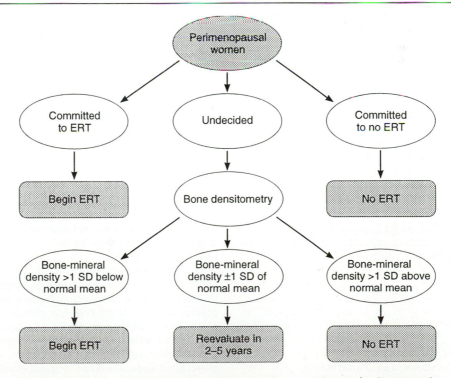

Figure 22–3. Algorithm for making decisions regarding estrogen replacement therapy for the prevention of osteoporosis. (Reproduced, with permission, from Johnston CC, Slemenda CW, Melton LJ: Clinical use of bone densitometry. N Engl J Med 1991;324:1105.)

Prevention & Treatment

At present there are several options available for both the prevention and the treatment of osteoporosis. Prevention should be attempted whenever possible. Table 22–3 summarizes the current treatment options and their mechanisms of action. The drugs for treatment and prevention of osteoporosis fall into two general categories: those that inhibit bone resorption and those that stimulate bone formation. Most of the drugs available fall into the antiresorptive category. Currently only estrogen and calcitonin are approved by the United States Food and Drug Administration (FDA) for use in osteoporosis.

A. Estrogen: Estrogen is currently the only agent that has been shown to maintain bone mass, reduce fractures, and treat established osteoporosis effectively. The mechanism of estrogen's effect on bone has not been elucidated fully, but the drug most likely works by increasing osteoblastic activity and thus decreasing bone resorption. Postmenopausal estrogen therapy should be started soon after menopause, because there is accelerated bone loss at that time. Beginning therapy within 3–5 years of natural menopause and within 6–12 months of surgical menopause should prevent bone loss. Estrogen given postmenopausally rapidly normalizes bone resorption and formation, thus reestablishing bone balance. The effective dosages of estrogen necessary to prevent bone loss are 0.625 mg/d of conjugated estrogen, 2 mg/d of 17-β-estradiol, or 50–100 µg/d of transdermal estrogen. Although there have been no definitive studies, it is believed that serum estradiol levels of 60 pg/mL represent the protective level for bone.

As previously mentioned, a study has shown that smokers using oral estrogen were afforded no protection against fractures to the degree that nonsmoking women were. Other studies show that smokers may need twice the normal dosages of nonsmokers to achieve the same serum estradiol concentrations. These data suggest that the percutaneous route may be appropriate in women who smoke and wish to take estrogen for the prevention of osteoporosis; higher dosages still may be required. Women should

Table 22–3. Drug therapy for osteoporosis.

Antiresorptive Drugs
  Estrogen
  Biphosphonates
  Calcium
  Calcitonin
  Vitamin D
  1,25-[OH]2D3
  Tamoxifen
Drugs that stimulate bone formation
  Sodium fluoride
  Low intermittent doses of parathyroid hormone
  Phosphate and calcitonin
  Growth hormone
  AFDR (coherence therapy)

be counseled to stop smoking both to decrease their risk of osteoporosis and to make therapeutic decisions less complicated.

The effect of estrogen on the maintenance of bone mass continues for as long as therapy is continued, and a positive effect has been shown up to age 75. After age 75, even long-term therapy may not be protective against fracture. Any time that estrogen is discontinued, bone loss proceeds at a rate similar to that of the early menopausal period. Studies have shown that 7 years of estrogen therapy is the minimal requirement for the effective maintenance of bone mass. Many studies have shown a 50% reduction in hip and wrist fractures and a 90% decrease in vertebral fractures with use of estrogen therapy.

In women with established osteoporosis, estrogen therapy increases vertebral bone mass by 5% and reduces risk of vertebral fractures by 50%. Thus, estrogen should be considered for all estrogen-deficient women for the prevention and treatment of osteoporosis.

B. Biphosphonates: The biphosphonates act as antiresorptives by inhibiting osteoclastic activity; etidronate is the currently available drug of this class. In two clinical trials, etidronate was shown to increase bone density in the spine by 1–2%/yr in women with established osteoporosis. Along with the increase in bone density, fractures were decreased by 50% at the spine. Currently, biphosphonates are given in a cyclic fashion with appropriate calcium intake; adequate calcium intake is essential to the success of the treatment. The regimen consists of 400 mg/d of etidronate for 2 weeks of every 12–14 weeks. For maximal absorption, the drug must be taken separately from meals, antacids, and calcium. There do not appear to be any major side effects.

Despite the encouraging results from the two studies, long-term therapy with biphosphonates has not been approved by the FDA; there are concerns over possible impairment of bone mineralization after long-term use. More recent data from studies of longer term use of etidronate continue to look encouraging.

Candidates for treatment with biphosphonates include women with documented osteoporosis who are unable to take estrogens and women who, despite estrogen therapy, continue to have a documented decrease in bone density.

C. Calcium: In numerous studies throughout the last decade, the effectiveness of calcium supplementation in the prevention and treatment of osteoporosis has been found to be inconclusive. This variability in results most likely is caused by the inclusion of women with varying menopausal status and varying calcium intakes. When studies are reevaluated and controlled for menopausal status and baseline calcium intake, it becomes clear that adequate calcium intake is essential to bone health in all age groups of women. It is important that adolescent women have adequate calcium intake so that they may achieve peak bone mass. A recent randomized, double-blind, placebo-controlled study of 94 adolescent white girls showed that increasing calcium intake from 960 mg/d (80% of RDA) to approximately 1300 mg/d (110% of RDA) resulted in increases in total bone density. The form of calcium used in this study was calcium citrate malate. This increase in bone density may serve as protection later against osteoporotic fractures.

In an important recent study of women who had been menopausal for more than 5 years with baseline calcium intakes of less than 400 mg/d, benefit was seen from calcium supplementation of 500 mg/d. These women, compared with a group treated with placebo, had no statistically significant bone loss at the spine, hip, and radius. The positive effect was not seen in women in the first 5 years of menopause, when bone loss is quite rapid. Two forms of calcium were used in the study, calcium carbonate and calcium citrate malate. Of the two forms, calcium citrate malate had more of a stabilizing influence on bone density than calcium carbonate, possibly because of variations in absorption.

In another confirmatory, placebo-controlled study, postmenopausal women with average calcium intakes of 750 mg/d showed slowing of bone loss by 43% over a 2-year period with calcium supplementation of 1000 mg/d. The form of calcium used in this study was calcium lactate-gluconate.

From the studies described in the preceding paragraphs of women of varying ages, the following conclusions can be drawn:

1. Appropriate calcium intake is important for women of all ages for maintenance of bone health.
2. The amounts of calcium necessary for bone health may vary by age, menopausal status, and pregnancy status.
3. Different forms of calcium may have different bioavailabilities.

Figure 22–4 shows the recommendations for calcium intake for women of various ages. An assessment of the dietary intake of calcium is an easy task during the history; one may use the guideline that each serving of dairy food contains approximately 300 mg of calcium. For women who do not have adequate calcium in their diet, supplemental calcium is an option. To ensure bioavailability of calcium supplements, it is recommended that they be taken with food, that chewable forms be used when possible for higher availability, and that amounts larger than 500 mg be taken in two doses. It may be appropriate to recommend the citrate form of calcium for patients who take H_2-blockers, elderly women who may have achlorhydria, and those with a history of nephrolithiasis. Unfortunately, the citrate form is considerably more expensive than other forms of calcium supplementation. Calcium citrate should be separated from meals for adequate absorption.

Although there has been mention of the risk of nephrolithiasis with increasing levels of calcium supplementation, the available data do not support this concern as a factor that should limit recommendations to women. All women should be counseled

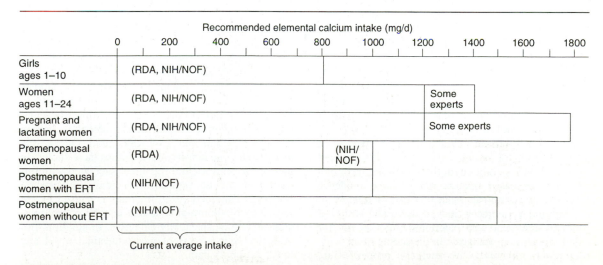

Figure 22–4. Recommended and current average calcium intakes in women of different ages. Although recommendations regarding intake vary, it is certain that the current average intake among adults in the USA of 550 mg/d falls well below recommended levels. RDA = recommended daily allowance; NIH = National Institutes of Health; NOF = National Osteoporosis Foundation. (Reproduced, with permission, from Utian WH et al: Calcium supplementation for the prevention and treatment of osteoporosis: A consensus opinion. Menopause Management Supplement, May/June 1994.)

about adequate calcium intake either in their diet or with supplementation.

D. Vitamin D: With the aging process, serum levels of vitamin D decline. The levels appear to be low enough to affect fracture thresholds in women over the age of 60. This decrease is secondary to decreased gastrointestinal absorption, decreased vitamin D synthesis by the skin, and renal deficiencies in the production of 1,25-[OH]2D3. There have been studies of nursing home populations that have shown reduced numbers of fractures with vitamin D supplementation. These data may not extend to the population of women who are not in nursing homes; therefore, recommendations for uniform use of vitamin D for treatment and prevention of osteoporosis have not been made. The dosage that has shown efficacy in women in nursing homes is 800 units/d of vitamin D or 150,000–300,000 units of intramuscular calciferol.

Another study of vitamin D revealed that in Boston at 42 degrees north latitude, perimenopausal women may lose bone mass in the winter months. Bone mass increased gradually during the summer months, but yearlong bone mass showed a slight decline. This decrease was presumed to be secondary to decreased sunlight, and therefore decreased vitamin D synthesis in the winter months. With supplementation of 400 units/d of vitamin D, the wintertime loss of bone density was slowed when compared with placebo. With vitamin D supplementation, there was a small but significant increase in bone density through the years; however, no correlation with decreased fractures was reported. This information may help physicians in recommending vitamin D supplementation to perimenopausal women in a similar geographic area, although it may not apply to all women.

E. Calcitonin: The action of calcitonin is to inhibit osteoclastic activity on bone, and it is effective in both the prevention and the treatment of osteoporosis. It is currently FDA-approved for use in osteoporosis. The form of calcitonin that is currently available in the USA is salmon calcitonin for parenteral use (intramuscularly or subcutaneously). Other preparations are available outside of the USA as nasal spray and suppository.

Studies of synthetic salmon calcitonin have shown a stabilization of bone density when administered over 2–3 years. Although these studies have not shown a decreased fracture risk, there is evidence from recent preliminary data that risk of fracture of the hip and vertebrae is indeed decreased with 1–2 years of treatment with calcitonin. Another use for calcitonin is as an analgesic in the setting of an acute osteoporotic fracture. The analgesic properties are thought to result from a release of beta-endorphins. Studies have found a 60% reduction in pain without the use of other pain killers such as narcotics. Dosages currently recommended for treatment of os-

teoporosis and for the analgesic effect are 100 units/d intramuscularly or subcutaneously.

One of the major disadvantages of the use of calcitonin is the need for parenteral administration, which is inconvenient for patients. Another major disadvantage is the cost. If the drug is used for treatment of osteoporosis at a dosage of 100 units/d, the annual cost is $2000. Although major side effects have not been noted in approximately 10 years of use, there may be mild nausea and facial flushing. There are ongoing studies of smaller dosages, doses given less frequently than daily, and cyclic regimens that may help to offset some of the concerns about cost and administration.

Candidates for therapy with calcitonin include women with documented osteoporosis that is not responding to other treatment, ie, estrogen or biphosphonates, and patients with acute fractures.

F. Tamoxifen: Tamoxifen, a drug used commonly in the treatment of breast cancer, appears to have both antiestrogenic and proestrogenic properties depending on the body site. It appears to act as an estrogen agonist on lipids, sex-binding hormones, and (as recently discovered), the skeleton. In a recent small study, 140 postmenopausal women with breast cancer received tamoxifen, 10 mg twice daily, or placebo. In the follow-up examination after 1 year, researchers found a 61% increase in bone density at the spine of women who received tamoxifen. Although this study did not document a decrease in fractures, it was encouraging that women with breast cancer may be protected from osteoporosis despite their inability to take estrogen. Further studies that document decreases in fractures with the increase in bone density will help to clarify the role of tamoxifen treatment of osteoporosis. At the present time, candidates for this therapy should probably be limited to women with breast cancer who are not candidates for estrogen therapy.

G. Sodium Fluoride: Because fluoride increases osteoblastic activity, it has been considered a possible therapeutic agent for osteoporosis. Studies have shown that flouride increases bone density in the spine but not at other sites containing trabecular bone. The increase in bone density depends also on adequate calcium intake of 1500 mg/d. Despite the increase in bone density, most studies have shown an increase in nonvertebral fractures associated with fluoride use and no significant decrease in vertebral fractures. This increase in fractures is caused by the formation of abnormal bone that may be poorly mineralized and mechanically defective. In addition, fluoride has side effects of gastrointestinal upset and lower extremity pain.

There is hope that fluoride may be more beneficial in decreasing fractures if given in a cyclic fashion or in a slow-release preparation. The previous studies were done with preparations that were not sustained release. A recent randomized, controlled trial of slow-release fluoride given in a cyclic fashion to women with documented osteoporosis showed encouraging results. When compared with placebo, the fluoride-treated group had an increase in bone mass of 4–6% and a decrease in fractures. Side effects for the two groups were similar.

Because of the concerns about safety and effectiveness and the questions about type of preparation and regimen, fluoride should not be considered effective treatment for osteoporosis.

H. Exercise: It is known that exercise is necessary for bone health: a sedentary life-style can increase the risk for osteoporosis. This fact has led to speculation that exercise might be viewed as a preventive measure for osteoporosis. From studies of exercise for prevention of osteoporosis, however, it is clear that exercise alone in the perimenopausal period does not maintain bone density. A regimen of aerobic exercise 3–5 days a week for cardiovascular fitness and for attainment of peak bone mass is still recommended for premenopausal patients.

In summary, first-line therapy in all patients should be appropriate calcium intake. In the perimenopausal period, estrogen therapy in addition to appropriate calcium intake should be considered. In women who cannot take estrogen or who have ongoing bone loss despite estrogen therapy, biphosphonates should be considered. Tamoxifen should be reserved for women with breast cancer for prevention and possibly treatment of osteoporosis pending further studies.

Referral to a Specialist

The primary care provider should ensure appropriate calcium intake and take menstrual histories in women of all age groups to assess the potential for osteoporosis. If there is a concern for osteoporosis, the primary care provider should begin the assessment and evaluation, provided he or she is able to do so. The specialists most commonly recognized as experts in metabolic bone disease and osteoporosis are endocrinologists. The following groups of patients may benefit from the input of a specialist:

1. Patients with documented osteoporosis who, because of personal preference or other diseases, eg, breast cancer, may not be a candidate for estrogen therapy. The specialist will discuss other options for treatment.
2. Women with documented osteoporosis who continue to have osteoporotic fractures despite treatment with estrogen. The specialist can help to ensure that secondary causes have been ruled out and discuss treatment options.
3. Women undergoing treatment for osteoporosis who have a considerable amount of related

disability. These patients might benefit from a multidisciplinary osteoporosis clinic to address rehabilitation, nutrition, exercise, and the psychosocial aspects of osteoporosis.

Controversies & Unresolved Issues

Although there has been tremendous progress in the prevention and treatment of osteoporosis, there are many unanswered questions. Most of these unresolved issues can be categorized as issues of either screening or treatment.

The major question concerning screening that has yet to be resolved is whether or not there is a role for mass screening with bone densitometry. This undertaking would be analogous to breast cancer screening with mammograms in an effort to decrease morbidity and mortality. Although computer models have predicted benefit, no cost analysis of this approach has been undertaken; it must be remembered, however, that osteoporosis is a costly disease.

Questions abound concerning the treatment of osteoporosis. Although it is clear that calcium is important at all ages, there are unanswered questions about the effectiveness of different preparations (carbonate versus citrate malate), the appropriate RDA in the adolescent group, and the risks of calcium supplementation including stone disease.

Although vitamin D supplementation appears to confer benefit in some groups of women, questions remain regarding who should have this supplementation, what form it should be in, and whether serum levels of vitamin D are helpful in predicting benefit.

Despite encouraging results of studies of biphosphonates, there is a need for data to ascertain whether long-term use is of benefit. It seems clear that short-term use is beneficial. Newer forms of biphosphonates are being evaluated that may avoid the potential abnormal bone mineralization that exists with etidronate.

The issues surrounding the use of fluoride are related to the abnormal mineralization that has been a problem with currently available preparations. Slow-release preparations and cyclic administration may improve its usefulness in osteoporosis.

Although calcitonin appears to be an effective agent, studies of optimal dosages, long-term benefit, and use in prophylaxis of osteoporosis are needed to clarify its role.

In conclusion, osteoporosis represents a preventable cause of considerable morbidity and mortality in women. With adequate education of women and their physicians regarding their roles in the prevention of the disease, one may hope for a decline in the medical complications related to osteoporosis.

REFERENCES

Cundy T et al: Bone density in women receiving depot medroxyprogesterone acetate for contraception. BMJ 1991;303:13.

Dawson-Hughes B et al: A controlled trial of the effect of calcium supplementation on bone density in postmenopausal women. N Engl J Med 1990;13:878.

Dawson-Hughes B et al: Effect of vitamin D supplementation on wintertime and overall bone loss in healthy postmenopausal women. Ann Intern Med 1991;115:505.

Felson DT et al: The effect of postmenopausal estrogen therapy on bone density in elderly women. N Engl J Med 1993;329:1141.

Hopper JL, Seeman E: The bone density of female twins discordant for tobacco use. N Engl J Med 1994;330:387.

Johnston CC, Slemenda CW, Melton LJ: Clinical use of bone densitometry. N Engl J Med 1991;324:1105.

Kiel DP et al: Smoking eliminates the protective effect of oral estrogens on the risk for hip fracture among women. Ann Intern Med 1992;116:716.

Lloyd T et al: Calcium supplementation and bone mineral density in adolescent girls. JAMA 1993;270:841.

Love RR et al: Effects of tamoxifen on bone mineral density in postmenopausal women with breast cancer. N Engl J Med 1992;326:852.

Melton LJ, Eddy DM, Johnston CC: Screening for osteoporosis. Ann Intern Med 1990;112:516.

Pak C et al: Slow-release sodium fluoride in the management of postmenopausal osteoporosis. Ann Intern Med 1994;120:625.

Riggs BL: Overview of osteoporosis. West J Med 1991;154:63.

Riggs BL, Melton LJ: The prevention and treatment of osteoporosis. N Engl J Med 1992;327:620.

Riggs BL et al: Effect of fluoride treatment on the fracture rate in postmenopausal women with osteoporosis. N Engl J Med 1990;322:802.

Rigotti NA et al: The clinical course of osteoporosis in anorexia nervosa: A longitudinal study of cortical bone mass. JAMA 1991;265:1133.

Schneider DL, Barrett-Connor EL, Morton DJ: Thyroid hormone use and bone mineral density in elderly women. JAMA 1994;271:1245.

Scientific Advisory Board of the National Osteoporosis Foundation: Clinical indications for bone mass measurement. J Bone Miner Res 1989;4(2):1.

Slemenda CW et al: Predictors of bone mass in perimenopausal women: A prospective study of clinical data using photon absorptiometry. Ann Intern Med 1990;112:96.

Utian WH et al: Calcium supplementation for the prevention and treatment of osteoporosis: A consensus opinion. Menopause Management Supplement, May/June 1994.

Watts NB et al: Intermittent cyclical etidronate treatment of postmenopausal osteoporosis. N Engl J Med 1990;323:73.

Section V.
Breast Disease

Evaluation of a Breast Mass

23

Richard C. Thirlby, MD

The evaluation of most patients with breast masses is straightforward. Although many breast masses are harmless, especially in young women, thorough evaluation of the patient is essential because, despite the increased use of screening mammography, the majority of breast cancers diagnosed in this country still present as palpable breast masses. The majority of palpable cancers are suspicious to experienced clinicians, whereas many breast masses, especially in young women, are harmless. Unfortunately, many women present with palpable abnormalities in the breast of unclear cause and significance. Cancer of the breast is diagnosed annually in approximately 180,000 women in the United States.

Essentials of Diagnosis
Pathophysiology
Incidence & Risk Factors
Signs & Symptoms
Clinical Findings & Diagnosis
Treatment
Referral to a Specialist
Issues of Pregnancy or Lactation

Essentials of Diagnosis
- Generally asymmetric masses, ie, not on opposite breast
- Lie within breast tissue

Pathophysiology
Breast masses are distinct from the surrounding breast tissue, are generally asymmetric when compared to the opposite breast, and lie within breast tissue. Other types of palpable masses that may be confused with breast masses include lipomas of the chest wall, dermal inclusion cysts, eg, sebaceous cysts, and low axillary lymph nodes. Also, normal structures frequently are mistaken for breast abnormalities, especially when they are tender. Tenderness at the costochondral junction, tenderness of a prominent tail of the breast, and tenderness of the pectoralis minor muscle, as well as symmetric ridges of firm tissue at the inframammary fold medially in the breast and ridges of tissue adjacent to previous excisional breast biopsies, frequently are mislabeled as breast masses.

Incidence & Risk Factors
Although many factors have been identified that increase the risk for breast cancer in individual women, most women with newly diagnosed breast cancers have no identifiable risk factors. For example, there is no family history of breast cancer in more than 90% of patients with breast cancer. Nevertheless, it is appropriate to increase the clinical suspicion in particular subsets of women. For example, women with mammary dysplasia, ie, fibrocystic disease of the breast, are at increased risk for breast cancer. However, this increased risk occurs only in women with biopsy-proven proliferative changes or atypical epithelial hyperplasia. It is inappropriate, therefore, to inform women with fibrocystic disease who have never had breast biopsies that they are at increased risk for cancer. Similarly, a recent study by Dupont et al suggested that women with fibroadenomas are at increased risk for breast cancer, especially if there was a family history of breast cancer and if the surrounding breast tissue had proliferative changes. Women who are at increased risk for development of breast cancer should be identified by their physicians, taught the techniques of breast self-examination, and followed carefully with physical examination and screening mammography. However, these guidelines are no different than those recommended in all women. When evaluating women with breast masses, one must recall that most women who develop breast cancer do not have significant identified risk factors. In my opinion, high-risk women and low-risk women with breast masses should be evaluated in an identical fashion.

The most common presentation of breast cancer is a single, nontender, firm immobile mass. Breast cancers rarely are tender to palpation and rarely cause pain. In contrast, benign masses frequently have discrete smooth margins and are mobile. They are frequently tender or painful.

Nipple discharge, unless bloody, rarely is caused by breast cancer. Other rare presenting signs noted by patients include eczematoid nipple changes (Paget's disease), dimpling, and skin thickening (peau d'orange).

Signs & Symptoms

Most palpable breast masses are identified by the patient during breast self-examination, by the clinician during routine physical examination, or by the clinician after a suspicious area is identified on screening mammography. Frequently, pain or tenderness prompts focused examination of the breast with subsequent identification of a possible breast mass. In general, breast cancers are neither painful nor tender. Occasionally, patients may note skin dimpling, retraction of the nipple, bloody nipple discharge, or unusual skin changes (peau d'orange). Most breast cancers, however, are asymptomatic palpable masses.

Clinical Findings & Diagnosis

A. Physical Examination: The clinical findings in most patient with palpable breast cancers are straightforward. Firm, asymmetric immobile masses in postmenopausal women are cause for suspicion and, when biopsied, are found to be malignant in more than three-fourths of cases. The clinical diagnosis in premenopausal women with palpable breast cancers is frequently less evident. Underlying cystic disease and nodular benign breast may make the presence of the cancer less evident. In a study by Boyd et al, there was agreement among experienced surgeons on the need for biopsy in patients with masses that subsequently proved to be cancer in only three-fourths of cases. In most prospective studies, experienced clinicians are found to predict the presence of cancer correctly in less than 85% of cases.

Factors that should guide the clinical examination are the impression of the patient and the symmetry of the breast. The patient's report of a change noted on breast self-examination should be taken seriously. Palpable abnormalities that are clinically benign but, according to the patient, have changed from previous examinations usually require biopsy. Finally, patients with distinctly asymmetric breast tissue should be followed more closely than those with palpable breast masses that are symmetric. A repeat breast examination in 3 months is appropriate in following a patient with asymmetric breast tissue.

B. Aspiration of Cysts: Needle aspiration of breast masses in which the physical findings are consistent with benign cystic disease should be a routine part of an evaluation of palpable breast masses. The technique is safe, inexpensive, diagnostic, and therapeutic. It immediately distinguishes cysts from solid masses and should cause complete disappearance of the breast mass if the mass is a benign cyst.

The two standard criteria for limiting the evaluation of women with breast cysts to continued observation of women with breast cysts are (1) a finding of nonbloody cyst fluid and (2) complete disappearance of the mass after cyst aspiration. Cyst fluid should not be submitted for cytologic examination unless it is bloody. Conversely, patients with cysts containing blood or residual masses after cyst aspiration should proceed immediately to open biopsy. Many cysts recur after initial aspiration. The management of patients with recurrent cysts is somewhat controversial. Although some authors state that cysts should be excised after two or three aspirations, there is no evidence in the literature that these lesions are more likely to be cancerous. It has been suggested that instillation of air into the cyst at the time of the fluid aspiration prevents cyst recurrence, but the efficacy of this technique has not been confirmed. In my opinion, multiple cyst aspirations are preferable to open biopsy in most patients. Cyst aspiration should be performed using an 18- to 22-gauge needle after anesthetizing the skin with dermal injection of a local anesthetic; nonbloody fluid can be discarded immediately.

C. Fine-Needle Aspiration Cytologic Examination: The role of fine-needle aspiration cytologic study in the evaluation of solid breast masses is controversial. Numerous reviews have established the sensitivity and specificity of this technique. In most series, there are no false-positive results; patients in whom aspiration shows malignant cells have breast cancer, and management decisions may be initiated before confirmation at the time of tumor excision. The sensitivity of fine-needle aspiration in patients with breast cancer, however, is only 35–95%. In the best series, at least 5% of patients with biopsy-proven breast cancer have falsely negative results of aspiration. The usefulness of this technique in the management of patients with dominant breast masses is unclear, therefore.

The advantages of cytologic examination are severalfold. The procedure can be performed quickly with little morbidity at an initial visit. The technique is much less expensive than excisional biopsies. If the test result is positive, showing malignant cells, treatment options, eg, breast conservation versus mastectomy, can be discussed with the patient without resorting to open biopsy. The disadvantages of the technique are that a skilled pathologist is required and that sampling errors result in false-negative results.

Most statistical reviews in the literature have concluded that the 5–15% false-negative rate for fine-needle aspiration precludes its use as a means of avoiding open biopsy of suspicious lesions. Experienced clinicians, however, have proposed that the combination of clinical, mammographic, and cytologic diagnostic techniques permits one to observe some breast masses without the need for open biopsy. In a study by Butler et al, 113 women with dominant breast masses were evaluated prospectively with clinical examination, mammography, and fine-needle biopsy cytologic examination. All patients underwent a subsequent biopsy; 46% of the women proved to have malignant masses. In cases of malignant disease, the sensitivities of physical examination, mammography, and fine-needle aspiration were 56%, 73%, and 93%, respectively. All patients in whom the results were benign in all three examinations had benign pathologic results, whereas the incidence of cancer in patients with one, two, or three suspicious test results was 6%, 64%, and 97%, respectively. The authors concluded that the combined triad of physical, mammographic, and fine-needle aspiration cytologic examinations is highly accurate in the diagnosis of breast masses and that patients in whom all three examinations are benign can be observed safely, obviating the need for open biopsy. However, authors of previous reviews of combined series including more than 31,000 aspirations have concluded that this technique is operator-dependent and that conclusions about its efficacy are problematic because of the differences in methods and different biases. One might conclude that the only proven value of aspiration cytologic examination is to confirm the diagnosis of breast cancer in women with highly suspicious lesions, thus obviating the need to perform an open biopsy prior to making treatment decisions. Therefore, the role of aspiration cytologic examination of breast in the evaluation of breast masses by nonspecialists is unclear.

Other authors have concluded that fine-needle aspiration cytologic examination may have a role in the diagnosis and management of young patients with apparent fibroadenomas of the breast. In a study by Walters et al, 75 patients with apparent fibroadenomas were evaluated prospectively. Ninety-five percent of the masses proved to be benign. The result of fine-needle aspiration examination was benign in three-fourths of the patients. In the remaining patients, inadequate, suspicious, or malignant tissue was obtained and treated appropriately. None of the 20 patients with a clinical diagnosis of fibroadenoma and benign cytologic examination was shown subsequently to have cancer. The authors concluded that the combination of clinical diagnosis and cytologic study was accurate in the diagnosis of fibroadenoma. They cautioned, however, that only 20 patients were studied to support this recommendation and that a nonexcisional policy should include prolonged follow-up and repeat biopsy.

D. Mammography: A mammogram should be obtained in all women with breast lumps in whom open biopsy is planned. The role of mammography is not only to characterize the size and location of the mass, but also to evaluate both breasts for synchronous lesions. There is little role for mammography, however, in the evaluation of breast masses in women under the age of 35 if biopsy is not anticipated.

E. Ultrasonography: Ultrasonography can be used to confirm that mammographically detected densities are cystic, thus avoiding the need to proceed with needle localization, open biopsy, or stereotactic biopsy. There is little or no role, however, for ultrasonography in the evaluation of palpable breast masses. Palpable breast masses should be aspirated in an effort to "normalize the breast examination." Readily apparent or palpable cysts should be aspirated to facilitate breast examination and to exclude the possibility that the cysts are masking the detection of adjacent neoplasms.

Treatment

The treatment of women with breast masses is summarized in Figure 23–1. Virtually all reviews of the subject have concluded that aspiration should be part of the initial evaluation of all breast masses. Ideally, aspiration should be performed before mammography because the cyst may mask a tumor or otherwise compromise the mammographic examination. If cyst fluid is nonbloody and the mass disappears, the patient should be observed. There is no evidence that cyst recurrence mandates excision, and patients should be reassured that repeat cyst aspiration is safe. Patients with bloody cyst fluid or persistent masses after cyst aspiration should have a mammography and excisional biopsy. Solid masses require diagnostic biopsy. As discussed previously, there is probably little role for fine-needle aspiration in the evaluation of breast masses by nonspecialists. In highly suspicious lesions, the diagnosis of cancer can be confirmed, thus expediting referral to and evaluation by breast specialists. If the aspiration is negative or nondiagnostic, however, there is little effect on management. However, benign results of aspiration and careful long-term follow-up may have a role in young women with the clinical diagnosis of fibroadenoma.

Prospective studies also have concluded that young patients with discrete, clinically benign breast lumps and benign fine-needle aspiration results can be followed without resorting to open biopsy. Sainsbury et al followed 112 women under the age of 35 years who had clinically and histologically benign breast lumps for up to 4 years (an average of 2 years). Four patients who were believed on a clinical basis to have benign lesions had malignant cytologic examinations, and six patients were lost to follow-up. The remaining 102 patients were evaluated prospectively. During an average follow-up period of 2 years, approximately 68% of patients experienced resolution of their breast lumps, including 30% who had clinical and histologically diagnosed fibroadenomas. These authors recommended that patients younger than 35 years with clinically and cytologically benign breast lumps be offered the option of nonexcision with reasonable expectation of resolution of their lesions.

There is little basis for recommending caffeine restriction or vitamin E supplementation in women with palpable breast lumps. Although many women report anecdotally that caffeine withdrawal or vitamin E supplementation improves breast tenderness or breast pain, clinical trials have not confirmed the ef-

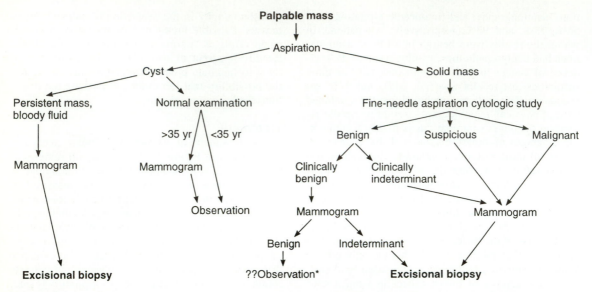

Figure 23–1. Proposed management of palpable breast masses. Note that virtually all masses require biopsy.* It is controversial whether lesions in women younger than 35 years of age that are benign clinically, cytologically, and radiographically may be observed.

ficacy of either of these methods in the resolution of breast masses. Clearly, there is no purpose in making these recommendations in women with painless or nontender breast lesions. It may be appropriate to recommend a trial of these measures in women with a primary complaint of breast tenderness or breast pain in whom incidental breast nodularity is present.

Unfortunately, most masses require open biopsy for definitive diagnosis (Fig 23–1). In many cases, this biopsy is performed under local anesthesia on an outpatient basis using frozen-section evaluation to provide immediate histologic diagnosis; this method enables one to perform appropriate tests, eg, hormone receptor analysis, and relieve the patient's anxiety. As mentioned previously, however, if an earlier fine-needle aspiration has been performed, a single-stage procedure can be performed after appropriate consultation with oncologists, radiation oncologists, and plastic surgeons.

Referral to a Specialist

Postmenopausal women with asymmetric solid breast masses require referral to a specialist. Women with breast cysts can be managed with careful observation and repeat cyst aspiration by nonbreast specialists. Women with breast pain or tenderness without definite palpable breast abnormalities do not require referral. Similarly, most women with nipple discharge do not require specialist referral (see Chapter 25). Women who have bloody nipple discharge or persistent nipple discharge from a single duct orifice also require specialist referral. Women with skin

changes of unclear causation usually require specialist referral.

Inflammatory carcinoma, which is rare, frequently is mistaken for an infectious process. If the physician suspects infection, but the skin changes do not respond rapidly to antibiotics, a specialist should be consulted and biopsy performed regardless of whether there is a palpable or mammographic abnormality.

Issues of Pregnancy or Lactation

The management of women with palpable breast masses during pregnancy or lactation is problematic. The proportion of breast cancers diagnosed during pregnancy is between 10 and 39/1000 pregnancies. Although only 1–2% of all patients with breast cancer are pregnant or in the postpartum period, the incidence of pregnancy in breast cancer patients younger than 40 years of age is at least 15%. Needle aspiration of masses readily differentiates cysts or galactoceles from solid tumors. Benign lesions during pregnancy, in decreasing order of frequency, include fibroadenomas, lipomas, papillomas, fibrocystic disease, galactoceles, and infections.

Patients with lesions that are benign clinically and cytologically, can be followed during pregnancy. This management option, therefore, requires fine-needle aspiration or core biopsies. However, there is no justification for postponing biopsy for most breast masses in pregnant women. Studies have found that less than 20% of patients with breast cancer during pregnancy were diagnosed and treated appropriately.

Unfortunately, biopsy of the breast in a pregnant or lactating woman is difficult. Careful hemostasis is required because of increased vascularity. Biopsy of a lactating breast requires meticulous attention to sterility, because milk provides a good culture medium. Local anesthesia is preferable, although general anesthesia is acceptable, especially in the second trimester of pregnancy. Because of the potential wound-healing problems after biopsy in lactating breasts, it is preferable to defer biopsy until lactation is terminated. If that delay is not possible, biopsy can be performed with the knowledge that healing may be poor.

REFERENCES

Boring CC, Squires TS, Tong T: Cancer statistics, 1992. CA 1992;42:19.

Boyd NF et al: Prospective evaluation of physical examination of the breast. Am J Surg 1981;142:331.

Butler JA et al: Accuracy of combined clinical-mammographic-cytologic diagnosis of dominant breast masses. Arch Surg 1990;125:893.

Ciatto S, Cariaggi P, Bulgaresi P: The value of routine cytology examination of breast cyst fluids. Acta Cytol 1987;31:301.

Donegan WL: Evaluation of a palpable breast mass. N Engl J Med 1992;327:937.

Dupont WD et al: Long-term risk of breast cancer in women with fibroadenoma. N Engl J Med 1994;331:10.

Ernster VL et al: Vitamin E and benign breast "disease": A double-blind, randomized clinical trial. Surgery 1985; 85:490.

Giard RW, Hermans J: The value of aspiration cytologic examination of the breast. Cancer 1992;69:2104.

Grant CS et al: Fine-needle aspiration of the breast. Mayo Clin Proc 1986;61:377.

Layfield LG, Glasgow BJ, Cramer H: Fine-needle aspiration in the management of breast masses. Pathol Annu 1989;24:23.

Layfield LJ et al: The palpable breast nodule. Cancer 1993;72:1642.

Leis HP Jr: Gross breast cysts: Significance and management. Contemp Surg 1991;39(2):13.

Meyer EC et al: Vitamin E and benign breast disease. Surgery 1990;107:549.

Parazzini F et al: Methylxanthine, alcohol-free diet and fibrocystic breast disease: A factorial clinical trial. Surgery 1986;99:576.

Sainsbury JRC et al: Natural history of the benign breast lump. Br J Surg 1988;75:1080.

Saunders G, Lakra Y, Libcke J: Comparison of needle aspiration cytology diagnosis with excisional biopsy tissue diagnosis of palpable tumors of the breast in a community hospital. Surg Gynecol Obstet 1991;172:437.

Vetrani A et al: Fine needle aspiration biopsies of breast masses. Cancer 1992;69:736.

Wallack MK et al: Gestational carcinoma of the female breast. Curr Probl Cancer 1983;7:1.

Walters TK et al: Fine needle aspiration biopsy in the diagnosis and management of fibroadenoma of the breast. Br J Surg 1990;77:1215.

Breast Cancer

Irene Kuter, MD, DPhil

ESSENTIALS OF DIAGNOSIS

- Preinvasive ductal carcinoma in situ detected by mammography because of associated microcalcifications.
- Five percent of cases have demonstratable genetic susceptibility; risk dependent on type of family history.
- Increased risk associated with early menarche, late menopause, late birth of first child, nulliparity, long-term (more than 15 years) use of exogenous estrogen, radiation exposure, and some proliferative lesions of the breast.
- Typical presentations: palpable breast lump or microcalcifications or occult mass on a screening mammogram. Less typical presentations: a diffuse area of breast-thickening, nipple inversion, dimpling, bloody nipple discharge, axillary lymphadenopathy, or diffuse swelling and erythema of the breast.

THE NORMAL BREAST

The mammalian breast, or mammary gland, consists of a specialized branching epithelial ductal system nestled in a specialized stroma; its purpose is to conduct milk from the alveoli to the nipple during lactation. Prepubescent girls already have a rudimentary ductal network, but during puberty the gland undergoes further growth and differentiation to become the adult virginal gland. During pregnancy and lactation, additional differentiation occurs accompanied by milk formation. After lactation ceases, the alveoli and ducts regress. The specialized stroma in which the ducts and lobules lie is composed largely of fat (Fig 24–1). The darkness of fat on an x-ray contributes to the visibility of abnormalities of the ductal network on a mammogram. With rare exceptions, eg, primary lymphomas and sarcomas of the breast, malignant tumors of the breast arise from the epithelial ducts or lobules.

TYPES OF BREAST CANCER

Figure 24–2 shows the sites of origin of the main subtypes of breast cancer. It is likely that the cells giving rise to the cancers are mostly in the terminal ducts. If the cancer cells migrate upward and fill the ducts, they are termed **ductal carcinomas** (85% of breast cancers), whereas if they migrate into the lobules, they are termed **lobular carcinomas** (14% of breast cancers). "Garden variety" breast cancer is invasive ductal carcinoma (IDC), not otherwise specified (NOS), which constitutes approximately 65% of all cases.

Breast Cancer In Situ
A. Atypical Hyperplasia and Lobular Carcinoma In Situ (LCIS): Some benign conditions of the breast confer significant risk of the future devel-

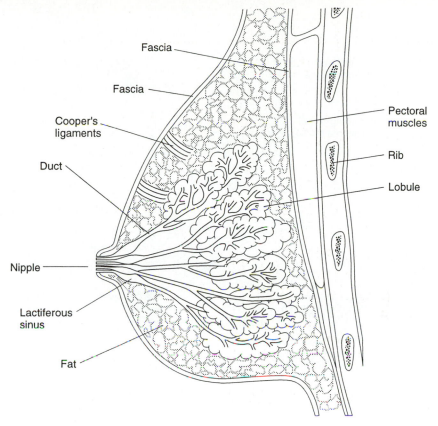

Figure 24–1. The normal breast.

opment of a cancerous growth. In general, these conditions involve excessive proliferation of the epithelial cells lining the ducts or lobules. Normally, this epithelial lining consists of a thin layer of cells. **Epithelial hyperplasia,** which there is proliferation of the epithelial lining (there are multiple layers of cells but the cells still appear normal), carries a moderately increased risk of breast cancer. If the cells in the multilayered epithelium have acquired histologic atypia, the condition is termed **atypical ductal hyperplasia** and carries an even higher risk of malignancy. Some pathologists believe that ductal hyperplasia represents a pathologic response to hormonal stimulation. It is most likely that the defect is at the level of the ductal cell.

Lobular carcinoma in situ, which most pathologists agree would be better termed **lobular hyperplasia,** frequently is found extensively throughout both breasts. Like atypical ductal hyperplasia, its presence confers an increased risk of future breast cancer but with LCIS the cancer can develop anywhere in either breast and can be of the ductal or the lobular subtype.

B. Ductal Carcinoma In Situ (DCIS): Unlike ductal hyperplasia or lobular carcinoma in situ, ductal carcinoma in situ is usually a focal process. It may arise in a breast with preexisting proliferative epithelial changes, or it may arise de novo. Pathologically, DCIS has the appearance of more advanced ductal cell proliferation, with the cells frequently filling the whole lumen of the affected ducts. There is often cellular necrosis and the laying down of calcium deposits. These calcium deposits are the microcalcifications seen on a mammogram. There are different subtypes of DCIS, eg, comedo or papillary, which have different propensities to recur after excision. Several lines of evidence suggest that DCIS is a precursor lesion to invasive ductal carcinoma. First, primary invasive breast cancers almost always have an area of DCIS within them. This may be a small area (less than 5% of the cancer), in which case the evolution to an invasive cancer probably occurred early in the growth of the cancer, or a large area (sometimes greater than 95%), in which case clonal evolution of an invasive cancer probably occurred later.

The second line of evidence that DCIS is a precursor to invasive ductal cancer is epidemiologic. Before the advent of screening mammography, pure

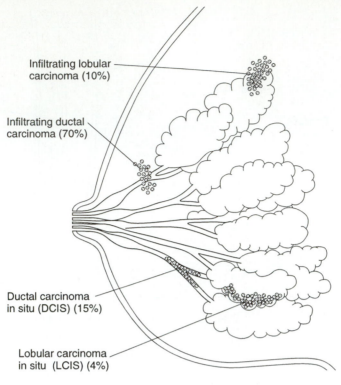

Infiltrating lobular carcinoma (10%)

Infiltrating ductal carcinoma (70%)

Ductal carcinoma in situ (DCIS) (15%)

Lobular carcinoma in situ (LCIS) (4%)

Figure 24–2. Subtypes of breast cancer.

DCIS was uncommon (less than 2% of breast cancers) and presented typically as a palpable lump. Mammography has allowed the detection of cancers at an earlier stage, and it is striking that the percentage of cancers that are pure DCIS has increased dramatically. (Currently, approximately 15–20% of all breast cancers are pure DCIS.) That this increase is not caused by the discovery of lesions that would never be detectable clinically is testified to by the simultaneous decrease in incidence of more advanced, invasive cancers. It is well accepted, therefore, that pure DCIS, if not detected early and removed, has a high probability of developing into an invasive cancer. When not discovered early, DCIS may continue to grow and spread through the branching ductal system of the breast in an insidious, indolent fashion rather than evolve into an invasive cancer. In the most extreme cases, almost the entire ductal network can be involved. In contrast to invasive cancer, however, even such extensive DCIS is not lethal; the lack of invasive properties ensures that the lesion is completely curable if a simple mastectomy is performed.

Paget's disease is a ductal carcinoma involving the nipple. Clinically, it resembles eczema of the nipple. It may be completely in situ, in which case the prognosis is excellent with local treatment, or it may be associated with an infiltrating component (which may form a mass in the breast), in which case the prognosis is that of the associated infiltrating carcinoma.

Invasive Breast Cancer

As previously noted, invasive ductal cancer is thought to arise from preexisting DCIS. It is called invasive, or infiltrating, because of the breaching of the basement membrane under the epithelial lining by the cancer cells, with resulting movement of the cells out of the duct or lobule and into the surrounding stroma. Cells that have become invasive have the ability to migrate into lymphatics and blood vessels and thus spread out of the breast to other parts of the body by the process of metastasis. There are some invasive ductal cancers that have characteristic histologic and clinical features such as mucinous carcinoma (which tends to metastasize less) and tubular carcinoma (which also has lower metastatic potential and tends to recapitulate ductal structure after spreading into the stroma).

Invasive lobular carcinoma spreads via lymphatic channels and blood vessels just as invasive ductal carcinoma does, but it has some characteristic features that differentiate it from invasive ductal carcinoma. First, essentially all invasive lobular carcinomas are estrogen-receptor-positive (ER-positive), whereas only two-thirds of invasive ductal carcinomas are ER-positive. Second, the lobular carcinoma cells characteristically invade the stroma in a single-file pattern without disrupting the architecture of the gland and without eliciting a scirrhous reaction. Third, as a result of the pattern of spread of lobular carcinoma, the disease presents clinically as a vague area of diffuse thickening in the breast rather than a discrete mass. For the same reason, lobular carcinomas are often missed on mammograms. Unlike infiltrating ductal carcinomas (often associated with DCIS), in which microcalcifications are found, lobular carcinomas characteristically do not lay down calcifications. Therefore, infiltrating lobular carcinomas are more difficult to diagnose than infiltrating ductal carcinomas and are a frequent cause of false-negative results on mammograms. Finally, infiltrating lobular carcinomas have a different pattern of metastasis from infiltrating ductal carcinomas; they have a tendency to grow on the serosal surface of the bowel or around the ureters with resulting bowel or ureteral obstruction.

Inflammatory breast cancer is a poorly differentiated infiltrating ductal carcinoma that extensively invades the dermal lymphatics. Clinically, the breast is swollen with peau d'orange changes in the skin (erythema, skin thickening with edema, and prominent pores), and the mammogram may show only a diffuse increase in the parenchymal pattern with or without a visible mass.

INCIDENCE

Carcinoma of the breast is the most common cancer in women in the United States (32% of cancers in women) and is exceeded only by lung cancer as a cause of death in women (18% of cancer deaths in women). It is projected that there will be 183,000 new cases of breast cancer and 46,300 deaths from breast cancer in women in the United States in 1994. At the present time, approximately one of nine women in this country, or about 11%, will be diagnosed with breast cancer during her lifetime. Although breast cancer is predominantly a disease of women, there will be approximately 1000 new cases and approximately 300 deaths from this disease in men in the USA in 1994. In most cases in men, there is either a hereditary (familial breast cancer), hormonal (hyperestrogenic state), or environmental (radiation exposure) risk that can be identified.

There is a striking variation in the incidence of breast cancer throughout the world (Table 24–1). The highest incidence is seen in Europe, Australia, and North America, and the lowest incidence is in Asia and Latin America. Although there are many possible reasons for this variation, it is known that racial susceptibility alone is not the explanation: women who migrate from low-risk countries such as Japan to high-risk countries such as the USA experience an increasing risk over the next two generations. It ap-

Table 24–1. Incidence of breast cancer around the world.*

Country	Age-Adjusted Death Rate per 100,000 Population	Rank (out of 46)
Argentina	20.9	19
Australia	20.7	21
Austria	22.0	17
Bulgaria	15.6	31
Canada	23.9	12
Chile	12.5	39
China	4.6	46
Costa Rica	12.9	38
Cuba	14.8	33
Czechoslovakia	19.8	22
Denmark	27.7	4
Ecuador	5.6	45
England and Wales	28.7	1
Finland	17.0	28
France	19.7	23
Germany (Federal Republic)	21.9	18
Greece	15.2	32
Hong Kong	8.6	41
Hungary	22.6	15
Iceland	23.7	13
Ireland	27.8	3
Israel	23.0	14
Italy	20.8	20
Japan	6.3	44
Luxembourg	25.4	10
Malta	28.1	2
Mauritius	6.7	43
Mexico	8.1	42
Netherlands	26.8	7
New Zealand	27.0	6
Northern Ireland	26.5	8
Norway	19.2	24
Poland	15.7	30
Portugal	17.8	26
Puerto Rico	14.2	35
Romania	14.8	34
Scotland	27.1	5
Singapore	12.9	37
Spain	17.1	27
Sweden	18.2	25
Switzerland	24.3	11
United States	22.4	16
Uruguay	26.4	9
USSR	13.6	36
Venezuela	9.6	40
Yugoslavia	15.9	29

*Reproduced, with permission, from Boring CC et al: Cancer Statistics, 1994. CA 1994;44:7.

pears more likely that environmental factors account for the worldwide variation.

In the USA, data from several sources, including the Connecticut Tumor Registry and the Surveillance, Epidemiology, and End Results (SEER) program of the National Cancer Institute, show a slow, gradual rise in incidence of breast cancer over the last several decades of approximately 1%/yr. The incidence now is approximately double what it was in 1940 (Fig 24–3), although the mortality rate has remained unchanged. Most oncologists have the uneasy feeling that they are seeing more cases of breast

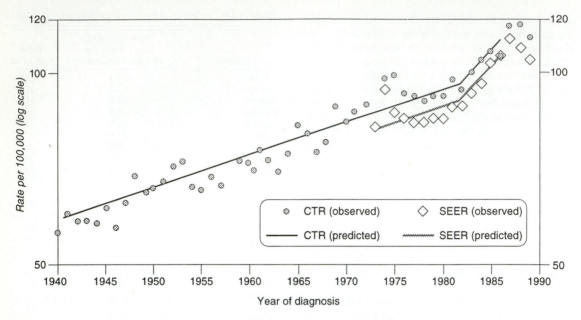

Figure 24–3. The changing incidence of breast cancer in the United States over time. (Reproduced, with permission, from Miller BA, Feuer EJ, Hankey BF: Recent incidence trends for breast cancer in women and the relevance of early detection: An update. CA 1993;43:27.)

cancer in premenopausal women, but in fact the baby boom has caused an absolute increase in the number of women younger than 50 years old. When the incidence of cancer per 100,000 women is calculated, the slow, gradual rise in incidence is confined to the postmenopausal group.

In looking for the reason for this increase in incidence, it must be remembered that breast cancer is largely a disease of older women; the decline in mortality from other causes (especially infections and cardiovascular disease) is allowing women to live longer, so that there a is greater percentage of women surviving to be at risk of development of breast cancer. It has been estimated that half of the increased incidence over the last 50 years is caused by increased longevity. Other factors that might contribute to the increased incidence include changes in life-style that have occurred in society since World War II. Children are better nourished, and the average age of a girl at menarche has dropped gradually as a result. Women are pursuing careers and delaying childbirth. Hormone replacement therapy has been used in postmenopausal women to decrease cardiovascular risk and osteoporosis. All of these factors are known to increase the risk of breast cancer (see the following section, Risk Factors). Use of oral contraceptive pills does not explain the increased incidence. To what extent environmental exposure to toxins such as organic pesticides can be implicated is not clear.

Since the early 1980s, there has been a steeper rise in incidence, which is believed to reflect increased detection of prevalent cancers through widespread acceptance and practice of screening mammography. There has been an increase in incidence of early-stage breast cancer (DCIS and small infiltrating carcinomas) and a decrease in incidence of larger tumors (greater than 2 cm) or those associated with positive lymph nodes or metastases. If this explanation for the recent accelerated increase in incidence is correct, one might anticipate a subsequent dip in incidence because most prevalent cancers would have been detected and treated. Since 1987 there has been a slight decrease in incidence consistent with this hypothesis. More important, with mammographic detection of earlier, more curable lesions, the mortality rate should decline after a lag of several years, and a drop in mortality is predicted for the mid-1990s.

RISK FACTORS

The number of risk factors suggested to predispose to breast cancer is a testimony to the fact that the cause of breast cancer is largely unknown. After factors of female gender and increasing age, it is not clear to what extent each of the leading risk factors (genetics, diet, environmental exposures, life-style, and hormonal factors) contributes to the incidence. Breast cancer, like other malignant diseases, is a genetic disease at the cellular level in the sense that mutations in the DNA (activation of oncogenes, deletion or inactivation of tumor-suppressor genes) seem to be essential for its development. However, the relative roles of carcinogens, which initiate these mutations, and promoters, which drive cellular proliferation and allow the expression of these mutations, is not clear. Risk factors can be categorized as either established or controversial.

Established Risk Factors

A. Race and Cultural Factors: The geographic variation in incidence clearly is caused by important life-style differences. The complexity of the analysis of such differences is underscored by the fact that there are many covariables. The average Japanese woman, compared with the average North American woman, not only eats a diet lower in fat but also eats a different spectrum of food entirely. Soybeans have been shown to contain a natural antiestrogen (which may be a cancer chemopreventive), so that there may be a protective effect of the Asian diet. Japanese women tend to mature later, to have a leaner body habitus, and to have a lower endogenous estradiol level than American women. Although geographic and cultural factors are definitely important, the underlying reason for the relative risks is not yet understood.

B. Heredity: Only about 5% of breast cancers in this country can be said to be hereditary inasmuch as there is convincing evidence for genetically transmitted susceptibility. In families in which the familial linkage is unquestionable, however, genetic susceptibility becomes the strongest risk factor known. When assessing an individual's risk of breast cancer based on a family history, it is important to recognize that there is an enormous variation in risk depending on the characteristics of the cancer of the affected relative or relatives. Usually only first-degree relatives are considered. If such a relative had unilateral breast cancer diagnosed after menopause, the individual's risk is minimal (relative risk [RR] approximately 1.2-fold). Even a positive family history of unilateral breast cancer in one first-degree relative before menopause gives a relative risk of only 1.8-fold. If the first-degree relative who had breast cancer postmenopausally had bilateral breast cancer, the risk jumps to 4.0-fold, and if a first-degree relative had bilateral breast cancer premenopausally, the risk escalates to 8.8-fold.

In some families in which more than one woman has bilateral premenopausal breast cancer, it is known that there is a faulty gene on the long arm of chromosome 17 that gives rise to the genetic susceptibility. The same gene seems to be linked to the familial syndrome of susceptibility to breast and ovarian cancer. This abnormal gene is inherited in an autosomal dominant mode, ie, each offspring of an affected individual has a 50:50 chance of inheriting the faulty gene. For a woman who inherits the gene, the lifetime risk of breast cancer is about 85%. For a woman in the same family who does not inherit the gene, the risk of breast cancer is that of the rest of population. A man who inherits the faulty gene probably will not develop breast cancer but will transmit the gene to 50% of his offspring. Even before this gene was identified, the chromosomal location was sufficiently well known that linkage analysis could predict with acceptable accuracy in some families whether an individual woman has inherited the flawed gene. Some such women are choosing to have prophylactic mastectomies. The gene (BRCA1) has recently been cloned and this will permit more accurate screening. A second breast cancer susceptibility gene, BRCA2, has recently been localized to chromosome 13.

There are a number of other rare familial syndromes associated with an increased risk of breast cancer. The Li-Fraumeni syndrome, characterized by a familial clustering of breast cancer in women, soft-tissue and bone sarcomas in children, acute leukemia, brain tumors, and adrenocortical carcinomas, is caused by a germline mutation in the p53 tumor-suppressor gene. Women in such families who inherit the faulty gene have a lifetime risk of breast cancer of greater than 50%; however, only about 1% of all breast cancers are caused by a germline mutation in the p53 gene.

In some families, there seems to be an associated susceptibility to breast, colon, and other epithelial tumors (Lynch syndrome type II). Recently it has been found that members of these families have an abnormal gene involved in DNA mismatch repair. There are other rare syndromes (Cowden's, Muir's) associated with increased risk of breast cancer, but the genes for these have not yet been identified.

C. Hormonal Factors: The breast epithelium is sensitive to stimulation by estrogen. Long-term (greater than 15 years) use of exogenous estrogens results in a small (approximately 1.3-fold) increased risk of breast cancer. Most physicians believe that the beneficial effects of replacement estrogen in postmenopausal women, with the attendant decrease in mortality from cardiovascular disease and osteoporosis, more than compensate for such a small increased risk of breast cancer. Women who used diethylstilbestrol (DES) in pregnancy also seem to have a small increased risk of breast cancer later in life.

Early menarche, late menopause, nulliparity, and delayed childbearing are associated with an increased risk of breast cancer. To what extent these risk factors are additive is not clear. It is stated commonly that early menarche and late menopause probably increase the risk by increasing the lifetime exposure of the breast epithelium to the proliferative effect of estrogen because of the increased number of menstrual cycles. It is interesting that the proliferative index of the breast epithelium is higher during the luteal phase of the menstrual cycle, when progesterone levels also are elevated. Progesterone, therefore, does not protect the breast in the way that it protects the uterine endometrium against the proliferative stimulus of estrogen. Thus, the relative roles of estrogen and progesterone levels in increasing risk are not clear.

Not only is delayed childbearing a risk factor, but an early full-term pregnancy is extraordinarily protective. Whereas a woman who delays childbearing until age 35 may have a relative risk of breast cancer of 1.2, a woman who has a child while in her early teens is protected significantly against breast cancer (relative risk 0.4). Oophorectomy at an early age is also protective. Lactation after pregnancy appears to confer a slight protection from breast cancer, but the protective effect is seen only in the premenopausal years and is lost after menopause.

D. Carcinogen Exposure: Exposure to ionizing radiation clearly is associated with an increased risk of breast cancer under certain circumstances. There was an increased incidence of breast cancer in women who survived the atomic bombing of Hiroshima. Young women who were treated with mantle radiation for Hodgkin's disease have been found to have a significantly increased risk of breast cancer later in life (often while they are still younger than 40). Reanalysis of old data on long-term consequences of exposure to fluoroscopy for tuberculosis showed that women who were under age 25 when they were exposed had a small increased risk of breast cancer, whereas older women did not. The radiation sensitivity of the breast epithelium clearly decreases with age. It should be emphasized that the risk of screening mammography in women older than 35 years is extremely small. It has been estimated that the risk of inducing a breast cancer is approximately one in one million. The risk of screening younger women is probably higher, which is one of the many reasons routine screening is not recommended for young women.

E. Proliferative Breast Disease: In a landmark study in 1985, Dupont and Page identified which histologic subtypes of benign breast lesions are associated with an increased risk of breast cancer. They looked at 10,542 consecutive breast biopsies performed because of a suspicion of breast cancer that turned out not to be cancer. They followed these women for a median of 17 years and compared the relative risk of breast cancer of these women with that of a population of case-matched normal women. Almost 70% of the women in the original group had disease that could be classified as "nonproliferative," including fibrocystic changes, ductal ectasia, and fibroadenomas. These women were at no increased risk of breast cancer compared with women in the control group. Slightly more than one-fourth of the women had "proliferative disease without atypia," ie, epithelial hyperplasia of the ducts or lobules (see the preceding section, Breast Cancer In Situ). These women had a relative risk of breast cancer of 1.6. There was a small group of women (close to 4%), however, who had proliferative disease with atypical

hyperplasia. This small group had a relative risk of breast cancer of 4.4, a highly significant elevation of risk. Of this high-risk group, those who had a first-degree relative with breast cancer were found to have a relative risk of 8.9. This study has been validated by others; not only did it point out the high risk of atypical hyperplasia, especially that associated with a positive family history, but also it laid to rest the idea that most women who have benign breast disease, especially fibrocystic mastopathy, are at increased risk of breast cancer. This conclusion should be reassuring to the 70% of women whose biopsy results fall in this category.

A recent study suggests, however, that women with complex fibroadenomas, those with fibroadenomas with surrounding benign proliferative disease, and especially women with both complex fibroadenomas and a family history of breast cancer are at increased risk of breast cancer. It should be noted, however, that two-thirds of the patients in this study had noncomplex fibroadenomas and no family history of breast cancer and did not have an increased risk.

F. Previous Breast Cancer: It should not be forgotten that a woman who has had one breast cancer has a risk of another breast cancer that is higher than the risk of a woman without risk factors of having a first breast cancer. Thus, annual mammography is one of the most important of the follow-up tests that women with a history of breast cancer should undergo.

When all the established risk factors are assessed, most women (approximately 75%) with breast cancer cannot be considered to have been at "high risk." The causes of the high incidence of breast cancer in the USA are still largely unknown.

Possible Risk Factors
A. Hormone Metabolism: Estrogen metabolism is extremely complicated. Estradiol, for example, can be metabolized along multiple different pathways, and some of the derivatives are more potent estrogens than estradiol itself. Some estrogen metabolites are even "genotoxic"; they form reactive quinone derivatives that can cross-link with DNA. Some investigators have hypothesized that variations in endogenous estrogen metabolism may contribute to breast cancer risk. Recently it has been found that exposure to some chemicals can affect hormone metabolism; this is an extremely active area of current research.

B. High-Fat Diet: The hypothesis that a high-fat diet is associated with an increased risk of breast cancer first came from epidemiologic studies showing that the incidence of breast cancer across the world correlated with the per capita fat intake in the countries studied (Fig 24–4). Although this hypothesis has been discussed for a long time, it never has been proved, and the theory has many protagonists

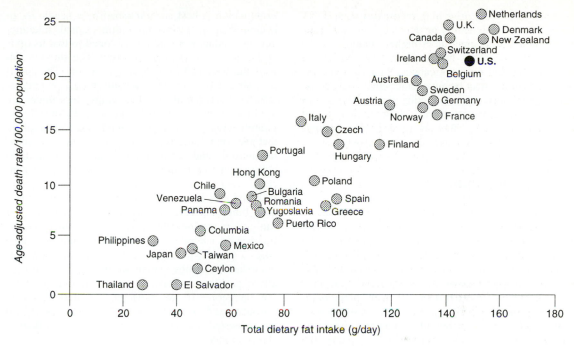

Figure 24–4. Breast cancer incidence in women around the world related to per capita fat intake. (Reproduced, with permission, from Carroll KK: Experimental evidence of dietary factors and hormone-dependent cancers. Cancer Res 1975;35:3374.)

and antagonists. It may be that total calorie intake, rather than fat consumption, is responsible for the increased risk, or it may be that the incidence is correlated with another variable linked to affluence. In the nurses' study conducted by the Harvard School of Public Health in which 89,000 nurses were surveyed about diet and other life-style factors, there was no increased risk of breast cancer associated with a high-fat diet. This study is not definitive, however, because the diet during childhood or adolescence may be the critical element, or the variation of fat intake in the women surveyed might not have been great enough to bring out a difference in risk. Attempts are being made to conduct a prospective study of diet modification through the Women's Health Initiative.

C. Alcohol: Several studies, including the nurses' health study mentioned previously, have looked at the role of alcohol intake in breast cancer. Although the finding is controversial, there seems to be a small increased risk associated with moderate alcohol intake. The small risk is seen mostly in young women, however, whose baseline risk is small, and the current thinking is that alcohol may work by elevating endogenous estrogen levels in these women. It is doubtful that alcohol intake is a major contributor to risk of breast cancer.

D. Oral Contraceptive: With the publication of the widely quoted report from the Cancer and Steroid Hormone Study in 1986, it was accepted that oral contraceptive pills were exonerated from a role in contributing to breast cancer risk. In recent years, multiple studies have been reanalyzed to determine whether any subsets of women who have taken oral contraceptives are yet at increased risk. Women who took high-estrogen pills (the first type available in the 1960s) when they were teenagers seem to have an increased risk of breast cancer later in life. Women who took oral contraceptive pills for prolonged intervals (longer than 12 years) also seem to be at a slightly increased risk, although the number of women in this risk group is small, and these statistics are not fully reliable. It appears reasonable to conclude that use of current oral contraceptive pills for several years has no known associated risk of breast cancer.

E. Progestins: Progesterone is a growth factor for breast epithelium. It is not known to what extent use of progestins contributes to the risk of breast cancer. Currently, there is no known elevation of risk associated with the use of progestin-based contraceptives; because of the known biologic effects of progesterone, however, breast cancer incidence should be assessed on a prospective basis in women taking these products in the coming years.

F. Environmental Carcinogens: There is increasing interest in exploring environmental carcinogens as possible etiologic agents in breast cancer. Recently, there was a disturbing report that some DDT derivatives, which tend to be deposited in fatty tissue in the body, were present in higher amounts in tissues from cancerous breasts than from breasts of women who did not have cancer. Some of these organic chemicals may be mutagenic; others may act as estrogen agonists or may modify the metabolism of estrogen in the tissues by affecting the activity of particular enzymes. There are no definitive findings to date from this major area of current research.

CLINICAL FINDINGS

As screening mammography is practiced more extensively, it is hoped that most breast cancers will be discovered as nonpalpable masses or preinvasive lesions associated with microcalcifications. Breast self-examination is encouraged, however, because interval cancers appear between mammograms, and there is a significant false-negative rate with mammography (approximately 10%). Invasive lobular carcinoma is particularly difficult to diagnose; it is not associated with microcalcifications and often does not form a mass visible on a mammogram. Even on physical examination, it often presents as a diffuse thickening of the breast rather than a discrete mass.

Other suspicious signs of cancer include nipple inversion, dimpling of the breast, bloody nipple discharge, and new axillary lymphadenopathy. Occasionally, breast cancer presents as diffuse swelling, pain, or erythema of the breast. This presentation is common in inflammatory breast cancer, in which the lymphatic channels are extensively invaded by cancer cells. This condition often is diagnosed incorrectly initially as infectious mastitis. Women who present with axillary lymphadenopathy that on biopsy proves to be adenocarcinoma but who do not have a palpable mass or a lesion detectable by mammography usually have occult breast cancer. The primary lesion is frequently high in the axillary tail. Occasionally, the primary lesion is in extramammary breast tissue in the axilla. The second most common adenocarcinoma to present as an axillary lymph node is lung cancer; chest computed tomography (CT) should be done to look for an occult primary tumor of the lung before definitive breast surgery is undertaken, although the finding of positive estrogen receptors strongly points to a primary tumor of the breast. Rarely, breast cancer presents with symptoms secondary to systemic metastases with a primary occult tumor of the breast.

DIAGNOSIS

Evaluation of a breast mass is discussed in Chapter 23. Evaluation of a mammographic abnormality suspicious for cancer but not palpable on physical examination is best accomplished by a needle localization biopsy. Using three-dimensional mammographic guidance, a wire is positioned so that its tip is at the site of the suspicious lesion. The surgeon follows the wire and excises around its tip. The specimen should be x-rayed to be sure the suspicious lesion has been removed. Other biopsy techniques are used under specific circumstances. A fine-needle aspiration biopsy is easy and quick and can confirm that a lesion is cancerous, but it gives cytologic information only and not histologic data. It can be difficult to decipher an invasive from a noninvasive cancer. Coring needle biopsy is becoming more popular. Although it is less invasive than needle-localized surgical biopsy, it gives a decent sample of tissue and can give much more histologic information than the fine-needle aspirate. An incisional biopsy is done when a (usually obvious) cancer is too big for a simple excisional biopsy under local anesthesia; it usually is performed to make a definitive diagnosis before surgery. At the time of the initial biopsy, estrogen- and progesterone-receptor studies should be requested because the results may influence choice of medical therapy.

STAGING

Breast cancer is staged by the internationally accepted tumor/nodes/metastasis (TNM) system. A simplified, current (1992) version of the staging system published by the American Joint Committee on Cancer is presented in Table 24–2. Stage I cancers must be less than 2 cm with negative lymph nodes. Stage II cancers either are larger or have involved axillary lymph nodes. Stage III cancers either are locally advanced (greater than 5 cm) tumors with positive axillary lymph nodes, have matted axillary lymph nodes, involve internal mammary lymph nodes, or extend to the chest wall or skin. Stage IV cancers have either supraclavicular lymph-node involvement or distant metastases.

The **clinical stage** applies to the extent of disease as assessed by physical examination and radiologic studies. The **pathologic stage** applies to the extent of disease found by examination of the breast tissue and lymph nodes removed at the time of surgery.

The reason for careful staging is twofold. First, staging has great prognostic value (see the following section, Prognosis). Second, accurate staging allows like patients to be enrolled in clinical trials with the assurance that they have a similar prognosis to each other.

PROGNOSIS

Figure 24–5 shows the survival rates (up to 6 years) of women with breast cancer as a function of

Table 24–2. The TNM staging system for breast cancer.

Primary tumor (T)
T0   No evidence of primary tumor
Tis   Carcinoma in situ
T1   Tumor 2 cm or less in greatest dimension
T2   Tumor between 2 and 5 cm in greatest dimension
T3   Tumor more than 5 cm in greatest dimension
T4   Tumor of any size with any of the following:
        Extension to chest wall
        Edema or ulceration of the skin of the breast
        Satellite skin nodules confined to the same breast
        Inflammatory carcinoma
Regional lymph nodes (N)
NX   Regional lymph nodes not assessed
N0   No regional lymph node metastasis
N1   Metastasis to movable ipsilateral axillary lymph
        node(s)
N2   Metastasis to ipsilateral axillary lymph node(s) fixed to
        one another or to other structures
N3   Metastasis to ipsilateral internal mammary lymph
        node(s)
Distant metastases
Mx   Presence of distant metastasis not assessed
M0   No distant metastasis
M1   Distant metastasis (includes metastasis to ipsilateral
        supraclavicular lymph node(s)
Stage grouping

Stage 0	Tis	N0	M0
Stage 1`	T1	N0	M0
Stage IIA	T0	N1	M0
	T1	N1	M0
	T2	N0	M0
Stage IIB	T2	N1	M0
	T3	N0	M0
Stage IIIA	T0	N2	M0
	T1	N2	M0
	T2	N2	M0
	T3	N1	M0
	T3	N2	M0
Stage IIIB	T4	Any N	M0
	Any T	N3	M0
Stage IV	Any T	Any N	M1

Reproduced, with permission, from Beahrs OH et al: *Manual for Staging of Cancer*, 4th ed. Lippincott, 1992.

their stage at diagnosis. Survival at 10 years is approximately 70% in patients with stage I breast cancer, approximately 50% in patients with stage II cancer, approximately 25% in stage III, and negligible in stage IV.

Carcinoma in situ (stage O) has no propensity to metastasize, and there is no significant death rate from this condition if the woman has a mastectomy. However, the delayed but continuing recurrence and death risk even from stage I breast cancer, which becomes apparent after a lag of about 3 years, has caused some clinicians to speculate that even early-stage breast cancer is a systemic disease. They hypothesize that because of its low volume at diagnosis, it takes longer to recur, but no one is ever cured, and if a woman with breast cancer lives long enough, she will have a recurrence.

Of all the prognostic factors available, the involvement of the axillary lymph nodes is the most important. Not only do women with involved axillary

lymph nodes have a worse prognosis than women with negative lymph nodes, but also the number and level of involved nodes are important factors. Microscopic involvement of only one lymph node carries a slightly worse prognosis than negative axillary nodes, and a finding of four or more positive lymph nodes carries a much worse prognosis than that of only one to three positive nodes. Women who have 10 or more positive lymph nodes have such a poor prognosis (less than 20% 5-year survival) that special protocols are being used currently to see whether early intensive treatment (autologous bone-marrow transplantation) will have a favorable impact on their survival.

For women with negative axillary lymph nodes, other prognostic factors attain more importance. Tumor size is one of the most important. Women who have a tumor that measures less than 1 cm with negative lymph nodes have a greater than 95% chance of a 10-year disease-free survival. As the tumor size approaches 2 cm, the chance of being disease free at 10 years drops to about 70%. Nuclear grade is also important. Only about 10% of breast cancers are grade 1, and women in this group have a better than average prognosis for their tumor size. Most breast cancers are grade II or III, and grade III carcinomas, often termed "poorly differentiated," tend to be more aggressive and faster growing. They also are commonly ER-negative.

Other prognostic factors that are used frequently include estrogen and progesterone receptors, mitotic index (or S phase), and the presence of lymphatic or blood-vessel invasion. When the lymph nodes are negative, women with estrogen-receptor-positive tumors have a disease-free survival at 4 years of 76%, compared with 67% for women with ER-negative tumors. Women who have cancers with a high mitotic rate have a poorer prognosis than those whose cancers have a low mitotic rate. Again, high mitotic index tends to be seen in the grade III, ER-negative tumors, so that these factors are not completely independent. Lymphatic or blood-vessel invasion, especially if extensive, connotes a poor prognosis with increased likelihood of systemic spread and increased chance of local recurrence.

Numerous other prognostic factors have been touted as important, especially in the group of women with negative nodes. Poor prognostic factors currently believed to be important include the expression or amplification of particular oncogenes (such as the expression of the growth-factor receptor HER-2/neu, seen in approximately one-third of breast cancers) and a high neovascularization index (thought to be related to the synthesis of angiogenesis factors). Aneuploidy was thought to be an important adverse prognostic factor a few years ago but is now out of favor, as is a high expression of cathepsin D, an enzyme that digests extracellular matrix. The list of prognostic factors is growing at an alarming rate, and

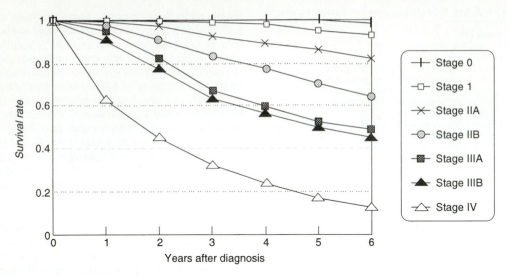

Figure 24–5. Survival rates of women with breast cancer by stage at presentation. (Reproduced, with permission, from Beahrs OH et al (editors): *Manual for Staging of Cancer,* 4th ed. Lippincott, 1992.)

what is desperately needed is an algorithm that gives appropriate relative weighting to each of the factors. Currently, most clinical decisions regarding the prognosis and therefore the need for adjuvant treatment are made on the basis of lymph-node status, grade, size, mitotic index, and estrogen-receptor status.

TREATMENT

Surgery

A. Invasive Breast Cancer: The Halsted radical mastectomy was an important advance in the treatment of breast cancer at the turn of the last century because it spared women from dying with fungating masses on the chest; however, it failed to prevent women with breast cancer from dying of systemic metastases. When it was understood that the lethality of breast cancer comes from its early systemic spread in the bloodstream and through embolization in the lymphatics, the goal of surgery was limited to providing adequate local control of the cancer. Although it took almost 80 years to learn this lesson, the equivalence of the modified radical mastectomy (in which the pectoralis major muscle is spared) to the radical mastectomy (in which the pectoralis major muscle is removed) in terms of both local control and the chance of a cure has been demonstrated clearly in multiple well-designed clinical trials. Furthermore, a partial mastectomy—"lumpectomy," "tylectomy," "quadrantectomy"—followed by radiation to the breast has been shown to be equivalent to mastectomy in terms of survival.

At the National Institutes of Health (NIH) Consensus Development Conference on Treatment of Early-

Stage Breast Cancer in June 1990, it was stated that breast conservation is appropriate for most women with stage I and II breast cancer and that breast conservation is preferable to mastectomy because it provides survival equivalent to mastectomy while preserving the breast. The recommended technique for breast conservation includes local excision of the primary tumor with clear margins, a level I and II axillary lymph-node dissection (sparing the higher, level III nodes), and breast irradiation to 4500–5000 cGy with or without a boost.

There are some women, such as those who have multiple foci of cancer within the breast, for whom breast conservation is not a good option because the likelihood of local recurrence is significantly higher than the (approximately) 5% achieved when lumpectomy and radiation are performed as previously outlined. When a cancer is central in the breast or the size of the lumpectomy would be unduly large considering the size of the breast, breast conservation may be a less attractive option because of poor cosmetic outcome. There are also women, such as those with connective tissue diseases, in whom breast conservation is not a good option because of an increased likelihood of scarring and fibrosis secondary to radiation therapy. Most other women can be reassured that they can choose between breast conservation and mastectomy with an equal likelihood of long-term disease-free survival. For very large cancers, chemotherapy given before surgery (neoadjuvant chemotherapy) results in tumor shrinkage and breast conservation in most patients. Although it is premature to conclude that the local control rate for these large tumors will be adequate, it is likely that the overall survival rate (influenced by distant spread) will be the same as it would have been if a mastectomy had been performed. In the USA, breast conservation generally is not advised for inflammatory breast cancer, although in France the primary treatment is chemotherapy and radiation, with reasonable results.

B. Ductal Carcinoma In Situ: With breast conservation for invasive breast cancer becoming more prevalent, it was natural to question whether mastectomy, the traditional treatment for (preinvasive) ductal carcinoma in situ, was necessary. Before the era of screening mammography, ductal carcinoma in situ was uncommon and presented as a palpable mass. Because of its propensity to spread extensively through the ductal tree, excision alone was associated with an unacceptably high recurrence rate (40–50% at 5 years); the rate continued to increase for at least a decade after the excision, reaching 75% in one series. What made this high local recurrence rate even more unacceptable was the fact that approximately half of the recurrences were invasive ductal carcinomas (more evidence that DCIS is a precursor of invasive ductal carcinoma). Although pure DCIS is cured by mastectomy 100% of the time, a recurrence of invasive ductal carcinoma is potentially life-threatening and would not be expected to have such a high cure rate. Rather, the prognosis would depend on the size of the invasive component and the lymph-node status. For this reason, DCIS has been treated until recently with a simple mastectomy (lymph-node dissection not required).

Studies such as the National Surgical Adjuvant Breast and Bowel Project (NSABP) B-17 study, reviewed in by Fisher and Anderson (1994), asked whether, in the modern era with a trend toward smaller tumors because of screening mammography, excision with or without radiation therapy would give adequate control of DCIS. Updated reports show that the local recurrence rate in the group having lumpectomy alone (at a median follow-up period of 4 years) is approximately 20%, with one-half of these recurrences presenting as invasive cancers. In the lumpectomy and radiation group, the recurrence rate is about 10%, but only one-fourth of these recurrences are invasive cancers. Only results from longer follow-up periods will reveal the true recurrence risk and the percentage of patients who die of recurrent invasive, metastatic disease. At the present time, mastectomy is still the standard treatment for all but the smaller lesions, although more and more women and their oncologists are willing to accept the recurrence risks because of the chance for breast conservation.

C. Lobular Carcinoma In Situ: LCIS would be better termed lobular hyperplasia. It is not considered a carcinoma in its own right but, like atypical ductal hyperplasia, is a marker of increased cancer risk throughout the breast epithelium. It is usually found incidentally at the time of a breast biopsy, and no specific treatment such as extensive excision is recommended. The risk of a future cancer in the ipsilateral breast is approximately 20–25% and is almost equally high in the other breast. In the past, some breast surgeons recommended bilateral mastectomy because of this high risk, but most women currently choose to be followed carefully by mammography and physical examination and have surgery only if a cancer occurs. There is no indication that cancers arising in a background of LCIS are more aggressive than other breast cancers. Careful breast examination by a physician every 6 months with annual mammography is a reasonable monitoring schedule for a patient with LCIS.

D. Inflammatory and Locally Advanced Breast Cancer: Inflammatory breast cancer traditionally has had an extremely poor prognosis. When primary mastectomy was performed, it was found that the surgeon was cutting across tumor because of the extensive invasion in the dermal lymphatics. Not only was there a high rate of systemic spread, but the local recurrence rates in the chest wall were unacceptably high. Preoperative radiation considerably improved the local recurrence rates but did nothing for systemic metastases. Currently, the accepted treatment for inflammatory breast cancer is initial chemotherapy—neoadjuvant chemotherapy—to shrink the tumor (often extremely successful) and provide early systemic protection. This treatment commonly is followed by mastectomy and then irradiation. Some centers give all the chemotherapy preoperatively; others give a "sandwich" regimen: chemotherapy, surgery, chemotherapy. With neoadjuvant chemotherapy as part of triple-modality treatment, the 5-year disease-free survival for inflammatory breast cancer now approaches 50%.

For locally advanced, unresectable breast cancer, neoadjuvant chemotherapy has also been successful in producing sufficient shrinkage to allow subsequent surgery (followed by radiation therapy). Again, disease-free survival at 5 years approaches 50% for this subgroup of women who traditionally had a dismal prognosis. Whether neoadjuvant chemotherapy has a role in operable locally advanced breast cancer is currently being debated. The advantage of neoadjuvant chemotherapy is that the patient receives the earliest possible systemic treatment; the main disadvantage is that the opportunity for accurate staging necessary for many protocols is lost. In addition, if the cancer grows despite chemotherapy there is a theoretical possibility that it may become inoperable due to the delay.

Radiation Therapy

If an invasive breast cancer is treated conservatively with lumpectomy, irradiation of the breast (with or without a boost, depending on the closeness of the margins) is part of the definitive treatment. If irradiation is not given, the chance of a local relapse within the breast is between 30 and 50%. With radiation therapy, the local recurrence rate is reported to be less than 5%. Radiation therapy without lumpectomy is not as effective in controlling the primary cancer.

If a mastectomy is performed as the primary definitive surgery, radiation treatment is not given routinely. Many studies have shown that radiation to the chest wall after mastectomy can reduce the local recurrence risk but does not affect survival, presumably because patients die of systemic metastases and not from a local recurrence. Therefore, radiation after mastectomy is given for specific indications only, eg, if a resection margin was positive, if the tumor was very close to the margin, if the original cancer was very large, or if there was extensive lymphatic invasion or chest-wall involvement. If more than four axillary lymph nodes were positive, irradiation of the chest wall and axilla often is recommended because the local recurrence risk in this subset of patients is high (approximately 30%). Finally, axillary irradiation commonly is given if there is extracapsular extension from involved axillary lymph nodes.

Adjuvant Chemotherapy

When it was realized that systemic spread of breast cancer cells can occur early, while the primary tumor is still small, clinical trials were initiated to see whether these micrometastases could be eliminated by chemotherapy before they grew to be well-established tumors. In the original studies, single drugs were given for short, perioperative courses with the rationale that the cells may be shed systemically at the time of surgery. As the trials evolved, multiple drugs were used for an extended number of cycles. In the initial studies, women who had a significant chance of a relapse—those with positive axillary lymph nodes—were enrolled and randomized to groups receiving either chemotherapy or no systemic treatment. By the time of the NIH consensus conference in 1985, it was clear that premenopausal women with positive lymph nodes gained a significant benefit from adjuvant chemotherapy, and it became standard practice to offer chemotherapy to this group. When the 10-year follow-up figures were published in 1985 for the regimen of cyclophosphamide, methotrexate, and 5-fluorouracil (5-FU), referred to as CMF, it was shown that premenopausal women with positive lymph nodes had an overall survival of 59% at 10 years in the CMF group compared with 45% in the control group. This 14% absolute increase in survival can be reported also as a 25% decrease in mortality. Most oncologists and patients recognize this difference to be a substantial benefit.

The same trial showed about a 2% absolute improvement in 10-year overall survival in postmenopausal women with positive lymph nodes; this benefit was thought to be too small to justify the standard use of chemotherapy in this group of older women. Since publication of the 1985 guidelines, therefore, premenopausal but not postmenopausal women with positive lymph nodes have been offered chemotherapy as standard treatment.

In 1992 the long-awaited meta-analysis by the Early Breast Cancer Trialists' Collaborative Group (EBCTCG) of all adjuvant chemotherapy trials (133 in number) that included treatment and control arms was published. This meta-analysis upheld the benefits of chemotherapy to premenopausal women with positive lymph nodes but showed some interesting new perspectives. When the postmenopausal group was broken down by age, it was noted that women between 50 and 59 benefited from the chemotherapy more than those who were 60–69 years old (although not as much as those who were less than 50 years old). In the past few years, therefore, more women in the 50- to 59-year-old group are being offered adjuvant chemotherapy if they had positive lymph nodes. Older women are encouraged to participate in clinical trials that are attempting to improve outcome with improved adjuvant regimens.

A second important finding from the meta-analysis was that women with negative lymph nodes derived a significant benefit from adjuvant chemotherapy, a result that was suspected for several years. In fact, in 1988 three ongoing trials were halted by the National Cancer Institute because the women in the treated groups were doing better than the controls. Premenopausal women with negative lymph nodes were found to experience the same percentage reduction in recurrence and mortality as women with positive lymph nodes, but because the absolute recurrence rates are smaller, the absolute benefit is also smaller (approximately half the benefit seen in the node-positive group).

Which patients with negative lymph nodes should receive adjuvant chemotherapy? Quite simply, women whose risk of recurrence is high enough to justify the toxicity with the promise of significant benefit. Most oncologists would agree that a woman with a 5-mm cancer with negative lymph nodes has a greater than 95% cure rate with surgery and radiation alone and that to attempt to improve outcome with chemotherapy (which might improve the cure rate to 96%) seems foolhardy. Young women with negative lymph nodes with tumors greater than 2 cm in size probably have a 10-year disease-free survival of only 70%, and most oncologists would treat this subgroup with chemotherapy, hoping to improve the disease-free survival rate to almost 80%. In between these two examples lies a gray area. Currently, most oncologists make decisions on whom to treat based on tumor size, grade, mitotic index, and ER status; one day there may be an algorithm that incorporates more of the biologic prognostic factors outlined previously.

Although CMF for 6 months is still regarded as standard adjuvant chemotherapy for breast cancer, in recent years there has been a trend toward using a regimen of cyclophosphamide, doxorubicin (Adriamycin), and 5-FU (CAF) instead of CMF. Because doxorubicin is more active against breast cancer than methotrexate, and because CAF gives a higher response rate than CMF when there is measurable metastatic disease, it was assumed that CAF would give improved results in the adjuvant setting. Rigorous proof of this advantage in direct comparisons has been hard to demonstrate, indicating that the increased effectiveness of CAF is probably small, but there is evidence that women who receive doxorubicin before other drugs have better outcomes than those who receive the same regimens without doxorubicin. More recently, a regimen of cyclophosphamide and doxorubicin without 5-FU (CA) has been gaining popularity.

Current clinical research in adjuvant chemotherapy regimens is focused on dose-intensity, with the hope that more dose-intensive regimens (often with growth-factor support) will improve the 10-year disease-free survival rate, on combination chemotherapy-hormonal therapy, and on neoadjuvant chemotherapy. (Some encouraging results have been obtained suggesting that the effects of chemotherapy and hormonal therapy may be additive.) Neoadjuvant chemotherapy is given before surgery and has become accepted treatment for locally advanced and inflammatory breast cancer, but its role in earlier stage breast cancer has not been defined. Finally, what role new drugs such as paclitaxel and docetaxel will have in the adjuvant setting still is to be defined.

Side effects of CMF include amenorrhea and infertility (age-related), partial alopecia, and a risk of secondary acute leukemia of approximately 1.3% at 7 years. With CAF there is total alopecia and a risk of cardiac toxicity of approximately 1%. Nausea used to be common with CAF, but with the improved antiemetics available today, nausea is well controlled in most cases.

Adjuvant Hormonal Therapy

At the NIH consensus conference of 1985, adjuvant tamoxifen was recommended for postmenopausal women with positive lymph nodes whose tumors were estrogen-receptor-positive. This group has been shown repeatedly to derive substantial benefit from hormonal therapy. The meta-analysis upheld this benefit, which is approximately equal to the benefit premenopausal women gain from chemotherapy (a 25–30% decrease in risk of recurrence) with a significant survival benefit. Premenopausal women with positive lymph nodes derive only a small benefit from tamoxifen, probably because they have a high endogenous estradiol level (which increases when tamoxifen is taken); therefore, chemotherapy remains the treatment of choice for that group. Whether tamoxifen after chemotherapy in the treatment of premenopausal women will give additional benefit over

that from chemotherapy alone has not been shown clearly and currently is being tested.

New information from the meta-analysis included the observation that postmenopausal women with positive axillary lymph nodes benefited substantially from tamoxifen even if their tumors were estrogen-receptor-negative. Although the magnitude of the benefit is only approximately half of that seen for women with ER-positive tumors, it is considered worthwhile. The current recommendation, therefore, is that postmenopausal women with positive axillary lymph nodes receive tamoxifen regardless of ER status; it is still debated whether these women also should receive chemotherapy, which is of lesser benefit. Premenopausal women with positive lymph nodes but negative estrogen receptors do not benefit from tamoxifen.

Node-negative patients also benefit from tamoxifen. As with chemotherapy, the benefit from adjuvant tamoxifen was the same as in node-positive women if expressed as a percentage reduction in recurrence; the benefit was considerably less in absolute terms because of the better prognosis of node-negative patients. The decision concerning which women with negative lymph nodes should receive adjuvant tamoxifen depends on a risk-benefit analysis. Because tamoxifen has fewer side effects than chemotherapy, it is prescribed more commonly when the benefit is likely to be marginal. Thus, postmenopausal women with ER-positive tumors 1.2 cm in size often receive tamoxifen even though their prognosis is already excellent.

Tamoxifen is not a pure antiestrogen. It has pro-estrogenic as well as antiestrogenic properties. Fortunately, this combination of qualities results in many positive side effects. It is proestrogenic in terms of its action on the cardiovascular system and bones. Tamoxifen has been shown to have a significant protective effect in postmenopausal women against death from cardiovascular disease (12% decrease in mortality, mostly from a decrease in strokes and myocardial infarctions), and the benefit of decreased osteoporotic bone loss also has been demonstrated. A further benefit is the reported reduction in risk of a new, contralateral breast cancer (2% risk in controls, 1.3% in the tamoxifen group). For these reasons, tamoxifen is liberally prescribed for postmenopausal women.

The side effects of tamoxifen are generally manageable. Hot flashes are common (approximately one-third of patients), decrease after a few weeks, and only rarely lead to cessation of the drug. Vaginal dryness can be made worse or, paradoxically, better (tamoxifen can act as an estrogen on the cervical glands and vagina). Postmenopausal women often notice a scant white or yellow mucoid discharge similar to that seen in mid cycle in premenopausal women. Recently, the slightly increased risk of endometrial cancer associated with tamoxifen use has been quantitated. In one European study (using 40 mg of tamoxifen daily), the incidence of endometrial cancer in the tamoxifen-treated group was 5%. However, the largest prospective study in this country, using a lower dosage of 20 mg of tamoxifen daily, showed a rate of endometrial cancer of 1.06% in the tamoxifen group compared with 0.14% in the placebo group, an overall increased risk of 7.6-fold. For patients in whom the benefit from tamoxifen is substantial, the small risk of endometrial cancer, although real, should not deter use of the drug; endometrial carcinoma usually presents with vaginal bleeding while still confined to the endometrium (stage I) and is highly curable with a prompt hysterectomy. Women taking tamoxifen should be made aware of the risk and counseled to seek prompt gynecologic evaluation for any vaginal bleeding.

Because tamoxifen has not been useful in premenopausal women, many current clinical trials are looking at the effectiveness of adjuvant treatment with luteinizing hormone-releasing hormone (LH-RH) agonists, which suppress ovarian function, given with and without tamoxifen. Furthermore, there is a renewed interest in oophorectomy because the EBCTCG's meta-analysis reported that oophorectomy in premenopausal women with positive lymph nodes gave benefits similar to those seen from chemotherapy. It is hoped that a combination of chemotherapy and ovarian ablation will be even more beneficial.

Treatment of Recurrent Disease

Recurrence of cancer in a breast treated conservatively with lumpectomy and irradiation, although unfortunate, is not a life-threatening event. Usually a "salvage" mastectomy is required, but prognosis is not altered, ie, women who choose lumpectomy have the same long-term prognosis as those who choose mastectomy regardless of whether there is a recurrence in the breast or not. A recurrence in the chest wall after a mastectomy has a worse prognosis. It is common for women with chest wall recurrences also to have systemic recurrences, and local treatment (excision, chest-wall radiation) probably yields a long-term disease-free survival rate of only about 20%. With modern CT, scanning, a small group of women with local recurrence and no synchronous distant spread can be selected for aggressive treatment, which may include chest-wall resection, with perhaps a 50% chance of long-term disease-free survival. Whether a course of chemotherapy at the time of such an isolated recurrence can improve these statistics is still speculative.

Unfortunately, most relapses are systemic. The most common sites of involvement are the bones, pleurae, lungs, and liver, but almost any part of the body can be affected. Although experimental therapies such as bone-marrow transplantation (see the following section) are being tried for curative purposes, the goal of treating metastatic disease should usually be palliation because standard treatments give no realistic chance of a cure. Breast cancer is usually responsive to systemic therapy, and there is no doubt that patients who respond benefit in terms of longevity and improvement in quality of life because of a significant reduction in complications secondary to metastases. Radiation therapy usually is reserved for palliation of pain, as prophylaxis for impending bony fractures or cord compression, or for brain metastases.

The two choices for systemic therapy are hormonal therapy and chemotherapy. Hormonal therapy usually is given first if the patient has an ER-positive cancer because it is gentler and yet can give as good a response rate as chemotherapy. Approximately two-thirds of women with ER-positive cancers respond to first-line hormonal treatment; the response rate is even higher (approximately 75%) if progesterone receptors are also positive but significantly lower (approximately 25%) if progesterone receptors are negative. Because it has the fewest side effects, tamoxifen is the usual first-line hormonal therapy. The mean time to an objective response is 2 months, and the mean duration of response is 1–2 years. Metastases in soft tissue and bone usually respond well, whereas visceral metastases (brain, liver, and lung) tend to respond poorly. If a patient has a good initial response to first-line hormonal therapy, there is a strong chance (50%) of a response to second-line hormonal therapy such as megestrol acetate or aminoglutethimide. The duration of response to hormonal therapy is quite variable, and it is not uncommon for an elderly patient with indolent breast cancer to be stable on hormonal therapy for many years and die of unrelated causes. In premenopausal women, tamoxifen has a reasonable response rate, but it is probably not as effective as oophorectomy. Newer hormonal therapies currently in clinical trials include use of aromatase inhibitors, LH-RH analogues, and progesterone antagonists. Regimens of high-dose progestins have significant toxicity and do not seem to be more effective than those of standard-dose progestins.

Chemotherapy is the next systemic treatment of choice for women who have progressed with hormonal therapy. It is the first treatment of choice for women with ER-negative cancers or who, despite having ER-positive cancers, experience rapid progression of their disease or are in "visceral crisis"; chemotherapy works faster than hormonal therapy and works more reliably on visceral metastases. Using common three-drug regimens such as CMF or CAF, response rates in the 50–75% range can be achieved easily. However, the complete response rate is low (approximately 10%), and the duration of response is short (6–12 months). Median survival time after institution of chemotherapy is $1\frac{1}{2}$–$2\frac{1}{2}$ years. Although more aggressive regimens can give higher response rates, longer survival does not result; therefore, regimens of moderate intensity remain the treatments of choice outside experimental protocols. After relapse from initial response to chemotherapy, response to second-line chemotherapy may be only 25% and to third-line chemotherapy only 10–15%. Clonal evolution and the development of drug resistance seem to be responsible for this poor responsiveness.

Role of Bone-Marrow Transplantation

Because there is a clear dose-response relationship in the treatment of metastatic breast cancer with chemotherapy, it has been speculated that metastatic breast cancer might be curable if the doses of the drugs could be escalated sufficiently. Autologous bone-marrow transplantation (ABMT) is a method of allowing otherwise lethal doses of chemotherapy to be given to a patient in an attempt to eradicate the cancer. The patient's own bone marrow is harvested and frozen while the high-dose chemotherapy is administered. After the body has excreted the drugs, the bone-marrow cells are infused and the patient's blood counts recover.

There have been dramatic improvements in techniques of transplantation in the last few years. Chemotherapy and growth factors are used now to stimulate the release of bone-marrow stem cells into the circulation from where they can be harvested by using a pheresis machine to skim off the white cells. This method allows harvesting to be done in the outpatient setting without the use of general anesthesia or an operating room. With peripheral stem cells and the use of growth factors such as G-CSF, recovery times for the blood counts can be quite rapid, sometimes as early as 9–10 days after stem cell infusion; the number of days in the hospital is reduced considerably as is the cost of the transplantation.

The first ABMTs for breast cancer were performed on women with advanced metastatic disease who had undergone many chemotherapy regimens. Although response rates to the high-dose chemotherapy were superb and rapid, these women relapsed within approximately 8 months of their transplants. Currently, the best candidates for bone-marrow transplantation are young women with limited metastatic disease who have had minimal previous chemotherapy and show a good response to "induction" chemotherapy (such as CAF), which is used to decrease the burden of disease. Bone marrow should be free of contamination by tumor cells. If a complete response or a good partial response is achieved, high-dose "consolidation" with ABMT may result in a 20% incidence of disease-free survival after 3 years. Whether any of these women are cured is not known yet; longer follow-up is needed. At the present time, randomized trials are ongoing to assess the role of "up-front" ABMT in the adjuvant setting for women who are at high risk of recurrence despite standard adjuvant chemotherapy, such as women who have 10 or more positive axillary lymph nodes. It will be important to compare results from these trials with results from trials of high-dose adjuvant chemotherapy with growth factors but without ABMT.

FOLLOW-UP

A patient who has had a lumpectomy for early-stage breast cancer needs to be followed for recurrence in the breast as well as for systemic recurrence. Usually the patient is seen and examined every 3 months for the first year, every 4 months for the second year, and every 6 months thereafter. A baseline mammogram often is requested 6 months after completion of radiation therapy, and bilateral mammograms are performed annually (occasionally every 6 months if the radiologist has a concern).

Mammography (looking for a recurrence in the breast or a new primary tumor) and physical examination (looking especially for local or regional recurrences) are the most important of the follow-up tests for patients with breast cancer because they may disclose lesions that are curable. Routine chest x-rays, bone scans, and liver scans are no longer recommended; they have not affected outcome in clinical trials, presumably because they detect systemic metastases that can be treated only with palliation. Noninvasive assessments for metastases include a detailed review of systems; a thorough general physical examination looking especially for adenopathy, chest-wall lesions, pleural effusions, hepatomegaly, bony tenderness, or neurologic dysfunction; and blood tests to screen for bone (alkaline phosphatase) and liver (liver function tests) abnormalities. These examinations and tests usually are performed every 4–6 months. Tumor markers are still investigational in breast cancer. Carcinoembryonic antigen (CEA) is neither sensitive nor specific enough to be reliable, and CA15.3, although more sensitive and specific, is not ideal. If ABMT proves to have a curative role in the treatment of metastatic disease, the routine use of scans and tumor markers to pick up metastatic disease at the earliest possible stage will have to be reassessed to give young women the best chance of a cure.

ISSUES OF PREGNANCY & BREAST CANCER

It was believed previously that breast cancer occurring during pregnancy had a worse prognosis than average; in fact, stage for stage the prognosis probably is not worse than that experienced by a nonpregnant woman. However, the breast swelling that accompanies pregnancy makes it more difficult to detect masses. Similarly, there has been a fear that pregnancy in a patient with a history of breast cancer might trigger a relapse because of the elevated hormone levels; again, this fear does not seem to be justified in practice. Advice to a woman who desires to become pregnant should be based on common sense; the assessment of the advisability of pregnancy depends on the statistical likelihood of recurrence, the decreased ability to detect a recurrence during pregnancy, and the dilemma posed by the possible need for systemic treatments for a recurrence during pregnancy.

HORMONE REPLACEMENT THERAPY AFTER BREAST CANCER

The conventional wisdom has been that hormone replacement therapy (HRT) after breast cancer is too dangerous to contemplate. However, it is important to consider all aspects of the woman and not just the woman as a cancer patient. For a woman with a history of DCIS 10 years previously who is now postmenopausal, has a strong family history of osteoporosis and heart disease, and herself has hypercholesterolemia, the risk-benefit ratio is almost certainly in favor of giving replacement estrogen and following her mammographically. A woman at higher risk of recurrence might be given tamoxifen for its proestrogenic effects. For women who have intolerable vaginal dryness making intercourse impossible even after the use of lubricants, low doses of topical estrogen cream seem reasonable, but if they are at moderate or high risk of breast cancer recurrence, concurrent systemic protection with tamoxifen is a wise precaution.

There has never been a prospective study addressing the impact of HRT on recurrence of breast cancer, and there is increasing circumstantial evidence that the recurrence risk may not be increased. Because of the enormous benefits of HRT on the cardiovascular system and bones, many experts are demanding randomized prospective trials to define the risk-benefit ratio of HRT in survivors of breast cancer.

CHEMOPREVENTION

Prevention of breast cancer is clearly desirable. Because the etiology is unknown, preventive efforts are aimed at inhibition of proliferation of the breast epithelium. In this country, the National Surgical Adjuvant Breast and Bowel Project (NSABP) protocol P-1 is randomizing 16,000 women deemed to be at high risk of breast cancer to groups that will receive tamoxifen or placebo for 5 years. Similar studies are ongoing in Europe, where fenretinide (a vitamin A derivative) also is in clinical trials. Because of the link between lifetime number of ovulatory cycles and incidence of breast cancer, a clinical trial is being conducted at the University of Southern California to see whether the risk of breast cancer can be reduced by chemical oophorectomy with LH-RH agonists. Young women participating in this trial are given low-dose replacement estrogen and pulse progesterone every 4 months.

Because of the concept of the "window of susceptibility," which seems to close with the first full-term pregnancy, reproductive endocrinologists have speculated that hormonal therapy designed to mimic pregnancy might induce similar changes in the breast epithelium and be protective. However, the ethical problems of performing such trials on teenage girls are forbidding. It is hoped that the next decade will see much more research into chemoprevention that will translate into a decrease in incidence of this feared disease.

REFERENCES

Beahrs OH et al (editors): *Manual for Staging of Cancer,* 4th ed. Lippincott, 1992.

Boice JD Jr et al: Frequent chest x-ray fluoroscopy and breast cancer incidence among tuberculosis patients in Massachusetts. Radiat Res 1991;125:214.

Boring CC et al: Cancer statistics. CA 1994;44:7.

Cobleigh MA et al: Estrogen replacement therapy in breast cancer survivors: A time for change. JAMA 1994;272:540.

Colditz GA: Epidemiology of breast cancer: Findings from the nurses' health study. Cancer 1993;71[4(Suppl)]:1480.

Dupont WD, Page DL: Risk factors for breast cancer in women with proliferative breast disease. N Engl J Med 1985;312:146.

Dupont WD et al: Long-term risk of breast cancer in women with fibroadenoma. N Engl J Med 1994;331:10.

Early Breast Cancer Trialists' Collaborative Group: Systemic treatment of early breast cancer by hormonal, cytotoxic, or immune therapy. (Meta-analysis.) Lancet 1992;339:1;71.

Fisher B, Anderson S: Conservative surgery for the management of invasive and noninvasive carcinoma of the breast: NSABP trials. National Surgical Adjuvant Breast and Bowel Project. World J Surg 1994;18:63.

Fisher B et al: Endometrial cancer in tamoxifen-treated breast cancer patients: Findings from the National Surgical Adjuvant Breast and Bowel Project (NSABP) B-14. J Natl Cancer Inst 1994;86:527.

Frykberg ER, Bland KI: Management of in situ and minimally invasive breast carcinoma. World J Surg 1994;18:45.

Harris JR et al (editors): *Breast Diseases,* 2nd ed. Lippincott, 1991.

Kagan AR, Steckel RJ: Routine imaging studies for the posttreatment surveillance of breast and colorectal carcinoma. J Clin Oncol 1991;9:837.

Kelloff GJ et al: Development of breast cancer chemopreventive drugs. J Cell Biochem [Suppl] 1993;17G:2.

Liehr JG: Genotoxic effects of estrogens. Mutat Res 1990;238:269.

Lynch HT et al: Hereditary breast cancer and family cancer syndromes. World J Surg 1994;18:21.

MacMahon B: Pesticide residues and breast cancer? (Editorial.) J Natl Cancer Inst 1994;86:572.

McCormick B: Radiation therapy for breast cancer. Curr Opin Oncol 1993;5:976.

Miki Y et al: A strong candidate for the breast and ovarian cancer susceptibility gene BRCA1. Science 1994; 266:66.

Miller BA, Feuer EJ, Hankey BF: Recent incidence trends for breast cancer in women and the relevance of early detection: An update. CA 1993;43:27.

Muss HB: Endocrine therapy for advanced breast cancer: A review. Breast Cancer Res Treat 1992;21:15.

Newcomb PA et al: Lactation and a reduced risk of premenopausal breast cancer. N Engl J Med 1994;330:81.

NIH consensus conference: Treatment of early-stage breast cancer. JAMA 1991;265:391.

Petrek JA: Pregnancy safety after breast cancer. Cancer 1994; 4(Suppl 1):528.

Pike MC, Spicer DV: The chemoprevention of breast cancer by reducing sex steroid exposure: Perspectives from epidemiology. J Cell Biochem [Suppl] 1993;17G:26.

Pike MC et al: Estrogens, progestogens, normal breast cell proliferation, and breast cancer risk. Epidemiol Rev 1993;15:17.

Proceedings of the NIH Consensus Development Conference, September 9–11, 1985. Adjuvant chemotherapy for breast cancer. Cancer Treat Res 1992;60:375.

Rosenberg L, Metzger LS, Palmer JR: Alcohol consumption and risk of breast cancer: A review of the epidemiologic evidence. Epidemiol Rev 1993;15:133.

Thomas DB: Oral contraceptives and breast cancer. (Commentary.) J Natl Cancer Inst 1993;85:359.

Vaughan WP: Autologous bone marrow transplantation in the treatment of breast cancer: Clinical and technologic strategies. Semin Oncol 1993;20;5[Suppl 6]:55.

Wong K, Henderson IC: Management of metastatic breast cancer. World J Surg 1994;18:98.

Wood WC: Integration of risk factors to allow patient selection for adjuvant systemic therapy in lymph node-negative breast cancer patients. World J Surg 1994;18:39.

Wynder EL et al: Dietary fat and breast cancer: Where do we stand on the evidence? J Clin Epidemiol 1994;47: 217; discussion 223.

Benign Breast Disorders

Joan E. Miller, MD

Breast symptoms, such as pain, tenderness, nipple discharge, swelling, nodularity, and lumps, are common reasons for a visit to a physician. Because breast cancer and benign breast disorders may present with the same symptoms, it is critical to rule out a malignant condition as the cause for the presenting symptom. Benign breast disorders comprise an array of symptoms and clinical and histopathologic diagnoses.

MASTODYNIA (Mastalgia)

Essentials of Diagnosis
- Pain in the breast. Often cyclic and worse during the luteal phase of the menstrual cycle.
- Rarely the sole presenting symptom of breast cancer.

Risk Factors
Mastodynia is common; most women experience some breast tenderness during the luteal phase of their menstrual cycle. Some women who take contraceptive pills or estrogen for hormone replacement therapy note an increase in breast pain. The most common age of presentation is 30–50 years.

Signs & Symptoms
Breast pain may occur alone or with other signs and symptoms such as nodularity, dominant lump, or breast swelling. It may be a component of the multi-symptom complex, premenstrual syndrome. It is usually cyclic; when it is persistent and noncyclic, it raises the suspicion of an underlying cancer.

Clinical Findings & Diagnosis
The history should include the location and character of the pain, the timing and relationship to the menstrual cycle, medications being taken (especially oral contraceptives or hormones), risk factors for breast cancer (family history, age at menarche, parity, past history of breast disease), and impact on lifestyle. A thorough breast examination must be performed to identify any dominant masses or other abnormalities. Mammography should be done if a suspicious abnormality is found on breast examination. The guidelines for mammography are contro-

Mastodynia (Mastalgia)
    Essentials of Diagnosis
    Risk Factors
    Signs & Symptoms
    Clinical Findings & Diagnosis
    Treatment
    Psychosocial Concerns
Mastitis
    Essentials of Diagnosis
    Risk Factors
    Signs & Symptoms
    Clinical Findings & Diagnosis
    Treatment
Nipple Discharge
    Essentials of Diagnosis
    Risk Factors
    Signs & Symptoms
    Clinical Findings & Diagnosis
    Treatment
    Prognosis
    Referral to a Specialist
    Special Issues of Pregnancy
Fibrocystic Breast Changes
    Essentials of Diagnosis
    Risk Factors
    Signs & Symptoms
    Clinical Findings & Diagnosis
    Treatment
    Prognosis—Risk of Subsequent Breast
        Cancer
    Referral to a Specialist
    Psychosocial Concerns

versial, but it is not unreasonable to perform mammography on women 35 years and older who present with mastodynia. Ultrasonography can be used to distinguish cysts from solid lesions; solid masses should be biopsied. Hormonal evaluation is usually not indicated.

The history and physical examination should exclude other causes of pain in the breast area such as musculoskeletal conditions, costochondritis, or angina.

Treatment

After an underlying malignant condition is ruled out, the patient can be reassured. Although most patients are satisfied with this assurance, a small subset of patients may experience pain that is severe or lasts for a prolonged period of time, so that some sort of treatment is desired. A pain chart or calendar is helpful in evaluating these patients (Fig 25–1). Most studies of treatment for mastodynia include only patients with severe cyclic mastodynia that has been present for more than 10 days of the monthly cycle for longer than 6 months.

Treatments for mastodynia have ranged from dietary therapy to hormonal manipulation. Physical factors such as wearing a properly fitted brassiere are important. Advocates for dietary therapy recommend a low-fat, high-fiber diet with beta-carotene, vitamin C, vitamin E, and selenium. Vitamin E supplementation has gained popularity as a treatment, although there are no studies to support its use. A randomized, controlled trial of 21 patients who had cyclic mastodynia for at least 5 years found that patients who followed a diet for 6 months that was low in fat (less than 15% of calories) and high in complex carbohydrates had a significant reduction in premenstrual breast swelling and tenderness. Avoidance of caffeine has been advocated; however, several studies have failed to find a relationship between caffeine intake, mastalgia, and fibrocystic breast changes.

Diuretics may be beneficial in treating cyclic mastalgia. Although no controlled studies specifically looking at diuretics have been reported, a study of weight and total body water changes during the menstrual cycle has been done. A comparison of women who have mastalgia with symptom-free age-matched controls showed no difference in premenstrual total body water: weight ratio.

Evening primrose oil, a natural product with a high content of essential fatty acids that is thought to act via prostaglandin mediators, has been recommended at a dose of 1000 mg orally 3 times daily. Pyridoxine, or vitamin B$_6$, 100 mg every day, had a 49% response rate in one retrospective study. Side effects of nausea and headache were seen in 2%. However, a double-blind controlled trial studying pyridoxine, 200 mg daily, found no significant difference compared to placebo.

Bromocriptine is a long-acting dopaminergic drug that suppresses prolactin. A European multicenter study (double-blind, parallel-group design) of bromocriptine, 2.5 mg orally twice daily, compared to placebo showed significant improvement in pain and tenderness in the group treated with bromocriptine. There were side effects in 41% of the treated patients (headache, nausea, vomiting) with a 26% dropout rate.

Tamoxifen, 10–20 mg orally daily for 3 months, has been shown to be beneficial in treating cyclic mastodynia but has many side effects including menorrhagia, hot flushes, nausea, headaches, depression, irritability, and alopecia.

Danazol has been shown to be effective in at least

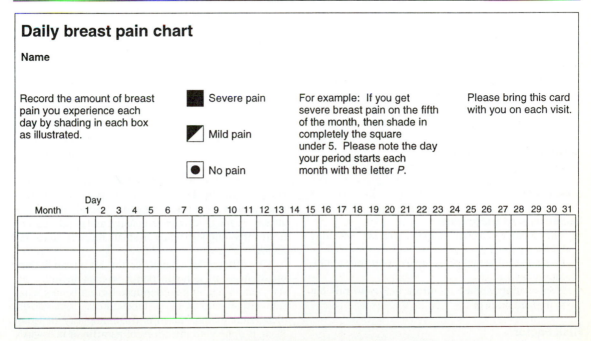

Figure 25–1. Daily breast pain chart.

two controlled trials, but side effects such as bloating, weight gain, menstrual irregularities, and nausea may make the treatment unacceptable. Dosages of 100–200 mg orally twice daily have been used. Some advocate tapering the dosage to arrive at a maintenance luteal-phase dosage (starting from 100 mg/d, days 14–28).

Nafarelin, an octapeptide analogue of gonadotropin-releasing hormone (GN-RH) used as a nasal spray, was not found to be significantly different from placebo and had side effects of vasomotor symptoms and menstrual irregularities. Long-term use may cause osteoporosis.

Micronized progesterone (100 mg) as a vaginal cream at bedtime on days 10–25 of the menstrual cycle for 6 months was effective in a placebo-controlled trial. No major side effects were reported.

An approach to management of patients with cyclic mastodynia used by a breast pain clinic is as follows:

1. Evaluate the patient and rule out cancer.
2. Reassure the patient of the benign nature of the condition.
3. After 2 months, if cyclic mastodynia is confirmed in a pain diary and the patient desires treatment, begin pyridoxine, 100 mg orally daily for 3 months.
4. If this treatment fails, prescribe oil of evening primrose, 3 g orally daily for 1 month, then 2 g orally daily for 2 months.
5. If this regimen fails, prescribe tamoxifen, danazol, or bromocriptine as a last resort.

Psychosocial Concerns

Mastodynia often causes anxiety in the patient, who fears that an underlying carcinoma is the cause of the pain. Some women experience pain that is sufficient to have an impact on their life-style and activities. They may avoid exercise, sexual activity or intimate contact because of breast pain. The physician should acknowledge the patient's fears and concerns. An open discussion of these issues leads to a better physician-patient relationship and improved patient satisfaction.

MASTITIS

Essentials of Diagnosis

• Inflammatory wedge-shaped area in lactating breast.
• *Staphylococcus* and *Streptococcus* are most commonly present.
• Nonlactating women require a biopsy to rule out malignant disease.

Risk Factors

Puerperal mastitis is thought to be a retrograde infection that results from disruption of the epithelial interface of the nipple-areola complex. Risk factors include nipple fissuring, milk stasis, skipped breast feedings, change in feeding patterns, and mechanical obstruction of a lobule, eg, because of tight brassiere straps. *Staphylococcus aureus* and streptococcal species are the most common bacteria associated with puerperal mastitis.

Mastitis in nonlactating women is rare. Duct ectasia, a benign condition affecting the major breast ducts, is associated with periductal mastitis, periareolar abscess, and mammillary fistula. The cause is unclear, but anaerobic infection is thought to play a role. Chronic infectious disorders (eg, tuberculosis) and inflammatory disorders (eg, inflammatory carcinoma and vasculitis) may present as mastitis.

Signs & Symptoms

Puerperal mastitis often presents as a tender, warm, swollen, wedge-shaped area of the breast associated with fever, chills, flulike aching, and systemic illness. Streptococcal infections often cause a diffuse cellulitis with no localization, whereas staphylococcal infections tend to be more localized and deeply invasive with acute and chronic abscess formation.

Signs of periductal mastitis or duct ectasia include noncyclic mastalgia, a periareolar breast mass, periareolar breast abscess, nipple discharge, nipple retraction, and mammillary fistula.

Clinical Findings & Diagnosis

A lactating woman who presents with signs and symptoms of breast inflammation, especially unilaterally and in a wedge-shaped pattern, most likely has mastitis. Purulent material may be expressed from the nipple and can be sent for culture. Milk can be cultured and a white blood cell (WBC) count determined. Infectious mastitis usually has a WBC count greater than 10,000,000 with bacterial colony counts greater than 10,000. Culture is not needed routinely. If point tenderness, erythema, and a fluctuant mass are present, abscess is suggested.

The differential diagnosis for puerperal mastitis includes engorgement, plugged duct, and all the causes for an inflammatory breast mass in nonlactating women. Engorgement occurs early in the postpartum period and involves both breasts in a generalized fashion. Fever and signs of systemic illness are absent. A plugged duct is usually unilateral and noticed after nursing when a small discrete mass remains.

The differential diagnosis for an inflammatory breast mass in a nonlactating woman includes inflammatory carcinoma, periductal mastitis/duct ectasia, inflammatory cyst, tuberculosis, sarcoidosis, oleogranulomatous mastitis (mammoplasty in Hong Kong is done with injections of paraffin or beeswax), parasitic infections (hydatid disease, filariasis), actinomycosis, blastomycosis, sporotrichosis, and giant cell arteritis. Mammography should be done, followed by drainage of any abscess and biopsy of indurated, viable tissue.

Treatment

Puerperal mastitis should be treated with the following:

1. Antibiotics that are active against *Staphylococcus* sp and *Streptococcus* sp and also safe for the nursing infant; good choices are amoxicillin clavulanate or a first-generation cephalosporin.
2. Drainage of milk from the breast by nursing or breast pump. Some recommend oxytocin nasal spray to enhance milk letdown.
3. Warm or cold compresses. If an abscess is present, surgical drainage is needed.

Periductal mastitis/duct ectasia usually requires surgical treatment, although some physicians recommend treatment with metronidazole and a first-generation cephalosporin because a mixture of anaerobic and aerobic bacteria is involved (*Bacteroides*, anaerobic *Streptococcus*, enterococcus). Surgery involves subareolar dissection and excision of the major duct system.

NIPPLE DISCHARGE

Essentials of Diagnosis

- Galactorrhea implies hyperprolactinemia, which can be due to pituitary adenoma, thyroid disease, medications, and excessive nipple stimulation.
- Associated palpable lump or discharge that is blood-stained and from a single duct raises the suspicion of an underlying cancer.
- Common causes of nipple discharge include normal lactation, galactorrhea (the spontaneous nipple discharge of milklike fluid as a result of stimulation of the breast by elevated secretion of prolactin from the pituitary gland), duct ectasia, intraductal papilloma, and carcinoma.

Risk Factors

Nipple discharge is more common in benign than in malignant lesions. In a study of women undergoing breast operations, it was reported that 7.4% presented initially for nipple discharge. It was the chief complaint in 9% of 6266 women with benign lesions and 3.4% of 2437 women with malignant disease.

In postmenopausal women, the most common cause of nipple discharge is duct ectasia, which is a benign condition affecting the major breast ducts. The second most common cause is intraductal papilloma; carcinoma is a rare cause.

Signs & Symptoms

Nipple discharge can be spontaneous or nonspontaneous (expressed), unilateral or bilateral, and from a single or multiple ducts. Discharge may be green, milky, serous, serosanguineous, sanguineous, or watery. A palpable mass may be present. With a single-duct discharge, a trigger point may be found; pressure at that point produces maximal discharge.

Clinical Findings & Diagnosis

Screening for nipple discharge is done by monthly breast self-examination and by the physician at an annual examination. If a palpable mass is present, a workup for a lump is indicated. If no palpable mass is present and the woman is older than 35 years, mammography should be considered. If discharge is milky, bilateral, and from multiple ducts, a workup for hyperprolactinemia should be initiated. Thyroid-stimulating hormone (TSH) and prolactin levels should be measured. The clinician should ask about medications taken, other medical problems, menstrual pattern, headaches, visual changes, sexual activity, and exercise—especially jogging. Some of the medications that may cause hyperprolactinemia include estrogen-containing oral contraceptives, phenothiazines, reserpine, opiates, H_2-receptor blockers, calcium channel blockers, tricyclic antidepressants, alpha-methyldopa, marihuana, and digoxin. Nipple stimulation from sexual activity or exercise such as jogging can raise prolactin levels. Chronic renal failure and tumors such as bronchogenic carcinoma or hypernephroma can cause hyperprolactinemia.

Patients with bilateral, multiduct discharge who have a normal breast examination and mammogram and normal TSH and prolactin levels should be treated conservatively. Patients with periductal mastitis/duct ectasia may have a unilateral or bilateral discharge, which can vary in color but is rarely blood-stained. They may also have mastalgia, nipple retraction, or a breast mass. A biopsy is the only way to make a definite diagnosis.

Patients with unilateral discharge, especially single-duct discharge, need evaluation for underlying malignant disease or intraductal papilloma. Bloody discharge (urine dipstick may be used for testing) can be seen with carcinoma, intraductal papilloma, duct ectasia, and near-term pregnancy. A bloody discharge in a prepartum woman is usually due to vascular engorgement and clears within weeks. If it persists, a biopsy should be performed.

Galactography, which is contrast mammography obtained by injecting a radiopaque dye into the discharging duct, may be used to visualize and localize an intraductal papilloma; however, it is time-consuming and uncomfortable for the patient. Cytologic study of the discharge is rarely useful; it is said to have a false-negative rate of 17.8% and a false-positive rate of 2.6%.

Treatment

Treatment, of course, depends on the cause of the nipple discharge. Cancers and intraductal papillomas require surgery. Duct ectasia sometimes can be treated by antibiotics, cleansing of the nipples and areolas with povidone-iodine (Betadine) or another antiseptic solution, and avoidance of nipple manipulation. However, the diagnosis is a histologic one. Most patients with duct ectasia are in the perimenopausal or postmenopausal age range and need a more aggressive workup for possible malignant disease, including surgical exploration and duct excision.

Patients with hyperprolactinemia need evaluation for a possible pituitary adenoma. In the absence of secondary causes of hyperprolactinemia, eg, medications, nipple stimulation, pregnancy, or hypothyroidism, patients with an elevated prolactin level should undergo pituitary gland imaging by computed tomography (CT) or magnetic resonance imaging (MRI). Prolactin elevations secondary to medications are generally less than 100 ng/mL.

Patients with nonbloody, bilateral, nonspontaneous discharge who have a normal examination and normal studies should be reassured and followed.

Prognosis

There is an increased likelihood of cancer when the nipple discharge is, in order of increasing frequency, (1) serous (5.9%), (2) serosanguineous (12.9%), (3) sanguineous (27.5%), or (4) watery (33.3%). High risk of cancer also is present when there is a lump, unilateral discharge, single-duct discharge, or abnormal cytologic or mammographic findings and when the patient is older than 50 years. In 13% of patients who had cancer as the cause of nipple discharge, no palpable mass was present.

Referral to a Specialist

Patients with a lump, unilateral discharge, single-duct discharge, bloody discharge, or abnormal mammogram should be referred.

Special Issues of Pregnancy

A bloody nipple discharge can be present in pregnancy, near term. It should clear within a few weeks, and if it persists, a biopsy is indicated.

FIBROCYSTIC BREAST CHANGES

Fibrocystic breast changes, formerly called fibrocystic disease, represent a controversial and confusing condition. Many clinical symptoms and various histologic diagnoses fall in this category. Two synonyms for fibrocystic change are **mammary dysplasia** and **chronic cystic mastitis**.

Clinically, fibrocystic change refers to a condition of lumpy breasts, which may be painful. Histologically, one may see cysts, hyperplasia, atypical hyperplasia, sclerosing adenosis, duct ectasia, fibrosis, or fibroadenoma. Because most women with lumpy breasts never have a breast biopsy, it is difficult to say what constitutes normal versus abnormal nodularity. Some advocate that the benign histopathologic and clinical changes that fall into the category of fibrocystic change be viewed as minor aberrations of normal processes. The concept of aberrations of normal development and involution (ANDI) provides a framework for understanding benign breast disorders. Normal development and involution of breast tissue is divided into 3 stages: (1) the early reproductive period, (2) the mature reproductive period, and (3) involution. Minor abnormalities or aberrations may occur during these stages, resulting in different clinical and pathologic conditions. More severe aberrations result in disease states. Table 25–1 summarizes the ANDI concept.

Essentials of Diagnosis

- Lumpy breasts that are often painful.
- Rapid appearance or disappearance of a breast mass is common with cysts.
- Cysts are rarely malignant.
- Dominant masses should be biopsied.
- Cysts, hyperplasia, atypical hyperplasia, fibrosis, sclerosing adenosis, duct ectasia, fibroadenoma, phyllodes tumor, and papilloma.

Risk Factors

Palpable nodularity is present in at least 50% of women. Autopsy studies have determined that 58% of patients had histologic changes associated with fibrocystic changes. Clinical studies estimate that 7–10% of women have breast cysts. In a study of 10,542 benign breast biopsies in 3303 women, 32% had microcysts and 23% had macrocysts (larger than 1 cm). Oral contraceptive use, especially before the first full-term pregnancy, decreases the risk of benign breast conditions. In a French study, the amount of estrogen in the pill and use of oral contraceptives after the first full-term pregnancy did not affect the risk. In addition, the effect was seen on the risk of nonproliferative changes; there was no effect on proliferative changes.

The effect of the interaction of caffeine and methylxanthines on fibrocystic breast changes is controversial.

Signs & Symptoms

Cyclic mastodynia, tenderness, nodularity, dominant lumps, inflammatory lesions, and nipple discharge may be seen.

Clinical Findings & Diagnosis

Benign causes of breast lumps include cysts, fibroadenomas, and sclerosing adenomas. Cysts are fluid-filled walled spaces which range in size from 1

Table 25–1. Aberrations of normal development and involution.*

| Stage (Peak Age in Years) | Normal Process | Aberration | | Disease State |
		Underlying Condition	Clinical Presentation	
Early reproductive period (15–25)	Lobule development	Fibroadenoma	Discrete lump	Giant fibroadenoma; multiple fibro-adenoma
Mature reproductive period (25–40)	Stroma formation Cyclic hormonal effects on glandular tissue and stroma	Juvenile hypertrophy Exaggerated cyclic effects	Cyclic mastalgia and nodularity— generalized or discrete	
Involution (35–55)	Lobular involution (including microcysts, apocrine change, fibrosis, adenosis)	Macrocysts Sclerosing lesions	Discrete lumps X-ray abnormalities Nipple discharge	Periductal bacterial infection and abscess formation
	Ductal involution (including, periductal round-cell infiltrates)	Duct dilatation		
	Epithelial turnover	Periductal fibrosis Mild epithelial hyperplasia	Nipple retraction Histologic report	Epithelial hyperplasia with atypia

*(Reproduced with permission from Hughes LE: Benign breast disorders: The clinician's view. Cancer Detect Prev 1992;16:1.)

mm to many centimeters. They are often multifocal and bilateral. Cysts can be diagnosed by fine-needle aspiration, ultrasonography, or both. Fibroadenoma is a benign tumor containing primarily fibrous tissue. Fibroadenomas usually arise between the ages of 15 and 25 but often are not diagnosed until later, when the breast is softer and drooping after pregnancy or from involution. A typical fibroadenoma is a mass that is between 1 and 2 cm round, firm, discrete, movable, and nontender. In women less than 25 years of age, a clinically typical fibroadenoma can be left alone, although there are newer data to suggest that it may be important to know the histology of the lesion as it may change the woman's risk for developing breast cancer. In women older than 25 years, biopsy is recommended, because fibroadenoma in this age group may be difficult to distinguish from carcinoma on clinical grounds. Phyllodes tumor is a variant of fibroadenoma that has a potential for malignancy. Sclerosing adenosis may present with mastodynia, a mass, or both. The term sclerosing adenosis is a histopathologic one, and a biopsy must be done to make the diagnosis. Pathologically, it is a nodular epithelial lesion in which fibrosis or myoepithelial proliferation is associated with a whorled distortion of the normal lobular pattern. It may be detectable by mammography; architectural distortion and microcalcifications that are similar to those seen in malignant disease can be seen.

The evaluation and diagnosis of mastodynia and nipple discharge are discussed in preceding sections. Duct ectasia is a condition of dilated ducts that presents as periductal mastitis and nipple discharge. Papilloma is a mass lesion of the large ducts usually in the subareolar region. It causes a bloody nipple discharge. Hyperplasia and atypical hyperplasia are di-agnosed by biopsy. Hyperplasia refers to an increased number of cells relative to a basement membrane. Atypical hyperplasia are lesions that show some but not all of the histologic features of carcinoma-in-situ. There are two types: atypical lobular hyperplasia (ALH) and atypical ductal hyperplasia (ADH).

Treatment

Once an underlying malignant condition is ruled out, many types of fibrocystic breast changes need no treatment. Treatment of mastodynia is discussed previously. Subcutaneous mastectomy is a treatment option for women who undergo multiple biopsies and suffer from severe mastodynia. Women with atypical hyperplasia need close follow-up with routine examinations and mammograms. There are no studies that help define the ideal intervals between checkups.

Cysts may be aspirated or followed. For women who need recurrent cyst aspiration, treatment with danazol may be considered. In one study, danazol, 100 mg 3 times daily for 3 months, decreased new cyst formation in treated women after 6 and 36 months compared to placebo controls. There was no significant difference after 60 months. Side effects of danazol include nausea, bloating, and menstrual irregularities.

Fibroadenomas are easily excised. Phyllodes tumors need a wide excision to prevent recurrence. Papillomas are usually found during the workup of nipple discharge and should be excised.

Prognosis—Risk of Subsequent Breast Cancer

The risk of development of breast cancer depends on the pathologic diagnosis. Dupont and Page showed that the relative risk for developing breast cancer was as follows: proliferative disease 1.9, atypical hyperplasia 4.4, atypical hyperplasia and a positive family history 4.8–17, cysts 1.2–1.9, and cysts and a positive family history 1.9–4.5. Other studies have confirmed that women with atypical hyperplasia have about a fourfold increased risk of breast cancer compared to women without proliferative changes. There is a synergistic effect of atypical hyperplasia and family history. Women with both these risk factors have a relative risk up to 20 times that of women without proliferative changes nor a positive family history. Studies of breast cysts and the relative risk of developing breast cancer have found relative risks to range from 1.7 to 4.0.

In 1986, a consensus statement was released concerning the pathologic diagnosis and risk of breast cancer. Apocrine metaplasia, sclerosing adenosis, cysts, duct ectasia, fibroadenoma, fibrosis, mild hyperplasia, and mastitis have no increased risk. There is a slight increased risk (1.5–2 times) with moderate or severe hyperplasia. Atypical hyperplasia (ductal or lobular) moderately increases the risk (5 times). There is a markedly increased risk (8–10 times) with carcinoma in situ (lobular or ductal).

Recent data on the long term risk of breast cancer in women with fibroadenoma contradicts the 1986 consensus statement. The histological features of the fibroadenoma influence the breast cancer risk. Fibroadenomas which contained cysts greater than 3 mm in diameter, sclerosing adenosis, epithelial calcifications or papillary apocrine changes were classified as complex. The relative risk of developing invasive breast cancer in women with complex fibroadenomas ranged from 2.24 to 3.10 (varying control groups). Having a positive family history of breast cancer or proliferative changes (with or without atypia) increased risk. Also the increased risk of breast cancer persists for greater than twenty years after the diagnosis of fibroadenoma.

Referral to a Specialist

Patients should be referred to a specialist if they have a discrete lump, recent nipple retraction, bloody nipple discharge, single-duct or unilateral nipple discharge, or any condition that is not clearly benign.

Psychosocial Concerns

There can be considerable anxiety regarding breast symptoms because of concerns about underlying breast cancer. Because of the fear of breast cancer, discovering any breast abnormality (lump, swelling, discharge, pain) can cause a great deal of anxiety. Some women may have so much fear that they may delay or avoid evaluation of the breast symptom. Women with lumpy painful breasts may avoid monthly breast self-examination because of the pain and\or because they feel they could not differentiate a "bad lump" from the other lumps they feel in their breasts. Education about breast self-examination and the need for routine examination by the physician is critical.

The medical literature on fibrocystic change is controversial and confusing. Therefore it is not surprising that the lay public is confused and often misinformed. Many women have been labeled as having "fibrocystic disease" just on the basis of palpable nodularity. Often they are led to believe they have an increased risk of developing breast cancer when they may not. Better methods for identifying those women at increased risk for developing breast cancer are needed.

REFERENCES

Benson EA: Management of breast abscesses. World J Surg 1989;13:753.

Boyd NF et al: Effect of a low-fat high-carbohydrate diet on symptoms of cyclic mastopathy. Lancet 1988; 2(8603):128.

Carpenter R, Adamson A, Royle GT: A prospective study of nipple discharge. Br J Clin Pract Symp [Suppl] 1989;68:54.

Charreau I: Oral contraceptive use and risk of benign breast disease in a French case-control study of young women. Eur J Cancer Prev 1993;2:147.

Consensus statement: Is "fibrocystic disease" of the breast precancerous? Arch Pathol Lab Med 1986;110:171.

Devitt JE: Benign breast disease in the postmenopausal woman. World J Surg 1989;13:731.

Devitt JE, To T, Miller AB: Risk of breast cancer in women with breast cysts. Can Med Assoc J 1992;147 (1):45.

Dixon JM: Periductal mastitis/duct ectasia. World J Surg 1989;13:715.

Dogliotti L, Mansel RE: Bromocriptine treatment of cyclical mastalgia/fibrocystic breast disease: Update on the European trial. Br J Clin Pract 1989;43(11):26.

Dupont WD et al: Long-term risk of breast cancer in women with fibroadenoma. N Engl J Med 1994;331:10.

Dupont WD, Page DL: Risk factors for breast cancer in women with proliferative breast disease. N Engl J Med 1985;312:146.

Fentiman IS et al: Studies of tamoxifen in women with mastalgia. Br J Clin Pract Symp [Suppl] 1989;68:34.

Hughes LE: Benign breast disorders: The clinician's view. Cancer Detect Prev 1992;16:1.

Hughes LE, Mansel RE, Webster DJT: Aberrations of normal development and involution (ANDI): A new perspective on pathogenesis and nomenclature of benign breast disorders. Lancet 1987;ii:1316.

Katz E, Adashi EY: Hyperprolactinemic disorders. Clin Obstet Gynecol 1990;33:622.

Lawrence RA: The puerperium, breastfeeding, and breast milk. Curr Opin Obstet Gynecol 1990;2:23.

Leis HP: Management of nipple discharge. World J Surg 1989;13:736.

Levinson W, Dunn PM: Nonassociation of caffeine and fibrocystic breast disease. Arch Intern Med 1986;146:1773.

Locker AP et al: Long-term follow up of patients treated with a course of danazol for recurrent breast cysts. Br J Clin Pract 1989;68:103.

London SJ et al: A prospective study of benign breast disease and the risk of breast cancer. JAMA 1992;267:941.

Love SM, Gelman RS, Silen W: Fibrocystic disease of the breast—a nondisease? N Engl J Med 1982;307:1010.

Lubin F et al: A case-control study of caffeine and methylzanthines in benign breast disease. JAMA 1985;253:2388.

Maddox PR, Harrison BJ, Mansel RE: Low-dose danazol for mastalgia. Br J Clin Pract Symp [Suppl] 1989;68:43.

Maddox PR, Mansel RE: Management of breast pain and nodularity. World J Surg 1989;13:699.

Mansel RE: The clinical assessment of mastalgia. Br J Clin Pract Symp [Suppl] 1989;68:18.

Minton JP, Abou-Issa H: Nonendocrine theories of the etiology of benign breast disease. World J Surg 1989;13:680.

Nappi C et al: Double-blind controlled trial of progesterone vaginal cream treatment for cyclical mastodynia in women with benign breast disease. J Endocrinol Invest 1992;15:801.

Ory H et al: Oral contraceptives and reduced risk of benign breast diseases. N Engl J Med 1976;294:419.

Parazzini F et al: Methyxanthine, alcohol-free diet and fibrocystic breast disease: A factorial clinical trial. Surgery 1986;99:576.

Preece PE et al: Mastalgia and total body water. Br Med J 1975;4:498.

Roberts JV: Experience in the use of nafarelin for treatment of benign breast disease. Br J Clin Pract Symp [Suppl] 1989;68:37.

Smallwood J et al: Vitamin B_6 in the treatment of pre-menstrual mastalgia. Br J Clin Pract 1986;40:532.

Section VI.
Urologic Disorders

26

Dysuria

Tamara G. Bavendam, MD & Laura J. Hart, MD

LOWER URINARY TRACT PAIN & ALTERED VOIDING

Millions of women present to health care providers each year with symptoms of pain or discomfort in their bladder, urethra, or both. The causes of these symptoms range from acute bacterial cystitis to pelvic floor myalgia. Sensations arising from the pelvic organs and supporting musculoskeletal tissue are poorly localized and travel via common pathways to the central nervous system. Consequently, impulses originating in the internal abdominal or pelvic organs or the bones, muscles, and nerves of the pelvis can generate impulses that are perceived as originating in the bladder or urethra.

These noxious sensations may be described as sharp, heavy, stabbing, aching, burning, or cramping, a severe sense of urgency, or an unrelenting awareness of the bladder. The most commonly recognized disorder associated with LUTP, excluding acute bacterial cystitis, is interstitial cystitis (IC). Although it once was thought to be a specific disease associated with progressive fibrosis and ulceration of the bladder, it currently is considered a constellation of symptoms that fall into the category of "sensory disorders of the bladder and urethra."

In this chapter, disorders associated with pain are viewed as dysfunctions rather than diseases. This approach allows the focus to be on symptom control rather than on disease cure; the result is a problem-solving approach to symptom management in which women take primary responsibility for their symptoms. The factors contributing to symptoms of LUTP are often multiple and additive and can be influenced by factors seemingly unrelated to the lower urinary tract. Figure 26–1 contains a depiction of the concept of "triggers" and "amplifiers" of symptoms of LUTP.

Essentials of Diagnosis
- Dysuria and pyuria may indicate bacterial cystitis.
- Dysuria without pyuria should not be diagnosed as an "infection."
- Gross hematuria without evidence of infection needs to be evaluated with intravenous pyelography and cystoscopy.

Lower Urinary Tract Pain & Altered Voiding
   Essentials of Diagnosis
   Lower Urinary Tract Function
   Pain: A Conceptual Overview
   Causes of Lower Urinary Tract Pain
   Other Causes of Lower Urinary Tract Pain
   Evaluation
   Physical Examination
   Laboratory Tests
   Treatment
Hematuria

Lower Urinary Tract Function

Normal functioning of the lower urinary tract (LUT) represents a delicate balance between the bladder and outlet and between the voluntary and involuntary control mechanisms through the autonomic and somatic nerve supply. Although the neurologic control of the LUT is incompletely understood, it generally is agreed that sympathetic innervation is responsible for urine storage and parasympathetic innervation for evacuation of urine. Somatic innervation is through the pudendal nerve to the pelvic floor muscles and the periurethral striated muscle. The bladder acts as a passive storage reservoir during filling and actively contracts during urination. During storage, the bladder outlet must maintain a pressure that exceeds bladder pressure. The role of the bladder neck smooth muscle is to maintain a constant tone or pressure during bladder filling (storage phase). With bladder muscle contraction during the emptying phase, the bladder neck muscle relaxes, which decreases the outlet resistance and promotes emptying.

The anatomic and neurologic forces that promote continence during the storage phase must be reversed for the emptying phase. The coordination between the bladder and outlet mechanisms in the transition phase between storage and emptying is poorly understood and difficult to evaluate in humans because of the significant voluntary (inhibitory and facilitory) influences involved in LUT function. Appreciating the delicate balance between bladder storage and emptying is crucial to understanding the symptoms associated with LUTP and how seemingly innocuous

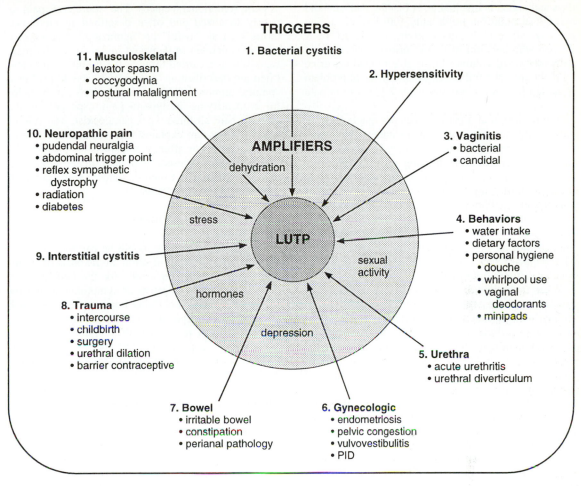

Figure 26–1. Factors triggering lower urinary tract pain (LUTP) with potential symptom amplifiers.

occurrences external to the urinary tract can contribute to its dysfunction.

Normal bladder capacity is considered to be in the range of 400–600 mL. Normally, an initial sense of bladder awareness occurs when the volume is approximately 250–300 mL, with gradually increasing awareness of fullness and the urge to urinate with progressive filling. In general, urination can be postponed indefinitely, and the bladder should never empty without intention. Once the toilet is reached, the outlet must relax and stay relaxed while the detrusor is generating and maintaining a contraction. When the volume in the bladder is less than 200–300 mL, the bladder may have difficulty generating and sustaining a contraction. Without a detrusor contraction, the outlet has difficulty maintaining relaxation. When there is a source of irritation in or around the LUT, the urge to urinate may occur at very low volumes (30–100 mL). At this low volume, coordinated detrusor contraction and outlet relaxation may not

occur, and urination may be hesitant, slow, and interrupted, with a sense of incomplete emptying. This condition can become exacerbated when the sense of urge is intense or painful at low volumes. Chronic straining to initiate or sustain urination against "tight" pelvic muscles can contribute further to the voiding dysfunction. In summary, increased bladder sensitivity can become associated quickly with a voiding dysfunction. Irrespective of what may have caused the irritation initially, the voiding dysfunction can be responsible for chronically maintaining the symptoms.

Most women with LUTP also note increased frequency of urination compared with their previous habits. Although urinating every 3 hours is not excessive, it may be bothersome for someone who used to urinate every 4–6 hours. The key is to determine what bladder volumes signal the urge to urinate and what happens if the signals are ignored. A voiding diary of time and volume of urination over several days and nights is invaluable. A bladder that can hold 600 mL at night but holds only 100–300 mL during the day suggests hypersensitivity of the LUT. A woman who gets out of bed to urinate several times with very small volumes but is able to hold her urine all night once she falls asleep has a different problem from someone who gets up every 2 hours to urinate 100 mL.

The reasons that a patient does not ignore the signals of urgency are important in understanding the cause of the problem. First, she may be afraid of being incontinent. Second, holding may be associated with severe pain, aching, or cramping. Third, the urge sensation may be annoying enough to impair concentration, although the urge can be ignored without fear of leakage or pain. Women may void frequently also because they have been told that holding after getting an urge can lead to bladder infections. This behavior can lead to voiding in progressively smaller volumes out of habit.

When incontinence is a woman's main symptoms, involuntary detrusor activity probably occurs. Young women with normal anatomic support may feel pain or discomfort during an involuntary detrusor contraction with bladder neck opening but not experience incontinence. Incontinence is avoided because voluntary contraction of strong pelvic floor muscles is able to prevent leakage. Severe pain with holding is suggestive of IC as the underlying problem. Annoying urgency is most suggestive of a hypersensitivity phenomenon. Pain during the act of urination is most consistent with acute bacterial cystitis. Pain after urination strongly suggests a muscular cause: the outlet muscles are relaxed during urination with increased activity after urination is complete.

Pain: A Conceptual Overview

Pain is a noxious sensation carried by nerve fibers from the site of tissue injury to the brain. Acute pain is beneficial when it alerts the person to the site of injury. Once injury is recognized, treated, and healed, persistent pain becomes chronic and is no longer beneficial. Chronic pain can severely affect quality of life by decreasing motivation, limiting physical activities, and disrupting sleep patterns. Chronic pain does not require the search for a source that acute pain requires, and it is rarely addressed by medical education. Too often, providers and patients believe that pain is acute and indicates a serious underlying problem.

There are three types of pain: somatic, visceral, and neuropathic. Somatic pain arises from skin, muscles, and bones. Rapid transmission by fibers to the cerebral cortex allows the source of pain to be localized quickly, yielding a fast response. Descriptions of somatic pain include "sharp," "stabbing," and "throbbing." Visceral pain arises from the internal organs and is carried on slower fibers through the limbic

system (emotional center). The source of pain is poorly localized and often described in emotional terms such as "awful" or "agonizing." Neuropathic pain is generated in damaged nerve fibers. Its messages also are carried through the limbic system and often are described as "electrical," "shocklike," or a "painful numbness." These descriptions can be helpful in identifying the type of pain, especially in the pelvis where all three types can coexist. The role of the limbic system explains why visceral and neuropathic pain (with afferent transmission through the limbic system) present with significant emotional overlay, which is not seen in somatic pain (in which the limbic system is bypassed).

Causes of Lower Urinary Tract Pain

Health care providers should be careful not to diagnose a urinary tract infection on the basis of symptoms alone. Confusion results for the patient when the culture returns negative or symptoms do not resolve with antibiotics. Using nonspecific terms such as "symptomatic episode" or "bladder inflammation" when a woman presents with symptoms is useful. When the word cystitis is used, there is an expectation that antibiotics are necessary for symptom relief. Antibiotics commonly improve symptoms even in patients who have a negative urinalysis and culture. One explanation is that most bottles of antibiotics instruct the patient to drink plenty of water with each dose. Once the course of antibiotics is completed, fluid intake returns to normal, which often includes negligible amounts of noncarbonated water; symptoms may return because of the hypersensitivity phenomenon discussed in the following section.

It is also important that the physician not localize the pain for the patient. If the patient describes vague, poorly localized symptoms, the physician should not suggest an organ to focus on by saying "that sounds like your bladder."

A. Lower Urinary Tract Hypersensitivity: This term has replaced others such as urethral syndrome, chronic trigonitis, chronic urethritis, and chronic nonbacterial cystitis. It refers to an overly sensitive bladder, which can contribute to the cascade of events leading to uncoordinated low-volume urination, voiding dysfunction, and eventually, pain before, during, or after urination. Usually, the pain is worse before or after urination, and patients often report that the pain feels different from that of a bacterial bladder infection. Comparing these symptoms to a sensitive stomach or a sore joint, such as tennis elbow, often helps the patient understand that these symptoms do not have to result from an infection. Identifying all the potential triggers and eliminating as many of them as possible, while increasing water intake, modifying the diet, and working with pelvic muscle relaxation, can alleviate symptoms and minimize the number of symptomatic episodes. A woman may be able to drink four cups of coffee, drink wine, and eat a chocolate dessert without triggering symptoms except premenstrually or on a day when she performs strenuous exercise. Exercise without increased water intake results in dehydration and concentrated urine.

B. Interstitial Cystitis: Women who have IC typically report frequency and urgency of urination (urinating as often as every 15 minutes both daytime and nighttime) as well as suprapubic, perineal, vulvar, or vaginal discomfort before, during, or after urination. Pain during or after sexual intercourse also is reported commonly. The diagnosis of IC is made based on symptoms, functional bladder data (cystometrogram), and cystoscopic criteria. There are no specific blood, urine, or bladder biopsy criteria to confirm the diagnosis.

The exact incidence of IC is not known. In the province of Uusimma in southern Finland, the incidence of IC was reported to be 103 of 974,305 adult inhabitants, with a prevalence of 10.6 per 100,000. In this series, 9.8% of the patients were men, which is consistent with most other series. In 1987, Held studied the epidemiology of IC in the United States; these data suggest a higher incidence in the USA than Finland by a factor of 4–5. In Helds study, the median age of onset of symptoms was 40 years, with 25% of the patients younger than 30 years old.

The social and economic costs of this syndrome are significant. Economic costs include direct medical costs, loss of productivity because of inability to work, or working at jobs with lower wages than other women of similar age and educational background. Even more profound are the social consequences of an overall decrease in quality of life, depression, increase in suicidal thoughts, inability to perform parental responsibilities, and inability to engage in activities such as exercise and sex that are important for overall physical and emotional well-being.

The cause is unknown, and there is no known cure. Etiologic concepts currently being considered include infectious, vascular, or lymphatic obstruction; psychologic factors; glycosaminoglycan alterations; reflex sympathetic dystrophy; toxic urinary agents; and immunologic factors. With the wide variety of potential etiologic factors, it is not surprising that no single intervention is uniformly successful and that often a combination of interventions is required to control symptoms.

C. Neuropathic Pain: The diagnosis of neuropathic pain rarely is considered in women who present with LUTP, but it should be considered first in women who describe their pain as "burning" or "electric shock-like" sensation. The mechanism of nerve injury may never be known; the injury can be perpetuated by local trauma, pelvic floor spasm, and repeated injury to the peripheral nerves. Trauma to the pudendal nerve has been attributed to events and

activities such as vaginal childbirth, horseback riding, and prolonged cycling. Reflex sympathetic dystrophy has been reported in women with chronic bladder pain. Exposure of the pelvic organs to radiation can damage the blood supply and the nerves, leading to symptoms of LUTP.

D. Musculoskeletal Pain: Musculoskeletal pain is probably the most frequently missed diagnosis in patients who present with pain in the pelvis and an altered voiding pattern. Typically, this pain is poorly localized, dull, and aching. Health care providers are not accustomed to thinking of the pelvic musculoskeletal system as a source of pain when patients attribute their discomfort to their internal organs. Musculoskeletal nociceptors are stimulated by mechanical stimuli (compression or stretching), chemical stimuli, inflammation, and metabolic disturbances. Intrapelvic muscle strain, imbalance between the trunk, hip, and abdominal muscles, poor posture, and strain injuries to abdominal, paravertebral and gluteal muscles (eg, compensation for a short leg) all can generate pain localized to the LUT and alterations in voiding function. Standard techniques of physiotherapy, such as applications of heat and cold, massage, and muscle stretching, strengthening, and relaxation, can be effective for this part of the body as well as for the extremities. The value of these techniques has been demonstrated in patients with extremely refractory chronic pain, and they now are employed early in the management of LUTP patients.

Other Causes of Lower Urinary Tract Pain

Urinary tract pain in women with vulvovaginal inflammation generally occurs during the act of urination, but it typically is felt as the urine contacts the external tissues rather than while it passes through the urethra. Chemical irritation of the external genitalia from soaps, douches, perfumes, and contraceptive preparations also is felt as pain on the external tissues. Urethral diverticula should be considered in women with recurrent lower urinary infections, pain during urination, painful coitus, and postvoid dribbling. On physical examination, there is usually a sense of fullness to palpation in the anterior vaginal wall. Endometriosis, pelvic inflammatory disease (PID), pelvic congestion, and vulvar vestibulitis (vulvodynia) are disorders that can present with symptoms primarily localized to the LUT and need to be considered in the differential diagnosis of LUTP of uncertain cause.

Women with symptoms of lower urinary tract pain commonly report disturbances in bowel function. Irritable bowel syndrome is a preexisting diagnosis in many of these women who present with LUT symptoms. Many women report long-standing problems with constipation, which may be an indicator of incomplete or imperfect neurologic structures that can affect both bowel and bladder function. The act of defecation triggers the pain complex in some patients. Many pharmacologic treatments for LUTP can increase the possibility of constipation.

Local trauma to the lower urinary tract can be caused by sexual activity, especially when it is aggressive, prolonged, or without adequate lubrication. Some positions may be uncomfortable for some women. It is not unusual for women to report partner-specific factors such as size of phallus, duration of intercourse, or variety of positions associated with their pain. Pain that begins hours to days after intercourse is highly suggestive of neuropathic pain.

Urethral dilation represents another form of trauma to the LUT. This treatment has been standard for many years for recurrent urinary tract infections, symptoms of obstructive voiding, frequency and urgency of urination, and urinary incontinence. Although there have been no prospective studies looking at the efficacy and potential harm of this form of treatment, it is commonly accepted by urologists and gynecologists who specialize in disorders of the LUT in women that the potential for physical and emotional harm far exceeds any benefit.

Evaluation

A. History: A complete history is the most important aspect of the initial evaluation of a patient with LUTP. Specific questions include:

1. *What are your current symptoms?* It is important to obtain specific answers to questions about daytime frequency and nocturia, an urgency rating on a scale of 0–10, and a pain rating on a scale of 0–10.
2. *Can you describe your pain?* The patient should be asked to be as specific as possible. Does the pain vary with how full or empty the bladder feels? Does sexual activity have an impact on the pain?
3. *Are the symptoms the same all the time?* For example, one may ask if the symptoms vary depending on time of day (morning versus evening) or with physical exercise.
4. *What were your bladder habits before this problem started?*
5. *Did you have infections, frequency, or daytime or nighttime incontinence as a child? If so, were any procedures performed such as a meatotomy, urethrotomy, or urethral dilation?* A history of such problems or procedures suggests that the patient may have a voiding dysfunction, possibly caused by the incomplete maturation of the nerve pathways to the LUT.
6. *Do symptoms vary with your menstrual cycle?*
7. *Do any of the following exacerbate your symptoms?*
   - Dehydration (increased physical activity and sweating or decreased fluid intake)
   - Dietary factors (coffee, carbonation, acidic foods, juices, spicy foods, sugar, aspartame)
   - Physical factors (sitting or standing for prolonged periods, car rides, lifting)
   - Emotional factors (stress, anxiety, depression, fatigue)
8. *What relieves your symptoms?*
9. *What is your normal daily fluid intake of the following:* coffee (include decaffeinated), tea, carbonated beverages (seltzer, sparkling water), fruit juices (especially citrus and cranberry), alcohol, water, milk.
10. *What was going on in your life at the time of the onset of symptoms?*
    - Becoming sexually active
    - Being with a new sexual partner
    - Using a new form of birth control
    - Experiencing hot weather
    - Injuring lower back or tail bone
    - Undergoing a pelvic operation or a minor gynecologic procedure
    - Suffering from a pelvic organ infection
    - Suffering from a perianal process, such as fissure or hemorrhoid
11. *What is your biggest fear concerning these symptoms?* Typically, women identify the following fears: cancer, an infection being passed back and forth with a sexual partner, kidney damage from undiagnosed infection, or that they will never get better or have a normal sexual relationship again.
12. *Do you have a history of physical, sexual, or emotional abuse that may have some significance for your current symptom complex?* If rapport with the patient has been difficult to establish, it may be best to avoid this question at the initial visit.

Physical Examination

Ensure the patient has voided shortly before the examination. It is important to explain the examination to the woman as it progresses. Having the woman positioned and draped in a manner allowing observation of facial expressions can be helpful in permitting her to feel like a participant in the process. First, the external genitalia are inspected visually for signs of irritation, discharge, and atrophic changes. A cotton-tipped applicator can be used around the introitus and urethral meatus to identify specific sites of pain reproduction. When the external part of the examination causes discomfort, the patient may be asked to relax and take some deep breaths before the clinician proceeds.

Next, one finger is introduced gently through the introitus, with pressure kept against the posterior vaginal wall. One should ask the patient to identify when she is having discomfort or pain and if the discomfort is the same as or different from her symptomatic episodes. Initially, the introitus is palpated circumferentially; the finger is introduced gently to the level of the cervix or vaginal cuff, with the pressure kept posteriorly. The levator muscles are palpated gradually following the arc of pubic bone, pushing up on the genitourinary diaphragm lateral to the bladder and urethra. This should be done on both sides, with the physician observing for symptom reproduction. The lateral pelvic sidewalls also are palpated, as is the anterior vaginal wall. The clinician begins with the urethra just proximal to the meatus and gently palpates toward the bladder neck. The urethra should feel like a midline spongy tube with a "gutter" on either side. These gutters may be obscured by a previous anterior colporrhaphy, anterior vaginal wall mass (cyst or infected glands), or urethral diverticulum.

Moving superiorly, the physician gently palpates the base of the bladder. A sense of urge is normal, but a sense of pain, burning, cramping, or aching is not. A bimanual examination is begun by gently putting downward pressure in the suprapubic area while pushing upward on the base of the bladder in the midline with the vaginal finger. Definite reproduction of symptoms with bimanual palpation of the bladder is suggestive of IC. Next, the clinician moves the vaginal finger lateral to the bladder and pushes up on the pelvic floor support immediately adjacent to the pubic bone. Pain in this area is consistent with myofascial pain. Bimanual examination of the uterus and ovaries is performed, again with careful assessment for pain reproduction. When pain is reproduced, the same spot should be assessed with abdominal and vaginal pressure independently to determine whether the pain is generated by abdominal or vaginal trigger points or the tissue in between.

A speculum examination is performed to look for signs of vaginitis or cervicitis. When there is concern about anatomic support, the examination is performed best with two separated posterior blades of a standard speculum. This part of the examination is described in detail in Chapter 27.

The final part of the examination is an assessment of the patient's ability to contract and relax the pelvic floor muscles. This muscle group should be supple and nontender at rest. There should be circumferential tightening of muscles around the vagina without lifting of the buttocks and immediate relaxation on command. It may be difficult to feel contraction if muscles are tight and in spasm. Verbal encouragement to relax or not to hold back often initiates relaxation. Once the muscles are relaxed, the tender areas are palpated again. Often, the pain decreases, which provides immediate feedback to the patient, indicating that at least part of the pain is related to tension in the pelvic muscles and can be lessened by muscle relaxation.

Laboratory Tests

A voided urinalysis always should be done. Microscopic examination of a spun specimen allows for immediate assessment of hematuria and infection (pyuria) and contamination. If the specimen appears contaminated with squamous epithelial cells, obtaining an immediate catheterized specimen can eliminate confusion about whether culture results are significant or whether the identified hematuria is in the bladder urine. Routine culture of a urine specimen that is chemically negative for leukocyte esterase, nitrates, and blood is not indicated unless the patient needs the additional reassurance that there is no bacterial infection requiring antibiotics.

A urine specimen collected with a small-caliber catheter (12 or 14 French) also provides an accurate determination of the postvoid residual (PVR), which is important in patients who have frequency and a sensation of incomplete emptying. Alternatively, an ultrasonographic estimation of the PVR can be done. A voided urine sample can be sent for cytologic study as an initial screen to rule out carcinoma in situ of the bladder, which can be present with symptoms of LUT irritation. This assessment is especially important in women with a present or past history of smoking. Urethral calibration or dilation is not indicated for diagnosis or therapy. When significant hematuria is found, an upper tract evaluation should be done before cystoscopy.

Treatment

A. General Considerations: Regardless of the cause of the symptom, treatment always begins with reassurance and education concerning the structure and function of the lower urinary tract and its interrelationship with the gynecologic, gastrointestinal, and musculoskeletal systems. Use of anatomic diagrams can be helpful in assisting the patient to understand the concepts being discussed. The patient should be helped to understand the interactions between the mind and body from the outset. She must be informed that the evaluation and treatment will not be based solely on her physical symptoms.

A working partnership between physician and patient needs to be established with the goal of obtaining symptom control and allowing the patient to get on with life. If the goal is to "cure" the disease, the patient is at risk for continual disappointment as one treatment after another fails to bring permanent symptom relief. Terms such as "dysfunctions" and "symptomatic episodes" or "flare-ups" are most accurate and do not lead to the expectation that antibiotics will help. It is crucial to ensure that the office personnel that patients deal with (in person or on the phone) understand the importance of terminology. Getting mixed messages from different persons fuels fear, frustration, and anxiety.

B. Behavioral Strategies: Common sense is important in using behavioral recommendations. Using a bladder diary to record time and volume of urination can be important in demonstrating objective improvement to the patient. Increasing the water intake to dilute the urine and flush out the lower urinary tract is important. The optimal volume varies, but it helps to start with four to six glasses of water per day and gradually increase the amount. Urine passed should be pale yellow; the water intake necessary to maintain dilute urine may vary from day to day. It is important to inform patients that frequency may worsen initially because of the increased intake. The pain and ease of urination are the first to improve; as it becomes more comfortable to hold larger volumes of urine in the bladder, the frequency decreases. Bladder-holding protocols can be helpful in decreasing frequency once pain is less severe. Avoiding particular foods or fluids also can relieve the discomfort. Although the rationale for this intervention is not known, it may be that some foods act as neuromodulators. Foods typically reported to exacerbate symptoms are coffee, tea (even decaffeinated), carbonation, and substances that are acidic and spicy.

Recognizing the potential of voluntary or involuntary pelvic muscle contraction in symptom generation, perpetuation, or exacerbation is important to the development of self-management strategies. Voluntary pelvic floor relaxation can ease symptoms. Many times patients need instruction in pelvic muscle localization and contraction before they can un-

derstand how to relax this muscle group. Anything that promotes generalized relaxation and stress management, eg, aerobic exercise or distraction, should be used when possible. To be accepted by the patient, these behavioral strategies must be presented as valid treatments by the provider. If a patient senses that the provider does not take these recommendations seriously, she is not likely to follow through with them.

C. Pharmacologic Management: A variety of medications can be used to treat LUTP syndromes. Often, a combination of drugs is needed. Table 26–1 lists the pharmacologic agents most commonly used and the symptoms that indicate various treatment plans. In particular, the use of alpha-blockers (eg, prazosin) can be helpful in patients with obstructive voiding symptoms that may be related to tension or spasm of the urethral smooth muscle. The list of medications should be regarded as a general guideline; in refractory conditions, a trial of one more agent or one more combination may be the key in breaking the pain cycle. Realistic expectations for treatment outcome are necessary, and patients must understand that medications have benefits and side effects that are particular to the individual and usually not predictable.

D. Physiotherapy: A comprehensive physio-

Table 26–1. Medications for treatment of LUTP.

Medication	Dosage	Symptom	Sign
1. Tricyclic Antidepressants • Amitriptyline • Doxepin • Trazodone • Fluoxetine	10–75 mg qhs HS* qhs 50 mg qhs HS* 20 mg PO q	Sleep disruption; sharp, burning, shock-like pain; bladder/urethral burning or constant awareness	Increased pelvic muscle tone; painful bladder
2. Alpha-blockers • Terazosin • Prazosin • Phenoxybenzamine	1–2 mg q HS (increase to TID as tolerated and necessary for symptom control)	Hesitancy; slow stream, sense of incomplete emptying. Postvoiding pain/spasm	Abnormal uroflow; ± tender pelvic muscles
3. Antispasmodics • Oxybutynin • Hyoscyamine • Flavoxate	½ tablet PO TID 1–2 tablet PO TID 1 tablet PO TID	Frequency; discomfort with full bladder; severe urgency	Involuntary detrusor contraction on CMG†
4. Skeletal muscle relaxants • Carisoprodol • Cyclobenzaprine • Methocarbanol	1 tablet PO TID " "	Postvoiding pain; dyspareunia	Increased tone of pelvic muscles; Pain reproduction with palpation
5. Anesthetics • Phenazopyridine • Lidocaine jelly 2% • Lidocaine ointment 5%	100–200 mg PO TID	Hypersensitivity; pain during urination; pain localized to meatal area during urination or intercourse	Tender introital area or perimeatal area
6. Anticonvulsants • Carbamazepine	200 mg PO BID, gradually increase to QID PRN	Neuropathic pain	Sensory deficits-perineum/lower extremity; dysesthesia

*gradually increase dosage; can use TID if sedation not a problem
†cystometrogram

therapy evaluation and treatment regimen is invaluable to women with LUTP. Patients with refractory symptoms who see physical therapists with a special interest in pelvic floor dysfunction can have surprising success. Most patients can be referred for physiotherapy assessment after their first or second visit. Patients almost universally report that they gain some improvement if not total symptom relief.

E. Treatments Specific to Interstitial Cystitis: Even patients with a confirmed diagnosis of IC may respond well to some of the simple behavioral strategies. It is best to start by reviewing what the patient knows about IC, what she knows about self-help strategies, and how well she has tried to incorporate these strategies into her life. Patients and their families can be reassured that most women arrive at a treatment strategy by combining behavioral, pharmacologic, and physiotherapeutic techniques, which allows them to have a reasonably pain-free, functional life. Current treatment for IC is aimed at symptomatic relief through a variety of means including dietary modification; intravesical instillations of various pharmacologic agents including dimethyl sulfoxide (DMSO), hydrocortisone, sodium bicarbonate, heparin, and oxychlorosene; and use of oral agents such as amitriptyline, hydroxyzine, nifedipine, and sodium pentosanpolysulfate. Other methods used to treat IC include transcutaneous nerve stimulation (TENS), neuromodulation (sacral nerve root stimulator), surgical enlargement of the bladder (augmentation cystoplasty), substitution cystoplasty, and cystectomy with urinary diversion.

HEMATURIA

Hematuria is the abnormal presence of erythrocytes in the urine and must be distinguished from myoglobinuria and hemoglobinuria. This distinction can be made by confirming the presence of red blood cells on microscopic analysis after a urine dipstick is found to be positive for blood. Hematuria, either macro- or microscopic, is frequently the first symptom of a significant urologic disease and warrants evaluation to determine its cause. In female patients, hematuria must be either localized to the urinary tract or established to have a gynecologic source. This distinction may be made by obtaining a catheterized urine specimen or by placing a tampon in the vagina. When the blood is found on the tampon, a gynecologic rather than a urologic source is likely.

When a patient presents with gross hematuria, whether painless or associated with abdominal or flank pain, a thorough investigation is imperative, even if only a single episode of bloody urine is reported. Evaluation should begin with a urine culture. If the urine culture is positive and hematuria resolves with treatment, further evaluation usually is not indicated unless a repeat urinalysis shows microscopic hematuria. In patients with culture-negative urine, further urologic evaluation is necessary. Evaluation typically includes cytologic study of the urine, intravenous pyelography (IVP), and cystoscopy. In some settings, renal ultrasonography has replaced IVP in the evaluation of microscopic hematuria.

Although the presence of a small number of red blood cells in the urine is normal and does not require extensive urologic evaluation, there is controversy concerning the degree of microscopic hematuria that requires evaluation. A widely accepted upper limit of normal is 5 RBC/hpf. Often hematuria is detected on dipstick only, and the patient is referred to a urologist before true hematuria is documented. Because dipstick tests generally are based on the peroxidase-like activities of red blood cells and hemoglobin, there may be false-positive results. Therefore, all patients who have dipstick-positive urine should have a microscopic evaluation of the urine sediment. In patients with a history of tobacco use or an occupational risk factor, a standard urologic evaluation is prompted by the findings of microscopic hematuria in two of three "clean-catch" uncatheterized specimens.

An issue of concern is how to manage hematuria in patients undergoing anticoagulant therapy. Studies have shown that approximately 20% of these patients have significant disease that will show up if appropriate studies are performed.

REFERENCES

Baker P: Musculoskeletal origins of chronic pelvic pain: Diagnosis and treatment. Obstet Gynecol Clin North Am 1993;20:719.

Bavendam T: A common sense approach to lower urinary tract hypersensitivity in women. Contemporary Urology 1992;4:25.

Brockoff D: Understanding pain and pain medications. Interstitial Cystitis Association, 1990.

Early experience with physical therapy in the management of pelvic pain in female urologic patients: 1992. In: Annual meeting of American Urological Society, Western Section. Maui, Hawaii.

Fleischmann J et al: Clinical and immunological response to nifedipine for the treatment of interstitial cystitis. J Urol 1991;146:1235.

Galloway N, Gabale D, Irwin P: Interstitial cystitis or reflex sympathetic dystrophy of the bladder? Semin Urol 1991;9:148.

Hanno P et al: *Interstitial Cystitis.* Springer-Verlag, 1990.

Hanno P, Buehler J, Wein A: Use of amitriptyline in the treatment of interstitial cystitis. J Urol 1989;141:846.

Held P et al: Epidemiology of interstitial cystitis. In: *Interstitial Cystitis.* Hanno P (editor). Springer-Verlag, 1990.

Koziol J: Epidemiology of interstitial cystitis. Urol Clin North Am 1984;21:7.

Krieger J: Urinary tract infections in women: Causes, classification, and differential diagnosis. J Urol 1990;35:4.

Leach G, Bavendam T: Female urethral diverticula. Urology 1987;30:407.

Mulholland S et al: Pentosanpolysulfate sodium for therapy of interstitial cystitis: A double-blind placebo-controlled clinical study. Urology 1990;35:552.

Oravisto K: Epidemiology of interstitial cystitis. Ann Chir Gynaecol Suppl 1975;64:75.

Parsons C, Koprowski P: Interstitial cystitis: Successful management by increasing voiding intervals. Urology 1991;37:207.

Perez-Marrero R et al: Prolongation of response to DMSO by heparin maintenance. Urology 1993;41(Suppl):64.

Petersen T, Husted S: Prazosin treatment of neurological patients with lower urinary tract dysfunction. Int Urogynecol J 1993;4:106.

Phillips H, Fenster H, Samsom D: An effective treatment for functional urinary incoordination. J Behav Med 1992;15:45.

Rapkin A, Mayer E: Gastroenterologic causes of chronic pelvic pain. Obstet Gynecol Clin North Am 1993;20:663.

Ratliff T, Klutke C, McDougall E: The etiology of interstitial cystitis. Urol Clin North Am 1994;21:21.

Schuster GA, Lewis GA: Clinical significance of hematuria in patients on anticoagulants. J Urol 1987;137:923.

Tanagho E, Schmidt R: Electrical stimulation in the management of the neurogenic bladder. J Urol 1988;140:1331.

Theoharides T: Hydroxyzine in the treatment of interstitial cystitis. Urol Clin North Am 1994;21:113.

Turner M, Marinoff S: Pudendal neuralgia. Am J Obstet Gynecol 1991;165:1233.

Wishard W, Nourse M, Mertz J: Use of chlorpactin WCS 90 for relief of symptoms due to interstitial cystitis. J Urol 1957;77:420.

Urinary Incontinence

27

Tamara G. Bavendam, MD, & Jane L. Miller, MD

Urinary incontinence (UI), or the involuntary loss of urine, is common in women. Wolin found that 50% of 4211 nulliparous women 18–25 years of age reported involuntary loss of urine with some type of activity, 16% on a daily basis. Although damp or wet underwear is assumed to be caused by urine by most women, it may not be. It is important for primary care providers to determine whether complaints of dampness are related to UI before initiating the evaluation, treatment, or referral. A history of chronic dampness without any inciting factor (activity or urge) suggests a gynecologic source (excessive vaginal secretions), vesicovaginal or ureterovaginal fistula, or an ectopic ureter. Use of a pharmacologic agent that colors the urine (phenazopyridine hydrochloride or methylene blue) can help distinguish a gynecologic from a urologic source.

The importance of UI is determined by the impact of the incontinence episodes on the woman's quality of life. Quality of life issues are different for each woman. Activity restriction, fluid restriction, and staying near bathrooms may eliminate accidents, making extra protection unnecessary, yet cause negative changes in the woman's quality of life. Questions that can help the patient and her provider understand the significance of the problem are "What have you done to minimize your episodes of urine leakage?" and "What impact have these changes had on your quality of life?" In other words, what has the woman given up to avoid UI?

Women may delay reporting UI because of embarrassment or because they fear surgery is the only treatment option. Primary care providers may not ask routinely about bladder control problems because they are not comfortable with the evaluation and initial treatment or satisfied with the available referral options. Education concerning UI is lacking at all levels of medical education from medical school through primary care and specialty residencies and postgraduate education programs. The educational material that is available often is so shrouded in confusing jargon and pharmacologic references that it is almost impossible to use the information clinically. Clinicians must have the basic information necessary to perform initial incontinence evaluations, institute treatment, and refer appropriate patients to specialists.

Essentials of Diagnosis
Terminology
Pathophysiology
Etiology
Clinical Findings & Diagnosis
Treatment
Referral to a Specialist
Case Study

Essentials of Diagnosis

- Involuntary loss of urine is common and treatable.
- Hypermobility of bladder and urethra.
- Pelvic muscle exercises are a useful treatment.
- A careful history is a key part of the evaluation.
- Many nonsurgical treatments can be effective.

Terminology

Incontinence is categorized based on the circumstances precipitating the involuntary loss of urine. **Stress incontinence** (activity-related) is the loss of urine coincident with an activity that increases the intra-abdominal pressure (coughing, sneezing, bending, lifting, or walking).

Urge incontinence is the loss of urine associated with a strong desire to urinate. Urgency can occur secondary to a sensory or motor dysfunction. With sensory urgency, the desire to urinate is so intense the person "lets go" of the urine to relieve the severe urgency. Motor urgency occurs with a bladder or detrusor contraction that cannot be suppressed voluntarily, referred to as an **involuntary,** or **uninhibited, detrusor contraction (UDC)**. The UDC is referred to as **detrusor hyperreflexia** when a specific neurologic cause can be identified and as **detrusor instability** when a specific cause cannot be identified.

Spontaneous, or **"unconscious," loss of urine** occurs without a specific pattern or inciting factors; it can be secondary to a UDC in a woman with severe sensory impairment of the bladder (no perceived urge), or it can result from a weak bladder outlet in which seemingly normal activity can cause urine loss.

Overflow incontinence occurs when the bladder

is at its maximal capacity and the intravesical pressure exceeds the pressure maintained by the outlet. The leakage occurs until enough urine has been released to lower the intravesical pressure temporarily until it is below the outlet pressure. The patient may experience this urine loss as stress, urge, or continuous incontinence. A history of continuous loss of urine suggests overflow incontinence; severe intrinsic urethral dysfunction, often referred to as type III incontinence; or an extraurethral source such as an ectopic ureter or fistula between the urinary tract and vagina. Ectopic ureters are congenital and often present in childhood with incontinence or recurrent urinary tract infections.

Another important type of incontinence is **functional incontinence,** which is the loss of urine secondary to factors extrinsic to the urinary tract such as (1) arthritis, stroke, or multiple sclerosis causing considerable mobility restriction; (2) heavy doors to toilets, poor wheelchair access, or other physical barriers; or (3) use of medications such as diuretics causing precipitous filling of the bladder over a short period of time. A patient often has more than one type of incontinence and more than one etiologic factor. A good history and working knowledge of the woman's overall health status are necessary for optimal outcome.

Pathophysiology

The function of the lower urinary tract in women is to provide a balance between the bladder and bladder outlet mechanism. Incontinence occurs when the bladder pressure exceeds the pressure maintained by the bladder outlet mechanism. In women, the bladder outlet mechanism is made up of the bladder neck muscle, the urethral mucosa and smooth muscle, and the skeletal muscle of the urethra and pelvic floor. Continence is maintained because of a low pressure storage capacity, intact structure and function of the urethra, the muscle and fascial support of the pelvic floor, and an intact autonomic (pelvic and hypogastric nerves) and somatic (pudendal) nerve supply.

The urethra has important functions in maintaining continence (intrinsic urethral factors) independent of its anatomic position. Normal urethral mucosa has abundant folds that provide complete apposition or mucosal seal, supplemented by the rich vascular supply of the submucosa. Normal estrogen levels are important for maintaining the folds of mucosa and the rich vascular network. Smooth-muscle connective tissue in the wall of the urethra also provides compressive forces toward maintaining urethral closure.

Normally, the bladder and proximal urethra occupy an intra-abdominal position above the level of the pelvic floor muscles. With strong anatomic myofascial support, the intra-abdominal position is maintained during activities that increase intra-abdominal pressure, providing equal transmission to the bladder and proximal urethra. With pressure equal at the bladder and the outlet, there is no loss of urine (Fig 27–1). Weakened anatomic support allows the proximal urethra and bladder neck to rest at or below the level of the pelvic muscles. Consequently, pressure increases are transmitted to the bladder but not to the proximal urethra. At times of increased intra-abdominal pressure, bladder pressure exceeds outlet pressure and leakage occurs (Fig 27–2).

Skeletal muscle dysfunction results in UI through

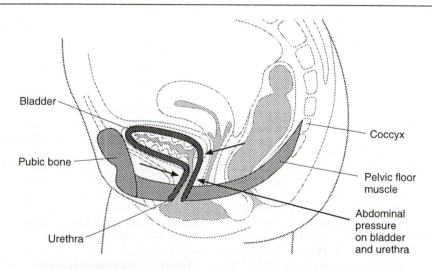

Figure 27–1. With normal support, the bladder neck and proximal urethra are maintained in an intra-abdominal position. During stressful maneuvers, the bladder and proximal urethra receive equal pressure transmission (arrows), and continence is maintained. (Reproduced, with permission, from Bavendam, TG. J. Enterostomal Therapy 1990;17:58.)

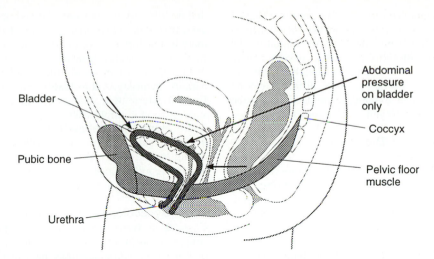

Figure 27–2. With weakened anatomic support, the bladder base sags (relaxes) into the vaginal space. Increased intra-abdominal pressure (arrows) is transmitted to the bladder but not to the proximal urethra. When the bladder pressure exceeds the outlet pressure, urinary leakage occurs. (Reproduced, with permission, from Bavendam, TG. J. Enterostomal Therapy 1990;17:59.)

loss of the reflex muscle contraction of the periurethral and pelvic floor muscles that normally occurs during increases in intra-abdominal pressure as well as through loss or decreased strength of voluntary contraction of these muscles. Voluntary contraction is an important adjunct to the reflex contraction and depends on the woman's awareness of how and when to use this muscle group effectively. The pelvic floor muscles are supplied by the pudendal nerve, which can be damaged by uncomplicated vaginal deliveries. This damage may not be apparent or relevant until the woman becomes older and begins to experience menopause or the generalized nerve and muscle deterioration that occurs with aging.

Etiology

The lower urinary tract has two functions: storage of urine and expulsion of urine. In women, UI is generally a storage abnormality secondary to increased bladder pressure, decreased outlet resistance, or a combination of the two. Increased bladder pressures can result from UDCs or from the inability of the detrusor muscle to increase capacity (volume) without increasing pressure, resulting in decreased compliance. When UDC or decreased compliance is suspected, it is important to determine whether there is an underlying neurologic cause that may be correctable or may progress with time, causing further deterioration in lower urinary tract function.

Impaired function of the female bladder outlet can result from (1) prolapse or relaxation of the bladder base and urethra into the vaginal space, commonly referred to as a **cystourethrocele;** (2) incompetence of the involuntary smooth muscle at the bladder neck, which may be iatrogenic or neurogenic; (3)

weakness of the skeletal muscle of the external sphincteric mechanism; or (4) intrinsic urethral damage. The cystourethrocele can be corrected by surgery, but if there are other contributing factors to the UI, the surgery may not result in perfect bladder control and normal voiding function.

The most common cause of failure to empty the bladder in women is previous anti-incontinence surgery resulting in an obstructed outlet. Primary bladder outlet obstruction in women is uncommon and is generally at the level of the bladder neck in young women and the urethral meatus in postmenopausal women. Impaired detrusor contraction can result in inability to empty the bladder and can result from a lifetime of infrequent voiding, diabetic sensory neuropathy, lower back injury, or surgery damaging the sensory or motor nerves to the bladder. Because the female outlet is short, many women can void by pelvic floor relaxation, and impaired contractility can be compensated for by outlet relaxation or Valsalva maneuver. Impaired contractility can result in prolonged urinary retention following anti-incontinence surgery when the outlet resistance is purposefully increased to prevent UI.

Although UI is not a normal part of the aging process, there are multiple changes that occur with aging that make UI more likely to develop. There is a gradual decrease in the bladder elasticity, resulting in smaller bladder capacity. There is gradual deterioration in the sensory nerves to the bladder, which seems to impair the early warning signal of bladder filling. The first sensation the person receives may be a strong urge and impending UDC. The detrusor muscle becomes less able to generate a voluntary contraction and to sustain the contraction until the bladder is empty, resulting in incomplete bladder emptying. The nerves supplying the lower urinary tract undergo the same gradual deterioration as the rest of the body. Mobility decreases, making it more difficult to get to the bathroom quickly. Extremity strength weakens, leading to more difficulty getting on and off the toilet. Nighttime production of urine increases, and the estrogen levels decrease.

Clinical Findings & Diagnosis
A. History:
1. Circumstances of the leakage–When UI occurs only with strong coughing or sneezing, correctable causes of chronic coughing or sneezing should be considered and investigated, eg, smoking, chronic bronchitis, or allergies. Life-style changes adopted because of the incontinence need to be identified to help the patient and provider understand the importance of the problem to the patient.

2. Daily pattern–Sporadic incontinence or incontinence with a specific pattern may be related directly to dietary factors. For reasons that are not clear, dietary substances such as spicy or acidic foods or beverages and carbonation can be irritating to the bladder and contribute to UI. The most common offenders are coffee and tea, even decaffeinated types; citrus fruits; tomatoes; and cranberries.

3. Illnesses–Diabetes, congestive heart failure, and venous insufficiency can increase the urinary output, especially at night when the patient is in a recumbent position. When the main complaint is of nocturia with or without urine loss at night, the volume of urine produced at night needs to be investigated first. Nighttime incontinence often is associated with the large volume of urine produced by the kidneys at night. Even in the absence of noticeable peripheral edema during the day, urine production during sleep increases with aging secondary to decreasing ability to concentrate the urine and is difficult to modify. It is important to recognize that this problem is not one of lower urinary tract function. If someone produces 2 L of urine at night, she would need to get up a minimum of 4 times under the best of circumstances.

4. Medications–Incontinence associated with a morning diuretic may be improved by changing to a lower dosage to be taken in both the morning and evening. Alpha-sympathomimetic blockers (prazosin, terazosin, and phenoxybenzamine) can precipitate incontinence by relaxing the bladder neck muscle and decreasing outlet resistance. Sedatives and hypnotics can decrease perception of the bladder signals and impair mobility, causing a delay in getting to the bathroom. Antidepressant medication may contribute to UI because of impaired bladder emptying secondary to the anticholinergic side effects.

5. Neurologic diseases, injuries, or symptoms–Back or neck injuries, surgeries, closed head injuries, strokes, multiple sclerosis, and Parkinson's

disease all need to be recognized and optimally managed before definitive management of the UI. When there is a history of urge incontinence or voiding difficulties and additional neurologic symptoms (visual disturbances, numbness, tingling, or lack of coordination), neurologic consultation should be sought. Even if intermittent, this symptom constellation is suggestive of multiple sclerosis.

6. Hormonal status–Many women find incontinence exacerbated premenstrually and nonexistent during the early part of their menstrual cycle. Some women report changes in their bladder function as one of their first symptoms of the perimenopausal period.

7. Gynecologic or urologic surgeries–Changes in vesicourethral function can occur after simple or radical hysterectomy. Internal urethrotomy or repeated urethral dilations have been performed commonly for a variety of complaints in women and young girls. Fortunately, this practice is decreasing. Although there may be no immediate effect on the continence mechanism, as the woman ages, the damage may become clinically significant.

8. Number of pregnancies–Pregnancy and delivery carry a risk of initiating persistent stress incontinence. A number of women experience incontinence for the first time during pregnancy. Most of these women regain continence during the first 3 months of the postpartum period; however, continence may continue to return for up to 12 months after delivery. The importance of obstetric factors such as episiotomy, length of labor, type of delivery, and type of anesthetic in the causation of incontinence remains controversial.

9. Radiation treatment–Radiation effects can occur years after the treatment was given and can cause decrease in bladder compliance and damage to the urethra and the nerves that supply the lower urinary tract.

10. History of urinary retention–Women with this history may have a very delicate balance between bladder storage and emptying functions and be at risk for increased postvoid residuals or urinary retention after anti-incontinence surgery or anticholinergic medication.

11. Sexual patterns–Pain, discomfort, or loss of urine associated with intercourse or climax may limit the frequency or pleasure associated with sexual activity. Hilton found that 24% of 324 sexually active women experienced UI with intercourse—two-thirds with penetration and one-third with orgasm. Loss of urine at climax is secondary either to a triggered detrusor contraction or to outlet relaxation. If the volume of urine lost is small or intermittent and the patient does not have UI at any other time, the likelihood of finding a solution or "cure" is low. The physician can provide an explanation to the patient such as the following: "Intercourse and orgasm provide a complex stimulation to the nerves of the pelvic organs. At times, the messages traveling to and from the brain and organs get confused or cross over to different organs, resulting in urinary incontinence. It is impossible to block the parts of the signals that trigger the urinary incontinence."

Position during intercourse, intensity of stimulation, and time during the menstrual cycle are factors that may contribute to the occurrence of this type of UI. It is important to reassure the woman that the condition is fairly common and will not necessarily get worse or begin to affect her during other activities.

B. Physical Examination: The physical examination includes an abdominal examination, a pelvic examination in the lithotomy position, a rectal examination, and a screening neurologic examination. The vaginal examination is important for assessing the degree of estrogenization of the external genitalia and vaginal tissues. Normal vaginal tissues are moist and rugose (containing folds of vaginal epithelium). Atrophic tissues are dry, thin, and friable. The urethral meatus often looks erythematous and prominent in the hypoestrogenic state. If the urethral mucosa has a fungating or friable appearance, the patient should be referred to a urologist for evaluation.

The vaginal vault is examined using two separate posterior blades of a standard vaginal speculum independently. One blade is placed posteriorly against the rectum with gentle downward pressure. The anterior vaginal wall is then examined in the resting and "stressed" positions. With normal anatomic support, the bladder base is "tucked up" behind the pubic bone and not readily visible when the posterior blade is placed. The woman is asked to cough strenuously while the physician observes for movement of the bladder base down into the space of the vaginal cavity. This movement is an indication of the hypermobility of the bladder and urethra (which generally move as a unit in women who have not had previous anti-incontinence surgery). A little movement with resumption of the normal "resting" position as soon as the cough is over should be considered normal. Movement or rotational descent half-way into the vaginal cavity is considered mild, and movement down to the level of the introitus is moderate. Prolapse of the bladder at rest or with stress through the introitus is considered severe.

A finding of significant bladder prolapse or a cystocele, however, does not mean the woman absolutely requires surgery. The need for surgery depends on what symptoms the woman is having and what her preferences for management are. Indications for surgical correction of cystocele are discussed in the section, Treatment. When minimal movement is observed during coughing, the patient should be asked to "bear down." It is important to assess the maximal degree of mobility the woman can generate, with the understanding that movement is even more pronounced in the erect position because

of the strenuous activities of daily living. A reasonably normal examination in the lithotomy position does not rule out activity-related incontinence during aerobic exercise or sports.

After examination of the anterior vaginal wall, the physician introduces the second blade against the top wall of the vagina and examines the apex during rest, cough, and Valsalva maneuver, observing for uterine descensus, enterocele formation, or vaginal vault prolapse (posthysterectomy). The posterior blade is removed, and the degree of rectocele is assessed during rest, cough, and bearing down. The integrity of the perineal body (perineum between the introitus and anus) is evaluated. It is important that all areas of potential anatomic weakness be identified and evaluated because of the overlapping nature of the symptoms of bowel and bladder function.

The rectal examination is an important part of the anatomic and neurologic examination and includes the following: (1) resting anal sphincter tone (lax sphincter is highly suggestive of neurologic impairment or damage to the external anal sphincter from birth trauma or rectal/anal surgery); (2) the degree of rectocele (thinning of the rectovaginal septum) and integrity of the perineum; (3) the ability to localize and contract the sphincteric mechanism; and (4) the bulbocavernosus reflex, which is an indication of intact pudendal afferent and efferent nerve supply. This reflex is elicited by squeezing firmly but gently over the clitoris and observing or feeling for any of the following: (1) contraction of the anal sphincter, (2) upward movement of the urethral meatus, or (3) contraction of the bulbocavernosus muscle around the introitus. The remainder of the neurologic examination includes lower extremity reflexes and sensory evaluation of the lower extremities, perineum, and buttocks. A patient with any obvious asymmetry or markedly diminished sensation should be referred for neurologic evaluation.

C. Laboratory Tests: A urinalysis is warranted, especially in patients who report an acute onset of UI. Urine culture is not warranted when there is no pyuria or bacteriuria on microscopic examination. When significant hematuria is identified (greater than 8 RBC/hpf) referral for hematuria workup is warranted. This evaluation usually includes an intravenous pyelogram and cystourethroscopy. Obtaining a first morning voided urine sample for cytologic examination in women with a current or past history of smoking can provide useful information for the urologist's evaluation for hematuria. When a urinary tract infection is identified (pyuria and positive urine culture), the patient should be treated for 3–5 days with appropriate antibiotics, with observation for improvement of UI while taking the antibiotics. When findings include bacteriuria without pyuria, no improvement in UI after antibiotic treatment, and no other symptoms of urinary tract infection, continuation of antibiotics is not indicated.

D. Functional Bladder Evaluation: A functional bladder evaluation of the lower urinary tract can be as simple as having the woman cough in a supine or erect position, obtaining a postvoid residual determination, performing uroflowmetry, and obtaining a patient record of time and volume of urination and occurrence of incontinence episodes (bladder diary); it may be as complicated as a multichannel videourodynamic evaluation. The primary care provider can obtain the bladder diary, the postvoid residual determination, and a simplified bladder function evaluation without having any expensive equipment. The main limiting factors are time and interest. Much of the evaluation can be accomplished with the help of trained nurses. The multichannel urodynamic evaluation is helpful in identifying significant urethral and detrusor dysfunction and may be indicated in women with the historical risk factors discussed in the section, Referring to a Specialist.

A simplified bladder function evaluation begins with voided volume and postvoid residual determinations using a 14 or 16 French urethral Foley catheter. The most useful information is obtained when the patient has a normal, "strong" urge to urinate. This information is often more accurate when the patient returns for a second visit after having completed the bladder diary. It is important to ask the patient whether she felt the urge to go, whether she thought she urinated normally in the bathroom, and whether she thought she emptied her bladder. Some people never are able to urinate normally in bathrooms outside of their home; this possibility needs to be taken into consideration when interpreting the results of the voided and residual volumes. The patient's total bladder capacity is equal to the voided plus the residual volume. A normal bladder capacity is 300–600 mL. A normal residual volume should be less than 100 mL; however, these numbers are relative. A residual volume of 100 mL is less significant in someone who voided 300 mL than in someone who voided 50 mL. The residual urine can be sent for culture in patients who had equivocal or confusing voided urine specimens.

The Foley balloon is inflated, and an open-ended syringe is attached to the end of the catheter and held straight up from the woman's body. The bladder is filled by placement of sterile saline or water (at 50-mL increments) into the open-ended syringe, filling the bladder by gravity. The volumes at which the patient has first awareness of bladder filling, first urge to urinate, and strong urge or severe urgency are recorded. The rate at which the fluid enters the bladder decreases as capacity is reached or before an episode of UDC. An episode of UDC can be identified by sudden leakage of urine around the Foley or rise in the fluid level in the open-ended syringe. Decreased bladder compliance is suggested by a decreased rate of filling as the bladder reaches capacity. When the bladder is full, the catheter is removed, and

the patient is asked to cough in the supine position. If no leakage is observed, the maneuver is repeated in the standing position. Leakage of urine per urethra coincident with a cough is consistent with stress UI. Continual leakage of urine around the catheter during filling or with minimal change in intra-abdominal pressure (normal inspiration or raising of the head off the table) suggests considerable intrinsic urethral dysfunction and need for referral to a specialist. When a sudden rise of fluid or leakage around the catheter is observed without the patient experiencing a sense of urgency, a significant sensory impairment is present and neurologic investigation may be warranted.

E. Cystoscopic Examination: Cystoscopy is necessary before treatment of urinary incontinence only if there is a finding of hematuria or if referral is indicated. Urethral calibration and dilation are not a necessary part of an incontinence evaluation or of cystoscopy, and women should have the option to request that these procedures not be performed as a part of a cystoscopic examination. A gently performed diagnostic cystoscopy with use of intraurethral 2% lidocaine jelly may be reported as uncomfortable with a sense of pinching or pressure but is rarely reported to be painful.

Treatment

Treatment begins after an accurate assessment of all factors contributing to the UI and after all contributing medical problems, environmental factors, and behavioral changes are addressed. Figure 27–3 displays the multiple factors that can contribute to UI and may need to be addressed simultaneously in devising the treatment strategy. In some patients, simultaneous treatment for bladder storage and emptying problems may need to be instituted (anticholinergic medication and clean intermittent catheterization).

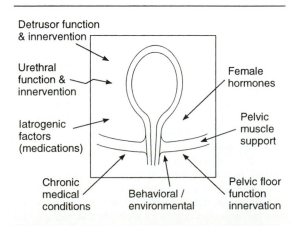

Figure 27–3. Pictorial representation of the multiple factors contributing to the urinary continence mechanism.

Multiple interventions are often necessary, especially in older women, and frequent changes in the treatment plan are common because of the balance that must exist between bladder storage and emptying (Fig 27–4).

A. General Therapeutic Considerations:

1. Estrogen–Estrogen replacement is important for the treatment of UI of any cause and should be recommended for all postmenopausal women with significant urinary tract complaints (infection, irritative voiding symptoms, or incontinence) who do not have significant contraindications to hormone replacement therapy. Women who are already on a regimen of oral or transdermal estrogen and continue to have atrophic changes on examination or complaints of vaginal dryness are likely to benefit from supplementation with vaginal estrogen replacement. Lower urinary tract symptoms respond more quickly to vaginal estrogens than to systemic replacement. Vaginal estrogen can be administered nightly for a short time (2–4 weeks), with the frequency of use decreased gradually to control symptoms and keep the tissues adequately estrogenized (often 1–2 times/wk). Many women find it more comfortable and less wasteful to apply the cream with their finger rather than the applicator. Usually, 1–2 inches of cream is recommended per application; some can be applied directly to the urethral meatus when it looks particularly erythematous or pronounced. Estrogen therapy usually is used in conjunction with other forms of treatment (pelvic muscle exercises, dietary changes, medication, or surgery).

2. Pelvic muscle exercises–Pelvic muscle exercises can be effective for the treatment of activity-related or urge UI. Muscle strengthening exercises can increase the resting tone of the striated muscles of the urethral and pelvic floor as well as increase the strength of the reflex muscle contraction that occurs during increases in intra-abdominal pressure. Exercise programs also increase the woman's awareness of her pelvic muscles and how to use voluntary pelvic muscle contractions to her benefit with stressful activities or episodes of urgency. A strong, well-localized pelvic muscle contraction at the time of a strong urge and impending leakage can abort the developing uninhibited bladder contraction reflexively and allow the woman time to walk to the bathroom without leakage. It is impossible to inhibit a UDC and run to the bathroom at the same time.

The main limiting factors for pelvic muscle exercises are the woman's ability to localize and contract the pelvic floor muscles and her motivation to learn the exercise regimen. Often the inability to contract the muscles arises from a difficulty in localizing the pelvic muscles as a separate entity from the thigh, buttock, and abdominal muscles. This form of treatment requires a lifelong commitment to the exercise program similar to that of other muscle rehabilitation and conditioning programs. Women who are successful with pelvic muscle exercises find the treatment regimen to be compatible with their life-style on a long-term basis.

Methods to improve pelvic muscle localization, which leads to more effective exercises, include verbal feedback from the examiner, biofeedback, and use of weighted vaginal cones. Verbal feedback is accomplished by inserting one or two fingers in the vagina or one finger in the anus while instructing the woman to squeeze on the finger or fingers, lift or pull in on the vaginal muscles, use the muscles she would use to stop the flow of urine, or hold back on rectal gas. Many women find it easier at first to localize the anal muscle than the vaginal muscles. At the time of muscle contraction, the physician observes for contraction of the abdominal, thigh, and buttock muscles. When inappropriate muscles are contracted, the woman is given verbal feedback and asked to repeat the contraction while relaxing the muscle she does not need to use. The only muscles that should be contracted are the pubococcygeus muscles around the examining fingers. Follow-up visits are important to ensure continued exercise of the proper muscles and provide reinforcement and motivation.

Biofeedback can be accomplished using surface electromyography (EMG) or a pneumatic compression device. Biofeedback training can be delivered by physicians, biofeedback therapists, nurses, social workers, psychologists, or physical therapists who have received training in pelvic muscle neuromuscu-

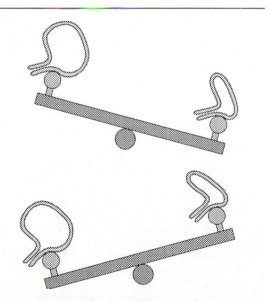

Figure 27–4. Pictorial representation of the balance between bladder storage and emptying functions. Treatments that increase storage can result in decreased emptying, and vice versa.

lar education. Provision of routine biofeedback training is probably not an efficient use of physician time. Each type of health care provider brings a slightly different form of expertise to a biofeedback treatment program. The best provider is one with experience and, most important, enthusiasm and interest in working with this patient population.

Weighted vaginal cones have been used in Europe and are currently available in the United States (Dacomed Corporation, Minneapolis, Minn). Women learn to isolate and properly contract their pelvic muscles by holding these tamponlike weights in the vagina. Studies have shown that UI decreases in 70% of women after use of the weights for 1 month and that women are able to strengthen their pelvic muscles using cones postpartum.

Whichever exercise plan is chosen, follow-up visits to review progress, provide positive reinforcement and encouragement, and possibly, change approaches are helpful in achieving treatment success. In general, exercises are a good therapeutic option for highly motivated women and worth a trial in any patient who is interested in nonsurgical therapy.

There have been many attempts to use electrical stimulation to strengthen the pelvic muscles passively. This form of therapy has been used for several years in Europe and is gradually gaining support in the USA. Specialists who offer a broad spectrum of treatment options may recommend transvaginal electrical stimulation for some women; it can be effective for both stress and urge incontinence.

3. Barrier methods–The contraceptive diaphragm and ring pessary have been used to support the bladder neck and limit its rotational descent during stressful activities. This treatment can be useful for women who have leakage with specific activities such as aerobics or sports. The goal is to keep the woman active with activities she enjoys while she begins a program of pelvic muscle exercises. With proper fit, the device should stop the leakage with activity but allow for comfort and normal urination. The goal is not to occlude the bladder neck but to support it and limit its movement. A small urethral occlusion "plug" currently is undergoing clinical trials. It is an 8 French stem with a small balloon that holds it in place and is disposable after one use.

B. Pharmacotherapy:
1. Urge incontinence–As discussed previously, urge incontinence usually is caused by diminished bladder storage capacity from either UDC or decreased bladder compliance. The mainstay of treatment is anticholinergic or smooth-muscle antispasmodic drugs. The goal of treatment is to abolish or delay the involuntary contractions during the storage phase while maintaining voluntary contraction during the emptying phase. To be most successful, the medications need to be combined with use of a timed voiding schedule and attempts to limit intravesical irritation (eliminate bacteriuria, replace estrogen, eliminate dietary irritants, and dilute the urine).

Table 27–1 lists the multiple anticholinergic and antispasmodic medications that can improve bladder storage capacity. Oxybutynin hydrochloride, propantheline bromide, imipramine hydrochloride, flavoxate hydrochloride, and hyoscyamine sulfate are probably the most widely used. A failure of one of these medications is not an indication that all drug therapy will be unsuccessful. The second or third drug tried may provide continence. In refractory cases, a combination of imipramine with propantheline or oxybutynin can be successful. A combination of lower dosages of two medications may provide equal or superior urinary control with fewer side effects than higher doses of one medication. Again, it must be emphasized that medical therapy needs to be combined with behavioral changes including timed voiding schedules.

It is important to obtain a postvoid residual measurement 1–2 weeks after the medication is started, especially in patients who had increased residual volumes before the medication was started. Residual volumes can be determined by catheterization or ultrasonography. When residual volumes start to increase, the options are to decrease the dosage or start the patient on clean intermittent catheterization in addition to the medication. A mildly elevated residual volume in the face of improved urinary control, absence of significant frequency of urination, and absence of infections does not need to be treated but should be monitored intermittently to make sure the amount of residual urine does not continually increase, putting the woman at risk for overflow incontinence and infection.

When patients have a preexisting problem with constipation, which is a common side effect of anticholinergics, it is important to start them on a bulking agent and monitor bowel function carefully. Other common anticholinegic side effects—dry mouth and blurred vision—can be managed by decreasing the dosage or changing medications. The keys to successful pharmacologic therapy are as follows:

1. Starting with a low dosage and increasing or decreasing the dosage as needed
2. Tailoring the timing and dosage of the medication to the patient's needs
3. Closely monitoring side effects such as constipation and incomplete bladder emptying
4. Scheduling frequent follow-up visits to make necessary changes in the timing and dosage of the medication
5. Monitoring the patient for new illnesses or medications that may compromise urinary control
6. Trying different drugs or combinations as needed

Table 27–1. Medications to promote continence.

Generic/Trade Name	Dose	Mechanism of Action	Side Effects
Oxybutinin hydrochloride/Ditropan	2.5 mg QD to TID	Musculotropic relaxant, anticholinergic, local anesthetic	Dry mouth, nausea, dizziness, constipation, blurred vision
Propantheline bromide/Probanthine	7.5 mg QD to TID	Anticholinergic	Dry mouth, nausea, dizziness, constipation, blurred vision
Imipramine hydrochloride/Tofranil	10 mg QD to TID	Direct smooth muscle inhibition, alpha adrenergic	Dry mouth, nausea, dizziness, constipation, blurred vision
Dicyclomine/Bentyl	20 mg QD to TID	Musculotropic relaxant	Dry mouth, nausea, dizziness, constipation, blurred vision
Hyosyamine sulfate/ Cystospaz, Anaspaz, Levsin	.125 mg QD to TID	Anticholinergic	Dry mouth, nausea, dizziness, constipation, blurred vision
Flavoxate hydrochloride/ Urispas	1 mg QD to TID	Musculotropic relaxant, anticholinergic, local anesthetic	Dry mouth, nausea, dizziness, constipation, blurred vision
17 β-Estradiol cream/Estrace	2 gram vaginally 1–3 × per week	Increased mucosal seal, increased vascular cushion	Menstrual bleeding, headache, fluid retention, breast tenderness, local irritation
Phenylproprolamine hydrochloriden Ornade/Entex	25 mg QD to BID 1 QD to BID	Alpha adrenergic	Hypertension, sedation, dizziness, dry mouth, headache, nervousness, nausea
Pseudoephedrine hydrochloride Sudafed/Actifed Rondec TR	30 mg QD to BID 1 QD to BID	Alpha adrenergic	Hypertension, sedation, dizziness, dry mouth, headache, nervousness, nausea

7. Referring appropriate patients for specialty evaluation early
8. Providing written instructions for the patient

2. Activity-related incontinence–For stress incontinence, pharmacologic therapy is aimed at increasing the tone or resistance provided by the bladder neck and proximal urethral smooth muscle, which is innervated by alpha-sympathetic receptors. Medications that stimulate alpha receptors are ephedrine, pseudoephedrine, and phenylpropanolamine. These drugs are the active agents in decongestants and antihistamines. Imipramine has the combined effect of relaxing the detrusor muscle and stimulating the bladder neck; it can be effective for stress and urge incontinence and is a reasonable first choice for a woman who presents with mixed UI. Estrogens increase the number of alpha receptors in the proximal urethra and thus are an important adjuvant to the alpha-sympathomimetic drugs in perimenopausal and postmenopausal women. One dose in the morning may be adequate, especially in the timed-released preparations such as Ornade, Entex LA, or Rondec TR. The main disadvantages are the potential side effects: drowsiness, dryness of the mucous membranes, elevation of the blood pressure, tachycardia, and palpitations. It is important to note that this medication is effective only when it is taken and does not solve the underlying problem. For women who are not motivated to do exercises and do not wish to have surgery, a trial of medication is worthwhile. Medication also can be used in conjunction with a pelvic muscle program to provide improved control while the muscles are being strengthened.

C. Surgical Intervention: Although surgical correction may be the best option for many women, patients should know that the continence mechanism is complex and that surgical repair corrects only one of the factors. The procedure may not be a permanent cure for UI and may cause additional problems.

This caution is particularly relevant for women who elect to undergo a bladder neck suspension at the time of a hysterectomy because they occasionally leak urine with coughing or sneezing. If the incontinence is not enough of a problem for them to seek treatment independent of their gynecologic problem, the risk-benefit ratio usually does not justify performing the procedure.

Women need to know there are both surgical and nonsurgical options for treatment. Many women are not motivated sufficiently to perform pelvic muscle exercises and elect surgery as the first treatment. They should be able to choose surgery as the first option without having "failed" nonsurgical treatment. Knowing the options and understanding the risk-benefit ratios are the keys to a successful surgical outcome.

1. Urge incontinence–Intractable urge incontinence can be managed by bladder enlargement procedures. A segment of small intestine is "patched" onto the bladder to increase its capacity. Urination is through the urethra, and bowel function returns to normal after the surgery. Under very specific circumstances, the native bladder may be abandoned with the creation of a bladder "substitute" from bowel. This substitute can be created in a way that does not require wearing an external appliance (continent urinary diversion). A small stoma located on the lower abdomen is catheterized by the patient to empty the new "bladder."

A few centers around the country are working with implantable sacral nerve root stimulators to control inappropriate bladder contractions and thus eliminate incontinence. The clinical use of this method will likely increase over the next 5 years.

2. Activity-related incontinence (urethral hypermobility)–The goal of surgical correction of urethral hypermobility is to elevate the bladder base and urethra to their normal resting position and limit their movement during stressful activities. Besides restoring continence, the surgery has the goal of maintaining the ability to urinate. Unfortunately, a woman may be "cured" of her stress incontinence but have difficulties initiating voluntary urination, have total urinary retention, or develop frequency and urgency of urination and possibly urge incontinence. The patient may trade one set of problems for another, which may be more debilitating than what she had to begin with. The longevity of surgical repairs is difficult to assess. Five years postoperatively, 50–60% of women report return of urinary incontinence. The surgical repair may be intact with UI now secondary to one of the many other potential causes such as medication, lack of estrogen, or gradual nerve deterioration with aging.

The surgical approach for correction of anatomic relaxation can be abdominal or vaginal. The choice of technique is based on surgeon and patient preference and factors individual to the patient. In general, the risks and outcome are similar. The vaginal approaches involve a shorter hospital stay and shorter recovery time, although heavy lifting (greater than 15 lb) is restricted after both approaches. The trend has been to develop minimally invasive techniques for bladder neck suspension such as the "no vaginal incision" and laparoscopic approaches. For women with isolated bladder neck—urethral hypermobility without other anatomic problems, these techniques may be the best option, although the longevity data are nonexistent at this time.

The most commonly used transabdominal procedures are the Marshall-Marchetti-Krantz (MMK) and Burch operations. The obturator shelf, or paravaginal repair, is another transabdominal approach that is gaining popularity. The Raz and Stamey needle endoscopic bladder neck suspensions are used most commonly used by urologists. Alternatives are the Gittes and Benderev "no vaginal incision" needle suspensions. Some surgeons place small suprapubic catheters for bladder drainage at the time of surgery until normal urination resumes, whereas others instruct patients on self-intermittent catheterization using a "clean" rather than sterile technique. Return of normal urination may take days to weeks.

Long-term success of surgical repairs can be enhanced by long-term follow-up and patient education concerning risk factors that may weaken the repair over time. Some of these risk factors include vaginal deliveries, Valsalva voiding, chronic coughing, significant weight gain, high-impact sports, menopause without hormone replacement therapy, and repeated heavy lifting. Common sense suggests a program of pelvic muscle exercises as an adjunct to surgical repair to enhance the longevity of the procedure by maintaining muscle tone and preventing the gradual weakness that occurs with aging.

3. Intrinsic urethral dysfunction (type III incontinence)–Procedures to correct intrinsic urethral dysfunction include sling procedures, the artificial urinary sphincter, and periurethral injection therapy. There are many variations of the sling procedure. A strip of autologous fascia, artificial material (Marlex or Gortex), or isolated segment of vaginal wall is placed between the proximal urethra and vaginal wall to act as a fixed "backstop" to prevent urethral movement and provide coaptation of the proximal urethral walls. Because of a higher incidence of postoperative urinary retention and onset of frequency or urgency after this repair than others, this technique is not generally a first-line repair even though it may last longer.

The artificial urinary sphincter can be placed through an abdominal or vaginal incision. This device consists of an inflatable cuff that surrounds the bladder neck and proximal urethra, a reservoir that is placed next to the bladder, and a pump positioned in the labia. Continence is maintained by fluid in the cuff. Urination is accomplished by "pumping" fluid from the cuff to the reservoir, which allows urine to flow through the urethra, after which the cuff reinflates over 1–2 minutes restoring continence. Because this device is artificial, the risks include infection, malfunction, and erosion of the cuff through the bladder neck tissue. The method virtually eliminates the possibility of urinary retention.

Periurethral injection therapy has the advantage of being a simple endoscopic procedure that can be performed with local anesthesia. Substances available in the USA for periurethral injection are autologous fat and cross-linked bovine collagen (marketed as Contigen). The goal is to increase periurethral compressive forces at the bladder neck and proximal urethra. It is not the treatment of choice for women who have activity-related leakage secondary to urethral hypermobility. The optimal candidates are women with normal urethral position, minimal mobility, but poor intrinsic urethral function. Most often, women require more than one injection to attain sustained dryness and are likely to require repeat injections over the years as the material is broken down gradually by the body. Although this procedure is not a permanent cure, the ease of the procedure and 1-day recovery period make it an appealing option for selected patients.

D. Cystocele Repair: The main indication for cystocele repair is patient discomfort from the prolapsing organ. Each woman's tolerance level is different, and comfort may depend on how gradually the prolapse develops. Cystoceles can be associated with voiding difficulties, incomplete bladder emptying, urinary incontinence, or recurrent urinary tract infections, or there may be no symptoms. Very large cystoceles can be associated with hydronephrosis from elongating and "kinking" of the distal ureters, and renal ultrasonography or intravenous pyelography is indicated before the decision is made to follow a large cystocele conservatively. Pessaries are a good option for many women who are not interested in surgery. Women can be instructed to insert and remove the pessaries themselves.

E. Summary of Treatment Strategy:
1. Patient education regarding lower urinary tract structure and function.
2. Discussion of potential role of diet and fluid intake.
3. Use of bladder diaries as appropriate.
4. Bladder retraining or "holding" protocols as appropriate.
5. Pelvic muscle awareness and strengthening programs: Written protocols can be tried for women with good muscle localization on examination; vaginal cones can be considered for women with some awareness of their muscles and those who think the cones would be easier for them to comply with; patients with minimal or no awareness of their pelvic muscles on examination can be referred for biofeedback training.
6. Initiation of hormone replacement therapy if appropriate.
7. Use of pharmacologic agents if appropriate, tailored to the patient's needs.
8. Referral to a specialist if treatment is considered unsuccessful by the patient.

The definition of treatment success is specific to the patient. For some patients, total dryness under all circumstances is necessary to meet their needs; unfortunately, this goal may not be realistic or possible. For other women, enough bladder control so that they can leave the house for social outings using external protection but without fear that they will leak through onto their clothing is sufficient. Physicians must keep in mind the complex nature of the continence mechanism and the multiple contributing causes of urinary incontinence, only some of which can be altered. The desire to cure should not interfere with listening to the patient and identifying what is important to her.

Referral to a Specialist

Historical factors that indicate the need for referral to a specialist in women's urologic problems (female urologist or urogynecologist) are as follows:

1. History of urinary retention or documented incomplete bladder emptying (increased postvoid residual)
2. Continuous incontinence
3. Spontaneous loss of urine or bed-wetting
4. History of possible neurologic diseases, injuries, or surgeries
5. History of repeated urethral dilation or internal urethrotomy
6. History of incontinence surgery that did not correct the problem or made it worse
7. History of radical pelvic surgery (radical hysterectomy or abdominal-perineal resection)
8. History of radiation to pelvic organs

Case Study

MB is an 88-year-old nulliparous woman who presents with a 5-year history of progressive activity-related, urge, and spontaneous UI. She rarely leaves her apartment. She manages her incontinence with superabsorbent commercially available pads and fluid restriction. She drinks 4–5 cups of coffee each day and minimal water.

MB has no significant medical illnesses, takes no medication on an ongoing basis, and has never undergone hormone replacement therapy. She has had no previous urologic or gynecologic surgeries. Her examination reveals atrophic external genitalia and vaginal tissues. She has normal anatomic support with minimal urethral hypermobility. She has fair awareness of her pelvic floor muscles and a weak but well-localized voluntary contraction of the muscle. Her postvoid residual is less than 50 mL, and her urinalysis is unremarkable.

The patient was instructed to decrease her coffee intake and increase her water intake. She was started on vaginal estrogen replacement 3 times/wk and given written instructions for a pelvic muscle exercise program. She was also started on low-dose anticholinergic therapy with oxybutynin, 2.5 mg morning and evening.

The patient returned 4 weeks later stating she was "99% improved." Her daily coffee intake was down to one cup, and she was drinking five glasses of water each day. Her postvoid residual remained below 50 mL. She now felt comfortable leaving her apartment with a small pad on for "psychologic protection." She indicated she was able to do her pelvic muscle exercises at least once daily. No changes were made in her treatment plan.

Although this case represents multiple simultaneous interventions, making it difficult to know which is most important, it is illustrative of what can be accomplished with simple, low-risk measures even in older women who have severely debilitating incontinence.

REFERENCES

Axelrod SL, Blaivas JG: Bladder neck obstruction in women. J Urol 1987;137:497.

Blaivas JG: Classification of stress urinary incontinence. Neurourol Urodynam 1984;2:103.

Bo K et al: Pelvic floor muscle exercise for the treatment of female stress urinary incontinence. III. Effects of two different degrees of pelvic floor muscle exercises. Neurourol Urodynam 1990;9:489.

Burgio KL, Robinson JC, Engel BT: The role of biofeedback in Kegel exercise training for stress urinary incontinence. Am J Obstet Gynecol 1986;154:58.

Fantyl JA et al: Diuretics and urinary incontinence in community-dwelling women. Neurourol Urodynam 1990; 9:25.

Hilton P: Urinary incontinence during sexual intercourse: A common, but rarely volunteered symptom. Br J Obstet Gynecol 1988;95:377.

Hilton P, Stanton SL: The use of intravaginal estrogen cream in genuine stress urinary incontinence. Br J Obstet Gynecol 1983;90:940.

Kegel AH: Progressive resistance exercise in the functional restoration of the perineal muscles. Am J Obstet Gynecol 1948;36:238.

Khan Z, Bhola A, Starer P: Urinary incontinence during orgasm. Urology 1988;31:279.

Lauberg S et al: Neurologic cause of idiopathic incontinence. Arch Neurol 1988;45:1250.

Lewis WH, Ilving AS: Changes with age in renal function in adult men. Am J Physiol 1938;123:500.

Norton P: Randomized prospective trial of vaginal cones vs Kegel exercises in postpartum primiparous women. 20th Annual Meeting of the International Continence Society, Aarhus, Denmark, 1990.

Parys BT et al: The effects of simple hysterectomy on vesicourethral function. Br J Urol 1989;64:594.

Peattie AB, Plevnik S, Stanton SL: Vaginal cones: A conservative method of treating genuine stress incontinence. Br J Obstet Gynecol 1988;85:1049.

Sugar EC, Firlit CF: Urodynamic biofeedback: A new therapeutic approach for childhood incontinence/infection (vesical voluntary sphincter dyssynergia). J Urol 1982; 128:1253.

Tanagho EA: Effect of hysterectomy and periurethral surgery on urethrovesical function. In: *Gynecological Urology and Urodynamics.* Ostergard DR (editor). Williams & Wilkins, 1985.

Viktrup L et al: The symptoms of stress incontinence caused by pregnancy or delivery in primiparas. Obstet Gynecol 1992;79:945.

Williams ME, Pannill FC: Urinary incontinence in the elderly. Ann Intern Med 1982;97:895.

Wolin LH: Stress incontinence in young, healthy nulliparous female subjects. J Urol 1969;101:545.

Urinary Tract Infections

28

Catherine S. Thompson, MD

Infections of the urinary tract occur in women of all ages and affect up to 20% of women during their lifetime. Many experience multiple or recurrent infections. Infections during the childbearing years are particularly common. In the United States, the annual cost of evaluation and treatment of urinary tract infections in women exceeds $1 billion. This significant health problem is reviewed with an emphasis on pertinent pathophysiology, a diagnostic approach that stresses differential diagnosis, and a discussion of therapeutic options.

DEFINITIONS

Urinary tract infections are caused most often by bacterial invasion of the urinary tract. Fungal and viral pathogens are much less common. **Bacteriuria** is defined as the presence of bacteria in the urine; however, this finding alone is never diagnostic of a urinary tract infection. Bacteria may be present in uninfected urine if contamination of the specimen with periurethral or vaginal flora occurs at the time of collection. The term **significant bacteriuria** is used to distinguish contaminated urine from true infection. Depending on the clinical setting and technique of collection, significant bacteriuria is defined in the following ways:

At least 10^2 coliforms per milliliter in a symptomatic woman
At least 10^5 noncoliforms per milliliter in a symptomatic woman
At least 10^5 bacteria per milliliter in an asymptomatic woman
At least 10^2 bacteria per milliliter in a woman with an indwelling bladder catheter.

Asymptomatic bacteriuria refers to significant bacteriuria in a woman with no symptoms of infection. Asymptomatic infections are particularly common during pregnancy and in older, postmenopausal women.

The term **lower urinary tract infection** includes **cystitis** and **urethritis**, which are infections of the urinary bladder and urethra, respectively. When the kidneys or upper urinary tracts are involved, the term **pyelonephritis** is used. Upper and lower tract infections can be difficult to distinguish on clinical grounds because of significant overlap in presenting symptoms and signs.

Urinary tract infections can be described as either uncomplicated or complicated. This broad division helps the clinician design treatment for the infection as well as make plans for follow-up. Complicated infections occur in women with anatomic or functional abnormalities of the urinary tract and often are associated with pathogens that are resistant to conventional antibiotics. The factors that suggest the presence of a complicated urinary tract infection are as follows:

Pregnancy
Indwelling bladder catheter
Recent urinary tract instrumentation
Functional or anatomic abnormality of the urinary tract

Diabetes mellitus
Immunosuppression
Recent antimicrobial use
Hospital-acquired infection
Symptoms for longer than 7 days at presentation.

PATHOGENESIS

Most urinary tract infections develop when fecal uropathogens colonize the vaginal introitus or urethra and ascend into the bladder. The usual result is an inflammatory host response characterized by specific symptoms and pyuria. Women with recurrent urinary tract infections may have an increased susceptibility to vaginal colonization with uropathogens. The risk of developing a urinary tract infection is enhanced by circumstances that propel bacteria from the introital area into the bladder. These include sexual intercourse, use of a contraceptive diaphragm or spermicidal jelly, urinary tract instrumentation, and poor perineal hygiene. The risk of infection also is influenced by intrinsic virulence factors unique to the organism.

Organisms that gain entry into the bladder and establish a lower tract infection may ascend into the upper urinary tract. The risk factors for the development of upper urinary tract infection are incompletely understood. Intrinsic virulence factors of the infecting organism as well as functional or anatomic abnormalities of the urinary tract in the host may increase the risk of upper tract infection.

The vast majority of urinary tract infections are caused by facultative anaerobic organisms that colonize the lower gastrointestinal tract. *Escherichia coli* is the most common of these organisms and accounts for 85% of all uncomplicated, community-acquired urinary tract infections. Other enteric gram-negative organisms such as the *Klebsiella* or *Proteus* species are less frequently observed. Gram-positive organisms such as *Staphylococcus saprophyticus* account for 10% of infections. Women with complicated urinary tract infections are infected with *E coli* in 50% of cases. In contrast to simple cystitis, however, in complicated urinary tract infections, there is a higher incidence of infection with other gram-negative organisms such as *Pseudomonas, Serratia, Proteus,* or *Klebsiella.* Gram-positive organisms including *Staphylococcus* and enterococci are also recognized pathogens in complicated infections, particularly after instrumentation of the urinary tract.

DIFFERENTIAL DIAGNOSIS

The symptoms of acute lower urinary tract infection (cystitis) are dysuria, urgency, and frequency with or without suprapubic or low back discomfort. Upper tract infection (pyelonephritis) is suggested by the presence of flank pain and a variety of systemic symptoms such as nausea, vomiting, or fever and chills. Differentiation of upper tract infection from simple cystitis may be difficult. Up to one-third of women with symptoms suggestive of simple cystitis may have unrecognized involvement of the upper urinary tract. The testing required to distinguish upper from lower tract infection includes such procedures as bladder washout, assay for antibody-coated bacteria (suggestive of upper tract involvement), and selective ureteral catheterization. These procedures are cumbersome and expensive and therefore have a limited role in the routine management of urinary tract infections. Fortunately, the confirmation of upper tract involvement is rarely necessary.

Dysuria does not necessarily imply a urinary tract infection. The differential diagnosis includes other conditions such as urethritis caused by *Neisseria gonorrhoea* or *Chlamydia trachomatis.* Urethritis is the likely diagnosis when pyuria without bacteriuria is detected in a woman with dysuria. Other conditions that may confuse the diagnosis include a variety of vaginal infections (*Candida* or *Trichomonas*), herpes simplex infection, genitourinary trauma, or the use of chemical irritants.

CLINICAL SYNDROMES

The approach to diagnosing a urinary tract infection is simplified by the identification of a specific syndrome that most likely accounts for the clinical presentation. Although there may be overlap in some cases, this approach is useful in evaluation and treatment. Urinary tract infections in women can be categorized broadly as follows:

Acute uncomplicated cystitis
Acute uncomplicated pyelonephritis
Complicated urinary tract infection
Pregnancy-associated urinary tract infection
Urinary tract infection in elderly women

ACUTE UNCOMPLICATED CYSTITIS

The acute, uncomplicated episode of cystitis constitutes the most common type of urinary tract infection in women. Women of childbearing age are most frequently affected. Sexual intercourse and the use of a contraceptive diaphragm with spermicidal jelly increase the risk of these infections.

Diagnosis

Most women are symptomatic with dysuria, frequency, or urgency; often there is suprapubic or low back discomfort. Pyuria and bacteriuria with or without hematuria are diagnostic findings on urinalysis. The leukocyte esterase dipstick can detect significant pyuria in up to 95% of cases. A urine culture is not necessary in nonpregnant women who present with typical symptoms and findings on urinalysis. A cost-effective approach is to confirm the presence of bacteria and pyuria and institute empiric treatment with oral antibiotics. A follow-up urine culture is not performed unless symptoms persist or recur after treatment. If a urine culture is performed in a symptomatic woman, a colony count of 100 or more (greater than 10^2) coliforms per milliliter of urine or of 100,000 or more (greater than 10^5) noncoliform organisms is considered diagnostic of significant bacteriuria (see the preceding section, "Definitions").

Treatment

The treatment of uncomplicated cystitis has been simplified by the use of shorter courses of oral antibiotics (Table 28–1). Single-dose therapy, which initially gained popularity, is no longer recommended because of lower rates of cure. A 3-day regimen is preferred and is associated with cure rates comparable with a 7-day regimen but without the added cost or drug side effects (rashes, monilial vaginitis, diarrhea) of the longer treatment. A variety of antibiotics can be used as outlined in Table 28–1. Although resistance to antimicrobials varies from region to region, resistance to trimethoprim and the combination trimethoprim-sulfamethoxazole is 5–15% and to the fluoroquinolone antimicrobials is less than 5%. These agents are the drugs of choice, therefore, for a 3-day regimen. The lower cost of trimethoprim and

trimethoprim-sulfamethoxazole makes these drugs the first-line agents, with fluoroquinolones generally reserved for refractory or more complicated cases.

Recurrent episodes of cystitis are a problem for many women and are almost always caused by reinfection. Only 10% of women have an anatomic or functional anomaly of the lower urinary tract that predisposes to recurrent, relapsing episodes of cystitis. Recurrent infections should be documented by urine culture and diagnosed as either a **relapse** (infection with the same organism occurring within weeks of initial therapy) or a **reinfection** (infection caused by a different bacterial strain, usually more than 2 weeks after the last course of antibiotic therapy).

A variety of interventions have been proposed to manage recurrent episodes of cystitis. A true relapse should be treated with a longer course of antibiotics, up to 2–6 weeks, and an anatomic or functional anomaly of the urinary tract should be considered in these cases. An intravenous urogram with or without cystoscopy may be helpful.

For most women, however, reinfection with a uropathogen is the problem; anatomic anomalies are rare. The treatment depends on the frequency of the recurrences. Women with fewer than two episodes of cystitis in 1 year might be managed with "patient-initiated" therapy. A 3-day regimen of antibiotics, generally trimethoprim-sulfamethoxazole, is initiated when classic symptoms of infection are recognized (Table 28–1). For women who have more than three infections per year, prophylactic antibiotic regimens can be considered as outlined in Table 28–2. Women who associate their recurrent infections with sexual activity may benefit from postcoital prophylaxis. Women whose recurrences are unrelated to coitus may benefit from daily or twice-weekly prophylaxis with a variety of low-dose oral antibiotics.

Postmenopausal women may be affected by recurrent urinary tract infections. Bladder or uterine prolapse may produce incomplete voiding and increase the risk of infection. Prophylactic antimicrobials in selected circumstances may be helpful (Table 28–2).

Table 28–1. Three-day oral regimens for the treatment of simple cystitis.*

Drug	Dosage
Trimethoprim-sulfamethoxazole DS	160 mg/800 mg q12h
Trimethoprim	100 mg q12h
Norfloxacin	400 mg q12h
Ciprofloxacin	250 mg q12h
Nitrofurantoin	100 mg q6h
Amoxicillin	250 mg q8h

*The specific choice and dosage of antibiotic may vary in patients with imparied renal and hepatic function.

Table 28–2. Prophylactic antibiotic regimens.*

Postcoital prophylaxis: single dose
  Trimethoprim-sulfamethoxazole, 40 mg/200 mg (one-half of a single-strength tablet)
  Cephalexin, 250 mg
  Nitrofurantoin, 50–100 mg
Daily or 3 times weekly prophylaxis
  Trimethoprim, 100 mg
  Trimethoprim-sulfamethoxazole, 40 mg/200 mg
  Nitrofurantoin, 50–100 mg
  Norfloxacin, 200 mg
  Cephalexin, 250 mg

*The specific choice and dosage of antibiotic may vary in patients with impaired renal or hepatic function.

ACUTE, UNCOMPLICATED PYELONEPHRITIS

Infection of the upper urinary tract (pyelonephritis) presents as a spectrum of illness. Many women have relatively mild symptoms suggestive of simple cystitis. Others have flank discomfort, fever, chills, or nausea and vomiting with or without lower tract symptoms. More than 80% of cases of pyelonephritis are caused by *E coli,* and the remainder of cases are attributed to other gram-negative organisms, enterococci, or *Staphylococcus.* Bacteremia occurs in 15–20% of cases of pyelonephritis.

Diagnosis

The unspun urine in women with pyelonephritis contains leukocytes and bacteria. A Gram stain of the urine may be helpful in selecting the antimicrobial therapy; most cases are caused by gram-negative organisms, but enterococcal infection is suggested by the presence of gram-positive cocci on Gram stain. A urine culture is advised in women with suspected upper tract infection. The distinction between simple cystitis and uncomplicated pyelonephritis may be difficult. A history of pyelonephritis or presence of unusually severe symptoms suggests upper tract infection.

Treatment

The management of pyelonephritis differs from that of simple cystitis in the selection and duration of antimicrobial therapy. Women with mild symptoms and no dehydration or gastrointestinal manifestations typically do well with oral antibiotics prescribed on an outpatient basis for 10–14 days. The antimicrobial agents of choice are the same as those used for treatment of simple cystitis (Table 28–1). Women with more severe illness should be hospitalized for hydration and intravenous antibiotics. Blood cultures should be obtained. Parenteral therapy as outlined in Table 28–3 is recommended until the patient is afebrile. Oral antibiotics are prescribed subsequently to bring the treatment course to 14 days. A follow-up

urine culture is recommended after completion of therapy.

The symptoms and signs of pyelonephritis should resolve within 72 hours of initiation of antibiotic therapy. Imaging studies of the urinary tract are indicated in women whose symptoms are slow to improve. Occult anatomic anomalies, intrarenal abscess, perinephric abscess, or obstruction may be identified in these settings. Renal ultrasonography, intravenous urography, or computed tomography (CT) of the kidneys may be helpful. Women in whom anomalies are detected on imaging studies are considered to have a complicated infection.

COMPLICATED URINARY INFECTIONS

In addition to anatomic anomalies, complicated infections can be associated with an indwelling bladder catheter or with multiresistant or unusual microbial agents. The clinical presentation of a complicated infection is variable, ranging from asymptomatic bacteriuria to life-threatening septicemia.

Diagnosis

The diagnosis of a complicated infection is largely one of recognition. As shown in the earlier section, "Definitions," women with one or more of the listed risk factors should be watched for development of a complicated infection and may require lengthier treatment or additional investigation. A complicated infection can be difficult to recognize if the presenting symptoms and signs are those of a simple, uncomplicated urinary tract infection (either cystitis or pyelonephritis). In other cases, more severe symptoms such as extreme flank discomfort or systemic signs of high fever, lethargy, or confusion provide the clue that a complicated infection may be present. Identification of the woman susceptible to a complicated infection is dependent on the recognition of the risk factors listed previously in this chapter.

Treatment

Treatment with antibiotics for a minimum of 10–14 days, selected on the basis of the results of a urine culture, is recommended. Parenteral treatment may be indicated, depending on the clinical setting (Table 28–4). Anatomic imaging of the urinary tract should be considered in patients who are slow to respond to treatment. A correctable abnormality such as obstruction or the detection of either a renal or perinephric abscess would affect duration and type of treatment. A urine culture obtained after completion of antibiotic therapy is advised in women with a complicated urinary tract infection.

Table 28–3. Intravenous treatment of pyelonephritis.*

Drug[†]	Dosage
Trimethoprim-sulfamethoxazole	160 mg/800 mg q12h
Ciprofloxacin	200–400 mg q12h
Gentamicin	1 mg/kg q8h, with or without ampicillin, 1 gm q6h
Ceftriaxone	1–2 g q24h

*The specific choice and dosage of antibiotic may vary in patients with impaired renal or hepatic function. Drug levels or other monitoring (eg, creatinine clearance) may be required.
[†]All drugs are given until the patient is afebrile and followed by oral antibiotics to bring the treatment course to 14 days.

Table 28–4. Treatment of complicated urinary tract infections.*

Intravenous[†]
  Ampicillin, 1 g q6h with gentamicin, 1 mg/kg q8h
  Ciprofloxacin, 200–400 mg q12h
  Ceftriaxone, 1–2 g q24h
  Aztreonam, 1 g q8–12h
  Imipenem-cilastatin, 250–500 mg q6–8h
Oral
  Norfloxacin, 400 mg q12h
  Ciprofloxacin, 500 mg q12h
  Trimethoprim-sulfamethoxazole, 160 mg/800 mg q12h

*The specific choice and dosage of antibiotic may vary in patients with impaired renal or hepatic function. Drug levels or other monitoring (eg, creatinine clearance) may be required.
[†]The course of treatment is 10–14 d for mild-to-moderate illness and 14–21 d for severe illness.

URINARY TRACT INFECTIONS IN PREGNANCY

The detection and treatment of asymptomatic bacteriuria during pregnancy is an important issue in obstetric care. Although asymptomatic bacteriuria complicates only 4–8% of all pregnancies, the infection progresses to a symptomatic urinary tract infection during gestation in 20–40% of these women. The relationship between asymptomatic bacteriuria and a variety of obstetric complications such as prematurity, preterm labor, growth retardation, and maternal hypertension is a controversial issue. There is agreement, however, that screening and treatment of women with asymptomatic bacteriuria during pregnancy is indicated, at least to prevent the development of overt symptomatic urinary tract infection.

The urinary tract undergoes significant change during pregnancy. Hormonal and mechanical factors allow for dilation of the renal collecting system and ureters. These changes predispose women to progression from asymptomatic bacteriuria to symptomatic, and often clinically severe, upper tract infection. Enteric gram-negative bacteria such as *E coli* are the most common organisms cultured from the urine. Less frequently, gram-positive organisms, *Gardnerella vaginalis,* or *Ureaplasma urealyticum* are identified.

Screening

Pregnant women should be screened early in gestation for asymptomatic bacteriuria. A quantitative urine culture done during the first trimester and no later than 16 weeks of gestation is recommended. A clean-catch midstream collection is preferred; bladder catheterization is not advised. Significant bacteriuria is defined by a colony count of greater than 10 bacteria per milliliter of urine.

Treatment

Treatment is recommended for 3–7 days with an appropriate antibiotic given orally. Amoxicillin has a long safety record and is preferred, but for resistant organisms or patients who are allergic to the drug, nitrofurantoin, sulfisoxazole, and cephalexin are alternatives (Table 28–5). A follow-up urine culture should be performed 1 week after antimicrobial treatment is completed. Persistent bacteriuria or relapse of infection during pregnancy can occur in up to 20–30% of women. Serial urine cultures may be needed at monthly intervals during pregnancy; the results guide further courses of oral antibiotic therapy. Women who require antibiotic therapy for the duration of pregnancy are likely to have infection of the upper urinary tract and should be evaluated for structural or functional anomalies in the postpartum period.

Symptomatic urinary tract infections develop in 1–2% of all pregnancies. The presentation most closely resembles acute pyelonephritis in nonpregnant women. The typical treatment is hospitalization for intravenous antibiotics, usually ampicillin and an aminoglycoside until culture results are known (Table 28–5). Conversion to oral antibiotics with a total duration of treatment of 2 weeks is advised. Suppressive antibiotics in lower doses usually are needed until delivery. Failure to respond to standard treatment suggests a complicated urinary infection. Sonography of the urinary tract may be necessary to exclude a renal or perirenal abscess or other anomaly.

URINARY TRACT INFECTIONS IN OLDER WOMEN

Bacteriuria in women older than 65 years is common; the prevalence increases with age and approaches 50% by age 80. The incidence of bacteriuria is highest in women living in nursing homes and

Table 28–5. Treatment of urinary tract infection in pregnancy.*

Asymptomatic bacteriuria: 3- to 7-d course
  Amoxicillin, 250–500 mg q8h
  Nitrofurantoin, 100 mg q6h
  Cephalexin, 250–500 mg q6h
  Sulfisoxazole, 1 g, followed by 500 mg q6h
Symptomatic infection: 14-d course[†]
  Intravenous
    Gentamicin, 1 mg/kg q8h and ampicillin, 1 g q6h
    Ceftriaxone, 1–2 g q24h
    Aztreonam, 1 g q8–12h
  Oral
    Amoxicillin, 500 mg q8h
    Cephalexin, 250–500 mg q6h
    Sulfisoxazole, 500 mg q6h

*The specific choice and dosage of antibiotic may vary in patients with impaired renal or hepatic function. Drug levels or other monitoring (eg, creatinine clearance) may be required.
[†]Mild, uncomplicated cases can be managed with oral antibiotics.

in women with incomplete bladder emptying, those with fecal incontinence, and those who require intermittent bladder catheterization. Bacteriuria in this population can occur sporadically and is often asymptomatic. There is no proven association between asymptomatic bacteriuria in the elderly and increased mortality.

An ascending route of infection via the urethra is the most common cause of bacteriuria in this population. Estrogen deficiency may allow enteric flora to populate the vaginal and periurethral areas, although treatment with exogenous estrogen does not reduce the incidence of urinary tract infection reliably in postmenopausal women. *E coli* continues to be the most common infecting organism in older women, with other enteric gram-negative rods and enterococci occurring more commonly than staphylococcal infection. Hospitalized elderly women are particularly prone to gram-negative infections other than *E coli.*

Diagnosis

The clinical features of urinary tract infections in elderly women are varied. Most women are entirely asymptomatic. Classic lower tract symptoms of dysuria, urgency, and frequency may occur and suggest simple cystitis. Upper tract infection may present with fever and flank discomfort; however, overwhelming sepsis, bacteremia, diminished mental status, and gastrointestinal or respiratory complaints may be the presenting features of pyelonephritis in this population.

Treatment

All symptomatic urinary tract infections should be treated. The selection of antimicrobial agents, duration of treatment, and route of administration should be guided by the clinical setting and whether the presentation most closely resembles simple cystitis; acute, uncomplicated pyelonephritis; or a complicated infection. Elderly women with suspected upper tract infection almost always require hospitalization and intravenous antibiotics. Lower tract infections can be managed with 3- to 7-day courses of oral antibiotics.

The management of asymptomatic bacteriuria in elderly women is controversial. The condition is defined as two successive urine cultures with greater than 10 organisms per milliliter. Depending on the clinical setting, either no treatment or no more than a 3-day course of oral antibiotics can be administered. A follow-up urine culture is not necessary, and routine screening for asymptomatic bacteriuria is not recommended in this population.

REFERENCES

Johnson JR, Stamm WE: Urinary tract infections in women: Diagnosis and treatment. Ann Intern Med 1989;111:906.
Kaye E (editor): *Urinary Tract Infections. Medical Clinics of North America.* Vol 75. Saunders, 1991.

Stamm WE, Hooton TM: Management of urinary tract infections in adults. N Engl J Med 1993;329:1328.

Section VII.
Gastrointestinal Disorders

Liver Disease

29

James E. Bredfeldt, MD

Liver disease in women may cause significant health problems, with clinical manifestations similar to those in men. There are, however, specific health issues related to liver diseases that are unique for women.

GENERAL CONSIDERATIONS

Liver disease is suspected when abnormalities in standard liver chemistry tests are uncovered. Often these abnormalities are identified inadvertently in women during the course of a routine health assessment. The most frequent abnormalities found are elevations of the serum aminotransferases: the aspartate aminotransferase (AST) and the alanine aminotransferase (ALT). The second most common abnormality revealed is an elevation of the serum alkaline phosphatase (SAP) level. In most instances, the degree of elevation is not great, and the first step is to confirm that these elevations are indeed arising from the liver. This step is of particular importance to avoid seeking a liver disease to explain an elevated AST that is caused by a muscle disease with an elevated creatine phosphokinase (CPK) level or an elevated SAP level that is of bone origin. Once it is determined that the abnormal elevations in AST, ALT, or SAP are of liver origin, disease-specific serologic testing is introduced to establish the cause.

The degree of AST or ALT elevation is important in the initial assessment and is best analyzed in terms of the normal limits of the AST and ALT values (Table 29–1). The degree of elevation can be mild (less than 2–3 times the upper limits of normal), moderate (2–20 times the upper limits of normal), or severe (greater than 20 times the upper limits of normal). This distinction is important because it may indicate the when to test for additional disease-specific markers (Table 29–2).

In asymptomatic patients with a mild elevation revealed for the first time, it is reasonable to repeat the tests in 4–6 weeks and obtain a CPK level before embarking on a more detailed evaluation. Further evaluation includes history of current medication use, alcohol ingestion, risk factors for acquiring chronic viral hepatitis (particularly injecting drug use, blood transfusions, or multiple sexual partners), changes in

General Considerations
  Hemochromatosis
  Wilson's Disease
  Liver Biopsy
  Serum Alkaline Phosphatase Elevations
Chronic Viral Hepatitis
  Essentials of Diagnosis
  Incidence & Risk Factors
  Clinical Findings & Diagnosis
  Treatment
  Prognosis
  Issues of Pregnancy & Viral Hepatitis
Autoimmune Liver Disease
  Autoimmune Hepatitis
    Essentials of Diagnosis
    Clinical Findings & Diagnosis
    Treatment
  Primary Biliary Cirrhosis
    Clinical Stages
    Diagnosis
    Treatment
    Prognosis
Alcoholic Liver Disease
  Essentials of Diagnosis
  Diagnosis & Treatment
Fatty Liver & Steatohepatitis
Hepatic Tumors
Hepatotoxicity Resulting from Vitamins &
  Herbal Agents
  Vitamins

health status (including obesity, diabetes, and hyperlipidemia), and family history. At this juncture, disease-specific markers to exclude chronic viral hepatitis B and C and hemochromatosis should be considered, because disclosing these diseases leads to further evaluation and recommendations.

Hemochromatosis

A diagnosis of hemochromatosis always should be sought, because it is the most common autosomal recessive genetic disorder in adults. The frequency of homozygotes in the hemochromatosis gene is approximately 1:350–1:500 in the Caucasian population. Hemochromatosis can be excluded by a combi-

Table 29–1. Differential diagnosis of elevated levels of aspartate aminotransferase and alanine transferase, in order of frequency.

Less than 2 × UNL*	2–20 × UNL	More than 20 × UNL
Fatty liver	Chronic viral hepatitis	Acute viral hepatitis
Chronic viral hepatits	Fatty liver	Acute drug toxicity
Alcoholic liver disease	Alcoholic liver disease	Autoimmune hepatitis
Hemochromatosis	Autoimmune liver disease	
Autoimmune liver disease	Drug hepatotoxicity	
Drug hepatoxicity	Wilson's disease	
Wilson's disease	Hemochromatosis	

*UNL = upper limits of normal.

nation of the following methods: (1) fasting serum iron level and iron-binding capacity, calculating the percentage of transferrin saturation, and (2) serum ferritin level. If the percentage of transferrin saturation exceeds 60% or the serum ferritin level is increased, one should suspect hemochromatosis. Evaluating iron levels of women of childbearing age may present problems in interpretation of the results as a consequence of chronic iron loss through menses or pregnancy. Identifying patients who have hemochromatosis is important, because treatment with therapeutic phlebotomy prevents irreversible organ damage from the iron overload and improves long-term survival.

Wilson's Disease

In patients younger than 35 years, Wilson's disease should be excluded. Wilson's disease is a rare disorder that may present with signs of liver disease or a neurologic disorder. If the serum ceruloplasmin level is low or borderline-low, additional studies are indicated, including a 24-hour urine collection for copper and a slit-lamp examination for Kayser-Fleischer rings. If the diagnosis is suspected, a liver biopsy is indicated to quantitate copper in the liver. This diagnosis is particularly important, because

treatment with D-penicillamine prevents many of the serious complications of Wilson's disease.

Liver Biopsy

If there is evidence for chronic hepatitis B or C or if testing indicates the possible presence of either hemochromatosis or Wilsons disease, a liver biopsy is indicated. The liver biopsy assists in staging the severity of chronic hepatitis B or C or in quantitating levels of iron or copper in hemochromatosis or Wilson's disease, respectively. If this initial serologic assessment does not identify a specific disease, however, it is justified to reassess the AST or ALT level in 3–6 months before proceeding further. In most patients with persistent and mild elevations of AST and ALT levels, fatty liver, related to obesity or an underlying hyperlipidemia, is the most common cause for the elevations.

In patients with a **moderate** elevation of AST and ALT levels, the presence of a significant liver disease is much more likely. In this setting, proceeding directly to disease-specific marker testing is justified. Patients with **severe** elevations of AST and ALT are more likely to have acute hepatitis, either viral or drug-induced. Serologic studies to exclude acute viral hepatitis should be obtained (Table 29–3).

Serum Alkaline Phosphatase Elevations

In patients with an elevated serum alkaline phosphatase level, particularly if it is an isolated abnormality, the initial approach should be to demonstrate that the alkaline phosphatase is derived from the liver (Table 29–4). This assessment can be made by test-

Table 29–2. Disease-specific markers.

Disease	Marker
Chronic viral hepatitis	
Hepatitis B virus	HBsAg
Hepatitis C virus	Hepatitis C antibody (ELISA* or RIBA)
	Hepatitis C virus RNA by polymerase chain reaction
Autoimmune liver disease	
Autoimmune hepatitis	Antinuclear antibody
	Smooth-muscle antibody
	Antiliver and kidney microsomal antibody
Primary biliary cirrhosis	Antimitochondrial antibody
Hemochromatosis	Serum iron, iron-binding capacity
	Serum ferritin
Wilson's disease	Serum ceruloplasmin

*ELISA = enzyme-linked immunosorbent assay.
†RIBA = recombinant immunoblot assay.

Table 29–3. Serologic diagnosis of acute viral hepatitis.

Hepatitis A virus
  IgM hepatitis A antibody
Hepatitis B virus
  Hepatitis B surface antigen (HBsAg)
  IgM Hepatitis B core antibody (anti-HBc)
Hepatitis C virus*
  Hepatitis C virus RNA by polymerase chain reaction

*Hepatitis C antibody usually is not detected for 2–6 months after the onset of the acute infection.

Table 29–4. Differential diagnosis of elevated alkaline phosphatase.

Hepatic
    Neoplasms (benign; malignant [primary, metastatic])
    Fatty liver
    Alcoholic liver disease
    Primary biliary cirrhosis
    Drug-induced hepatotoxicity
    Hepatic granulomas
Biliary tract
    Bile duct obstruction (stones, strictures, neoplasms)
    Primary sclerosing cholangitis
Nonhepatic
    Paget's disease
    Bone metastases
    Physiologic (pregnancy, puberty)

ing for either gamma glutamyl transpeptidase (GGTP) or the 5′ nucleotidase. Hepatic neoplasms require exclusion in this setting, and liver ultrasonography or computed tomography (CT) definitely is indicated. Biliary tract disease often is present, and endoscopic retrograde cholangiopancreatography (ERCP) is performed to exclude a vast array of disorders, including choledocholithiasis, primary sclerosing cholangitis, ampullary stenosis, and neoplasms of the bile duct and the head of the pancreas. Because primary biliary cirrhosis is a common disorder in women, an antimitochondrial antibody often is obtained.

CHRONIC VIRAL HEPATITIS

Chronic hepatitis as a consequence of hepatitis B or C virus may lead to serious health consequences. In women, several health issues are present that require review. First, vertical transmission of the infection from the mother to the neonate may occur. Second, viral hepatitis may be sexually transmitted. Third, chronic viral hepatitis may affect the overall health of the woman.

Essentials of Diagnosis
- AST/ALT elevations are present for longer than 6 months
- Specific serologic testing (eg, a positive hepatitis B surface antigen [HBsAg])
- Confirmation of a chronic hepatitis C antibody (EIA) requires additional testing by hepatitis C antibody (RIBA) or hepatitis C virus-RNA by polymerase chain reaction.

Incidence & Risk Factors
Both hepatitis B and C virus infections should be considered possibly sexually transmitted; the risk appears to be greater if the infected partner is male. Evidence for heterosexual transmission of hepatitis B may occur in at least 25% of regular sexual partners of persons known to have a hepatitis B infection.

Persons having multiple sexual partners, five or more within 6 months, have a prevalence greater than 20% for exposure to hepatitis B. The incidence of heterosexual transmission of hepatitis C is less well defined. Epidemiologic studies have suggested that sexual transmission of non-A, non-B hepatitis, which represents hepatitis C in most cases, is responsible for 10–15% of sporadically occurring disease, in the absence of a known parenteral exposure. Most studies to date have demonstrated a low transmission rate for hepatitis C—usually less than 10%. A recent study from Japan indicated, however, that 27% of spouses of patients with chronic hepatitis C infections had evidence of the infection, and 16% demonstrated hepatitis C viremia.

The potential for heterosexual transmission of both hepatitis B and C probably can be lessened through the use of condoms. Transmission of hepatitis B can be prevented through vaccination of the uninfected partner, using the series of three hepatitis B vaccine injections. This recommendation is contingent on demonstrating that the vaccine recipient is HBsAg-negative when vaccination is initiated. Unfortunately, a similar recommendation cannot be made for hepatitis C, because no vaccine is currently available.

Chronic hepatitis B and C are lifelong infections, and as a consequence, they may lead to severe and fatal liver disease. In the United States, chronic hepatitis C is identified more often than hepatitis B. A subset of patients with chronic hepatitis C infections currently is emerging. These persons, now in their 30s and 40s, well-educated, and most often middle-class, had transient periods of injecting drug use 10–25 years in the past.

Clinical Findings & Diagnosis
Chronic viral hepatitis is established when the presence of the infection is demonstrated for 6 months or longer. The infection usually is identified by the presence of abnormally elevated levels of AST and ALT, and the cause of the infection is established by specific serologic tests for the viral hepatitis agent. The diagnosis of chronic hepatitis B is relatively straightforward. The presence of HBsAg is diagnostic for hepatitis B infection. Demonstrating the presence or absence of additional antigens or antibodies against the core or "e" subunits is not required in this setting. If it is necessary to determine whether the infection is active (the replicative phase) or inactive (nonreplicative phase), the hepatitis B virus DNA is the most specific determinant and is present during the replicative phase.

The diagnosis of chronic hepatitis C infection is less straightforward. The initial screening test is the hepatitis C antibody, measured by EIA techniques. A reactive hepatitis C antibody should be interpreted with some reservations. Certainly, most persons with a reactive hepatitis C antibody have an ongoing hepatitis C infection. The antibody also may be reactive as a false-positive result or may represent evidence for a past exposure to hepatitis C. Additional confirmatory testing is required using one or two methods; the first test is for the hepatitis C virus antibody measured by RIBA, and the second is for the hepatitis C virus RNA (HCV-RNA) by PCR. Presently, the RIBA antibody is more readily available, whereas the HCV-RNA is a more specific indicator of an active infection.

Currently, blood bank centers are using a second-generation hepatitis C antibody EIA test, which has eliminated a significant number of false-positive results. Additional and confirmatory testing with HCV-RNA, if available, is recommended. HCV-RNA testing is particularly valuable in persons who have a negative hepatitis C antibody but have abnormal levels of AST and ALT and risk factors for acquiring hepatitis C, namely, a history of blood transfusion or injecting drug use.

Treatment

Even though a chronic hepatitis B or C infection can be readily identified, eradication of these infections is difficult. The only available treatment for either infection is the use of interferon alfa. In patients infected with hepatitis B, the initial assessment is whether hepatitis B virus DNA is present in the serum, because interferon treatment is indicated in these patients only. When used in dosages of 5 million units subcutaneously daily for 16 weeks, approximately 30–40% of patients have a sustained therapeutic response that leads to the loss of both HBeAg and HBV-DNA from the serum, and one-half of those patients become HBsAg-negative. Patients who have no detectable levels of HBV-DNA in the serum have a poor response to interferon and are not candidates for treatment.

Hepatitis C patients respond less well to interferon. Only 15% of patients with chronic hepatitis C have a sustained response to interferon treatment, defined by the normalization of AST and ALT levels and the loss of HCV-RNA from the serum. The greatest problem is identifying the hepatitis C patients who would benefit from treatment. Preliminary information suggests that patients respond better to interferon if they have minimal elevations of ALT, a shorter duration of infection, less severe histologic changes on liver biopsy, low titers of HCV-RNA in the serum, and specific HCV subtypes.

Prognosis

Two significant liver problems may result from chronic hepatitis B or C. First, cirrhosis may develop, and the ensuing complications of portal hypertension may result. These complications include esophageal varices with hemorrhage, ascites, portal-systemic encephalopathy, and renal failure. Second, having a chronic hepatitis B or C infection increases the po-

tential for the development of hepatocellular carcinoma (HCC).

Although it has been known for a long time that a chronic hepatitis B infection markedly increases the risk for developing HCC, it has been recognized recently that a similar risk is present in patients chronically infected with hepatitis C. The risk for developing HCC is related to the duration of the infection and the presence of cirrhosis.

Despite these dire predictions of cirrhosis and hepatocellular carcinoma in patients with chronic hepatitis B or C, most patients with chronic hepatitis B or C have a relatively normal life expectancy. The histologic stage at the time of initial diagnosis has importance: lower grades of chronic hepatitis have a favorable 10- to 15-year prognosis. Sequential histologic analysis of liver biopsy in patients with hepatitis C has shown a slow rate of progression when evaluated over a 10- to 20-year interval. A long-term follow-up study of patients with posttransfusion hepatitis C revealed only a small increase in liver disease-related deaths.

Issues of Pregnancy & Viral Hepatitis

Vertical transmission of hepatitis B or C from an infected mother to her infant at the time of birth is an important phenomenon, because the infant develops a lifelong infection. It has been known for many years that hepatitis B virus is readily transmitted in this fashion. A hepatitis B infection in an infant may not be recognized and often leads to an asymptomatic chronic infection that manifests in adulthood as chronic hepatitis, cirrhosis, or HCC. Most infants born to women who are positive for both HBsAg and HBeAg become chronically infected with hepatitis B virus. This represents a major health issue in geographic regions where nearly 10% of the population may have a chronic hepatitis B infection. In the USA, where the prevalence of chronic hepatitis B infections is less than 1%, approximately 22,000 infants, are born each year to mothers who have chronic hepatitis B. Vertical transmission is probably the most common means for transmitting hepatitis B infection within the population.

In the USA, many pregnant women with chronic hepatitis B infections do not have overt clinical or laboratory findings that reveal the presence of the infection. The current obstetrics policy of recommending universal prenatal screening was devised to ensure that all women with hepatitis B infection would be identified. Although most screening takes place in the first trimester, it might be preferable to delay the HBsAg testing until the third trimester to ensure that mothers have not become infected during the course of pregnancy.

Once a hepatitis B-infected pregnant woman is identified, the infant can be provided with immunoprophylaxis using a combination of hepatitis B immune globulin and hepatitis B vaccine, initiated within 24 hours of birth. This regimen has proved to be highly effective in preventing transmission of hepatitis B to infants.

Vertical transmission of hepatitis C appears to be less common than of hepatitis B. The reported risk ranges from as low as 1% to as high as 13%. Several factors may increase the risk for vertical transmission. A coexisting HIV infection appears to be additive. It has been suggested that higher titers of hepatitis C RNA in the blood increase the potential risk. Unfortunately, no effective immunoprophylaxis can be offered to the infant. Counseling concerning the risk of transmission may be provided to the mother so that a decision can be made whether to evaluate the infant for signs of the infection. The preferred method for this assessment is through HCV-RNA by PCR testing, because hepatitis C antibody results may be falsely positive through passive transplacental transmission of maternal antibodies.

AUTOIMMUNE LIVER DISEASE

Autoimmune hepatitis, formerly described as chronic lupoid hepatitis, is a chronic liver disorder characterized by moderate elevations of AST and ALT, hepatosplenomegaly, the presence of autoantibodies, and abnormal findings on liver biopsy demonstrating features of chronic active hepatitis (Table 29–5). Autoimmune hepatitis is identified most often in women, who represent approximately 80% of cases. Manifestations range from mild fatigue to serious, life-threatening illness with jaundice. Levels of AST and ALT are likely to be moderately elevated, although the levels may exceed 1000 U/mL and mimic the picture of an acute viral hepatitis. A polyclonal hypergammaglobulinemia is a characteristic finding. The liver biopsy reveals features of chronic active hepatitis with varying stages of severity.

Table 29–5. Diagnosis of autoimmune hepatitis.

Female sex (80% of cases)
Jaundice
Hepatosplenomegaly
Hypergammaglobulinemia
Autoimmune markers
　Type 1: Antinuclear antibody, smooth-muscle antibody
　Type 2: Antiliver and kidney microsomal antibody
　Type 3: Antisoluble liver antigen antibody
Histologic findings compatible with chronic hepatitis

AUTOIMMUNE HEPATITIS

Essentials of Diagnosis
- Elevations of AST and ALT
- Liver biopsy showing histologic features of chronic active hepatitis
- Presence of autoantibodies

Clinical Findings & Diagnosis
The key to the diagnosis is the presence of autoantibodies, particularly the antinuclear antibody, smooth-muscle antibody, and liver-kidney microsomal antibodies. Because hepatitis C also may be associated with a high frequency of these autoantibodies, it should be excluded initially by testing, preferably by HCV-RNA by PCR. Additionally, drug-induced chronic hepatitis should be excluded. Some commonly used medications, particularly the nitrofurantoins, may lead to a chronic hepatitis with the presence of autoantibodies.

Three types of autoimmune hepatitis have been identified. The classic disease, called **type I,** is associated with a positive antinuclear antibody or smooth-muscle antibody titers of 1:80 or greater. Historically, this type was linked with the presence of a positive lupus erythematosus (LE) preparation, hence the older term **chronic lupoid hepatitis.** This type may be identified in all age groups. **Type 2** autoimmune hepatitis is associated with the antiliver and kidney microsomal antibodies and is identified most often in adolescent or young adult women. This type is a particularly aggressive disease that can lead readily to fulminant liver failure. **Type 3** disease is linked with an antibody to soluble liver antigen, a serologic test that is not readily available.

Treatment
Identification of autoimmune hepatitis is especially important, because treatment is recommended using prednisone alone or in combination with azathioprine. This treatment regimen prevents death from liver failure and results in improved 5- and 10-year survival rates, although progression to cirrhosis is not prevented in these patients. These patients should be treated for at least 1 year. Because most patients experience a relapse of their disease after withdrawal of immunosuppressive agents, a liver biopsy should be repeated before stopping the drugs, because the presence of ongoing inflammation may weigh against drug withdrawal.

PRIMARY BILIARY CIRRHOSIS

The second autoimmune-related liver disease is primary biliary cirrhosis (PBC). Ninety percent of patients with PBC are women.

Clinical Stages

Three clinical stages of PBC can be defined.

A. Symptomatic Stage: The symptomatic stage occurs in the presence of jaundice, pruritus, and fatigue. The serum alkaline phosphatase level may be quite elevated, and the histologic state of the liver often includes the presence of bridging fibrosis or cirrhosis (histologic stage 3 or 4). This clinical stage is the classic presentation for PBC but rarely is encountered today.

B. Asymptomatic Stage: The asymptomatic stage most often is uncovered during the evaluation for elevated serum alkaline phosphatase when a positive AMA is identified. No symptoms of jaundice or pruritus are present, and the liver biopsy most often shows early histologic abnormalities, similar to those of chronic persistent hepatitis or a mild case of chronic active hepatitis (histologic stage 1 or 2). This presentation is the one most commonly seen.

C. Preclinical Stage: The preclinical stage is identified in patients who have no symptoms; the serum alkaline phosphatase level is normal. Because PBC is associated with other autoimmune-related disorders in more than 80% of patients, this stage often is identified by an elevated antimitochondrial antibody (AMA) found during the course of serologic assessment; symptoms develop in one-third of these patients over the next 5 years.

Diagnosis

A diagnosis of PBC is made most often in the course of evaluating an elevated serum alkaline phosphatase level. PBC is associated with an autoantibody, the AMA, which is highly specific for the disease when present in titers exceeding 1:40. A liver biopsy is recommended to confirm the diagnosis and to define the histologic stage.

Treatment

A definitive treatment for PBC that arrests the disease process has not been discovered. Ursodiol, 10–15 mg/kg/d, may be effective in improving biochemical parameters and may slow histologic progression. Liver transplantation may be quite successful in suitable candidates in whom liver failure has developed.

Prognosis

The natural history of PBC is long and may be measured more accurately in decades than in years from the time of initial onset and clinical appearance. The prognosis of PBC depends on the combination of symptoms and histologic and biochemical parameters, particularly levels of serum bilirubin, prothrombin, and albumin. For example, patients with a normal serum bilirubin level, histologic stage 1, and with no clinical symptoms are expected to have a near-normal 10-year survival rate for their age. Once symptoms develop or the serum bilirubin levels begin to rise, 5-year survival is greatly modified.

ALCOHOLIC LIVER DISEASE

Although alcoholic liver disease in women is similar to its counterpart in men, important differences exist. Women appear to be more susceptible to liver injury from alcohol; the amount of alcohol consumed per day required to produce serious alcoholic liver injury is less in women than in men. Consumption of 40 g or more of alcohol per day appears to increase the potential of significant alcoholic liver injury leading to cirrhosis. Forty grams of alcohol is roughly equivalent to 120 mL of distilled spirits, 400 mL of beer, or 1000 mL of wine. Women's greater susceptibility may be related to size and gender differences in alcohol metabolism. Women have a smaller volume of distribution for alcohol, which leads to higher blood levels. There also may be differences in the peripheral metabolism of alcohol in women, who have lesser concentrations of alcohol dehydrogenase in the stomach. The duration of heavy daily alcohol ingestion is also important; significant injury rarely is found with less than 5 years of abuse, and the risk markedly escalates with 20 years or longer of abuse.

The natural history of alcoholic hepatitis also may be different in women. A recent study suggested that women are more likely than men to progress from alcoholic hepatitis to cirrhosis, even if they remain abstinent from alcohol.

Finally, women are less likely than men to be suspected of alcohol abuse. This factor may delay the diagnosis of alcoholism in women and allow the liver injury to develop to a more advanced stage before it is diagnosed.

Essentials of Diagnosis

- Risk of alcohol liver disease increases when more than 40 g of alcohol are consumed daily.
- AST:ALT ratio exceeds 1.5.
- Steatohepatitis identify by liver biopsy.

Diagnosis & Treatment

The diagnosis is suspected when evidence for liver disease is found in a patient with alcohol abuse. One key biochemical abnormality is the AST:ALT ratio, which exceeds 1.5, whereas in other chronic liver disorders the ratio is usually less than 1. A liver biopsy assists in the diagnosis when it reveals features of a severe alcoholic liver injury, steatohepatitis, the so-called alcoholic hepatitis. When alcoholic hepatitis is particularly severe with the presence of portal-systemic encephalopathy, the use of corticosteroids may be lifesaving.

Patients with chronic viral hepatitis B or C should be cautioned that the abuse of alcohol potentiates the liver injury from viral hepatitis. Minimal use of alcohol, 10 g/d, is not deleterious in this setting.

FATTY LIVER & STEATOHEPATITIS

The most common cause for asymptomatic and mild-to-moderate elevations in the serum AST and ALT is fatty infiltration of the liver (steatosis). Testing for disease-specific markers can exclude the vast majority of other causes for the abnormally elevated liver enzymes. Once these are ruled out, a clinical diagnosis of steatosis can be made with a high degree of confidence in patients with a combination of obesity, hyperlipidemia (particularly hypertriglyceridemia), or glucose intolerance. When liver ultrasonography reveals increased echogenicity, steatosis is the most likely diagnosis, and it may not be necessary to recommend a liver biopsy to confirm the clinical impression.

More recently, it has been recognized that a liver disorder resembling alcoholic liver disease may be identified in some patients with severe steatosis. This disorder, termed **nonalcoholic steatohepatitis (NASH) syndrome,** is found most often in middle-aged obese women who have type II diabetes mellitus. Histologic study of the liver shows steatosis with necrosis, an inflammatory infiltrate with polymorphonuclear leukocytes, and the presence of alcoholic hyaline, all features resembling alcoholic hepatitis. A careful history of alcohol ingestion, obtained from the patient and her close friends and relatives, reveals the absence of significant, or any, alcohol use. The clinical importance of identifying this liver disorder is that an increased amount of liver fibrosis often is present, and features of cirrhosis also may be noted. The exact natural history of the NASH syndrome is not clearly defined, although the syndrome may be one cause for the development of cryptogenic cirrhosis.

HEPATIC TUMORS

Most often, tumors of the liver are identified during the course of an imaging study of the liver, usually ultrasonography, employed to evaluate abnormal liver enzyme elevations or other abdominal symptoms. These incidentally identified lesions are often solitary in nature and may appropriately be called "incidentalomas." When these lesions are small (less than 2–3 cm), solitary, and noncystic and found when metastatic liver disease is not suspected, they are most often benign; it is reasonable to follow these abnormalities with serial ultrasonography in 3–6 months to ascertain that no growth has occurred. If any significant change in size has occurred, the lesion requires a reevaluation and a directed biopsy for diagnosis.

The great majority of these incidental lesions are hemangiomas, which are found in up to 5% of the population. When specific criteria are met, hemangiomas of this size range can be identified and followed. Liver hemangiomas that present greater difficulties in their evaluation are those greater than 5–6 cm with inhomogeneous internal structures. On the initial view, these hemangiomas often lead to a high suspicion for malignant lesion. The best and most specific way to establish the nature of these lesions is through a ^{99m}Tc-tagged red blood scan. Hemangiomas typically exhibit a delayed and increased uptake of the radionuclide that is highly specific for these lesions. For reasons that remain unclear, the larger, cavernous hemangiomas are found more often in women, possibly because of hormonal influences on their growth.

A second liver neoplasm identified more frequently in women is liver cell adenoma. More than 90% of these lesions are identified in women; in most instances, they are related to the use of oral contraceptives. The duration of use may be as short as several months, but more typically the neoplasm develops several years of continuous ingestion. Most of these lesions are revealed during an evaluation for right upper quadrant abdominal pain by ultrasonography or CT scanning. When they are identified as having characteristics of liver cell adenomas in the setting of abdominal pain, these lesions should be considered for immediate surgical resection, because there is a high risk for spontaneous rupture with an ensuing serious intraperitoneal hemorrhage. Alternatively, these lesions may be uncovered in a relatively asymptomatic patient. Once a diagnosis of liver cell adenoma is established in this setting, a dilemma arises. Although there are reports of regression in size of these lesions after cessation of oral contraceptives, these instances are probably the exception rather than the rule. Additionally, liver cell adenomas have been identified as undergoing transformation into hepatocellular carcinoma. Although this occurrence is distinctly unusual, a recommendation should be made to resect these lesions.

HEPATOTOXICITY RESULTING FROM VITAMINS & HERBAL AGENTS

Recent studies have indicated a high prevalence in the general population for using alternative health measures such as vitamins and herbal agents. Although most of these products are safe when used in normal amounts, a potential for hepatotoxicity is present if they are ingested in greater than normal doses.

Vitamins

Vitamin A has been advocated for its use in preventing aging and cancer. When ingested in normal quantities, it has little potential for developing hepatotoxicity. Megavitamin doses, however, may lead to a serious and irreversible liver injury. Daily ingestion of amounts as low as 20,000–25,000 units for 5–6 years or 50,000 units for 2 years can cause hepatotoxicity. Vegetarians, who may supplement their diet with vitamin A, may be at greater risk for development of hypervitaminosis A. Vitamin A is a fat-soluble vitamin and is stored within the peristellate sinusoidal (Ito) cells that line the sinusoidal space of Disse in the liver. These cells are particularly important for their role in collagen formation within the liver and the sinusoidal space. As a consequence of vitamin A toxicity, hepatic collagen is increased with the subsequent development of a noncirrhotic form of portal hypertension and its complications of ascites and bleeding from gastroesophageal varices. The toxicity can be avoided if the clinician is aware of the doses of vitamin A required for hepatotoxicity.

Another vitamin compound readily obtained over the counter is nicotinic acid (niacin). Although this agent is prescribed commonly for its cholesterol-lowering properties, patients may take it on their own to achieve a similar effect. Nicotinic acid is available in both an immediate-release and a sustained-release preparation. Although most cases of hepatotoxicity are reported with the use of the sustained-release formulation, toxicity can occur also with the immediate-release form. Hepatotoxicity can occur with doses in the range of 2–4 g/d using the sustained-release form for 2–4 weeks. The liver damage may be a combination of a hepatocellular injury with elevations of the ALT and AST with prolonged cholestatic features. Fatalities from liver failure have occurred from the use of nicotinic acid.

Less commonly known is the hepatotoxic potential of easily obtained herbal agents. It is often assumed that these agents are innocuous and have little potential for toxicity to the liver. Consequently, a history of herbal ingestion should be obtained from anyone presenting with unexplained abnormalities of liver enzymes. Comfrey tea (*Symphytum officinale*), a frequently used herbal agent, has been recognized as a cause for hepatic venoocclusive disease. This disorder leads to fibrosis and occlusion of hepatic veins with the development of ascites and liver failure. The clinical picture resembles the Budd-Chiari syndrome. Comfrey tea is a derivative of pyrrolizidine alkaloids, which are acknowledged as being hepatotoxic; senecio teas are the classic example. Of greater concern is that these substances can be transmitted transplacentally with the development of hepatic venoocclusive disease in the neonate.

Another herbal substance, chaparral leaf (*Larrea tridentata)*, is derived from the leaves of the creosote bush. Chaparral leaf has been recommended for the treatment of various types of infections and as a free-radical scavenger. Several reports of hepatotoxicity have been made, with a description of an acute hepatocellular injury resulting in marked elevations of ALT and AST greater than 1000 U/mL. Evidence of liver failure may be found in an elevated serum bilirubin level and a prolonged prothrombin time. Recovery from the liver injury is expected following withdrawal of the inciting agent.

Hepatotoxicity also has occurred after the ingestion of germander (*Teucrium chamaedrys*), used to promote weight loss. This agent has led to an acute liver injury with marked elevations of AST and ALT, jaundice, and prolongation of the prothrombin time. This injury is reversible after discontinuance of the herbal agent, with recovery occurring within 1–2 months.

Recently, a significant liver injury was reported after ingestion of a traditional Chinese herbal agent, Jin Bu Huan, which is used as a sedative and analgesic agent. An acute icteric hepatitis was reported with an uneventful recovery occurring once the agent was identified.

The experience with these agents serves to illustrate that easily obtained over-the-counter products may lead to significant hepatotoxicity. The potential of these agents for causing abnormalities in liver enzymes may not be apparent unless a careful history is obtained.

REFERENCES

GENERAL CONSIDERATIONS

Edwards CQ, Kushner JP: Screening for hemochromatosis. N Engl J Med 1993;328:1617.

Ludwig J et al: Liver biopsy diagnosis of homozygous hemochromatosis: A diagnostic algorithm. Mayo Clin Proc 1993;68:203.

Maddrey WC: Chronic hepatitis. Dis Mon 1993;39:53.

Niederau C et al: Survival and causes for death in cirrhotic and noncirrhotic patients with primary hemochromatosis. N Engl J Med 1985;313:1256.

Reichling JJ, Kaplan MM: Clinical use of serum enzymes in liver disease. Dig Dis Sci 1988;33:1601.

Sherman KE: Alanine aminotransferase in clinical practice. Arch Intern Med 1991;151:260.

Walshe JM: Diagnosis and treatment of presymptomatic Wilsons disease. Lancet 1988;ii:435.

Walshe JM: Wilson's disease presenting with features of hepatic dysfunction: A clinical analysis of eighty-seven patients. Q J Med 1989;70:253.

CHRONIC VIRAL HEPATITIS

Akahane Y et al: Hepatitis C virus infection in spouses of patients with type C chronic liver disease. Ann Intern Med 1994;120:748.

Alter MJ et al: The changing epidemiology of hepatitis B in the United States. JAMA 1990;263:1218.

Alter MJ et al: Hepatitis B virus transmission between heterosexuals. JAMA 1986;256:1307.

Alter MJ et al: The natural history of community-acquired hepatitis C in the United States. N Engl J Med 1992;327:1899.

Davis GL et al: Treatment of chronic hepatitis C with recombinant interferon alfa. N Engl J Med 1989;321:1501.

DiBisceglia AM et al: Recombinant interferon alfa therapy for chronic hepatitis C. N Engl J Med 1989;321:1506.

Gretch D, Lee W, Corey L: Use of aminotransferase, hepatitis C antibody, and hepatitis C polymerase chain reaction RNA assays to establish the diagnosis of hepatitis C virus infection in a diagnostic virology laboratory. J Clin Microbiol 1992;30:2145.

Hsu H-M et al: Efficacy of a mass hepatitis B vaccination program in Taiwan. JAMA 1988;260:2231.

Lynch-Salamon DI, Combs CA: Hepatitis C in obstetrics and gynecology. Obstet Gynecol 1992;79:621.

Ohto H et al: Transmission of hepatitis C virus from mother to infants. N Engl J Med 1994;330:744.

Osmond DH et al: Risk factors for hepatitis C virus seropositivity in heterosexual couples. JAMA 1993;269:361.

Perrillo RP et al: A randomized, controlled trial of interferon alfa-2b alone and after prednisone withdrawal for treatment of chronic hepatitis B. N Engl J Med 1990;325:295.

Rubin RA, Falestiny M, Malet PF: Chronic hepatitis C: Advances in diagnostic testing and therapy. Arch Intern Med 1994;154:387.

Seeff LB et al: Long-term mortality after transfusion-associated non-A, non-B hepatitis. N Engl J Med 1992;327:1906.

Tsukuma H et al: Risk factors for hepatocellular carcinoma among patients with chronic liver disease. N Engl J Med 1993;328:1797.

Wejstad R et al: Mother-to-infant transmission of hepatitis C virus. Ann Intern Med 1992;117:887.

AUTOIMMUNE LIVER DISEASE

Amontree JS, Stuart TD, Bredfeldt JE: Autoimmune chronic active hepatitis masquerading as acute hepatitis. J Clin Gastroenterol 1989;11:303.

Culp KS et al: Autoimmune associations in primary biliary cirrhosis. Mayo Clin Proc 1982;57:365.

Czaja AJ: Chronic active hepatitis: The challenge for a new nomenclature. Ann Intern Med 1993;119:510.

Homberg J-C et al: Chronic active hepatitis associated with antiliver/kidney microsomal antibody type 1: A second type of "autoimmune" hepatitis. Hepatology 1987;7:1333.

Kaplan MM: Primary biliary cirrhosis. N Engl J Med 1987;316:521.

Keating JJ et al: Influence of aetiology, clinical and histological features on survival in chronic active hepatitis: An analysis of 204 patients. Q J Med 1987;62:59.

Maddrey WC: Subdivisions of idiopathic autoimmune chronic active hepatitis. Hepatology 1987;7:1372.

Mitchison HC et al: Positive antimitochondrial antibody but normal alkaline phosphatase: Is this primary biliary cirrhosis? Hepatology 1986;6:279.

Poupon RE et al: Ursodiol for the long-term treatment of primary biliary cirrhosis. N Engl J Med 1994;330:1342.

Powell FC, Schroeter AL, Dickson ER: Primary biliary cirrhosis and the CREST syndrome: A report of 22 cases. Q J Med 1987;62:75.

ALCOHOLIC LIVER DISEASE

Diehl AM, Goodman Z, Ishak KG: Alcohol-like liver disease in nonalcoholics: A clinical and histologic comparison with alcohol-induced liver injury. Gastroenterology 1988;95:1056.

Frezza M et al: High blood alcohol levels in women: The role of decreased gastric alcohol dehydrogenase activity and first-pass metabolism. N Engl Med 1990;322:95.

Lee RG: Nonalcoholic steatohepatitis: A study of 49 patients. Hum Pathol 1989;20:594.

Morgan MY, Sherlock S: Sex-related differences among 100 patients with alcoholic liver disease. Br Med J 1977;i:939.

Norton R et al: Alcohol consumption and the risk of alcohol related cirrhosis in women. Br Med J 1987;295:80.

Pares A et al: Histologic course of alcoholic hepatitis: Influence of abstinence, sex and extent of hepatic damage. J Hepatol 1986;2:33.

HEPATIC TUMORS

Conter RL, Longmire WP Jr: Recurrent hepatic hemangiomas: Possible association with estogen therapy. Ann Surg 1988;207:115.

Gordon SC et al: Resolution of a contraceptive-steroid-induced hepatic adenoma with subsequent evolution into hepatocellular carcinoma. Ann Intern Med 1986;105:547.

Gyorffy EJ, Bredfeldt JE, Black WC: Transformation of hepatic cell adenoma to hepatocellular carcinoma due to oral contraceptives. Ann Intern Med 1989;110:489.

Leese T, Ferges D, Bismuth H: Liver cell adenomas. Ann Surg 1988;208:558.

Marks WH, Thompson N, Appleman H: Failure of hepatic adenomas (HCA) to regress after discontinuance of oral contraceptives. Ann Surg 1988;208:190.

Reading NG et al: Hepatic haemangioma: A critical review of diagnosis and management. Q J Med 1988;67:431.

Reddy KR, Schiff ER: Approach to a liver mass. Semin Liver Dis 1993;13:423.

HEPATOTOXICITY RESULTING FROM VITAMINS & HERBAL AGENTS

Bach N, Thung SN, Schaffner F: Comfrey herb tea–induced hepatic venoocclusive disease. Am J Med 1989;87:97.

Bioulac-Sage P et al: Chance discovery of hepatic fibrosis in patient with asymptomatic hypervitaminosis A. Arch Pathol Lab Med 1988;112:505.

Katz M, Saibil F: Herbal hepatitis: Subacute hepatic

necrosis secondary to Chaparral leaf. J Clin Gastroenterol 1990;12:203.

Larrey D et al: Hepatitis after germander (*Teucrium chamaedrys*) administration: Another instance of herbal medicine hepatotoxicity. Ann Intern Med 1992;117:129.

MacGregor FB et al: Hepatotoxicity of herbal agents. Br Med J 1989;299:1156.

McKenney JM et al: A comparison of the efficacy and toxic effects of sustained- vs intermediate-release niacin in hypercholesterolemic patients. JAMA 1994;271:672.

Ridker PM, McDermott WV: Comfrey tea and hepatic venoocclusive disease. Lancet 1989;i:657.

Roulet M et al: Hepatic venoocclusive disease in a newborn infant of a woman drinking herbal tea. J Pediatr 1988;112:433.

Woolf GM et al: Acute hepatitis associated with the Chinese herbal product Jin Bu Huan. Ann Int Med 1994;121:729.

Section VIII.
Cardiovascular Disorders

Risk Factors for Coronary Artery Disease & Their Treatment

30

Edward F. Gibbons, MD

Coronary artery disease is the leading cause of death in the United States. Despite a lower overall population prevalence of coronary artery disease in women, women die from coronary artery disease in equal numbers with men. The death rate from cardiovascular disease is nearly twice the death rate from all cancers in women. Risk factors for coronary artery disease in women include the postmenopausal state, hyperlipidemia, hypertension, diabetes, smoking, obesity, family history, and use of oral contraceptives in smokers and older women. In addition, a low level of formal education is associated with a higher risk for coronary disease in women.

A progressive decline in the death rate from cardiovascular disease has occurred over the past 25 years, but the slower rate of decline in women compared with men serves to underscore the lethal nature of established coronary disease in women. Modification of risk factors for coronary disease in women is an emerging science; thus far, only cessation of cigarette smoking and probably postmenopausal estrogen use have been shown to confer benefit to women.

Essentials of Diagnosis
- Ischemic coronary disease
- Stroke
- Congestive heart failure

Incidence
Cardiovascular disease (CVD) is the foremost cause of death in women. Yearly, more than 2.5 million women in the USA are hospitalized for cardiovascular disease. Five hundred thousand of these women die annually. Nearly one-half of these deaths are caused by ischemic coronary disease and the remaining number by stroke, congestive heart failure, or a combination of the three.

Cardiovascular disease as a public health problem in women has been underemphasized when compared with other gender-specific and general diseases. When compared to cancers, coronary artery disease and stroke claim almost twice as many lives (Fig 30–1). Fortunately, the overall incidence of coronary artery disease and stroke in the general population has fallen progressively over the past 25

Essentials of Diagnosis
Incidence
Risk Factors
Clinical Findings
Treatment of Modifiable Risk Factors
Primary Prevention of Coronary Artery Disease

years: the coronary death rate has fallen nearly 50% from 1970 to 1990, and the stroke death rate has fallen 57% during the same time period (Fig 30–2). Women as well as men have benefitted from this decline in overall age-adjusted mortality, but white women have benefitted somewhat less than white men, and black women have benefitted less than white men or women or black men (Fig 30–3). The reasons for this general decline in cardiovascular mortality are not clear, but the drop has been attributed to the effects of blood pressure control, reduction of dietary fat, decline in cigarette smoking, and improved care of established coronary disease in myocardial infarction.

The incidence of coronary artery disease (CAD) follows a different pattern in men and women. Although the diagnosis of CAD increases decade by decade in both sexes, women acquire the disease approximately 6–10 years later than men. Because women live longer than men, by the time they reach their eighth or ninth decade of life, their death rate from coronary disease equals that of men of the same age (Fig 30–4). The Framingham Heart Study, from its earlier publications over the past 30 years, emphasized the gender differences in presentation with coronary disease. Not only were the women 10 years older than their male counterparts when presenting with any manifestation of CAD, but also they were 20 years older than their male cohorts when they had their first myocardial infarction. Women in this group were more likely than men to present with the clinical syndrome of angina (69 versus 30%). Yet within 5 years of the development of angina, myocardial infarction developed in 25% of men and only 14% of women. Even the most recent update from

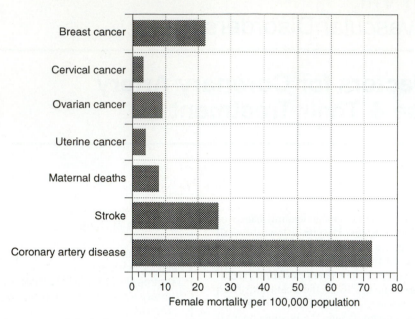

Figure 30–1. Major causes of death in women in the United States, 1989. (Courtesy of American Heart Association Stroke and Death Facts, 1993.)

Framingham shows similar gender differences (14.3% 2-year and 33.4% 10-year myocardial infarction rates after angina onset for men, 6.2% 2-year and 17.8% 10-year myocardial infarction rates for women).

Several key observations must be emphasized in interpreting these data: (1) the Framingham data for clinical presentation of CAD represented all age groups including both pre- and postmenopausal women; (2) the diagnosis of angina was a clinical one and not correlated initially with more objective measures of ischemia or coronary atherosclerosis; (3) the slower progression of angina to infarction in women led to the general clinical impression that angina in women conveyed a more benign prognosis than in men, despite similar or worse functional limi-

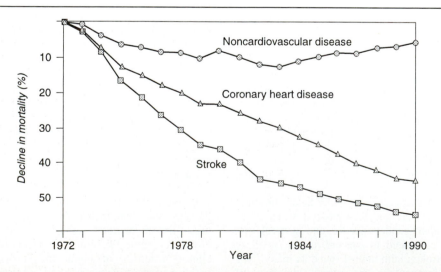

Figure 30–2. Decline in age-adjusted mortality from cardiovascular disease and stroke in the United States since 1972. (Courtesy of National Center for Health Statistics and the National Heart, Lung, and Blood Institute.)

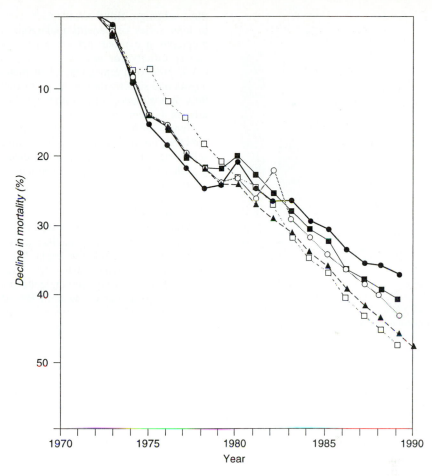

Figure 30–3. Decline in age-adjusted mortality for coronary artery disease by race and gender since 1972. ▲ = total mortality; ■ = black men; ● = black women; □ = white men; ○ = white women. (Courtesy of National Center for Health Statistics and the National Heart, Lung, and Blood Institute.)

tation; and (4) the same Framingham population of women in fact had a worse prognosis than men after myocardial infarction. The 1-year mortality rate after symptomatic myocardial infarction was 45% for these women versus 10% for men. The reinfarction rate within 1 year was 40% for women and 13% for men. The in-hospital mortality rate for myocardial infarction in women then and now is substantially higher than in men (see Chapter 31).

The general tone of earlier studies of gender and CAD gave the impression that CAD in women was an insignificant problem in all but diabetic and elderly women who had reached a degree of disease severity and comorbidity that inexorably led to a poor outcome at the end of life. Yet the data just presented do not indicate a clear threshold at which CAD in women becomes a major clinical threat other than the onset of menopause. CAD incidence in women rises decade by decade and kills just as many women per year as men; in fact, the disease is more

lethal for women than men in every age category. In addition, the annual health care expenditure for cardiovascular disease for women and men is approximately the same, despite the perceived lower overall incidence of the disease in women. Because the doubling and tripling of CAD incidence occurs with age after menopause, it must be concluded that the incidence of true ischemic CAD, as opposed to nonischemic clinical angina, must rise as women age and "angina" becomes more specifically related to the pathogenesis of atherosclerotic coronary disease as occurs in men. The Coronary Artery Surgery Study (CASS) correlated coronary angiographic patterns with CAD risk factors, symptoms, and treadmill testing in men and women younger than 65 years; the study found that women with clinical angina (typical or atypical) had significant obstructive CAD only 50% of the time, whereas men with angina had significant CAD 83% of the time. This observation buttressed the clinical impression that angina in women

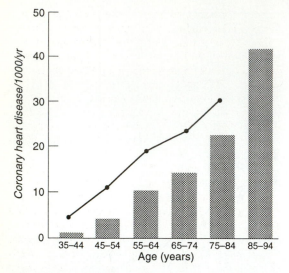

Figure 30–4. Yearly incidence of coronary artery disease in men (indicated by line) and women (indicated by bars) by decade of onset. (Reproduced, with permission, from Castelli W: Cardiovascular disease in women. Am J Obstet Gynecol 1988;158:1552.)

often is benign. However, the Cleveland Clinic found in their series of patients undergoing coronary angiography a marked difference in menopausal state and specificity for angina in women as a sign of CAD: 50% of premenopausal women with clinical angina had significant coronary obstruction, whereas 90% of postmenopausal women with angina had significant angiographic CAD.

Gender differences in the epidemiology of CAD are clear, but their underlying determinants require a fuller analysis for the purpose of developing an approach to both primary prevention and secondary treatment of the disease.

Risk Factors

Women and men share most of the risk factors for coronary artery disease established by the Framingham study: hypercholesterolemia, hypertension, diabetes, obesity greater than 30% over ideal body weight, family history, and cigarette smoking. Fortunately, the National Cholesterol Education Program (NCEP) has added the postmenopausal state without estrogen replacement to their list of risk factors for coronary disease in women. The additive effects of these Framingham risk factors apply to both men and women; Figure 30–5 illustrates their multiplicative

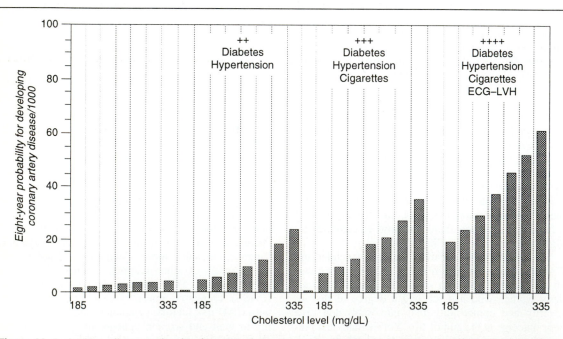

Figure 30–5. Additive effects on the development of coronary artery disease of multiple risk factors: elevated cholesterol, diabetes, hypertension, cigarette smoking, and left ventricular hypertrophy on ECG. The data are derived for 35-year-old men followed for 18 years in the Framingham Study, expressed as the 8-year probability of developing coronary heart disease. (Adapted, with permission, from Castelli WP: Epidemiology of coronary heart disease: The Framingham Study. Am J Med 1984;76:4.)

effect in the Framingham study. Male gender by it-self conveys a 3.5-fold increased risk and acts synergistically with the other risk factors. Just as women benefit from their inability to have male gender as a risk factor for CAD, their manifestations of CAD may be influenced by gender-specific hormonal-metabolic factors, use of oral contraception, pregnancy, menopause (natural or surgical), and post-menopausal estrogen-progestin use.

Clinical Findings

A. Hyperlipidemia: Women demonstrate cholesterol profiles that vary as they age and are significantly different from those of men. Women and men have similar total cholesterol levels up to ages 20–25, after which the levels diverge. Men demonstrate a rise of total cholesterol over the next 20 years, with a subsequent plateau. Women demonstrate a slower increase of total cholesterol, but at ages 45–50, their levels exceed the male average by 20–25 points for the duration of life (Fig 30–6). As it has for men, total cholesterol level in women has been correlated with risk for CAD. The Framingham study reported that a direct relationship appears to exist between total cholesterol level and annual coronary event rate such that women with cholesterol levels exceeding 265 mg/dL had double the risk of CAD of women with cholesterol levels under 205 mg/dL. Data from the Israeli Donolo-Tel Aviv Study show a similar pattern: coronary artery disease incidence triples in women with cholesterol levels greater than 265

mg/dL, compared with those whose cholesterol was less than 200 mg/dL. The national Lipid Research Clinics (LRC) study found that women with a total cholesterol of 235 mg/dL had a 70% higher risk of coronary disease than women whose total cholesterol fell below 200 mg/dL.

The total cholesterol level may not be a reliable index of risk for many women, however. Women have a substantially different lipoprotein profile from men, and authors of recent studies place far greater emphasis on these differences.

Cholesterol and triglyceride, the major plasma lipids, are solubilized in the bloodstream in envelopes of water-miscible proteins. These lipids are the products of digestion and tissue synthesis, and their concentration in the bloodstream is influenced by both genetic synthetic profiles and dietary intake of cholesterol and fat. In addition, a variety of endocrine and metabolic forces may alter the relative size of these lipid-laden lipoprotein particles. This size differential appears to affect their biochemical activity in that "small" particles appear more active and exert a greater net effect (either atherogenic or atherolytic). The relevant lipoprotein fractions for discussion of coronary risk in women are shown in Table 30–1. It should be emphasized that the measurement of each of these fractions may vary from laboratory to laboratory; unless a clinical laboratory follows national guidelines for the measurement of these lipoproteins, significant errors, particularly in the measurement of high-density lipoprotein (HDL)

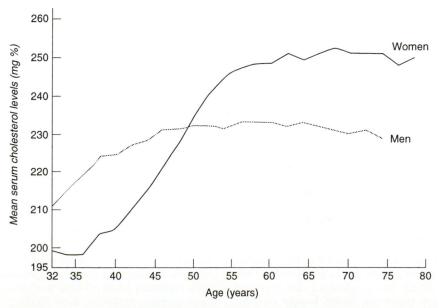

Figure 30–6. Relationship of age to serum cholesterol level in men and women. (Data from the Framingham Heart Study, Examinations 1–10. Department of Health, Education, and Welfare Publication No. [NIH] 74-478, 1973.)

Table 30–1. Lipoprotein fraction terminology.

Total cholesterol: total of all lipoprotein cholesterol
High-density lipoprotein (HDL) cholesterol: lipoprotein
  fraction affecting atherolysis
Very low-density lipoprotein (VLDL) cholesterol: lipoprotein
  fraction rich in triglycerides
Low-density lipoprotein (LDL) cholesterol: atherogenic
  lipoprotein fraction
Apolipoprotein A-1: "favorable" lipoprotein subunit of HDL
Apolipoprotein B: "unfavorable" lipoprotein of LDL

cholesterol, may occur and lead either to misdiagnosis or to an inability to determine the effects of treatment.

Although total cholesterol levels are higher in men than women after age 20, HDL cholesterol levels are higher in women than men from puberty until menopause, when they may show a decline, along with a rise of total cholesterol. Generally, HDL is higher for women than men throughout life. Thus, with the rise of total cholesterol and a trend for HDL to decrease following menopause, the total cholesterol:HDL ratio in postmenopausal women rises toward that of men. Triglyceride levels in women and men are similar at puberty and rise slowly with age, but they rise more slowly in women than men. By ages 65–70, triglyceride levels are similar in women and men, although they appear to convey a higher risk for women.

The Framingham study has shown that HDL cholesterol is inversely correlated with coronary risk in both men and women and suggests that a low HDL cholesterol level is a more powerful predictor of CAD in women than in men. These studies have suggested that for every 10 mg/dL fall in HDL cholesterol, CAD risk rises by 40–50%. The Israeli Donolo–Tel Aviv Study found that women with a total cholesterol:HDL ratio of greater than 4.3, regardless of the total cholesterol level, had a two- to fivefold increase in CVD risk; this increase occurred even in those with total cholesterol levels less than 200 mg/dL. In addition, women with elevated triglyceride levels have a higher CAD risk independent of total cholesterol; in the Framingham women, triglyceride level tended to be a better predictor for CAD than the level of low-density lipoprotein (LDL) cholesterol. This finding appears to reflect a true gender difference. Of course, an elevated triglyceride level in a patient should prompt an investigation to see if there is an underlying glucose intolerance needing primary attention (see preceding section, "Hyperlipidemia").

Based on Framingham data and treatment data for hypercholesterolemia from the Lipid Research Clinics trial, the NCEP has emphasized diet and drug therapy for hyperlipidemia based largely on male lipid risk profile. The Framingham data have shown that total cholesterol, high LDL, and low HDL (below 35 mg/dL) are CAD risk factors in men; therefore, therapy has been directed toward a reduction of total cholesterol and LDL and increase of HDL, with minor emphasis on reduction of triglyceride. These recommendations may not be directly applicable to women, however, because the risk profile is different for women.

Recent evidence of the magnitude of this difference came from the follow-up study of the Lipid Research Clinics. In this study, 1405 women ages 50–69 were followed for an average of 14 years to observe the relationship between lipoprotein levels and cardiovascular disease death rates (heart disease and stroke). The study presented strong evidence that CVD risk is increased in women with HDL levels less than 50 mg/dL and with triglyceride levels of 200–399 mg/dL; the risk is still higher in women with triglyceride levels greater than 400 mg/dL. CVD risk with total cholesterol level was driven largely by HDL level, ie, only women with HDL less than 50 mg/dL had an increased CVD risk with total cholesterol greater than 240 mg/dL. Also, LDL cholesterol was a poor predictor of CVD risk in women: at all levels of LDL, an HDL level less than 50 mg/dL was a greater risk predictor than was LDL level. HDL and triglyceride levels commonly vary reciprocally in men and in some women (estrogen can increase both). In women with low HDL (less than 50 mg/dL), the triglyceride level is a progressive risk such that women with triglyceride levels greater than 400 mg/dL have a nearly eightfold increase in risk over women with low HDL and triglyceride levels less than 200 mg/dL. When the risk is adjusted for age, hypertension, diabetes, smoking, history of heart disease, and estrogen use, women still have independent CVD risks with low HDL and high triglyceride and not necessarily with a high total cholesterol level (Table 30–2).

It should be emphasized that these figures are from one large study. Other studies investigating the influence of high levels of triglyceride in a general population have found that the risk is of borderline significance in women. Reciprocally low HDL and high triglyceride levels tend to occur in patients with diabetes and with obesity. Therefore, primary treatment of this lipid abnormality is directed at the treatment of diabetes and obesity.

The influence of LDL on CVD risk in women remains controversial. The Framingham study found a positive association of LDL cholesterol with CVD in women. The Israeli Donolo–Tel Aviv study did not directly evaluate the effect of LDL on CVD rate. Yet both earlier and later analyses of LRC data show little influence of LDL level on CVD mortality in women. Evidence in men for significant CVD risk with increased levels of both total and LDL cholesterol persists, however; these findings seem to represent a poorly understood gender difference in lipoprotein atherogenicity or susceptibility. Hyperin-

Table 30–2. Lipid Research Clinics follow-up study of coronary heart disease (CHD) risk in women.*

Lipoprotein Fraction	Relative Risk for CHD
Total cholesterol	
< 200 mg/dL	1.0
200–239 mg/dL	1.11
≥ 240 mg/dL	1.42
High-density lipoprotein cholesterol	
< 50 mg/dL	1.74[†]
≥ 50 mg/dL	1.0
Low-density lipoprotein cholesterol	
< 130 mg/dL	1.0
130–159 mg/dL	0.54
≥ 160 mg/dL	0.80
Triglycerides	
< 200 mg/dL	1.0
200–399 mg/dL	1.65[†]
≥ 400 mg/dL	3.44[†]

*Adapted, with permission, from Bass KM: Arch Intern Med 1993;153:2209. Based on Lipid Research Clinics follow-up study analysis of female participants' risk of CHD in 14 years of follow-up.
[†]Result is statistically significant.

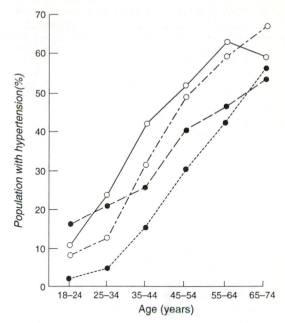

Figure 30–7. Prevalence of hypertension by race and gender analyzed by decade of onset. Hypertension is defined as a systolic blood pressure of 140 mmHg or higher, or a diastolic blood pressure of 90 mmHg or higher, or both. ●—● = white men; ●------● = white women; O——O = black men; O–·–·–O = black women. (Reproduced, with permission, from Rowland M, Roberts J: National Health and Nutritional Examination Survey (NHANES) I Data, Vital Health Statistics, 1982.)

sulinemia has been targeted as a promoter of atherogenesis in men but not in women and may facilitate LDL deposition to a greater degree in men. There may be subpopulations of women with what has been termed "small dense" LDL, which predisposes, with other constitutional CVD risks, to a higher CVD incidence (see the section, "Obesity").

B. Hypertension: Hypertension is defined as a systolic blood pressure of 140 mmHg or greater or a diastolic blood pressure of 90 mmHg or greater. The 1990 Census and the Third National Health and Nutrition Examination survey project that 50 million people in the USA are hypertensive. High blood pressure prevalence increases with age, is more common blacks than whites, and is more common in persons with a lower level of education and a lower socioeconomic status. Hypertension is more common in men than women up to middle age, but in late middle age and the elderly years, women are more likely to be hypertensive than men (Fig 30–7). Hypertension is positively associated in both men and women with both fatal and nonfatal cardiovascular disease, including coronary artery disease, stroke, congestive heart failure, peripheral vascular disease, and renal failure. Morbidity and mortality rise with progressive elevations of both systolic and diastolic blood pressure. Moreover, for any given diastolic blood pressure, CVD risk is higher the higher the systolic blood pressure.

In the Framingham study, diastolic blood pressure was emphasized. In women, diastolic blood pressure of 90–109 mmHg was associated with a 1.5-fold excess of CVD events, and diastolic blood pressure of greater than 110 was related to a 4-fold excess of CVD events. It is true, however, that women (at least in middle age) tolerate hypertension better than men,

with a longer delay in onset of cardiovascular complications. It is probably for this reason that treatment effects for hypertension in women appear to be less than for men.

The Fifth Report of the Joint National Committee of Detection, Evaluation, and Treatment of High Blood Pressure (JNC V) includes recommendations for high blood pressure as a national public health program. These recommendations serve as a useful framework for discussion of hypertension as a risk factor in women. The classification of high blood pressure (Table 30–3) emphasizes both systolic and diastolic blood pressure levels; "high normal" blood pressure readings also are targeted and require serial observation to avoid over- and undertreatment of hypertension. The detection and evaluation of hypertension requires much more "hands on" evaluation by the primary physician than does the assessment of hyperlipidemia: the physical examination and physical blood pressure measurement must assess the presence and degree of hypertension, signs of target organ damage, and secondary causes of hypertension or failure of treatment.

1. Measurement–Despite its elementary nature, blood pressure measurement is subject to some

Table 30–3. Classification of blood pressure for adults aged 18 years and older.*†

Category	Systolic (mmHg)	Diastolic (mmHg)
Normal‡	< 130	< 85
High normal	130–139	85–89
Hypertensive§		
Stage 1 (mild)	140–159	90–99
Stage 2 (moderate)	160–179	100–109
Stage 3 (severe)	180–209	110–119
Stage 4 (very severe)	≥ 210	≥ 120

*Reproduced, with permission, The Fifth Report of the Joint National Committee on Detection, Evaluation and Treatment of High Blood Pressure. Arch Intern Med 1993;153:154.
†Not taking antihypertensive drugs and not acutely ill. When systolic and diastolic pressures fall into different categories, the higher category should be selected to classify the individual's blood pressure status. For instance, 160/92 mmHg should be classified as stage 2, and 180/120 mmHg should be classified as stage 4. Isolated systolic hypertension is defined as a systolic blood pressure of 140 mmHg or more and a diastolic blood pressure of less than 90 mmHg and staged appropriately, eg, 170/85 mmHg is defined as stage 2 isolated systolic hypertension.
   In addition to classifying stages of hypertension on the basis of average blood pressure levels, the clinician should specify presence or absence of target-organ disease and additional risk factors. For example, a patient with diabetes and a blood pressure of 142/94 mmHg plus left ventricular hypertrophy should be classified as having stage 1 hypertension with target-organ disease (left ventricular hypertrophy) and with another major risk factor (diabetes). This specificity is important for risk classification and management.
‡Optimal blood pressure with respect to cardiovascular risk is less than 120 mmHg systolic and less than 80 mmHg diastolic. However, patients with unusually low readings should be evaluated to determine clinical significance.
§Based on the average of two or more readings taken at each of two or more visits after an initial screening.

common errors. Blood pressure measurements should be obtained initially in both arms after 5 minutes of rest with appropriate cuff size with a calibrated sphygmomanometer. The diastolic reading should correspond to phase V "disappearance of Korotkoff sounds." To diagnose hypertension, multiple readings should be obtained, which should coincide within 5 mmHg. "White coat" hypertension can be documented by having the patient, a relative, or another health care provider measure the blood pressure using similar criteria. At times, ambulatory blood pressure monitoring may be necessary to get an accurate measurement.

Errors in blood pressure measurement may be related to any of the following:

1. Defective equipment: bulb cuff mercury level leakage or cuff size too big or too small.
2. Patient physiology: pain, anxiety, caffeine or cigarette use within 30 minutes, irregular heart rhythm accentuating systolic blood pressure after an extrasystolic pause, or "rigid vessels" causing overestimation of blood pressure.

3. Observer error and bias: improper use of stethoscope over the brachial artery, incorrect speed of inflation or deflation, or improper recording of the figures owing to inability to see the mercury column accurately or to bias in rounding numbers.

The patient's physiologic characteristics may dictate more detailed measurement. Elderly women may have "stiff" arterial vessels that are palpable even with the cuff inflated above systolic blood pressure. "Palpation" of blood pressure here is probably not accurate. Young women, pregnant women, and women with a higher cardiac output (eg, caused by anemia, thyrotoxicosis, or sepsis) have a diastolic blood pressure that corresponds more closely to phase IV "muffling" of Korotkoff sounds.

2. History–A directed medical history should include (1) a family history of high blood pressure, early CAD, stroke, congestive heart failure, diabetes, or hyperlipidemia; (2) a patient history of prior hypertension, onset in relation to puberty, pregnancy, oral contraception, pelvic surgery, and menopause; (3) a history of drug treatment; cardiac, neurologic, or kidney disease; hyperlipidemia, diabetes, or gout; fluid overload; or claudication; (4) a patient profile of weight gain or loss; activity and exercise level; smoking or tobacco chewing; (5) a dietary profile of sodium intake, alcohol use, and fat and cholesterol intake; (6) symptoms that suggest a secondary cause of hypertension; and (7) psychosocial stresses at work and home and from the financial burden of medical care.

3. Physical examination–Physical examination should include (1) blood pressure seated and after standing for 2 minutes; (2) measurement of height and weight and observation or measurement of the approximate waist:hip ratio; (3) fundoscopic examination to assess arterial narrowing, hemorrhage, exudate, and papilledema; (4) neck examination for jugular venous distention, carotid bruits, or thyroid enlargement; (5) cardiac examination for rate, rhythm, S3, S4, murmur of mitral or aortic insufficiency, cardiac enlargement, or apical heave; (6) abdominal examination for vascular bruits, renal enlargement, masses, or aneurysm; (7) peripheral pulse profile and identification of trophic or venous disease; and (8) neurologic examination.

4. Laboratory tests and procedures–For the initial workup of hypertension, the tests to be considered include complete blood cell count (CBC), electrolytes, creatinine, urinalysis, uric acid, calcium, fasting blood sugar, cholesterol, HDL and triglycerides, and if indicated, T4 and thyroid-stimulating hormone (TSH). An electrocardiogram is indicated for assessment of left ventricular hypertrophy (LVH) and prior infarction. Optional treadmill testing (with echocardiography or nuclear perfusion imaging is indicated [see Chapter 31]) if cardiovascular target organ damage is suspected. If labile or borderline blood pressure is present, measurement of left ventricular mass index by echocardiography is indicated to identify a higher risk "borderline" hypertensive condition with left ventricular mass index greater than 125 g/m^2 of body surface area (BSA). At each stage of evaluation, the clinician must be alert to the discovery of target organ damage (Table 30–4).

5. Secondary hypertension–Although 90–95% of hypertension in women is idiopathic or "essential" and often familial in nature, 5–10% of women with hypertension have a secondary, potentially correctable or specifically treatable cause for hypertension. Some of these causes have a predilection for women over men and thus deserve special attention. They should be sought for in women with a negative family history, in children, or in patients with an accelerated or a difficult-to-control pattern of high blood pressure.

6. Renovascular hypertension–Renovascular hypertension resulting from renal artery stenosis is responsible for 2–4% of cases of hypertension. Fibromuscular dysplasia (FMD) is the underlying cause in 20–50% of cases of renovascular hypertension, more often in younger women; the remainder of cases in older women are attributed to atherosclerotic obstruction in the renal arteries. Medial FMD shows an 8:1 female-to-male predominance and is found in middle age (35–52 years), is often bilateral, and causes moderate-to-severe hypertension. Older women account for 40% of cases of atherosclerotic renal vascular hypertension. The diagnosis may be suspected with identification of a flank or epigastric bruit or deterioration of creatinine level with angiotensin converting enzyme (ACE) inhibitors, frequently in com-

bination with a negative family history for high blood pressure. The diagnosis is confirmed with captopril challenge testing and renin sampling and with subsequent direct or magnetic resonance angiography. Treatment with balloon angioplasty or surgical reconstruction is helpful.

7. Renal parenchymal disease–Renal parenchymal disease caused by hypertension, nephritis, chronic urinary infection, or diabetic nephropathy may not be curable, but control of hypertension with ACE inhibitors or calcium channel blockers may slow progression of chronic renal failure. A history of a single episode of eclampsia during pregnancy does not necessarily predispose to subsequent chronic hypertension, although eclampsia in multiple pregnancies can (see Chapter 55).

8. Aortic coarctation–Although aortic coarctation has a 2:1 male-to-female predisposition, it is the most common congenital cardiac anomaly of Turner (XO) syndrome in women. Any young woman with upper extremity hypertension should have a leg (popliteal) blood pressure measurement to exclude this diagnosis.

9. Endocrine causes–Mineralocorticoid excess with hypertension, virilization, and hypokalemia caused by 11-β-hydroxylase deficiency is a rare cause of hypertension in young women. The hypertension and hypokalemia are correctable with corticosteroids. On the other hand, deficiency of 17-α-hydroxylase does not produce virilization, appears at puberty, and is not associated with hypertension or hypokalemia; this condition usually presents with primary amenorrhea.

Aldosterone excess, usually due to an adenoma, results in hypokalemic hypochloremic alkalosis, frequently with glucose intolerance; symptoms are referable to the hypertension, hyperglycemia, and alkalosis. Drug or surgical therapy can be effective in eliminating hypertension.

Glucocorticoid excess (Cushing's syndrome) usually results from a pituitary adrenocorticotropic hormone (ACTH)—producing adenoma, occurs 6 times more often in women than men, and occurs in the third and fourth decades of life. Less common causes include primary adrenal tumors or malignant tumor—associated ectopic ACTH production. The decision to use drugs, radiotherapy, or surgery depends on consultation with a specialist.

Catecholamine excess caused by pheochromocytoma may be part of a familial multiple endocrine disorder and occurs more frequently in women than men. The manifestations relate to the specific catecholamines produced. Patients may present with flushing, cardiac arrhythmias, chest pain, headache, or syncope. Chronic weight loss; myocardial infarction; cardiomyopathic presentation; "myocarditis," or ECG abnormalities may be forms of presentation in the absence of discrete "spells." The diagnosis of pheochromocytoma depends on a high index of sus-

Table 30–4. Manifestations of target-organ damage in patients with high blood pressure.*

Organ System	Manifestations
Cardiac	Clinical, electrocardiographic, or radiologic evidence of coronary artery disease; left ventricular hypertrophy or "strain" by electrocardiography or left ventricular hypertrophy by echocardiography; left ventricular dysfunction or cardiac failure
Cerebrovascular	Transient ischemic attack or stroke
Peripheral vascular	Absence of one or more major pulses in extremities (except for dorsalis pedis) with or without intermittent claudication; aneurysm
Renal	Serum creatinine ≥ 130 μmol/L (1.5 mg/dL); proteinuria (1+ or greater); microalbuminuria
Retinopathy	Hemorrhages or exudates, with or without papilledema

*Reproduced, with permission, from The Fifth Report of the Joint National Committee on Detection, Evaluation and Treatment of High Blood Pressure. Arch Intern Med 1993;153:154.

picion and documentation of metanephrine excess in a urine sample, an elevated catecholamine level from an intravenous sample at the time of a "spell," or an elevated plasma chromogranin A level.

Growth hormone excess caused by pituitary adenoma results in hypertension or congestive heart failure in approximately 50% of cases, with other organ manifestations of growth hormone excess or separate endocrine pituitary insufficiency resulting from a tumor compressive effect. The approach to treatment (surgical, chemical, radiation) depends on how advanced the disease is and its morphologic status in the pituitary.

Hyperthyroidism occurs more commonly in women than in men and is associated with hypertension, usually systolic blood pressure elevation from increased cardiac output. Hypothyroidism also results in hypertension, often diastolic blood pressure elevation, caused by elevated peripheral vascular resistance, fluid and sodium retention, and lower cardiac output in the face of elevated peripheral resistance. Hyper*para*thyroidism is associated with hypertension 60–70% of the time, although removal of the adenoma and normalization of the serum calcium level do not necessarily correct the hypertension completely. When any of these more unusual secondary causes of hypertension are suspected, it is appropriate to refer such a patient to an endocrinologist, nephrologist, or cardiologist, depending on the suspected diagnosis.

C. Diabetes: Established symptomatic or asymptomatic glucose intolerance is a well-known, ominous, and influential risk factor for coronary disease in women. The Framingham study found that women with diabetes have a fivefold increase in risk for coronary artery disease and stroke. The Nurses Health Questionnaire Study noted that diabetes conveyed a six- to sevenfold, age-adjusted, increased risk of nonfatal myocardial infarction and total cardiovascular mortality and a threefold risk of all-cause mortality. The CVD risk is independent of other cardiac risk factors in women and remains a strong risk factor even with diabetes of short recognized duration. But the overall risk of diabetes is magnified threefold when hypertension, cigarette smoking, or obesity is present.

Diabetes appears to be a more important risk factor for CVD in women than in men. The Framingham study found that female diabetics had twice the CVD risk of male diabetics. Because of this expressed risk and the higher incidence of obesity, hypertension, and dyslipidemia in female diabetics, therefore, even premenopausal diabetic women lose the protective effect of their premenopausal status. Diabetic women without these risks have a lower CVD rate, but their risk is elevated above that of the general population. The CVD risk in diabetics manifests in an excess incidence of myocardial infarction, congestive heart failure, stroke, and cardiovascular death. The complication rate with myocardial infarction, coronary angioplasty, cardiac surgery, and peripheral vascular surgery also is significantly increased (see Chapter 32).

D. Cigarette Smoking: The Framingham study early on defined cigarette smoking in men as a major risk factor for CAD. Smoking was not defined as a risk in early profiles of Framingham women, probably because smoking incidence in the older woman who manifests CAD was low at the outset of the study in the early 1950s. Since that time, however, cigarette smoking in women has become more common and is associated with excess CVD risk in virtually every population study.

The percentage of men who smoke exceeds that of women (32 versus 26%). Although the rates of smoking have declined since the 1964 Surgeon General's report, the rate of decline in women has not been nearly as encouraging as in men (6% in women versus 21% in men). Also, the number of women who begin the habit exceeds that of men, and women's average cigarette consumption has doubled in number. The CAD incidence in women who smoke is particularly enhanced in the premenopausal woman who would otherwise have a low incidence of the disease. The Kaiser-Permanente Walnut Creek Study documented a threefold increase in CVD death in premenopausal women who smoke. The Nurses Health Study and other studies have found that the cardiovascular morbidity of smoking is dose-dependent: the risk of premenopausal, nonfatal myocardial infarction is 3 times higher in women who smoke more than 25 cigarettes per day than in those who smoke 15–24 cigarettes per day. Smoking as few as one to four cigarettes per day increases the risk of CVD death and nonfatal myocardial infarction by a factor of 2.5 over nonsmokers. All health care providers should realize that the risk of nonfatal myocardial infarction in women who both use oral contraceptives and smoke is markedly increased. In women who smoke more than 25 cigarettes per day, the relative risk of nonfatal myocardial infarction has been calculated at 23 versus 4.8 for women who smoke but do not use oral contraceptives.

Similar to the pattern observed in men, cessation of smoking in women reduces the risk of heart disease. The risk of myocardial infarction diminishes to near baseline within 2–3 years of abstinence, and it recently has been shown that the risk reaches baseline by 10 years after cessation of smoking. There is no benefit to switching to low-tar and low-nicotine cigarettes. Based on these observations, it should be a major emphasis of primary care to encourage both middle-aged and young women to stop smoking, and their risk needs to be placed in context with other risks for coronary disease evolving with age and with the use of oral contraceptives.

E. Obesity: Heart disease and obesity have not always been linked statistically. Early studies eliminated overweight as an independent risk factor. Long-term longitudinal analysis of Framingham study women associated obesity with a more than twofold increase in CAD, however. In fact, only hypertension and age have been assigned greater risk values in these women. The Nurses Health Study identified obesity of greater than 30% of ideal body weight by Quetelet index to be associated with a relative risk of 3.3 for nonfatal myocardial infarction and CVD death. This risk was only slightly less when adjusted for presence of diabetes, hypertension, or hypercholesterolemia.

In both women and men, the distribution of body fat may be more relevant to CVD risk, especially CAD risk. Women with truncal fat (android habitus) as opposed to hip and thigh fat (gynoid habitus) seem to be at greater risk for CVD complications. The waist:hip ratio has been used to quantify fat distribution (Fig 30–8). The risk of CVD increases as this ratio increases, with a ratio of 0.8 defined as a threshold for possible aggressive treatment of obesity along with the associated risk factors. The waist:hip ratio also has been used as the criterion for a component of the so-called **metabolic syndrome X,** or "insulin-resistant syndrome," in women. This syndrome is defined as an association of obesity, increased waist:hip ratio, hypertension, and glucose intolerance, with hyperinsulinemia, hypertriglyceridemia, low HDL, and hypercholesteremia. It comes as no surprise that patients with this syndrome have an excess of CVD and CAD. That this "phenotype" may be in part genetic and in part acquired has been evaluated by the Women's Twin Study. This study looked at monozygotic twins of which one twin showed signs of the metabolic syndrome X and found that the clinical expression of the disorder was closely linked to a subclass "phenotype B" of LDL cholesterol. This small, dense LDL cholesterol particle is believed to be more atherogenic and, in association with hypertriglyceridemia and lower HDL, its presence appears to accelerate CAD risk markedly. This manifestation in discordant twins was felt to be acquired with obesity, which magnifies a genetic predisposition to the LDL phenotype B of LDL receptor abnormality. Whether "small, dense LDL" accounts for other manifestations of CVD in women and whether treatment of the obesity specifically alters this risk remain to be investigated. It is clear, however, that women with central (android) obesity are at a substantial disadvantage in their risk of acquiring premature CAD.

Approximately 30–35% of white men and women in the USA are considered overweight, an increase from 25% between 1981 and 1990. But 50% of black women and 30% of black men may be overweight,

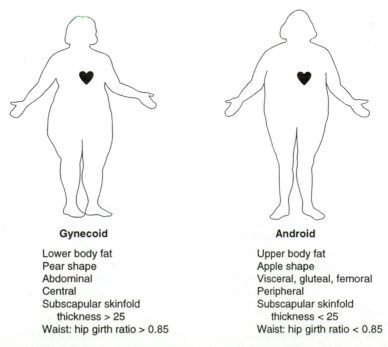

Gynecoid

Lower body fat
Pear shape
Abdominal
Central
Subscapular skinfold
    thickness > 25
Waist: hip girth ratio > 0.85

Android

Upper body fat
Apple shape
Visceral, gluteal, femoral
Peripheral
Subscapular skinfold
    thickness < 25
Waist: hip girth ratio < 0.85

Figure 30–8. Characteristics of central and peripheral obesity, defined by the pattern of fat distribution: central "android" obesity markedly increases the risk of development of coronary artery disease. (Reproduced, with permission, from Kaplan NM: The deadly quartet: Upper body obesity, glucose intolerance, hypertriglyceridemia, and hypertension. Arch Intern Med 1989;149:1514.)

and Hispanics and Pacific Islanders in the USA also are overrepresented in the obese population. Like cigarette smoking, the control of obesity as a public health problem needs to address multiple layers of psychosocial as well as socioeconomic problems.

F. Family History: The influence for women of a history of premature coronary disease in a first-degree relative is variable. In small population studies, the proportion of women with CAD having relatives with CAD ranges from 29–48%. The Cleveland Clinic retrospective study identified a 54% rate of family history of CAD in women with CAD who presented for first-time coronary angiography. The Nurses Health Study reported that a parental history of premature CAD conveys a 2.8-fold age-adjusted relative risk of nonfatal myocardial infarction and a 5-fold risk of fatal CAD in women. This risk was not diminished by adjustment for other risk factors. Family history of premature CAD appears to be an independent CAD risk factor for women, and premature CAD in a female relative (onset under age 65) has been recognized by the NCEP as a risk factor for both men and women.

G. Use of Oral Contraceptives: In this discussion, use of oral contraceptives is considered a CAD risk factor, and postmenopausal estrogen replacement is considered a CAD treatment.

Early reviews of complications of oral contraceptive pills (OCPs) found a disturbingly strong association between the use of these agents and the incidence of myocardial infarction, stroke, and thromboembolic disease. There appeared to be a dose-dependent relationship between the estrogen component and thrombotic potential in women using OCPs. In fact, higher dose estrogens cause significant elevations of plasma fibrinogen and factor 7 and reductions of antithrombin III. The relative risk in the 1970s of OCPs for cardiovascular death appeared to be related both to the age of the woman and to whether or not she smoked (Table 30–5). Older women and women who smoke have a greatly increased risk of CVD when they use oral contraceptives.

In addition to the procoagulant effect (venous effect) of higher dose estrogen, lipid effects and the induction of hypertension may play a role. Estrogen increases HDL and triglycerides and decreases LDL, whereas progestins in OCP decrease HDL and increase LDL, with a net effect varying by specific formulation. Most OCPs raise LDL levels. Progestins also may bring out glucose intolerance and hypertension, ie, via arterial disease, in susceptible women. Frank hypertension caused by OCPs is uncommon and is usually mild and reversible within several months of OCP cessation. It is more common in the older or obese OCP user. As a result of earlier adverse CVD effects of OCP, manufacturers have reduced estrogen content from 50–150 μg to 30–35 μg. More recent longitudinal study of women using OCPs with a lower estrogen content and less androgenic progestins suggests that the CVD risk for OCP use has diminished significantly. However, perimenopausal women and women who smoke may still be at increased risk and may need to avail themselves of other methods of contraception. Once OCPs are stopped, prior use does not appear to be a long-term risk factor for the development of CVD.

Although the lower estrogen OCPs appear to have a lower thrombotic potential, individual susceptibility to thromboembolic disease exists, for example, in smokers. Premenopausal women with other CAD risk factors may heighten their risk of CAD with OCPs.

Postmenopausal estrogen replacement likely has a net CVD risk-reduction potential of 45–50%, although the dosing effect and duration of risk reduction may vary from woman to woman. For some women, there may be a heightened thrombotic potential with even 1.25 mg of estrogen per day. There are insufficient data to evaluate this effect properly. The Women's Health Initiative is planning to randomize postmenopausal women to groups taking estrogen, estrogen in combination with progesterone, and placebo to evaluate the effect on coronary and other thrombotic events prospectively.

H. Psychosocial Factors: A review of social patterns since World War II had led some observers to speculate that the increased recognition of CAD in women might be related to their assumption of "male" roles and that women in the workforce may develop more CAD than women who stay home. The Framingham study data lead to an opposite interpretation. In 14 years of follow-up, CAD was found to be unassociated with a woman's fact of employment (at home or commercially). Blue collar working women tended to have more CAD than white collar women, but analysis did not show a statistically significant difference. Marital status or spouse's occupation also did not predict CAD. Educational level has an inverse relationship to the development of

Table 30–5. Risk of age and cigarette smoking in promoting cardiovascular death in women who used oral contraceptives.[*][†]

Age Group (yr)	Nonsmoking Women	Smoking Women
25–34	1.6	3.4
35–44	3.3	4.2
> 45	4.6	7.4

[*]Reproduced, with permission, from: Layde PM, Beral V: Further analysis of mortality in oral contraceptive users. Royal College of General Practitioners Oral Contraception Study. Lancet 1981;1:541.
[†]Shown is the adjusted relative risk of cardiovascular death from age and cigarette smoking in women who used oral contraceptives with higher dose estrogen (50–150 μg) and more androgenic progestin components in Great Britain.

CAD, however, such that women with an eighth grade educational level or less appear to have a fourfold excess incidence of CAD, independent of age, cholesterol level, smoking, blood pressure, weight, or diabetes. This finding deserves further study in a larger cohort, which may be forthcoming from the Women's Health Initiative.

"Type A" personality in men was suggested and then refuted as a CAD risk factor. Women in the Framingham study with type A personality also exhibited an excess incidence of CAD. Some researchers believe that the disruptive type A personality, who is critical, impatient, demeaning, self-important, and somewhat socially isolated, may have a true disposition to CAD, but the causal link remains obscure.

Treatment of Modifiable Risk Factors

The vast majority of women who develop CAD do so in the postmenopausal years. As mean survival time of women continues to increase and to exceed that of men, the amount of time a woman spends in the postmenopausal years is clearly increasing. A women who lives until the age of 85 spends more than one-third of her life in the postmenopausal state. Little is known concerning the reasons women under the age of 50 are so well protected against cardiovascular disease, and less is known about how the deterioration of this protection after the age of 50 occurs. There is even less information concerning how to retard or prevent the clinical development of CVD in women. Clinical trials of risk-factor intervention prior to myocardial infarction, eg, the MILIS Study, have excluded women by design. Younger women most often are excluded from drug or life-style modification studies because of "considerations of childbearing" and because CVD incidence in the short term is so low that statistical design would require enormous numbers of women in treatment arms to provide evidence of a significant risk or benefit. Elderly potential victims of CVD (presently, men and women in near equal numbers) may be excluded because of comorbidity or "advanced disease." For these and other reasons, including bias, evidence showing that CAD risk-factor intervention in women might be effective is far less than for men. However, some guidance data that are available are reviewed here.

A. Hormone Replacement Therapy: The understanding of the protective effect of estrogen against CAD in women has continued to evolve. In the 1970s, data regarding the cardiovascular risk of OCPs in women were used to argue that hormone administration promoted the disease. The Coronary Drug Project showed an excess of CVD morbidity with estrogen administration after myocardial infarction in men. In the Framingham Study, the initial analysis of postmenopausal estrogen use suggested an excess of CVD morbidity in women who reported estrogen use and that this excess in mortality correlated with level of serum estradiol. Because this result contradicted results of other studies, which showed an estrogen benefit, flaws in statistical formulation were uncovered, and a small estrogen benefit was calculated.

As discussed earlier, the expectation is that the lipid effects of estrogen are beneficial and protective against CAD in women. Used alone, estrogen increases the HDL level 20–30% and reduces LDL 10–15%. Triglycerides rise slightly on average, but this potential adverse effect is generally dose-dependent, and some authors believe it does not contribute to atherosclerosis. However, this triglyceride effect requires further study in light of the data on hypertriglyceridemia and coronary disease in women. The postmenopausal deterioration of a woman's protective profile appears to correlate with the net rise of LDL, total cholesterol, and triglyceride and with the rise in the total cholesterol:HDL ratio. The Donolo–Tel Aviv Study showed that the HDL level and a total cholesterol:HDL ratio greater than 4.3 predicted cardiovascular complications. Recently, angiographic CAD in women was found to be predicted best by the total cholesterol:HDL ratio; a rise in the ratio may be a sign of loss of the protective effect of estrogen. Four studies of women undergoing angiography have demonstrated that women taking estrogen are far less likely (by 60–70%) than estrogen nonusers to have angiographically significant CAD. Physiologic studies in women and studies in laboratory animals have suggested that the protective effect of estrogen may be more complex than its effect on lipoprotein levels. There is also evidence that estrogen may retard uptake of oxidized LDL cholesterol and other atherogenic lipoprotein components into the intimal layers of coronary vessels and that estrogen may inhibit tonic arterial vasoconstriction. Thus, there may be short-term dynamic physiologic vasodilation effects, metabolic effects, and long-term synthetic biochemical effects, all of which create a protective profile for women who take estrogen postmenopausally.

Despite these speculations, no randomized prospective trial of postmenopausal estrogen use has been completed, although several are under way, the largest of which is the Women's Health Initiative. The bulk of evidence favoring estrogen as primary protection against CAD has come from case-control and cohort studies. Both the Lipid Research Clinic Study (2269 women) and the Nurses' Health Study (32,317 women) suggested a marked reduction of CAD risk with postmenopausal estrogen use. A meta-analysis of all extant studies has led to the proposal that estrogen use results in a highly significant reduction in CAD risk of approximately 40–50%. However, there is no convincing evidence yet that estrogen use significantly reduces overall stroke risk. The beneficial effect of estrogen appears to be independent of the cause of menopause (surgical versus natural), duration of estrogen use, or age, at least as defined in the Nurses' Health Study.

In individual women the risk of estrogen therapy must be considered and balanced with its potential benefits. Women with a uterus have a three- to five-fold higher risk of endometrial cancer with estrogen therapy than without therapy. Progestins appear to reduce that risk when their addition is coordinated with endometrial sampling. No long-term follow-up information is available to judge the safety of combined therapy or its potential additional benefit. However, several studies suggest that estrogen and medroxyprogesterone can exert a net beneficial effect on the lipid profile of users of combined therapy. The Framingham study of women who are daughters of the original Framingham cohort and who were either present or past users of postmenopausal estrogen therapy or of combined therapy has evaluated participants for their lipid status based on their hormone use. A statistical analysis adjusted for age, body mass index, smoking, alcohol use, and use of beta-blockers and diuretics has been completed. Both estrogen and combined hormone therapy raised HDL levels and levels of the beneficial apolipoprotein A1 of HDL significantly, but only the users of combined hormonal therapy had a potentially beneficial and significant reduction of LDL level and total cholesterol:HDL ratio, when compared to nonusers of postmenopausal hormone therapy. Of course, the theoretic benefit of the lipid response to combined therapy must be studied clinically; this assessment also is part of the Women's Health Initiative for prospective randomized study.

The unresolved issues regarding postmenopausal hormonal therapy are many; they involve not only the type of therapy (estrogen versus combined) but the following additional questions:

1. What is the optimal duration of use?
2. When is it too late to start estrogen therapy?
3. Is estrogen or combined hormonal therapy helpful in secondary prevention in patients with established CAD?
4. Which lipid effects of hormone replacement are valuable?
5. Are the effects that are considered to be from estrogen partially representative of factors in the lives of healthier, more motivated women who may have a lower CAD incidence because of other beneficial behaviors?

The decision to use postmenopausal hormonal therapy must be individualized with the risk of endometrial carcinoma, possible higher risk of breast carcinoma, and side effects of the medications. A woman with a low-to-moderate risk of CAD, with a family history of breast carcinoma or endometrial atypia, might be advised to forgo hormone replace-

ment therapy. A hypertensive woman with low HDL and glucose intolerance, with a normal breast examination and mammogram, may benefit significantly from estrogen-progestin therapy. Decision making must involve the patient and other health care providers to reduce anxiety, promote compliance, and maximize risk reduction in all areas. Despite all these considerations, the American College of Physicians recommends that every woman be advised of the potential benefit of postmenopausal hormone replacement therapy and that this discussion be part of a comprehensive primary program.

B. Hyperlipidemia: The relationship between cholesterol level as a risk factor and treatment risk reduction is generally accepted, although public health issues of cost-effectiveness and population targeting continue to be controversial. Both the Lipid Research Clinic Study and the Helsinki Study have shown that lipid-lowering drug therapy in high-risk men reduces CAD incidence but not all-cause mortality. Women have been excluded from, or included in insufficient numbers in, primary prevention studies of lipid therapy. It is impossible to prescribe treatment based on proven benefit because of the lack of prospective, controlled studies of women.

No convincing study has demonstrated efficacy of dietary therapy alone in primary CAD prevention in either men or women. Secondary prevention of CAD morbidity and mortality with lipid-lowering therapy, however, may be valid in both women and men. Angina and recurrent infarction appear to be lessened in degree in men and in the small numbers of women with established CAD who have been treated aggressively with lipid-lowering drug therapy. In one small study, women with CAD treated with combined lipid-lowering drug therapy had a 40% reduction in LDL level equivalent to the male participants, with a far greater area of reduction in angiographic stenosis than the men. Curiously, this effect occurred without a rise in the level of HDL cholesterol. This study was done in patients with severe familial hypercholesterolemia. Whether women with other types of hyperlipidemias such as hypertriglyceridemia or low HDL cholesterol also will respond remains to be determined. There are preliminary data from small studies in Europe that women in an age group with a high incidence of coronary disease have a moderate reduction in coronary disease end points with reduction of LDL and total cholesterol. The role of pharmacologic management of lipids separate from hormone replacement therapy needs further study.

The National Cholesterol Education Program, Second Report, places somewhat greater emphasis on CAD in women as a problem, postmenopausal state as a risk factor, and female family member with CAD under the age of 65 as a separate risk factor. Unfortunately, the report is limited to urging justifiable caution against treatment of premenopausal women and promoting estrogen treatment as an initial approach to therapy for LDL excess (Fig 30–9). No specific guidelines for treating hyperlipidemia above a threshold level of LDL or triglyceride in women are provided. The report still lists HDL less than 35 mg/dL as a threshold applicable to men but fails to list HDL less than 50 mg/dL as a risk factor differential for women.

Clinicians must make individual treatment decisions for hyperlipidemia in women on their own, therefore. Although lipoprotein fraction risks have a gender difference, overall CAD risk factors are nearly identical (Table 30–6), and coronary artery disease complications and infarction mortality rates are higher in women. Because risk represents a continuum from primary to secondary prevention, a plan must be formulated to stratify and treat hyperlipidemia in women.

Table 30–6. Coronary artery disease (CAD) risk factor profile in women with hyperlipidemia.

Age >55 or premature menopause without estrogen therapy
Family history of premature CAD in a male first-degree relative before age 55 or in a female first-degree relative before age 65
Current cigarette smoking
Hypertension, treated or untreated
Low high-density lipoprotein cholesterol (<50 mg/dL)
Diabetes mellitus

Personal responsibility for health and recognition of CAD risk factors for women should be emphasized. Diet, exercise, weight reduction, and elimination of cigarette smoking are all to be encouraged, whether or not lipid-lowering drug therapy is initiated. The comprehensive approach that includes diet

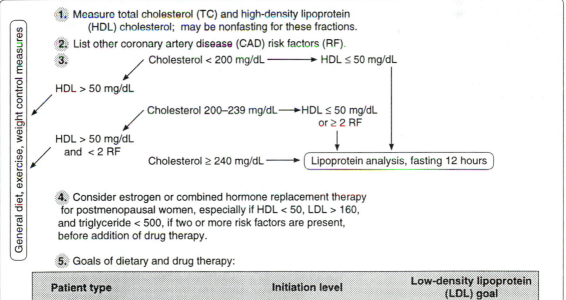

Figure 30–9. Modification of National Cholesterol Education Program treatment guidelines for hyperlipidemia in women.

and exercise is particularly important in women's lipid profile. Dietary change alone may reduce LDL and raise HDL in men, but dieting alone in women often results in reductions of both LDL and HDL, with a rise of triglyceride. This potentially adverse pattern is exaggerated with rapid acute weight loss and fat restriction. Dietary modification with exercise, however, allows a more favorable lowering of triglyceride and LDL levels and a modest rise of HDL in women according to small studies that have evaluated this process.

Cholesterol treatment in women may be initiated following the scheme outlined in Figure 30–9. Although this proposal has no prospective validation, it is a conservative approach emphasizing early introduction of estrogen and optimizing the total cholesterol:HDL ratio; LDL reduction in documented CAD has considerable support from small angiographic studies that have included women. As in any hyperlipidemia workup, secondary causes of hypercholesterolemia should be assessed and, if possible, reversed. Secondary causes include the following:

Nephrotic syndrome
Obstructive liver disease
Hypothyroidism
Diabetes mellitus
Beta-blockers
Thiazide diuretics
Alcohol excess
Cyclosporine, corticosteroids
Anabolic steroids, androgenic progestins
Retinoid cream for acne

In addition, several months of diet and exercise therapy should be initiated before drug therapy is considered in the asymptomatic patient.

A detailed review of drug therapy for hyperlipidemia is beyond the scope of this chapter. However, based on the preceding recommendations related to lipoprotein profile, several drugs and drug combinations may be considered in addition to diet and exercise in women. No drugs should be initiated without obtaining at least one, and preferably two, fasting lipoprotein profiles after a trial of dietary therapy, because drug therapy should be tailored to lipoprotein profile.

1. High LDL–The "statin" drugs—lovastatin, simvastatin, and pravastatin—can be the most effective per dose in lowering LDL. At 10–40 mg daily, they result in marked reductions of LDL and total cholesterol, moderate reductions in triglyceride, and a concomitant elevation of HDL. They are expensive but generally better tolerated than the resins or niacin, which is less expensive. Both the resins (cholestyramine and colestipol) and niacin reduce LDL in a dose-related fashion. Intolerance is high early on, but the persistent patient gains tolerance. Resins can increase very low-density lipoprotein

(VLDL) and thus triglyceride to high levels in some women and interfere with estrogen absorption as well. Niacin at low dosages (1000–1500 mg daily) raises HDL and lowers triglyceride and at higher dosages (3000–12,000 mg daily) also lowers LDL. Its vasomotor side effects are frequently intolerable, but some individuals find relief by taking aspirin before each dose. Resins and niacin are additive in their effect on LDL, and they can be combined for mixed hyperlipidemias at a lower dose of each to improve compliance and acceptability. Sustained-release niacin should not be used, because hepatotoxicity is much more common (80%) than with simple-release niacin.

2. Low HDL–Niacin can be effective in raising HDL also. Fibric acid derivatives (gemfibrozil) can raise HDL and lower triglyceride markedly, but the risk of cholelithiasis is increased. When the goal of treatment is to reduce LDL levels, and HDL is in the 40–50 mg/dL range with triglyceride less than 400 mg/dL, the "statin" drugs may produce a better overall effect in reducing cholesterol. There is no sense in continuing a drug to raise HDL if the HDL level fails to rise. Low HDL with total cholesterol under 200–240 mg/dL is often resistant to much elevation; in this situation, the total cholesterol:HDL ratio may be the best target for treatment. Ideally, this ratio should fall below 3.8, a target that may be more meaningful for risk-factor reduction in women.

3. High triglyceride–As an isolated phenomenon without a secondary cause, hypertriglyceridemia is uncommon. In patients with triglyceride greater than 500 and certainly above 800 mg/dL, drug therapy is necessary. Gemfibrozil or niacin, sometimes in combination, can be effective and should be used to prevent pancreatitis as well. Some women who begin to take estrogen have a marked rise of serum triglyceride; as in all instances of treatment of hyperlipidemia in women, the fasting lipid profile should be obtained pre- and posttreatment to document significant beneficial or detrimental effects of combined treatment. High triglyceride levels may be exacerbated by alcohol use, and thus alcohol abstention and dietary restriction of simple carbohydrates must be emphasized in the treatment of hypertriglyceridemia.

Occasionally, mixed hyperlipidemias occur with high triglycerides and LDL, often with low HDL, and require combined therapy. Niacin and bile-acid resins in combination may not be tolerable or desirable (especially in diabetics, in whom glucose control worsens with niacin). Gemfibrozil in combination with one of the "statin" drugs must be used with caution, as hepatotoxicity and myopathy may occur more frequently with this combination. Pravastatin, a second-generation drug, has been associated with a low incidence of myopathy and would be a logical choice to combine with gemfibrozil. In general, with all drugs except resins, it is essential to monitor liver function serum glutamic-oxaloacetic transaminase (SGOT) for signs of liver toxicity.

C. Hypertension: Although women tolerate hypertension for a longer time than men before they show signs of CVD complications, their hypertension accelerates the atherosclerotic process and the risk of myocardial infarction, stroke, and congestive heart failure. The general benefit of antihypertensive therapy has been demonstrated in several large trials. However, the significant reduction in cardiovascular mortality and morbidity has applied most specifically to patients with severe hypertension. Men, who have more atherosclerotic disease, and black women, whose hypertension takes a more accelerated course, appear to benefit from blood pressure treatment more than white women. White women thus far have appeared to achieve marginal if any reduction in CAD or mortality risk with treatment of mild hypertension. Because the effects of their hypertensive disease take a longer time to become evident, in the treatment trials done so far, the low number of (albeit excess) CAD end points in treated white women may be as much a reflection of treatment toxicity as treatment benefit. The major impact in studies to assess CVD risk reduction in hypertensive treatment, however, is in the reduction of incidence of stroke. The fact that stroke risk reduction is significant in all groups is the major justification for therapy of moderate and severe hypertension in women. In addition, the older woman, who frequently has isolated systolic hypertension, has been shown in the Systolic Hypertension in the Elderly Trial to benefit from antihypertensive therapy. In this study, treatment of systolic hypertension (systolic blood pressure above 160 mmHg) was associated with a 36% reduction in total and nonfatal stroke and a 27% reduction in fatal and nonfatal myocardial infarction.

Nonpharmacologic therapy for borderline or mild hypertension, and in combination with drug therapy for severe hypertension, can have beneficial blood pressure lowering effects. These factors include the following:

Salt restriction to less than 6 g NaCl daily. This modification is more efficacious in blacks, the elderly, and patients with established hypertension.

Weight loss to within 10% of ideal weight.

Restriction of alcohol to no more than 1 oz daily of ethanol (8 oz of wine, 24 oz of beer, 2 oz of whiskey).

Moderate exercise (as little as 30 minutes 3–5 times weekly of brisk walking).

Balanced diet for an adequate potassium, calcium, and magnesium intake. Supplements are unnecessary if serum levels are normal and not perturbed by diuretic use.

"Wellness" programs, smoking cessation, and "heart smart" dieting.

In mild hypertension, 3–6 months of such a program may obviate the need for drug therapy.

The choice of drug therapy for hypertension is a matter of continued debate. The fifth report of the Joint National Committee on Detection, Evaluation, and Treatment of High Blood Pressure (JNC V) has recommended that beta-blockers and diuretics remain first-line therapy for hypertension based on population studies demonstrating hypertension mortality reduction with these drugs. Because some studies have shown an increase in morbidity with diuretic use for hypertension and also a heterogeneous response to beta-blockade, whether these drugs are the best first-line treatment is still subject to varied interpretation. This issue is largely unsettled, particularly for women, in light of the preceding data on treatment effects for women. Therapy should be individualized based on the patient's physiologic status, response to sensible therapy, and minimization of side effects. For example, elderly women with systolic or combined hypertension often have a lower cardiac output with age, higher peripheral resistance, and lower intravascular volume. In addition, they may have depressed autonomic function and reduced renal function with a reduced creatinine clearance. Beta-blockers can reduce cardiac output further and contribute to fatigue, lethargy, and depression. In this instance, vasodilators and ACE inhibitors or calcium channel blockers may produce better blood pressure control with fewer side effects. If combination therapy is necessary, the addition of a low-dose diuretic to a vasodilator regimen may be useful.

Young women with mild hypertension tend to have higher cardiac output than older women. They often have normal peripheral resistance and blood volume and increased sympathetic activity. They tend to have a more compliant circulation than men of their age. If a woman's profile fits this clinical description, blood pressure may be treated easily with a low dose of a beta-blocker or a sustained-release calcium channel blocker. Consideration of the tendency of beta blockers to lower HDL and raise triglyceride and to promote glucose intolerance should enter into the decision process.

Black women tend to have an expanded plasma volume and accelerated organ damage, particularly of the kidney, from their hypertension. These women often respond best to diuretics and calcium channel blockers. Blacks in general tend to respond poorly to beta-blockers, with the exception that some may respond better to labetalol, a beta-blocker with both alpha-vasodilating and (weak) beta-blocking properties.

Obese women tend to have a higher cardiac output because of their increased body surface area, and they tend to have a higher blood volume with normal peripheral resistance. They may be particularly subject to fluid retention with unopposed vasodilation, and as a result, calcium channel blockers and ACE inhibitors may need to be combined with a diuretic. In these patients, beta-blockers may worsen lipid and glucose profiles and slow attempts at weight loss because of their tendency to decrease metabolic rate.

Women with coronary artery disease and hypertension may require selective therapy with calcium blockade, beta-blockers, or both, targeted to the control of heart rate, blood pressure, and symptoms.

Women with congestive heart failure, whether or not hypertension exists, may benefit from ACE inhibitors, especially after a myocardial infarction and particularly if their ejection fraction is below 40%. As is discussed in Chapters 32 and 34, there is more of a dissociation between ejection fraction and congestive heart failure risk in women than in men. More study needs to be done to evaluate drug treatment of this condition, particularly in diabetics and patients with both diabetes and hypertension.

Primary Prevention of Coronary Artery Disease

A. Aspirin: The Nurses' Health Study has reported a correlation between the use of one to six aspirins per week and a lower CAD risk compared with nonusers of aspirin. In this nonrandomized study, there was a 32% reduction in the incidence of a first myocardial infarction based on this intervention. Although this benefit extended to women who reported taking one to six aspirins per week, it disappeared in women who took more than seven aspirin per week. Moreover, those who reported taking more than 15 aspirin per week had a statistically insignificant but nonetheless increased incidence of hemorrhagic stroke. The benefit was limited to women older than 50 years and was greatest among women who smoked and women with hypertension or hypercholesterolemia. There is little evidence, therefore, to recommend prophylactic aspirin use to premenopausal women who do not have risk factors for coronary disease. In women who do have risk factors for coronary disease, including postmenopausal state in combination with diabetes, hypertension, or hypercholesterolemia, the use of one aspirin per day may be beneficial. The conclusion of the Physician's Health Study that one-half aspirin per day may be beneficial cannot be extended to women, because women were not included in that study.

B. Alcohol: The Nurses' Health Study, based on a questionnaire completed by 87,526 female nurses, ages 34–59 years, reported that moderate alcohol consumption appeared to be protective against the risk of nonfatal myocardial infarction, cardiovascular death, and ischemic stroke. Approximately one to two drinks per day was found to reduce the risk of CAD and ischemic stroke by 40–60%. Other studies have indicated that this finding is likely to be related to the increase in synthesis of subfractions 1 and 2 of HDL cholesterol. However, there was a statistically nonsignificant but worrisome increased risk of subarachnoid hemorrhage in female nurses who consumed three or more drinks per day. It is not recommended that women who do not currently consume alcohol initiate this habit to ameliorate their CAD risk. Those who do drink should be cautioned against excess alcohol consumption and be monitored in relation to its effect on weight, hypertriglyceridemia, and hypertension.

C. Vitamin E, Beta-Carotene, and Other Antioxidants: Only vitamin E intake, dietary as well as oral supplementation, has been associated with the reduction of CVD events in both men and women. In women, this finding comes from a questionnaire derived from the Nurses' Health Study. Nurses who reported increased vitamin E intake had a 30–40% reduction in risk of coronary events. This reduction appeared to be independent of age, smoking status, or other risk factors for coronary disease. This finding needs to be tested specifically, however; cause and effect cannot be construed from the data. It may be that women who reported vitamin E use were exhibiting a healthier life-style profile. The safety and efficacy of vitamin E in established coronary disease needs to be evaluated as well. Other antioxidants, such as selenium and beta-carotene, have yet to be associated with a significant risk reduction of coronary disease in women. The Women's Health Initiative will address this issue for beta-carotene and indirectly for other antioxidants.

D. Smoking Cessation, Exercise, and Diet: Because cigarette smoking is the only reversible CAD risk factor in women besides estrogen replacement that has a proven beneficial effect, cessation of smoking should be emphasized. A program of exercise coupled with diet and weight reduction should be part of a long-term approach to health maintenance.

REFERENCES

GENERAL

Arnold A, Underwood D. Coronary artery disease in women: A risk factor analysis. Cleve Clin J Med 1993;60:387.

Castelli W: Cardiovascular disease in women. Am J Obstet Gynecol 1988;158:1552.

Castelli WP: Epidemiology of coronary heart disease: The Framingham Study. Am J Med 1984;76:4.

Eaker E, Packard B, Thom T: Epidemiology and risk factors for coronary heart disease in women. In: *Heart Disease in Women.* Douglas P (editor). Davis, 1989.

Eysmann S, Douglas P: Coronary heart disease: Therapeutic principles. In: *Cardiovascular Health and Disease in Women.* Saunders, 1993.

Kuhn F, Rackley C: Coronary artery disease in women. Arch Intern Med 1993;153:2626.

Manson J et al: A prospective study of aspirin use and primary prevention of cardiovascular disease in women. JAMA 1991;266:521.

Manson J et al. A prospective study of maturity-onset diabetes mellitus and risk of coronary heart disease and stroke in women. Arch Intern Med 1991;151:1141.

Wenger N: Coronary heart disease: Diagnostic decision making. In: *Cardiovascular Health and Disease in Women.* Douglas P (editor). Saunders, 1993.

Wenger N: Coronary heart disease in women: A "new" problem. Hosp Pract (Nov 15) 1992;59.

Wenger N, Speroff L, Packard B: Cardiovascular health and disease in women. N Engl J Med 1993;329:247.

HYPERLIPIDEMIA

Bass K et al: Plasma lipoprotein levels as predictors of cardiovascular death in women. Arch Intern Med 1993;153:2209.

BIP Study Group: Lipids and lipoproteins in symptomatic coronary heart disease: Distribution, intercorrelations, and significance for risk classification in 6700 men and 1500 women. Circulation 1992;86:839.

Brunner D et al: Relation of serum total cholesterol and high-density lipoprotein cholesterol percentage to the incidence of definite coronary events: Twenty-year follow-up of the Donolo-Tel Aviv prospective coronary artery disease study. Am J Cardiol 1987;59:1271.

Burris J: Beta-blockers, dyslipidemia, and coronary artery disease. Arch Intern Med 1993;153:2085.

Gaziano J et al: Moderate alcohol intake, increased levels of high-density lipoprotein and its subfractions, and decreased risk of myocardial infarction. N Engl J Med 1993;329:1829.

Kane J et al: Regression of coronary atherosclerosis during treatment of familial hypercholesterolemia with combined drug regimens. JAMA 1990;264:3007.

LaRosa J: Lipoproteins and lipid disorders. In: *Cardiovascular Health and Disease in Women.* Douglas P (editor). Saunders, 1993.

Romm P et al: Relation of serum lipoprotein cholesterol levels to presence and severity of angiographic coronary artery disease. Am J Cardiol 1991;67:479.

Selby J et al: LDL subclass phenotypes and the insulin resistance syndrome in women. Circulation 1993;88:381.

Stampfer M et al. A prospective study of moderate alcohol consumption and the risk of coronary disease and stroke in women. N Engl J Med 1988;319:267.

Stampfer M et al: Vitamin E consumption and the risk of coronary disease in women. N Engl J Med 1993;328:1444.

Summary of the Second Report of the National Cholesterol Education Program (NCEP) Expert Panel on Detection, Evaluation and Treatment of High Blood Cholesterol in Adults (Adult Treatment Panel II). JAMA 1993;269:3015.

Wood P et al: The effects on plasma lipoproteins of a prudent weight-reducing diet, with or without exercise, in overweight men and women. N Engl J Med 1991;325:461.

HYPERTENSION

Bittner V, Oparil S: Hypertension. In: *Cardiovascular Health and Disease in Women.* Douglas P (editor). Saunders, 1993.

The Fifth Report of the Joint National Committee on Detection, Evaluation and Treatment of High Blood Pressure. Arch Intern Med 1993;153:154.

Hall P: Hypertension in women. Cardiology 1990;77(Suppl 2):25.

NHBPEP Working Group: National High Blood Pressure Education Program Working Group report on primary prevention of hypertension. Arch Intern Med 1993;153:186.

Perloff D. Hypertension in women. In: *Heart Disease in Women.* Douglas P (editor). Davis, 1989.

Tifft C, Chobanian A: Are some antihypertensive therapies more efficacious than others in preventing complications and prolonging life? Hypertension 1991;18 (Suppl I):I-146.

DIABETES

Spelsberg A, Ridker P, Manson J: Carbohydrate metabolism, obesity, and diabetes. In: *Cardiovascular Health and Disease in Women.* Douglas P (editor). Saunders, 1993.

Stone P et al: The effect of diabetes mellitus on prognosis and serial left ventricular function after acute myocardial infarction: Contribution of both coronary disease and left ventricular diastolic dysfunction to the adverse prognosis. J Am Coll Cardiol 1989;14:49.

CIGARETTE SMOKING

Kawachi I et al: Smoking cessation and time course of decreased risks of coronary heart disease in middle-aged women. Arch Intern Med 1994;154:169.

Palmer J, Rosenberg L, Shapiro S: "Low yield" cigarettes and the risk of non-fatal myocardial infarction in women. N Engl J Med 1989;320:1569.

Rosenberg L, Palmer J, Shapiro S: Decline in the risk of myocardial infarction among women who stop smoking. N Engl J Med 1990;322:213.

OBESITY

Denke MA, Sempos CT, Grundy SM: Excess body weight: An underrecognized contributor to dyslipidemia in white American women. Arch Intern Med 1994;154:401.

Freedman DS et al: Body fat distribution and male/female differences in lipids and lipoproteins. Circulation 1990;81:1498.

Kaplan NM. The deadly quartet: Upper body obesity, glucose intolerance, hypertriglyceridemia, and hypertension. Arch Intern Med 1989;149:1514.

Manson J et al: A prospective study of obesity and risk of coronary heart disease in women. N Engl J Med 1990;322:882.

Modan M et al. Hyperinsulinemia, sex, and risk of ather-osclerotic cardiovascular disease. Circulation 1991; 84:1165.

HORMONE REPLACEMENT THERAPY

American College of Physicians: Guidelines for counseling postmenopausal women about preventive hormone therapy. Ann Intern Med 1992;117:1038.

Barrett-Connor E, Bush T: Estrogen replacement and coronary heart disease. In: *Heart Disease in Women.* Douglas P (editor). Davis, 1989.

Hong M et al: Effects of estrogen replacement therapy on serum lipid values and angiographically defined coronary artery disease in postmenopausal women. Am J Cardiol 1992;69:176.

Nabulsi A et al: Association of hormone-replacement therapy with various cardiovascular risk factors in postmenopausal women. N Engl J Med 1993;328: 1069.

Stampfer M et al: A prospective study of past use of oral contraceptive agents and risk of cardiovascular diseases. N Engl J Med 1988;319:1313.

Stampfer M et al: Postmenopausal estrogen therapy and cardiovascular disease: Ten year follow-up from the Nurses' Health Study. N Engl J Med 1991;325:756.

Stampfer M, Colditz G: Estrogen replacement therapy and coronary heart disease: A quantitative assessment of the epidemiologic evidence. Prev Med 1991;20:47.

Vaziri S et al: The impact of female hormone usage on the lipid profile. Arch Intern Med 1993;153:2200.

Evaluation of Chest Pain

31

Edward F. Gibbons, MD

The epidemiology of coronary artery disease in women attests to its neglect as a public health problem, because of both the large number of women affected and the incomplete understanding of the evolution of serious coronary artery disease in women. Because the mortality rate of myocardial infarction is higher in women than in men, earlier diagnosis and treatment of the manifestations of coronary disease in women are needed. The clinical manifestations of ischemic coronary disease in women must be understood and placed in perspective alongside an understanding of the pitfalls of diagnostic testing for coronary disease, testing that has been designed largely for the diagnosis of coronary disease in men.

MANIFESTATIONS OF CAD

Angina

Women are much more likely than men to present with angina as their initial clinical manifestation of coronary artery disease (CAD). The 30-year follow-up of men and women in the Framingham Study continues to reflect this earlier trend of the study. Stable and unstable angina account for 54% of initial presentations in women but only 38% of initial presentations in men (Table 31–1). The earlier Framingham data suggested that men were twice as likely as women to have a myocardial infarction within 5 years after the onset of angina. The 30-year data give the same impression: men who present with angina have 2-year and 10-year myocardial rates that are double those in women. CAD death rates and overall mortality rates have been 40–50% higher in men than women at 2 and 10 years after the development of angina. However, survival in women is highly dependent on the age at which angina begins. Women in whom angina begins in their 50s live longer than their male counterparts. Women in whom angina begins in their 60s have a mortality rate comparable to age-matched men (Fig 31–1).

It is not clear whether this stepwise worsening of prognosis is related to aging itself or to the specificity of the diagnosis of coronary artery disease from the clinical diagnosis of angina pectoris. Women with angina who were enrolled in the registry of the Coronary Artery Surgery Study (CASS)

Manifestations of CAD
  Angina
  Unstable Angina
  Myocardial Infarction
  Sudden Death
  Left Ventricular Dysfunction
Diagnosis of CAD
  Clinical Diagnosis
  ECG Treadmill Testing
  ECG Stress Testing With Cardiac Imaging
  Coronary Angiography
Evaluation of Chest Pain in Women Without
    Atherosclerotic CAD
  Coronary Artery Spasm
  Microvascular Angina
  Left Ventricular Hypertrophy
  Myocardial Bridging
  Aortic Valve Disease
  Aortic Dissection
  Mitral Valve Prolapse
  Pulmonary Hypertension
  Miscellaneous Noncardiac Causes
Diagnostic Algorithm

had a mean age of 54 years, similar to the men, but they were much more likely to have atypical or nonexertional chest pain than men (Table 31–2). Thus, it is not particularly surprising that 50% of these women had no or minimal coronary artery disease by angiography, whereas only 17% of the men had trivial coronary disease at angiography (Table 31–3). The pathophysiology of angina in women without angiographic evidence of significant disease has not been adequately explained. Even in women with a high risk-factor profile for CAD or with typical exertional angina, the incidence of angiographically significant CAD is lower than in men (70 versus 90%). However, if postmenopausal status is added to these features of typical angina pectoris in women, the Cleveland Clinic has shown in their large angiography series that 90% of such women are found to have significant coronary artery disease.

These observations call into question the validity of angina as a clinical marker for CAD in women. Moreover, if angina is used as a clinical marker with-

Table 31–1. Initial clinical presentations of coronary heart disease.*

Presentation	Men No.	Men %	Women No.	Women %	Total No.	Total %
Angina	291	32	319	47	610	39
Coronary insufficiency[†]	52	6	50	7	102	6
Recognized myocardial infarction (MI)	267	30	118	18	385	25
Unrecognized MI	140	16	96	14	236	15
Death	145	16	91	14	240	15

*Reproduced, with permission, from Framingham Heart Study Follow-up Data. Courtesy of J Murabite and the American Heart Association, 1993.
[†]Coronary insufficiency is synonymous with unstable angina.

out the discrimination of other factors, such as quality of pain, menopausal status, and functional limitation, its presumed benign course may result in underdiagnosis and undertreatment of significant CAD in women. The prognosis of angina becomes diluted when women without significant CAD are included in studies (as in the CASS study), which makes the true prognosis of women with angiographically significant CAD less clear. Also, the migration from atypical to typical symptoms in some women presents a diagnostic dilemma, because population studies have shown that atypical chest pain syndromes appear to be associated with a fivefold excess of long-term morbidity even in the initial absence of documented coronary artery disease. Thus, the distinction between chest pain and clinical exertional

angina must be made at the outset; further research is needed to be able to interpret other signs and symptoms of ischemia to allow a more precise diagnosis of CAD in women.

Unstable Angina

The Framingham Study found no gender differences in unstable angina (prolonged rest pain without myocardial infarction), referred to as "coronary insufficiency," as an initial CAD manifestation (see Table 31–1). The CASS enrolled similar numbers of men and women with unstable angina, but of those proceeding to coronary artery surgery, a higher proportion of women than men had a diagnosis of unstable rest angina. Thus, women entered the surgical arm of the study with more advanced disease, which partially explains their higher surgical mortality (see Chapter 32). Unstable angina in the Framingham Study was associated with slightly higher 2-year and much higher 10-year myocardial infarction and late mortality rates in men than in women. However, these men had a higher incidence of diabetes, smoking, and hypertension than the women at the outset. Other observational surgical and angiographic studies report a higher incidence of women coming to surgery and angiography with unstable angina. Whether this finding reflects a gender-specific predisposition to an unstable pattern or a delay in diagnosis is not certain. A potential delay in angiography

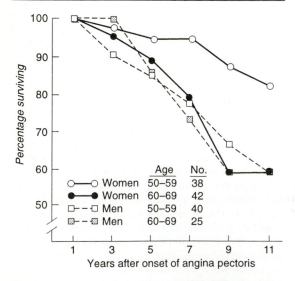

Figure 31–1. Survival of men and women after the onset of angina. The postmenopausal state and age greater than 60 years are associated with a worse angina prognosis. (Reproduced, with permission, from Kannel WB, Feinleib M: Natural history of angina pectoris in The Framingham Heart Study. Am J Cardiol 1972:29;154.)

Table 31–2. Classification of angina at entry into the Coronary Artery Surgery Study (CASS).*

Classification	Male (%)	Female (%)
Definite angina	46	28
unstable	41	52
Probable angina	29	35
unstable	27	31
Probably not angina	9	25
Definitely not angina	2	4
No chest pain	15	7

*Reproduced, with permission, from CASS Principal Investigators (authors). The National Heart, Lung, and Blood Institute Coronary Artery Surgery Study (CASS). Circulation 1981;63(Suppl):I–23.

Table 31–3. Extent of coronary artery disease (CAD) of participants in the Coronary Artery Surgery Study.*

Extent of CAD[†]	Male (%)	Female (%)
None	12	40
Mild	5	10
Moderate	4	5
Significant (> 70%)		
1 VD	21	17
2 VD	25	14
3 VD	24	15
Left main (> 50%)	9	4

*Reproduced, with permission, from CASS Principal Investigators (authors). The National Heart, Lung, and Blood Institute Coronary Artery Surgery Study (CASS). Circulation 1981;63(Suppl I):I–23.
[†]Extent of disease determined by angiography.

for women with unstable angina also may be fueled by the impression that more women than men with unstable angina are found on angiography to have normal coronary vessels. Again, this dilemma requires that more specific diagnostic strategies be developed to define true coronary disease in women with chest pain syndromes.

Myocardial Infarction

Recognized and unrecognized myocardial infarction (MI) in the Framingham Study accounted for 46% of initial CAD events in men but only 32% of initial events in women (see Table 31–1). However, an MI as an initial manifestation of CAD is more likely to be fatal in a woman than in a man. Recognized MI accounts for 66% of MI in men, but recognized MI make up only 50–55% in women. Both categories of MI are associated with an excess of early and late recurrences of MI, as well as of cardiovascular and all-cause mortality in women. The recognition and timely treatment of MI in women may be compromised by women's tendency to have (1) less ST-segment deviation with MI, (2) non–Q wave infarction, and (3) more atypical symptoms. One series of clinical syndromes with MI studied in Germany suggested that women were significantly more likely than men to present with neck and shoulder pain and nausea and vomiting. Other aspects of potential gender bias or gender underdiagnosis are discussed in Chapter 32.

When MI occurs in women, the following adverse variables appear to affect prognosis:

- Higher rate of non–Q wave infarction
- Higher rate of reinfarction at 1 and 2 years
- Higher rate of prior and subsequent congestive heart failure
- Higher rate of myocardial lateral wall and mitral valve rupture (likely age-related)
- Higher rate of post-MI stroke
- Higher 1-year CAD mortality rate (45 versus 10% for men)

- Higher 2-year CAD mortality rate after MI (33 versus 20% for men)
- Higher 10-year overall mortality rate after MI (69 versus 53%, likely age-related)
- Similar 10-year cardiovascular mortality rate (49 versus 41% for men).

Mortality for MI is higher across all age groups in women; the age-adjusted risk of post-MI death across study groups is 40–45% higher for women than men. Diabetes compounds this risk independent of the size of infarction. Several authors have examined this gender-related difference in mortality and have suggested it can be explained completely on the basis of age and prior comorbidities of diabetes, hypertension, and congestive heart failure. Authors of other studies, in particular the Multicenter Investigation of Limitation of Infarct Size (MILIS) Study, argue for an independent gender-related risk. Whichever interpretation is correct, the average woman with an MI is 40% more likely than a man to die in the hospital.

Sudden Death

Sudden death accounts for approximately two-thirds of coronary deaths and is the single manifestation in 11% of men and 8% of women. The risk of sudden death occurring as a complication of chronic CAD is twice as likely in men as women, but its risk in women may be heightened by cigarette smoking and alcohol abuse; possibly concomitant with the greater likelihood of development of CAD, sudden death as a manifestation of initial CAD occurs more commonly in women in their 70s compared with men in their 50s. Complex ventricular ectopy after MI has a worse prognosis for men but not consistently for women. These features have yet to be scrutinized in larger studies set up specifically to look at gender as a risk for sudden death. This topic is discussed in greater detail in Chapter 34.

Left Ventricular Dysfunction

Several features of MI complication rates in women may relate to women's underlying risk factors for CAD. Female patients with CAD appear to have more diabetes, hypertension, and hypercholesterolemia than men with CAD. Congestive heart failure complicating MI is more common in women, particularly in black women. Black women have a higher short- and long-term post-MI mortality rate than white women. Curiously, women tend to have a higher left ventricular ejection fraction (LVEF) than men after MI, and for both men and women, the LVEF is an accurate predictor of survival after MI. However, the higher incidence of symptomatic left ventricular dysfunction suggests diastolic dysfunction related to left ventricular hypertrophy and diastolic noncompliance from chronic hypertension and diabetes. Whether this is a sign of myocardial lack of reserve, increased subendocardial ischemia from left ventricular hypertrophy, or silent myocardial ischemia remains to be addressed. If women are more likely than men to have unrecognized MI, the risk of silent ischemia may be greater also. The therapeutic implications of these unanswered questions are likely to have a direct impact on post-MI morbidity and mortality in women.

DIAGNOSIS OF CAD

Because the prevalence of CAD is lower in women than men, any diagnostic test useful for the diagnosis of CAD in men is likely to have less value in women. Even when a test is specifically evaluated for women, the population of women studied can strongly influence the reliability of the test. For example, tests for CAD in women with typical angina who are postmenopausal or post-MI are bound to have greater sensitivity and specificity than the same tests in an unselected population. The diagnostic task of the primary care provider, therefore, is more difficult than that of the cardiologist; a broad, comprehensive strategy is needed to elicit symptoms and reliably find coronary disease in the women at risk for this disease.

Clinical Diagnosis

Of course, a careful history and physical examination in a women with the described CAD risk factors should be a part of general health care. Women should be asked not only about chest pain, but also about exercise stamina; exertional dyspnea; and exertional neck, throat, and arm tightness or interscapular pain. If such symptoms are present, they may represent true exertional angina. **Probable angina** refers to a symptom similar to exertional angina but varying in position, precipitant, or duration of pain. **Nonischemic chest pain** refers to a symptom complex of nonexertional chest pain of atypical duration, association, and precipitation so inconsistent as to raise major doubt concerning its cardiac source. The angiographic prevalence of CAD for each of these categories of chest pain is much lower in women than men even if angina is typical and exertional (Fig 31–2). Even with typical angina, only 62% of women on average have significant CAD on angiography, as opposed to 90–93% of men. The yield is even lower with less typical pain. Multivessel disease or left main coronary disease is seen to occur in only 50% of women with typical angina, 19% of women with probable angina, and 2% of women with nonischemic chest pain. Thus, the clinical history of angina in women has a higher false-positive rate than in men.

ECG Treadmill Testing

All protocols for ECG treadmill testing rely on the assessment of the electrocardiographic response to

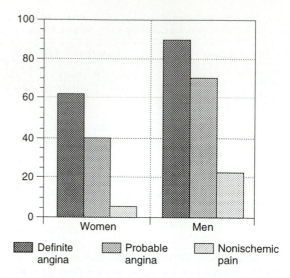

Figure 31–2. The percentage of men and women with angiographically significant CAD, by gender and type of chest pain symptoms. (Reproduced, with permission, from the American Heart Association: CASS registry data. Circulation 1981;63[Suppl I].)

exercise. A response is called positive if the ST segment is depressed 1 mm or more when measured 0.06–0.08 seconds after the J point of the QRS deflection. If baseline ST depression is present, interpretation is more difficult and specificity is lower, but sometimes the result is considered positive if at least 2 mm of ST-segment depression beyond the baseline is seen. Exercise ECG testing was performed as part of the large CASS registry. Although the sensitivity for detecting CAD by this test was similar in men and women (84 versus 80% typical angina), the specificity suffered (71 versus 57% in women) (Table 31–4). Indeed, the less typical the pain, the greater the likelihood that an exercise ECG will be falsely positive (Fig 31–3).

In general, ECG exercise testing is marred by false-positive results in women and false-negative results in men. In the CASS registry, when patients were matched for age, sex, and degree of coronary artery disease, sensitivity and specificity were similar for men and women. However, other studies looking at the sensitivity of exercise testing (and therefore the percentage of false-negative results) in women have found sensitivity to be 20–30% less for women than men, even when angiographic CAD incidence is comparable. The lower sensitivity of treadmill testing for the diagnosis of CAD in women in several studies may reflect a lower maximal heart rate achieved by women and the lower sensitivity to single-vessel CAD under these circumstances.

For these reasons, there may be a problem in detecting coronary disease in women beyond the differ-

Table 31–4. Sensitivity and specificity of ECG treadmill testing.*

Test	Clinical Pattern	Men		Women	
		Sensitivity (%)	Specificity (%)	Sensitivity (%)	Specificity (%)
Treadmill ECG	Definite angina	84	71	80	57
Normal resting ECG	Probable angina	72	80	67	69
	Nonangina	46	79	22	81
Abnormal resting ECG	Definite angina	90	29	96	22
	Probable angina	85	45	88	33
	Nonangina	90	66	50	41

*Reproduced, with permission, from CASS Principal Investigators (authors). The National Heart, Lung, and Blood Institute Coronary Artery Surgery Study (CASS). Circulation 1981;63(Suppl I):I–24.

ence accounted for by a decreased overall population prevalence, ie, a non-bayesian pattern. In general, the clinician can have the greatest confidence in a negative ECG treadmill test in a woman with typical exertional angina who achieves high workload on treadmill testing. A considerable number of women in whom a false-positive result is suspected need to be evaluated by additional testing, however. Concern over cost and yield of testing have given rise to several formulas that define exercise treadmill testing as positive when a stratification score is applied to women based on ST-segment depression and exercise performance. The formulation by Robert et al, which integrates ST depression with workload and peak heart rate, increases sensitivity from 59% to 70% and specificity from 72% to 89% and probably deserves wider application. In addition, computer methods for calculating ST heart rate slope have been applied specifically to women and found to achieve a higher specificity with maintenance of sensitivity. The adverse prognostic value of exercise-induced ST-segment depression alone is greater for men than for women, because such a pattern is more likely to represent myocardial ischemia in most men but only in women who are postmenopausal and have CAD risk factors. However, when exercise duration is factored in with ST depression and exercise-induced angina, prognosis can be reliably graded, such that an ischemic pattern with angina at a low workload predicts a poor prognosis and by itself is an indication for coronary angiography. The higher rate of false-positive results in women with atypical pain has yet to be explained. The ST segment is known to be sensitive to metabolic variables. Left ventricular hypertrophy, thiazide diuretics, digoxin, and hyperventilation can exaggerate the ST segment. The steroid nucleus of estrogen, which is similar to that of digoxin, may account in part for the nonischemic exaggeration of the ST segment in some women.

ECG Stress Testing With Cardiac Imaging

A. Thallium Treadmill Testing: When thallium perfusion imaging is added to ECG stress test-

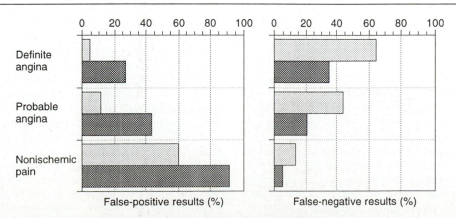

Figure 31–3. Percentage of false-positive and false-negative ECG treadmill tests by type of symptom and gender. (Reproduced, with permission, from the American Heart Association: CASS registry data. Circulation 1981;63[Suppl I].)

ing on treadmill, sensitivity remains in the range of 70–85%, for both men and women, but specificity in women rises in some studies from 60–65% to 80–90%. The test is most useful for "probable" angina or when the baseline electrocardiographic ST segment is abnormal at rest, and it is less useful for nonischemic pain. Studies of more representative general populations than seen in referral centers have shown a disappointing deterioration of specificity in women down to 70%. This result appears to apply to both planar and single photon emission computed tomography (SPECT) imaging, but it may improve with greater general recognition of breast attenuation artifact. It is important to note that single-vessel disease is diagnosed less often in women (50–60%) than in men (75–85%). The reduced sensitivity appears to be related to a lower heart rate achieved. In some series, single-vessel disease is diagnosed almost equally in women and men, but patients in these series have had a predominance of anterior ischemia, to which thallium has a higher sensitivity in both men and women. The diagnostic yield of thallium imaging in defining multivessel disease is improved if multiple perfusion defects are found and thallium lung uptake (indicative of left ventricular dysfunction) is seen.

B. Dipyridamole Thallium Imaging: By using a pharmacologic "stress" to magnify myocardial perfusion differences, dipyridamole thallium imaging without exercise avoids the heart rate response problem and is applicable to women unable to exercise adequately because of cardiac or noncardiac limitations. Sensitivity and specificity are somewhat higher for this method than for thallium treadmill testing, depending on the population studied. However, women with single-vessel disease are still underdiagnosed compared with men.

C. Stress Echocardiography: ECG treadmill testing combined with pre- and postexercise imaging of left ventricular regional and global wall motion by echocardiography assesses left ventricular ischemia and infarction in a way that is complementary to thallium perfusion imaging. In general, the sensitivity and specificity of stress echocardiography are comparable to thallium imaging for CAD detection. In women particularly, this technique shows some promise; single-vessel disease sensitivity and specificity in one series have both been reported to be 80–90%, similar to that of multivessel disease. Although significantly less expensive than thallium imaging, stress echocardiography is technically demanding for the average cardiac ultrasonography laboratory. The study has the potential also to assess coexisting valvular heart disease and define left ventricular hypertrophy in patients with hypertension and a false-positive exercise ECG; also, the method does not involve intravenous infusion or radiation exposure.

D. Dobutamine Stress Echocardiography: This diagnostic tool is an alternative to dipyridamole thallium imaging with similar indications. Instead of magnifying flow differences with dipyridamole, dobutamine uses its inotropic stimulus in a graded dosing protocol to bring out regional ischemic wall motion abnormalities indicative of coronary artery stenosis. Dobutamine echocardiography provides greater accuracy in predicting CAD in men than treadmill stress cardiography and is a promising but unproven method for diagnosing CAD in women.

E. Radionuclide Blood Pool Imaging: Radionuclide blood pool imaging with stress uses global and some regional left ventricular assessment to diagnose significant CAD. The test is much less sensitive in women than men for the detection of CAD, apparently because the diagnostic usefulness of the test is in identifying multivessel disease by a fall in or failure to increase the LVEF. Men without coronary disease usually raise their LVEF by 20–24%. Normal women do not have this pattern but maintain stroke volume by increasing left ventricular end-diastolic volume with graded exercise. Thus, even normal women by these criteria have a "positive test." This is a pertinent problem, because the large Thrombolysis in Myocardial Infarction-II (TIMI-II) study used exercise blood pool scanning to define ischemia remote from the infarct in evaluating indications for coronary angiography after thrombolytic therapy. Because this approach may be invalid in women, an important aspect of women's post-MI care is uncertain. Dipyridamole thallium imaging appears to have the greatest usefulness for this purpose, and screening exercise ECG in this high-risk population also has some prognostic usefulness, although its sensitivity is poorly studied.

F. Chest Fluoroscopy: Calcification of the coronary vessels may be identified by fluoroscopy of the cardiac shadow and is a useful marker of underlying atherosclerosis. In women, the reported sensitivity of chest fluoroscopy in identifying CAD is 75–80%, and the specificity is 83%. Thus, the test might be used for risk stratification of women who have a positive exercise ECG. However, the chest fluoroscopy gives no indication of site or degree of ischemia, prior infarct, or left ventricular (LV) dysfunction (as with thallium or stress echocardiography). Its usefulness would be highest with normal results in a woman with "probable" angina and a positive treadmill test. Although it is potentially useful in the workup, the test is not commonly used.

Coronary Angiography

Coronary angiography is generally regarded to be the clinical standard for identifying significant CAD. The test is invasive and more expensive than noninvasive testing, but in large centers, it is safe and reliable. The most common measure of coronary stenosis severity is a visual estimate of luminal narrowing.

Quantitative computer program measurements of coronary stenosis have become more common, and seem to have a closer relationship to the physiologic significance of a lesion as measured by perfusion imaging or positron emission tomography (PET) than do mere "visual estimates." Although the method of quantitative stenosis measurement has not been studied in a large series of women, it may provide more objective assessment of significant coronary disease than visual estimation, because a woman's coronary diameter is significantly smaller than a man's and luminal narrowing may be more difficult to perceive. The recorded threshold of coronary narrowing by angiography is believed to be at least 50% for moderate disease. Severe CAD is defined as one or more stenoses of at least 70–75% or greater than 50% of the left main coronary trunk. Normal or minimal coronary narrowing conveys an excellent prognosis. Moderate coronary narrowing of 50–70% may not be correlated with a worse prognosis unless left main or proximal left anterior descending disease is found, the patient has limiting angina, or thallium perfusion deficit is evident. Also, because coronary stenoses are not uniformly circular and vary in length, an apparent mild stenosis may be hemodynamically important and vice versa. In the coronary angiography descriptions in CASS, women had similar degrees of coronary disease to men, but they had more "tubular, long" stenoses than men. The significance of this difference in terms of women's tendency to present with unstable angina is a provocative aspect that needs further evaluation.

Significant CAD sometimes requires both angiography and stress imaging to define prognosis and suggest treatment. When coronary angiography shows only moderate narrowings of 50–70%, the functional correlates—patient symptoms and treadmill performance—coupled with thallium or echocardiography should take priority over anatomic findings in clinical decision making. Thus, the greatest risk to the patient is a positive thallium treadmill test and significant coronary disease by angiography. It has been demonstrated in men that any other combination of results of thallium testing and angiography is associated with excellent long-term survival (Table 31–5). Moderate CAD in an individual with a normal maximal thallium treadmill test or an abnormal thallium test in a patient with convincingly mild CAD on angiography are both associated with a greater than 95% 2- to 3-year survival rate. When both studies are abnormal, long-term survival suffers, and the rates of revascularization and nonfatal MI rise as well. Despite an overall excellent prognosis, each discordant combination is associated with a 2–3% risk of nonfatal MI, likely related to coronary plaque hemorrhage or in situ thrombosis rather than progression of trivial luminal narrowing. This type of nonfatal MI in a patient with a history of mild coronary disease by angiography is more likely to be seen in women who

Table 31–5. Likelihood of survival based on angiography and thallium perfusion imaging.*

Thallium Perfusion Scan Results	Normal Coronary Vessels	Abnormal Coronary Vessels
Normal	96% 7-year survival	98% 2-yr survival (1% nonfatal myocardial infarction (MI)
Abnormal	97% 3-year survival	86% 5-yr survival (12% nonfatal MI, 35% CABG†/PTCA)‡

*Compiled from data of Brown, 1963; Cannon, 1992; Kaul, 1988; and Raymond, 1988.
†CABG = Coronary artery bypass grafting.
‡PTCA = percutaneous transluminal coronary angioplasty.

smoke or take oral contraceptives. Clinicians should recognize that any chest pain syndrome is a morbidity marker, and patients should be instructed to seek attention for a change in symptoms that may herald such an event even when they have been told in the past that they had trivial coronary disease.

EVALUATION OF CHEST PAIN IN WOMEN WITHOUT ATHEROSCLEROTIC CAD

Each year in the United States, more than 1.5 million people undergo cardiac catheterization, usually with coronary angiography. This procedure is done most often for the evaluation of chest pain. Most cardiac laboratories report normal coronary anatomy in up to 30% of patients, with a higher percentage in women for reasons outlined in the preceding section. These individuals have an excellent prognosis from a coronary standpoint; however, even after the reassuring knowledge of normal coronary anatomy is obtained, chest pain morbidity continues. Up to 70–80% of such individuals continue to have chest pain and to see a physician for this pain. Twenty to seventy percent of these individuals may curtail their activity or employment because of the symptom. Although patients who undergo coronary angiography early in their evaluation are more likely to go back to work on finding out that coronary anatomy is normal, pain complaints often persist. Subsequent evaluation may be more directed and less expensive, however, once the coronary anatomy has been defined as normal. Long-term, unjustified anti-ischemic medications often can be eliminated.

Such patients require from their clinicians a careful ear in history taking and a proper understanding of the differential diagnosis of chest pain syndromes. Women are more likely than men to have atypical chest pain and thus to need such support and insight.

Coronary Artery Spasm

Coronary blood flow is regulated by coronary

smooth muscle tone, with input from the central nervous system and neuroendocrine stimuli as well as from local factors. **Prinzmetal's angina,** strictly defined, refers to focal spasm of a coronary vessel at the site of a mild atherosclerotic narrowing. This condition may produce angina at rest, at night, or with exercise; it is more common in men than women as classically described. **Variant angina** is a syndrome of rest, nocturnal, and exertional chest pain with normal epicardial coronary anatomy. This syndrome is more common in individuals aged 40–60 years, and it is more common in women than men. Cigarette smokers and women with migraine headaches and Raynaud's phenomenon are more likely to have coronary spasm as well. These individuals describe nocturnal awakening with chest pain, a variable onset of effort angina, and angina with cold exposure. Treadmill testing may be positive for ischemia; it is more likely to be so if testing is done in the morning rather than in the afternoon. This difference likely reflects the diurnal variation of coronary artery tone. Holter monitoring or ECG done during pain may show ST-segment elevation or depression and suggest the diagnosis. Nitroglycerin typically relieves the chest pain. Myocardial infarction is uncommon, and the prognosis is generally better than that of fixed atherosclerotic coronary disease if the symptoms are controlled. Coronary angiography is frequently necessary to distinguish spasm from fixed CAD, and spasm may be provoked and proved by graded injection of ergonovine maleate during angiography for both variant and Prinzmetal's angina. Strict criteria must be applied by the cardiologist to define focal spasm; it should not be used as a "wastebasket" diagnosis. Therapy includes chronic nitrates, calcium channel blockers (diltiazem, verapamil) administered at moderate-to-high dose, cessation of smoking, and avoidance of cold. Beta-blockers may promote coronary spasm in some individuals, just as they exacerbate Raynaud's phenomenon. Their use in such patients for hypertension or arrhythmias should be limited, and the response of chest pain should be judged empirically.

Microvascular Angina

First described in 1967, microvascular angina became known as syndrome X. This term is still sometimes used, but it should not be confused with the "metabolic syndrome X" of insulin resistance, obesity, hypertension, and hyperinsulinemia. The National Institutes of Health has defined a population of patients with microvascular angina, more commonly women, who have exertional angina, normal epicardial coronary arteries, no focal spasm with ergonovine provocation, and no left ventricular hypertrophy. Their angina is nitrate-responsive and often associated with ST-segment depression. Treadmill testing, even with thallium, is inconsistent and often negative in women with this syndrome. Research studies have shown regional or global microvascular coronary flow reserve deficit in some patients. A variety of sophisticated techniques using coronary sinus blood sampling and PET have indicated that in some patients with the clinical syndrome, there is a documented change in such indicators of ischemia with episodes of pain. Because of the subtlety of this diagnosis, it is often made clinically and based on normal angiographic findings. Support for the diagnosis may be strengthened if ergonovine produces typical chest pain with ECG changes but no focal spasm. Some researchers believe that microvascular angina is a disorder of coronary pain perception rather than coronary ischemia and should be treated symptomatically. Sensitivity to endogenous adenosine, which is felt to be a mediator of perceived myocardial ischemia, has been suggested as a mechanism. However, a subset of patients with microvascular angina who have intermittent or constant left bundle-branch block appear to suffer from a cardiomyopathic process as well, with left ventricular dysfunction appearing after months to years of anginal pain. These individuals should be treated for ischemia and monitored for congestive heart failure and arrhythmias to avert major morbidity and mortality. High-dose calcium channel blockade, nitrates, and occasionally, beta-blockers to limit heart rate appear to be the most useful for symptom relief, even in patients without left bundle-branch block.

Left Ventricular Hypertrophy

Coronary perfusion to the left ventricular myocardium may be compromised with congenital or acquired left ventricular hypertrophy, elevated left ventricular end-diastolic pressure, or both in combination. Chronic systemic hypertension may lead to both phenomena and compromise subendocardial blood flow. This process may become symptomatic with exertion or tachycardia and cause a form of angina pectoris in the absence of fixed coronary disease. This physiologic picture also may magnify the ischemic potential of mild-to-moderate coronary disease in women with uncontrolled hypertension. Evaluation should be directed toward documenting the uncontrolled exertional hypertension, quantifying any fixed coronary disease, and controlling hypertension. This angina pattern usually responds to beta-blockade, calcium channel blockade, or both in combination.

Asymmetric septal hypertrophy (formerly called IHSS) can exist in women either as a congenital anomaly and familial process or as an acquired process as a result of chronic hypertension. Any obstructive component is exacerbated by dehydration or afterload reducing agents. With marked hypertrophy, anginal chest pain may occur with exertion or arrhythmias and may even be associated with thallium perfusion abnormalities without associated fixed coronary disease. This phenomenon is diagnosed most easily by cross-sectional and Doppler echocardiography. Hypertension is better managed with beta-blockers or verapamil rather than vasodilators or diuretics. Over diuresis can provoke or exacerbate the obstructive component of asymmetric septal hypertrophy.

Myocardial Bridging

A myocardial bridge consists of a zone of epicardial myocardium through which a coronary artery dips and by which blood flow may be partially compromised at rapid heart rate during systole. To be considered a cause for angina, the stenosis of the dynamic bridge should be long (10–15 mm) and severe (greater than 70%). Ideally, the ischemic consequences of a bridge should be documented by perfusion imaging (thallium). Both beta-blockers and verapamil, which decrease exercise heart rate and contractility, are effective treatment.

Aortic Valve Disease

Aortic stenosis of a severe-to-critical degree has angina as one of its cardinal symptoms. Angina results from increased afterload, as described for left ventricular hypertrophy; in this instance, however, it is related to a fixed obstruction from a narrowed aortic valve orifice. This diagnosis is important to make prior to treadmill testing, because such testing in patients with critical aortic stenosis can result in circulatory collapse. Echocardiography is the best method for making this assessment. Occasionally, severe or acute aortic insufficiency can cause rest angina, but it is often associated with other signs of heart failure and is an indication for urgent surgery.

Aortic Dissection

Dissection of the thoracic aorta results from a disruption of aortic intima with medial dissection of varying length along a false lumen. Typically, the chest pain produced is acute, severe, and "ripping" in nature as the trajectory of the tear proceeds. Women with Marfan's syndrome can develop aortic dissection in the third trimester of pregnancy and are called the "young dissectors"; it is important to note that dissection can occur in young women with uncontrolled hypertension or Marfan's syndrome even in the absence of pregnancy. Men in their 50s and 60s with hypertension and atherosclerosis are the largest group of dissectors; in the elderly, however, women predominate in aortic dissection, with the same risk factors of hypertension and atherosclerosis. These elderly women (for example, Lucille Ball) may present acutely with chest pain or chronically with a secondary aortic aneurysm and heart failure. Acute aortic dissection is a surgical emergency if the ascending aorta is involved. Prompt cardiologic and cardiac surgical referral is essential. The diagnosis is made most quickly and reliably with transesophageal echocardiography. If this method is unavailable, chest computed tomography (CT) with contrast should be performed.

Mitral Valve Prolapse

Mitral valve prolapse (MVP) is a common congenital anomaly discussed in detail in Chapter 33. MVP is an overused diagnosis to explain chest pain, particularly in young women. Careful epidemiologic study argues against chest pain as specific to the true congenital MVP independent of documented tachyarrhythmias. Older studies suggesting focal thallium perfusion deficits with MVP have not stood the test of time. Unfortunately, the clinical practice of diagnosing MVP when a young woman has atypical chest pain has led to a false epidemic of MVP, with cases often unsupported by echocardiographic diagnosis. Other causes for chest pain should be sought in women with both undiagnosed murmurs and classic structural MVP.

Pulmonary Hypertension

Pulmonary hypertension caused by chronic thromboembolic disease, chronic obstructive pulmonary disease (COPD), collagen vascular disease, or primary pulmonary hypertension may be associated with exertional and rest angina. This anginal syndrome appears to be the result of increased right ventricular afterload and right ventricular hypertrophy. The pain sometimes responds to nitrates, control of systemic hypertension, treatment of hypoxia, and attempts to treat the underlying cause of pulmonary hypertension. This syndrome is discussed in more detail in Chapter 34.

Miscellaneous Noncardiac Causes

In clinical practice, both the primary clinician and the cardiologist must evaluate noncardiac chest pain in women. Esophageal spasm may produce substernal chest pain radiating to the neck and upper arm, and it may be relieved by nitrates. The pain may be associated with dysphagia for solid foods and cold fluids. Ideally, the diagnosis should be made using strict criteria of esophageal manometry. Diltiazem can be effective treatment. Gastroesophageal reflux can be exertional, particularly in the postprandial time period. Specific questioning and response to treatment with antacids often lead to the diagnosis. Cholelithiasis may result in radiated substernal or epigastric pain that mimics angina in some individuals but is usually nonexertional. This diagnosis may complicate the course in women with CAD or with CAD risk factors; when suspected, it should be documented by ultrasonography and treated. Musculoskeletal, costochondral, or cervical radicular pain or large pendulous breasts may mimic atypical angina, but the pain in these cases is usually positional or manipulable on examination. Finally, panic disorders can be associated with a multitude of cardiac symptoms including chest pain, palpitations, dyspnea, and dizziness. This disorder should be diagnosed and treated according to strict criteria (see Chapter 12).

DIAGNOSTIC ALGORITHM

From the preceding discussion, it is evident that the diagnosis of CAD in women is a stepwise process, requiring the input of both clinical pretest diagnostic assessment and posttest likelihood of disease with a positive test result. The clinician's goals are the relief of symptoms, avoidance of MI, and avoidance of unnecessary treatment. The diagnostic algorithm shown in Figure 31–4 synthesizes the concepts explored earlier in the chapter. The rationale for treatment is elaborated on in Chapter 32. Several aspects should be emphasized:

1. Simple ECG treadmill testing is unlikely to improve diagnostic yield with probable angina; thallium treadmill or stress echocardiography is the best first test.
2. Medical therapy should be justified by signs of ischemia.
3. Nonischemic chest pain has a narrow margin of diagnostic yield; even thallium imaging was found to increase CAD likelihood only from 7 to 25%; the latter figure is approximately the same as the false-positive rate of thallium imaging in women. If nonischemic chest pain is limiting the patient's life-style, coronary angiography may be necessary to refute or confirm the presence of significant coronary disease, particularly in postmenopausal women.

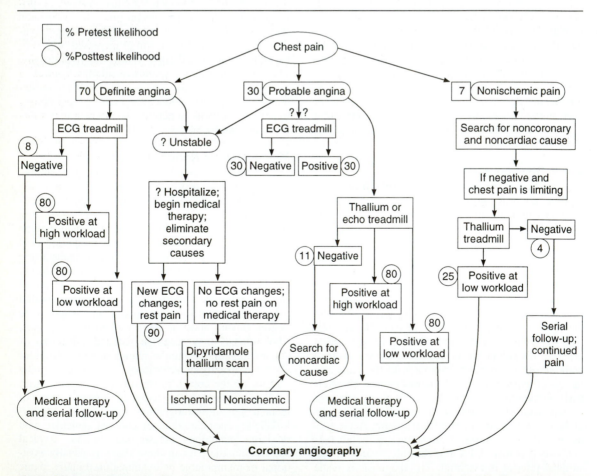

Figure 31–4. Diagnostic algorithm for the evaluation of chest pain in women. Pretest and posttest likelihoods determine the extent of workup.

REFERENCES

Assey M: The puzzle of normal coronary arteries in the patient with chest pain: What to do? Clin Cardiol 1993;16:170.

Brown K, Rowen M: Prognostic value of a normal exercise myocardial perfusion imaging study in patients with angiographically significant coronary artery disease. Am J Cardiol 1993;71:865.

Cannan C et al: Prognosis with abnormal thallium images in the absence of significant coronary artery disease. Am J Cardiol 1992;70:1276.

Chae S et al: Identification of extensive coronary artery disease in women by exercise single-photon emission computed tomographic (SPECT) Thallium imaging. J Am Coll Cardiol 1993;21:1305.

Cupples L et al: Preexisting cardiovascular conditions and long-term prognosis after initial myocardial infarction: The Framingham Study. Am Heart J 1993;125:863.

Edlavitch S et al: Secular trends in Q wave and non-Q wave acute myocardial infraction: The Minnesota Heart Survey. Circulation 1991;83:492.

Goldberg R et al: A community wide perspective of sex differences and temporal trends in the incidence and survival rates after acute myocardial infarction and out-of-hospital deaths caused by coronary heart disease. Circulation 1993;87:1947.

Greenland P et al: In-hospital and 1-year mortality in 1,524 women after myocardial infarction: Comparison with 4,315 men (SPRINT). Circulation 1991;83:484.

Kaul S et al: Superiority of quantitative exercise Thallium-201 variables in determining long-term prognosis in ambulatory patients with chest pain: A comparison with cardiac catheterization. J Am Coll Cardiol 1988;12:25.

Kong B et al: Comparison of accuracy for detecting coronary artery disease and side-effect profile of dipyridamole Thallium-201 myocardial perfusion in women versus men. Am J Cardiol 1992;70:168.

Mancini G et al: Prognostic importance of quantitative analysis of coronary cineangiograms. Am J Cardiol 1992;69:1022.

Mark D et al: Exercise treadmill score for predicting prognosis in coronary artery disease. Ann Intern Med 1987;106:793.

Murabito J et al: Prognosis after the onset of coronary heart disease: An investigation of differences in outcome between the sexes according to initial coronary disease presentation. Circulation 1993;88:2548.

Okin P, Kligfield P: Identifying coronary artery disease in women by heart rate adjustment of ST-segment depression and improved performance of linear regression over simple averaging method with comparison to standard criteria. Am J Cardiol 1992;69:297.

Opherk D et al: Four year follow-up study in patients with angina pectoris and normal coronary arteriograms ("Syndrome X"). Circulation 1989;80:1610.

Raymond R et al: Myocardial infarction and normal coronary arteriography: A 10 year clinical and risk analysis in 74 patients. J Am Coll Cardiol 1988;11:471.

Robert A, Melin J, Detry J-MR: Logistic discriminant analysis improves diagnostic accuracy of exercise testing for coronary artery disease in women. Circulation 1991;83:1202.

Sawada S et al: Exercise echocardiographic detection of coronary artery disease in women. J Am Coll Cardiol 1989;14:1440.

Shaw L et al: Gender differences in the noninvasive evaluation and management of patients with suspected coronary artery disease. Ann Intern Med 1994;120:559.

Taylor P, Becker R: Noninvasive diagnosis of coronary heart disease in women. Cardiology 1990;77(Suppl 2):91.

Wenger N: Coronary heart disease in women: Clinical syndromes, prognosis and diagnostic testing. In: *Heart Disease in Women.* Douglas P (editor). Davis, 1989.

Willich S et al: Unexplained gender differences in clinical symptoms of acute myocardial infarction. J Am Coll Cardiol 1993;21:238A.

Treatment of Coronary Artery Disease

Edward F. Gibbons, MD

Women live longer with angina than men do before myocardial infarction develops, and symptomatic coronary disease develops at an older age. Yet when women do develop infarction, their complication and mortality rates in most series appear to be higher than in men. Even studies that find no survival disadvantage after age and comorbidity adjustment must be examined in light of the fact that women with CAD are more difficult to treat. Many studies on primary prevention and secondary treatment of CAD have excluded women or excluded sicker women on the basis of age or coexisting diseases. The current approach to therapy of CAD in women is based on the few studies in which gender is addressed and, by default, on studies in which women appear to do no worse or better than men. An approach to primary prevention of CAD in women is presented in Chap- ter 30.

Established Coronary Artery Disease
    Angina Pectoris
Acute Coronary Syndromes
    Unstable Angina Pectoris
    Myocardial Infarction
    Postinfarction Ischemia
Cardiac Rehabilitation
Gender Bias

ESTABLISHED CORONARY ARTERY DISEASE

Angina Pectoris

A. Medical Therapy:

1. Antianginal drug treatment–There is no information to suggest that one form of antianginal therapy is more useful in the treatment of women than another form. Thus, beta-blockers, calcium channel blockers, and nitrates are used in standard practice. The Coronary Artery Surgery Study (CASS) included women treated either surgically or medically, but the study design did not allow for specific evaluation of women. The medical arm of the study had significantly more women than the surgical arm, but this fact probably was related to the lower overall severity of angiographic CAD in the women enrolled. A higher percentage of women than men had normal or mildly diseased coronary arteries. Thus, it is not surprising that men received surgical therapy more often than women. It can only be inferred that women at high risk for poor outcomes with chronic coronary artery disease (CAD) (ischemic at low workload on treadmill testing with left main stenosis, or three-vessel CAD and left ventricular dysfunction) should be directed toward surgery rather than medical therapy.

If it is true that women are more sensitive than men to fluctuations in coronary vasomotor tone and that this predisposition might be exacerbated with the loss of the protective effect of estrogen, calcium channel blockers and nitrates would be expected to be first-line medical therapy. However, effective management must account for angina pattern, heart rate, and blood pressure response to exercise for symptom relief and functional improvement with these agents to be evaluated. Beta-blockers may be useful and should be added to other medical therapy to effect symptom relief, especially in women with hypertension, a resting relative tachycardia, or atrial arrhythmias.

2. Hormone replacement therapy–There is strong evidence that estrogen replacement in postmenopausal women is associated with a 40–50% reduction in development of CAD. Although this benefit must be balanced with the risks of adverse effects, estrogen is likely to become a mainstay of primary prevention of CAD in women. There is also evidence that estrogen replacement is beneficial in secondary prevention of complications of angiographic CAD. In a study by Sullivan of 2268 postmenopausal women, those with severe CAD (greater than 70% stenosis in at least one coronary artery) had a 10-year survival rate of 97% if they had ever used estrogen and a 60% survival rate if they had never used estrogen. The survival benefit of estrogen in women with less severe CAD also was significant but less marked: with mild-to-moderate CAD, the rate was 96% for users versus 85% for nonusers; the benefit was still less in patients with no angiographic CAD. It is not known yet whether these findings imply that estrogen therapy is beneficial after CAD is diagnosed, that estrogen-progestin combination therapy is as useful, or that the hormones must be used for a specific duration to be effective.

3. Risk factor modification and atherosclerotic regression–Angiographic regression of atherosclerotic plaque in coronary arteries has been used as an index of treatment benefit in several studies of hypercholesterolemia. Although the studies are small, they have shown that significant reductions in low-density lipoprotein (LDL) cholesterol with diet and drug treatment are associated with angiographic regression of disease. A study by Kane that included slightly more women than men, all with familial hypercholesterolemia, showed that both women and men have a significant response to hypolipidemic agents including niacin, bile acid resins, and lovastatin. With these hypocholesterolemic treatments, reduction of LDL, increase of HDL, and regression of angiographic disease were noted. In fact, regression of disease was more pronounced in women than men in this small series.

Studies of "life-style" programs of exercise, vegetarian diet, meditation, and smoking cessation have shown that women have at least as great a potential for atherosclerotic regression as men in this highly motivated population. However, the numbers of women studied have been quite small. Because these effects have been documented in high-risk younger patients, their application to older women needs further study.

B. Surgical Therapy:
1. Coronary artery bypass grafting (CABG)–Clinical practice and consensus from surgical studies in the United States and Europe now dictate that CABG is useful for symptomatic relief of limiting angina and for long-term survival when significant left main coronary disease is discovered or significant three vessel-disease is associated with left ventricular dysfunction. The largest European cooperative study has shown a survival benefit in three-vessel CAD at all levels of left ventricular function, but this study included men only.

Short-term and long-term follow-up data of women undergoing CABG are now available from several large centers. In general, women have a higher operative mortality than men, with equivalent long-term survival. The features that result in these gender patterns are useful to examine, both to understand risk and to forestall treatment bias.

a. Preoperative profile–In the CASS, as well as in studies conducted in Portland, Atlanta, and Cleveland, women coming to CABG were older than men, were more likely to have unstable angina, and if stable, had more limiting angina than men. Women also had more diabetes, hypertension, and congestive heart failure than men before their operation. Men

had a higher rate of previous myocardial infarction, more angiographic CAD, and lower left ventricular ejection fractions than women. Therefore, men had more angiographic risks, and women had more comorbid clinical risks. Men were more likely to be referred for CABG after a positive treadmill test, and women were more likely to be referred based on symptoms refractory to medical therapy and later in the course of their clinical disease and functional deterioration.

b. Operative mortality and graft patency–In separate studies from 1969 to 1991, operative mortality for CABG was found to be consistently higher in women (1.3–8.8%) than men (0.9–3.0%). The relative risk of CABG mortality in women is 2.2-fold higher than in men. It appears, however, that gender does not play an independent role in CABG mortality; rather, women undergoing CABG are more likely to have clinical and physical predictors of surgical mortality (Table 32–1). These predictors are not contraindications to CABG but factors that increase the risk of postoperative death. When these risk factors are used to explain the higher mortality rate in women, it is found that smaller coronary size, short stature, and severity and instability of clinical disease play a greater role then gender. Despite these considerations, operative mortality is higher for women at all ages studied.

Serial study of CABG mortality at the Cleveland Clinic has shown that, as the general population has aged, so has the CABG population; the CABG mortality rate also has reflected this population trend. In this referral center, women are older, they have more left main and three-vessel disease than women in earlier surgical series and they require more urgent surgery. These features generally are related to a more severe clinical profile. It should be noted that left main coronary stenosis occurs equally in men and women; because it is the most ominous angiographic sign, it almost always requires bypass surgery for survival. However, the surgical mortality of left main coronary disease is twice as high in women as in men.

Both acute and long-term graft patency appear to be lower in women than men, which may be related

Table 32–1. Predictors of mortality from coronary artery bypass grafting.

Age > 70 years
Functional class 3–4 symptoms
Short stature; body surface area < 1.8 m^2
Unstable angina
Postinfarction angina
Congestive heart failure
Diabetes
Emergency surgery
Angiographic severity of coronary artery disease, especially
left main artery > 50%

to the size of coronary vessels bypassed (smaller in women) and to a lower percentage of women undergoing left internal mammary artery (LIMA) bypass to the left coronary system. In general, these factors would be expected to reduce symptomatic benefit and short-term survival, but they appear to explain only partially the increased in-hospital mortality rate for CABG in women. Men with small blood vessels and short stature also have an increased incidence of graft closure and a higher mortality rate after bypass surgery. Gender appears not to be a separate risk factor for CABG when age, diabetes, urgency of surgery, and comorbid noncardiac diseases are factored into the analysis; yet these factors are more common in women.

c. Long-term survival–Despite the lower survival rate for women undergoing CABG, women who survive the hospitalization have long-term survival rates nearly identical to those of men. In the CASS, the 6-year mortality rate was 7.9% for men and 8.7% for women. The 10-year mortality rate from the Cleveland Clinic study was 22% for men and 21% for women. A study conducted in Portland, Oregon, of 1979 women and 6927 men after CABG found similar survival rates in men and women at 10, 15, and 18 years. Survival was lower with three-vessel CAD and left ventricular dysfunction in this series for both men and women. Women tend to die of myocardial infarction after bypass surgery and from congestive heart failure. Men are more likely than women to die of sudden death or of cancer.

d. Symptomatic status–Just as women have angina longer than men before myocardial infarction and have limiting angina more frequently than men prior to bypass surgery, they are more likely than men to have angina postoperatively. At 2, 5, and 10 years, women are more likely to have angina than men (40–45 versus 30–35%). However, women report angina to be more manageable than men do and respond in life-style questionnaires that they feel their life has been improved after bypass surgery. The fact that, according to most studies, women are less likely to return to work full-time and more likely to retire after CABG may be related to age, financial needs, and other social features rather than anginal status.

2. Percutaneous transluminal coronary angioplasty (PTCA)–
a. Patient profile–Indications for PTCA are less well defined for mortality reduction and level of ischemia than they are for CABG. PTCA has grown tremendously over the past 16 years in the USA, and its technical success and refinements appear to have benefited women. PTCA is used for partial or complete coronary revascularization for chronic stable angina, unstable angina, acute myocardial infarction, postinfarction ischemia, and ischemia after CABG in grafts and native vessels.

A review of early (1978–1981) experience with PTCA in the USA by the National Heart, Lung, and Blood Institute indicated that women have a lower angiographic success rate and higher in-hospital mortality and complication rates than men. Procedural and technical problems were more likely to occur in women than men and seemed to be related to women's higher risk of acute coronary occlusion, myocardial infarction, and hypotension with bradycardia. Surviving women had a higher risk of recurrent angina, but they appeared to have lower rates than men of restenosis, mortality, and CABG/PTCA. The higher initial mortality rate and chronic angina recurrence rate may have led cardiologists to reduce their enthusiasm for PTCA in women.

Although early mortality remains higher in women based on more recent experience, the overall trend is toward a more encouraging benefit profile. The 1985–1986 National Heart, Lung, and Blood Institute PTCA registry of 1590 men and 546 women has followed patients for more than 4 years. In this series, women were older than men once again, and twice as many women as men were older than 65 years. Women had significantly higher rates of hypertension, diabetes, hypercholesterolemia, and prior congestive heart failure, and twice as many women as men had severe coexisting noncardiac disease or were believed to have an inoperable or high-risk surgical profile based on clinical and angiographic features. Women had a higher rate of unstable angina; surprisingly, however, most of this subset of women were under the age of 65. Men had a higher rate of prior myocardial infarction and bypass surgery and, as a result, a lower ejection fraction than women. The angiographic degree of coronary disease was similar in men and women in this series.

b. Acute results and complications–According to more recent study, a successful result of coronary dilation appears equal in men and women (89 versus 88%), and the clinical success rate (dilation successful with no death, myocardial infarction, or CABG) is identical at 79%. Complications in the National Heart, Lung, and Blood Institute (NHLBI) series were more common in women (29 versus 20%), however. Major events occurred more commonly in women, with death in 2.6% of women versus 0.3% of men. Women older than 65 had a 5.3% mortality rate. Adverse outcome as defined by death, myocardial infarction, or emergency CABG was more common in women (9.7 versus 6.3% for men). Nonfatal myocardial infarction and elective bypass surgery showed no gender difference. Multivariate risk factor analysis showed that age, history of congestive heart failure, diabetes, or multivessel disease conferred a three- to fivefold increase in risk; however, women appeared to have a four- to fivefold increase in risk based on gender alone. Body size was a risk only regarding short stature and presented a similar risk for men.

The Mayo Clinic review of its PTCA experience

between 1988 and 1990 showed no independent risk of PTCA for 860 women, despite a rise in complications and mortality when comparing the results from the 1979–1987 data with the newer data. Several shifts in their PTCA population appeared to account for the rise in PTCA mortality in women from 2.9 to 5.4%. First, both men and women were older, and there was a consistently greater number of risk factors for women, 75% of whom had unstable angina. Second, women had more multivessel disease than in the previous era and matched the men in this regard. Third, and most important, 15% of women and 18% of men had PTCA within 24 hours of an acute myocardial infarction, representing an expanded, almost routine, application of the procedure. When acute myocardial infarction patients were excluded, women had a 3% mortality rate overall, still double that of men in the same series; however, disease severity, congestive heart failure, age, and proximal left anterior descending and multivessel disease were more important predictors of mortality than gender.

c. Long-term outcome and restenosis–Initially, it appeared that restenosis was less common in women (20 versus 30% in men), but with improvements in technique and equipment for both men and women, initial success rates for women have risen, and restenosis rates for men appear to have fallen. Current estimates of restenosis for men and women are similar at 20–30%. It remains to be seen whether risk-factor modification differentially affects this rate. Newly introduced antiplatelet and tissue growth factor inhibitors to retard stenosis are under investigation. In addition, new approaches to the treatment of unstable angina with more thrombin-specific agents (hirudin) may lower the short-term thrombotic risk in patients requiring angioplasty and make angioplasty a safer and more durable procedure.

Long-term results after PTCA are nearly comparable for men and women. Although women have slightly lower rates of myocardial infarction, repeat PTCA, or CABG, their 4-year mortality rate is higher than that of men (10.8 versus 6.6%). This higher rate is related to age, coexisting congestive heart failure, and other premorbid conditions as listed previously. Like the situation after bypass surgery, women are more likely than men (30 versus 18%) to have angina and to require medication. However, women are more likely than men to rate their angina as less severe and as improved compared to their pre-PTCA angina. Despite a higher initial PTCA risk for women, therefore, the benefit for symptom relief and long-term maintenance of improvement appears secure and similar to that of men. The absolute risk of PTCA remains low given the clinical severity of disease in women and is somewhat but not dramatically lower than the risk of CABG in elderly women. Risks for CABG and PTCA in women are similar for in-hospital morbidity and mortality, so that the potential benefit of revascularization must be evaluated

using short- and long-term benefit figures and considering symptoms, degree of multivessel coronary disease, and left ventricular dysfunction.

d. Device development–Recent developments in directional coronary atherectomy, intracoronary stent placement, and a variety of laser applications have not shown superior clinical benefit in either men or women. Perhaps in relation to women's smaller coronary size, higher complication and lower success rates have appeared in women with these new applications. Technical refinements and pharmacologic improvements in antithrombotic drugs may change this adverse picture.

ACUTE CORONARY SYNDROMES

Unstable Angina Pectoris

Because women present with unstable angina resulting in necessity for CABG and PTCA more commonly than men do, it is important to emphasize the role of initial medical therapy prior to or in lieu of revascularization for unstable angina in women.

The syndrome of unstable angina may range from recent onset of limiting chest pain and an acceleration of angina to rest angina refractory to standard medical therapy. Women may present later in the clinical course of angina and are overrepresented in PTCA and CABG series with more severe forms of unstable angina. Unstable angina with ST-segment depression or T-wave inversion is associated with a higher risk of infarction and is an indication for aggressive anticoagulation and antianginal therapy. Although no specific gender difference has been reported in the clinical course or in therapeutic response in women with unstable angina, a careful review of the two studies in which women were included in the assessment of treatment of unstable angina reveals a nonsignificant higher rate of infarction in women treated either with standard anti-ischemic therapy or with the more effective regimens of aspirin with or without heparin. Nonetheless, women appeared to respond to aggressive antithrombotic therapy in these series in a similar manner to men, with a 50–70% reduction in infarction rate after the development of unstable angina with rest pain.

Unfortunately, the impression that women are more likely to have normal coronary anatomy by angiography in the setting of unstable angina may not benefit women who have angiographic CAD. With a higher mortality rate postinfarction, therefore, women need careful and timely diagnosis and treatment of ischemia if it exists. Their appropriate clinical triage to PTCA or bypass surgery in other series appears related primarily to the knowledge of their coronary anatomy by angiography. This issue is discussed further in the section Gender Bias.

Any initial evaluation of unstable angina must include a clinical and laboratory survey to exclude the secondary causes of unstable angina, eg, fever, hypoxia, anemia, arrhythmias, uncontrolled hypertension, hyperthyroid state, and volume overload. In the absence of anterior ischemic ECG changes, the therapy of an underlying precipitant to unstable angina frequently allows a delay in or even eliminates entirely the need for more aggressive measures such as angiography, PTCA, or CABG. In the absence of a major secondary cause, primary unstable angina should be treated with systemic heparinization, aspirin, nitrates, and beta-blockers. Calcium channel blockers may be added to control blood pressure further and reduce ischemic episodes. Patients with rest angina with electrocardiographic changes should be treated in a similar manner and most likely will require coronary angiography; this pattern of disease is frequently refractory to continued medical therapy. Aspirin usually is continued with and after heparin therapy to avoid a rebound hypercoagulable state with rebound angina and its risk of infarction. There is no apparent gender difference in response to these agents.

The decision to proceed to angiography is an individual clinical one. Primary unstable angina with rest pain within 48 hours of admission, continued rest pain on medical therapy, or angina with ischemic ECG changes, particularly in the anterior septal leads, usually warrants angiography. The decision to proceed with PTCA or CABG depends on the identified anatomy, degree of multivessel disease, and left ventricular function. Women with considerable left ventricular dysfunction and multivessel disease are more likely to need CABG, although their morbidity and mortality rates after surgery are higher than in men. In this setting, however, PTCA is believed to carry too high a risk to apply safely with a favorable long-term outcome.

Myocardial Infarction

Most large studies have demonstrated that women have a higher mortality rate than men with myocardial infarction (see Chapters 30 and 31). Even studies that have not found an independent gender risk for women with myocardial infarction have shown that in-hospital mortality unadjusted for age is higher in women. Furthermore, mortality in women with myocardial infarction appears higher than in men at all ages studied. All these data precede the era of intravenous thrombolysis, however. At best, only 30–40% of patients in community hospitals receive thrombolytic therapy, with the national average only slightly more than 20%. Moreover, thrombolytic therapy is given less frequently in women. The result is a large population of women without the benefit of this therapy, with a persistently high in-hospital mortality rate.

A. Thrombolytic Therapy: Thrombolytic therapy has been shown in large international trials to promote significant reduction in in-hospital and long-

term mortality (Fig 32–1). There is no apparent gender difference in the pharmacologic effects, biochemical response, infarct vessel patency rate, or clinical reperfusion rate. As would be expected, women made up 20–25% of the patients studied in thrombolysis trials. Women in the thromolysis trials tended to be older and to have more diabetes, hypertension, and antecedent angina as well as a slightly higher rate of prior myocardial infarction than men. Women also had a higher Killip class of left ventricular dysfunction on admission and received thrombolytic therapy slightly later than men. Women had a higher rate of major and minor hemorrhage than men by a factor of 50–90%. As a consequence, their transfusion requirement was also higher. In most series, women had a higher risk for hemorrhagic and total stroke (by two- to threefold) and a trend toward a higher risk of reinfarction. When corrected for worse

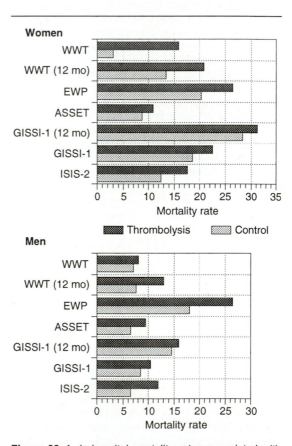

Figure 32–1. In-hospital mortality rates associated with acute myocardial infarction in the major trials of thrombolytic therapy, charted by gender response. WWT = Western Washington Trial; EWP = European Working Party; ASSET = Anglo-Scandinavian Study of Early Thrombolysis; GISSI = Gruppo Italiano per lo Studio Della Streptochinasi Nell'Infarto Miocardico; ISIS = International Study of Infarct Survival.

baseline clinical characteristics, hemorrhagic stroke is still an independent risk factor for women, probably somewhat greater for tissue plasminogen acivator (t-PA) than for streptokinase.

Mortality rate reduction with thrombolytic therapy is significant for women; it ranges from 19 to 31% for in-hospital zmortality and from 10 to 37% at 1 year postinfarction in the published series of thrombolysis trials (Fig 32–1). Although the absolute reduction in acute mortality is the same in women and men (5–5.5%), the relative reduction in mortality compared to control women is less than in men, ie, more women than men die in the hospital even after thrombolysis. In the largest study to date (13,125 men and 3945 women received streptokinase and aspirin [International Study of Infarct Survival (ISIS-2) study]), women had a mortality of 17.5% (control) versus 12.2% (streptokinase), whereas men had a mortality of 12% (control) versus 6.7% (streptokinase). This persistent excess in mortality for women despite treatment with thrombolysis, appears to hold for t-PA as well, with its attendant risk of hemorrhagic and fatal stroke.

This excess in mortality in women even after thrombolysis holds at every age group and is doubled in insulin-dependent diabetic women. Because the control populations in these studies have mortality rates similar to women's statistics in the earlier era, the higher mortality rate after thrombolysis in women has been explained in terms of risk associated with coexisting factors of age, Killip class, reinfarction risk, and stroke risk. There is no gender difference in left ventricular function, infarct vessel site, degree of complex coronary disease, or infarct vessel patency on early angiography. Dosing of t-PA is an issue to be addressed, because the standard dose of 100 mg of front-loaded t-PA for all body weights may be an overdose for small women. Hemorrhagic stroke risk is known to be higher for individuals who in earlier trials received 150 mg of t-PA. Weight-adjusted dosing of thrombolytic therapy is now being studied. Current gynecologic opinion is that thrombolytic therapy is not contraindicated in menstruating women, because vaginal bleeding in this setting should be manageable with appropriate gynecologic intervention.

B. Direct PTCA: In large centers with active coronary angiography laboratories, immediate PTCA for acute myocardial infarction has been feasible. When PTCA was compared to t-PA in the Primary Angioplasty in Myocardial Infarction (PAMI) trial, 107 women and 288 men were randomized to one of the two groups. PTCA candidates were treated with balloon inflation within 1 hour of presentation of their myocardial infarction. Overall, there was a nonsignificant trend to lower mortality with PTCA and a marked (0 versus 3.5%) stroke risk reduction with PTCA over t-PA. In women, however, the in-hosptial mortality rate was 4% for PTCA and 14% for t-PA

(p = .06), and the rate of stroke was 5.3% for t-PA and 0% for PTCA (nonsignificant). Enthusiasm for this response must be tempered by the fact that the excess mortality related to thrombolytic therapy appeared to be related to the hemorrhagic stroke risk, which was significantly higher in this series than in most other published series. Whether PTCA, even in this ideal setting, is preferable to t-PA is therefore still open to question.

Although these data are encouraging and help justify the use of PTCA in women and the elderly (who have contraindications to thrombolytic therapy, or fail to improve with thrombolytic therapy), the results cannot be applied universally. Time is of the essence in achieving reperfusion after myocardial infarction is diagnosed; most community and tertiary centers do not have immediate PTCA capacity 24 hours a day. Therefore, when it is the only option, thrombolytic therapy should be given to women with acute myocardial infarction, because it is still associated with a significant short- and long-term mortality rate reduction.

C. Drug Therapy: Because the majority of women with myocardial infarction currently are not treated with thrombolysis or direct PTCA, adjunctive therapy should be given when appropriate.

1. Aspirin–Aspirin given after myocardial infarction has not been shown to reduce overall mortality in women. Aspirin after myocardial infarction does reduce the rate of reinfarction and overall cardiovascular mortality by 15%, however, when it is used for cerebrovascular symptoms, unstable angina, or myocardial infarction. Whether this effect applies equally to women has not been studied. The ISIS-2 study showed that aspirin alone reduced mortality by 23% compared with thrombolysis and reduced reinfarction and stroke risk for men and women combined. Thus, aspirin should be given on presentation to the emergency room with suspected myocardial infarction and continued after discharge in women who suffer an infarction until new data argue to the contrary.

2. Beta-blockers–Both the Timolol Myocardial Infarction Study and the Beta-Blocker Heart Attack Trial (BHAT) included women and reported reductions as great as or greater than those found in men in mortality and recurrent myocardial infarction. This finding has applied most convincingly to women with Q-wave infarctions and to individuals whose early course has been complicated by arrhythmia, transient left ventricular dysfunction, or ischemia. The benefit seems to persist for at least 1 year after myocardial infarction in these higher risk patients, with a 43% mortality rate reduction with continued use of the beta-blocker. The mortality rate in women in this trial was doubled by poor compliance with the medication regimen.

3. Angiotensin converting enzyme (ACE) inhibitors–The Survival and Ventricular Enlargement (SAVE) trial enrolled men and women with left ventricular dysfunction after myocardial infarction. Patients were randomized to receive captopril therapy or standard therapy for congestive heart failure and were followed for complications. Captopril therapy resulted in a 35% reduction of recurrent myocardial infarction, cardiovascular death, and hospitalization for congestive heart failure. It is not clear whether women benefit more than men with this therapy or at what level of left ventricular ejection fraction the drug begins to have a significant effect. Because women have more congestive heart failure at a higher left ventricular ejection fraction than men after a myocardial infarction, women who have any degree of global left ventricular dysfunction may benefit from ACE inhibitor therapy early after myocardial infarction. This finding is most pertinent in the population of women with diabetes and hypertension.

4. Warfarin–Stroke risk after myocardial infarction is higher in women than men, even without thrombolytic therapy. The stroke risk is related to intracavitary thrombosis in the left ventricle and left atrium rather than hemorrhagic stroke in the group of women who are not given thrombolytic therapy. There has been no gender-specific study of warfarin use after myocardial infarction despite many studies proposing its general benefit. Warfarin is used currently for women with significant anteroapical hypokinesis or dyskinesis of the left ventricle after myocardial infarction, and it is used for 2–3 months or indefinitely in the presence of leftventricular aneurysm. In addition, individuals with left ventricular ejection fractions less than 30%, particularly with atrial fibrillation or with class IV heart failure, should be treated with warfarin after myocardial infarction. In this setting, chronic warfarin use with an International Normalized Ratio (INR) goal of 2–3 is felt to reduce the risk of cardioembolic stroke and of venous thromboembolism. It should be noted that estrogen supplements tend to increase the daily warfarin requirement through their stimulation of hepatic synthesis of procoagulant cofactors.

Postinfarction Ischemia

Reduced left ventricular ejection fraction and postinfarction ischemia are the major predictors for mortality and complications in the years after myocardial infarction in both men and women. Early mortality is greater when ischemia is symptomatic soon after infarction. The detection of post-MI ischemia in women is of great importance, therefore, but has not been rigorously studied. The Thrombolysis in Myocardial Infarction (TIMI-II) study recommended and used exercise radionuclide ventriculography to detect early ischemia after myocardial infarction in men given t-PA. As discussed in Chapter 31, however, this test may be too insensitive in women to detect ischemia remote from a myocardial

infarction. Therefore, dipyridamole thallium or dobutamine echocardiography after myocardial infarction needs to be performed in women and the results compared to treadmill testing. This is particularly important after non-Q-wave myocardial infarction, in which the reinfarction rate in the first year after myocardial infarction is high, and subsequent mortality in women is excessive. At present, many clinicians perform standard treadmill testing within 3–6 weeks after myocardial infarction, dipyridamole thallium scanning prior to discharge, or direct coronary angiography for angina recurrence in both men and women after myocardial infarction.

In a series of 164 women and 341 men studied by Welty et al, PTCA performed for post-MI ischemia produced similar, excellent results for both sexes. Women in this series were older, more likely to have a non-Q-wave myocardial infarction, and less likely (15 versus 25%) to have received thrombolytic therapy than men. At PTCA, a 90% success rate was achieved, with equivalent low CABG, myocardial infarction, and death rates (0.6–0.9%). Three-year follow-up showed only a 19% repeat PTCA rate, a 3.6% death rate, and identical reinfarction rates with no differential gender effect. Although this trend is encouraging, patient subsets appropriate for such intervention need to be defined.

CARDIAC REHABILITATION

Formal cardiac rehabilitation is beneficial in men in promoting early return to work after myocardial infarction and bypass surgery, promoting life-style changes to reduce primary risk factors, and identifying and treating these risk factors. Meta-analysis has suggested a trend in men for cardiac rehabilitation to reduce fatal reinfarction rates and cardiac mortality rates. No such data are evident for women. However, fewer women are referred to rehabilitation programs after myocardial infarction or bypass surgery, and dropout rates are greater and compliance lower for women. Women are excluded more often from rehabilitation programs for cardiac or medical reasons, yet they have a lower exercise capacity and employment rate 1 year after myocardial infarction or CABG than men. Psychological studies have shown that lack of emotional support after myocardial infarction increases the 6- to 12-month mortality risk after MI more for men than for women. Cardiac rehabilitation should be explored for its potential to identify women at higher risk for post-MI ischemia and congestive heart failure and to facilitate a greater functional capacity after myocardial infarction.

GENDER BIAS

Although angina is the most common presenting form of CAD in women, women are less likely than men to undergo diagnostic study for angina. One large series reported that even when nuclear perfusion studies were done, men were 10 times more likely to have coronary angiography than women (40 versus 4%) after a positive scan. At the time of that series, studies were not necessarily corrected for a woman's potential to exhibit breast thallium attenuation; therefore, current interpretation and appropriate referral may be somewhat better. Regardless, the studies were ordered and interpreted for the purpose of looking for ischemia. The authors of this report conclude that when pre- and posttest likelihood analysis was performed on this population of patients, they would have anticipated only a 2:1 ratio of referral for men versus women based on the positivity of the scan.

In the SAVE trial mentioned previously, coronary angiography was required for participation. Yet women were excluded on this basis more often than men, because angiography was performed, even for postinfarction angina, only half as often in women as in men. Perhaps for similar reasons, women appear to present for CABG and PTCA later and sicker in their course than men, which may contribute to their higher mortality rate with these interventions. However, women do appear to undergo revascularization with PTCA or CABG in equal numbers with men once they have undergone coronary angiography and have "as much disease as a man."

The false impression of the "benign" nature of angina in women may stem from skewed clinical experience or misleading interpretation of the early Framingham and CASS data (Chapter 31). Similarly, thrombolytic therapy has been given less often to women than men, both in the 1987–1988 and 1991–1992 series studied. This undertreatment was not accounted for by contraindications to thrombolysis, and bias appeared greatest in women under the age of 50 who had a nonanterior myocardial infarction. A women was more likely to receive thrombolytic therapy if her myocardial infarction was anterior, if she had a history of cardiac disease, or if she had a family history of coronary artery disease, in which case there was no gender bias. Patient education programs for women should identify which symptoms are to be interpreted as ischemic or indicative of infarction. Women should be aware of their past history, CAD risk factors, and family history so that they may receive effective treatment if they have the misfortune to present with a myocardial infarction. Simply giving a lucid history may be lifesaving.

It is important to recognize that gender bias may not be malevolent nor universally detrimental. If it is true that men undergo CABG more often on the basis of a positive treadmill test, and women undergo the procedure more often for angina and unstable angina symptoms, it may be that men are overtreated with aggressive revascularization. However, women will be served best when the diagnosis of CAD is made properly and securely and the timing of medical or surgical intervention maximizes survival and functional capacity and minimizes morbidity and mortality.

REFERENCES

MEDICAL THERAPY

Berkman L, Leo-Summers L, Horwitz R: Emotional support and survival after myocardial infarction: A prospective, population-based study of the elderly. Ann Intern Med 1992;117:1003.

Eysmann S, Douglas P: Coronary heart disease: Therapeutic principles. In: *Cardiovascular Health and Disease in Women.* Douglas P (editor) Saunders, 1993.

Gallagher E, Viscoli C, Horwitz R: The relationship of treatment adherence to the risk of death after myocardial infarction in women. JAMA 1993;270:742.

Kane J et al: Regression of coronary atherosclerosis during treatment of familial hypercholesterolemia with combined drug regimens. JAMA 1990;264:3007.

O'Toole M: Exercise and physical activity. In: *Cardiovascular Health and Disease in Women.* Douglas P (editor). Saunders, 1993.

Sullivan J: Estrogen replacement and coronary artery disease. Arch Intern Med 1990;150:2557.

Theroux P et al: Aspirin, heparin, or both to treat acute unstable angina. N Engl J Med 1988;319:1105.

Theroux P et al: Reactivation of unstable angina after the discontinuation of heparin. N Engl J Med 1992;327:141.

Viscoli C, Horwitz R, Singer B: Beta-blockers after myocardial infarction: Influence of first-year clinical course on long-term effectiveness. Ann Intern Med 1993;118:99.

Willard J, Lange R, Hillis L: The use of aspirin in ischemic heart disease. N Engl J Med 1992;327:175.

CABG

Eaker E et al: Comparison of the long-term, postsurgical survival of women and men in the coronary artery surgery study (CASS). Am Heart J 1989;117:71.

O'Connor G et al: Differences between men and women in hospital mortality associated with coronary artery bypass graft surgery. Circulation 1993;88(part 1): 2104.

Rahimtoola S et al: Survival at 15 to 18 years after coronary bypass surgery for angina in women. Circulation 1993;88(part 2):71.

Weintraub W et al: Changing clinical characteristics of coronary surgery patients. Circulation 1993;88(part 2):79.

PTCA

Bell M et al: The changing in-hospital mortality of women undergoing percutaneous transluminal coronary angioplasty. JAMA 1993;269:2091.

Kahn J et al: Comparison of procedural risks of coronary angioplasty in men and women for conditions other than myocardial infarction. Am J Cardiol 1992;69:1241.

Kelsey S et al: Results of percutaneous transluminal coronary angioplasty in women: 1985–1986 National Heart, Lung, and Blood Institute's coronary angioplasty registry. Circulation 1993;87:720.

Stone G et al: Primary angioplasty is the preferred therapy for women and the elderly with acute myocardial infarction: Results of the primary angioplasty in myocardial infarction (PAMI) trial. J Am Coll Cardiol 1993;21:330A.

Welty F et al: Similar results of percutaneous transluminal coronary angioplasty for women and men with postmyocardial infarction ischemia. J Am Coll Cardiol 1994;23:35.

THROMBOLYTIC THERAPY

Eysmann S, Douglas P: Reperfusion and revascularization strategies for coronary artery disease in women. JAMA 1992;268:1903.

Lincoff A et al: Thrombolytic therapy for women with myocardial infarction: Is there a gender gap? J Am Coll Cardiol 1993;22:1780.

White H et al: After correcting for worse baseline characteristics, women treated with thrombolytic therapy for acute myocardial infarction have the same mortality and morbidity as men except for a higher incidence of hemorrhagic stroke. Circulation 1993;88:2097.

Zuanetti G et al: Influence of diabetes on mortality in acute myocardial infarction data from the GISSI-2 study. J Am Coll Cardiol 1993;22:1788.

GENDER BIAS

Ayanian J, Epstein A: Differences in the use of procedures between women and men hospitalized for coronary heart disease. N Engl J Med 1991;325:221.

Bickell N et al: Referral patterns for coronary artery disease treatment: Gender bias or good clinical judgment? Ann Intern Med 1992;116:791.

Healy B: The Yentl syndrome. (Editorial.) N Engl J Med 1991;325:274.

Khan S et al: Increased mortality of women in coronary artery bypass surgery: Evidence for referral bias. Ann Intern Med 1990;112:561.

Maynard C et al: Underutilization of thrombolytic therapy in eligible women with acute myocardial infarction. Am J Cardiol 1991;68:529.

Steingart R et al: Sex differences in the management of coronary artery disease. N Engl J Med 1991;325:226.

Valvular Heart Disease

33

Edward F. Gibbons, MD

Prior to the twentieth century epidemic of athero-sclerotic coronary artery disease and its recognition as a major cause of cardiac death, valvular heart disease occupied most of medicine's diagnostic and therapeutic attention to cardiac illness. With the steep decline in incidence of rheumatic fever and rheumatic heart disease over the past 75 years, and with heightened awareness of and attention to coronary artery disease in men, attention to valvular heart disease may have waned. Its importance in the area of women's heart disease deserves emphasis, both to outline functional and morbidity risks for women and to dispel some myths about how valvular heart disease presents. Diseases of mitral and aortic valves are discussed, whereas right-sided valve and childhood congenital anomalies are not reviewed because of their uncommon nature and the scarce data regarding gender impact.

Gender appears to exert an important influence on the manifestations of valvular heart disease. Women are hospitalized more frequently than men for valvular heart disease and have more valvular cardiac surgery than men. Discharge coding of hospitalizations for heart disease reveals that more than 70% of hospital discharges for aortic or mitral valve disease in 1987 were for woman, compared with 39% of discharges for myocardial infarction for women. Rheumatic valve disease affects women 1.5-fold more commonly than it does men, but with rheumatic fever on the decline, women's risk of valve disease appears to be more strongly related to degenerative and calcific disease of aortic and mitral valves and to the late complications of mitral valve prolapse. Of approximately 50,000 heart valve replacements or repairs done yearly in the United States, 60% are performed in women. This figure contrasts strikingly with the fact that less than 30% of coronary bypass operations or angioplasty procedures are performed in women.

Certainly, the recognition and appropriate management of valvular heart disease in women must be emphasized. Yet a proper clinical perspective must be brought to patient care: to avoid overdiagnosis of disease from trivial or functional murmurs or noncardiac symptoms and to direct proper attention to overall cardiovascular health when a mild valvular abnormality has been identified. It is important to note that

Rheumatic Fever & Rheumatic Heart
    Disease
  Mitral Stenosis
  Mitral Regurgitation
  Aortic Valve Disease
Mitral Valve Prolapse
  Diagnosis
  Complications
Nonrheumatic Mitral Valve Disease
  Mitral Annular Calcification
  Nonrheumatic Connective Tissue
    Disorders
  Antiphospholipid Antibody Syndrome
Nonrheumatic Aortic Valve & Thoracic Aortic
    Disease
  Aortic Stenosis
  Aortic Insufficiency
  Marfan Syndrome with Aortic Dissection
Pregnancy & Valvular Heart Disease .
  The Normal Examination in Pregnancy
  Preexisting Heart Disease in Pregnancy:
    Risk Assessment
Antibiotic Prophylaxis for Surgical
    Procedures

the complications and mortality rates from non-rheumatic valvular heart disease remain greater for men with these diseases. The origins of these differences are discussed in Chapter 34.

RHEUMATIC FEVER & RHEUMATIC HEART DISEASE

Although the incidence of acute rheumatic fever has become so low that many younger clinicians cannot recall ever having seen a case, primary clinicians must be able to recognize both acute and chronic manifestations of rheumatic heart disease. In Third World countries, rheumatic heart disease is the leading cause of cardiac illness; it is estimated that 15–20 million cases of acute rheumatic fever occur in these countries each year. Overcrowding, lack of access to medical care, and exposure and susceptibility to group A beta-hemolytic *Streptococcus* all appear to predispose to the disease in these populations. More recent outbreaks in the USA have not followed these socioeconomic boundaries and may reflect rheumatic fever outbreaks caused by a more virulent streptococcal serotype. Moreover, in some series, less than one-third of affected individuals had a history of pharyngitis.

With migration of populations from Southeast Asia, Central and South America, and Africa to urban centers in the USA, with the increase in child care outside the home, and with a lower clinical index of suspicion for rheumatic fever and chronic rheumatic heart disease, the potential for an increased incidence of rheumatic heart disease exists.

Susceptibility to acute rheumatic fever in childhood and the teenage years is greater for white boys than white girls by a factor of 2:1–3:1. There is no gender difference for nonwhite young people. The manifestations of acute rheumatic fever are similar for males and females (Table 33–1), except that females may develop pure "chorea" and chronic rheumatic heart disease without other acute signs. The mortality rate of acute rheumatic heart disease is higher for females by 20–30% despite the lower incidence of rheumatic fever in females. The increased severity of rheumatic heart disease in women carries over to its chronic manifestations as well.

Whereas mitral valve disease is 2.3 times more common in women, aortic valve disease is 3.6 times more common in men. Combined valve disease is approximately equal in incidence in men and women. The overall prevalence of rheumatic heart disease is 1.2–1.5 times higher for women, but the death rate for all chronic rheumatic heart disease (1984 data) is twofold higher for women. Up to 20% of individuals with rheumatic heart disease have no history of rheumatic fever.

Mitral Stenosis

Mitral stenosis exhibits a 3:1 female:male predominance. Women are more likely than men to progress

Table 33–1. The Jones Criteria for the diagnosis of acute rheumatic fever.*

Major Manifestations	Minor Manifestations
Carditis	Fever
Polyarthritis	Arthralgia
Chorea	History of rheumatic fever or rheumatic heart disease
Sucutaneous nodules	Elevated erythrocyte sedimentation rate, C-reactive protein, or white blood cell count
Erythema marginatum	Prolonged PR interval on ECG

*Two major or one major and two minor manifestations, with supporting evidence of a recent streptococcal infection, indicate the probable presence of rheumatic fever.

to significant mitral stenosis after acute rheumatic fever, even in the absence of recurrent rheumatic fever. Once mitral stenosis becomes clinically significant, prognosis is slightly worse for men. Males tend to develop more calcification of the valve apparatus, which may lead to more complex surgery and to poor valve repair and commissurotomy results. Women, on the other hand, are far more likely to have fatal and nonfatal arterial emboli with mitral stenosis, with an excessive 9:1 risk over men. Newer approaches to mitral valve surgery may benefit women more than men. In younger women, less valvular calcification appears to lead to more successful open commissurotomy and closed balloon valvuloplasty. Indeed, earlier intervention of this kind may forestall the need for prosthetic valve replacement. A woman of child-bearing age who wishes to plan a family and who has significant mitral stenosis may do well to elect a valve repair or valvuloplasty while in sinus rhythm to avoid the difficulty and risks of anticoagulation during pregnancy as well as the higher risk of untreated mitral stenosis during pregnancy.

Mitral Regurgitation

Rheumatic mitral regurgitation with trivial stenosis is more common in men, with a male:female ratio of 1.5:1. Even in men with a history of rheumatic fever, however, stenosis is more common than severe regurgitation. Mitral regurgitation may become the predominant hemodynamic lesion if mitral endocarditis develops, if chordal rupture occurs, or if valvulotomy is unsuccessful in preserving valve integrity. In general, severe mitral regurgitation is 4–20 times more common from mitral valve prolapse than from rheumatic disease.

Aortic Valve Disease

Aortic regurgitation is the predominant aortic valve lesion after rheumatic fever; aortic stenosis is rare. Men are more likely than women to have significant aortic regurgitation, with a ratio of 3:1. Symptoms of early congestive heart failure or signs of left ventricular dysfunction on echocardiography or angiography are indications for aortic valve replacement, and this surgery appears to be equally successful in men and women.

MITRAL VALVE PROLAPSE

Mitral valve prolapse (MVP) is defined anatomically (and by echocardiography) as the systolic displacement of both mitral leaflets superiorly and posteriorly above their usual position at the mitral annulus. Most cases of MVP are associated with leaflet thickening, chordal elongation, and excess leaflet tissue and are "primary" cases of MVP. Other connective tissue disorders may result in MVP, such as Marfan's syndrome, and are associated with other cardiovascular manifestations, as discussed in Chapter 31. Also, MVP may appear if the mitral annulus is "undersized" for the mitral leaflets, as in atrial septal defect, or in volume-depleted states such as anorexia nervosa.

Primary MVP appears to be genetically determined. The genetic transmission is likely to be autosomal dominant with incomplete expression, such that as few as 10–20% and as many as 50% of first-degree relatives of MVP index cases are affected. The overall incidence of MVP varies according to the population studied and the definition used. The Framingham study found 7.6% of women and 2.5% of men to have M-mode echocardiographic evidence of MVP. The strictest study using cross-sectional echocardiographic criteria found MVP in 5.4% of women and 3% of men. Women are more likely to have recognized MVP, therefore, as are their female first-degree relatives. The expression of MVP appears to vary with age; it is highest in first-degree relatives of women 20–49 years old (49%) and falls after age 50 to only 27% in first-degree relatives. This decline after age 50 may be related to age-associated valve stiffening and concomitant development of mitral valve calcification.

Diagnosis

Because MVP is a common anatomic entity, its presence has been considered in some population studies to be the cause of a variety of signs and symptoms to which it only appears closely associated. The higher incidence of MVP in women appears to have led to what is now believed to be a misguided view of MVP symptoms and to an unfortunate overuse of MVP as a diagnosis to explain atypical cardiac symptoms in young women. It is important, therefore, to be precise and objective in diagnosing MVP and its consequences.

The physical diagnosis of MVP requires the auscultation of an early- to midsystolic click. This click is to be distinguished from a normal split S1 and from the fixed early click of a bicuspid aortic valve. The click of MVP should move closer to S1 with a reduction of preload on standing and closer to S2 on assuming a supine posture or squat. An associated mitral regurgitation murmur should move in parallel to the click and become louder with isometric hand grip. It is possible for the murmur to be heard only intermittently or only with excitement and then very late in systole. A holosystolic, coarse murmur of mitral regurgitation is most often hemodynamically important and places the patient at higher risk of complications.

When other clinical traits are examined in individuals with MVP and their first-degree relatives, it is clear that some components of the "MVP syndrome" are unlikely to be related to MVP. For example, it is true that click murmurs, thoracic bony abnormalities (pectus excavatum, scoliosis, straight spine), and palpitations are associated statistically with true MVP; however, other, less specific components of the so-called syndrome are not statistically associated with true MVP. These less specific components include atypical chest pain, dyspnea, panic attacks, high anxiety score, and inferior ECG lead ST-T wave abnormalities. If these symptoms or signs appear in the absence of significant mitral regurgitation, attributing their existence to MVP is not justified. Moreover, individuals with these symptoms should not be assigned a diagnosis of MVP in the absence of firm auscultation or echocardiographic evidence of MVP. The fact that atypical chest pain is more common in women than men has perpetuated the false clinical impression that MVP and atypical chest pain are closely linked. Atypical chest pain is better evaluated as outlined in Chapter 31.

An additional confounding factor that has led to overuse of MVP as a diagnosis for cardiac disease is the former lack of strict echocardiographic criteria for the diagnosis of MVP. In the 1970s and early 1980s, criteria of low specificity from M-mode and cross-sectional echocardiography were used to make the diagnosis of MVP. Since that time, the criteria of mitral leaflet displacement and thickening on multiple views, characteristics and timing of regurgitation and abnormalities of the subvalvular apparatus, appear to be more specifically diagnostic of the abnormality and to stratify risk for complications of MVP more appropriately. Echocardiography is indicated when the physical examination is unclear or atypical, when the patient's symptoms or the examination suggests more than mild mitral regurgitation, when Marfan's syndrome is suspected (to assess aorta and aortic valve), or when a previous diagnosis of MVP is held in question.

Complications

The long-term risk factors for complications of mitral valve prolapse include severe mitral regurgitation requiring valve surgery, endocarditis, congestive heart failure from valvular regurgitation, arterial emboli, and stroke, particularly with atrial fibrillation. The risk of sudden death in association with MVP appears closely linked to the severity of mitral regurgitation. MVP as a major risk factor is evident from the fact that 25% of instances of mitral valve replacement or repair are in patients with mitral valve prolapse and that 13–15% of instances of endocarditis involve valves afflicted with mitral valve prolapse.

Despite a higher prevalence of MVP in women than men, the risks for its most serious complications are higher in men. In multiple studies of MVP and severe mitral regurgitation, 67% of patients with severe regurgitation were men. This finding may be related to the higher average blood pressure in men and the higher blood pressure in both men and women with complicated MVP with severe mitral regurgitation. Endocarditis is more common in men than women; when endocarditis occurs with MVP, an average of 58% of cases have been in men. Antibiotic prophylaxis is warranted with any degree of mitral regurgitation and documented mitral valve prolapse. Risk stratification is useful clinically, therefore, for patient counseling and management.

The patients with the highest risk include those with moderate-to-severe mitral regurgitation, particularly those with hypertension. Such patients should be followed at least annually for signs of congestive heart failure, cardiac enlargement, or worsening mitral regurgitation or left ventricular dysfunction so that valve surgery can be considered when appropriate. Optimal treatment of increased blood pressure is essential, ideally with afterload-reducing agents to lessen the hemodynamic impact of mitral regurgitation. Clear instructions regarding antibiotic prophylaxis must be given.

Patients with a moderate risk are those with mild mitral regurgitation and intermittent murmurs. Antibiotic prophylaxis is warranted, and treatment of hypertension should be pursued. As in the high-risk group, signs of worsening mitral regurgitation should be followed up with echocardiography, with a search for signs of chordal rupture, left ventricular enlargement, endocarditis, or left ventricular dysfunction.

Patients at low risk are those with no murmur or echocardiographic-Doppler regurgitation, especially young women. Antibiotic prophylaxis is not clearly indicated. Serial clinical follow-up is indicated.

NONRHEUMATIC MITRAL VALVE DISEASE

Mitral Annular Calcification

Calcification of the mitral annulus and mitral valvular apparatus is an age-related phenomenon that is more common in women than men with a gender ratio of 2:1. Rarely, this pathologic calcification can lead to mitral regurgitation or mitral stenosis. More commonly, however, mitral calcification is a radiographic or echocardiographic finding that may be a marker for age-related cardiovascular risk. Specifically, mitral annular calcification has been statistically associated with a higher risk of cardiogenic embolic stroke. This association is strongest in hypertensive women and those with a history of atrial fibrillation or sick sinus syndrome. Thus, the presence of mitral calcification should prompt a survey for these other cardiovascular risks, rather than considering the calcification a risk factor.

Nonrheumatic Connective Tissue Disorders

Systemic lupus erythematosus (SLE) affects women primarily, particularly black women. Acute noninfectious inflammatory nodules may develop on aortic and mitral valves (Libman-Sacks vegetations) and result in moderate-to-severe valvular regurgita-

tion. Chronic immunosuppression has been reported to result in fibrosis of these lesions, resulting in a secondary phenomenon of mitral or aortic stenosis.

Antiphospholipid Antibody Syndrome

Patients with SLE and other connective tissue diseases may have a peripheral embolus and stroke syndrome because of the development of in situ intracardiac and valvular thrombus. This syndrome has been related to the development of antiphospholipid antibody (formerly called anticardiolipin antibody) and requires warfarin anticoagulation for an indefinite period of time. This syndrome and Libman-Sacks endocarditis may be diagnosed with serologic testing and transesophageal echocardiography.

Radiation valvulitis may occur 10–30 years after mediastinal or breast irradiation for the treatment of lymphoma or breast cancer. Although the present technology of radiation oncology is likely to avoid this situation, patients cured of their cancer decades ago may present with signs and symptoms of radiation heart disease, aortic and mitral stenosis, pericardial constriction, or radiation coronary artery disease. When the condition is hemodynamically important, surgery may be necessary and quite successful.

NONRHEUMATIC AORTIC VALVE & THORACIC AORTIC DISEASE

Aortic Stenosis

Bicuspid aortic valve is the most common adult congenital anomaly; it occurs in from 0.5 to 1.5% of the general population. Men are much more likely than women to develop hemodynamically important aortic stenosis or insufficiency caused by bicuspid aortic valve disease (75–80% of persons in such surgical series are men). An important subset of patients with bicuspid aortic valve, however, are women who have Turner syndrome. These individuals commonly develop cardiac congenital anomalies including aortic coarctation. The aortic coarctation is associated with upper extremity hypertension, and 40–50% of affected patients with coarctation have a bicuspid aortic valve. Women of short stature with upper extremity hypertension should be evaluated for aortic valve disease.

Women older than 65 are more likely to represent the population with senile calcific aortic stenosis of a trileaflet aortic valve. Thus, women needing aortic valve replacement are more likely to be older and may have concomitant hypertension or coronary artery disease. A diagnosis of aortic stenosis is made by auscultation of a holosystolic, coarse, often high-pitched murmur at the base of the heart, radiating to the neck. Often, the carotid impulse is delayed and diminished. Quantification of the degree of stenosis is done reliably with Doppler echocardiography.

Valve replacement should be considered if symptoms of angina, heart failure, or syncope develop. It is not uncommon for elderly patients to withdraw gradually from activities to avoid symptoms. A careful history is necessary, therefore, followed by the appropriate workup when significant aortic stenosis is suspected.

Aortic Insufficiency

Aortic insufficiency in men is more likely to be caused by bicuspid aortic valve. In women, idiopathic aortic root dilatation without intrinsic valvular disease may result in aortic annulus enlargement and progressive insufficiency. Echocardiography is useful in defining valve pathology, and excluding endocarditis and chronic aortic dissection. Treatment of systemic hypertension is indicated in asymptomatic individuals to reduce the chronic volume overload of insufficiency. There is evidence that use of angiotensin converting enzyme inhibitors for hypertension in this setting may slow the progression of cardiac dilatation with aortic insufficiency. Individuals with heart failure symptoms or left ventricular dysfunction should be considered for valve replacement.

Marfan Syndrome
With Aortic Dissection

The Marfan syndrome is an inheritable autosomal connective tissue disorder linked to a synthetic defect of the protein "fibrillin." As a consequence, cardiac, vascular, ocular, skeletal, and pulmonary complications develop. Most deaths from untreated Marfan syndrome are caused by cardiac complications. The early natural history of Marfan syndrome led to death by the age of 40 in men and 50 in women. The cardiovascular manifestations of Marfan syndrome include aortic root and sinus Valsalva dilatation, with secondary aortic insufficiency, as well as mitral valve prolapse and regurgitation. Aortic root complications (aortic insufficiency and aortic dissection) are more common in men, whereas MVP complications (mitral regurgitation) are more common in women.

There is currently evidence that prophylactic treatment of affected individuals with Marfan syndrome using beta-blockers, to decrease blood pressure and the force of contractility of the left ventricular outflow, slows the progression of aortic root dilatation and perhaps the risk of aortic dissection. Women with Marfan syndrome should be followed serially with echocardiographic measurement of aortic root dimension. The risk of aortic dissection or rupture appears to accelerate as the aortic root dimension rises above 55 mm. Most tertiary care centers follow the practice of elective aortic root and aortic valve replacement when the aortic root diameter exceeds 55 mm in the setting of significant aortic insufficiency and when the root exceeds 60 mm without significant aortic insufficiency. The current success rate for surgery exceeds 97%, far better than the survival rate with emergency surgery.

A major consideration in treatment of young women with Marfan syndrome is the planning of pregnancy. In older studies, an excess number of aortic dissections in late pregnancy or early in the postpartum period were reported in women with Marfan syndrome. It appears that the risk of dissection in this setting rises with increasing root diameter in the short term. A woman with marked root dilatation or aortic insufficiency may wish to defer pregnancy. Recently, the association of aortic dissection and pregnancy has been called into question. Oskovi and Lindsay reviewed a total of 1253 cases of aortic dissection (385 women) and found no association with pregnancy in the 12 patient groups. Hypertension was the most common predisposing disease overall and in women younger than 40. The overall incidence of Marfan syndrome was not reported. It is prudent not to minimize the risk of Marfan dissection in pregnancy and also to realize that the risk of aortic dissection in a susceptible young woman remains substantial apart from pregnancy.

Another concern regarding Marfan syndrome and pregnancy is the risk of transmission of the disease to offspring. Because the condition is autosomal dominant by linkage, the risk of transmission from either parent is 50%. The severity of expression of the condition is variable, however. As yet, no fetal testing can identify the trait; progress in molecular biology is likely to make such a test available in the future.

PREGNANCY & VALVULAR HEART DISEASE

The Normal Examination in Pregnancy

The hemodynamic and neurohumoral adjustments of pregnancy produce a "volume overload" state with a rise in cardiac output, stroke volume, and heart rate, only partly alleviated by a marked decrease in peripheral vascular resistance. These changes are evident initially in the first trimester and are quite marked in the second and third trimesters. The progressive demands of the circulatory adjustments often result in symptoms that appear to represent cardiac disease but that are more often normal: dyspnea, fatigue, hyperventilation, palpitations, and edema. Exaggeration of the following normal signs is potentially representative of cardiac disease and should prompt further investigation: syncope, hemoptysis, chest pain, paroxysmal nocturnal dyspnea, or anasarca with or without proteinuria.

The hyperdynamic circulation of pregnancy also may produce physical findings of volume overload that are most often normal: jugular neck vein fullness, sustained left ventricular impulse, and relative tachycardia are to be expected. Basilar pulmonary rales may be heard owing to atelectasis of the lower lung fields from the abdominal distention. More than

50% of women have an audible S3 sound by the end of the second trimester, and more than 80% have that sign by the end of the third trimester.

Systolic murmurs are the rule rather than the exception in pregnancy, and they are audible in more than 90% of pregnant women. The origin of these murmurs is usually increased flow across pulmonic or aortic valves or mild degrees of mitral or tricuspid insufficiency. These murmurs are typically audible in early to mid systole. Holosystolic, continuous, and diastolic murmurs are not normal and may require investigation with echocardiography. Diastolic rumble mimicking mitral stenosis or tricuspid stenosis may be caused by increased flow. This question also can be resolved by noninvasive imaging with echocardiography. Because of the sharp reduction in peripheral vascular resistance in pregnancy, regurgitant murmurs may become less prominent during the progress of pregnancy owing to physiologic afterload reduction. This is certainly the case with mitral valve prolapse; however, the clinician should not mistake the late systolic click and murmur of mitral valve prolapse as a diastolic murmur by mistiming the second heart sound during an episode of relative tachycardia.

Preexisting Heart Disease in Pregnancy: Risk Assessment

In general, women with a history of mild-to-moderate valve disease, congenital malformations, and ventricular dysfunction who are asymptomatic prior to pregnancy tolerate pregnancy reasonably well. Specifically, women with mild-to-moderate aortic insufficiency or mitral regurgitation or with congenital left-to-right shunts (atrial septal defect, ventricular septal defect, patent ductus arteriosus) have a reduction in volume of regurgitation or shunting while pregnant. If supraventricular arrhythmias develop, however, they may become symptomatic and require drug treatment. Mild-to-moderate pulmonic stenosis and hypertrophic cardiomyopathy with or without obstruction are generally well tolerated, because volume expansion reduces the obstruction potential in individuals who are asymptomatic with these cardiac diseases. However, these patients should be monitored closely to avoid volume depletion during and after delivery.

Cardiac conditions that women tolerate less well and that place women at a higher risk of heart failure, circulatory compromise, arrhythmias, and fetal demise include prior symptomatic heart failure, marked obstructive lesions, and Marfan syndrome. Prior cardiomyopathy with congestive heart failure symptoms is likely to become worse with pregnancy. Significant aortic or mitral stenosis poses a high risk of arrhythmias, congestive heart failure, and respiratory compromise at term and in the first 48 hours post partum. Congenital right-to-left shunting is worsened during pregnancy in the Eisenmenger syndrome and carries an extremely high risk to both mother and fetus. Women with primary pulmonary hypertension may become severely symptomatic during or after pregnancy when the increased blood volume of pregnancy heightens the pulmonary pressure in a fixed-resistance vascular bed. These patients should be advised to avoid becoming pregnant.

Echocardiography is the most reliable and safest radiation-free method for assessing the presence and severity of the preceding conditions during pregnancy, if a new diagnosis is in question. Echocardiography may be indicated during pregnancy in the presence of the following:

1. Symptoms such as cardiogenic syncope, paroxysmal nocturnal dyspnea, hemoptysis, chest pain, or anasarca
2. Holosystolic murmur, diastolic murmur, or continuous murmur that is not caused by a venous hum
3. Suspicion of Marfan syndrome, cyanotic shunt, cardiomyopathy, or pulmonary hypertension

Flow murmurs, as previously described, do not warrant echocardiography in the absence of the pathologic symptoms outlined. It should be emphasized, however, that when a high degree of suspicion exists, for the safety of the woman and her child, radiation-associated testing should be performed to define risks clearly; effective fetal shielding must be provided, and the radiographic testing must be performed efficiently and in a highly directed manner.

ANTIBIOTIC PROPHYLAXIS FOR SURGICAL PROCEDURES

The most recent recommendations for antibiotic prophylaxis by the American Heart Association were published in 1990. These guidelines are generally simpler to follow than previous ones and place a greater emphasis on oral rather than intravenous antibiotic prophylaxis for most indications. Parenteral antibiotics are still recommended for high-risk patients, such as those with prosthetic heart valves or prior history of endocarditis. This recommendation is particularly important for oral or genitourinary instrumentation in the presence of infection. The reader is directed to these guidelines for a complete outline of indications.

Several points deserve emphasis in considering antibiotic prophylaxis in women. Because endocarditis is less common in women than men, the justification for antibiotic prophylaxis must be considered cautiously, particularly with the risk of antibiotic side effects, allergic reaction, and potential for vaginal *Candida* infection. Mitral valve prolapse without regurgitation (or documentation) does not mandate antibiotic prophylaxis, nor does cesarean delivery. Vaginal uncomplicated delivery in the absence of infection does not require prophylaxis either. Some practitioners do use prophylaxis in high-risk women, however, such as those with prosthetic valves, a history of endocarditis, or surgical vascular conduits.

Prophylaxis is recommended for vaginal hysterectomy, for urethral dilatation, and for urinary catheterization in the presence of infection. Women should be cautioned that penicillin, amoxicillin, and erythromycin may interact with oral contraceptives, making the contraceptive inactive. All patients requiring antibiotic prophylaxis should be given written instructions regarding the technique and justification. Wallet-sized cards for this purpose may be obtained from the American Heart Association. Reprints of guidelines may be obtained from the following address:

The Office of Scientific Affairs
American Heart Association
7320 Greenville Avenue
Dallas, Texas 75231

REFERENCES

Burge D, DeHoratius R: Acute rheumatic fever. In: *Valvular Heart Disease: Comprehensive Evaluation and Treatment,* 2/e. Frankl W, Brest A (editors). Davis, 1993.

Cole P, Sutton M: Cardiovascular physiology of pregnancy. In: *Cardiovascular Health and Disease in Women.* Douglas P (editor). Saunders, 1993.

Dajani A et al: Prevention of bacterial endocarditis: Recommendations of the American Heart Association. JAMA 1990;264:2919.

Devereux R: Valvular heart disease. In: *Cardiovascular Health and Disease in Women.* Douglas P (editor). Saunders, 1993.

Devereux R, Kramer-Fox R, Kligfield P: Mitral valve prolapse: Etiology, clinical manifestations and management. Ann Intern Med 1989;111:305.

Dollar A, Roberts W: Morphologic comparison of patients with mitral valve prolapse who died suddenly with patients who died from severe valvular dysfunction or other conditions. J Am Coll Cardiol 1991;17:921.

Farb A, Tang A, Atkinson J: Comparison of cardiac findings in patients with mitral valve prolapse who die suddenly to those who have congestive heart failure from mitral regurgitation and to those with fatal noncardiac conditions. Am J Cardiol 1992;70:234.

James K: Heart disease arising during pregnancy. In: *Cardiovascular Health and Disease in Women.* Douglas P (editor). Saunders, 1993.

Marzo K, Herling I: Valvular disease in the elderly. In: *Valvular Heart Disease: Comprehensive Evaluation and Treatment,* 2nd ed. Frankl W, Brest A (editors). Davis, 1993.

Oskovi R, Lindsay J: Aortic dissection in women < 40 years of age and the unimportance of pregnancy. Am J Cardiol 1994;73:821.

Rutherford J, Hands M: Pregnancy and preexisting heart disease. In: *Cardiovascular Health and Disease in Women.* Douglas P (editor). Saunders, 1993.

34

Congestive Heart Failure & Arrhythmias

Edward F. Gibbons, MD

CONGESTIVE HEART FAILURE

Congestive heart failure is a clinical syndrome of dyspnea and fatigue with effort intolerance caused by left-sided valvular or ventricular dysfunction and subsequent activation of neurohumoral mechanisms that promote and perpetuate fluid retention. Isolated right heart failure is uncommon and requires a differential diagnostic and therapeutic approach (see the section Primary Pulmonary Hypertension).

Incidence

Congestive heart failure (CHF) is a distressingly common clinical syndrome that frequently represents the final stage of several cardiac disease processes. In the United States, more than 3 million people are affected by CHF. The new case incidence of CHF exceeds 400,000 individuals per year. In fact, CHF is the most common cardiac discharge diagnosis in the elderly. In 1990, more than 750,000 discharges listed CHF as the primary diagnosis, accounting for more than 5 million hospital days and almost $8 billion in expenditures. CHF is time-intensive for patient and physician alike, and it is second only to hypertension in requiring outpatient physician visits for cardiovascular disease. The mortality rate for CHF remains high despite increased treatment options; little impact has been made over the past 40 years in reduction of CHF mortality. Indeed, CHF is the only major cardiac condition that continues to increase in overall mortality, incidence, and prevalence; stroke and coronary artery disease (CAD), in contrast, continue to decline.

The incidence of congestive heart failure varies in populations depending on the incidence of underlying cardiovascular diseases and the method of ascertainment. Serial outpatient examinations, as used in the Framingham Heart Study, are more likely to reveal mild cases of CHF than in-hospital records, such as reported by the Mayo Clinic. These studies generally find that CHF occurs at a rate of 1–2% in the general population; up to age 75, it is 30–50% more common in men than women, whereas after age 75, the incidence of CHF for women meets and then exceeds that of men. The prevalence of CHF is simi-

Congestive Heart Failure
  Incidence
  Risk Factors
  Clinical Findings
  Diagnosis
  Treatment
  Prognostic Indicators
  Summary
Arrhythmias
  Asymptomatic Ventricular Arrhythmias
  Atrial Fibrillation
  Summary

larly greater for men than women according to several population studies. However, the National Health and Nutrition Examination Surveys (NHANES I & II) data suggest that milder cases of CHF should be included to estimate total prevalence. When this is done, the gender gap in prevalence is somewhat narrower.

CHF in the USA can be attributed to CAD, hypertensive heart disease, valvular heart disease, or "idiopathic cardiomyopathic" causes. The Framingham Heart Study evaluated the causes of CHF by gender. Coronary heart disease was significantly less common in women with CHF (odds ratio 0.55), whereas valvular heart disease was significantly more common in women with CHF (odds ratio 1.88) (Table 34–1).

The development of CHF carries a particularly poor prognosis, with short- and long-term mortality rates as dismal as those in many forms of cancer. The immediate short-term survival rate after the onset of CHF is ominous: the 90-day mortality rate for CHF was 22 and 27% for the Rochester and Framingham cohorts, respectively. Acute mortality is steepest for men with valvular heart disease and for women with CAD.

After adjustment for age, survival after the onset of CHF is better for women than men. Overall mortality for men and women is equal at 90 days (Fig 34–1), but higher for men at 1, 2, and 5 years after the onset of CHF (Fig 34–2). Survival decreases

Table 34–1. Causes of congestive heart failure by gender.*

	Coronary Heart Disease		Valvular Heart Disease		Hypertensive Heart Disease		Other†	
	No.	%	No.	%	No.	%	No.	%
Men	195	56	40	38	71	46	24	53
Women	154	44	64	62	83	54	21	47

*Reproduced, with permission, from Ho et al: Survival after the onset of congestive heart failure in Framingham Heart Study Subjects. Circulation 1993;88:107.
†Other = idiopathic and unknown.

steadily with age after the acute onset of CHF, but at a steeper rate for men than women in each age category (Fig 34–3). Despite technologic and pharmacologic advances in the acute treatment of CHF, long-term survival with CHF remains dismal both now and compared with 40 years ago (Fig 34–4). Whereas in men, valvular and idiopathic causes for CHF carry a particularly poor outcome, long-term survival in women was not particularly affected by any of the causes (see Fig 34–2). However, diabetic women and women with left ventricular hypertrophy (LVH) by prior ECG had a poorer survival rate than women without these risk factors in the Framingham Heart Study.

Risk Factors

It is evident from the preceding discussion that the aging process itself is a risk factor for the development of CHF. This predisposition may be manifest only in the presence of other physiologic stresses such as bleeding, anemia, volume overload, or surgical or psychological stress. CHF develops in women at a considerably older age than in men. Systemic hypertension, particularly systolic hypertension in women, predisposes to the development of congestive heart failure.

CAD increases the risk of CHF two- to eightfold over age-matched population controls. The risk of developing CHF after myocardial infarction (MI) is higher for women than men (35 versus 23% in the Framingham Study). Also, patients who suffer a silent MI are at equally high risk of developing CHF, at rates nearly equal for men and women.

Diabetes mellitus is strongly associated with a risk of CHF, in large part because of its association with CAD and hypertension. The impact of diabetes is greatest in women and the relatively young (under age 65), in whom it is an independent risk factor. In addition, there is new structural evidence from the echocardiographic data derived from the Framingham Heart Study that diabetes may induce additional hypertrophy of the left ventricle out of proportion to the degree of associated hypertension. This phenomenon is likely to worsen diastolic dysfunction and to enhance the manifestations of CHF. The phenomenon is most evident in the women rather than the men in the Framingham Heart Study.

Other patient factors have a statistical association with the development of CHF. An elevated heart rate is a risk factor for men but not for women, despite a subjective complaint of such in women. Obesity, especially in women with associated glucose intolerance and hypertension, and a reduced or falling measured vital capacity, increase the risk of CHF. Cigarette smoking also independently increases the CHF incidence in older women. In women but not in men, both a high (above 40–42%) and a low hematocrit are associated with an increased CHF risk. It seems logical, therefore, that ECG evidence for LVH, particularly with secondary ST- and T-wave abnormalities, also is a separate risk factor for the development of CHF. In particular, women with CAD and LVH with ST-T-wave changes on ECG have a particularly poor short-term survival rate after the onset of CHF. It remains to be proved, however, that

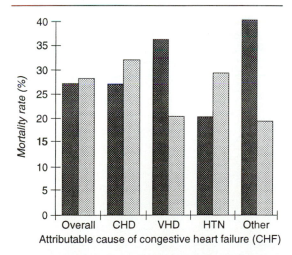

Figure 34–1. The 90-day mortality rate after the onset of congestive heart failure (CHF) is stratified by gender and cause of CHF. CHD = coronary heart disease; VHD = valvular heart disease; HTN = hypertensive heart disease; other = idiopathic or unknown. (Data from Ho et al: Survival after the onset of congestive heart failure in Framingham Heart Study subjects. Circulation 1993;88:107.)

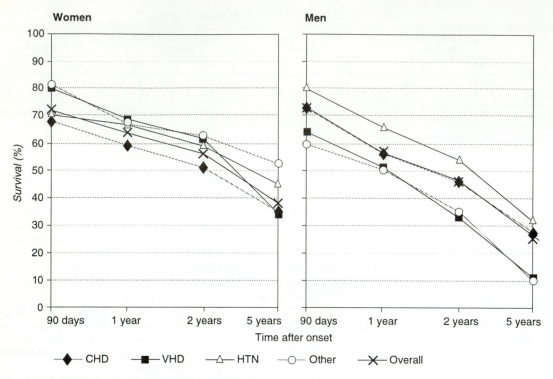

Figure 34–2. Survival by gender and cause of congestive heart failure (CHF) over 5 years after onset. (Data from Ho et al: Survival after the onset of congestive heart failure in Framingham Heart Study subjects. Circulation 1993;88:107.)

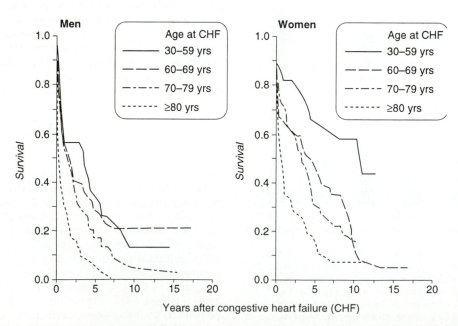

Figure 34–3. Survival by gender and age over 30 years after onset of congestive heart failure (CHF). (Data from Ho et al: Survival after the onset of congestive heart failure in Framingham Heart Study subjects. Circulation 1993;88:107.)

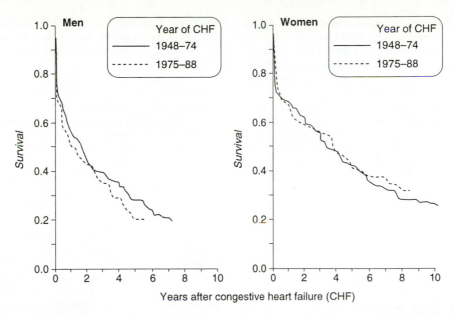

Figure 34–4. Age-adjusted survival by gender and era of treatment of CHF, early (1948–1974) versus recent (1975–1988). (Data from Ho et al: Survival after the onset of congestive heart failure in Framingham Heart Study subjects. Circulation 1993;88;107.)

modification of these correctable risk factors reduces the incidence or severity of CHF.

Clinical Findings

Often, CHF is manifested by pulmonary and other systemic venous congestion, but it may present with symptoms of a low cardiac output (cool skin, fatigue, mental depression, and azotemia). This picture is typical of systolic dysfunction. Diastolic dysfunction more typically causes pulmonary venous congestion and signs of inadequate cardiac output with effort. There is such a great overlap of symptoms and signs of systolic and diastolic dysfunction, however, that the distinction cannot be made easily on clinical or radiographic grounds. Yet the distinction has such clear prognostic and therapeutic importance that further diagnostic testing is necessary.

The distinction is made fairly easily by radionuclide ventriculography (multiple gaited acquisition [MUGA] scan) or by echocardiography. Echocardiography has the advantage of being able not only to quantify ejection fraction, but also to measure cardiac chamber sizes, quantify hypertrophy, recognize valvular and pericardial dysfunction, and estimate pulmonary artery pressure. Because symptomatic CHF has such a poor prognosis, identification of systolic function is essential in evaluation for CHF. Moreover, identification of systolic dysfunction in asymptomatic or minimally symptomatic individuals is now an indication for treatment (see discussion of SOLVD and SAVE trials in the section "Treatment").

A. Gender Differences in Left Ventricular Performance and Hypertrophy: Women have a significantly lower left ventricular mass compared with age-matched men, even when the figure is corrected for total body mass. But women also demonstrate a more exaggerated response to hypertension than men, with a greater degree of left ventricular hypertrophy. Women have a steeper age-related increase in LV mass compared with men, even when healthy men and women are compared. In addition, women demonstrate a divergent pattern of LV response to exercise compared with men. Whereas men increase left ventricular ejection fraction (LVEF) in response to exercise, women increase LV diastolic volume to enhance exercise cardiac output, typically at a lower systolic pressure and a higher peak heart rate. Although these differences probably account for a woman's lower exercise oxygen consumption capacity, the interaction of this factor with the pathophysiologic factors of CHF remains obscure.

B. Influence of Diabetes and Hypertension: As discussed in Chapters 30 and 31, women with heart disease have a higher incidence of diabetes and hypertension than men. Not only is a woman's response to hypertrophy exaggerated in hypertension, diabetic women appear to have a hypertrophic response that is also out of proportion to the degree of hypertension. Thus, the combination may predispose to diastolic dysfunction at high ejection fractions but be complicated by ischemic CAD as the vascular effects of diabetes and hypertension affect the coronary circulation. Systolic dysfunction may ensue, with an abrupt worsening of prognosis and shift in therapeutic emphasis as more severe CHF develops.

C. Coronary Artery Disease: Heart failure in women with severe coronary disease poses difficult therapeutic challenges. Even coronary artery bypass surgery has little impact on survival in women who have heart failure. Data are available for patients in the Coronary Artery Surgery Study (CASS) registry who had LVEF above 45% but who also had clinical heart failure. These patients were more likely to be women; were older; and had more hypertension, diabetes, and lung disease (reduced vital capacity) as well as more severe angina and prior MI than matched controls without CHF. The 6-year survival rate for CHF patients with three-vessel CAD was 68%, whereas it was 92% for patients without coronary disease. Also, patients who underwent surgical revascularization had no improvement in survival compared with those treated medically. This finding underscores the debilitating and lethal nature of ischemic heart disease in women, particularly with the development of a combination of severe ischemic disease with heart failure.

Diagnosis

A. Cardiomyopathy: The term **cardiomyopathy** is best reserved for characterizing primary myocardial dysfunction in the absence of significant primary CAD, valvular heart disease, or pericardial disease. Cardiomyopathies appear to be better tolerated in women than men and to convey a better prognosis than other causes of heart failure. A number of gender-specific cardiomyopathies are worthy of mention.

1. Peripartum cardiomyopathy–Peripartum cardiomyopathy (PPCM) belongs to the class of dilated cardiomyopathies characterized by generalized cardiac chamber enlargement and systolic dysfunction. As its name implies, PPCM presents in the last month of pregnancy or in the first 5 months after delivery, in the absence of any preexisting heart disease. The disease is rare, with a frequency in the USA of between 1 in 1300 and 1 in 4000 deliveries. Risk factors for the development of PPCM include toxemia, older maternal age, twin or multiple births, and multiparity. Women with prior signs of PPCM are more likely to suffer a recurrence, and rare familial cardiomyopathies may present in the peripartum period.

Women with PPCM present with dyspnea, cardiomegaly, orthopnea, and tachycardia. Signs of pulmonary congestion with hemoptysis and rales, atypical chest pain, and palpitations also are reported. With cardiac chamber enlargement and systolic dysfunction, left atrial and left ventricular mural thrombi may form. Thromboembolic episodes, both right- and left-sided, can complicate the clinical course of heart failure. The ECG is nonspecific, but bundle-branch block, ST-T-wave abnormalities, and LVH

have been reported. It is essential to exclude valvular and coronary ischemic causes by echocardiography or angiography before assigning a diagnosis of PPCM.

The cause of PPCM is unknown. Histologic findings of myocarditis have been reported and are most likely to be found by biopsy soon after symptoms develop. Immunosuppressive treatment may play a role in treatment, but spontaneous recovery and the rarity of the disease make proof of the efficacy of immunosuppression unconvincing. The mortality rate of PPCM ranges from 25 to 50%; death is most likely to occur in the first year after diagnosis and in women with recurrent and progressive heart failure. At least 27% of patients who become pregnant again suffer a recurrence. Women die from this disorder as the result of refractory heart failure, arrhythmias, or thromboembolic phenomena, and outcome worsens if a low ejection fraction or cardiomegaly persists after 6 months. At least 50% of women with PPCM have a spontaneous recovery, and resolution of cardiomegaly on chest x-ray at 1 year after onset of symptoms is a favorable prognostic sign.

Treatment for PPCM is currently the same as for any symptomatic dilated cardiomyopathy: digoxin, diuretics, angiotensin converting enzyme (ACE) inhibitors, and warfarin anticoagulation. The role of immunosuppressive therapy is uncertain. Refractory CHF in PPCM has been treated successfully with cardiac transplantation. The age and prior health of these women typically make them appropriate candidates for this aggressive treatment.

2. X-linked cardiomyopathies–Both Duchenne and Becker muscular dystrophy are X-linked recessive disorders. Duchenne muscular dystrophy is caused by a mutation of the dystrophin protein gene and results in severe peripheral myopathy in affected males. The associated cardiomyopathy contributes to the cardiopulmonary mortality of affected men, but it is often overshadowed by the crippling skeletal myopathy. The ECG in affected males often shows a pattern of a *pseudo*posterolateral MI with tall R waves in leads V1–V3 and Q waves in the lateral leads. Heterozygous carrier women may have a milder form of Duchenne dystrophy and may present in their 30s or 40s with a cardiomyopathy, similar ECG findings, systolic dysfunction, and an elevated level of muscle creatine phosphokinase (CPK) in peripheral blood.

Becker muscular dystrophy presents in a milder form in males later in life and only rarely in heterozygous females. An ECG pattern of a pseudoinfarct in the anteroseptal region has been reported.

Treatment of CHF from these disorders does not differ from standard treatment of dilated cardiomyopathy with systolic dysfunction.

B. Primary Pulmonary Hypertension: Primary pulmonary hypertension (PPH) is defined as a mean pulmonary arterial pressure exceeding 25 mmHg at rest, in the absence of congenital shunt, thromboembolic disease, pulmonary disease, left-sided organic heart disease, or systemic illness such as connective tissue disease. PPH occurs most commonly in women of childbearing age (60–90% of cases) and has an average survival time of only 2–3 years. Like the pulmonary hypertension of Eisenmenger's syndrome in congenital cardiac shunts, PPH is associated with high (at least 40%) perinatal maternal mortality. PPH occasionally is discovered late in pregnancy or at delivery. Women with PPH should be discouraged from becoming pregnant.

The presenting symptoms of PPH include dyspnea, exertional syncope, and atypical chest pain. Later, signs of right heart failure may appear. The diagnosis of PPH rests on a high index of suspicion based on age, gender, and symptoms. A chest x-ray showing prominent central pulmonary arteries, with right atrial or right ventricular enlargement, contributes to the diagnosis. The findings of right ventricular hypertrophy (RVH) and right ventricular enlargement with pulmonary hypertension may be confirmed by echocardiography. Adverse prognostic hemodynamic variables include right heart failure, right atrial pressure elevation above 10 mmHg, a low cardiac index (below 2.5 L/min/m^2 body surface area), and a high pulmonary vascular resistance (above 1000 dyne-seconds-cm^{-5}). Mean pulmonary artery pressure is a better prognostic indicator than systolic pulmonary pressure. Secondary causes of pulmonary hypertension should be excluded as stated previously.

Although therapy is disappointing, high-dose calcium channel blockade with nifedipine or diltiazem has been shown to prolong survival in PPH patients who respond to a drug challenge with a significant reduction in pulmonary mean pressure and pulmonary vascular resistance. Responders to calcium channel blockade therapy had a 94% 5-year survival rate compared with a 55% 5-year survival rate in nonresponders, according to Rich et al.

It should be emphasized that high-dose calcium channel blockade therapy must be initiated in the hospital after placement of a pulmonary artery (PA) catheter and intensive care unit (ICU) cardiac monitoring to evaluate the response to successive doses of the drug with appropriate hemodynamic improvement. Cardiologic referral is indicated. It should be noted as well that all patients treated with calcium channel blockade in the research study by Rich et al were pretreated with therapeutic doses of digoxin.

Warfarin anticoagulation probably plays a role in PPH; the patients who failed to respond to calcium blockade had a significant 1- (91 versus 52%) and 5- (47 versus 31%) year survival advantage over those who were not anticoagulated. Nonresponders may be candidates for lung or heart-lung transplantation; promising results have been reported from several centers.

Treatment

The first order of business in treating CHF is to make the diagnosis and define its cause. Diastolic dysfunction should be distinguished from systolic dysfunction, and coronary ischemia should be defined by provocative testing (see chapter 31). Valvular heart disease should be characterized, and cardiologic consultation should be obtained to discover causes for CHF that may be treated surgically: aortic and mitral valve disease, pericardial constriction, severe CAD with systolic dysfunction, congenital shunts, and atrial myxomas.

A. General Management: Certain general principles apply, none of them gender-specific, to the treatment of fluid retention and heart failure. Patient education is required concerning the origin of heart failure, the need for daily or thrice-weekly weight measurement, sodium restriction, and fluid restriction, if appropriate. Regular light aerobic exercise has proved beneficial for the reduction of muscle deconditioning and respiratory complications and to provide the patient and physician with a measurement of functional capacity and potential deterioration. Warfarin anticoagulation for class IV CHF patients reduces the risk of both venous and arterial thromboembolism.

B. Drug Treatment: None of the pharmacologic treatments presently used for CHF appear to be gender-specific. CHF is the end product of decompensated cardiac disease and must be approached based on symptoms and underlying physiologic factors. Recent reviews provide an excellent summary of these principles and are listed in the reference section. Each of the classes of drugs used for CHF treatment deserves some emphasis.

1. Diuretics–Diuretics are useful to relieve pulmonary and systemic venous congestion and are appropriate when these findings are present in both systolic and diastolic dysfunction. However, the complaint of dyspnea alone may not be sufficient to judge the need for diuresis, particularly in elderly women with diastolic dysfunction and hyperdynamic LVH. "Hyperdynamic hypertrophic cardiomyopathy of the elderly" frequently and usually involves women. These patients initially are treated effectively for pulmonary congestion with diuretics, but overdiuresis may result in an even greater hyperdynamic state—functional left ventricular outflow tract obstruction with an acquired physiologic state similar to that of idiopathic hypertrophic subaortic stenosis (IHSS). After initial diuresis, these patients are best treated with either a calcium channel blocker such as verapamil or a beta-blocker to reduce hyperdynamic contractility.

2. Calcium channel blockers–Calcium channel blockers have no proven role in systolic dysfunction, and all calcium channel blockers, with the possible exception of amlodipine, depress LV contractility. In diastolic dysfunction with incomplete

LV diastolic relaxation, the aim is to improve filling at a lower heart rate; diltiazem and verapamil are preferable to the dihydropyridines such as nifedipine and amlodipine (which produce a relative tachycardia).

3. Beta-blockers–Beta-blockers also can improve diastolic performance, especially in hypertension with coronary ischemia. If supraventricular tachycardia or ventricular arrhythmias are to be treated, beta-blockers are more effective than calcium blockers for overall treatment. Some patients with systolic dysfunction, hypertension, tachycardia, diaphoresis, and other signs of hyperadrenergic state may respond to beta-blockers at carefully escalated doses with improvement in systolic function and CHF symptoms.

4. Digoxin and other inotropes–Digoxin appears to have a role in the treatment of systolic dysfunction and has been shown recently to have an additive effect in improving CHF symptoms at exercise capacity, even when diuretics and ACE inhibitors are already being used. Digoxin dosing should be adjusted to therapeutic range by appropriate blood testing. It has been shown in national surveys that digitalis toxicity is more common in women and that appropriate dosing may reduce this excess risk.

Other inotropes (amrinone and milrinone) may improve symptoms in the short term in patients with class IV heart failure, but at a cost of shorter survival times. These drugs as well as intermittent dobutamine infusion may be used as a bridge to cardiac transplantation or for palliation of symptoms to minimize hospitalization. Outpatient dobutamine infusion may be provided as a palliative therapy in selected cases of severe CHF, after inpatient titration, in coordination with outpatient pharmacy services.

5. ACE inhibitors and vasodilators–ACE inhibitors as a class appear to provide the greatest survival benefit for CHF patients with systolic dysfunction, with no apparent gender difference in response. Based on studies of their use (Table 34–2), ACE inhibitors appear to be indicated for symptomatic LV systolic dysfunction and for asymptomatic individuals with LVEF below 40%. The benefit appears to be in survival time, reduction in symptoms of congestion, improvement in functional capacity, and reduced incidence of hospitalization for CHF.

For patients who have had MI with reduced LVEF, whether Q wave or non–Q wave infarct has occurred, ACE inhibitors have improved survival, reduced incidence of symptomatic CHF in asymptomatic MI survivors, and reduced the incidence of recurrent MI. However, timing and dose escalation of ACE inhibition may be critical, because the CONSENSUS II study showed that early hypotension with enalapril had a deleterious effect when the drug was given in the first 24 hours after MI. However, the GISSI-3 study found that there was a survival

Table 34–2. Summary of drug trials for left ventricular dysfunction.*

Study	Women (%)	Drugs	Left Ventricular Ejection Fraction	CHF/NYHA[†] Class	End Points
VHeFT-I	None	Isosorbide DN Hydralazine	Unknown	Yes/III–IV	Improved short-term survival 34%
VHeFT-II	None	Enalapril versus ISDN-hydralazine	Unknown	Yes/II–III	Enalapril improved survival over ISDN-H 28% at 2 yr
CONSENSUS I	30	Enalapril	Unknown	Yes/IV	Improved survival 41% at 6 mo, 31% at 1 yr
CONSENSUS II	27	Enalapril (early post-MI)	Unknown	Possible	Less need for CHF therapy change; low blood pressure after first dose adverse
SOLVD	19	Enalapril	≤ 35%	Yes/II–III	Improved survival at 2 yr by 28%, fewer CHF hospitalizations
SOLVD Prevention	12	Enalapril	≤ 35%	No	Reduced risk of combined death/CHF by 29%
SAVE	17	Captopril (3–16 days post-MI)	≤ 40%	No	Improved survival by 19%; reduced risk of second MI by 25%; fewer admissions
AIRE	26	Ramipril (3–10 days post MI)	Unknown	Yes/II–III	Improved survival by 27% at 15 mo
GISSI-3	22	Lisinopril, nitrates, or both (day 1 of MI)	Unknown	Possible/not class IV	Improved survival at 6 wk by 11%; reduced death+CHF by 21% in women, 17% in men

*Drugs used were angiotensin converting enzyme (ACE) inhibitors and vasodilators.
[†]CHF/NYHA = congestive heart failure/New York Heart Association.

benefit in MI patients when lisinopril was given in adjusted doses within 24 hours of MI. Also, the GISSI-3 study showed that the reduction of early mortality was significant for women and that the combined enhancement of survival and reduction of CHF incidence (21%) met and exceeded that of the men in the study (17%) with the combined use of lisinopril and transdermal nitrates.

The application of these studies to patients with symptomatic or asymptomatic systolic dysfunction requires appropriate dosing. The use of subtherapeutic doses of ACE inhibitors is common and should be avoided. For instance, the standard dosage of enalapril is at least 10 mg twice daily; the dosage may be increased if blood pressure tolerates. Similarly, the therapeutic dosage of captopril is 50–100 mg 3 times daily. Also, ACE inhibitors complement and do not replace digoxin and diuretics in symptomatic systolic dysfunction.

Patients who are unable to tolerate ACE inhibitors because of renal insufficiency or side effects may benefit from vasodilation therapy. The combination of nitrates (isosorbide dinitrate, 10–20 mg 3 times daily) and hydralazine (25–100 mg 3 times daily) has been shown to improve symptoms of severe heart failure and to improve survival over placebo. The survival benefit is somewhat less than with ACE inhibitors, however.

Prognostic Indicators

Despite the fact that women generally have a better prognosis with CHF than men, the prognosis is poor when compared to that of many other chronic illnesses. Six general categories of mortality predictors have been described. Their application to women has been explored only partly.

A. Functional Status: With the onset of CHF, a patient's functional capacities are a predictor of 1-year mortality. Those with New York Heart Association (NYHA) class IV symptoms (dyspnea or discomfort with any activity) have a 1-year mortality rate of 50–75%. Those with class III symptoms experience only half that mortality rate. Patients with even milder symptoms have death rates of only 6–16% per year, depending on their degree of functional impairment. Improvement in exercise capacity with treatment in most instances improves both short-term survival and sense of well-being.

B. Hemodynamic Factors: Although women tend to develop CHF at a higher LVEF than men, diminished systolic performance, particularly LVEF below 40%, predicts mortality for both men and women. With each 10-point decline in LVEF, the 1-year mortality rate doubles; with LVEF below 20%, the 1-year mortality rate exceeds 25%, even in patients with mild-to-moderate symptoms of CHF. The clinical and invasive hemodynamic indices of left ventricular (LV) failure (S_3 gallop, cardiac index reduction, systemic vascular resistance excess, right atrial pressure increase, pulmonary vascular resistance elevation, and reduced right ventricular ejection fraction) all have prognostic value. No gender difference is apparent.

C. Neurohumoral Factors: Activation of the sympathetic nervous system and its neuroendocrine arms in CHF is a manifestation of physiologic distress. Elevated plasma norepinephrine, plasma renin activity, atrial natriuretic polypeptides, and arginine vasopressin are associated with a higher mortality rate when significantly elevated in heart failure. A depressed serum sodium level (below 133) also carries an adverse prognosis with CHF, but it is not as powerful as the atrial natriuretic polypeptide level as a prognostic indicator.

D. Arrhythmias: A true gender difference appears to exist for the prognostic significance of ventricular arrhythmias in CHF. Whereas asymptomatic complex ventricular ectopy and frequent premature ventricular contractions (PVCs) in men are predictive of sudden death after MI, these arrhythmias have little prognostic value for women in CHF or after MI. Even allowing for the lower incidence of CAD in women, ventricular arrhythmias do not have the same mortality association they exhibit in men. This issue is discussed in more detail in the section "Arrhythmias."

E. Cause of Heart Failure: Acute mortality in women with CHF clearly is related to the cause of CHF, according to the Framingham Heart Study. Other studies suggest that ischemia is a major determinant and that its presence doubles the 1-year mortality rate of patients with CHF; this finding is inconsistent, however. The Studies of Left Ventricular Dysfunction (SOLVD) found no difference in mortality rate between patients with ischemic and those with nonischemic cardiomyopathy. The definition of ischemic may need to be more specific, however; the term may need to be applied to ongoing active ischemia rather than to simple MI without postinfarction ischemia. In women, CAD and CHF have a significantly worse mortality association than other causes of CHF.

F. Systolic Versus Diastolic Dysfunction: With the publication of several large studies on the natural history and treatment of CHF has come a keener recognition of the incidence of diastolic dysfunction as a cause of heart failure. Diastolic dysfunction (CHF signs and symptoms with LVEF above 45–45%) is usually attributable to left ventricular hypertrophy caused by hypertension. Although mortality in patients with diastolic dysfunction exceeds that of patients with asymptomatic hypertensive heart disease, mortality is significantly lower in patients with systolic dysfunction, ie, LVEF below 40–45%. The Veterans Heart Failure Trial-I (VHeFT-I) study found that diastolic dysfunction in men was associated with an 8% yearly mortality rate, whereas systolic dysfunction in men with CHF carried a 19%

yearly mortality rate. It has been estimated that 20–30% of all CHF patients may have diastolic dysfunction as the proximate cause for heart failure and that women may be affected disproportionately. There are no large-scale studies to evaluate gender-specific patterns, but the distinction of diastolic from systolic dysfunction and the concomitant association with CAD has important prognostic and treatment implications.

Summary

CHF is a lethal clinical syndrome that requires early diagnosis to effect functional improvement and survival. Although women tolerate the pathophysiologic processes of CHF better than men, the short- and long-term mortality rate of CHF in women is worse than most forms of breast cancer and rivals the mortality rate of ovarian cancer. CHF associated with CAD is more devastating, more difficult to manage, and, even when associated with operable three-vessel disease and relatively preserved systolic function, is helped little by surgical revascularization. Perhaps the key to preventing or delaying CHF in women with CAD is the early introduction of ACE inhibitor therapy in asymptomatic women at higher levels of LV ejection fraction than 35–40%, particularly in diabetic and hypertensive women and after MI.

ARRHYTHMIAS

Women report a subjective sense of palpitations and irregular heart action somewhat more frequently than men. Often, there is little correlation between a sense of palpitations and a documented cardiac arrhythmia. Although women in their 20s and 30s are in fact more likely than men to have atrial and ventricular ectopic beats on ambulatory and exercise continuous monitoring, the prognostic significance of such ectopy, even complex ventricular ectopy, with nonsustained, asymptomatic ventricular tachycardia, must be judged by both gender and the presence or absence of organic heart disease.

Asymptomatic Ventricular Arrhythmias

Ventricular arrhythmias, both isolated PVCs and complex ventricular ectopic beats, increase in frequency with age in men and women. In the Framingham Heart Study, asymptomatic frequent or complex ventricular ectopy was more common in men than women at each age group, but it was more common in both men and women in each age group if CAD was also present. However, only in men without CAD was the presence of complex ectopy predictive of future cardiac events (mortality, infarction, or sudden death). In women, the presence of asymptomatic complex ventricular ectopy had no useful prognostic value. Also, exercise-induced complex ventricular ectopy in clinically normal women on treadmill testing was not associated with an excess of cardiac mortality or morbidity. This was true even though the frequency of such ectopy increased in women older than 60 years.

A. Sudden Death—Gender Differences: Although the data on asymptomatic ventricular arrhythmias in women without evident organic heart disease are reassuring, women still are subject to sudden death from ventricular arrhythmias. The epidemiology of sudden death in women is both interesting and puzzling.

The Framingham Heart Study provides gender-specific data on ventricular arrhythmias. **Sudden death** is defined in the study as death occurring within 1 hour of the onset of symptoms. Most individuals who experience sudden death are men; sudden death accounts for 32% of deaths in men aged 20–64 years. In association with CAD, sudden death accounts for 46% of deaths in men and 34% of deaths in women. The total incidence of sudden death in women is reported as only one-third that of men. Although the risk of sudden death doubles for each decade of life, the risk for women is delayed 20 years behind that of men. Even adjusting for the lower incidence of CAD in women, the rate of sudden death is disproportionately lower in women. The majority of sudden deaths in women with coronary disease (64%) occur without prior manifestations of ischemic heart disease.

In patients without previous clinical evidence for CAD, traditional risk factors for CAD (age, weight, cholesterol level, LVH on ECG, smoking) are not predictive for sudden death in women, although they all are in men. In women, only an elevated hematocrit and a decreased vital capacity (as predictive for CHF) are associated with an increased risk for sudden death. With prior diagnosed CAD, women have an eightfold increased risk of sudden death over asymptomatic women.

Because asymptomatic ventricular ectopy in women is poorly predictive for sudden death, other epidemiologic information must be used to study risk profiles in women. Left ventricular hypertrophy on the electrocardiogram (ECG-LVH) has been shown to increase the risk for sudden death in both men (3-fold) and women (3.4-fold) over 30 years of follow-up in the Framingham Heart Study. Echocardiography is more sensitive than ECG for the detection of LVH, but the finding of LVH on echocardiography is predictive for sudden death in men only. LVH as a continuous variable in echocardiographic measurement of LV mass also is associated with a stepwise increase in simple and complex ventricular ectopy, but only in men with LVH is this ectopy predictive for sudden death. Also, ECG-LVH does not have a strong association with measured ventricular arrhythmias in women despite its signal importance in marking risk for sudden death in women.

After MI, the prognosis for survival in women is generally as bad as or worse than for men. However, after symptomatic infarction, women have a sudden death rate that is less than half that of men. Despite similar 1- and 2-year postinfarction death rates reported by the Multicenter Postinfarction Research Group (MPRG), only in men did ventricular ectopy predict death. The same study found left ventricular dysfunction to predict death in men and women with equal frequency. The Norwegian Multicenter Study Group (20% women) reported that the beta-blocker timolol reduced postinfarction mortality by 39% and sudden death by 44%; the Beta Blocker Heart Attack Trial showed mortality rate reductions with propranolol to be similar in men and women. Thus, clinical markers other than ambient ventricular ectopy are likely to be operative for women in predicting sudden death, and additional features in ischemic and nonischemic disease besides ECG-LVH remain to be discovered.

Left ventricular dysfunction is nearly the sine qua non marker for sudden death risk in women, apart from the less common Wolff-Parkinson-White syndrome, obstructive hypertrophic cardiomyopathies, and the rare mitral valve prolapse associated with sudden death. Both asymptomatic left ventricular systolic dysfunction and symptomatic CHF with systolic or diastolic dysfunction are associated with a high risk for sudden death. Nonetheless, even with clinical CHF, women are less likely than men to suffer sudden death. Of patients with CHF in the Framingham Heart Study, 25% of men suffered sudden death, whereas only 13% of women were so affected.

B. Symptomatic Ventricular Arrhythmias: There is no doubt, despite the dissociation of asymptomatic ventricular ectopy with sudden death in women, that women develop sustained ventricular tachycardia (VT) and ventricular fibrillation (VF), experience cardiovascular collapse, and die or are resuscitated. Women with coronary disease (evident or occult), single women, alcoholic women, and women with psychiatric illnesses are more likely to develop VT or VF. According to some reports, women have a lower defibrillation threshold and a higher rate of resuscitation from VT or VF than men; however, it appears that time to effective DC countershock has the greatest impact on successful resuscitation, regardless of gender.

Symptomatic VT, with syncope or presyncope, or cardiac arrest, requires a full examination of the contributing features to the event. This workup should include cardiac consultation, an electrolyte battery, magnesium level, thyroid function, oxygen level, left ventricular morphologic study, and assessment of ischemic potential by echocardiography, radionuclide imaging, or cardiac catheterization.

The evaluation of symptomatic ventricular arrhythmias in women presents more problems than in men. Whereas programmed stimulation or prolonged ambulatory monitoring can be used to predict recurrent arrhythmias and sudden death in men, these studies have less value in women. In the series of programmed stimulation reported by Freedman et al, men with prior MI had a 95% probability of arrhythmia inducibility by electrophysiologic testing, and women with this history had a success rate of 77%. In women without prior MI, only 19% had rhythm inducibility that could be used to predict future events, compared with 72% of men; in addition, the predictive ability was lower in women than men. Even in women who have suffered a cardiac arrest, therefore, electrophysiologic testing is less sensitive and less specific than in men.

1. Drug treatment–The approach to the treatment of symptomatic ventricular arrhythmias in women has not yet achieved the level of sophistication found in the treatment of men. It is disappointing that the time-honored methods of electrophysiology fail to help predict drug efficacy in women; however, current drug treatment of ventricular arrhythmias in both men and women has a troubled record concerning efficacy and safety.

In congestive heart failure and after MI, there is no proof that empirical or directed therapy of asymptomatic ventricular arrhythmias improves survival; it may in fact promote sudden death through a proarrhythmic drug effect. Several large studies of proarrhythmic drug effects caused by a variety of antiarrhythmic medications, including quinidine, disopyramide, amiodarone, bepridil, and sotalol, have shown a significant excess of the proarrhythmic polymorphous ventricular tachycardia known as torsades de pointes. This proarrhythmic effect is overrepresented in women, with up to 70–75% of all cases reported in women. Only procainamide had equal gender specificity for this proarrhythmic effect. Because women appear to be at higher risk for prolonged QT-syndrome arrhythmias, both congenital and drug-induced, the drug treatment of symptomatic VT and VF may be particularly unreliable and unpredictable in women. In women without a prolonged QT syndrome, only amiodarone, sotalol, and procainamide in moderate doses are now commonly used, and such women who are survivors of VT and VF are still at risk for sudden death without an automatic implantable cardiodefibrillator (AICD).

2. AICD treatment–AICD implantation for out-of-hospital cardiac arrest survivors has been shown in nonrandomized studies to be far superior to the use of any drug in effectively treating sudden death; therefore, AICD therapy has become the mainstay of prevention of sudden death. AICD devices appear equally effective in both men and women who are candidates for implantation. With the development of transvenous AICD devices, the risk of implantation will likely be reduced, and the benefit will be extended to sicker women and men. AICD therapy is the treatment of choice for appropriate female survivors of sudden death, given the difficulties of drug treatment. It is hoped that women with asymptomatic ventricular ectopy or organic heart disease at high risk for sudden death will be included in sufficient numbers in the current ongoing studies of prophylactic AICD implants to judge the efficacy of this treatment in these high-risk patient populations.

Atrial Fibrillation

Atrial fibrillation (AF) is a common arrhythmia that accounts for a significant expenditure of hospital and outpatient time for its evaluation and treatment. AF is more common in men than women in all age groups. Nonvalvular AF (NVAF) is associated with a history of hypertension, ischemic heart disease, diabetes, thyrotoxicosis, and CHF. NVAF incidence increases with age (Table 34–3), as seen in the Washington State Medicare hospital population. Outpatient incidence is likely to be 25–30% higher, according to population studies from Framingham and Australia.

Like valvular AF, NVAF is associated with an increased risk for cardioembolic stroke. Stroke risk with NVAF varies with clinical risk factors, including increasing age, ischemic heart disease, hypertension, diabetes, CHF, prior embolic event, and left atrial dilatation or significant systolic dysfunction (LVEF below 40–45%) on echocardiography. Although embolic risk with NVAF in patients younger than 60–65 years who have few or none of these risk factors is as low as 0.5–1%, the stroke risk in patients older than 65 years with multiple risk factors is as high as 18–19% per patient year. This stroke risk is as high as the risk of atrial fibrillation with rheumatic mitral stenosis.

The five published studies of anticoagulation for NVAF and their meta-analysis confirm that treatment with warfarin or aspirin significantly reduces stroke risk. There appears to be a surprising gender difference in response to warfarin over aspirin for stroke risk reduction. In the five studies, 20% of patients were women. Although women randomized to placebo treatment had a slightly higher stroke risk than men, this difference was not statistically significant. In women, warfarin reduced the NVAF stroke risk by 84% compared with a 60% stroke risk reduction in men. Women treated with aspirin had a stroke

risk reduction of only 23%, versus a 44% stroke risk reduction in men (Fig 34–5). The marginal benefit seen with aspirin in women may reflect the older age of women in the studies, the small dose of aspirin used [75 mg compared with 325 mg in the study with the largest number of women, the Copenhagen Atrial Fibrillation Aspirin Anticoagulation Trial (AFASAK) Study], and the higher rate of ischemic CHF in women taking lower dose aspirin. The gender difference also may reflect the benefit in men of aspirin in atherosclerotic stroke risk reduction.

Warfarin anticoagulation is not without risk, however. The major bleeding risk of warfarin in these studies was approximately 1% per patient year, and the risk of intracranial bleeding was 0.2% per patient year. Intracranial bleeding has been reported at 1.8% per patient year in the age group above 75 years in the Stroke Prevention in Atrial Fibrillation (SPAF)-II study, but methodologic problems and the high anticoagulation range in the SPAF-II study make this high intracranial bleed rate questionable. A meta-analysis of the five studies mentioned previously found that the subgroup of patients older than 75 years had only a 0.3% intracranial bleeding rate.

A careful evaluation of both risk and benefit in an individual patient must be based on age, degree of clinical risk of stroke and bleeding, and reliability of the patient for testing and maintenance of chronic warfarin anticoagulation. Although the SPAF-I study argued that aspirin was not effective in patients older

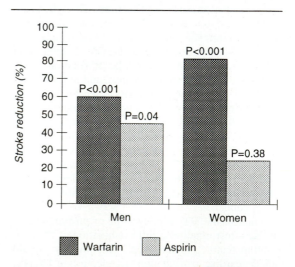

Figure 34–5. Stroke risk reduction in atrial fibrillation with antithrombotic therapy using warfarin or aspirin, analyzed by gender. P values represent stroke risk comparison of placebo with warfarin or aspirin. (Reproduced, with permission, from Risk factors for stroke and efficacy of antithrombotic therapy in atrial fibrillation: Analysis of pooled data from five randomized controlled trials. Arch Intern Med 1994;154:1449.)

Table 34–3. Atrial fibrillation in hospitalized Medicare patients, Washington State, 1992.*

Age Group	Male (%)	Female (%)
65–69	1.8	1.1
70–74	3.2	2.2
75–79	5.2	3.6
80+	8.1	6.5

*Data from PRO-West, Seattle, Washington, Dr John C Peterson III, personal communication.

than 75 years, further analysis of individuals who may benefit from aspirin or a low-dose combination of aspirin and warfarin will clarify the issue.

Summary

Women may report more symptoms of palpitations, but they have fewer documented arrhythmias than men at older ages, when the risks for sudden death and stroke are greatest. Documentation of an arrhythmia, definition of associated structural heart disease and clinical risks, and directed therapy for symptomatic arrhythmias are vital to appropriate treatment. Because of the increased risk in women for proarrhythmic drug effects with medications commonly used to suppress both ventricular arrhythmias and paroxysms of atrial fibrillation, caution should be used in choosing therapy. The control of

signs and symptoms of CHF, blood pressure, electrolyte abnormalities, and oxygenation, and the abstention from caffeine and alcohol should be first-line treatments. The use of beta-blockers when appropriate for hypertension and arrhythmias post-MI should be emphasized. In women with atrial fibrillation who tolerate the rhythm well, with a controlled ventricular response rate, the cautious clinician must decide when to anticoagulate with warfarin, attempt to reduce stroke risk, and avoid the potentially life-threatening proarrhythmic side effects of potent antiarrhythmic polypharmacy prescribed in the effort to maintain sinus rhythm. Because many women fear stroke more than CHF or MI, the clinician should direct cost-effective therapy toward allaying these fears and maximizing the benefits of treatment.

REFERENCES

The Acute Infarction Ramipril Efficacy (AIRE) Study: Effect of ramipril on mortality and morbidity of survivors of acute myocardial infarction with clinical evidence of heart failure. Lancet 1993;342:821.

Benjamin E et al: Independent risk factors for atrial fibrillation in a population-based cohort. The Framingham Heart Study. JAMA 1994;271:840.

Bikkina M, Larson M, Levy D: Prognostic implications of asymptomatic ventricular arrhythmias: The Framingham Heart Study. Ann Intern Med 1992;117:990.

Bonow R, Udelson J: Left ventricular diastolic dysfunction is a cause for congestive heart failure: Mechanisms and management. Ann Intern Med 1992;117:502.

Brophy J: Epidemiology of congestive heart failure: Canadian data from 1970 to 1989. Can J Cardiol 1992;8:495.

Busby M, Shefrin E, Fleg J: Prevalence and long-term significance of exercise-induced frequent or repetitive ventricular ectopic beats in apparently healthy volunteers. J Am Coll Cardiol 1989;14:1659.

Carvalho A et al: Prognosis in peripartum cardiomyopathy. Am J Cardiol 1989;64:540.

Cody R, Pickworth K: Approaches to diuretic therapy and electrolyte imbalance in congestive heart failure. Cardiol Clin 1994;12:37.

Cohn J et al: A comparison of enalapril with hydralazine–isosorbide dinitrate in the treatment of chronic congestive heart failure (VHeFT-II). N Engl J Med 1991;325:303.

Dahlberg S: Gender differences in the risk factors for sudden cardiac death. Cardiology 1990;77(Suppl 1):31.

Deedwania P: Ventricular arrhythmias in heart failure: To treat or not to treat? Cardiol Clin 1994;12:115.

Effect of enalapril on mortality and the development of heart failure in asymptomatic patients with reduced left ventricular ejection fractions. N Engl J Med 1992;327:685.

Effect of enalapril on survival in patients with reduced left ventricular ejection fractions and congestive heart failure. N Engl J Med 1991;325:293.

Eichhorn E: Do beta-blockers have a role in patients with congestive heart failure? Cardiol Clin 1994;12:133.

Freedman R et al: Clinical predictors of arrhythmia inducibility in survivors of cardiac arrest: Importance of gender and prior myocardial infarction. J Am Coll Cardiol 1988;12:973.

Gaasch W: Diagnosis and treatment of heart failure based on left ventricular systolic or diastolic dysfunction. JAMA 1994;271:1276.

Galderisi M et al: Echocardiographic evidence for the existence of a distinct diabetic cardiomyopathy (The Framingham Heart Study). Am J Cardiol 1991;68:85.

Ghali J et al: Impact of left ventricular hypertrophy on ventricular arrhythmias in the absence of coronary artery disease. J Am Coll Cardiol 1991;17:1277.

GISSI-3: Effects of lisinopril and transdermal glyceryl trinitrate singly and together on 6-week mortality and ventricular function after acute myocardial infarction. Lancet 1994;343:1115.

Gradman A, Deedwania P: Predictors of mortality in patients with heart failure. Cardiol Clin 1994;12:25.

Greene H: Clinical significance and management of arrhythmias in the heart failure patient. Clin Cardiol 1992;15(Suppl I):I13.

Ho K et al: Survival after the onset of congestive heart failure in Framingham Heart Study subjects. Circulation 1993;88:107.

Judge K et al: Congestive heart failure symptoms in patients with preserved left ventricular systolic function: Analysis of the CASS registry. J Am Coll Cardiol 1991;18:377.

Kimmelstiel C, Goldberg R: Congestive heart failure in women: Focus on heart failure due to coronary artery disease and diabetes. Cardiology 1990;77(Suppl 2):71.

Klapholz M, Buttrick P: Myocardial function and cardiomyopathy. Pages 105–115 in: *Cardiovascular Health and Disease in Women.* Douglas P (editor). Saunders, 1993.

Lee W, Cotton D: Peripartum cardiomyopathy: Current concepts and clinical management. Clin Obstet Gynecol 1989;32:54.

LeJemtel T et al: Peripartum cardiomyopathy: A human

model of reversible left ventricular dilatation. Heart Failure 1993;9:63.

Makkar R et al: Female gender as a risk factor for torsades de pointes associated with cardiovascular drugs. JAMA 1993;270:2590.

Myerburg R, Kessler K, Castellanos A: Sudden cardiac death: Epidemiology, transient risk, and intervention assessment. Ann Intern Med 1993;119:1187.

Packer M et al: Withdrawal of digoxin from patients with chronic heart failure treated with angiotensin-converting-enzyme inhibitors (RADIANCE Study). N Engl J Med 1993;329:1.

Parmley W: Pathophysiology of congestive heart failure. Clin Cardiol 1992;15(Suppl I):I5.

Pfeffer M et al: Effect of captopril on mortality and morbidity in patients with left ventricular dysfunction after myocardial infarction: Results of the Survival and Ventricular Enlargement trial (SAVE). N Engl J Med 1992;327:669.

Rich S, Kaufmann E, Levy P: The effect of high doses of calcium-channel blockers on survival in primary pulmonary hypertension. N Engl J Med 1992;327:76.

Risk factors for stroke and efficacy of antithrombotic therapy in atrial fibrillation: Analysis of pooled data from five randomized controlled trials. Arch Intern Med 1994;154:1449.

Rodehofer R et al: The incidence and prevalence of congestive heart failure in Rochester, Minnesota. Mayo Clin Proc 1993;68:1143.

Schocken D et al: Prevalence and mortality rate of congestive heart failure in the United States. J Am Coll Cardiol 1992;20:301.

Swedberg K et al: Effects of the early administration of enalapril on mortality in patients with acute myocardial infarction (CONSENSUS II). N Engl J Med 1992;327:678.

Venous Thromboembolism

35

James Simmons, MD

Venous thromboembolism (VTE) is the most common preventable cause of death in hospitals. Acute deep venous thrombosis (DVT) is the primary disease, typically beginning in the veins of the leg. The complications of DVT can be classified as acute or chronic and as local or distant (Table 35–1). Pulmonary embolization (PE) is the most feared complication because it can cause death within minutes in a patient without clinical findings of DVT. Every clinician sees women at risk for DVT; prevention is the top priority. Every clinician sees women with symptoms and signs that could be due to VTE; prompt objective diagnosis allows effective and safe treatment.

```
Essentials of Diagnosis
Incidence & Risk Factors
Screening
Prevention
Diagnosis
Treatment
Prognosis
Consultation With a Specialist
Issues of Pregnancy & VTE
Psychosocial Concerns
Current Controversies & Unresolved Issues
```

Essentials of Diagnosis

- Objective diagnostic testing is mandatory to manage suspected VTE appropriately.
- Used alone clinical judgment is neither sensitive enough to exclude VTE in a patient with clinical markers, nor specific enough to justify a definitive course of treatment. Clinical findings are helpful in deciding who needs objective testing.
- Deep venous thrombosis is suspected on the basis of unilateral inflammation in an extremity. The most reliable predictors of DVT in the history are known cancer, recent surgery, recent prolonged immobilization, or recent trauma to the symptomatic leg. The physical finding which is the most reliable predictor of DVT is a difference between the circumference of the legs 3 cm in the calves or 4 cm in the thighs.
- Pulmonary embolization is suspected in patients presenting with otherwise unexplained new symptoms of dyspnea, pleuritic chest pain, or cough. Less common reasons to suspect pulmonary embolization include otherwise unexplained hemoptysis, syncope, resistant congestive heart failure, or cardiac arrhythmia.

Incidence & Risk Factors

Estimates of the annual incidence of VTE vary widely. A population-based study in acute care hospitals in the northeastern United States found an average DVT incidence extrapolating to 270,000 recognized cases of VTE in US hospitals annually. This figure underestimates the true incidence, because many cases occur outside hospitals.

A. Risk Factors for DVT: The blood is always in a dynamic equilibrium between forming and lysing clots. Over a century ago, Virchow postulated a triad of conditions favoring clotting in the venous system: stasis, hypercoagulability, and venous injury (Table 35–2). At the time of diagnosis, patients with DVT can be divided into those with or without obvious risk factors. Those without apparent risk factors are said to have **idiopathic DVT.** The term **thrombophilia** often is applied to patients with an increased tendency to thrombosis, either inherited or acquired. The diagnosis of thrombophilia is made on clinical grounds. The most important criteria are (1) a family history of thrombosis; (2) a personal history of recurrent thrombosis; (3) thrombosis before age 40 or 45; (4) idiopathic thrombosis; (5) thrombosis in an unusual site; and (6) thrombosis after minimal provocation such as during pregnancy, while taking low-dose estrogen-based oral contraceptives (OCPs), or after immobilization during a prolonged trip. Some thrombophilic patients are found to have one of the known hypercoagulable conditions listed in Table 35–2.

The inherited risk factors are not sex-linked. In reported series of patients with congenital hypercoagulability, the women often suffered VTE when they were exposed to additional risk factors such as use of OCPs, or pregnancy, surgery, trauma, or immobility.

The risk factors that differentially affect women are acquired: pregnancy and the postpartum period, estrogen therapies, the antiphospholipid syndrome, gynecologic tumors and surgery, and adjuvant chemotherapy for breast cancer.

Table 35–1. Complications of deep venous thrombosis.

Acute complications
  Local
    Propagation: calf to thigh is ominous
    Inflammation: pain and swelling
  Distant
    Pulmonary embolization (PE) can cause death in
      minutes
Chronic complications
  Local
    Recurrent deep venous thrombosis
    Postphlebitic syndrome: pain, swelling, stasis dermatitis
      and ulcers, recurrent bacterial cellulitis
  Distant
    Recurrent PE
    Chronic pulmonary hypertension
    Thromboneurosis

1. Pregnancy and the postpartum period–
Symptomatic VTE is uncommon in women of child-bearing age and remains so in pregnancy. Women who develop VTE during pregnancy should be evaluated for a familial or acquired hypercoagulable syndrome such as ATIII deficiency or antiphospholipid syndrome.

VTE is much more likely to occur in the postpartum period than during pregnancy. A placental anticoagulant factor may be protective during pregnancy. The risk of postpartum VTE is higher with cesarean than vaginal delivery. Although it is uncommon, PE remains a leading cause of maternal death.

Table 35–2. Risk factors for venous thromboembolism.

Venous stasis
  Congestive heart failure
  Immobility
  Obesity
  Obstruction: mass in leg, groin, or pelvis; prior deep
    venous thrombosis
Hypercoagulable state
  Congenital
    Deficiency of antithrombin III
    Deficiency of vitamin K–dependent anticoagulants:
      protein C or S
    Resistance to activated protein C
  Acquired
    Age over 40
    Surgery, especially for cancer in the abdomen or pelvis
    Cancer and chemotherapy for cancer
    Antiphospholipid syndrome
    Pregnancy and the puerperium
    High-dose estrogen therapy
    Medical problems: disseminated intravascular
      coagulation, nephrosis, inflammatory bowel disease,
      polycythemia, hemolysis, sickle cell disease
    Trauma
Venous injury
  Hip fracture or hip replacement surgery
  Major surgery (causes venous distention remote from the
    surgical site)
  Trauma to a limb
  Indwelling venous catheter

2. Estrogen therapy–High-dose estrogen therapy, as was used in early OCPs, is probably a risk factor for VTE. The threat to the average, healthy user of modern, low-dose OCPs (estrogen doses under 50 μg) appears slight, especially the risk of death from PE. An autopsy study in Finland done when the under 50 μg estrogen pills were being used, found the relative risk of death from PE in OCP users to be 1.2, compared to the nonuser risk of 1. That figure extrapolated to an absolute risk of one excess PE death annually for every 1 million pill users. A case-control study of risk factors for fatal VTE in young women in England in the late 1980s found no significant excess of OCP use among the cases. There was an increased relative risk of 2.1 among the women with idiopathic VTE; again, the absolute risk was small. The risk of death during pregnancy or delivery appears higher than the risk of death from OCPs in the average woman.

Women who desire to begin taking estrogen-based OCPs should be questioned about a personal or family history of VTE and personal risk factors for VTE such as systemic lupus erythematosus (SLE). Women under the age of 40–45 who have had a prior VTE, regardless of the circumstances, should be suspected of having a familial syndrome or the antiphospholipid syndrome and be considered for screening for these conditions. Women with significant risk factors for VTE should be encouraged to use effective non-estrogen-based contraception such as progestin-only hormonal methods or intrauterine devices (IUDs).

Contemporary estrogen replacement therapy (ERT) provides less estrogen than even the lowest dose estrogen-based OCP. The risk-benefit analysis generally comes out in favor of ERT, even in women known to have risk factors for VTE. Consideration can be given to using transdermal estrogen in women with prior VTE or high risk for VTE. Transdermal delivery avoids estrogen's first-pass hepatic effect of increasing production of procoagulant proteins. However, this method also precludes oral estrogen's potentially beneficial first-pass effect of raising high-density lipoprotein (HDL) cholesterol levels.

3. Antiphospholipid syndrome (APS)–The antiphospholipid syndrome is defined by the clinical features of recurring arterial or venous thrombosis or recurring fetal loss and the laboratory findings of persisting circulating antibodies to negatively charged phospholipids. Antiphospholipid antibodies are identified by coagulation tests that provide evidence for a circulating lupus anticoagulant or by enzyme-linked immunosorbent assay (ELISA) for anticardiolipin antibodies. The syndrome may occur in women with SLE or related autoimmune diseases or alone as primary APS.

4. Gynecologic surgery–The DVT risks in gynecologic surgery are comparable to those of general surgery; they are highest for patients undergoing cancer surgery (35%), less in patients having abdominal hysterectomy (12%), and lower still for patients having vaginal hysterectomy (7%).

5. Cancer and cancer chemotherapy– Known cancer has long been recognized as a potent risk factor for VTE, which is often recurrent and may be difficult to treat with anticoagulants in that setting. The association is generally thought to be greatest for adenocarcinoma of the gastrointestinal tract, especially the pancreas, but the relative VTE risk for women with stage 4 breast cancer undergoing chemotherapy is nearly as high. Adjuvant chemotherapy for early-stage breast cancer has been shown to increase the risk of VTE during periods that the patient undergoes therapy compared to periods off chemotherapy. Use of tamoxifen increases the risk of thrombosis in stage II breast cancer patients.

Clinicians have long worried that patients presenting with VTE without obvious risk factors might have occult cancer. Recent studies have shown that 5–10% of patients presenting with idiopathic VTE have clinically apparent cancer within several years. The most common occult cancers affecting women with idiopathic VTE are of the lung, breast, colon, ovary, and uterus.

B. Risk Factors for PE in Patients With Venous Thrombosis:

1. Distal DVT–Distal DVT is confined to the calf veins below the popliteal fossa. Calf vein DVTs are unlikely to cause clinically important PE. The greatest risk is that they will propagate to larger caliber, more proximal veins, which occurs 20–30% of the time in untreated patients. Proximal DVT is a potent risk factor for PE.

2. Proximal DVT–Proximal DVT occurs in the popliteal veins and above and is the most important risk factor for clinically significant PE. Proximal DVT usually results from propagation of calf DVT. DVT often begins proximally in women with recent hip fracture or total hip replacement. DVT may begin in the pelvic veins in pregnant women and in women with pelvic tumors or recent pelvic surgery. In studies of patients with symptomatic proximal DVT but no symptoms of PE, routine lung scanning is compatible with a high probability of PE 50% of the time. About 50% of patients with PE confirmed by pulmonary angiography but no symptoms of DVT are found to have proximal DVT if objective testing is done.

3. Upper extremity DVT of axillary or subclavian veins–Significant PE occurs in enough patients with upper extremity DVT to warrant standard anticoagulation therapy. The most common risk factor for upper extremity DVT is presence of an indwelling central-access venous catheter. Another cause is so-called effort thrombosis, occurring after strenuous use of the arms.

4. Superficial thrombophlebitis–Superficial thrombophlebitis does not cause significant PE unless there is propagation into the proximal deep venous system, which is more likely to occur near the popliteal fossa or above.

Screening

A. Screening for Risk Factors for DVT:

1. Congenital hypercoagulable states–Indications for screening for a congenital thrombophilia include VTE with a family history of such, VTE that is recurrent, VTE occurring prior to age 40 or 45, and thrombosis in uncommon sites such as the mesenteric or cerebral veins. Screening for familial hypercoagulable states should be done in women with VTE that began during pregnancy or while using low-dose estrogen OCPs. Consider screening women without prior VTE if their family history suggests thrombophilia and the patient wishes to achieve pregnancy or begin estrogen-based OCPs or is considering elective surgery.

Studies of consecutive patients with DVT seen in two thrombosis centers in Europe found 6–7% rates of one of three familial deficiencies: ATIII, protein C, or protein S. VTE patients under the age of 45 had about a 15% chance of diagnosis of one of these three familial syndromes. Patients with three cardinal markers of familial VTE (first VTE before age 45, recurrent VTE, and family history of VTE) still had only a 30% chance of having one of these deficiencies found when tested for all three. Recently, a new familial syndrome, resistance to activated protein C, has been reported, and it appears to be much more common than any previously discovered familial hypercoagulable state.

If a familial syndrome is diagnosed, other family members should be screened for it. Patients diagnosed with a familial hypercoagulable state should not be treated in the absence of a documented VTE. They should receive information about the signs and symptoms of VTE and be told to seek medical care immediately should they experience any. They should be considered at high risk for VTE with surgery and should receive special attention to ensure effective DVT prophylaxis. Women should be considered at risk for VTE during pregnancy and at high risk in the postpartum period. Women with a diagnosed familial hypercoagulable state should be encouraged to choose contraceptive methods other than estrogen-containing OCPs.

The appropriate screening battery for familial hypercoagulability includes a determination of serum activity levels of ATIII and levels of protein C and free protein S. Testing for resistance to activated protein C is not generally available clinically at the present time. The optimal time to test for any of these familial deficiencies is several months after an acute VTE or a pregnancy and with the patient off anticoagulation therapy. However, testing can be done at less than optimal times if the effects of treatment are kept in mind. ATIII can be checked with the patient undergoing therapy with the understanding that low levels while taking heparin should not be taken as diagnostic of a familial problem and that normal levels while taking warfarin cannot be taken as conclusively ruling out familial ATIII deficiency. Deficiencies of protein C or S cannot be proved by the usual testing while the patient is undergoing warfarin therapy. Levels of ATIII and protein S are decreased in normal women during pregnancy.

2. Acquired hypercoagulable states–Women diagnosed with idiopathic VTE should be suspected of having occult cancer or the antiphospholipid syndrome. Cancer case-finding and screening should be emphasized in the history, physical examination, and radiologic and laboratory evaluations of such patients. A careful review of systems should be done with questions directed toward symptoms that might point to systemic effects of or a site of cancer. A thorough physical examination with special attention to breast, pelvic, and rectal areas is needed. Routine laboratory investigation should include a complete blood cell count (CBC), erythrocyte sedimentation rate (ESR), alkaline phosphatase level, serum glutamic-oxaloacetic transaminase (SGOT), and urinalysis.

Cancer screening should be considered; tests include a chest film, mammography, cervical Papanicolaou (Pap) smear, and fecal occult blood testing. Serial fecal occult blood tests done in the months that the patient is undergoing anticoagulation therapy should increase the yield of cancer detection while increasing the safety of the therapy. If fecal occult blood tests become positive, investigation should be done. If the patient is asymptomatic, the colon should be investigated first with either flexible sigmoidoscopy followed by air contrast barium enema or colonoscopy. If no tumor is found, the upper gastrointestinal tract should be investigated by esophagogastroduodenoscopy (EGD). It seems prudent to decide in advance not to perform biopsies and to keep the patient fully anticoagulated while doing the studies. If tumor is seen, a plan needs to be devised that will ensure protection against PE as well as a safe and timely biopsy.

Screening for the APS should be done in women with VTE without other risk factors. Testing for anticardiolipin antibodies can be done while the woman is undergoing anticoagulant therapy, although testing for a lupus anticoagulant cannot be done at that time. Women without prior VTE who have SLE or a history of multiple pregnancy losses should be screened before starting estrogen OCPs or before elective surgery. Women are not treated with anticoagulants simply because of the presence of antiphospholipid antibody, but they should be protected against VTE at the time of elective surgery, and protection should be considered in the postpartum period.

B. Screening for VTE: Screening even high-risk asymptomatic patients for DVT and treating only those with positive findings is not cost-effective. In-

stead, efforts should be directed to identifying high-risk situations and patients and providing appropriate preventive measures. This strategy has been shown to decrease death rates from VTE and to be cost-effective.

Screening patients diagnosed with symptomatic proximal DVT or PE for concomitant asymptomatic VTE is not usually done in clinical situations because therapy is not altered. Some authorities advocate obtaining routine lung scans in patients with proximal DVT to have for comparison purposes if the patient develops symptoms suggesting PE, but there is no compelling evidence for adopting such a policy.

Prevention

When DVT is prevented, so are the morbidity and mortality caused by it and its complications. Clinicians should evaluate all hospitalized patients for risk for DVT (Table 35–3) and need for prophylaxis. A safe and effective method can be found for almost any patient at risk (Table 35–4). Hospital staffs should develop policies for DVT prophylaxis and monitor compliance with them.

The question arises whether estrogen therapy should be stopped as part of DVT prophylaxis in hospitalized patients. For estrogen replacement therapy at the usual dose in a menopausal women, the treatment need not be interrupted. For estrogen-based OCPs, the issue is more controversial because strong evidence is lacking. There is some evidence supporting concern even with contemporary, low-dose estrogen pills. Four of the five women in the Prospective Investigation of Pulmonary Embolism Diagnosis (PIOPED) study who took OCPs in the 3 months prior to surgery had documented PEs; this finding was statistically significant. The most recent prospective study directly addressing this issue showed double the relative risk of postoperative VTE in pill users compared to nonusers, but it showed only a slight ab-

Table 35–3. Risk of deep venous thrombosis (DVT) in unprotected hospital patients.

Low Risk: proximal DVT < 1%; fatal pulmonary embolization (PE) .01%
  Minor surgery (< 30 min); no risk factor (RF) except age
  Major surgery (> 30 min); age < 40; no other RF
  Less than 3 days of immobilization
Moderate risk: proximal DVT 1–10%; fatal PE 0.1–1%
  Minor surgery on patient with prior DVT or hypercoagulable state
  Major surgery; age > 40; other RF
  Major trauma
  Major medical illness: cancer, cardiopulmonary disease
High risk: proximal DVT 10–30%; fatal PE 1–5%
  Hip fracture
  Major leg surgery: joint replacement or amputation
  Leg paralysis: stroke or paraplegia
  Major pelvic or abdominal surgery for cancer
  Prior venous thromboembolism or hypercoagulable state with major surgery or medical illness

Table 35–4. Methods of prophylaxis for venous thromboembolism.

Mechanical methods
  Early ambulation
  Graduated compression stockings (GCS)
  Intermittent pneumatic compression (IPC)
  Inferior vena cava filter
Pharmacologic methods
  Standard heparin
    Miniheparin or low-dose heparin (LDH)
    Adjusted-dose heparin (ADH)
  Low-molecular-weight heparin (LMWH)
  Warfarin
    Miniwarfarin or low-dose warfarin (LDW)
    Adjusted-dose warfarin (ADW)
Combination methods

Table 35–5. Prophylaxis for deep venous thrombosis.

Low-risk patients
  Early ambulation
  Consider graduated compression stockings (GCS)
Moderate-risk patients: consider GCS for all
  Bleeding complication risk acceptable: low-dose, heparin (LDH) or low-molecular-weight heparin (LMWH) or low-dose warfarin (LDW)
  Bleeding complication risk unacceptable: intermittent pneumatic compression (IPC)
High-risk patients: all get GCS
  Bleeding complication risk unacceptable: IPC
  Bleeding complication risk acceptable: consider adding IPC
    Adjusted-dose warfarin (ADW)
    Adjusted-Dose heparin (ADH)
    LMWH
    LDH (not as effective as ADW, ADH, or LMWH)

solute risk (0.96%). This small increase in absolute VTE risk must be compared to the risk of pregnancy or termination of pregnancy for the woman and of surgery and anesthesia for any fetus conceived in the month or more that the patient is off the pill (some authors recommend stopping OCPs for that length of time before elective surgery).

A reasonable policy is to counsel a woman taking estrogen OCPs about these considerations prior to elective surgery. If she decides to stop the pill before surgery, effective alternative contraception must be ensured until the pill is resumed. For the woman who decides to remain on the pill prior to elective surgery or who requires emergency surgery while on the pill, a decision must be made concerning the use of active methods of prophylaxis. There is a difference of opinion about this issue; some clinicians differentiate between elective surgery and emergency surgery, because the VTE risk is greater after emergency surgery. It seems prudent at least to use graduated compression stockings or pneumatic compression prophylaxis in patients having surgery while taking estrogen OCPs. Low-dose heparin seems a better choice, especially in emergency surgery, if there are no contraindications. In clinical trials, low-dose heparin has been shown to reduce the incidence of fatal PE, whereas the mechanical methods have to date been documented to reduce postoperative DVT only. Although the risk of fatal PE is low in young women taking estrogen OCPs with or without surgery, the possibility of so many lost years of life mandates caution. The recommendations for DVT prophylaxis are given in Table 35–5.

A. Mechanical Prophylaxis: Mechanical methods include early ambulation, graduated compression stockings (GCS), and intermittent pneumatic compression (IPC). They work largely by preventing venous stasis. IPC has some additional protective mechanism, perhaps an augmentation of fibrinolysis.

Graduated compression stockings have their highest pressure at the ankle with a decreasing gradient up the leg. They are made in both above- and below-the-knee styles. Below-the-knee GCS are cheaper, less likely to be worn incorrectly, and more acceptable to patients and nurses. They are not recommended for patients having total hip replacement surgery, however; these patients should use the above-the-knee style. GCS must be fitted and worn properly. A tourniquet effect could occur if the stockings were partially rolled down. Contraindications to GCS use are skin disease and severe arterial insufficiency.

Intermittent pneumatic compression is comparable to miniheparin in preventing DVT and carries no bleeding risk. IPC should be considered in patients having surgery on the central nervous system or the eye and in patients with bleeding diatheses or with active potential bleeding sites such as peptic ulceration, trauma, or CNS hemorrhage. IPC is the recommended first-line DVT prophylaxis in patients undergoing total knee replacement. In surgical patients, it is best to start IPC at the time of induction of anesthesia and to continue it until the patient is discharged. IPC can be removed temporarily so that the patient can ambulate or go to the bathroom. The contraindications are the same as for GCS.

B. Anticoagulant Prophylaxis: Anticoagulation methods of DVT prophylaxis include the use of warfarin and standard and low-molecular-weight heparin. Acetylsalicylic acid (ASA) has not been shown to be highly effective in DVT prevention and could increase the risk of bleeding if given concurrently with heparin or warfarin during DVT prophylaxis or treatment. It is preferable that ASA be stopped 5–7 days before anticoagulation prophylaxis is started and that other nonsteroidal anti-inflammatory drugs (NSAIDs) be stopped 1–2 days before elective surgery.

Low-dose heparin (LDH), or miniheparin, has been shown to reduce death from PE in patients having general, orthopedic, or urologic surgery and in medical patients. For surgical patients, the dose is 5000 units given subcutaneously 2 hours before surgery and every 8–12 hours thereafter, with possible advantage to the thrice daily dose without any increased bleeding risk. Major bleeding is not increased, but the frequency of wound hematomas is. It is not the most effective method available for high-risk patients, such as those undergoing total hip replacement.

LDH is also effective in medical patients. In one provocative study, it was found to reduce mortality from all causes by 30% when given to all medical inpatients over the age of 40 without a contraindication. It should be considered for all patients without a contraindication who will be immobilized 3 or more days. There is no need to monitor any test of coagulation when using LDH. Patients receiving LDH longer than 5 days should have platelets monitored every 3 days, with the therapy stopped if counts under 100,000 occur.

Adjusted-dose heparin is more effective than LDH in patients undergoing total hip replacement. It is given in a dose of 5000 units subcutaneously 2 hours before surgery and every 8 hours postoperatively. The heparin dose is adjusted to keep the activated partial thromboplastin time (APTT) near the upper limits of normal.

Low-molecular-weight heparins (LMWHs) have been studied in a variety of situations. One preparation, enoxaparin, is currently approved for use in the USA but only after total hip replacement surgery. It is started as soon after surgery as is practical within the first 24 hours, and it is given subcutaneously in a fixed dosage of 30 mg twice daily. Although there is no need for monitoring tests of anticoagulation, platelet counts should be monitored every 3 days if therapy is continued beyond 5 days, with LMWH discontinued if counts fall below 100,000.

Warfarin, like heparin, can be given for DVT prophylaxis in mini- or adjusted doses. Low-dose warfarin has been shown to prevent thrombosis in central-access indwelling catheters when used in a dosage of 1 mg daily started 3 days before insertion. Adjusted-dose warfarin (ADW) is effective in high-risk patients such as those with hip fracture or total hip replacement. Five to ten milligrams can be given the night before elective hip replacement surgery or the evening of admission for patients with hip fracture. The prothrombin time (PT) should be monitored daily until it is stable, with the international normalized ratio (INR) goal of 2–3. An INR of 1.5 is considered minimally effective. The optimal duration of DVT prophylaxis after hip fracture or total hip replacement has not been determined by experimental studies. Continuing DVT prophylaxis for a period of 4–6 weeks after the surgical therapy is advocated by some.

C. Combination Methods of Prophylaxis: Combining mechanical and anticoagulant methods may provide an added benefit over using either method alone. For example, the combination of GCS and LDH was found to be superior to LDH alone in general surgery patients. In a study of patients having total hip replacement, the trend was in favor of adding IPC to ADW, although the difference was not statistically significant.

Diagnosis

A. Diagnostic Tests for DVT: Diagnostic tests' efficiency are quantified by calculating their sensitivity and specificity. SnNout and SpPin are pneumonics for remembering the clinical usefulness of these test characteristics. A highly sensitive test that is negative rules out a diagnosis (SnNout). A highly specific test that is positive rules in the diagnosis (SpPin).

It is important to distinguish a suspected first episode of DVT from suspicion of a recurrent episode in the same leg. The diagnosis of a first episode usually can be accomplished readily. A reliable diagnosis of a recurrent DVT in the same limb remains a challenge.

1. Clinical diagnosis–Although the clinical diagnosis of DVT is not reliable—it is neither highly sensitive nor highly specific—clinical criteria can be used to decide which patients need objective study, and they may be helpful in deciding when a negative study can be relied on. DVT usually is suspected on the basis of unilateral signs of inflammation in an extremity—pain, swelling, or increased heat. The most reliable predictors of proximal DVT in the history are a known cancer, recent prolonged immobility, surgery, or trauma to the symptomatic leg. The most useful clinical finding for predicting proximal DVT is swelling of the leg. A difference between the circumferences of the legs of 3 cm in the calves or 4 cm in the thighs is significant.

2. Contrast venography–Contrast venography has been the gold standard for DVT diagnosis for over 20 years. A definitively positive test is one that shows filling defects in well-opacified veins. Advantages of venography are that it is reliable for diagnosing both proximal and distal and both symptomatic and asymptomatic DVT. Recurrent DVT often can be diagnosed with certainty if a previous study is available for comparison. Disadvantages are that it cannot be done or interpreted in 5–20% of patients; it requires experts to perform and interpret (and they disagree on the interpretation about 10% of the time); and it must be done in the radiology department. The contrast agent can cause problems such as allergic reactions, renal failure, congestive heart failure from osmotic load, pain, skin slough if extravasation occurs, and DVT in 1–2% of studies.

3. Real-time B-mode ultrasonography (U/S): This test is currently the best choice for noninvasive diagnosis of an initial symptomatic proximal DVT. A positive study is one that shows inability to compress a vein with gentle pressure. **Duplex ultrasonography** combines B-mode ultrasonography and Doppler in the same instrument. A color duplex translates flow information into colors, making identification of veins easier. The reliability of the study is operator-dependent.

The advantages of U/S include high sensitivity for symptomatic proximal DVT, high specificity, the fact that it can be done outside the radiology department, and its ability to diagnose a non-DVT cause of the presenting symptoms (such as a popliteal cyst, hematoma, or abscess) in 10–20% of patients. The fact that compression U/S is highly sensitive for proximal DVT in symptomatic patients means that a negative study makes proximal DVT unlikely. In asymptomatic patients in high-risk situations, such as after total hip or knee replacement, the sensitivity is not high enough to use the test for screening for DVT. The high specificity makes confirmatory studies unnecessary before treatment after a positive study in a patient without prior DVT in the same leg.

Disadvantages of U/S are that the sensitivity is low for calf vein DVT, so that a single negative study cannot exclude calf DVT, which might propagate and put the patient at risk for a significant or even fatal PE. A vein that has had DVT may remain non-compressible in over 50% of cases for a year or more after an initial positive compression ultrasound. A positive compression ultrasound alone cannot be relied on to make the diagnosis of recurrent DVT unless a negative study has been obtained since the initial positive one.

4. Plethysmography–Plethysmography is a noninvasive way to diagnose symptomatic proximal DVT; it measures venous flow indirectly. The most commonly used method has been impedance plethysmography (IPG). A thigh cuff is inflated to permit arterial filling but occlude venous return. When the cuff is deflated, the rate of venous drainage is reflected in the change in impedance that is recorded.

The sensitivity is low for calf DVT and in asymptomatic, high-risk patients after hip surgery. Initial studies reported sensitivities in the 90% range for proximal DVT in symptomatic patients. A more recent, uncontrolled study has raised doubts, reporting only a 66% sensitivity when venography was done despite negative IPG in symptomatic patients with a high clinical suspicion for DVT. The specificity of IPG is too low to rely on to commit to long-term treatment without a more specific confirmatory test, such as a compression ultrasound or contrast venography. An advantage of IPG may be in the management of patients with suspected acute recurrent DVT. IPG reverts to normal after a positive study much more rapidly and reliably than U/S: 65% of cases are normal by 3 months, 85% by 6 months, and 95% by 1 year. A negative study following an initial positive study is still required to accept positive IPG results as indicating acute recurrent DVT.

5. Magnetic resonance imaging (MRI)–MRI and the recently described magnetic resonance venography (MRV) are highly sensitive and specific for the diagnosis of DVT when compared to contrast venography. The clinical role of MRI in managing DVT still is being defined. MRI may prove to be the best diagnostic method when a patient is suspected of having acute recurrent DVT or pelvic DVT.

B. Diagnostic Strategies for a Suspected First Episode of DVT: If a patient will not be available for serial follow-up over a 1-week period, the first study done should be one with a high sensitivity for all DVT; ascending contrast venography is the test of choice. If there is a contraindication to contrast use, such as renal failure, obvious infection in the foot, or history of contrast reaction, MRI is an effective second choice. Any DVT that is found is treated in the usual fashion.

If a patient will be available for follow-up, noninvasive tests sensitive only for proximal DVT may be chosen. Compression U/S has been shown to be more specific than IPG in evaluating symptomatic outpatients and is the noninvasive test of choice. If the first U/S evaluation is positive, the patient needs long-term treatment. If the first U/S study is negative, the patient should be instructed to return immediately if there is any sign or symptom of PE so that appropriate study may be done. Follow-up U/S should be done over the next week to exclude propagation of an undiagnosed calf DVT. Two prospective studies including about 600 patients have demonstrated the safety of withholding therapy from symptomatic outpatients with serial negative compression U/S studies done 1 and 7 days after the initial negative study.

The only study using serial compression U/S in hospitalized patients with a clinically suspected first episode of DVT suffered from small numbers and patient dropout during long-term follow-up. The high sensitivity of U/S for the diagnosis of proximal DVT in symptomatic outpatients predicts that this should be a safe strategy.

The question remains whether serial studies are needed in all patients whose U/S studies are initially negative. If the patient's symptoms have resolved totally and there have been no symptoms of PE in the interval, some clinicians choose not to do further testing. This strategy is not as strongly supported by evidence as the serial testing approach.

The clinical safety of withholding therapy in symptomatic patients with serially negative IPG has been shown in several studies with large numbers of patients. The schedule of repeat testing is the same as for U/S. If the IPG result is positive, the specificity is low enough in most centers that further testing is done before long-term therapy is undertaken. Any more specific test could be used: U/S, MRI, or venography.

Serial compression U/S has been found to be more useful clinically than IPG in managing symptomatic patients with suspected DVT when compared in the same experimental studies; therefore, it is preferred over IPG as a diagnostic tool for diagnosis of an initial episode of DVT.

C. Diagnostic Strategies for Suspected Acute Recurrent DVT: Patients with prior DVT are at risk not only for recurrent DVT, but also for nonspecific symptoms and signs such as swelling and pain that might be due to recurrent acute DVT, might be sequelae from the first DVT, or might be unrelated to DVT. The diagnosis of recurrent DVT has important clinical implications. Anticoagulation therapy usually is longer for a second episode of DVT than for a first. If the recurrence occurs while the patient is taking warfarin with a therapeutic INR, some change in therapy has to be made, either setting the INR goal higher, with an increased risk of bleeding; changing to chronic heparin anticoagulation, with the inconvenience and discomfort of parenteral therapy and the risk of osteopenia and fracture; or insertion of a vena caval filter. Recurrent DVT in patients without obvious risk factors should lead to increased concern for an undiagnosed occult cancer, familial hypercoagulable syndrome, or the antiphospholipid syndrome. Given these crucial clinical implications, an easily applicable and reliable method for diagnosing acute recurrent DVT is important yet this diagnosis remains a difficult challenge.

If a comparison venogram is available, a repeat venogram can make the diagnosis of recurrent acute DVT if new intraluminal filling defects are found. Unfortunately, even with a comparison study, a venogram done at the time of suspected acute recurrent DVT can be inconclusive.

If the patient has had documented DVT, positive results on U/S or IPG in the same leg cannot be taken as evidence for recurrent acute DVT unless reversion to normal has been documented. If an intervening normal compression U/S or IPG result has been obtained since the original diagnosis of DVT, diagnosis can proceed as in a suspected first occurrence of DVT, with therapy unchanged if serial studies remain negative for a week. If results of serial compression U/S that included measurements of the maximal diameter of the noncompressible vein are available, an increase of 2 mm or more since the last measurement is evidence in favor of an acute recurrence of DVT.

MRI may have a useful, even first-line role in demonstrating the inflammation associated with acute DVT and the contraction associated with chronic DVT; theoretically, therefore, it can distinguish between the two without the necessity of having a previous study for comparison. At this time, there are no studies demonstrating the clinical usefulness of MRI diagnoses to make therapeutic decisions in the setting of possible acute recurrent DVT.

D. Diagnostic Tests for Pulmonary Embolization:

1. Clinical diagnosis–The clinical manifestations of PE range from no symptoms to sudden cardiovascular collapse and death within an hour. Patients with proximal DVT and no symptoms of PE have lung scans compatible with a high probability of PE about 50% of the time. Symptomatic PE can be grouped into several clinical syndromes: (1) transient dyspnea and tachycardia with no other clinical manifestations; (2) pulmonary infarction or ischemic pneumonitis with pleuritic chest pain, cough, hemoptysis, rales, pleural effusions, and pulmonary infiltrates; (3) right heart failure with severe dyspnea and tachypnea; and (4) cardiovascular collapse with hypotension, syncope, or coma. PE also may present with a variety of less common and even less specific clinical features including confusion, fever, wheezing, resistant congestive heart failure, and unexplained arrhythmia.

The likelihood of PE can be estimated clinically from the presence of risk factors for VTE (see Table 35–2), presenting symptoms and signs, and results of nonspecific tests such as chest film, ECG, and measurements of arterial oxygenation. Clinical judgment is neither sensitive enough to exclude PE in a patient with clinical markers, nor specific enough to justify a definitive course of treatment. In autopsy series, fatal or significant PE is suspected ante mortem only about 30% of the time. More than 50% of patients whom clinicians suspect of having a PE have negative pulmonary angiograms. Combining clinical information with the results of specific tests for VTE allows for better management decisions as discussed in the following section, "Diagnostic Strategies for Suspected PE."

In recent studies diagnosing PE by pulmonary angiogram, the most common symptoms have been dyspnea in approximately 80%, pleuritic chest pain in about 60%, and new cough in about 40%. Hemoptysis was present in only about 15% of PE patients, and blood streaking was the most common type of hemoptysis among PIOPED patients. The most common signs in patients with PE diagnosed by pulmonary angiogram have been tachycardia over 90 beats/min in about 80%, tachypnea with a respiratory rate of 20 or more in about 75%, and rales on auscultation of the chest in about 60%.

Chest films, ECGs, and arterial blood gas measures are nonspecific when done in patients suspected of PE. They can be helpful in confirming other diagnoses, such as pneumothorax or acute myocardial infarction. A chest film is needed to interpret a lung scan.

Chest film abnormalities were seen in over 70% of the PE patients in PIOPED; dyspnea with a normal chest film was an uncommon presentation. The chest x-ray findings included atelectasis, an elevated hemidiaphragm, small pleural effusions, and parenchymal abnormalities.

ECG abnormalities occurred in 70% of patients with PE who had no prior history of cardiopulmonary disease. Nonspecific ST-segment and T-wave abnormalities were the most common findings.

Arterial hypoxemia with a pO_2 below 80 occurs in only about 80% of patients with PE, so that a normal pO_2 or O_2 saturation can not be relied on to exclude PE. An argument can be made for avoiding an arterial puncture in a patient who may soon be anticoagulated. An O_2 saturation obtained noninvasively can be used to guide decisions about oxygen therapy in most patients.

In PIOPED, combinations of clinical findings were sensitive for the diagnosis of PE: 99% sensitivity was found using the combination of dyspnea, or tachypnea, or pleuritic pain or a chest film showing atelectasis or a parenchymal abnormality; 91% sensitivity was achieved if the patient had either dyspnea or tachypnea with a respiratory rate of 20 or more. Clinical findings are most helpful, therefore, in deciding who needs further study.

2. Pulmonary angiography–Although it is the gold standard for the diagnosis of PE, pulmonary angiography is less than perfect. The risk of pulmonary angiography is almost always much less than the risk of inappropriate management based on inconclusive diagnosis. A positive test is one showing a constant filling defect in a pulmonary artery or the abrupt cutoff of a large or medium-sized pulmonary artery. The sensitivity is over 99%. All patients cannot be studied adequately, and interobserver agreement is less than perfect, with more differences in the reading of negative than of positive studies.

3. Perfusion lung scans–Perfusion lung scans measure pulmonary blood flow by scanning the distribution of radioactive macroaggregated albumin particles injected intravenously. The sensitivity is over 99%, so that a negative study virtually excludes PE (SnNout). The specificity is not sufficient to justify treating patients whose test results are positive; other studies must be done.

4. Ventilation-perfusion lung scans (VPS)–This test combines a perfusion scan of pulmonary circulation with a radioactive aerosol scan of pulmonary ventilation. The theory was that a PE would cause perfusion defects in areas that were ventilated and that a mismatch between perfusion and ventilation would make the diagnosis of PE and matched ventilation and perfusion defects would exclude it. Two large prospective studies using pulmonary angiography and clinical follow-up as the gold standards have not confirmed this theory.

The results of a VPS usually are reported as being compatible with a high, intermediate, or low probability of PE. In prospective studies, 85% of patients with a high probability based on VPS had pulmonary angiograms showing PE, but 15% had negative angiograms. PIOPED found the high probability scan to be accurate 91% of the time if the patient had no prior PE but only 74% of the time if there had been previous PE. If the VPS interpretation was of a low

probability of PE, there was still a significant chance (15–30%) that the pulmonary angiogram would be positive. An intermediate probability of PE is the most common VPS result and is no help in deciding if a patient has had PE; further testing always is needed.

E. Diagnostic Strategies for Suspected PE: Heparin treatment should be started if the clinical suspicion of PE is high, there are no contraindications to its use, and definitive objective testing cannot be performed quickly. If massive PE is suspected, pulmonary angiography is a reasonable first test if it is readily available.

A diagnostic strategy for deciding on definitive treatment or no long term treatment for patients presenting with suspected submassive PE is presented in Table 35–6. If a perfusion lung scan is negative and there is no clinical suspicion of DVT, the patient does not need treatment or further testing for VTE.

If the perfusion lung scan is not negative, a VPS is needed. The addition of clinical impressions formed before the VPS was done increases the accuracy of decisions made using the results of VPS if there is congruence, with both being either high or low probability of PE. A patient with clinical features compatible with PE with no other obvious cause and who has one or more of the risk factors for VTE listed in Table 35–2 can be judged on clinical grounds to have a high probability of PE. A clinical impression of a high probability of PE combined with a high-probability VPS was accurate 96% of the time in predict-

Table 35–6. Diagnostic strategies for suspected pulmonary embolization (PE).

Perfusion lung scan is first test
  If negative, no further testing and no treatment
  If not negative, further testing is needed
Ventilation-perfusion lung scan (VPS) is next test
  High-probability VPS
    Clinical probability high and no prior PE: treat
    Clinical probability not high or prior PE: test further
      If proximal deep venous thrombosis (DVT) found, treat
      If proximal DVT not found, obtain pulmonary angiogram
  Low-probability VPS
    Clinical probability low: consider test for DVT versus no treatment without further testing
    Clinical probability not low: test for proximal DVT
      If DVT found: treat
      If initial noninvasive test for proximal DVT negative: serial studies, treat if become positive
  Intermediate-probability VPS: always test further, start with test for DVT
    Test for DVT positive: treat
    Test for DVT negative: test further
      Patient with poor cardiopulmonary reserve: obtain pulmonary angiogram
      Patient with adequate cardiopulmonary reserve options are
        Serial testing for DVT if patient available for follow-up and consents
        Pulmonary angiogram if preceding criteria not met

ing a postive pulmonary angiogram in two prospective studies. A patient with a highly unusual prsentation for PE, with none of the recognized risk factors for VTE and with an obvious alternative explanation for the clinical manifestations, would be judged on clinical grounds to have a low probability of PE. A clinical impression of a low probability of PE combined with a low-probability VPS was accurate 91–98% of the time.in predicting a negative pulmonary angiogram. Any other combination of clinical impression and VPS results other than both being high or both being low probability is not accurate enough to base definitive management on, and further testing is always required.

The usual specific treatment for VTE is prophylactic, aimed at preventing propagation or embolization, and is the same for PE and DVT. Fifty percent of patients with proved PE are found to have proximal DVT if studied. If a patient with suspected PE has nondiagnostic results of clinical evaluation combined with VPS, the next study can be a test such as compression U/S in a search for proximal DVT. If the U/S is positive, the patient is treated for VTE. If the U/S is negative, further testing is needed. The decision concerning how to proceed with further testing can be aided by classifying patients into those with and those without cardiopulmonary reserve adequate to withstand additional PE without suffering serious morbidity or death. Adequate cardiopulmonary reserve has been defined as the absence of pulmonary edema, right ventricular failure, systolic blood pressure below 90, syncope, acute tachyarrhythmias, or respiratory failure (FEV_1 below 1, pO_2 below 50, or pCO_2 above 45).

If the patient has inadequate cardiopulmonary reserve and thus is at high risk for death or serious clinical deterioration if PE occurs again, the appropriate next test is pulmonary angiography.

If the patient has adequate cardiopulmonary reserve, is available for follow-up, and provides informed consent, a strategy of performing serial noninvasive testing for proximal DVT over an 8- to 15-day period and not treating those whose tests remain negative has been shown to be safe. The longer sequence of serial testing for proximal DVT is suggested for patients with risk factors for VTE. If the patient is not available for serial testing for DVT, either pulmonary angiography or contrast venography should be done, with definitive treatment for those with positive studies and no treatment for those with negative studies.

Treatment

Treatment for VTE can be classified by type or phase. Types of treatment for VTE are general, anticoagulant, thrombolytic, and mechanical. Phases of treatment for VTE are initial and long-term.

A. General Treatment: Bed rest is not required after therapeutic levels of heparin anticoagulation are achieved, preferably within the first 24 hours of treatment. Aspirin and other antiplatelet drugs should be avoided in patients anticoagulated for VTE, as should intramuscular injections. Constipation should be prevented actively. The Valsalva maneuver and release that occur with straining to have a bowel movement can create the effect of a plumber's plunger, which in theory promotes embolization.

B. Anticoagulant Treatment: Anticoagulation therapy of VTE is prophylactic. The purpose is the prevention of clot propagation, embolization, and recurrent thrombosis. The use of anticoagulation therapy requires the determination that the potential benefit outweighs the risk of serious bleeding. The usual therapy for VTE is initial heparin for 4 or more days, given as a continuous intravenous infusion or subcutaneously every 12 hours, followed by long-term anticoagulation for at least 3 months with oral warfarin or, less commonly, subcutaneous heparin.

1. Laboratory monitoring of anticoagulation therapy–The theory is that monitoring anticoagulation therapy with a test of coagulation can maximize the benefit of treatment while minimizing the risk of bleeding complications. The most commonly used tests are the APTT to monitor standard heparin therapy and the PT to monitor warfarin therapy. Both tests were developed to evaluate patients with bleeding disorders and do not directly measure the antithrombotic properties of the drugs. There are situations in which the APPT or PT results might mislead clinicians. This problem can occur for the APTT in patients with the antiphospholipid syndrome being treated with heparin and in patients with subtherapeutic APTTs despite high doses of heparin. PT results might be misleading in the first few days of combined warfarin and heparin administration, when the clinician considers the safety of stopping heparin, or when a very high INR is obtained from a laboratory using an insensitive thromboplastin reagent, and the decision must be made concerning the appropriate response in a patient who is not bleeding.

For both the APTT and the PT, the absolute result in seconds depends on the thromboplastin reagent the laboratory adds to the sample of the patient's blood, as well as on the properties of the blood. There is no standardization of thromboplastin reagents. The same blood tested with different brands of thromboplastin or even different batches of the same brand may give significantly different absolute results.

Fortunately, PT results for monitoring warfarin therapy can be standardized by using the INR, which converts the results using any thromboplastin to those of a standard reagent. Clinicians should insist on receiving PT results for monitoring warfarin therapy in the form of an INR. The currently recommended INR for warfarin prophylaxis and treatment of VTE is 2–3.

Differences in INR results with different thromboplastins are probably not clinically significant when the INR is in or near the therapeutic range of 2–3. A problem could arise when a very high INR (10–20) is obtained in a patient receiving warfarin whose blood was tested in a laboratory using a very insensitive thromboplastin. The true INR may be far below the reported one, and the clinical action taken based on the less accurate result may be exaggerated. Clinicians should encourage laboratories to use PT thromboplastin reagents with sensitivities as close as possible to the international sensitivity index (ISI) for international standard reagents of 1.

Experimental animal and clinical studies have shown that the effective range of APTT for treating VTE occurs with plasma heparin levels of 0.2–0.4 units/mL measured by the protamine titration method at least 4 hours after a dose of heparin has been given. Unfortunately, no reporting standardization exists to take into account the effect of using different thromboplastins to measure the APTT. Before clinicians accept an APTT range as a therapeutic goal for heparin therapy, they should be sure that the target APTTs correspond to plasma heparin levels of 0.2–0.4 units/mL. Until a standard reporting system for APTT results is adopted, local laboratories should establish a therapeutic range of APTT for each new batch of thromboplastin reagent and report this along with the absolute result.

Heparin therapy also can be monitored by plasma heparin assays done by protamine titration or by antifactor Xa levels. The therapeutic range for treating VTE includes plasma heparin levels of 0.2–0.4 units/mL by protamine titration or 0.35–0.7 units/mL by automated chromogenic antifactor Xa levels. Heparin assays are more expensive than APTTs and are not necessary for routine clinical use. They can be helpful in monitoring heparin therapy when the APTT response is dissociated from the plasma heparin level. This situation occurs in the antiphospholipid syndrome, in which there are prolonged APTTs before heparin therapy is started. Dissociation between heparin assay and APTT results also can occur in patients receiving high doses of heparin, 50,000 units per 24 hours or more, who still have subtherapeutic APTTs. Most such patients have therapeutic plasma heparin assay results despite the subtherapeutic APTT and can be treated effectively without escalating the dose of heparin. A minority of patients with subtherapeutic APTT results despite high doses of heparin have true heparin resistance and require even higher doses to achieve therapeutic heparin levels.

2. Initial heparin anticoagulation–Heparin is available either as a standard, unfractionated preparation (SH) or as a low-molecular-weight (LMWH) preparation. LMWH has not been approved for use in treating VTE in the USA, although it may well supplant standard heparin in the future. The following discussion applies to the use of standard heparin.

Adequate initial heparin therapy is associated with a major reduction in morbidity and mortality from VTE. Initial therapy for DVT with oral anticoagulants alone has been shown to produce unacceptable outcomes. Failure to achieve effective levels of heparin anticoagulation in the first 24 hours of treatment has been found to increase the risk of recurrent VTE up to 15-fold for up to 3 months after such a failure. Although the importance of achieving the minimal therapeutic levels of heparin within the first 24 hours and maintaining them for the duration of therapy is widely accepted, controversy exists concerning the importance of staying below the upper limits of the therapeutic range. In experimental clinical studies, the risk of major bleeding during heparin therapy has been predicted more accurately by patient factors such as recent surgery or other significant medical problems than by the level of the APTT. There is, nonetheless, some evidence that bleeding complications are related to the dose of heparin and to heparin levels. The ideal heparin dosing method would rapidly exceed minimal therapeutic plasma heparin levels and avoid prolonged excessive heparin administration. Heparin requirements differ considerably among patients. In one study using a dosing nomogram based on actual body weight, this factor accounted for approximately one-third of the variability, with the remainder caused by multiple other interacting factors.

Heparin should be begun when there is significant suspicion of PE or proximal DVT; contraindications to heparin include a high risk of serious bleeding and a prior episode of heparin-associated thrombocytopenia. Heparin acts directly on the patient's ATIII, increasing its anticoagulant activity. Onset of therapeutic action is immediate after an adequate intravenous bolus, but it is delayed for 1–2 hours after an initial subcutaneous dose. The usual intravenous bolus dose is 5000 units. Because heparin clearance is increased in patients with PE, some clinicians give a higher initial bolus to these patients, up to 10,000 units.

The most widely used method of heparin administration for initial anticoagulation of VTE in the USA is continuous intravenous infusion following a bolus. Heparin dosing usually is empirical, with audits showing wide variations in practices and generally poor records in achieving and maintaining therapeutic APTT goals. Recent studies have shown improved performance using nomogram protocols for continuous intravenous heparin therapy. These protocols dictate not only the doses of heparin, but also the timing of APTT monitoring. A published heparin dosing schedule based on APTT results should not be adopted for local use unless it is ascertained that the APTT results in the study are comparable to those currently being reported by the local laboratory. Ideally, nomograms should be revised locally each time the laboratory starts using a new batch of thromboplastin and validated by monitoring how they are performing in clinical use, with adjustments made in the dosing recommendations as dictated by this empirical approach.

These published studies of nomogram dosing can help to guide heparin therapy even in the absence of a locally validated nomogram. Compared with the usual empirical dosing by physicians, effective nomograms used more heparin for the initial infusion (at least 1300 units/h or 18 units/kg actual body weight), obtained more APTTs early in therapy (up to four in the first 24 hours), had shorter times to the first heparin dose adjustment (4–6 hours) and had quicker responses to subtherapeutic APTT results. If the APTT fell too far below the lower limit of the therapeutic range, patients were given another bolus along with an increase in their infusion rate. If the APTT was too far above the upper limit of the therapeutic range, the infusion was held no more than an hour before the dose was lowered. APTTs always were checked 4–6 hours after a change in the infusion rate. The current evidence suggests that the risk to patients is greater if their APTTs fall below the lower limit of the therapeutic range than if they exceed the higher limit. After the first 24 hours of therapy and when the dose of heparin has been stable, APTT monitoring can be done once each morning.

Subcutaneous heparin administration is as safe and effective as continuous intravenous heparin for initial anticoagulation therapy of VTE, if a high enough dose is given. The initial subcutaneous dose of heparin should be 17,500–20,000 units every 12 hours. If immediate onset of action is desired, an intravenous bolus of 5000 units should be given along with the first dose of subcutaneous heparin. An APTT is checked 6 hours after the initial injection, and any needed changes in the heparin dose are made in the next dose. Once a stable dose is achieved, the APTT is checked daily 6 hours after the morning injection.

Initial heparin therapy should be continued for 4–10 days and discontinued only when there have been at least 3 or 4 days of combined heparin and warfarin therapy and when the PT is therapeutic from the effects of warfarin alone. The shorter course of heparin depends on warfarin being started on the first afternoon of heparin therapy. Two studies have shown 4 or 5 days of heparin to be as effective as 9 or 10 days when treating patients with submassive VTE. Safety of the shorter courses of heparin has not been proved for patients presenting with massive DVT (a tensely swollen, shiny, purplish leg) or PE (persisting hypotension or severe dyspnea). The major complications of heparin therapy are bleeding, heparin-associated thrombocytopenia (HAT), and osteopenia.

In experimental studies, Hull stratified patients on clinical grounds for bleeding risk and gave less heparin in the initial infusion to those with high bleeding risk. Patients with high bleeding risk were defined as those with (1) surgery or major trauma

within 14 days; (2) a stroke within 14 days; (3) a current platelet count under 150,000; (4) a history of gastrointestinal or genitourinary bleeding; (5) a history of peptic ulcer; and (6) serious concomitant medical problems such as hepatic, renal, or cardiac failure. Such patients received an initial heparin infusion of 1240 units/h, whereas low-risk patients got 1680 units/h. Serious bleeding complications correlated with clinical bleeding risk and not with supratherapeutic APTT results.

If a patient on heparin therapy has bleeding that threatens life or function by virtue of its location or briskness, the treatment must be stopped and the effects of heparin reversed immediately by infusing protamine sulfate. If the bleeding is less threatening, it can be managed by stopping the heparin and letting the APTT drift down to normal. This takes only hours if the route of heparin administration has been intravenous, but it may take more than 24 hours if the subcutaneous route has been used. Patients in whom heparin must be stopped or reversed because of serious bleeding should be protected against PE by the insertion of a vena caval filter.

The current recommendation is that a platelet count be checked before therapeutic heparin is begun and once daily during its administration. Minor drops in the count are common and should not lead to stopping heparin. Heparin must be stopped if the platelet count falls below 100,000 or if it decreases by 50% or more over a 24- to 48-hour period. These significant declines may be a sign of HAT, believed to be caused by formation of an IgG-heparin immune complex that activates platelets, causing them to aggregate. Rarely, this can result in devastating arterial thrombotic events causing death, stroke, or the need for limb amputation. Bleeding is an even rarer complication of HAT. In patients who were not previously exposed to heparin, HAT does not occur until after 3 or more days of heparin therapy. For previously exposed patients, it can occur sooner, even within the first few hours of therapy. The diagnosis of HAT can be confirmed by a sophisticated coagulation laboratory and should be obtained to guide future decisions about heparin therapy; however, clinical response to the immediate situation cannot await the results. Platelet transfusion should not be considered unless the patient is bleeding and then only if all the heparin has been cleared as verified by the coagulation laboratory with a normal thombin clotting time (TCT).

Attention must be turned to protecting the patient against PE. If warfarin has been started and the INR is in or near the therapeutic range of 2–3, this measure can be relied on. There are case reports of patients being switched to low-molecular-weight heparin safely, but this course is potentially dangerous because immunologic cross-reactivity with standard heparin occurs. The most certain protection against PE in a patient with pelvic or lower extremity DVT who is not anticoagulated is provided by the insertion of an inferior vena caval (IVC) filter. The platelet count generally returns to baseline levels within about 4 days of stopping heparin if HAT was the cause of the thrombocytopenia. Patients who have had HAT should not be exposed to heparin in the future—not even in the form of heparin flushes to maintain the patency of intravenous lines. Indeed, an argument can be made that all hospitals should change to the routine use of saline flushes to maintain intravenous patency to avoid unnecessary exposure to heparin.

3. Long-term warfarin anticoagulation—Warfarin is the most commonly used oral anticoagulant in North America. Its anticoagulation effect occurs by interference with the liver's manufacture of the vitamin K-dependent procoagulants, factors II (prothrombin), VII, IX, and X. Warfarin also inhibits the hepatic synthesis of at least two vitamin K-dependent anticoagulants, proteins C and S. The antithrombotic effect of warfarin depends on the balance between the reduction in pro- and anticoagulant vitamin K–dependent proteins.

Unlike the effects of heparin, the antithrombotic effects of warfarin are delayed. The anticoagulant activity of warfarin is reflected in prolongation of the PT, which is sensitive to reductions in procoagulant factors VII, X, and II. Time is required for the preexisting normal vitamin K–dependent procoagulants to be cleared from the blood and be replaced by their warfarin-altered, inactive analogues. Factor VII has the shortest half-life, about 6–7 hours. Factors X and II have much longer half-lives, 3–5 days. The anticoagulant protein C has a short half-life, comparable to that of factor VII. It is theoretically possible in the first 24–48 hours of combined heparin and warfarin therapy for the PT to be prolonged and the blood to be hypercoagulable but for the effect of heparin. This situation might occur when the PT is prolonged mainly because of reduction in factor VII levels but the anticoagulant effect is overbalanced by the thrombogenic effect of the parallel reduction in protein C. This possibility is the reason for the recommendation that heparin and warfarin therapy overlap by at least 3–4 days before a therapeutic PT is taken as a sign that the patient will be protected by the antithrombotic effects of warfarin alone.

Warfarin can be started on the first day of heparin administration in patients with submassive VTE, with the goals of a therapeutic PT and safely stopping the heparin in 4–5 days. The safety of short-term heparin therapy has not been demonstrated in patients with massive VTE; they probably should receive 7–10 days of heparin therapy with warfarin started on day 4 or 5.

Warfarin is usually given at about 5 PM, so that blood for PT monitoring can be drawn about 16 hours later, in the morning. Recommendations for initial warfarin dosing vary. Some of the older recommendations, such as 10 mg for all patients for the first few days, lead to overshooting of PT goals in a significant percentage of patients. Because bleeding risk clearly increases with increasing INR levels, avoiding excessive anticoagulation with warfarin is important. Initial warfarin dosing probably should depend on whether the patient is judged on clinical grounds to be likely to be warfarin-sensitive. Warfarin sensitivity is suggested if the patient is (1) age 80 or older, (2) malnourished (albumin under 3.0 or by clinical assessment), (3) given nothing orally for longer than 3 days, (4) recently postoperative, (5) suffering from uncompensated congestive heart failure, (6) suffering from a prolonged major illness, or (7) taking interacting drugs that increase the PT.

The initial dose of warfarin can be 5 mg in patients predicted to be warfarin-sensitive and 10 mg in others. Doses after the first day are based on PT results. PTs should be obtained daily until the INR goal of 2–3 is achieved and the level is stable (confirmed by two consecutive daily PTs). Heparin can be stopped when combination heparin and warfarin therapy has overlapped by at least 3 or 4 days and when the INR of 2 or more is due to the effects of warfarin. Heparin does lengthen the PT, although this effect is usually slight if the APTT is not supratherapeutic. Because the minimal known effective level of warfarin anticoagulation for VTE is reflected by an INR of 2, it is prudent to be sure that the PT will not be subtherapeutic when heparin is stopped. If the INR is near or above the midrange INR goal on therapeutic heparin and warfarin, the INR is likely to remain therapeutic when heparin is stopped. If the INR is near 2 on combined therapy, the laboratory can remove heparin from blood samples before doing the PT to be sure that the INR will be therapeutic from the effects of warfarin alone before the heparin is stopped.

After a stable maintenance dose of warfarin has been found, dosage adjustments should be based on the weekly warfarin dose (eg, 5 mg/d = 35 mg/wk). Every-other-day or skipped-day regimens should be avoided because they interfere with patient compliance. Instead, the patient should be given a schedule that provides for any variation in warfarin dose to be coupled with a day of the week. For example, instruct the patient to take 5 mg on Monday and Friday and 2.5 mg the rest of the days of the week. Warfarin dosage adjustments should be made in weekly dose increments or decrements of 10–15%. A sample warfarin-adjustment nomogram and approach to adjustment is included in Appendix C.

Warfarin therapy should be continued for at least 3 months after an initial episode of VTE. Warfarin should be continued indefinitely if the patient has a continuing stimulus to VTE, such as continuing cancer or chemotherapy, or an identified familial predisposition to VTE. Patients with a first recurrence of VTE even in the absence of a known predisposing cause should have a year of warfarin therapy. Patients with a life-threatening recurrence of VTE or a third recurrence should be offered lifelong warfarin anticoagulation.

If objectively documented VTE recurs when the INR is in the range of 2–3, the patient should be protected by another course of initial heparin therapy, after which several treatment options are available: (1) maintenance warfarin anticoagulation can be resumed with a higher INR goal, such as 2.5–4; (2) long-term subcutaneous heparin therapy can be used to keep the APTT in the therapeutic range; or (3) an IVC filter could be inserted.

The major risk of warfarin therapy is bleeding, which increases with supratherapeurtic INRs, the coadministration of certain drugs, and serious comorbidity such as uncompensated congestive heart failure or active ulceration of the gastrointestinal tract.

When INR levels are kept in the therapeutic range of 2–3, the rate of major bleeding reported in experimental studies has been under 4%. Supratherapeutic INRs are a major risk factor for bleeding complications of warfarin therapy. Adequate frequency of INR monitoring should reduce the risk of bleeding related to excessive anticoagulation. A recommended schedule of monitoring depends on demonstrating stability, defined as therapeutic PTs for two consecutive tests, over increasingly longer intervals. Initial warfarin therapy for VTE given along with heparin therapy should be monitored daily. Subsequent monitoring should be twice weekly, followed by weekly, every 2 weeks, monthly, and every 4–6 weeks. The interval between tests should not exceed 6–8 weeks no matter how long the patient has had stable PTs on a stable warfarin dose. If dosage adjustments are required after a period of stability, the PT should be rechecked in a week and the sequence of demonstrating stability repeated. If drugs that significantly interact with warfarin are added or discontinued, the INR should be checked 3–7 days after the change in regimen is made. When drugs with long half-lives such as amiodarone or rifampin are discontinued after the warfarin dosage has been stabilized, the increased frequency of INR monitoring should continue until the drug effect is gone.

The response to a supratherapeutic INR depends on whether the patient is having significant bleeding or needs emergency surgery as well as on the level of the INR. The first response to an unexpectedly greatly prolonged INR in a patient who is not bleeding should be to repeat the PT. The options for managing a bleeding problem or a threatening prolongation of the INR include replacing vitamin K–dependent anticoagulation factors with plasma infusions, giving parenteral vitamin K, or both, along with withholding warfarin administration. For life-threatening bleeding or emergency surgery, all three methods are used. If the patient is judged to be at high risk for serious pulmonary embolism during the

period when anticoagulation is contraindicated, a vena caval filter should be inserted. For minor prolongations of the INR without a clinical need to reverse the warfarin effect, withholding the warfarin for one or more doses while monitoring the INR and the patient's status is sufficient.

Concomitant therapy with a variety of drugs can interfere with the efficacy and safety of warfarin therapy. NSAIDs are especially dangerous. They not only interfere with platelet function, they also increase the chances of upper gastrointestinal tract ulceration. Some antibiotics are common offenders in adverse drug interactions with warfarin. Special care should be taken to avoid carelessly giving a "routine" prescription for sulfamethoxazole-trimethoprim to a woman taking warfarin. This drug can greatly prolong the PT and lead to serious bleeding complications in patients who were previously stable. Telephone prescriptions can be especially dangerous. A useful habit is to consider all drugs as potentially complicating to warfarin and check any being added to or deleted from the regimen of a patient on a stable warfarin regimen for possible interaction. Without reliable information that a drug does not affect warfarin therapy, the PT should be checked 3–7 days after a drug is initiated or stopped.

Patient education is important in achieving efficacy and safety of warfarin therapy. The patient should understand the critical importance of compliance with prescibed warfarin doses and of regular PT monitoring. She should be aware of the risks of other drugs and instructed to discuss any changes in prescribed medicines with a physician who will consider the possibility of an adverse interaction. She should not take any nonprescription drugs without being sure there is no potential for adverse interaction with warfarin. Acetaminophen can be used for pain or fever. She should be aware that major dietary changes, especially those made in an attempt to lose weight, can interfere with effective anticoagulation with warfarin. The major dietary source of vitamin K is green leafy vegetables, and these are often increased greatly in the diets of women trying to lose weight. Alcohol should be avoided completely or used regularly in moderation during warfarin therapy. Patients should be taught the symptoms and signs of bleeding that they might not recognize. Examples include new-onset severe headache, abdominal or flank pain, melena or coffee-ground emesis, and orthostatic symptoms.

4. Long-term subcutaneous heparin anticoagulation—Therapeutic doses of subcutaneous heparin can be used for long-term anticoagulation in patients who should not take warfarin such as pregnant women or women who live in remote areas without access to PT monitoring. Patients in whom warfarin therapy fails may benefit from long-term therapeutic heparin.

Heparin is given subcutaneously every 12 hours in

a dose sufficient to give a therapeutic APTT 6 hours after the morning dose. For people who will not be available for periodic APTT monitoring, satisfactory results can be achieved for up to 3 months using an individually adjusted, fixed dose of heparin. The fixed dose is determined during a 3-day period at the start of subcutaneous heparin therapy during which the dose is adjusted to maintain the APTT in the therapeutic range 6 hours after the morning dose.

In addition to the bleeding and thrombocytopenic complications of shorter term heparin therapy, long-duration therapeutic heparin treatment carries some risk of osteoporosis. This effect can be asymptomatic or can cause debilitating clinical events such as vertebral compression fractures. The determinants of heparin-induced osteoporosis are not well understood. Patients who receive doses of heparin of 15,000 units or more daily for more than 1 month have some risk of demonstrable osteopenia. The majority of reports of heparin-associated osteoporosis have been in patients treated with at least 20,000 units daily for at least 6 months. Fortunately, fractures have been uncommon.

C. Thrombolytic Therapy: At present, thrombolytic therapy for VTE should be reserved for patients with a life-threatening presentation of pulmonary embolus such as refractory shock or right heart failure. For other patients with PE, studies have shown increased bleeding complications with no significant clinical benefit in patients treated with any currently available thrombolytic agent compared with the usual initial heparin therapy.

The hope of thrombolytic therapy in patients with DVT has been to prevent the postphlebitic syndrome, but studies have not shown a clinical benefit and have shown problems with bleeding.

D. Inferior Vena Caval Filters: The best indication for insertion of an IVC filter is in a patient who cannot be anticoagulated safely and who remains at risk for significant PE from DVT in the pelvis or legs. Failure of adequate anticoagulation to prevent embolization is another indication. The Greenfield filter is preferred. Patency rates of 90–98% are reported. Rates of confirmed PE (about 2%) or death from PE (less than 1%) after filter placement have been quite low in uncontrolled series. Recently, a modified version, the titanium Greenfield filter, has been used; it makes percutaneous insertion in the internal jugular or femoral vein less traumatic because a smaller dilator can be used. The filter usually is advanced to an infrarenal location, but it can be placed above the renal veins if necessary, with the expectation that renal function will not be compromised. Suprarenal placement should be considered in pregnant women or women anticipating pregnancy. There is considerable experience in patients treated with Greenfield filters without anticoagulation, because many of the patients who need this therapy cannot tolerate anticoagulation. There re-

mains a theoretic advantage of preventing morbidity from DVT by maintaining anticoagulation therapy during the patient's period of continued risk, which must be considered along with the need for continued monitoring of anticoagulation therapy and bleeding risk. Many patients and physicians opt for no anticoagulation therapy once the filter is in place. A case can be made for using a vena caval filter as primary therapy for patients with advanced cancer, reserving anticoagulation with its bleeding risks and need for intense medical management for patients with symptomatic DVT after filter placement.

Prognosis

Untreated calf DVT is unlikely to cause clinically significant PE in the absence of propagation. Death from calf DVT has not been reported in clinical series involving large numbers of patients. The bleeding risk of standard 3-month anticoagulation treatment of DVT confined to the calf seems at least as great as the risk of clinically recognized PE. The incidence of postphlebitic syndrome after calf DVT is uncertain but appears to be approximately 15%. The major risk of calf DVT is propagation into the proximal leg veins, which has been reported to occur in up to 23% of untreated patients in clinical series.

Untreated proximal DVT carries a high risk of clinically apparent PE—approximately 50%. Before anticoagulation therapy was available, mortality from PE was about 10% in hospitalized patients with clinically diagnosed DVT. Adequate heparin therapy reduces the PE rate in patients with proximal DVT to about 5% and the rate of fatal PE to about 0.5%. A 5–7% symptomatic recurrence rate has been reported during a 3-month course of anticoagulation therapy for patients wth a first episode of proximal DVT. Inadequate treatment of proximal DVT results in about a 25% recurrence rate of VTE. Inadequate heparin dosing in the first 24 hours of therapy is an especially potent risk factor for recurrence within 3 months.

The longer term recurrence rate of adequately treated VTE depends considerably on the patient's risk factors and general health. Patients in whom DVT results from surgery or trauma have less than a 2% recurrence rate of VTE in the following year. Medical patients have a 5–10% recurrence rate in the first year after stopping anticoagulation therapy. Recurrences are more likely in patients with a known continuing risk factor such as carcinoma, as well as in patients with idiopathic VTE. Patients with a recurrent VTE who are treated for 3 months have a 20–25% recurrence rate in the following year, with up to a 5% mortality. The incidence of the postphlebitic syndrome after proximal DVT is not well known, but it appears to be high despite anticoagulant treatment. Thrombolytic agents have not shown unequivocal benefit in preventing postphlebitic syndrome and cause an increase in bleeding complications of VTE therapy when compared to standard therapy.

Untreated clinically apparent PE was reported to have a 30% hospital mortality rate before the introduction of anticoagulation therapy. In the PIOPED study, the death rate for treated PE was 2.5%. Half the deaths from PE occurred on the first day of therapy, 80% within the first week, and 90% within the first 2 weeks. Ninety percent of these deaths were attributed to recurrent PE.

Chronic pulmonary hypertension is a rare complication of pulmonary emboli. The diagnosis usually is made when evaluating patients with unexplained dyspnea on exertion; patients may have no history of known VTE. A lung scan shows one or more segmental or larger perfusion defects, and a pulmonary angiogram shows evidence of proximal pulmonary emboli. Selected patients get satisfactory results from surgical endarterectomy.

Consultation With a Specialist

All clinicians should recognize patients in their practice who are at risk for VTE and know when and how to provide prophylaxis. All clinicians should know when to suspect VTE, how to initiate objective diagnostic testing, and how to protect the patient until a decision is reached. Primary care providers should be able to rule in or out a suspected first episode of VTE in consultation with diagnostic radiologists experienced in interpretation of compression U/S and lung scans. Consultation with physicians who perform and interpret contrast venography or pulmonary angiography or insert vena caval filters is needed less often.

Primary care providers should be able to manage most episodes of VTE without additional consultation. Improved outcomes can be shown both in hospital and outpatient settings when institutions provide guidelines and protocols for anticoagulation or organized anticoagulation services.

Primary care providers should seek consultative help for patients with uncommon problems, especially if the evidence available in the medical literature is inconclusive. For VTE, this could include patients with suspected recurrent DVT when the diagnosis is not straightforward. Patients with suspected or proved thrombophilia should have the chance to be seen by a physician with interest and experience in that area; often this is a hematologist. Significant complications of anticoagulation therapy such as HAT or complicated anticoagulation reversal problems benefit from the attention of a coagulation specialist. Patients with chronic pulmonary hypertension from PE should be seen in a medical center with a medical and surgical team experienced in their care. Pregnant patients with prior or current VTE or with known or suspected thrombophilia benefit from consultation with a physician with experience and expertise in their care.

Issues of Pregnancy & VTE

The significance of VTE in pregnancy depends not on its frequency but on its potential for tragic outcomes. Pulmonary embolus was found to be second only to trauma as a cause of maternal death in Massachusetts. Many obstetric services now report pulmonary embolism as the leading cause of maternal death, with the majority of deaths occurring during the postpartum period.

Management of a pregnant patient involves balancing maternal and fetal needs and seems a daunting task to the inexperienced. The overriding principle is that fetal well-being depends on maternal well-being. Appropriate diagnostic or therapeutic intervention for the mother should not be withheld for fear of adverse fetal effects, when the risk of doing so endangers both. The reported mortality in untreated VTE in pregnancy is high; the diagnosis must be confirmed or refuted when clinical suspicion is raised. The risk to the fetus of the most radiation-intensive strategy to diagnose DVT or PE can be held to a theoretically slightly increased risk of developing childhood cancer, estimated to be on the order of 0.2%. The risk of properly managed anticoagulation treatment throughout pregnancy is low, but a reported side effect of prolonged therapeutic doses of heparin in pregnant women has been debilitating vertebral compression fractures; therefore, long-term treatment must not be based on clinical diagnosis.

The care of pregnant women with management issues concerning VTE is complicated by the scarcity of reliable evidence regarding the best course of action. Pregnant women typically were excluded from the clinical trials that produced the evidence on which informed practice in nonpregnant patients is based. Even the recent literature in this area remains filled with citations of studies done on patients in whom the diagnosis of VTE was made on clinical grounds. Randomized trials of therapy are rare. Recruiting enough patients for conclusive clinical trials is difficult because VTE in pregancy, although a significant cause of maternal morbidity and mortality, is uncommon. Shared decision making with the patient after discussion of the issues and uncertainties is often the best course of action. This is especially true when trying to decide whether and how to offer VTE prophylaxis in a woman thought to be at risk of VTE while pregnant.

Pregnancy might be expected to put all women at high risk for VTE. Much has been written about the possibility of a pregnancy-induced hypercoagulable state because several procoagulant plasma factors are increased and anticoagulant factors ATIII and protein S are decreased. As pregnancy progresses, the gravid uterus promotes venous stasis by compression of pelvic veins. Evidence is accumulating that pregnancy alone is a minor risk factor for VTE and that a woman in whom VTE develops during pregnancy should be considered for investigation of a preexisting hypercoagulable state. A recent small series found approximately a 20% incidence of diagnosable deficiencies of ATIII, protein C, and protein S in patients with confirmed DVT during pregnancy. This was a much higher prevalence than found in similarly studied patients with DVT beginning in the postpartum period.

The incidence of DVT during pregnancy is not known. The best evidence comes from series using objective diagnostic methods in symptomatic pregnant women. The reported rate of confirmed DVT is under 1 in 1000 deliveries, with a range of 0.13–0.8. The rate of postpartum DVT is reported to be about 5 times higher than the rate during pregnancy, and cesarean delivery further increases it. DVT occurs with equivalent frequencies during all trimesters of pregnancy. Because leg pain and swelling occur commonly in later stages of uncomplicated pregnancies, the likelihood of demonstrating DVT should be increased in women presenting with symptoms in the first 2 trimesters. There is a striking predominance for DVT during pregnancy to occur in the left leg, although confirmed cases have occurred in the right leg. Risk factors for DVT in pregnancy include immobility, obesity, maternal age over 35, parity over 4, and familial and acquired hypercoagulable states.

A. Prophylaxis of VTE During Pregnancy: The question of VTE prophylaxis during pregnancy in women with prior VTE or a hypercoagulable disorder is controversial and difficult. Reliable evidence is lacking concerning the important variables that could be used to guide decisions, ie, the likelihood of a recurrent or first-time VTE with pregnancy, the dose of heparin to use, and the management of anticoagulation at the time of delivery.

The risk of recurrence of VTE during pregnancy is likely to be in the range of 5–15%. It is unclear whether the circumstances of the first episode help predict the likelihood of recurrence in pregnancy. Because VTE is uncommon in women of childbearing age, any history of prior documented VTE should lead to consideration of a hypercoagulable condition and a risk of recurrence in pregnancy. Some evidence appears to show risk of recurrence to be greater if the first episode occurred during pregnancy as opposed to the postpartum period. A first episode when the patient was taking OCPs also has been thought to increase the risk of recurrence in pregnancy. Among the familial hypercoagulable states, ATIII deficiency is believed by many to be especially likely to cause a first episode of VTE during pregnancy, with deficiencies of protein C or S less likely to do so.

Because warfarin has adverse fetal effects, heparin, which does not cross the placenta, is used for prophylaxis and treatment of VTE in pregnancy. Fetal risk appears to be minimal. Because prophylactic therapy may be for the duration of pregnancy, maternal risk of heparin-induced osteoporosis is a concern. The management of heparin at the time of delivery is

problematic if anticoagulating doses are used. The safe and effective prophylactic heparin dose in pregnancy is much more a matter of opinion than of evidence. A bewildering array of dosing suggestions have been published. Expert consultation should be sought when the question of need for DVT prophylaxis in pregnancy arises.

The postpartum period is one of increased risk for VTE. Although the risk is greatest shortly after delivery, it persists for up to 6–8 weeks after delivery. Warfarin can be used for treatment or prophylaxis of DVT after delivery. Clinicians who are content to withhold prophylaxis during pregnancy may start it after delivery in women with a prior episode of DVT or a hypercoagulable condition without prior VTE. Initial therapy can be with fixed low-dose heparin, and the patient can be switched to warfarin with an INR goal of 2–3 for the duration of the prophylaxis, which is generally 6 or more weeks.

B. Diagnosis of DVT During Pregnancy: The diagnosis of DVT during pregnancy must be confirmed by objective testing. The previous discussion of these diagnostic methods applies to pregnant patients with the following comments:

- Pressure on pelvic veins from the gravid uterus has been reported to cause false-positve results on ascending contrast venography, IPG, and MRI. This explanation usually can be confirmed by repeating the test with the patient in a different position and finding no evidence for DVT.
- Noninvasive testing remains preferred, with compression U/S preferred over IPG. Theoretic concerns of missing isolated iliac thrombosis have been expressed, but case reports suggest that this condition can be suspected using published criteria. Confirmation could come from MRI if necessary.
- Two prospective cohort series have shown the safety of withholding treatment in pregnant women suspected of DVT as long as their IPGs remained negative on serial studies over a 1- or 2-week period. No such study has been reported yet for compression U/S, but there is no theoretic reason to believe that outcomes would be different if decisions were based on serial U/S.
- Venography can be done safely if needed, for example, in a woman with a negative noninvasive study who will not be available for follow-up. A limited venogram with pelvic shielding can be obtained with fetal radiation exposure of under 50 mrads. Without shielding, a full unilateral venogram can be done with fetal radiation exposure under 350 mrads. Both doses are well below exposure levels that are considered teratogenic.

C. Diagnosis of Pulmonary Embolus During Pregnancy: The suspicion of pulmonary embolus in pregnancy mandates objective testing. The patient should be protected with intravenous heparin until the results are known. The methods and strategies for evaluating a pregnant patient suspected of PE are the same as those previously discussed for nonpregnant patients with the following comments:

- A pefusion lung scan can be done with fetal radiation exposure of under 20 mrads; a combination ventilation-perfusion lung scan can be done with under 60 mrads. Fetal radiation exposure can be reduced by having the patient void shortly after the studies because some exposure comes from isotope in bladder urine. If the ventilation-perfusion scans are not conclusive (results are other than a negative perfusion scan or a high-probability VPS), compression U/S should be done, looking for DVT in the legs; any woman with positive results should be treated. If VTE cannot be confirmed by noninvasive testing of the legs, a pulmonary angiogram should be obtained.
- If pulmonary angiography is done through a brachial rather than a femoral approach and abdominal shielding is employed, the fetal radiation exposure should be under 50 mrads. If the femoral approach is used with abdominal shielding, the fetal exposure should be about 400 mrads.

D. Treatment of VTE During Pregnancy, Labor, and Delivery: When VTE is diagnosed during pregnancy, treatment differs from that of the nonpregnant woman in several ways:

- Maternal oxygen saturation should be maintained above 95% because fetal hypoxemia may occur when maternal pO_2 is near 70.
- Initial treatment with continuous intravenous heparin is the same, but long-term treatment differs. Warfarin is not used before delivery because of adverse fetal effects.
- Long-term treatment is with subcutaneous heparin given every 12 hours in doses sufficient to keep the APTT in the therapeutic range 6 hours after the morning dose. The heparin requirements can be expected to increase in the third trimester. If the dose exceeds 50,000 units daily, consideration should be given to monitoring therapy with heparin levels.
- Given the choice, many women prefer self-administration of subcutaneous heparin twice daily via an indwelling catheter made of polytetrafluoroethylene (Teflon) rather than the usual method of twice-daily subcutaneous injection using an insulin syringe with a 25-gauge needle. The catheter can be left in the subcutaneous tissues of the abdomen for 1 week at a time. The indwelling catheter method costs more, and urticarial reactions at the injection site may be more bothersome than with the usual method.

- Heparin management at the time of labor and delivery can be problematic, and recommendations vary among experts. Women in whom the APTT is prolonged are not candidates for epidural or spinal anesthesia. The risk of bleeding during or after vaginal or cesarean delivery must be balanced against the risk of a complication of VTE during a period off anticoagulation. In the usual case, subcutaneous heparin should be stopped when the patient goes into active labor, and APTT or heparin levels should be monitored. For a planned delivery, one option is to stop the subcutaneous heparin 24 hours or more beforehand, use continuous intravenous heparin in full therapeutic doses up to 4–6 hours before delivery, and stop the intravenous heparin at that time. Because it is not certain how long it is safe to leave a woman at high risk for recurrent VTE off anticoagulants, some experts recommend continuing low-dose continuous intravenous heparin during labor and delivery, maintaining levels of 0.1–0.2 units/mL by protamine titration. Women with a new episode of VTE within the preceding month are candidates for such continuous low-dose heparin therapy during labor and delivery. It has been reported that this method does not increase the rate of postpartum hemorrhage in normal delivery. A slight increase in risk of episiotomy hematoma and an increase in blood loss in patients with uterine atonia and retained placenta may occur. Another recommendation for women at high risk of recurrent VTE is to continue the usual dose of heparin intravenously until the woman is 8–9 cm dilated and then reverse with protamine sulfate for delivery.
- There are case reports of successful thrombolytic therapy of pregnant patients with massive PE who continued in shock despite therapy.
- Indications for Greenfield filter insertion are the same as in nonpregnant women. Favorable results with suprarenal placement have made this an acceptable choice in pregnant women or in women anticipating pregnancy. Placement above the renal vein avoids compression by the enlarged uterus and prevents emboli from the ovarian veins, which can bypass an infrarenal filter.

E. Treatment of VTE in the Postpartum Period: Protection against VTE is especially important in the postpartum period because the risk of new or recurrent VTE is heightened for up to 8 weeks after delivery.

For women treated during pregnancy, heparin can be resumed in full therapeutic doses as early as 2–4 hours after delivery if there are no contraindications. Warfarin can be started the first afternoon after delivery and heparin discontinued when the INR is therapeutic and after a 3- to 4-day overlap with heparin therapy. Alternatively, the patient can continue taking therapeutic doses of subcutaneous heparin; however, the risk of osteoporosis probably increases with increasing duration of treatment, and there is no reason to prefer heparin after delivery unless the woman lives in a remote area and cannot have appropriate laboratory monitoring of warfarin therapy. Both heparin and warfarin can be used in nursing mothers without adverse effects on the infant.

Full-dose anticoagulation therapy is continued for a minimum of 3 months from the time of diagnosis, but it is continued for at least the first 6–8 weeks post partum regardless of the duration of full-dose anticoagulation during the pregnancy.

Treatment of a VTE diagnosed during the postpartum period does not differ from that previously described. Initial heparin therapy is followed by at least 3 months of long-term anticoagulation.

Psychosocial Concerns

One of the chronic complications of a diagnosis of VTE is a clinical syndrome labeled **thromboneurosis.** Patients with this syndrome live in fear of PE and DVT and interpret trivial symptoms or signs as possible manifestations. Such patients often are treated for VTE without an objective diagnosis ever having been made. If there were an initial objective diagnosis, recurrent episodes of VTE have been diagnosed without using reliable criteria. In many patients, the condition may be considered to be iatrogenic.

The best way to prevent thromboneurosis is to base the diagnosis of VTE on objective tests. The symptomatic patient who is appropriately investigated with negative findings can be reassured with confidence. The patient who receives an objective diagnosis of VTE should be educated concerning the positive prognosis with appropriate treatment. On follow-up visits, signs and symptoms of the postphlebitic syndrome should be sought and explained.

The best treatment of an established case of thromboneurosis is to have the patient's history and any available records and studies reviewed by a physician who is knowledgeable in the objective diagnosis of VTE. If there is not sufficient evidence for recurrent VTE and the patient is undergoing chronic anticoagulation therapy, the treatment can be stopped and the patient followed with appropriate responses to symptoms or signs causing concern.

Controversies & Unresolved Issues

A. Risk Factors for VTE: Resistance to activated protein C can be expected to draw attention from investigators who can provide evidence concerning how to integrate this new finding into clinical practice. Much is unclear regarding the strength of pregnancy and estrogen-containing OCPs as risk factors for VTE.

B. Prophylaxis for VTE: How best to manage patients at high risk for DVT after hospital discharge needs study. It seems likely that patients are discharged after hip fracture or total hip replacement at a time when their risk of VTE is substantial. Should they all get outpatient anticoagulation prophylaxis and, if so, for how long? Would routine venography before discharge be a better approach?

The issue of how best to deal with pregnant women at special risk for VTE has long called for a multicenter, controlled trial.

C. Diagnosis of VTE: It is possible that D-dimer blood levels done by ELISA will prove to be useful in excluding VTE in symptomatic patients. D-dimer is a fragment that is specific for the degradation of fibrin. The ELISA assay (but not the latex agglutination assay) has a high sensitivity for VTE, so that a negative result may help rule out acute VTE. If the safety of this strategy is demonstrated in clinical trials, patients with suspected acute DVT with an initial negative compression ultrasound and a low D-dimer level may not require serial testing. A preliminary study found that about 40% of patients could be managed without serial study if initial testing produced a negative U/S scan of the legs and a low level of D-dimer by ELISA assay. Patients with suspected PE but nondiagnostic lung scans and normal D-dimer assay results might be managed safely without other studies.

More clinical trials are needed on how best to manage patients with suspected acute recurrent DVT.

D. Treatment of VTE: The promise of LMWH is to simplify the prophylaxis and treatment of VTE while maintaining efficacy and decreasing further the risk of bleeding complications. It is hoped that one day patients will be taught to self-inject a once-daily dose of LMWH to prevent DVT in high-risk situations or to treat VTE uncomplicated by other problems. Many questions remain to be answered by clinical trials before this can be considered for routine practice.

REFERENCES

Anderson DR et al: The use of an indwelling teflon catheter for subcutaneous heparin administration during pregnancy. A randomized crossover study. Arch Int Med 1993;153:841.

Carpenter JP et al: Magnetic resonance venography for the detection of deep venous thrombosis: Comparison with contrast venography and duplex Doppler ultrasonography. J Vasc Surg 1993;18:734.

Ginsberg JS, Hirsh J: Use of antithombotic agents during pregnancy. Chest 1992;102:385S.

Heijboer H et al: A comparison of real-time compression ultrasonography with impedance plethysmography for the diagnosis of deep-vein thrombosis in symptomatic outpatients. NEJM 1993;329:1365.

Hirvonen E, Idanpaan-Heikkila J: Cardiovascular death among women under 40 years of age using low-estrogen oral contraceptives and intrauterine devices in Finland from 1975 to 1984. Am J Obstet Gynecol 1990;163:281.

Hull RD et al: Optimal therapeutic level of heparin therapy in patients with venous thrombosis. Arch Int Med 1992;152:1589.

Hull RD et al: A noninvasive strategy for the treatment of patients with suspected pulmonary embolism. Arch Int Med 1994;154:289.

Hyers TM, Hull RD, Weg, JG: Antithrombotic therapy for venous thromboembolic disease. Chest 1992;102:408S.

PIOPED Investigators: Value of the ventilation/perfusion scan in acute pulmonary embolism. Results of the Prospective Investigation of Pulmonary Embolism Diagnosis (PIOPED). JAMA 1990;263:2753.

Prins MH, Lensing AWA, Hirsh J: Idiopathic deep venous thrombosis. Is a search for malignant disease justified? Arch Int Med 1994;154:1310.

Quinn DA et al: A prospective investigation of pulmonary embolism in women and men. JAMA 1992;268:1689.

Salzman EW, Hirsh J: The epidemiology, pathogenesis, and natural history of venous thromboembolism. In: *Hemostasis and Thrombosis: Basic Principles and Clinical Practice,* 3/e. Colman RW et al (editors). Lippincott, 1994.

Stein PD et al: Clinical, laboratory, roengenographic, and electrocardiographic findings in patients with acute pulmonary embolism and no preexisting cardiac or pulmonary disease. Chest 1991;100:598.

Thromboembolism Risk Factors (THRIFT) Consensus Group: Risk of and prophylaxis for venous thromboembolism in hospital patients. BMJ 1992;305:567.

Turpie AGG: Principles of thromboprophylaxis in pregnancy and after gynaecological surgery. In: *Haemostasis and Thrombosis in Obstetrics and Gynaecology.* Greer IA, Turpie AGG, Forbes CD (editors). Chapman & Hall Medical, 1992.

Section IX.
Infectious Diseases

HIV Infection

36

Roger W. Bush, MD

The human immunodeficiency virus (HIV) epidemic has brought sharp focus to the social, economic, and medical conditions of women. Heterosexual contact and drug use, alone and in combination, expose women to HIV, often without their awareness of risk at the time of exposure or clinical presentation. Providers must be vigilant for HIV risk and manifestations, because HIV infection is increasing faster in women than in any other group. High transmission rates in adolescents and young adults, vertical transmission, and social conditions that promote high-risk behaviors guarantee continuation of the HIV epidemic into the next century. As the HIV epidemic continues beyond the risk behaviors, geographic areas, and demographic groups initially described, health care providers will be confronted with HIV infection, including its prevention, treatment, and continuing care.

Incidence

In the years before 1988, 7% of AIDS cases reported in the United States occurred in women, a figure that increased to 10% in 1988. By June 30, 1993, women and teenage girls (older than 13 years) constituted 12% of all adults and adolescents with AIDS. However, AIDS cases and deaths probably exceeded these figures. Worldwide, one-third of approximately 10 million HIV-infected adults are women. Globally, by the year 2000, the number of women with HIV infection will equal that of men.

AIDS is the sixth leading cause of death in women ages 25–44 in the USA. Women constitute the fastest growing group of new AIDS cases in the USA. Early in the epidemic, women with AIDS were few in number and usually were infected through injection drug use rather than heterosexual contact. Since 1992, however, more women with AIDS have acquired infection through heterosexual activity than through injection drug use. Although these AIDS statistics are ominous, HIV seroprevalence data, which aresketchier, are more foreboding. HIV seroprevalence data probably reflect recent patterns of HIV infection better than AIDS data and have been related to heterosexual contact for much longer, particularly in women younger than 30 years, who often are infected as adolescents.

Incidence
Risk Factors for HIV Transmission
HIV Testing
Gender Differences
Prevention
Clinical Spectrum
Clinical Evaluation & Monitoring
Treatment
Psychosocial Concerns

Risk Factors for HIV Transmission

Race and ethnicity are not risk factors, but they serve as markers of socioeconomic status and access to medical care; therefore, they identify groups at high risk for HIV infection such as blacks and Hispanics. Rates of infection for black and Hispanic women are 13 and 6 times higher, respectively, than for whites. Three-fourths of women infected with HIV are black or Hispanic.

The social blights of crack cocaine and injection drug use often are associated, directly or indirectly, with HIV, especially in the Northeast and in women older than 30. In 1992, injection drug use was the predominant mode of HIV transmission for women in the Northeast. Of HIV infections attributed to heterosexual contact, most (56.8%) involved sex with an injection drug user. Risk factors such as anal intercourse, genital ulcers, syphilis, sex without condoms, multiple sexual contacts, oral contraceptive use, and advanced disease state of male contacts increase the male-to-female transmission rate. Sex with high-risk men and survival sex (trading sex for money, shelter, food, or drugs) are also important risk behaviors. Unfortunately, many women with HIV and their health care providers are unaware of their condition, because women often are diagnosed with HIV at or near their death. To make an early diagnosis of HIV infection, it is imperative for providers to ask patients about drug use and sexual behaviors that have taken place since 1978. Because many women are unaware of their risk even when questioned, risk-based screening may miss 50–60% of infected women.

HIV Testing

Women who have been determined to be at risk

should be counseled concerning how tests are performed and the meaning of positive and negative tests results. Issues of confidentiality, anonymity, and voluntary disclosure should be addressed frankly. After careful risk assessment and pretest counseling, a screening enzyme-linked immunosorbent assay (ELISA) should be offered, and a time should be arranged for test results to be delivered in person. Pre- and posttest counseling sessions are strategic opportunities for advice on modifying behaviors to avoid additional exposures and transmission; these sessions require expert communication skills.

If the initial ELISA is positive, the test should be repeated and then confirmed with a Western blot. If the test result is indeterminate, it is unexpectedly positive or negative, or there is any doubt about test validity, it should be repeated with a new sample.

Gender Differences

Expansion of the HIV epidemic to women has not yet been addressed by major studies, although concerted efforts have been made to include women in clinical trials. In 1993, the multisite, large-scale, four-year Women's Interagency HIV Study (WIHS) was launched to assess the impact of HIV and AIDS on women. This study investigates signs and symptoms of HIV infection in 1700 women, describe the pattern and rate of their immune system decline, explore cofactors that affect their disease progression, and study the effect of therapies on survival and quality of life. Until such rigorous studies produce useful information, clinicians must rely on small observational studies and retrospective series to guide decisions.

In addition to facing gynecologic and pregnancy-related problems, women with AIDS get the same opportunistic infections as men. Risk behaviors that result in HIV infection dictate opportunistic diseases; the gender does not. For example, Kaposi's sarcoma is rare in women and limited to those who have had sex with bisexual men. Herpes simplex virus and cytomegalovirus infection, wasting, and esophageal candidiasis may be more common in women than men. *Pneumocystis carinii* pneumonia (PCP) is still the most common opportunistic illness in both genders. When the data are controlled for race, ethnicity, and mode of transmission, most AIDS-defining conditions are of equal prevalence in women and men. Although the clinical course of PCP is similar in women and men, women may have greater hospital mortality from the disease than men, possibly because of inadequate access to providers experienced in its treatment.

Prevention

The low socioeconomic status of many women at risk for HIV makes prevention difficult. Elimination of risk behaviors is the only available definitive prevention strategy. Knowledge of what motivates and influences behavior and effective counseling practices are the fundamental tools of prevention. Most communities can provide substance abuse treatment, detection and treatment of all sexually transmitted diseases, needle exchange programs for injection drug users, frank sexual safety education, prenatal care for expectant HIV-infected mothers, and promotion of condom use.

In Washington state, women with class IV HIV infection generally were tested because of illness, sexual contact, or blood donation; most did not perceive that they were at risk. Most of these women were infected during heterosexual contact (56%), never used condoms in the 5 years prior to diagnosis (85%), and either injected drugs or had a sexual partner who injected drugs. In 1990, between 15 and 30% of heterosexuals reported an HIV risk factor. Only 17% of those with multiple sex partners and 11% of those with high-risk sex partners used condoms all the time. HIV prevention programs have failed to reach women as well as male heterosexuals at risk for HIV infection. Few prevention messages are specifically targeted at women, many messages are too euphemistic to be effective, and women often are not in control of condom use or their sexual exposures. Ideally, methods for prevention of HIV and other sexually transmitted diseases would be controlled by women and of high efficacy. Condoms have the highest theoretic preventive efficacy, but diaphragms and spermicides are controlled by women and therefore likely to be more effective. Only 18% of women reported that their male partners used condoms for any reason. Intravaginal pouches (female condoms), which are now available, may offer a level of protection similar to condoms, are woman-controlled, and appear to be acceptable in use; however, they cost approximately $2.50 each. All these methods should be promoted, along with limiting and carefully selecting partners. Women must do their best to persuade male sexual partners to use condoms. If for any reason sex without condoms occurs, a spermicide and latex barrier should be used.

Clinical Spectrum

The occurrence of AIDS-indicator diseases is strongly associated with degree of immune suppression but not with gender or risk group. Major infectious illnesses that are not in the 1987 AIDS case definition (see Table 36–1) are related to immune compromise as well, but they also are related to injection drug use, probably caused by ongoing needle use, alcohol use, and poor living conditions. The most common and serious infections are pneumococcal pneumonia, sepsis, and tuberculosis. For people with an AIDS-indicator disease, two more receive care for serious HIV-related conditions that are not in the 1987 definition.

Gynecologic care may present a problem for women who receive care at medical facilities dedi-

Table 36–1. CDC classification of HTLV-III/LAV infection.

Group I: Acute infection
Mononucleosislike syndrome associated with seroconversion

Group II: Asymptomatic infection
Positive HTLV-III/LAV antibody or viral culture. May be subclassified on basis of laboratory evaluation (CBC, platelet count, T-cell subset studies)

Group III: Persistent generalized lymphadenopathy
Palpable lymphadenopathy (> 1 cm) at two or more extrainguinal sites for more than three months in the absence of a concurrent illness or infection to explain the findings. May be subclassified on the basis of laboratory evaluation (see above)

Group IV—Other HTLV-III/LAV disease
  Subgroup A: Constitutional disease
    One or more of the following: fever or diarrhea persisting more than one month or involuntary weight loss greater than 10% of baseline; and absence of a concurrent illness or infection to explain the findings
  Subgroup B: Neurologic disease
    One or more of the following: dementia, myelopathy, or peripheral neuropathy; and absence of a concurrent illness or condition
  Subgroup C: Secondary infectious diseases
    Infectious disease associated with HTLV-III/LAV infection and/or at least moderately indicative of a defect in cell-mediated immunity
    Category C-1
      Symptomatic or invasive disease due to one of 12 specified diseases listed in the surveillance definition of AIDS: *Pneumocystis carinii* pneumonia, chronic cryptosporidiosis, toxoplasmosis, extraintestinal strongyloidiasis, isosporiasis, candidiasis (esophageal, bronchial, or pulmonary), cryptococcosis, histoplasmosis, mycobacterial infection (*Mycobacterium avium* complex or *M. kansasii*), cytomegalovirus infection, chronic mucocutaneous or disseminated herpes simplex virus infection, and progressive multifocal leukoencephalopathy
    Category C-2
      Symptomatic or invasive disease due to one of six other specified diseases: oral hairy leukoplakia, multidermatomal herpes zoster, recurrent Salmonella bacteremia, nocardiosis, tuberculosis, and oral candidiasis (thrush)
  Subgroup D: Secondary cancers
    Diagnosis of one or more cancers known to be associated with HTLV-III/LAV infection as listed in the surveillance definition of AIDS and at least moderately indicative of a defect in cell-mediated immunity: Kaposi sarcoma, non-Hodgkin's lymphoma (small, noncleaved lymphoma or immunoblastic sarcoma), or primary lymphoma of the brain
  Subgroup E: Other conditions in HTLV-III/LAV infection
    Clinical findings or diseases, not classifiable above, that may be attributable to HTLV-III/LAV infection and are indicative of a defect in cell-mediated immunity; symptoms attributable to either HTLV-III/LAV infection or a coexisting disease not classified elsewhere; or clinical illnesses that may be complicated or altered by HTLV-III/LAV infection. These include chronic lymphoid interstitial pneumonitis and constitutional symptoms, secondary infectious diseases, and neoplasms not listed above

From CDC: Classification system for human T-lymphotropic virus type III/lymphadenopathy-associated virus infections. MMWR 35:334, 1986

cated to HIV care; the women may not have gynecologic care available to them at those sites and therefore may not have any access to such care. Gynecologic conditions are common HIV-associated clinical problems and often occur before the patient is aware of her HIV infection or exposure. Cervical dysplasia and cancer became AIDS-defining illnesses in January 1993. Nearly half (49%) of HIV-infected women have evidence of human papillomavirus (HPV) infection compared with 25% in high-risk HIV-negative women. Women with both HIV and HPV infection have an increased risk of cervical disease, and cervical cancer is more aggressive when accompanied by HIV infection. HIV infection is often otherwise asymptomatic in women who present with cervical cancer.

Candida vulvovaginitis is the most common gynecologic problem of HIV-infected women and was the initial clinical manifestation of 38% of women in one series. It can cause painful ulcerations that are refractory to topical treatment, particularly in severely immunocompromised hosts. Similarly, herpes genitalis can be severe, widespread, and refractory to treatment. Syphilis is increasing in incidence, and coinfection with HIV is common. The clinical course of syphilis in HIV-infected patients is telescoped in that neurosyphilis can occur early after infection. Such genital ulcers are common in those at risk for HIV, can be signs of HIV infection, and can increase sexual transmission of HIV.

Clinical Evaluation & Monitoring

After diagnosis of HIV infection, baseline clinical and laboratory data should be obtained. The clinician's goal is to collect a comprehensive database, provide staging and prognostic information, and formulate a treatment plan. The patient, however, often needs counseling, empathy, and reassurance. With a simple structure to follow and with practice, both agendas can be met.

One way to start an initial interview is with an open-ended question as to why the patient took the test, followed by some exploration of her social milieu. An explicit history of risks and current practices, an estimate of the likely duration of infection, identification of contacts and children who may be infected, and a review of symptoms may follow. Disclosure to children, other family members, and child care providers as well as reproductive counseling are features of HIV care for women that are foreign to many HIV care providers. These are difficult tasks that may elicit fears of rejection and loss. Once women understand the risks that their loved ones may bear and the benefit of early medical intervention, however, they are usually eager to cooperate.

The presence of HIV-related symptoms may have important prognostic implications; therefore, the review of systems should include early symptoms of

HIV infection, such as fevers, night sweats, diarrhea, weight loss, lymphadenopathy, thrush, vaginitis, and skin changes, as well as all the following items:

Past or present sexually transmitted diseases
Past or present pelvic inflammatory disease
Recurrent or severe vulvovaginal candidiasis
Sepsis or recurrent bacterial pneumonia
Herpes zoster
Tuberculosis
Unexplained persistent constitutional symptoms
Hepatitis B markers
Autoimmune thrombocytopenic purpura
Cervical dysplasia or genital warts
Genital ulcers
Unexplained diarrhea

Fever and thrush are independent predictors of early progression to PCP and should lead to prophylactic antibiotic therapy for the disease. The medical history should determine if the patient has been diagnosed with tuberculosis or sexually transmitted diseases (eg, genital warts, cervical dysplasia, herpes, and syphilis) at any time; reproductive history should include the determination of contraception method. Immunization history, travel, diet, drug and alcohol history, and a review of urgent social needs and supports are also important issues to be addressed.

Advance directives regarding life-sustaining treatments, durable power-of-attorney for health care, and guardianship of dependent children should be addressed as soon as rapport allows. Most patients appreciate the affirmation of control over their own care and are glad to have the opportunity to discuss treatment goals, although negative emotional responses such as fear and hopelessness can occur initially.

The initial physical examination should be comprehensive, with particular attention to the weight, mouth, pelvic examination, and mental status examination. Weight trends provide a useful index of progression of disease and response to therapy, and weight loss greater than 10% of body weight constitutes "wasting syndrome," an AIDS-defining illness particularly common in women. Thrush, oral ulcers, and oral hairy leukoplakia are common findings, whereas Kaposi's sarcoma is unusual in women. These examinations should be performed at each visit. A fundoscopic examination should be done every 3–6 months, with the clinician looking for the hemorrhage and yellow-white spots commonly seen in cytomegalovirus (CMV) retinitis. Papanicolaou (Pap) smears should be done at least every 6 months, with early gynecologic referral if atypia, dysplasia, or squamous intraepithelial lesion (SIL) is found, or if there is a history of untreated SIL. The clinician should remain vigilant for mental disorders; depression, dementia, encephalopathy, CNS toxoplasmosis,

lymphoma, and drug or alcohol abuse are encountered frequently.

The laboratory evaluation must be tailored to the patient, practice circumstances, and laboratory capabilities. The following list of initial tests and vaccines for HIV-infected women provides a guideline for the clinician:

Complete blood cell count (CBC) and platelets
Purified protein derivative (PPD-5TU) and anergy panel (yearly if patient is positive for PPD and not anergic)
CD4 lymphocyte count—absolute and percentage—(every 3–6 months if no symptoms are present and no PCP prophylaxis is indicated yet)
Serologic test for syphilis (yearly)
Toxoplasma IgG
Hepatitis B serologic study (hepatitis B core antibody)
Pap smear (every 6 months)
Vaccinations: pneumococcus once, influenza yearly, diphtheria-tetanus every 10 years, hepatitis B if not immune
If symptomatic, chest x-ray and chemistry panel

T-cell subsets are useful prognostically, but they are notoriously variable from day to day and laboratory to laboratory. Every reasonable effort should be made to have serial subsets drawn at the same time of day, at the same menstrual stage, and not during or immediately after an acute illness. Many HIV-related infections are reactivation illnesses; therefore, tuberculin testing, syphilis serologic tests, and *Toxoplasma* antibody status can guide the practitioner diagnostically when an acute illness occurs. CD4 lymphocyte counts are the most prognostically useful laboratory index, yet similar levels do not necessarily reflect identical risk of progression. Opportunistic diseases usually do not occur in patients with CD4 lymphocyte counts greater than 0.25×10^9/L. Although these counts are incomplete in their predictive value, they help the clinician to anticipate progression of disease and survival.

In general, asymptomatic patients with CD4 counts greater than 0.50×10^9/L should be monitored every 6 months; symptomatic patients with CD4 counts between 0.20 and 0.50×10^9/L should be seen every 3–6 months, and patients with fewer than 0.20×10^9/L CD4 cells should be monitored according to their disease activity.

Treatment

Management of women with HIV infection should be in the context of comprehensive, longitudinal, patient-centered care given by primary care providers. Patients who require fiberoptic bronchoscopy, cancer treatment planning, or treatment for complex, rare infectious complications often require subspecialty consultation, but the value of a close doctor-patient relationship cannot be overstated. Multidisciplinary teams may include social workers, mental health professionals, nutritionists, rehabilitation specialists, and pharmacists.

A. Antiretroviral Treatment: Antiretroviral therapy is an area of active controversy. Each of the currently available antiretroviral agents (the nucleosides zidovudine (ZDV), didanosine, and zalcitabine) has a role in the treatment of HIV infection, but they are weak, frequently toxic treatments that should be used carefully in the context of comprehensive primary care with patients sharing in decision making. These choices must be made with awareness of benefits, toxicities, limited effectiveness, uncertainty, and expense. Patients must be educated about treatment options and their impact on quality of life. Clear, validated algorithms are not feasible, although broad, evidence-based guidelines are available.

Initiation of antiretroviral therapy should be considered for symptomatic patients with CD4 cell counts less than 0.50×10^9/L and for all patients with CD4 cell counts less than 0.20×10^9/L; antiretroviral therapy may delay progression to AIDS, reduce incidence of opportunistic infections, and prolong life in many patients. Zidovudine, 600 mg daily in three divided doses, is recommended for initial therapy. Although combination therapy often is offered to those with CD4 counts less than 0.20×10^9/L, data on its effectiveness are inconclusive, particularly when the benefits are balanced with the increased toxicity and expense.

Antiretroviral therapy is not recommended for patients with stable CD4 counts of more than 0.50×10^9/L and is of uncertain, temporary (12–24 months or less) benefit for asymptomatic patients with CD4 counts of $0.20–0.50 \times 10^9$/L.

Patients who tolerate zidovudine therapy but have progressive immunodeficiency (CD4 cell counts fall to less than half of pretreatment levels, below 0.30×10^9/L) or therapeutic failure (new HIV-related events, loss of functional status, or other clinical deterioration) while taking ZDV should consider alternative antiretroviral monotherapy; therapy is available with didanosine tablets (100 mg twice daily if weight is less than 45 kg, 200 mg twice daily if more than 45 kg) or zalcitabine (0.75-mg tablet, 3 times daily). Patients who are intolerant of ZDV and desire ongoing antiretroviral treatment are also candidates for these alternatives.

The primary adverse effects of ZDV include headache and nausea; however, myopathy and anemia also occur and can result in intolerance and discontinuation. Although treatment of anemia with erythropoietin or transfusions is possible, patients with persistent symptomatic or severe anemia (hemoglobin less than 80–90 g/L) usually are switched to alternative drugs or have the dosage of ZDV reduced to 100 mg 3 times daily.

B. Gynecologic Care: Vaginal symptoms and sexually transmitted diseases often herald HIV infection and must be taken seriously in all women. HIV testing should be offered to all sexually active women and promoted for women with any risk factors or suggestive clinical problems, such as severe yeast vaginitis, cervical dysplasia, or invasive cervical carcinoma. As mentioned, HIV-infected women should receive Pap smears every 6 months, with prompt referral to gynecologic specialists if SIL is identified, because cervical dysplasia progresses rapidly in these patients.

Standard therapies for yeast vaginitis are often effective, and they can be used as periodic maintenance treatment when frequent recurrences are a problem. Unusually severe or recalcitrant cases usually can be controlled with systemic ketoconazole or fluconazole.

Fertility and reproductive issues are complex and difficult for women with HIV infection. Because most children are infected perinatally and prenatal care may reduce vertical transmission, prenatal testing has been advocated. Contraception and abortion decisions are complicated by increased risk of pregnancy for the mother, the likelihood she would not live to raise the child, and the frequent absence of other suitable child care. HIV-infected women may want to continue a pregnancy but fear potential outcomes so much that they seek termination, which may be difficult to arrange.

C. Pregnancy Care: Because pregnancy does not appear to accelerate progression of HIV disease in the mother, treatment of pregnant women should not be significantly different from that of nonpregnant women. CD4 lymphocyte counts should be determined at the time of presentation for prenatal care or at delivery for women who receive no prenatal care. Pregnant women with CD4 cell counts less than 0.20×10^9/L usually should be offered zidovudine treatment, without repeated counts during the pregnancy. When the CD4 count is between 0.20 and 0.50×10^9/L, the decision to treat can be based on the woman's preference, with counts repeated each trimester. With CD4 counts of 0.60×10^9/L or greater, treatment usually is withheld.

In February 1994, the National Institute of Allergy and Infectious Diseases (NIAID) released results from ACTG 076, a randomized, double-blind, placebo-controlled clinical trial of zidovudine treatment for pregnant women with CD4 counts of 0.20×10^9/L or greater and no clinical indications for antepartum zidovudine therapy. The study found an 8.3% vertical (mother to child) transmission rate when the mother took ZDV, 500 mg/d orally, initiated in the second or third trimester, and 1 mg/kg/h intravenously during labor; the vertical transmission rate in the placebo group was 25.5%. No significant short-term side effects were seen in mothers or infants. On the basis of this study, it is reasonable to offer second- and third-trimester antepartum and intrapartum zidovudine therapy, even though long-term risks to exposed infants are unknown. A substantial (8.3 ± 4.5%) risk of transmission persists even with treatment, so women must be counseled that this intervention does not make pregnancy free of risk for the infant. Although the effect of ZDV on the fetus is unknown, delaying treatment may put the fetus at increased risk for HIV infection and put the mother at increased risk for progression, which could endanger both mother and fetus. These women also should receive prophylaxis for PCP with trimethoprim-sulfamethoxazole until 32 weeks of gestation; at that point they should receive inhaled pentamidine for the last 2 months because of the risk of kernicterus in premature infants exposed to sulfamethoxazole.

D. Prevention of Opportunistic Illness: Primary (for those with CD4 count less than 0.20×10^9/L) and secondary PCP prophylaxis is justified by strong evidence of reduced incidence and prolonged survival at a reasonable cost. Trimethoprim-sulfamethoxazole is the first-line, most effective agent and should be promoted actively, even if only as small a dose as three double-strength tablets a week can be tolerated. It also may prevent *Toxoplasma* and gram-positive bacterial infection. Dapsone rarely cross-reacts in patients allergic to sulfa and is more effective as well as much less expensive than inhaled pentamidine (Fig 36–1).

Secondary prophylaxis (maintenance therapy) of *Cryptococcus, Toxoplasma,* recurrent herpes simplex, and cytomegalovirus infections, as well as tuberculosis prophylaxis for 12 months, is imperative in all PPD-positive patients. Early pneumococcal and annual influenza vaccination may be useful, and hepatitis B vaccination for unexposed women is advised. In addition to preventing the psychologic and physiologic stress of opportunistic disease, prevention and early detection of treatable complications may slow HIV disease progression.

Psychosocial Concerns

Psychosocial support is crucial to effective care. Testing positive for HIV is a dramatic event for anyone. Additional social and psychologic burdens for women with HIV include pregnancy and motherhood, rejection as marital or romantic partners, and loss of security and income. It also usually means a child, husband, lover, or other significant person is infected. Female users of injectable drugs are likely to be the sole support person for young children; treatment centers are proportionally less available to clients with children, and most centers will not accept women who are pregnant or have children. Most HIV-infected women in North America are mothers with dependent children, a problem that will escalate with time. The increase in AIDS among women has led to in an increase in cases among children ages 0–4 years, most (95%) of whom are infected perinatally. Adolescent women, in addition to being at high risk for heterosexual HIV transmission, are also in their peak childbearing years.

The risk of vertical HIV infection (mother to child) is 13–15% in Europe, 15–30% in the USA, and 25–52% in developing countries. The risk of increased vertical transmission is correlated with high p24 antigen levels, high CD8 lymphocyte levels, low CD4 lymphocyte levels, placental inflammation, anemia, fever, and premature birth. Some experts suspect that 50% of vertical transmission occurs perinatally; therefore, all infants should be regarded as uninfected while in labor and be protected from maternal secretions. Women in the USA should avoid breast-feeding if they can afford bottle-feeding, because breast-feeding increases vertical transmission risk by 14%. Issues of economics and water purity make bottle-feeding less desirable in the developing

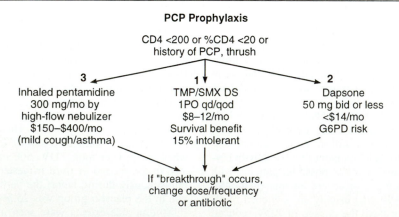

Figure 36–1. Comparative cost and efficacy of three common prophylaxis regimes.

world. Prenatal care may reduce the rate of vertical transmission.

Conservatively estimated, 45,600 children will be orphaned secondary to HIV by 1996, and the figure will be 82,000 by the year 2000; most are living in poverty. Whether or not they are infected, more than 80,000 children in the USA are expected to see their mothers die of HIV infection by the year 2000. These children may be ill themselves, and they may depend on ill parents or on grandparents, relatives, friends, or foster parents for their care. Bearing the burden of care for her family and dependents often is the major barrier to the patient's medical care.

Clinicians who work with HIV-infected women must determine social, psychologic, medical, and economic ramifications; actively identify other family members who have HIV; and arrange entry into the health care system.

Women often care for others with AIDS and then find themselves to be infected. While ill, a woman may have to arrange for the care of her dependents after her death. These women often defer their own care to provide for the care of their children. Because women with AIDS are more likely to be black or Hispanic, they are likely to be poor and have less access to health care. Primary care physicians may not

recognize HIV in women, and HIV clinics may not be well suited to the care of women. Loss of employment, rejection by family and friends, and impoverishment are frequent, as is the remorse of feeling responsible for transmission of HIV to a child.

Disclosing one's HIV infection to a child is difficult, but openness and early disclosure often allow a child better psychosocial adjustment. A proper setting, telling the oldest child first, judicious timing, and use of comprehensive family social support services make disclosure less painful. Uninfected women also carry a disproportionate burden of caring for men with HIV, because men are often less supportive than women of sons or brothers with homosexually transmitted AIDS. Mothers of hemophiliacs may feel responsible for transmitting both a defective gene and HIV, a burden that weighs heavily on a woman who cares for an adolescent denied his adulthood. Elderly mothers may feel isolated from the lives and communities of adult children dying in their care.

The time, energy, and skills required of providers to help women cope with these issues must be safeguarded, because emotional suffering is often the most difficult to bear and psychosocial issues are often the most challenging for clinicians to manage.

REFERENCES

EPIDEMIOLOGY

Bastian L et al: Differences between men and women with HIV-related *Pneumocystis carinii* pneumonia: Experience from 3,070 cases in New York City in 1987. J Acquir Immune Defic Syndr 1993;6:617.

Buehler JW et al: The reporting of HIV/AIDS deaths in women. Am J Public Health 1992;82:1500.

Campbell CA: Women and AIDS. Soc Sci Med 1990; 30:407.

Centers for Disease Control: Characteristics of, and HIV infection among, women served by publicly funded HIV counseling and testing services—United States, 1989–90. MMWR 1991;40:195.

Centers for Disease Control: Classification system for human T-lymphotrophic virus type III/Lymphadenopathy associated virus infections. MMWR 1986; 35:334.

Centers for Disease Control and Prevention: Update: Acquired immunodeficiency syndrome—United States, 1992. MMWR 1993;42:547;557.

Clark R et al: HIV: What's different for women? Patient Care (Sept 15) 1993;119.

de Bruyn M. Women and AIDS in developing countries. Soc Sci Med 1992;34:249.

Dunn DT et al: Risk of human immunodeficiency virus type 1 transmission through breastfeeding. Lancet 1992;340:585.

Farizo KM et al: Spectrum of disease in persons with human immunodeficiency virus infection in the United States. JAMA 1992;267:1798.

Fleming PL et al: Gender differences in reported AIDS-indicative diagnoses. J Infect Dis 1993;168:61.

Fullilove MT et al: Black women and AIDS prevention: A view towards understanding the gender rules. J Sex Res 1990;27:47.

Gwinn M et al: Prevalence of HIV infection in childbearing women in the United States: Surveillance using newborn blood samples. JAMA 1991;265:1704.

Hankins CA, Handley MA: HIV disease and AIDS in women: Current knowledge and a research agenda. J Acquir Immune Defic Syndr 1992;5:957.

Jones L, Catalan J: Women and HIV disease. Br J Hosp Med 1989;41:526.

Padian N: Epidemiology of AIDS and heterosexually transmitted HIV in women. AIDSFILE 1991;5:1.

Padian N et al: Male-to-female transmission of human immunodeficiency virus. JAMA 1987;258:788.

Schoenbaum EE, Webber MP: The underrecognition of HIV infection in women in an inner-city emergency room. Am J Public Health 1993;83:363.

Selik RM, Chu SY, Buehler JW: HIV infection as leading cause of death among young adults in U.S. cities and states. JAMA 1993;269:2991.

Vermund SH: Rising HIV-related mortality in young Americans. JAMA 1993;269:3034.

PREVENTION

Catania JA et al: Prevalence of AIDS-related risk factors and condom use in the United States. Science 1992;258:1101.

Norris-Walczak L, Frederick M: Prevention of HIV: Are women getting the message? Washington State Seattle-King County HIV/AIDS Report 1992; 4th quarter:20.

Rosenberg MJ, Gollub EL: Commentary: Methods women can use that may prevent sexually transmitted disease, including HIV. Am J Public Health 1992;82:1473.

Stein ZA: Editorial: The double bind in science policy and the protection of women from HIV infection. Am J Public Health 1992;82:1471.

CLINICAL EVALUATION & MONITORING

Allen MA: Primary care of women infected with the human immunodeficiency virus. Obstet Gynecol Clin North Am 1990;17:557.

Allen MH, Marte C: HIV infection in women: Presentations and protocols. Hosp Pract (March 15) 1992;155.

Minkoff HL, DeHovitz JA: Care of women infected with the human immunodeficiency virus. JAMA 1991;266:2253.

THERAPY

Bermon N: Family and reproductive issues: Reproductive counseling. AIDS Clin Care 1993;5:45.

Boyer PJ et al: Factors predictive of maternal-fetal transmission of HIV-1: Preliminary analysis of zidovudine given during pregnancy and/or delivery. JAMA 1994;271:1925.

Carpenter CCJ et al: Human immunodeficiency virus infection in North American women: Experience with 200 cases and a review of the literature. Medicine (Baltimore) 1991;70:307.

Cu-Uvin S, Flanigan TP, Carpenter CCJ: Routine gynecologic monitoring of HIV-seropositive women: Research and recommendations. The AIDS Reader (July/Aug) 1993;133.

Ellerbrock TV et al: Heterosexually transmitted human immunodeficiency virus infection among pregnant women in a rural Florida community. N Engl J Med 1992;327:1704.

European Collaborative Study: Risk factors for mother-to-child transmission of HIV-1. Lancet 1992;339:1007.

Feingold AR et al: Cervical cytologic abnormalities and papillomavirus in women infected with human immunodeficiency virus. J AIDS 1990;3:896.

Jewett JF, Hecht FM: Preventive health care for adults with HIV infection. JAMA 1993;269:1144.

Lipson M: Disclosure within families. AIDS Clin Care 1993;5:43.

Maiman M et al: Human immunodeficiency virus infection and invasive cervical carcinoma. Cancer 1993;71:402.

Michaels D, Levine C: Estimates of the number of motherless youth orphaned by AIDS in the United States. JAMA 1992;268:3456.

Nicholas SW, Abrams EJ: The "silent" legacy of AIDS: Children who survive their parents and siblings. JAMA 1992;268:3478.

St. Louis ME et al: Risk for perinatal HIV-1 transmission according to maternal immunologic, virologic, and placental factors. JAMA 1993;269:2853.

Sande MA et al: Antiretroviral therapy for adult HIV-infected patients: Recommendations from a state-of-the-art conference. JAMA 270;21:2583.

Sperling RS, Stratton P: Treatment options for human immunodeficiency virus–infected pregnant women. Obstet Gynecol 1992;79:443.

Sperling RS et al: A survey of zidovudine use in pregnant women with HIV infection. N Engl J Med 1992;326:857.

Vermund SH et al: High risk of human papillomavirus infection and cervical squamous intraepithelial lesions among women with symptomatic human immunodeficiency virus infection. Am J Obstet Gynecol 1991;165:392.

Sexually Transmitted Diseases & Pelvic Inflammatory Disease

37

David E. Soper, MD

Sexually transmitted diseases (STDs) affect more than 12 million people in the United States each year. Current figures suggest that one of four and perhaps as many as one of two people will contract an STD at some time in their lives. The groups most affected by STDs include women, teenagers, the poor, and members of minority groups, especially blacks.

Women are more susceptible to STD infection and have a harder time being diagnosed than men because the diseases are often asymptomatic in women. Serious problems can result including pelvic inflammatory disease (PID), infertility, ectopic pregnancy, cervical cancer, and transmission of STD to offspring during pregnancy or childbirth. Perinatal and neonatal STD infections can cause spontaneous abortion, stillbirth, infant death, premature delivery, mental retardation, blindness, and low birth weight. The annual cost associated with just three STDs—*Chlamydia,* gonorrhea, and herpes—has been estimated to be more than $5 billion.

The female genital tract is contiguous from the vulva to the fallopian tube. Division of the genital tract into four levels (vulva, vagina, cervix, and upper genital tract [endometrium and fallopian tube]) is helpful in the evaluation approaching the of STDs. The clinical manifestations of STDs are due to the ability of most pathogens to elicit an inflammatory response from the host. For this reason, the primary clinical sign of infection with an STD is the presence of pus. Pus, an accumulation of polymorphonuclear inflammatory cells, is almost always present in patients with symptomatic STDs. The detection of this inflammation is the clinical challenge.

It should be noted that HIV infection modifies the presentation and response to therapy of patients with STDs. All patients with STDs should be offered serologic testing for HIV infection.

SEXUALLY TRANSMITTED DISEASES

Incidence & Risk Factors

The World Health Organization estimates that at least 250 million sexually transmitted infections occur annually worldwide, with a large percentage oc-

---

Sexually Transmitted Diseases
  Incidence & Risk Factors
  Screening
  Signs & Symptoms
  Clinical Findings & Diagnosis
  Treatment
  Referral to a Specialist
  Issues of Pregnancy & Sexually
    Transmitted Diseases
  Psychosocial Concerns
Pelvic Inflammatory Disease
  Signs & Symptoms
  Clinical Findings & Diagnosis
  Treatment
  Referral to a Specialist
  Issues of Pregnancy & Pelvic Inflammatory
    Disease

---

curring in young adults between the ages of 20 and 24. Trichomoniasis is the most common STD; Table 37–1 presents the numbers of cases per year of common STDs.

In the USA, approximately 12 million cases of STDs were reported in 1990. Approximately 4–4.5 million people in the USA acquire chlamydial genital infections, and nearly 1.4 million cases of gonorrhea occur annually. Epidemic syphilis reached an all-time high for the last 30 years, increasing more than 100% in major urban centers during the past few years. Many of these diseases had significant impacts on minority groups, women, and infants.

It is estimated that more than 100,000 infants currently die or suffer birth defects because of STDs transmitted during pregnancy or birth. Approximately 3 million teenagers are infected with an STD annually, and HIV infection rates are increasing dramatically among heterosexuals within inner-city minority-group populations.

Traditional STD risk factors appear to be correlates of the probability of encountering an infected partner; others influence the probability of infection if exposed or the probability of manifesting disease if

Table 37–1. Sexually transmitted diseases worldwide.*

Disease	Number of cases (millions)
Trichomonas	120
Chlamydia	50
Genital warts	30
Gonorrhea	25
Genital herpes	20
HIV infection	9
Syphilis	4
Hepatitis B	3
Chancroid	2

*Data from the World Health Organization, 1991.

infected. At the present time, major sexual behavioral risk factors for STDs appear to include (1) multiple sex partners, (2) high rates of acquisition of new sexual partners within specific time periods, (3) high rates of partner change, (4) contact with casual sexual partners, and (5) risky sexual practices (eg, rectal intercourse). Alcohol and drug abuse produce situational modification of sexual behavior or health care behavior. Health care behaviors that can reduce the risk of acquiring STDs or prevent complications include the use of condoms for prophylaxis, early consultation for diagnosis and treatment, compliance with therapy, and partner referral. Absence of such behaviors can be regarded as risk factors for STDs. Douching represents a behavior that, although undertaken for "feminine hygiene," may increase the risk of PID and its sequelae.

Other indicators of risk include young age, single marital status, membership in particular ethnic groups, and urban residence. These risk indicators are correlates of sexual behavior and of disease prevalence in sex partners. Age also may affect host susceptibility in that the prevalence of cervical ectopy is higher in young women and may increase a woman's susceptibility to particular STD pathogens such as *C trachomatis*.

Screening

Many, if not most, women with STDs are asymptomatic. For this reason, screening for selective STDs is important. The prevalence of STDs in a patient population should influence the decision to screen. It should be remembered that women with one STD often are infected with others.

The screening of women for chlamydial infections is a critical component in a *Chlamydia* prevention program, because many women are asymptomatic and the infection may persist for extended periods of time. Many women of reproductive age undergo pelvic examination during visits for routine health care or because of illness. During these examinations, specimens can be obtained for screening tests for *Chlamydia*.

Women who should be screened for chlamydial infection include adolescents, those undergoing induced abortion, those attending STD clinics, and women in detention facilities. Screening at family planning and prenatal care clinics is particularly cost-effective because of the large numbers of sexually active young women who undergo pelvic examinations. Other groups of women who should be tested for *Chlamydia* include those who have MPC and those who are sexually active and younger than 20 years of age. In addition, women between 20 and 24 years of age who meet either of the following criteria and women older than 24 years who meet both of the criteria should be screened: (1) inconsistent use of barrier contraception and (2) having a new sex partner or more than one sex partner during the last 3 months. Screening should be repeated at least annually.

Gonococcal infections also are often asymptomatic in women. For this reason, a primary measure for controlling gonorrhea in the USA has been the screening of high-risk women. Because gonorrhea tends to be spread by a core group, screening the general population is not as effective as screening women with specific risk factors for the infection. Women with a prior history of gonorrhea, prostitutes, young women, and homeless are considered at greater risk for gonorrhea.

With syphilis increasing to epidemic proportions, screening for this disease must be increased. Screening with the low-cost nontreponemal tests such as the rapid plasma reagin (RPR) is appropriate for women who are likely to have had multiple sex partners for short periods of time and patients seen for STDs other than syphilis. Pregnant women should undergo routine serologic screening as a means of preventing congenital syphilis.

The Papanicolaou (Pap) smear is not an effective screening test for STDs. However, a significant proportion of abnormal Pap smears are representative of subclinical genital human papillomavirus (HPV) infection. Whenever a woman has a pelvic examination for STD screening, the health care provider should inquire about the result of her last Pap smear and should emphasize the importance of yearly Pap smears. A Pap smear should be performed for any woman has not had one during the previous 12 months.

Signs & Symptoms

A. Vaginitis: Symptoms associated with vaginitis include an abnormal vaginal discharge, vulvar itching or irritation, and a foul vaginal odor. The three common diseases characterized by vaginitis are vaginal candidiasis, bacterial vaginosis, and trichomonas vaginitis.

B. Genital Ulcer Disease: Genital ulcers are common manifestations in women who present with an STD. Genital herpes, the most common cause of genital ulcer disease in the USA, is characterized by a prodrome of paresthesias 12–48 hours before the appearance of blisters. The mean incubation period is 7 days. Grouped vesicles on an erythematous base are the hallmark of genital herpes. These vesicles rupture, leaving multiple shallow and painful ulcerations. The severity of first episodes of genital herpes varies, depending on whether the patient has been exposed previously to herpes simplex virus (HSV). Primary first-episode disease (no preexisting antibody to HSV) is severe, with multiple painful vesicles and associated lymphadenopathy, myalgia, headache, and fever. The lesions last 2–3 weeks. Nonprimary first-episode and recurrent genital herpes (preexisting antibody to HSV present) present a much milder clinical picture. These patients have many fewer vesicles usually clustered unilaterally on the vulva and disappearing within 3–4 days. No systemic signs are noted in patients with preexisting antibody to HSV.

A common symptom accompanying an outbreak of genital herpes is dysuria. This dysuria is external in nature (splash dysuria). Patients failing to respond to urinary tract antiseptics for a presumptive diagnosis (many times prescribed over the phone) of lower urinary tract infection should be examined to rule out genital herpes.

Despite the association of genital herpes with the symptoms described, most infected women never recognize symptoms suggestive of genital herpes. Some have symptoms shortly after infection and then never again. Most infected women never have recurrent genital lesions.

Syphilis is the second most common cause of genital ulcer disease. The mean incubation period is 3 weeks, and primary disease is characterized by a solitary ulcer called a **chancre.** This chancre is surprisingly painless; it has smooth margins and a firm, palpable (indurated) border. The ulcer base is clean with a serous, not purulent, exudate. Atypical ulcers are common , especially when associated with secondary infection. In women, the external genitalia are the most common site for ulcers. Ulcers may occur in the vagina and on the cervix. Bilateral lymphadenopathy is common.

Secondary syphilis usually occurs about 4–10 weeks after the chancre appears and may manifest as a flulike syndrome and generalized lymphadenopathy. The most prominent feature of secondary syphilis is a generalized maculopapular rash affecting the trunk and limbs, including the palms of the hands and soles of the feet. Condylomata lata, fleshy lesions with a pearly gray appearance, may occur on the genitalia.

Chancroid is rare in the USA. This genital ulcer disease tends to be limited to prostitutes and other women who are at very high risk of STDs. Lesions are usually few (one to three) and are associated with unilateral, tender lymphadenopathy. The ulcers are painful and tend to be deep, "beefy," and purulent; they usually have an irregular, undermined border.

These ulcers have a ragged appearance and can reach the size of a quarter. Lymphadenitis may result in local suppuration and rupture of a lymph node with drainage of pus unilaterally.

Lymphogranuloma venereum (LGV) is also rare in the USA. The ulcer associated with this disease is transient, shallow, and painless and precedes the appearance of bilateral inguinal lymphadenopathy by 7–30 days. Most patients do not notice this subtle ulcer, which may be described better as a fissure. The inguinal lymphadenopathy occurs as a result of multiple enlarged, matted, and tender nodes, which coalesce and result in what has been referred to as the groove sign.

C. Genital Warts: Exophytic genital and anal warts are benign growths most commonly caused by HPV types 6 and 11. Studies from family planning clinics suggest a prevalence of 6%. The incidence of genital warts in a population of patients who have an STD is twice that figure. The total incidence in the USA of HPV infection is much higher: most women with HPV are asymptomatic, with so-called flat condyloma. HPV types 16, 18, 31, 33, and 35 have been associated with squamous intraepithelial lesions of the cervix and cervical cancer.

Most genital warts are seen in young adults. The mean age of onset for women is between 16 and 25 years. Condylomata (warts) generally occur first at the posterior fourchette and adjacent labia; they also may appear on the perineum or perianal area. Occasionally, exophytic condylomata can be seen on the cervix.

D. Pubic Lice and Scabies: Patients with pediculosis pubis (pubic lice) usually seek medical attention because of pruritus or because they notice lice on pubic hair. In addition, many women present for treatment because their sex partners are suspicious of infection. The predominant symptom of scabies is also pruritus.

E. Urethritis: Urethritis, or inflammation of the urethra, is caused by infection characterized by the discharge of mucoid or purulent material and by burning during urination. In women, dysuria is the most common symptom; urethral discharge may be noticed as a vaginal discharge or may be asymptomatic. Although the most common cause of acute dysuria or urgency in women is bacterial cystitis secondary to coliform bacteria, 65% of women with a negative urine culture have a chlamydial infection. Urethral infection with *N gonorrhoeae* is another cause of acute dysuria in women.

F. Mucopurulent Endocervicitis: MPC is characterized by a yellow or green endocervical exudate. The condition is asymptomatic among many women, but some experience an abnormal vaginal discharge, abnormal vaginal bleeding especially after coitus, and pelvic cramping. MPC can be caused by *Chlamydia trachomatis* or by *N gonorrhoeae*, although in most cases neither organism can be isolated.

Clinical Findings & Diagnosis

A. Vaginitis: The diagnosis of vaginitis is made with four clinical tests. These tests include an assessment of the appearance of the vaginal discharge, the pH of the vaginal secretions, microscopy of the vaginal secretions, and the whiff test. The whiff test is positive when the addition of potassium hydroxide to the vaginal secretions results in the volatilization of organic amines, causing a fishy odor.

Patients with vaginal candidiasis have a cottage cheese-like discharge and a normal pH of less than 4.5. Microscopy of the vaginal secretions may show the presence of fungal elements. The whiff test is negative.

Women with bacterial vaginosis have a homogeneous discharge, a pH greater than 4.5, microscopy showing clue cells, and a positive whiff test.

Women with vaginal trichomoniasis commonly show evidence of concurrent BV. Diagnosis of trichomoniasis is based on the appearance of motile trichomonads during microscopy of the vaginal secretions.

B. Genital Ulcer Disease: Diagnostic efforts traditionally are directed at excluding syphilis because of the consequences of inappropriate therapy (the development of tertiary syphilis or, in pregnant women, congenital syphilis). Therefore, a serologic test for syphilis should be obtained in all women with genital ulcer disease. Despite the imprecision of the clinical diagnosis of genital ulcer disease, several presentations are highly suggestive of specific diagnoses: (1) A nonpainful and minimally tender ulcer that is not accompanied by inguinal adenopathy is likely to be syphilis, especially if the ulcer is indurated. (2) Grouped vesicles mixed with small ulcers, particularly in a patient with a history of such lesions, are almost pathognomonic of genital herpes. (3) One to three extremely painful ulcers, accompanied by tender inguinal lymphadenopathy, are unlikely to be anything except chancroid; if the adenopathy is fluctuant, the diagnosis is secured. (4) An inguinal bubo accompanied by one or several ulcers is most likely to be chancroid; if there is no ulcer, the most likely diagnosis is LGV.

In addition to a serologic test for syphilis, a test for herpes simplex virus should be performed in all patients with genital ulcer disease. In areas where chancroid is common, a Gram stain of ulcer exudate may suggest the diagnosis by showing gram-negative rods in a "school of fish" arrangement. These lesions also should be cultured for *Haemophilus ducreyi*. If buboes are present, a diagnostic and therapeutic aspiration through intact skin (not through inflamed skin, for fear of fistula formation) should be performed. The aspirate should be cultured for *H ducreyi* and *C trachomatis*.

C. Genital Warts: Condylomata acuminata are soft, fleshy, vascular lesions first noticed on the vulva. They must be differentiated from condylomata lata, a manifestation of secondary syphilis. In addition, there are epithelial papillae and small sebaceous glands common on the vulva as well as fibroepithelial polyps that can be confused with condylomata acuminata. Consideration of vulvar intraepithelial neoplasia, especially in women with persistent lesions, is important. Vulvar biopsy and serologic testing for syphilis should be performed when there is a question concerning the diagnosis.

D. Pubic Lice and Scabies: Both adult lice and their eggs (nits) are seen easily by the naked eye. On examination of the vulva, lice may be perceived as scabs over what first appear to be excoriations. Nits may be seen on the hairs. Microscopic analysis of the pubic hair can confirm the presence of both adult lice and nits.

Scabies most commonly affect the hands, with characteristic lesions occurring mainly on the finger webs. Women may have eczematous lesions on the breasts or papular lesions on the abdomen, particularly around the umbilicus, and on the lower buttocks in the crease where they join the thigh. The diagnosis can be confirmed by skin scrapings of the unexcoriated papules or burrows. Microscopy confirms the presence of the mite. A shave biopsy of a suspicious papule also may be performed to obtain material for microscopy.

E. Urethritis: The diagnosis of urethritis is based on the clinical symptoms of internal dysuria and urgency. A urinalysis shows evidence of pyuria. Urine culture rules out acute urethral syndrome caused by coliform bacteria or *Staphylococcus saprophyticus*. In high-risk patients and those with a negative urine culture, urethral infection with either *C trachomatis* or *N gonorrhoeae* should be considered and tests for these organisms performed.

F. Mucopurulent Endocervicitis: MPC is characterized by a yellow or green endocervical exudate. Gram stain confirms a predominance of leukocytes, usually greater than 10–30 per oil immersion field. The cervix may be friable (bleeds easily when touched with a cotton swab), erythematous, and edematous. Tests for *C trachomatis* and *N gonorrhoeae* should be performed.

Treatment

A. Vaginitis: The principal goal of therapy is to relieve vulvovaginal symptoms and signs. In patients with trichomoniasis, prevention of transmission is also a goal of therapy. Treatment regimens for vaginitis are noted in Table 37–2.

B. Genital Ulcer Disease: Genital herpes is a viral disease that can be recurrent and has no cure. Systemic acyclovir provides partial control of symptoms and signs of a first clinical episode and may suppress recurrences. Acyclovir does not prevent the

Table 37-2. Regimens for the treatment of vaginitis.*

Bacterial vaginosis
  Recommended:
    Metronidazole, 500 mg orally 2 times daily for 7 days
  Alternatives:
    Metronidazole, 2 g orally in a single dose
    or
    Clindamycin 2% cream, one full applicator (5 g)
      intravaginally at bedtime for 7 days
    Metronidazole 0.75% gel, one full applicator (5 g)
      intravaginally 2 times daily for 5 days
    Clindamycin, 300 mg orally 2 times daily for 7 days
Trichomoniasis
  Metronidazole, 2 g orally in a single dose
  or
  Metronidazole, 500 mg twice daily for 7 days

*Data from MMWR 1993;42:69.

establishment of latent infection and therefore does not prevent recurrent episodes of genital herpes. Topical therapy is substantially less effective than oral therapy, and its use is discouraged. Most women with recurrent genital lesions receive no benefit from intermittent therapy for recurrent episodes unless therapy can be initiated during the prodrome or within 2 days of the onset of lesions. Because recurrent disease tends to be associated with a milder and shorter course of lesions, acyclovir generally is not recommended for women with recurrent disease except for use in suppression.

The recommended regimens for treatment of genital herpes are noted in Table 37-3. Patients desiring therapy for recurrent episodes receive shorter courses of acyclovir than those having a first episode. Daily suppressive therapy reduces the number of recurrences by 75% in patients who have frequent recurrences. Intravenous therapy should be offered to patients with severe disease or with complications of infection necessitating hospitalization, eg, disseminated infection, hepatitis, pneumonitis.

Table 37-3. Acyclovir treatment regimens for genital herpes.*

Episode	Dosage[†] and Duration of Therapy
First	200 mg 5 times daily for 7–10 days[‡]
Recurrent	200 mg 5 times daily for 5 days
	or
	400 mg 3 times daily for 5 days
	or
	800 mg 2 times daily for 5 days
Suppressive	400 mg 2 times daily
	or
	200 mg 3–5 times daily[§]
Severe[‖]	5–10 mg/kg every 8 hours for 5–7 days[‡]

*Data from MMWR 1993;42:23.
[†]Oral administration.
[‡]Or until clinical resolution is attained.
[§]Administer lowest effective dose.
[‖]Intravenous administration.

Patients should be advised to refrain from sexual contact while lesions are present and be informed of the natural history of the disease and risk for subsequent transmission. Transmission usually occurs from an asymptomatic sexual contact who may be unaware that he is infected. The use of condoms should be suggested for future sexual exposures. Women should alert their obstetricians concerning a history of genital herpes so that strategies for the prevention of neonatal transmission can be considered.

Parenteral penicillin G is the preferred drug for treatment of all stages of syphilis. The preparations used (eg, benzathine penicillin), the dosage, and the length of treatment depend on the stage and clinical manifestations of the disease. Parenteral penicillin is the only therapy with documented efficacy for neurosyphilis and for syphilis during pregnancy. Patients with neurosyphilis and pregnant women with syphilis in any stage who report penicillin allergy almost always should be treated with penicillin, preceded by desensitization if necessary. Skin testing for penicillin allergy is helpful since most patients with a history of penicillin allergy are skin-test-negative.

The Jarisch-Herxheimer reaction is an acute febrile reaction, accompanied by headache, myalgia, and other symptoms, that may occur within the first 24 hours after any therapy for syphilis. This reaction is common among patients with early syphilis. Antipyretics are recommended, but there is no proven method for prevention. Recommended regimens for the treatment of the various stages of syphilis are listed in Table 37-4. Quinolones are not active against *Treponema pallidum*. Persons exposed to a patient with syphilis should be evaluated clinically and serologically and treated, even if they are seronegative.

Successful treatment of chancroid cures infection, resolves clinical symptoms, and prevents transmission to others. Recommended regimens for the therapy of chancroid are listed in Table 37-5.

Treatment of LGV cures infection and prevents ongoing tissue damage, although the tissue reaction can result in scarring. Buboes may require aspiration

Table 37-4. Treatment regimens for syphilis.*

Stage	Treatment Regimen
Primary, secondary, or early latent[†]	Benzathine penicillin, 2.4 million units IM
Late latent[‡] or late	Benzathine penicillin, 2.4 million units IM for 3 doses at 1-week intervals (total = 7.2 million units)
Neurosyphilis	Aqueous penicillin G 12–24 million units daily administered as 2–4 million units IV every 4 hours, for 10–14 days

*Data from MMWR 1993;42:30.
[†]Asymptomatic syphilis of less than 1 year in duration
[‡]Asymptomatic syphilis of greater than 1 year in duration

Table 37–5. Treatment regimens for chancroid.*

Recommended:
  Azithromycin, 1 g orally in a single dose
  or
  Ceftriaxone, 250 mg IM in a single dose
  or
  Erythromycin base, 500 mg orally 4 times daily for 7 days
Alternatives:
  Amoxicillin, 500 mg, plus clavulanic acid, 125 mg, orally 3
    times daily for 7 days
  or
  Ciprofloxacin,† 500 mg orally 2 times daily for 3 days

*Data from MMWR 1993;42:21.
†Contraindicated in pregnant and lactating women, children,
and adolescents younger than 18 years of age.

or incision and drainage through intact skin. Doxycycline is the preferred treatment (Table 37–6).

C. Genital Warts: The goal of therapy is removal of exophytic warts and eradication of the signs and symptoms of infection. No therapy has been shown to eradicate HPV infection. It is speculated that HPV infection may persist throughout a patient's lifetime in a dormant state and become infectious intermittently. It has been suggested that genital warts are more infectious than subclinical infection and that the risk of subsequent transmission of HPV can be decreased by removal of the warts. Recurrences of genital warts result more commonly from reactivation of subclinical HPV infection than from reinfection by a sex partner. The effect of treatment on the natural history of genital warts is unknown.

Treatment of genital warts should be guided by patient preference. Expensive therapies, toxic therapies, and procedures that result in scarring should be avoided. Limited numbers of external genital and perianal warts can be treated with cryotherapy with liquid nitrogen or cryoprobe or with electrodesiccation or electrocautery. Topical therapy with podophyllin 10–25%, podofilox 0.5%, and trichloroacetic acid 80–90% also can be used. These chemical treatments should be repeated weekly for as long as lesions persist or for six applications. Lesions persisting for longer than 6 weeks should be treated with other therapies; biopsy should be considered in such patients to rule out intraepithelial neoplasia.

Examination of sex partners is not necessary because the role of reinfection is believed to be minimal. However, sex partners with obvious warts should be counseled to seek treatment because the disease is contagious. The use of condoms may reduce the chance of transmission to new partners who may be uninfected.

D. Pubic Lice and Scabies: The recommended regimens for the treatment of lice and scabies are noted in Tables 37–7 and 37–8, respectively. Sex partners within the past month should be treated.

E. Urethritis and MPC: Urethritis, MPC, and PID can be caused by *C trachomatis* or *N gonorrhoeae* infections. Regimens for the treatment of these pathogens are noted in Tables 37–9 and 37–10, respectively. Because of the high prevalence of coinfection with *C trachomatis* among patients with gonococcal infection, presumptive treatment for *Chlamydia* in patients being treated for gonorrhea is appropriate, particularly if no diagnostic test for *C trachomatis* infection has been performed.

Many antibiotics are safe and effective for treating gonorrhea—eradicating *N gonorrhoeae,* ending the possibility of further transmission, relieving symptoms, and reducing the chances of sequelae. Recommended regimens for the treatment of uncomplicated gonococcal infections are listed in Table 37–10. Selection of a treatment regimen for *N gonorrhoeae* infection requires consideration of the anatomic site of infection, resistance of *N gonorrhoeae* strains to antimicrobials, possibility of coinfection with *C trachomatis,* and side effects and costs of the various treatment regimens. In clinical trials, the recommended regimens cured more than 95% of anal and genital infections; any of the regimens may be used for uncomplicated anal or genital infection. Published studies have indicated that both ceftriaxone, 125 mg, and ciprofloxacin, 500 mg, can cure more than 90% of pharyngeal infections.

Ciprofloxacin or ofloxacin are quinolones and can be used as oral agents for the treatment of gonorrhea. They are less expensive than ceftriaxone. Both agents are contraindicated for pregnant or nursing women and for persons younger than 18 years of age, on the basis of information from animal studies.

Women with gonorrhea should be screened for

Table 37–6. Treatment regimens for lymphogranuloma
venereum (LGV).*

Recommended:
  Doxycycline, 100 mg orally 2 times daily for 21 days
Alternatives:
  Erythromycin, 500 mg orally 4 times daily for 21 days
  or
  Sulfisoxazole, 500 mg orally 4 times daily for 21 days

*Data from MMWR 1993;42:27.

Table 37–7. Treatment of pediculosis pubis.*

Lindane 1% shampoo applied for 4 minutes and then
  thoroughly washed off (not recommended for pregnant or
  lactating women)
or
Permethrin 1% cream rinse applied to affected areas and
  washed off after 10 minutes
or
Pyrethrins with piperonyl butoxide applied to the affected
  area and washed off after 10 minutes

*Data from MMWR 1993;42:94.

Table 37–8. Treatment of scabies.*

Recommended:
  Permethrin cream (5%) applied to all areas of the body
    from the neck down and washed off after 8–14 hours
  or
  Lindane 1% 1 oz of lotion or 30 g of cream applied thinly to
    all areas of the body from the neck down and washed off
    thoroughly after 8 hours
Alternative:
  Crotamiton (10%) applied to the entire body from the neck
    down nightly for 2 consecutive nights and washed off 24
    hours after the second application

*Data from MMWR 1993;42:96.

Table 37–10. Treatment for gonococcal infections.*

Ceftriaxone, 125 mg IM in a single dose
or
Cefixime, 400 mg orally in a single dose
or
Ciprofloxacin, 500 mg orally in a single dose
or
Ofloxacin, 400 mg orally in a single dose
PLUS
A regimen effective against possible coinfection with
  Chlamydia trachomatis, such as doxycycline, 100 mg orally
  2 times daily for 7 days

*Data from MMWR 1993;42:57.

syphilis by serologic study when gonorrhea is first detected. Gonorrhea treatments that include ceftriaxone or a 7-day regimen of doxycycline or erythromycin may cure incubating syphilis, but few data relevant to this topic are available.

A test of cure is not necessary for women treated with the recommended regimens. Women with persistent symptoms should be evaluated by culture for *N gonorrhoeae,* and any gonococci isolated should be tested for antimicrobial susceptibility. Infections following therapy with the regimens mentioned usually are due to reinfection. Persistent symptoms also may be caused by *C trachomatis.*

Sex partners should be evaluated and treated for uncomplicated lower genital tract infection with *N gonorrhoeae* and *C trachomatis.* Patients should be instructed to avoid coitus until both the patient and partner or partners are cured. In the absence of a test of cure, abstinence should continue until treatment is completed and the patient is asymptomatic.

It is not uncommon for clinicians to treat women with acute dysuria and pyuria with antimicrobial therapy appropriate for an uncomplicated lower urinary tract infection. Many of these antimicrobials such as nitrofurantoin have insufficient activity against *Chlamydia* and the gonococcus. It is appropriate to consider the STD pathogens as a cause of these symptoms, especially in high-risk women.

Ideally, patients with MPC should have cervical specimens tested for *Chlamydia* and gonorrhea before they are treated. Treating such women empiri-

Table 37–9. Treatment for chlamydial infections.*

Recommended:
  Doxycycline, 100 mg orally 2 times daily for 7 days
  or
  Azithromycin, 1 g orally in a single dose
Alternatives:
  Ofloxacin, 300 mg orally 2 times daily for 7 days
  or
  Erythromycin base 500 mg orally 4 times daily for 7 days
  or
  Erythromycin ethylsuccinate, 800 mg orally 4 times daily
    for 7 days

*Data from MMWR 1993;42:51.

cally without testing is a reasonable approach, but one must remember that sex partners need to be treated as well. It may be more difficult to involve the sex partner in the treatment program without proof of an STD.

Referral to a Specialist

Two situations suggest the need for specialty consultation when dealing with STDs. First, when the clinician is unsure of the diagnosis, referral is appropriate. Second, when the patient fails to respond to a treatment regimen initiated by the clinician, suggesting either misdiagnosis or antimicrobial resistance, referral is appropriate. Two examples of situations requiring referral follow:

1. A patient with a genital ulcer fails to respond to antimicrobial therapy. Referral results in a biopsy of this ulcer, which reveals squamous cell carcinoma.
2. A patient with trichomonas vaginitis fails to respond to antimicrobial therapy with metronidazole. Reinfection has been ruled out. The possibility of metronidazole-resistant trichomonas is present, requiring vaginal cultures and susceptibility studies. Subsequent therapy is based on the degree of metronidazole resistance in the isolate.

Issues of Pregnancy & Sexually Transmitted Diseases

Genital herpes has special relevance in pregnancy. Active lesions found when a patient presents in labor are an indication for cesarean section. This method of delivery prevents exposure of the neonate to viral shedding and therefore prevents vertical transmission of herpes. Antepartum cultures to detect asymptomatic viral shedding no longer are recommended.

All women should be screened serologically for syphilis during the early stages of pregnancy. Testing should be repeated in the third trimester in high-risk populations. Women delivering stillborn infants after 20 weeks of gestation should be tested for syphilis. Penicillin is effective for preventing transmission to the fetus and for treating established fetal infection.

Pregnant women treated for syphilis in the second half of pregnancy are at risk for preterm labor and fetal distress if their treatment precipitates a Jarisch-Herxheimer reaction. Any change in fetal movement or the onset of uterine contractions should be evaluated.

Pregnant women with pubic lice or scabies should not be treated with lindane. Permethrin or crotamiton regimens are acceptable during pregnancy.

Treatment options for chlamydial endocervicitis during pregnancy do not include the use of doxycycline or ofloxacin. The safety and efficacy of azithromycin among pregnant and lactating women have not been established, but preliminary data are promising. Repeat testing is recommended after therapy with one of the regimens noted in Table 37–11 is completed. Frequent gastrointestinal side effects of erythromycin may discourage a patient from complying with these regimens.

Psychosocial Concerns

Psychological variables are closely associated with STDs. Specific behaviors, such as multiple partners, risky sexual practices, and the context in which sex occurs, are related to STD risk. It is well known that substance abuse can be associated with an increased risk for STD. This abuse is generally thought to be associated with street drugs. However, an important but poorly recognized high-risk behavior involves the use of alcohol in socially acceptable situations such as college mixers. Alcohol abuse can lower one's inhibitions and lead to high-risk sexual behavior.

PELVIC INFLAMMATORY DISEASE

Pelvic inflammatory disease is a major complication of STDs in women. Nearly 150,000 women annually become infertile as a complication of PID. An estimated 50% of 88,000 cases of ectopic pregnancy in 1990 were caused by an STD-related PID.

Table 37–11. Treatment of chlamydia endocervicitis during pregnancy*†

Recommended:
  Erythromycin base, 500 mg orally 4 times daily for 7 days
Alternatives:
  Erythromycin base, 250 mg orally 4 times daily for 14 days
  or
  Erythromycin ethylsuccinate, 800 mg orally 4 times daily for 7 days
  or
  Erythromycin ethylsuccinate, 400 mg orally 4 times daily for 14 days
  or
  Amoxicillin, 500 mg orally 3 times daily for 7–10 days

*Data from MMWR 1993;42:52.
†Test of cure cultures suggested.

Signs & Symptoms

Traditionally, the diagnosis of PID has been applied to patients presenting with lower abdominal pain. It is now well recognized that pain is not necessarily present in patients with PID. Any of the genitourinary symptoms previously described that lead the clinician to consider the presence of *Chlamydia* or gonorrhea should be considered symptoms compatible with a diagnosis of PID. Lower genital tract symptoms of dysuria, urgency, and abnormal vaginal discharge may herald the onset of PID. In addition, symptoms suggesting peritoneal irritation such as pelvic pain should be considered suggestive of PID. Abnormal uterine bleeding, especially breakthrough bleeding in patients taking oral contraceptives, may indicate the presence of endometritis and therefore also is suggestive of PID. Classic symptoms associated with clinically severe PID include fever and lower abdominal pain.

It is important to appreciate the clinical signs associated with the diagnosis of PID. These signs result from the ascending inflammation present in patients with PID. The most important sign is leukorrhea, which is present when a wet mount of the vaginal secretions reveals a predominance of inflammatory cells, namely polymorphonuclear leukocytes. Cervical motion tenderness and adnexal tenderness, usually bilateral but possibly unilateral, reflect the presence of inflammation in the upper genital tract.

If an adnexal mass is found during bimanual pelvic examination and other criteria for the diagnosis of PID are present, the patient should be presumed to have a tuboovarian abscess (TOA). Ultrasonography can be used to characterize the adnexal mass.

Clinical Findings & Diagnosis

PID should be considered in women presenting with any genitourinary symptoms. The finding of leukorrhea in addition to pelvic organ tenderness noted on bimanual pelvic examination suggests the diagnosis of PID. Endometrial biopsy can be used to confirm the presence of upper genital tract inflammation (endometritis). Additional findings of elevated temperature, abdominal tenderness with or without rebound, leukocytosis, and positive tests for *Chlamydia,* gonorrhea, or both, help to increase the specificity of the diagnosis.

Treatment

PID treatment regimens must provide empiric, broad-spectrum coverage of likely pathogens. Antimicrobial coverage should include *N gonorrhoeae, C trachomatis,* gram-negative facultative bacteria, anaerobes, and streptococci (Tables 37–12 and 37–13). Because PID may be due to a polymicrobial flora, a longer duration of therapy is needed than for single infections. Generally speaking, women with mild clinical disease who are able to tolerate oral

Table 37–12. Outpatient treatment for pelvic inflammatory disease.*

Regimen A:
  Cefoxitin, 2 g IM, plus probenecid, 1 g orally in a single
    dose, or ceftriaxone, 250 mg IM, or other parenteral
    third-generation cephalosporin (eg, ceftizoxime or
    cefotaxime)
  PLUS
  Doxycyline, 100 mg orally 2 times daily for 14 days
Regimen B:
  Ofloxacin, 400 mg orally 2 times daily for 14 days
  PLUS
  Clindamycin, 450 mg orally 4 times daily, or metronidazole,
    500 mg orally 2 times daily for 14 days

*Data from MMWR 42:1993.

Table 37–13. Inpatient treatment for pelvic inflammatory disease.*

Regimen A:
  Cefoxitin, 2 g IV every 6 hours, or cefotetan, 2 g IV every
    12 hours
  PLUS
  Doxycycline, 100 mg IV or orally every 12 hours
Regimen B:
  Clindamycin, 900 mg IV every 8 hours
  PLUS
  Gentamicin, loading dose IV or IM (2 mg/kg of body
    weight) followed by a maintenance dose (1.5 mg/kg)
    every 8 hours

*Data from MMWR 42:1993.

therapy can be treated as outpatients. Patients with severe clinical disease should be admitted for observation. Outpatients should be reevaluated in 72 hours to ensure that there is clinical improvement. Hospitalized patients should be treated as inpatients until their fever has lysed, the white blood cell count has normalized, and abdominal and bimanual pelvic examinations reveal marked amelioration of pelvic organ tenderness with the absence of rebound tenderness. Failure to respond to antibiotic therapy requires further diagnostic workup, surgical intervention, or both.

Patients with TOA should be admitted to the hospital for observation and parenteral antibiotic therapy. Either of the inpatient regimens given in Table 37–13 is acceptable. Failure to respond to therapy suggests the need for surgical drainage.

Sex partners of women with PID should be evaluated and treated for lower genital tract infection by *N gonorrhoeae* and *C trachomatis*.

Referral to a Specialist

As in the STDs discussed in this chapter, referral for PID is warranted when the diagnosis is uncertain or treatment is unsuccessful. For example, a patient is treated as an outpatient for PID, but her symptoms persist. A review of her chart reveals that this is her third case of PID, and in no instance was either *N gonorrhoeae* or *C trachomatis* cultured. Referral and diagnostic laparoscopy to confirm the diagnosis and rule out endometriosis are appropriate in this situation.

Issues of Pregnancy & Pelvic Inflammatory Disease

PID is an uncommon complication of pregnancy. Ectopic pregnancy should be ruled out as the most important alternative diagnosis. Laparoscopy should be considered to confirm the diagnosis. This disorder occurs only in the first trimester before fetal membranes have occluded the internal cervical os, thus preventing ascending infection. Doxycycline should not be used to treat pregnant women with PID.

REFERENCES

Centers for Disease Control and Prevention: 1993 Sexually transmitted diseases treatment guidelines. MMWR 1993; 42.
Centers for Disease Control and Prevention: Recommendations for the prevention and management of *Chlamydia trachomatis* infections, 1993. MMWR 1993;42.
Holmes KK et al: *Sexually Transmitted Diseases,* 2nd ed. McGraw-Hill, 1990.
Martin DH (editor): Sexually transmitted diseases. Med Clin North Am 1990;74.
The Alan Guttmacher Institute: Testing positive: Sexually transmitted diseases and the public health response. 1993;4.

Section X.
Musculoskeleton Disorders

38 Fibromyalgia & Myofascial Pain

Faren H. Williams, MD, MS, & Matthew P. Kaul, MD

Musculoskeletal pain has a significant impact on society in terms of personal suffering, cost of health care, and lost productivity. A major portion of visits to physicians involve musculoskeletal complaints, most of which are focal and responsive to treatment. Chronic myofascial pain syndromes, which affect up to 5% of patients seen in a general medicine practice, are complex conditions that are not well understood by many practitioners. These syndromes are characterized by chronic aches, pains, and stiffness in multiple areas of the musculoskeletal system, including articular and periarticular areas, muscles, ligaments, tendon insertions, subcutaneous tissues, and bony prominences. Treatment should be specific for the identified problem and often interdisciplinary in nature. A disproportionate number of patients with chronic myofascial problems apply for disability compensation compared with individuals with other chronic conditions such as rheumatoid arthritis.

Most myofascial pain was referred to as fibrositis until 1978. The term **fibrositis** was coined by Sir William Gowers in 1904, in an article about lumbago. Stockman found edema in muscle biopsies of tender areas of these patients, but others have not found inflammatory cells microscopically. Myofascial pain can be local, regional, or widespread; the diffuse form is referred to as **fibromyalgia.**

FIBROMYALGIA

Because fibromyalgia is a disease without a unifying cause, it is better referred to as a syndrome. Women are affected 10 times more frequently than men, and the course is often chronic with functional disability. Up to 6 million people in the United States are affected by fibromyalgia. Synonyms for fibromyalgia in the older literature include fibrositis, generalized tension myalgia, generalized nonarticular rheumatism, and generalized soft tissue rheumatism.

Essentials of Diagnosis
- History of widespread pain
- Tenderness in at least 11 of 18 tender point sites on digital palpation

---

Etiology & Associated Conditions

Although the cause of fibromyalgia is unknown, in one-fourth to one-half of cases there appears to be an antecedent event. Such events may include injury sustained in a motor vehicle accident or unusual physical activity, recent surgery, other medical problems, a viruslike illness, and emotional or psychological stress. When symptoms occur after a recognizable event, the syndrome is referred to as **reactive fibromyalgia.** Patients with reactive fibromyalgia are more disabled, have more reduced physical activity, are less likely to work, and apply for disability compensation more often than those without a precipitating event.

The presence of fibromyalgia may be concomitant with other medical conditions such as sleep disturbance, chronic fatigue, depression, irritable bowel syndrome, headaches, Raynaud's phenomenon, and mitral valve prolapse. Some patients have an autosomal dominant hereditary disposition to development of the muscle tender points associated with fibromyalgia. Generalized joint hypermobility is associated, especially in children. There may be mechanical or systemic perpetuating factors that encourage involvement of additional muscles and inhibit recovery of those already involved. Fibromyalgia may have an increased incidence in women with hyperprolactinemia.

There is some association between fibromyalgia and infectious agents. Fibromyalgia has been reported after infection with coxsackievirus and parvovirus and after Lyme disease. Eleven to twenty percent of patients with HIV have fibromyalgia. It is detected commonly in patients with chronic fatigue syndrome, which may be caused by a virus. Infectious agents may directly invade tissues releasing cytokines, which can cause severe myalgias, fatigue, and neurocognitive disturbances; however, Buchwald found that the antibody titers to Epstein-Barr virus in patients with those symptoms were no different from those in controls. The infectious episode does not explain why the symptoms of fibromyalgia persist for months or years after the "triggering event." Because persons with chronic infections may become anxious and be advised to rest, avoidance behaviors may follow, leading to inactivity, time loss, sleep disturbances, mood disturbances, and tense muscles. Others who develop fibromyalgia and its associated symptoms remain active and continue working.

Pathophysiology

Patients with fibromyalgia do not have chronically increased levels of muscle enzymes; there are no distinctive electromyographic findings; and biopsies do not show any distinctive histopathologic changes. Metabolic studies have shown that these patients reach an anaerobic threshold at a reasonable workload; their reason for limiting their activity is musculoskeletal pain rather than exhaustion of oxygen uptake. When their muscles are electrically stimulated, patients are found to have normal muscle strength.

Tender areas in the trapezius muscle in patients with fibromyalgia were found to have reduced levels of high-energy phosphates. Pain-free tibialis anterior muscles had normal phosphate levels. In blind muscle biopsy studies, no histochemical and immunoenzymatic abnormalities were found, but nonspecific degenerative changes were detected with electron microscopy. These findings can be seen in other

muscle and rheumatic diseases, with neurogenic atrophy, and with aging.

There appears to be an important peripheral component to the musculoskeletal pain in fibromyalgia. Patients with fibromyalgia experience additional pain for 24–48 hours after activity to which they are unaccustomed. This pain may reflect muscle microtrauma, which may be especially evident at the muscle-tendon junction where there is less capillary perfusion. Other ultrastructural studies have demonstrated shortening of both extra- and intrafusal fibers, resulting in excessive firing of spindle afferents, which may lead to muscle stiffness. If there is a sleep disturbance, the muscles become fatigued and are more susceptible to microtrauma and associated pain.

Serotonin is a recognized chemical mediator of deep sleep and of pain perception by the thalamus and the peripheral nervous system. It alters the function of substance P with reference to interpretation of sensory stimuli. Tryptophan is a precursor to serotonin, and lower postfasting plasma free tryptophan levels have been found in some studies of patients with fibromyalgia. Substance P levels may be elevated in the cerebral spinal fluid.

Low levels of somatomedin C have been reported in patients with fibromyalgia. Somatomedin C is the mediator of the anabolic effects of growth hormone and is involved in muscle homeostasis. It is secreted primarily during stage 4 sleep; therefore, disrupted stage 4 sleep may lead to low levels of somatomedin C and changes in muscle homeostasis, which lead to susceptibility to muscle microtrauma (Fig 38–1).

Signs & Symptoms

In addition to widespread pain and muscle tenderness, the most characteristic symptoms of fibromyalgia are sleep disturbance, fatigue, and morning stiffness. Although these three symptoms are present in 75% of patients with fibromyalgia, the simultaneous presence of the three is not required for diagnosis. Other symptoms include axial pain involving the neck and shoulders, diffuse musculoskeletal pain, paresthesias, frequent headaches, anxiety, sicca symptoms (dry eyes and mouth), diarrhea, constipation, and abdominal cramps. Symptoms are modulated by external factors including noise, fatigue, stress, activity, anxiety, humidity, warmth, cold, poor sleep, and weather changes. Pain is usually worse in the morning or evening; after inactivity; or after vigorous, unaccustomed activity.

Fatigue is experienced by 90% of patients with fibromyalgia. Many patients are light sleepers and awaken "unrefreshed." Sleep electroencephalograms of these patients show an intrusion of alpha waves during stage 4 (non-REM, delta wave) sleep. Because alpha activity is a part of arousal, one experiences a wakeful arousal pattern during periods of what should be deep, restful sleep. This pattern provokes nonrestorative sleep, which may influence the

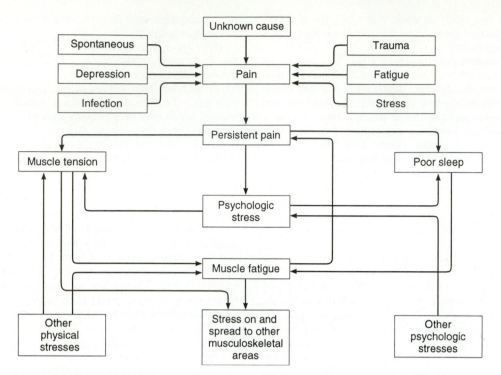

Figure 38–1. "Pathogenesis" for patients. The connecting arrows do not imply cause and effect. The figure serves as an aid for physicians in helping their patients understand and cope with their symptoms. (Reproduced, with permission, from Block SR: Fibromyalgia and the rheumatisms: Common sense and sensibility. Rheum Dis Clin North Am 1993;19:No. 1. 61–78.)

ability to modulate pain, contributing to a lower pain threshold. A stage 4 sleep anomaly is reported in patients with depression, night terror, rheumatoid arthritis, and postaccident pain. It may be related to other factors that are associated with fibromyalgia (Fig 38–2). Insomnia (difficulties falling asleep or maintaining sleep, early morning awakening), tiredness, mood and cognitive disturbances, and muscular pain all have been reported more commonly by patients with fibromyalgia than controls. Fifty-six to ninety-two percent of patients with fibromyalgia report insomnia, compared with 10–30% in a healthy population.

Diagnosis

Widespread pain and tenderness of joints, muscles, or both are the presenting complaints of fibromyalgia. **Widespread pain** is defined by the following criteria: presence of pain for longer than 3 months; presentation above and below the waist as well as on the right and left side of the body; and presence of axial pain (cervical or anterior chest, thoracic spine, or lower back).

The diagnosis requires the finding of tenderness in 11 of 18 tender point sites on digital palpation (Fig 38–3). The most common tender points are bilateral in the following areas: the occiput (at the suboccipital muscle insertions); the low cervical area (at the

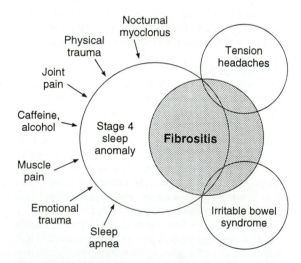

Figure 38–2. An etiologic paradigm for fibrositis. Many initiating factors are hypothesized to impinge on a final common pathway—the induction of a stage IV sleep anomaly. (Reproduced, with permission, from Fan PT, Blanton ME: Clinical features and diagnosis of fibromyalgia. J Musculoskel Med (April) 1992;9(suppl 4):24.)

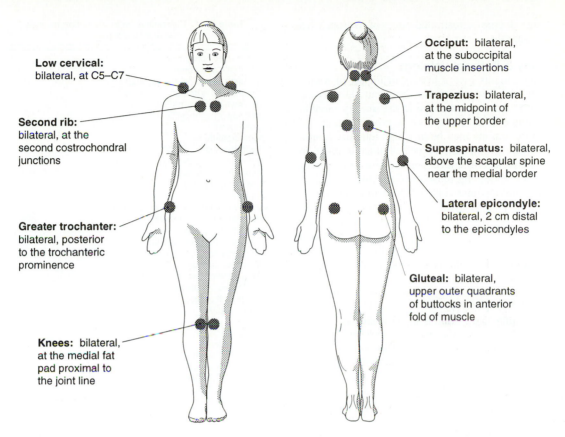

Low cervical: bilateral, at C5–C7

Second rib: bilateral, at the second costrochondral junctions

Greater trochanter: bilateral, posterior to the trochanteric prominence

Knees: bilateral, at the medial fat pad proximal to the joint line

Occiput: bilateral, at the suboccipital muscle insertions

Trapezius: bilateral, at the midpoint of the upper border

Supraspinatus: bilateral, above the scapular spine near the medial border

Lateral epicondyle: bilateral, 2 cm distal to the epicondyles

Gluteal: bilateral, upper outer quadrants of buttocks in anterior fold of muscle

Figure 38–3. Anatomic location of tender points according to the American College of Rheumatology 1990 classification criteria for fibromyalgia. (Reproduced, with permission, from Bennett RM: Fibrositis: Evolution of an enigma. (Editorial.) J Rheumatol 1986;13:4.)

anterior aspects of the intertransverse spaces at C5–7); the trapezius muscle (at the midpoint of the upper border); the supraspinatus muscle (at its origins above the scapular spine near the medial border); the second rib (at the second costochrondral junctions, just lateral to the junctions on the upper surfaces; the lateral epicondyle (2 cm distal to the epicondyle); the gluteal area (in the upper outer quadrants of the buttocks in the anterior fold of muscle); the greater trochanter (posterior to the trochanteric prominence); and the knee (at the medial fat pad proximal to the joint line).

Although these criteria must be satisfied for diagnosis, the presence of a second clinical disorder does not exclude the diagnosis of fibromyalgia. The elicitation of 11 (or more) of 18 possible tender points, together with diffuse pain, discriminates patients with fibromyalgia from those with other soft-tissue problems. The tender point sites are thought to reflect a state of pain amplification or a pain modulation disorder. Patients with fibromyalgia have lower pressure and pain thresholds and tolerances on both muscle and bone than controls. For a tender point to be considered positive, the patient must state that tender-

ness is experienced on palpation with sufficient pressure that causes the examiner's fingernail to turn white.

MYOFASCIAL PAIN SYNDROME

Myofascial pain syndrome (MPS), in contrast to fibromyalgia, affects men and women equally and is more of a regional condition. The term **myofascial** was coined by Dr. Janet Travell after she observed a muscle fiber twitch in response to light stroking of the muscle fascia at open biopsy. MPS tends to have a more sudden onset than fibromyalgia, and the pain is of musculoskeletal origin.

Essentials of Diagnosis
• Complaint of regional pain
• Report of pain or altered sensation in the expected distribution of referred pain from a myofascial trigger point (TrP)
• Taut band palpable in an accessible muscle
• Exquisite spot tenderness at one point along the length of the taut band

- Some degree of restricted range of motion, when measurable

Etiology & Pathophysiology

Many patients give a history of impact or trauma of sufficient force to cause acute muscle overload and subtle structural damage to the sensory modulation pathways in the central nervous system. Although the trauma may be of a high intensity (contusions, strains, or sprains), repeated, microtraumas are more frequent. As the condition progresses, it involves the remaining muscles of the functional muscle unit and becomes regional. Structural abnormalities can perpetuate myofascial syndromes. Examples include a short leg, a small hemipelvis, a short arm, or relatively long second and short first metatarsal bones. MPS may be confused with other regional pain syndromes including sciatica, tennis elbow, and cervical root irritation.

Signs & Symptoms

Fatigability and morning stiffness are not as common in MPS as in fibromyalgia, and tender points occur within an area of regional pain. Trigger points, or sites that refer pain, may be identified on examination. Muscle trigger points are locally tender regions in taut bands of muscle that usually refer pain, tenderness, and dysesthesias to distant areas. Myofascial pain syndrome tends to be less chronic than fibromyalgia, and it often remits with limited therapy.

Diagnosis

Besides the major criteria for diagnosis of myofascial pain, which are listed in the section preceding, Essentials of Diagnosis, there are three minor criteria: (1) reproduction of the clinical pain or altered sensation by pressure on the tender spot; (2) elicitation of a local twitch response by transverse snapping palpation at the tender spot or by needle insertion into the tender spot in the taut band; and (3) alleviation of pain by elongation (stretching) of the muscle or by injecting the tender spot.

DIFFERENTIAL DIAGNOSIS

Fibromyalgia and regional myofascial pain syndrome may represent different ends of a spectrum; because there is much overlap between the two problems, the approach to differential diagnosis outlined in Table 38–1 needs to be considered when patients are evaluated for either problem.

A classification of soft-tissue problems into localized, regional, and generalized groups, as shown in Table 38–2, helps to illustrate the similarities and differences among different pain syndromes. The features distinguishing a regional pain syndrome from generalized fibrositis (fibromyalgia) are listed in Table 38–3.

Table 38–1. Differential diagnosis of fibromyalgia and myofascial pain.

Inflammatory conditions
  Sjogren's syndrome
  systemic lupus erythematosus
  rheumatoid arthritis
  polymyalgia rheumatica
  ankylosing spondylitis
  polymyositis
Endocrinopathies
  hypothyroidism
  hyperparathyroidism
  hyperprolactinemia
Metabolic myopathy
Viral infections
Human immuodeficiency virus (HIV)
Paraneoplastic syndromes
Somatoform disorders
  Psychogenic pain disorder
  Conversion disorder
  Hypochondriasis
  Somatization disorder
Neurological problems
  Peripheral neuropathy
  Radiculopathy
  Sciatica
  Myopathy
Enthesopathies
Bursitis, Tendonitis
Widespread osteoarthritis
Osteopenia, Osteomalacia
Parkinson's disease

Table 38–2. Classification of soft-tissue problems.

Localized
  Bursitis and tendinitis (pathologically well defined)
    Acute, eg, gout
    Subacute, eg, trauma
    Chronic, eg, rheumatoid
  Chronic bursitis and tendinitis-like syndromes
    Repetitive motion
    Cumulative trauma
    Functional
    Overuse
Regional
  Acute and subacute regional musculoskeletal painful
    events
  Chronic
    Chest wall pain-costochondritis
    TMJ syndrome
    Myofascial pain syndromes
    Tension headaches
    Pelvic pain
Generalized
  Transient events
  Chronic
    Fibromyalgia
    Chronic fatigue syndrome
    Irritable bowel syndrome
    Postviral syndromes
    Premenstrual syndrome

Table 38–3. Features distinguishing a regional pain syndrome from generalized fibrositis.*

Feature	Myofascial Pain (Local Fibrositis)	Fibrositis (Generalized Fibrositis)
Sex	M:F ratio	M:F ratio 1:10
Site of pain	Regional	Widespread
Easy fatigability	Unusual	Prominent
Morning stiffness	Regional	Generalized
Trigger points (ie. a tender area causing referred pain)	Invariable, a necessity for the diagnosis	May occur as part of an associated myofascial pain syndrome
Tender points (ie. a tender area without referral of pain)	Occur in a limited area within the area of regional pain	Widespread—a necessity for the diagnosis
Response to therapy	Responds to local anesthetic injections and the technique of "spray and stretch"	Seldom responds to any single therapeutic method
Natural course	Usually remits, often causes dysfunction for a limited period of time	Seldom remits, pursues a chronic course of waxing and waning pain with functional disability

*(Reproduced, with permission, from Bennett RM: Fibrositis: Evolution of an enigma (Editorial). J Rheumatol 1986;13:676.)

CLINICAL FINDINGS

The following sections address the workup and treatment of patients with either fibromyalgia or regional myofascial pain. Because the two conditions appear to represent points on a continuum, with myofascial pain at one end and fibromyalgia at the other, their medical and psychological assessments and treatment are similar. Making the definitive diagnosis is more difficult than treating the symptoms and not as important as it is in diagnosing a life-threatening illness. It is crucial, however, that the physician rule out other diagnoses that may have a worse prognosis and require different treatment.

Medical History

The medical history should focus on pertinent questions regarding function and pain. Open-ended questions allow patients to describe their pain in their own words. Any initiating event should be described in detail. Specific symptoms such as anxiety, headaches, numbness or tingling, and dizziness should be included, and location of pain should be documented. A pain diagram can be helpful (Fig 38–4). When there are multiple sites of pain, these should be localized, and the patient should be asked which is the most painful. Other neuromusculoskeletal illness can occur in patients with fibromyalgia or myofascial pain, and questions that help rule out other problems are important.

Pain may be experienced with activity (postexertional pain) or worsen 24–48 hours after activity. Factors that perpetuate or exacerbate the pain should be identified. The physical and postural issues of daily activities, including work, household chores, and avocational activities, should be addressed. Ongoing stressors, both at work and home, should be discussed. These may include issues concerning relationships, children, or finances. The patient's sleep habits, including difficulties falling asleep and maintaining sleep and early morning awakening, are im-

portant. The patient should be asked whether she feels refreshed in the morning. A drug history including medications (types, dosages, and frequency), smoking, and alcohol consumption needs to be obtained. Other associated conditions such as irritable bowel syndrome and tension headaches should be described in detail (see Fig 38–2).

Physical Examination

A. Inspection: The patient with trigger points (TrPs) often shows asymmetries of the body, postural deviations, reduced mobility of one or more joints, and typical postural attitudes of protective antalgic character. The examiner should look for muscle symmetry or asymmetry and atrophy. Any erythema or edema over muscles or joints should be noted.

B. Muscle Palpation: It is beneficial to begin palpating the muscles in a gentle, less painful area first to put the patient at ease and help establish rapport. Muscles harboring TrPs should be palpated using either a flat hand or a pincer motion, depending on the configuration of the muscle. Sufficient pressure must be used with palpation to produce whitening of the examiner's fingernail. The clinician should search for taut bands within the muscles and try to localize the TrPs within the bands (Fig 38–5). There are characteristic sites where myofascial TrPs are found, and there are established tender point (TeP) sites; of the nine established TeP sites, all but two are located over a TrP site in a muscle. The only non-TrP tender sites are the greater trochanter and the medial fat pad of the knee. When trigger points are palpated, they produce referred pain. These patterns do not follow the usual pathways of peripheral nerves, dermatomes, blood vessels, or sclerotomes. Palpation may cause the patient to jump, which is termed a positive "jump sign," and may produce localized erythema.

C. Joint Palpation: With myofascial pain, active synovitis is not found. The surface temperature of muscles and joints should be noted. Any tempera-

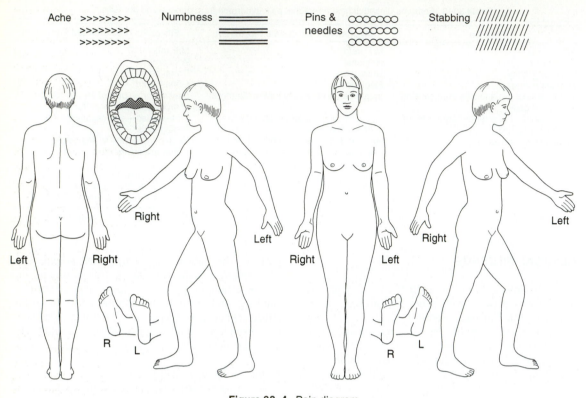

Figure 38–4. Pain diagram.

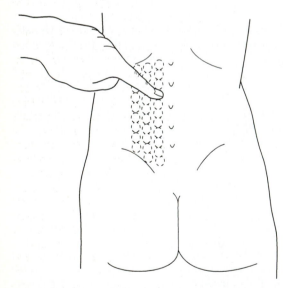

Figure 38–5. Method of palpating one side of the back in a patient in whom a myofascial syndrome is suspected. The second finger is pressed forcefully and deeply to detect trigger points in the deep muscles. The entire area of pain should be palpated systematically as indicated by the confluent circles above, below, and to the side of the palpating finger. (Reproduced, with permission, from Bonica JJ (editor): Pain in the low back, hips and lower extremities. In: *The Management of Pain*. Lea & Febiger, 1990.)

ture differences should be described, because an inflammatory process may be suggested.

D. Range of Motion: Both active (how far the patient can move on her own) and passive (the amount of motion the examiner can obtain) range of motion (ROM) of painful joints should be measured. Neck, back, and hip ROM are especially important to obtain, because limitations may occur in different planes.

Muscle strength should be evaluated carefully because weakness may occur secondary to chronic muscle overload. Some weakness may be related to muscle atrophy from disuse. A standardized manual muscle test should be done for all major muscle groups. The commonly accepted terms for the evaluation of muscle strength are as follows:

0/5	No muscle contraction
1/5	Trace contraction
2/5	Less than antigravity strength
3/5	Antigravity strength
4/5	Limited resistance possible
5/5	Normal muscle strength

With myofascial syndromes, muscle strength is usually in the 4/5–5/5 range. There may be evidence for "giveway weakness," which is a feeling of jerkiness that is associated commonly with functional problems. Circumferential measurements of muscles provide objective evidence for muscle atrophy.

Neurologic Examination

A detailed examination should include deep tendon reflexes (DTRs) and other tests to rule out an upper motor neuron problem. A detailed sensory examination including vibration and proprioception should be performed. The neurologic examination is normal in patients with both fibromyalgia and myofascial pain syndrome.

A. Gait: Abnormalities of gait should be sought, from the shoulder, to the trunk, to the hips, and to the foot placement during the gait cycle. Posture is important to describe in a variety of positions, including sitting, standing, and walking.

B. Waddell's Signs: These signs are associated with functional problems more than with physiologic abnormalities and help to differentiate organic disease from conditions that may have an organic component but should also be evaluated for psychological impairment. These signs are as follows:

1. Superficial nonanatomic tenderness.
2. Positive simulation response–Light axial loading of the head should not increase lower back pain significantly.
3. Distraction–Leg pain elicited with straight leg raising should be present whether the patient is sitting or supine.
4. Nonphysiologic regional disturbances of sensation, distribution of pain, or weakness.
5. Overreaction–Responses such as excessive verbalization, facial grimacing, and other pain behaviors out of proportion to the test stimulus and the findings of the history and physical examination.

Eliciting three or more of these signs warrants psychosocial assessment.

Laboratory Tests

Laboratory tests should be obtained if there is suspicion of an underlying systemic problem. Commonly ordered tests include the following:

Erythrocyte sedimentation rate
Antinuclear antibody test (ANA)
Rheumatoid factor
Thyroid-stimulating hormone
Muscle enzymes
Prolactin level (if there is breast discharge or infertility)

Although these tests are usually normal in patients with myofascial syndromes, a subset of patients with Raynaud's phenomenon may have a positive ANA; it may be a low titer with a nonspecific pattern. The

test results provide the patient with reassurance that she does not have a more serious illness.

Electrodiagnostic studies and muscle biopsies do not reveal abnormalities and are not indicated, except to help exclude other muscle problems. Figure 38–6 provides an algorithm for the diagnosis of fibromyalgia.

Imaging

X-rays usually are not indicated because they do not reveal any acute or structural abnormalities other than age-related degenerative changes or chronic problems such as scoliosis. Reviewing available x-rays with the patient or obtaining x-rays in difficult cases helps to reassure and educate the patient.

Magnetic resonance imaging (MRI) is not helpful except to rule out underlying pathologic conditions. Again, reviewing available scans with the patient helps to reassure her. The low yield of these relatively expensive tests needs to be explained to the patient.

Psychological Findings

Because most of the psychological literature predates the 1990 classification by the American College of Rheumatology, the term fibrositis commonly is found. The patients studied were more likely than others to have chronic psychological problems. It is generally accepted, however, that patients with fibromyalgia have similar psychopathologic profiles to patients with other chronic pain conditions.

The most common comorbid psychiatric disorder is major depression, which is found in 20% of patients. Depression is 3–4 times more prevalent in patients with fibromyalgia than in the general population. Other comorbid disorders include somatization disorder, panic disorder, and obsessive-compulsive disorder. Within the general population of patients with chronic pain, women with fibromyalgia are more likely to have current depression than those with other pain syndromes. Women are as likely as men to have current depression with fibromyalgia.

Some patients have major affective disorders associated with fibromyalgia. Minnesota Multiphasic Personality Interview (MMPI) scores of fibromyalgia patients are higher on the hysteria, hypochondriasis, and depression scales than controls, but the variability in these scores is great. Other investigators have identified a sense of helplessness in fibromyalgia patients; the patients believed their symptoms depended on uncontrollable events and that they could not influence their disease.

A detailed psychosocial history including sexual abuse and physical or emotional trauma or neglect should be obtained. If any specific problems are noted, further evaluation by a psychologist is helpful to determine the need for psychological intervention.

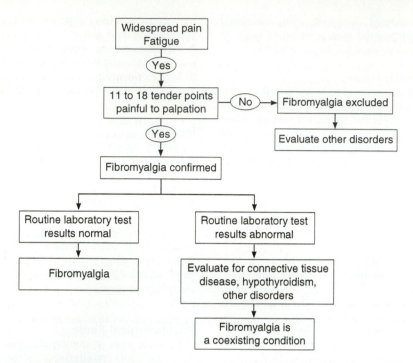

Figure 38–6. Algorithm for the diagnosis of fibromyalgia. (Reproduced, with permission, from Fan PT, Blanton ME: Clinical features and diagnosis of fibromyalgia. J Musculoskel Med (April) 1992;9(Suppl 4):24.)

TREATMENT

Differences in treatment of patients with fibromyalgia and myofascial pain syndrome are related to the acuteness of the problem rather than the specific diagnosis. As in most medical problems, the key to successful medical management is treatment of the symptoms.

Treatment of fibromyalgia should be individualized depending on symptoms and their effects on the individual. Unaccustomed physical activity and stress exacerbate symptoms universally and need to be identified. Strategies useful in chronic pain management may be applied in fibromyalgia. Because a substantial placebo response has been reported in drug trials with fibromyalgia patients, evaluation of interventional studies is difficult.

Education

Education is the first and most important facet of treatment. Patients should know the theories about underlying pathophysiologic mechanisms and be informed of the chronic but nonprogressive nature of the syndrome. Spouses and close members of the patients' support network need to be educated so that they can help identify what activities exacerbate or alleviate symptoms. It is important for patients to know that fibromyalgia may be associated with other rheumatologic conditions but that it usually is not associated with the development of other pathologic conditions. The patient should understand the symptoms associated with fibromyalgia but be instructed not to assume that all symptoms are specific for fibromyalgia. For example, hand numbness may occur with fibromyalgia, but it could be carpal tunnel syndrome or a cervical radiculopathy and may require further evaluation by a physician. Many patients with fibromyalgia have had extensive workups including MRI, and their symptoms have been attributed incorrectly to a degenerated or herniated disk. Patients need to understand that 20–30% of pain-free persons have abnormal MRI scans that show herniations or disk degeneration.

Exercise

Exercise has modest effects on some symptoms of fibromyalgia. Although exercise may not affect pain scores, a marked improvement in symptoms was found to be more likely in those who exercised compared with those in a control group who mainly stretched. Exercise does increase tender point pain threshold, but it may not correlate with symptomatic improvement. Fibromyalgia symptoms could be induced more readily in unfit than in physically fit patients. Clearly, exercise reduces pain in some patients who have fibromyalgia.

Clinicians generally recommend some type of low-impact exercise such as walking, biking, or swimming for 20–30 minutes between 3 and 5 times per week for patients suffering from fibromyalgia. In myofascial pain or asymmetric fibromyalgia, stretching and strengthening may be indicated to reduce tissue hypertonus, reduce the threshold for symptom exacerbation, and improve restrictions in range of motion. Progressive resistive exercises, in which weights are increased slowly and repetitively, may help some patients but may not be tolerated by others. The key is to start slowly and make small, incremental advances in weight and repetitions over time. In patients who must maintain static work positions, a regular stretching program throughout the day every 1–2 hours is advised.

Sleep Hygiene

Sleep hygiene begins with improved habits. Patients should go to sleep and wake up at the same time every day. Caffeine should be used sparingly, especially at night. The bedroom should be quiet, and the bed should be used for sleeping, not for watching television.

If noise is a problem, the patient should use earplugs or sleep in a quieter room. Antidepressants that improve non-REM sleep should be considered. Drugs that may disrupt sleep should be avoided. These include appetite suppressants, antiemetics, and sedative hypnotics, which can exacerbate sleep apnea. Potentially addicting drugs such as benzodiazepines should not be prescribed.

Smoking

Smoking may contribute to a higher frequency of many types of musculoskeletal problems. Although the mechanism of action is not entirely clear, it is known that cigarettes cause constriction of blood vessels, which may lead to some muscle ischemia. Patients should be encouraged to quit smoking, and appropriate interventions should be suggested.

Alcohol Use

Excessive alcohol use adversely affects sleep stages, increases the risk of depression, may interact with medications prescribed for fibromyalgia, and leads to stress within relationships. All of these factors may lead to an exacerbation of fibromyalgia. Therefore, it is recommended that alcohol be used in moderation. Substance abuse programs should be considered first-line treatment if indicated.

Medications

The most commonly prescribed and studied medications for these conditions are the tricyclic antidepressants. Cyclobenzaprine is a muscle relaxant with a chemical structure similar to that of the tricyclics and can be equally effective. The dosages are usually lower than those effective for treatment of depression. If taken consistently, this drug is associated with clinical improvement in 25–45% of fibromyalgia patients. Typical dosages for tricyclics are 10–50 mg or more at bedtime; for cyclobenzaprine, a typi-

cal dosage is 10–40 mg/d in single or divided doses. Improvement in sleep is more common than reduction of pain, but decreasing fatigue allows the patient to be more active, which in time leads to a healthier, less stressful life-style. If there are adverse side effects such as morning tiredness, the patient should be directed to take these medications 1–2 hours before bedtime. In most cases, the side effects subside after 1–2 weeks of daily drug use. Therefore, patient education is extremely important for compliance with prescribed drugs.

Serotonin uptake inhibitors have been found useful for fibromyalgia in preliminary studies in Europe, but they have not been studied systematically yet. They are prescribed frequently for fibromyalgia, nevertheless, and some patients appear to obtain an analgesic response.

Nonsteroidal anti-inflammatory drugs (NSAIDs) and steroids provide little benefit, except for acute conditions. Long-term use of these drugs should be discouraged because of their limited effectiveness and their potential for adverse side effects.

The role of narcotic analgesics in chronic pain is controversial. There may be a role for their use in circumstances such as occasional exacerbations. Escalating doses, addiction, depression, and poor ability to function in society are causes for concern about narcotic use. A history of substance abuse is a relative contraindication to their use.

Injections

Trigger point injections usually are not helpful in fibromyalgia, but they are an accepted treatment for myofascial pain. The key concepts in this therapy are the local twitch response (LTR) and the taut band. The latter is an area in muscle with decreased tissue compliance in which resides the **trigger point.** Needle insertion in this area can elicit an LTR and reproduce pain symptoms. After injecting the trigger point with 1 mL of 0.5% procaine (or a similar agent), the LTR no longer can be elicited and symptoms are relieved. Both short- and long-term pain relief frequently are obtained, with the best response from the regions that have fewer (two to four) trigger points. Naloxone reverses the short-term analgesic effects of injections. Cortisone is not recommended for injection because of myotoxicity. Contraindications to trigger point injections include acute trauma, allergy to the anesthetic injected, bleeding diathesis, and presence of cellulitis. Another contraindication is unfamiliarity of the clinician with the anatomy of the area. Injection near the occiput could cause vertebral artery damage. Injection into the chest may cause a pneumothorax.

Biofeedback

Biofeedback is a form of relaxation therapy. Surface recorded electromyographic signals from muscles are displayed on a monitor and used to help the patient learn how to reduce muscle tension voluntarily. Patients receiving biofeedback may demonstrate significant improvements in symptoms. A significant benefit is maintained when patients are assessed 6 months later.

PROGNOSIS

Patients with fibromyalgia often are more debilitated than those with myofascial pain because of its chronic and diffuse nature. The literature on natural history varies; some authors have reported that 85% of patients continue to meet the criteria for fibromyalgia and 60% have worse symptoms 4 years after initial diagnosis. Others have found remission in up to 24% and that up to 47% no longer meet the American College of Rheumatology criteria for fibromyalgia 2 years after diagnosis. In the latter study, in which a more favorable outcome was reported, regular physical exercise rather than drugs or specific physical therapies correlated highly with decreased symptoms. The differences described also may reflect differences in severity of disease.

REFERRAL TO A SPECIALIST

Physiatrist

Patients who have symptoms consistent with fibromyalgia or myofascial pain should be referred to a physiatrist (physical medicine and rehabilitation specialist) when they do not respond to appropriate treatment within a few weeks. Patients whose symptoms began after a motor vehicle accident or work-related injury may benefit from earlier referral, because physiatrists are familiar with issues related to litigation and worker's compensation. Patients who receive specialized treatment may be able to return to gainful employment sooner than otherwise, and more chronic problems may be prevented. Physiatrists are leaders of multidisciplinary teams that include physical, occupational, and speech therapists; psychologists; and vocational counselors; they can prescribe the most appropriate exercises and arrange for vocational evaluations. They reevaluate the treatment plan with the various therapists as therapy progresses and work with the patient to minimize disability by suggesting possible modifications in the home environment or workplace that may allow the patient to function with less pain. If the patient does not respond to the usual treatment, the physiatrist can make further recommendations for medical evaluation.

Psychotherapist

Psychological assessment and treatment may be helpful in patients who have severe symptoms, those with poor coping skills, and those with anger and hostility. Pain management techniques that can be learned include various coping and relaxation techniques, pacing, and identification of activities that exacerbate symptoms. Because interpersonal relationships may be affected, the involvement of relatives or partners in counseling is recommended. Many of the psychological aspects of fibromyalgia are the sequelae of chronic pain rather than of significant psychopathologic conditions.

Treatment of uncomplicated depression involves appropriate counseling and use of antidepressants. The low doses of antidepressants frequently used for their analgesic or sleep modulating effects are not adequate treatment for depression, although they help alleviate some of the symptoms of fibromyalgia. Higher dosages of tricyclics or use of other antidepressants may be helpful. Successful treatment of depression frequently is accompanied by decreased pain levels in patients with chronic pain, but pain relief may not occur in fibromyalgia even with treatment of the depression.

Patients who have **reactive fibromyalgia,** in which symptoms develop after a specific traumatic event, frequently harbor resentment toward another person. Because these patients become more disabled, the problem should be identified and dealt with early. A multidisciplinary management approach should be instituted at the earliest sign of dysfunction in the social, vocational, psychological, or medical area.

CONCLUSION

Chronic problems such as those associated with fibromyalgia require an intense, coordinated, multidisciplinary approach to treatment, whereas the myofascial pain syndromes can be treated more focally. Worry about illness or sense of vulnerability to illness is correlated with physical disability in patients with chronic disease. Patients may limit their activity beyond what is reasonable because of their uncertainty with regard to the diagnosis and the relative lack of reassurance from their physicians. This inactivity coupled with ongoing worry may lead to depression and more somatic symptoms.

Education is the most important aspect of any treatment program and may need to be reinforced by direct patient-physician communication, provision of reading material about fibromyalgia and myofascial pain, and referral to support groups. Without these adjuncts, patients may overuse the health care system looking for a more definitive diagnosis and undergo expensive, time-consuming, and unnecessary tests.

REFERENCES

Bennett RM: Fibromyalgia and the facts: Sense or Nonsense. Rheumatic Disease Clinics of North America. 1993;19:45.

Bennett RM: Fibrositis: Evolution of an enigma. (Editorial.) J Rheumatol 1986;13:676.

Block SR: Fibromyalgia and the rheumatisms: Common sense and sensibility. In: Rheumatic Disease Clinics of North America, 1993; 19, No.1., 61-78.

Bonica JJ (editor): *The Management of Pain.* Lea & Febiger, 1990.

Buchwald D, Komaroff AL: Review of laboratory findings for patients with chronic fatigue syndrome. Rev Inf Dis 1991;13(Suppl 1):45.

Fan PT, Blanton ME: Clinical features and diagnosis of fibromyalgia. J Musculoskel Med (April) 1992;9(Suppl 4):24.

Greenfield S, Fitzcharles JA, Esdaile JM: Reactive fibromyalgia syndrome. Arthritis Rheum 1992;35:678.

Mikkelsson M et al: Muscle and bone pressure pain threshold and pain tolerance in fibromyalgia patients and controls. Arch Med Rehabil 1992;73:814.

Robbins JM, Kirmayer LJ: Illness worry and disability in fibromyalgia syndrome. Int J Psychiatry Med 1990; 21:49.

Russell IJ, Orr MD, Littman B: Elevated cerebral spinal fluid levels of substance P in patients with fibromyalgia. Arthritis and Rheumatism 1994;37:1593.

Travell JG, Simons DF: Myofascial pain and dysfunction: The trigger point manual. Williams & Wilkins, 1992.

Wolfe F et al: The American College of Rheumatology 1990 Criteria for the Classification of Fibromyalgia. Report of the Multicenter Criteria Committee. Arthritis Rheum 1990;33:160.

Yunus M et al: Primary fibromyalgia (fibrositis): Clinical study of 50 patients with matched normal controls. Semin Arthritis Rheum 1981;11:151.

39

Sports Medicine

Margot Putukian, MD

The history of women in sport certainly has been interesting. In 1908, the New York Times reported that the United States Olympic Committee was "opposed to women taking part in any event in which they could not wear skirts." Thankfully, time has proved that women can participate and excel in sport at every level.

More and more girls and women are becoming physically active, taking part in organized athletics, and enjoying a healthy, active life-style. Involvement in sport is beneficial not only for improving health and decreasing risk factors for disease, but also for personal development and mental well-being. Although the medical care of athletes does not differ significantly from that of the general population, there are some considerations that make athletes a special population. Female athletes have specific issues to deal with such as exercise in pregnancy, menstrual dysfunction, and eating disorders as well as nutritional and musculoskeletal factors.

Exercise can play a role in decreasing the risk factors for coronary heart disease, with its effect on the lipid profile, body mass index, and diabetes mellitus. Because coronary heart disease is the leading cause of death in women, accounting for 28% of all fatalities, an exercise program is an essential component of preventive and rehabilitative medicine for women. For many individuals, exercise also provides an opportunity for social interaction and personal growth.

The physiologic responses to strengthening and conditioning are the same in women and men, as are the types of muscle fibers utilized and the ability to metabolize fat. Although there is an absolute difference in some of these variables, such as maximal oxygen uptake, these differences disappear when related to lean body weight. Similarly, although the absolute increase in muscle size in response to strength training is larger in men than women, it is the same when lean body mass is taken into account. Relative changes in other physiologic variables in response to exercise, such as heart size, volume, and metabolism, are similar in men and women.

Although it is clear that the benefits of exercise and competitive athletics transcend gender, it is unclear what the effects are of competitive exercise on the female reproductive, endocrinologic, and musculoskeletal systems. Most of the information used in

---

Preparticipation Physical Examination
  History
  Physical Examination
Clinical Musculoskeletal Problems

---

the field of sports medicine has been gleaned from studies of men; however, there is new information being obtained that relates specifically to active women. Examples of these issues are exercise in pregnancy and the **female athlete triad,** which includes menstrual dysfunction, eating disorders, and osteoporosis (see Chapters 9 and 10, respectively).

PREPARTICIPATION PHYSICAL EXAMINATION

A warning is found on many pieces of exercise equipment to consult a physician before beginning any exercise program. In addition, most school-age children are required to obtain a physical examination before participating in their sport. The focus of the chapter is on the examination for participation in sports or exercise, with emphasis on concerns of female athletes.

The preparticipation physical examination for girls in school is different from that of older women, and health care providers need to be familiar with the problems and issues that face each age group. In addition, different activities have different demands, which must be taken into account when making recommendations. For example, the demands on a competitive cross-country runner are different from those on a soccer player and certainly different from those on an obese individual who wants to initiate an exercise program such as walking. To be effective, the health care provider needs to understand the goals of the individual, attain a thorough medical history, and perform a complete physical examination. At that point, recommendations regarding activity can be individualized and allow for safe and enjoyable participation in sport.

The preparticipation physical examination is one of the most important responsibilities for physicians, yet in many instances it receives little attention.

School-age children often are seen in a group setting where loud gymnasium rooms do not allow for appropriate cardiac examinations or discussions of personal health issues such as sexuality, drug use, and weight control. On the other hand, individual examinations with a physician who is not familiar with the demands of the contemplated activity are not adequate either. Both office and group (or "station") settings for the preparticipation examination have their advantages and disadvantages, but both can be effective if done properly.

The timing of the preparticipation examination is also important. It should be done early enough to allow for follow-up tests, rehabilitation, and consultations, if necessary, yet close enough to the start of participation to be relevant. In general, a time frame of 2–6 weeks before the beginning of the activity is recommended. For school-age athletes, repeat examinations often are performed when a new level of school is reached, eg, middle school, high school, or college. In addition, a repeat examination is indicated if there is a new medical problem, significant injury has occurred, or the student has requested one. An interim physical examination form can be used. Examples of forms suitable for a university setting are shown in Appendices D and E.

History

The history component of the preparticipation physical examination should target the cardiovascular, neurologic, and musculoskeletal systems. The history also should obtain information about any ongoing or previous medical problems, prior surgery, medications, and allergies; emergency contacts should be noted. Additional questions are often helpful in targeting issues that pertain to specific age groups. For older girls and women, questions that relate to menstrual function, osteoporosis, pulmonary and cardiovascular risk factors, medical problems, and medications are important. For younger girls, questions that relate to sexuality, recreational drug use, and the components of the female athlete triad are important. Asking these questions demonstrates to the young athlete that the physician feels these issues are important and appropriate to discuss. For many athletes, the preparticipation physical examination can serve as an introduction to the health care system and provide the basis of a physician-patient relationship that can help foster the behaviors of a healthy life-style.

Other areas of importance in the preparticipation physical examination include history of an absent organ that is supposed to be paired (ie, one kidney, one ovary), seasonal allergies, medication use, and medical problems that may have an impact on the proposed exercise regimen. For example, exercise can be beneficial in the management of diabetes and asthma, but precautions are necessary to optimize participation. It is important to emphasize the benefits of being involved. At times, people have exercise goals that are not realistic, such as an older patient with degenerative arthritis and osteoporosis who wants to start roller-blading because her grandchildren enjoy it. The recommendations given to the patient must be individualized, realistic, and geared to the person's goals.

Tailoring the preparticipation physical examination to female athletes requires an understanding of the issues that are important and unique to this group, such as nutrition as it relates to health and performance, the effect of exercise on the menstrual cycle, and the high incidence of eating disorders among athletes.

A. Nutrition: The field of sports nutrition has gained increased interest. Athletes are seeking the advice of nutritionists in an attempt to maximize their performance, and a great deal of research is going on in the area. The specific nutritional needs of women should be addressed in the preparticipation physical examination, including total caloric intake and intake of calcium, protein, fat, and iron. It is also important to consider nutrition when an athlete presents with symptoms of fatigue, burnout, and recurrent minor injuries. Constant dieting unfortunately has become acceptable for girls and women, and athletes often attempt to lose weight to improve performance. Numerous studies have demonstrated the poor eating behavior of athletes, particularly female athletes.

Ideally, nutritional intake should include 6–10 g of carbohydrate per kilogram of body weight, 0.8–1.5 g of protein per kilogram, and the rest of the calories from fat. These levels translate into a diet of 60–70% carbohydrate, 10–15% protein, and 25–30% fat. More recently, the protein recommendation has been increased to 20–25% and the fat decreased to 10–15%. Clark has stated that "theoretically, women who eat more than 1200–1500 calories from a variety of wholesome foods can obtain most nutrients necessary for top athletic performance (with the possible exception of iron)." This information is important to relay to female athletes, especially young girls, who may restrict their intake and attempt to meet their nutritional needs by supplementation. The use of a daily multivitamin preparation, and for some individuals iron and calcium supplements, is reasonable; however, female athletes should understand that no supplement can take the place of proper food selection.

1. Iron—Iron deficiency is common entity in young athletes, especially female athletes. Iron deficiency or decreased iron stores can occur without anemia in as many as 9.5–57% of this population. Girls take in significantly less than the recommended daily allowance (RDA) of 18 mg of iron. Because there is often an increase in plasma volume of 6–25% with training, the hemoglobin and hematocrit levels can appear falsely low with resultant "pseudoanemia." A screening hemoglobin level with follow-up ferritin determination is reasonable for assessing iron deficiency in female athletes. Ferritin is the storage form of iron, and its determination can be helpful in differentiating pseudoanemia from true iron deficiency. In some situations, such as acute infection, the level of ferritin can be increased; additional studies, as well as clinical correlation, are then necessary. Iron loss can be caused by hemolysis with hemoglobinuria, gastrointestinal losses, and loss of iron through excessive sweating. Female athletes are at increased risk because of the additional iron loss that occurs with menses. Correction of iron deficiency anemia can improve performance, and therapy should include intake of iron-rich foods and adequate vitamin C and supplementation.

2. Calcium–Another important nutritional concern for female athletes is calcium intake; as with iron, the intake is often far less than the RDA. Various studies of female athletes have demonstrated that 40% of gymnasts, 42% of ballet dancers, and 51% of cross-country runners consume less than two-thirds of the RDA for calcium. Calcium, along with adequate estrogen, is necessary for normal bone acquisition; if calcium stores are depleted, a lower bone density may result. Because peak bone density is reached early in life, in the 20s and 30s, ensuring adequate intake is especially important in early childhood and adolescence. Poor acquisition of bone density contributes to the development of stress fractures and premature osteoporosis, which is one of the final outcomes of the female athlete triad (see Chapter 10).

3. Calories–One of the most important nutritional concerns for young female athletes is ensuring adequate total caloric intake. Many athletes do not consume adequate calories to meet their energy needs. In an attempt to "eat healthy," many athletes restrict their fat intake such that the fat-soluble vitamins are at risk for being deficient. Risks of a diet that contains less than 10% fat include low energy intake and low levels of protein, iron, zinc, and vitamin E. Deficiencies also have been noted in zinc; magnesium; folate; and vitamins B_6, C, A, and B_{12}. Many athletes experiment in restricting their intake, often as part of a "diet" plan to lose weight, even though they may not be overweight. Distorted body image and the displeasure that young women often have with their body can result in pathogenic weight control behavior.

B. Pathogenic Eating Behaviors: The female athlete triad of disordered eating, menstrual dysfunction, and osteoporosis have become known as the female athlete triad; is probably one of the biggest challenges facing the sports medicine community. Pathogenic eating behavior is especially difficult to treat for several reasons: (1) weight and body image are sensitive issues to discuss; (2) as in alcoholism, it is difficult to detect normal from abnormal behavior; and (3) the individual often denies there is a problem. Although most commonly seen in sports such as figure skating, gymnastics, cross-country running, and

swimming, eating disorders are present in every sport. Sports that select for a lean body weight or are judged subjectively put athletes at particular risk. The origins of eating disorders are multifactorial and beyond the scope of this chapter (see Chapter 10); they include issues of identity, self-esteem, family dynamics, control, and alterations in body image. Often there is a history of sexual or physical abuse and a sense of self-worth based on appearance. Unfortunately, societal pressures are such that a thin body is considered desirable, and constant dieting is the norm. Some of the characteristics associated with the best athletes—perfectionism, goal-setting, overachievement—may put the athlete at additional risk for developing eating disorders. Some of the features that can help distinguish athletes from people with disordered eating are shown in Table 39–1.

Because eating disorders are difficult to identify, a team approach is often necessary for proper treatment. The treatment team usually includes a physician, a psychiatrist, and ultimately, a nutritionist. Others involved with treatment include the family, the athletic trainer, the team, and the coach. The fact that treatment is often unsuccessful highlights the importance of early identification and prevention. Education is one of the most important tools in preventing eating disorders, and the preparticipation physical examination is an appropriate time to start the process.

C. Menstrual Function and Dysfunction: Menstrual dysfunction is another common entity for the female athlete. The exact mechanisms through which exercise-associated menstrual dysfunction occurs are not well known. Most athletes understand that their menses can be affected by their exercise patterns, yet many do not understand that oligomenorrhea and amenorrhea may have long-standing, harmful consequences. A shortened luteal phase, anovulation, oligomenorrhea, and amenorrhea all have been demonstrated to occur in response to chronic exercise and in association with decreased bone mineral density. These disorders are associated with an increased risk for both stress fractures and premature osteoporosis. It is important for athletes, parents, and coaches to understand the significance of menstrual dysfunction, the risks involved with amenorrhea, and the importance of complete evaluation of symptoms. Because athletes are not immune from other medical problems, one cannot assume that the menstrual cycle has stopped because of exercise. Again, the preparticipation examination offers the opportunity to discuss this issue.

The effects of the menstrual cycle on performance have been reviewed, and the data remain controversial. In 37–63% of the studies to date, no change in performance has been found during different phases of the cycle. In 13–29% of the studies, an improvement was noted during menstruation. The best performances occurred shortly after and the worst just

Table 39–1. Characteristics of anorectics and athletes.*

	Anorectics	Athletes
Distinguishing features	Aimless physical activity Poor or decreasing exercise performance Poor muscle development Flawed body image Body fat below normal level Electrolyte abnormalities if abusing laxatives or diuretics Cold intolerance Dry skin Cardiac arrhythmias Lanugo hair Leukocyte dysfunction	Purposeful training Increased exercise tolerance Strong muscular development Accurate body image Body fat level within defined normal range Increased plasma volume Increased 2 extraction from blood Efficient energy metabolism Increased high-density lipoprotein–2
Shared features	Dietary faddism Controlled caloric consumption Specific carbohydrate avoidance Low body weight Resting bradycardia and hypotension Increased physical activity Amenorrhea or oligomenorrhea Anemia (sometimes)	

*Reproduced, with permission, from McSherry JA: The diagnostic challenge of anorexia nervosa. Am Fam Physician 1988;29:144.

before menstruation. There appear to be no changes in strength during various phases of the menstrual cycle when assessed by isokinetic knee extension and flexion.

There are many variables to consider when evaluating for menstrual dysfunction in an athlete. Exercise-related changes in the stress and sex hormones, nutrition, body composition changes, and "energy drain" have been proposed as important factors that warrant consideration. Exercise-related increases in estradiol, progesterone, testosterone, prolactin, catecholamines, and cortisol all occur with acute exercise. Beta-endorphin and beta-lipotropin levels also increase. If an individual is amenorrheic or oligomenorrheic, careful assessment including gynecologic examination; pregnancy test; and workup to rule out prolactin-secreting tumors, hypothyroidism, and adrenal or ovarian dysfunction should be pursued. An algorithm for workup of amenorrhea is given in Chapter 47.

If menstrual dysfunction is determined to be secondary to exercise, treatment includes decreasing training intensity or quantity if possible, weight gain if appropriate, and estrogen and progesterone therapy. There are some researchers who believe that progesterone, not estrogen, is the important factor in bone acquisition and that optimal therapy includes progesterone for this reason and to protect against the risks of unopposed estrogen therapy. Because estrogen therapy in postmenopausal women has been shown to protect the bone loss that normally occurs, estrogen therapy is used also in exercise-associated amenorrhea (EAA). The data addressing estrogen supplementation in EAA is in its early stages, however, and early results have been controversial. A re-

cent study by Prior et al revealed a positive effect on bone density as measured by dual-energy x-ray absorptiometry in patients with EAA treated with progesterone. The extremely low estrogen levels appear to warrant treatment, and one of the easiest therapeutic interventions is the use of the oral contraceptive pill along with calcium supplementation. This approach is especially useful in sexually active women, and because of its few side effects, it often yields a higher compliance than other forms of estrogen.

It is important to address the issues of menstrual function, stress fractures, nutrition, and body image. Questions about dysmenorrhea, missed periods, and amenorrhea are important in detecting abnormalities but also in opening up discussion concerning the importance of maintaining a normal menstrual cycle, including the relationship to bone health. Asking questions about anemia, fatigue, burnout, and depression can highlight the relationship of proper nutrition to performance enhancement. Questions regarding stress fractures, family history of osteoporosis, smoking, and alcohol consumption can help young athletes to understand how these risk factors relate to the risks of eating disorders and menstrual dysfunction. Many young athletes do not understand the consequences of low bone density or osteoporosis, but they may have friends who have had eating disorders and they understand the effect of stress fractures on their ability to train and perform. Explaining the components of the female triad in a positive manner that relates to the young athlete is the key to combating the increasing incidence of the triad. An example of a supplemental history form for female athletes is given in Appendix F.

D. Cardiovascular System: Sudden cardiac

death occurs in 1 in 200,000 athletes, and studies have shown that exercise increases the risk; attempts should be made to detect those at risk. The major causes for sudden death in athletes age 30 or younger and in those older than 40 years are given in Table 39–2. In individuals younger than 30, hypertrophic cardiomyopathy, anomalous coronary arteries, and ruptured aorta secondary to Marfan's syndrome are important congenital disorders to consider, whereas in athletes older than 40, the leading cause of sudden death is atherosclerotic heart disease. It is important to attempt to identify individuals with hypertrophic cardiomyopathy during the preparticipation examination, because their presentation is often sudden death. Maron et al found in a series of 78 patients that 40% were involved in exercise before their death. Because hypertrophic cardiomyopathy is an autosomal dominant disorder, family history is important. Maron found that 25% of the patients with sudden death secondary to hypertrophic cardiomyopathy had a family history of sudden nontraumatic death in at least one parent or sibling younger than 50 years of age.

Marfan's syndrome, another autosomal dominant disorder, also is a cause of sudden cardiac death, and family history is important in detecting those at risk. A family history is present in 85% of patients with Marfan's syndrome, and it is one of the four criteria needed to make the diagnosis. The major features of Marfan's syndrome are given in Table 39–3.

Table 39–3. Major features of Marfan's syndrome.

1. **Family history**
2. **Cardiovascular abnormalities**
   Cystic medial necrosis
   Aortic dilatation
   Aortic aneurysm
   Aortic dissection
   Aortic insufficiency
   Mitral valve prolapse
   Mitral regurgitation
3. **Musculoskeletal abnormalities**
   Kyphoscoliosis
   Anterior thorax deformities: pectus excavatum, pectus carinatum
   Tall, with limb length greater than trunk length
   Arachnodactyly
   Spina bifida
   Spondylolisthesis
4. **Ocular disorders**
   Ectopia lentis
   Myopia
   Iridodonesis

Table 39–2. Causes of sudden death in athletes.

Age 30 or Younger

Condition	Total (%)
Hypertrophic cardiomyopathy	20 (24)
Coronary artery abnormalities	15 (18)
Coronary artery disease	12 (14)
Myocarditis	10 (12)
Marfan's syndrome	3 (4)
Dysrhythmias	2 (2)
Mitral valve prolapse	3 (4)
Other (include idiopathic concentric cardiac hypertrophy or rheumatic heart disease	9 (11)
No cause identified	10 (12)

Adapted from McAffrey et al: Sudden cardiac death in young athletes; A review. AJDC, 1991;145:177.

Age 40 or Older

Condition	Incidence (%)
Coronary artery disease (CAD)	88.7
Anomalous coronary arteries	4.2
Myocardial infarction without CAD Hypertrophic cardiomyopathy Myocarditis Mitral valve prolapse Mitral stenosis with left ventricular hypertrophy	7.1

Adapted from Chillags et al: Sudden Death; Myocardial infarction in a runner with normal coronary arteries. Phys and Sportsmed 1990;18(3):89.

Questions should be asked about a history of chest pain, dizziness, syncope, presyncope, and extreme fatigue or shortness of breath with exertion. Any history of a heart murmur, rheumatic fever, or structural heart disease is important. If there are any symptoms, a careful history often can differentiate between benign and pathogenic causes. If an athlete has had syncope after completion of exercise at rest, or on standing quickly, the symptom is more likely to be neurocardiogenic in origin. If a syncopal episode occurs during intense exercise, there should be concern for hypertrophic cardiomyopathy or another form of outflow obstruction, some form of dysrhythmia, or seizure. The patient may warrant immediate evaluation by echocardiography and other tests before clearance is given for participation in an exercise program.

Other cardiac concerns that do not relate specifically to sudden cardiac death include arrhythmias, atherosclerotic heart disease, and hypertension. Previous or family history of arrhythmia, hypertension, or hypercholesterolemia and diabetes are important to ascertain. If there are multiple cardiac risk factors, additional testing may be necessary before the patient begins an unsupervised exercise regimen. Cardiac risk factors and an algorithm for further testing based on risk factors and patient history are given in Chapter 30.

E. Neurologic System: Important questions for the neurologic history include any history of concussion, neck or spinal injury, or epilepsy. If an individual has had any of these conditions, obtaining detailed information is important. For head concussions, it is useful to determine the mechanism, whether there was loss of consciousness, results of any diagnostic tests performed, and the presence of persistent symptoms. If there is a history of spinal injury, one should obtain diagnostic tests results and information concerning treatment. A history of seizure or family history of epilepsy, along with treatment, medication use, and control of seizure activity, should be obtained. This information can be useful in providing risk stratification for the various exercise activities in which the patient is interested.

The natural history of head concussions and other neurologic injuries in sport has yet to be elucidated fully. The guidelines used to treat individuals with head injuries are based on anecdotal and common sense practices, with few objective data to support them. Nonetheless, it is important to quantitate previous head injuries and the exact details of each event, as well as when they occurred. After a player sustains a first concussion, the chance of incurring a second one is more than 4 times greater than in a player who has never sustained a concussion. In addition, the "second impact syndrome" is always a concern; this phenomenon involves the occurrence of a second brain impact before recovery from a previous one is complete, which can lead to edema of the brain and sometimes death.

For individuals who have had previous spinal injury, careful assessment is important in determining the risk for further injury. In addition, ensuring that proper rehabilitation has occurred is important, although this is often difficult to ascertain. Conditions such as disk degeneration with herniation, spondylolysis or spondylolisthesis, and prior fracture or fusion may require further diagnostic studies. On determining that any of these abnormalities is present, the health care provider should make recommendations for exercise that will not put the individual at risk for further injury.

A seizure disorder that is under control should not prevent an individual from participating in an exercise program; participation in all sports, including contact sports such as football and soccer, is possible. There is debate concerning at what point a seizure disorder is considered controlled, however; this determination often is an individual matter. Epilepsy should be differentiated from other causes of seizure including febrile seizures associated with infection, seizures associated with tumor, seizures secondary to vascular abnormalities, and seizures secondary to alcohol withdrawal or cocaine toxicity.

After testing is done and diagnosis has been made, careful monitoring of medication is important. The recommended time before return to activity remains controversial; it ranges from 1 month to 1 year. There is additional concern for individuals who wish to engage in underwater sports such as snorkeling. These individuals should be given information regarding the severity of the risk if seizure occurs, and they should not be instructors in these sports.

F. Musculoskeletal System: There are aspects of the preparticipation physical examination of the musculoskeletal system that relate specifically to

women. Although upper extremity injuries are similar in men and women, lower extremity injuries appear to be slightly different. Women tend to have a wider pelvis than men, femoral neck anteversion, and varus at the hip and valgus at the knee. The result may be compensatory external rotation of the tibial tubercle with pronation at the hindfoot. These factors contribute to an increase of the Q angle, which is the angle between the femoral shaft and a line drawn from the center of the patella to the tibial tubercle. Women also have a lower center of gravity than men; it is at 56.1% of height in women and 56.7% in men.

It is important to obtain information regarding prior musculoskeletal problems, their treatment, and their rehabilitation. It is not uncommon to detect ligamentous laxity in athletes who never sought medical attention for what they thought was a minor injury. It is important to screen for the presence of scoliosis, alignment abnormalities, and general ligamentous laxity, strength, and flexibility. This process can help to identify areas for which exercise recommendations can be made specific to the individual's goals.

Physical Examination

The areas of particular interest are the cardiovascular, neurologic, and musculoskeletal systems. Height and weight measurements, assessment of vital signs, and evaluation of visual acuity are important also. Attention to preexisting pupil size asymmetry can be useful in evaluating later head concussions.

The preparticipation physical examination should be sport-specific. Otitis can be a particular problem for swimmers, whereas it presents only minor problems for tennis players. A skin abnormality such as herpes gladiatorum is more important to recognize in someone who plays a contact sport such as basketball than in a golfer. The thyroid should be palpated, and any thyromegaly assessed. If the individual has given any history of exercise-induced cough, wheezing, or shortness of breath (consistent with exercise-induced asthma), attention to the lung examination is helpful; often, provocative testing is necessary. The abdominal examination is important for detecting hepatosplenomegaly, polycystic kidney disease, or other organomegaly or gastrointestinal disorders. The examination should include instruction regarding self-examination of the breast. A gynecologic examination may be indicated, such as in an athlete with menstrual dysfunction or amenorrhea.

The cardiovascular examination begins with an assessment of blood pressure and heart rate and rhythm. The health care provider should be familiar with **athlete's heart,** which results from the physiologic adaptations to exercise that allow the heart to work more effectively. Functional murmurs and extra heart sounds are not uncommon in athletes and must be differentiated from those seen in pathologic conditions. The changes seen in association with athlete's heart depend on the type of exercise performed; they can include enlargement of the ventricle and thickening of the ventricular walls. The ECG and chest x-ray can demonstrate changes that correspond to athlete's heart. Sinus bradycardia, junctional rhythms, and first-degree and type I second-degree heart block all have been seen more frequently in athletes than in sedentary individuals; voltage changes and ST segment and T wave abnormalities also are common in athletes. Premature ventricular contractions (PVCs), ventricular couplets, and bigeminy are common, although most of these benign rhythm disturbances tend to disappear with the onset of exercise. The history is crucial in determining whether these findings are functional or pathologic. It is often difficult to determine whether a murmur is pathologic or not. A murmur that increases on going from the standing to the squatting position is likely to be physiologic, because the increased venous return augments functional murmurs. If the murmur increases when going from squatting to standing, however, concern for hypertrophic cardiomyopathy or other outflow obstruction is raised. Further testing is indicated if there is any doubt about the nature of a murmur, if there is a history of cardiac symptoms with exertion, or if there is a family history of sudden cardiac death or premature atherosclerotic disease. Physical findings that are associated with some of the major causes of sudden cardiac death in athletes are given in Table 39–4.

Further diagnostic testing is based on the results of the history and physical examination. An echocardiogram is a useful and noninvasive tool to assess wall motion, chamber size, ejection fraction, valvular abnormalities, and wall thickness. It is probably the most important tool in assessing for the presence of hypertrophic cardiomyopathy, ruling out aortic dilatation, and assessing murmurs and other structural abnormalities. In thin individuals, echocardiography may help detect anomalous coronary arteries. For conduction and rhythm disturbance, an ECG in conjunction with 24- to 48-hour Holter or event monitoring and exercise treadmill testing with monitoring are useful. For more complicated preexcitation disturbances, an ECG and electrophysiologic study (EPS) may be necessary. Exercise stress testing is often helpful in assessing for anomalous coronaries and papillary dysfunction; in conjunction with echocardiography or thallium, it can be even more sensitive and specific. These procedures may reduce the need for angiography, which is a more invasive test. Angiography remains the gold standard for assessing for anomalous coronaries, however.

One of the newest tests available for evaluation of syncope is tilt table testing, which has been used to assess for neurocardiogenic syncope. There has been debate, however, concerning the usefulness of tilt table testing in athletes, in whom there may be a high rate of false-positive results because of the high vagal tone often seen. If the echocardiogram, ECG, and stress testing are all negative but tilt testing is positive in an athlete with syncope, the origin is most likely neurocardiogenic. If syncope occurs during exertion, however, further evaluation is indicated.

The neurologic examination is important is evaluating general strength, reflexes, and sensory abnormalities. Pain along the spinous processes, pain with atlantoaxial compression, and any deficit in motion or strength of the cervical spine should be assessed to rule out instability or preexisting neurologic injury. For older individuals, it is also important to assess balance, stability, and proprioception. Deficits secondary to prior concussion, injury, or cerebrovascular accident are important to assess in ensuring that the contemplated exercise regimen is realistic and safe.

The musculoskeletal examination must be done in an organized fashion. Different areas of the musculoskeletal system are more important for different activities. For example, swimming is often an excellent exercise for an older individual who may be at risk of falling and for whom knee osteoarthritis is a problem. If such a patient plans to begin rock climbing, however, careful assessment of the hip, leg, spine, and shoulders becomes more important. General

Table 39–4. Physical examination findings in conditions causing sudden cardiac death.

Condition	Finding
Hypertrophic obstructive cardiomyopathy (HOCM) or idiopathic hypertrophic subaortic stenosis (IHSS)	Jugular venous pulse with prominent a wave Carotid pulse: short duration, brisk upstroke, often bifid (67%) Double or triple apical impulse Systolic ejection murmur at left lower sternal border (classic); murmur increases with standing, expiration, and second and third phases of Valsalva; murmur decreases with squatting and inspiration Fourth heart sound at apex
Marfan's syndrome	Early ejection sound Aortic regurgitant murmur at right upper sternal border Mitral valve prolapse with mitral regurgitant murmur
Aortic stenosis (AS)	Large a wave with severe AS Narrow pulse pressure (late) Systolic thrill at base of heart Apex beat displaced inferiorly and laterally (left ventricular hypertrophy) Early systolic ejection murmur (crescendo-decrescendo) Paradox splitting S_2 (severe AS) Fourth heart sound
Anomalous coronary artery	Mitral regurgitation sometimes present secondary to papillary muscle ischemia or infarction Examination often normal

strength and flexibility should be assessed, along with gait and alignment abnormalities. Scoliosis is always a concern, especially for younger athletes. Leg length discrepancies should be sought. Ligamentous laxity in the knee, shoulder, and ankle is important to assess, especially if there is a history of previous injury with little or no rehabilitation. In these situations, a careful examination can detect laxity that may put the athlete at risk for further injury. The identification of deficits can lead to the institution of a rehabilitation program before the season begins or may lead to disqualification until some kind of intervention is made. Surgery may be necessary prior to participation if rehabilitation alone is not sufficient. In making these difficult decisions, it is important to consider the risks of the sport involved and the patient's risk of injury.

CLINICAL MUSCULOSKELETAL PROBLEMS

In recent years, there have been advances in the training regimens and fitness levels and increases in the opportunities available for girls and women in sport. No longer can clinical differences between men and women be attributed to inferior strength or training; it is important for thorough assessment to be made so that problems can be detected early and rehabilitation initiated.

Iliotibial friction syndrome, patellofemoral dysfunction, reflex sympathetic dystrophy, greater trochanteric bursitis, and ankle and anterior cruciate ligament (ACL) sprains appear to occur more commonly in women than men. It remains unclear whether these clinical differences arise from differences in biomechanics and musculoskeletal structures, muscle imbalances, or unknown factors. More studies are needed of girls and women who are active in sport; the data are sparse and do not represent women who are active at increasingly competitive levels.

The occurrence of patellofemoral dysfunction (PFD) is potentiated by an increased Q angle, genu valgum, and genu recurvatum. PFD is characterized by anterior knee pain, often made worse by climbing or descending stairs or prolonged sitting (the "theater sign"). Individuals with PFD often have deficient vastus medialis obliquus (VMO) musculature or tight vastus lateralis musculature; these conditions can combine to cause an abnormal tracking pattern of the patella with resultant patellofemoral irritation and pain. The static and dynamic orientation of the patella are important for an understanding of the biomechanics of the patellofemoral dysfunction and to plan rehabilitation. The presence of an effusion is also important; a grade 2 effusion has been shown to affect adversely the strength of the quadriceps muscle complex by as much as 10–40% by isokinetic testing. The presence of an effusion should expand the differential diagnosis to include meniscal lesions, ligamentous injury, articular surface defects, and osteochondral defects.

Strengthening of the VMO is one of the mainstays of therapy for PFD. Various taping techniques have been developed to allow the patella to track more normally and facilitate pain-free strengthening of the VMO. Closed-chain kinetic exercises, such as partial squats or one-legged squats, are excellent rehabilitative exercises. Newer rehabilitative tools include a harness system that can decrease an individual's body weight while doing exercises or running on a treadmill. As the athlete's condition improves, more weight is gradually added until they are carrying all of the their body weight again. This system allows an athlete to continue the sport-specific nature of her exercise as part of her rehabilitation. Open-chain kinetic exercises such as knee extensions and straight leg raises are used less often because they are not sport-specific; however, they may play an important role in sports such as soccer and karate that use open-chain kinetic skills.

Another clinical problem seen commonly in female athletes is trochanteric bursitis. Although it is unclear why this condition occurs more commonly in women than men, it may be because of structural differences. Tightness of the lateral structures often compress the bursa and cause an irritative force to occur with repetitive sliding of the iliotibial band over the greater trochanter. Pain is elicited with both passive and active abduction of the leg as the bursa is compressed but not with resisted abduction at the neutral position (unless there is a concomitant tendonitis or strain). Treatment with a nonsteroidal anti-inflammatory agent, ice massage, iliotibial band stretching, and, occasionally, phonophoresis or iontophoresis usually suffices. Corticosteroid injection can be useful. It is also important to assess for biomechanical problems or leg length discrepancies as a potential cause, along with training pattern errors.

An area of increasing concern is the higher number of ACL injuries in women than in men. In almost every sport that is represented in the National Collegiate Athletic Association (NCAA), women have more ACL injuries than men. A 2-year study of knee injuries in NCAA soccer and basketball athletes demonstrated a higher ACL injury rate in both sports in women compared with men. These statistics are demonstrated in Table 39–5. The female basketball and soccer players had an ACL injury rate 6 times greater and 2 times greater, respectively, than the men. The 4-year data have not yet been reviewed, but they appear to follow the same trend. These statistics are worrisome given the increased number of girls and women participating in both sports.

The explanation for this increased incidence of ACL injuries remains unclear. An initial idea was that women lacked the muscular development necessary to supplement joint stability. However, another

Table 39–5. Knee injuries in collegiate basketball and soccer athletes.*

Basketball (more than 400,000 A-E†)	Men	Women
Knee injuries (% all injuries)	12%	19%
Knee injury requiring surgery (% all injuries)	20%	39%
Knee injury rate (per 1000 A-E)	0.7	1.0
ACL injury rate (per 1000 A-E)	0.05	0.3*

Soccer (more than 180,000 A-E)	Men	Women
Knee injuries (% all injuries)	16%	18%
Knee injury requiring surgery (% all injuries)	15%	22%
Knee injury rate (per 1000 A-E)	1.3	1.3
ACL injury rate (per 1000 A-E)	0.14	0.29‡

*Reproduced, with permission, from Arendt EA, Dick RW: Gender Specific Knee Injury Patterns in Collegiate Basketball and Soccer Players. National Collegiate Athletic Association: NCAA Injury Surveillance System. NCAA, 1991–1992.
†A-E = athlete-exposure: one athlete participating in one practice or game.
‡Significantly greater than M value (p < .05).

study looked at ACL injuries in Olympic-caliber male and female basketball players and found a much higher incidence of injuries in women compared with men (53 versus 13%). In addition, the severity of injuries and the need for surgery were higher in women than men. Other factors that might explain the increased incidence of ACL injuries include muscle imbalances, trochlear groove size or configuration, biomechanical differences in jumping and landing technique, and alignment differences. More information is needed to answer this question.

As women have begun to excel in sport, the field of sports medicine has grown and more research is being done on issues related to women. It is not uncommon to see a primary care physician taking on the role of "team physician." As more information is gained about the physiologic adaptations that occur with exercise and the risk factors for health, efforts at prevention of injury and disease will be improved.

REFERENCES

Balaban EP: Sports anemia. Clin Sports Med 1992;11:313.

Cann CE et al: Decreased spinal mineral content in amenorrheic women. JAMA 1984;251:626.

Caselli G, Piovano G, Vernando A: A follow-up study of abnormalities of ventricular repolarization in athletes. In: *Sports Cardiology*. Lubich T, Vernando A (editors). Aulo Gaggi, 1980.

Chillag S et al: Sudden death: Myocardial infarction in a runner with normal coronary arteries. Phys Sports Med 1990;18(3):89.

Clark N: Nutritional problems and training intensity, activity level, and athletic performance. In: *The Athletic Female*. Pearl AJ (editor). Human Kinetics, 1993.

Costill D: Carbohydrates for exercise: Dietary demands for optimal performance. Int J Sports Med. 1988;9:1.

Drinkwater BL, Bruemmer B, Chestnut CH III: Menstrual history as a determinant of current bone density in young athletes. JAMA 1990;263:545.

Drinkwater BL et al: Bone mineral content of amenorrheic and eumenorrheic athletes. N Engl J Med 1984;311:277.

Drinkwater BL et al: Bone mineral density after resumption of menses in amenorrheic athletes. JAMA 1986;256:380.

Emans SJ et al: Estrogen deficiency in adolescents and young adults: Impact on bone mineral content and effects of estrogen replacement therapy. Obstet Gynecol 1990;76:585.

Epstein SE, Maron BJ: Sudden death and the competitive athlete: Perspectives on preparticipation screening studies. J Am Coll Cardiol 1986;7:220.

Ettinger B, Genant HK, Cann CE: Postmenopausal bone loss is prevented by treatment with low-dosage estrogen with calcium. Ann Intern Med 1987;106:40.

Gerberich SG et al: Concussion incidence and severity in secondary school varsity football players. Am J Public Health 1983;73:1370.

Huston TP, Puffer JC, Rodney WM: The athletic heart syndrome. N Engl J Med 1985;313:24.

Jaffe R: History of women in sports. In: *Medical and Orthopedic Issues of Active and Athletic Women*. Agostini R (editor). Hanley & Belfus, 1994.

Lebrun CM: Effect of the different phases of the menstrual cycle and oral contraceptives on athletic performance. Sports Med 1993;16:400.

Lindberg JS et al: Exercise-induced amenorrhea and bone density. Ann Intern Med 1984;101:647.

Malone TR, Sanders B: Strength training and the athletic female. In: *The Athletic Woman*. Pearl AJ (editor). Human Kinetics, 1993.

Mansfield MJ, Emans SJ: Anorexia nervosa, athletics, and amenorrhea. Pediatr Clin North Am 1989;36:533.

Marcus R et al: Menstrual function and bone mass in elite women distance runners: Endocrine and metabolic features. Ann Intern Med 1985;102:158.

Maron BJ, Roberts WC, Epstein SE: Sudden death in hypertrophic cardiomyopathy: A profile of 78 patients. Circulation 1982;65:1388.

Metka M et al: Hypergonadotrophic hypogonadic amenorrhea (World Health Organization III) and osteoporosis. Fertil Steril 1992;57:37.

Myburgh KH et al: Low bone density is an etiologic factor for stress fractures in athletes. Ann Intern Med 1990;113:754.

National Collegiate Athletic Association: *NCAA Injury Surveillance System*. NCAA, 1991–1992.

Pearl AJ (editor): *The Athletic Female*. Human Kinetics, 1993.

Prior JC et al: Cyclic medroxyprogesterone treatment increases bone density: A controlled trial in active women with menstrual cycle disturbances. Am J Med 1994;96:521.

Putukian M: The female triad: Eating disorders, amenorrhea, and osteoporosis. Med Clin North Am 1994;78: 345.

Putukian M, McKeag DB: The preparticipation physical examination. In: *Sports Medicine and Physical Examination: A Sport-Specific Approach.* Buschbacher RM, Braddom RL (editors). Hanley & Belfus, 1994.

Rosen LW et al: Pathogenic weight control behaviors in female athletes. Phys Sports Med 1986;14:79.

Saunders RL, Harbaugh RE: The second impact in catastrophic contact-sports head trauma. JAMA. 1984;252: 538.

Selby GB, Eichner ER: Endurance swimming, intravascular hemolysis, anemia, and iron depletion: New perspective on athlete's anemia. Am J Med 1986;81:791.

Yeager KK et al: The female athlete triad: Disordered eating, amenorrhea, osteoporosis. (Commentary.) Med Sci Sports Exerc 1993;25:775.

Zehender M et al: ECG variants and cardiac arrhythmias in athletes: Clinical relevance and prognostic importance. Am Heart J 1990;119:1378.

Zeppilli P et al: Ventricular repolarization disturbances in athletes: Standardization of terminology, ethiopathogenetic spectrum, and pathophysiologic mechanisms. J Sports Med Phys Fitness 1981;21:322.

Section XI.
Other Common Disorders

40

Hematologic Complications
of Pregnancy

David M. Aboulafia, MD

Essentials of Diagnosis
- Anemia (ie, iron deficiency and sickle cell)
- Leukocytosis
- Thrombocytopenia
- Preeclampsia and eclampsia-related abnormalities
- Disseminated intravascular coagulation
- von Willebrand's disease

Hematologic abnormalities account for greater than half of the medical complications diagnosed during pregnancy. Under normal conditions, the quantities of circulating blood cells, platelets, and plasma proteins are regulated within a relatively narrow physiologic range. Pregnancy represents a challenge to the body's homeostatic reserves. The hematologic consequences of this challenge may be negligible, as in mild-to-moderate iron deficiency or the induction of an asymptomatic hypercoagulable state. The consequences are more serious when the woman is faced with anemia-induced high-output cardiac failure, pulmonary embolism, or life-threatening thrombocytopenia.

One difficulty in evaluating hematologic abnormalities during pregnancy is distinguishing normal physiologic changes that occur routinely from uncommon pathologic events that occur only occasionally. This challenge is heightened because of the fact that common laboratory values change in pregnancy, and their interpretation requires an understanding of the hematologic changes of pregnancy (Table 40–1). In this chapter, the clinical features, diagnosis, and management of the most commonly encountered blood disorders of pregnancy are reviewed. The hypercoagulable state induced by pregnancy and the treatment of pregnancy-associated thrombosis are discussed in Chapter 35.

ANEMIA

Anemia is the most common hematologic problem in pregnancy. The physiologic expansion of the expectant mother's blood volume consists of an increase in plasma volume (25–60%) beginning at approximately 6 weeks of gestation and continuing until the twenty-fourth week, at which time there is a

Table 40–1. Hematologic laboratory values.

Test	Nonpregnant Women	Pregnant Women
White blood count	4–10.5/µL	9–15,500/µL
Hemoglobin	12.5–14 g/dL	10–13 g/dL
Platelets	150,000–400,000/µL	125,000–400,000/µL
Reticulocyte count	0.5–1%	1–2%
Total iron-binding capacity	250–300 µg/dL	280–400 µg/dL
Transferrin saturation	25–35%	15–30%
Serum ferritin	75–100 µg/L	55–70 µg/L
Serum folate	6.5–19.6 µg/mL	4–10 µg/mL

more gradual rise. The red blood cell (RBC) mass also increases during this time but at a slower rate (20–30%); this "hydremia" of pregnancy results in a decline in hematocrit (HCT) to the 30–32% range, necessitating a revision downward in the limits of a normal hemoglobin level to 10 g/dL (Table 40–1). The precise stimuli leading to the increase in plasma volume and RBC mass are unknown, although alterations in various hormones, eg, progesterone and erythropoietin, and the development of placental vascular shunts may be important in this process. The decline in blood viscosity results in decreased peripheral resistance and may offset the effects of increased levels of fibrinogen and enhanced RBC aggregation during the later stages of pregnancy.

IRON DEFICIENCY ANEMIA

The most common type of anemia in pregnancy, iron deficiency anemia (IDA), occurs when there is insufficient iron to support normal RBC production. In some developing countries, as many as 83% of anemic pregnant women have iron deficiency; in inner-city pregnant women in the United States, 50% may have IDA even though prenatal iron is prescribed. The average menstruating woman requires 15–20 mg of absorbable iron in her daily diet to compensate for the loss of approximately 2 mg/d (from urine, stool, and skin); more is lost if she is pregnant. These figures translate into an average daily requirement of 4 mg of iron during the early stages of pregnancy; the requirement reaches 6.6–8.4 mg/d at term. Because this amount is more than can be supplied by even the most iron-rich diets, supplements are necessary if iron deficiency is to be avoided.

For many women, dietary sources are especially iron-poor. A variety of social, economic, and cultural factors are important in determining the quantity and quality of the food supply. Even among fairly homogeneous groups, factors such as menstrual blood loss and amount of animal protein consumed are variable.

Clinical Findings & Diagnosis

Because the symptoms of mild IDA are insidious and nonspecific, they are not of great value. When the hemoglobin level falls below 9 g/dL, however,

IDA should be suspected. Careful physical examination may detect pallor, glossitis, stomatitis, splenomegaly, or koilonychia. Congestive heart failure may be seen rarely with extreme anemia. As with all patients, a rectal examination and stool guaiac test are performed to rule out occult fecal blood loss.

In pregnant patients, a diagnostic evaluation begins with morphologic classification using the RBC mean corpuscular volume (MCV) and the blood smear. In clear-cut instances of IDA, a peripheral blood smear demonstrates small hypochromic RBCs of various sizes and shapes. It is worth emphasizing, however, that the microcytosis that typically is seen in uncomplicated IDA may not be seen in mild IDA associated with pregnancy, because the MCV usually rises slightly in pregnancy. Laboratory diagnosis of IDA in pregnancy is complicated further by the observation that total iron-binding capacity (TIBC) increases in pregnancy even when iron stores are normal (Table 40–1). To enable a better interpretation of laboratory indices of anemia, serum iron, TIBC, and ferritin levels should be drawn and reviewed together. Serum iron levels less than 30 µg/dL, TIBC greater than 450 µg/dL, and plasma ferritin levels less than 10 µg/L are the most reliable laboratory indicators of IDA. A direct and indirect Coombs' test and levels of urine hemosiderin and serum haptoglobin are useful if hemolysis is suspected. For complex cases or those not responding to iron therapy, bone-marrow examination for stainable iron is the "gold standard" for assessing iron stores and for ruling out much more unusual causes of reticulocytopenia, such as myelodysplasia, aplastic anemia, leukemia, or lymphoma.

Differential Diagnosis

Folate deficiency also may complicate pregnancy because of a similar increase in demand for this essential cofactor in nucleic acid synthesis. Total body folate stores are small and short-lived, and nausea and vomiting may significantly impair the intake of folate. Drugs interfering with the absorption and metabolism of folic acid, such as phenytoin, trimethoprim, and nitrofurantoin, can aggravate folate deficiency further.

The assessment of folate status in pregnancy, like that of iron, must take into account the expected decline in serum folate levels occurring in normal pregnancy; at term, the levels are only one-half of the early pregnancy values. The observed decline in serum folate levels is believed to be, in part, a dilutional effect caused by plasma volume expansion. A normal serum folate level is helpful in ruling out folate deficiency as a cause of anemia, and a fasting serum folate level of less than 3 ng/mL is considered diagnostic of folic acid deficiency. Pure folate deficiency typically leads to a macrocytic anemia, but the expected elevation in RBC MCV may be masked by the contribution of a concomitant IDA. A deficiency of both these nutrients produces a normocytic, normochromic anemia, although the presence of hypersegmented polymorphonuclear cells may be a clue to diagnosing folate deficiency. Finding a dimorphic population of small and large RBCs on peripheral blood smear should alert the clinician to a possible combined nutritional deficiency.

Folate deficiency in pregnancy is accompanied by a three- to fourfold increase in occurrence of spina bifida in the fetus. In a recent study by Rosenberg, 4753 pregnant women were randomized in groups to receive vitamin supplements with or without folic acid. In the group that did not receive folic acid (n = 2052), there were six infants born with neural-tube defects. In the group that routinely received complete vitamin supplementation (n = 2014), no infants with neural-tube defects were found. Most prenatal vitamins contain folate in addition to iron. Pregnant women should receive 0.5–1.0 mg/d of folate. The salutary effects of vitamins and the importance of obtaining an accurate dietary history are underscored by a study by Suharno, indicating that vitamin A ameliorates IDA—an additional reason that all pregnant women should take multivitamin supplements.

During pregnancy, there is a progressive decline in the serum cobalamin (B_{12}) level, but the availability of maternal stores and the low fetal requirement for this vitamin mean that pregnancy has little effect on overall cobalamin status. Pernicious anemia is usually a disease of older women, and women who have significant cobalamin deficiency are often infertile. Cobalamin deficiency should not be considered an important cause of anemia during pregnancy.

Among the most common nonnutritional causes of hypoproliferative anemia encountered in pregnant women is the anemia associated with chronic disease, eg, rheumatoid arthritis, or an inflammatory process, eg, osteomyelitis. Recognition of the presence of an underlying disorder is generally the only diagnostic maneuver in this circumstance. Erythropoietin is effective in ameliorating the anemia of chronic disease, and its use may be a preferred alternative to blood transfusions in nonemergent situations.

Patients with thalassemia trait commonly develop a more exaggerated decrease in hemoglobin during pregnancy compared with that of normal controls.

This decrease is attributable to an expansion in plasma volume and has no ill effects on the mother or fetus. The workup of heterozygous thalassemia, which is common in some Mediterranean, Asian, and African populations, may provide a diagnostic challenge and usually requires the assistance of a hematologist.

Treatment

Because IDA is the most common type of anemia in pregnancy, some authors recommend empirical iron therapy without further testing if no other cause is suggested by review of the peripheral smear and physical examination. Three to four 325-mg ferrous sulfate tablets per day (60–180 mg of elemental iron) is sufficient to ensure maximal hemoglobin regeneration. Within 4–6 weeks of treatment, the HCT should normalize to a level expected as a result of blood volume expansion, with the increase beginning at 2 weeks. An increase in the reticulocyte count 5–10 days after the initiation of iron therapy provides even earlier evidence for improved RBC production. If there is minimal or no rise in the HCT in 4–6 weeks or the reticulocyte count remains depressed after 10 days, further investigation is necessary. For patients who are intolerant of oral therapy, parenteral iron is an acceptable alternative. Intravenous iron is not without risk, however; the product insert should be read and a hematologist consulted before it is used.

Controversies & Unresolved Issues

The recommendation to provide all pregnant women with iron supplements is based largely on the following assumptions:

1. IDA in the mother is potentially harmful to the mother, fetus, and newborn.
2. The use of iron supplements can reduce perinatal morbidity.
3. The potential benefits of iron supplements outweigh their adverse effects.

A critical review of the available literature, however, does not show clearly that routine iron supplementation during pregnancy improves clinical outcomes for the mother, fetus, and newborn. The United States Preventive Services Task Force (USPTF) stated in a 1993 policy statement that "the evidence is insufficient to recommend for or against routine iron supplements during pregnancy." Rather than providing the clinician with specific recommendations, the USPTF has called for further research, including randomized, controlled trials with adequate sample size before definitive conclusions can be reached about the effectiveness of routine iron supplementation.

SICKLE CELL ANEMIA

Sickle cell disease is endemic to black people of both northern and sub-Saharan African descent and is the most common inherited form of anemia complicating pregnancy. In the USA, approximately 8% of the black population carries the sickle hemoglobin (Hgb S) gene; 0.15% of black newborns are homozygous (Hgb S-S) and suffer from sickle cell anemia (SCA). The most common heterozygote sickle genotypes are Hgb S-A (sickle cell trait), Hgb S-B thal (sickle-beta thalassemia), and Hgb S-C.

The biochemical basis for the abnormal, premature sickling of RBCs in Hgb S-S is a genetic point mutation resulting in the substitution of valine for glutamic acid on the beta-hemoglobin chain. This single beta-globulin alteration results in RBC membrane distortion with resultant obstruction of capillary blood flow as well as the characteristic electrophoretic mobility that allows for ready laboratory distinction between the various hemoglobinopathies.

Obstruction of blood vessels leads to worsening hypoxemia that serves to perpetuate and aggravate RBC sickling. Patients with this condition experience painful vasoocclusive crises resulting in severe skeletal, abdominal, and chest pain syndromes often associated with fever. The spleen is the most susceptible organ to sickle-induced injury because of its highly vascularized tissue. Because of repetitive microinfarcts, the spleen eventually is rendered fibrotic and without function. Other organs at risk for ischemic damage include the heart, lungs, kidneys, eyes, long bones, and brain. Hypoxemia, acidosis, and dehydration are just a few factors that can precipitate a painful crisis and trigger end-organ damage.

Clinical Findings & Diagnosis

Although morbidity and mortality among patients with SCA has improved substantially over the past 2 decades, there is still a higher incidence of pneumonia, cholecystitis, pulmonary emboli, retinal hemorrhage, preeclampsia, and pyelonephritis compared to the general population. Hyposplenism, decreased serum IgM, reduced opsonization activity, impaired phagocytosis, and, not infrequently, poor general nutrition contribute greatly to the increased risk of infection. Similarly, the fetus faces an increased risk of spontaneous abortion, preterm delivery, intrauterine growth retardation, and stillbirth.

Because of routine screening hemoglobin electrophoresis in families known to be at risk as well as the development of clinical complications at an early age, most women with sickle cell disease are diagnosed before pregnancy. Rarely, patients become symptomatic for the first time during pregnancy with painful crisis, infection, or overt infarction. Anemia is typically normocytic, with HCT below 25% and a reticulocyte count greater than 10%. On peripheral blood smear, characteristic sickle cells, target cells, and, because of splenic hypofunction, Howell-Jolly bodies can be seen. A total bilirubin value between 3 and 5 mg/dL is primarily unconjugated, reflecting the presence of brisk RBC hemolysis. An elevation in alkaline phosphatase and conjugated bilirubin should trigger an evaluation to rule out choledocholithiasis.

It is important to screen all black patients by hemoglobin electrophoresis to detect the asymptomatic carrier state and arrange for genetic counseling. With the availability of prenatal diagnosis, all patients at risk for delivering a newborn with hemoglobinopathy should be counseled. Testing the father for carrier status allows for better risk assessment of the fetus. Amniocentesis, chorionic villus sampling, and cordocentesis allow for in utero diagnosis with the aid of new advances in molecular biology.

Treatment

The enthusiasm for prophylactic exchange transfusions for all pregnant women with sickle cell disease has waned and given way to watchful anticipation of the patient's course by hematologist and obstetrician in consultation. The advantage of exchange transfusion is that it increases the level of hemoglobin A in the blood, thereby improving oxygen-carrying capacity and decreasing the percentage of sickled hemoglobin. Disadvantages include the risks of viral infection (ie, HIV, hepatitis B and C, cytomegalovirus [CMV], and human T-cell leukemia/lymphoma virus [HTLV-I-II]), transfusion reaction, and allosensitization.

Many series have documented a high risk of stillbirth, abortion, and fetal growth retardation in pregnancies of hemoglobin S-S patients who have not been transfused, but some investigators have speculated that poor prenatal care in this often socioeconomically deprived group may be a more important factor leading to fetal morbidity and mortality. Because of the increase in fetal morbidity, fetal assessment, biophysical profiles, or contraction stress tests should begin at 32 weeks of gestation. Serial ultrasonography is performed to assess for intrauterine growth retardation.

Pain crisis in pregnancy is managed as in nonpregnant patients with oxygen, hydration, and adequate analgesia. Transfusions are reserved for any acceleration of the sickling disorder itself, worsening anemia (HCT below 18%), or obstetric complications. Because of ongoing hemolysis, folic acid is given routinely to avoid a reticulocytopenic megaloblastic crisis. Iron therapy also is needed because these young women usually have meager iron stores. Newer strategies aimed at preventing vasoocclusive complications such as pain crisis include the use of butyrate preparations, hydroxyurea, high-dose intravenous methylprednisolone, and bone-marrow transplantation. The most extensively studied of these treatments, hydroxyurea, decreases intracellular hemoglobin polymerization and erythrocyte sickling by increasing the levels of fetal hemoglobin. None of these strategies has been attempted in pregnant patients, however.

Management of women with sickle cell disease during delivery is controversial. Many physicians continue to advocate exchange transfusions if general anesthesia is contemplated; the potential for an anesthetic accident with hypoxemia is the rationale for this recommendation. Epidural anesthesia reduces this risk, but hypotension secondary to venous pooling may develop. Attention to adequate fluid repletion, use of pneumatic stockings or pressure leg wraps, and left-sided positioning of the mother to reduce inferior vena cava compression are reasonable strategies to minimize blood pressure fluctuations. Routine care includes frequent monitoring for fetal distress. Oxytocin and conduction anesthesia are safe during labor, and early ambulation is introduced post partum to reduce the risk of thromboembolism.

For patients who wish to terminate pregnancy, most abortion methods are well tolerated. Hypertonic saline injections are contraindicated because they may precipitate RBC sickling, but hypotonic urea can be used. If abortion is to be performed, it is best done early in pregnancy.

Potential complications and concerns that are relevant for pregnant women with sickle cell disease are applicable to individuals with other interacting hemoglobins that can participate in the sickling process, ie, Hgb S-C, Hgb S-B-thal, and Hgb S-E. In contrast, sickle cell trait poses no increase in maternal morbidity with the exception of a higher incidence of kidney and bladder infections and, rarely, splenic infarction. These patients should be screened for asymptomatic bacteriuria.

LEUKOCYTOSIS

Total leukocyte counts rise in pregnancy mainly because of an absolute increase in the number of neutrophils. Neutrophilia usually is discovered during the second month and progresses gradually before plateauing in the second or third trimester. The average peak is at the upper limits of nonpregnant normal, with white blood cell counts of approximately 9000/μL; however, leukocyte counts of up to 18,000/μL occasionally are noted in normal pregnant women during the third trimester. Total leukocyte counts within the normal range of nonpregnant women are to be expected by the sixth postpartum day, provided no complications supervene.

Clinical Findings & Diagnosis

Plasma cortisol, which is known to stimulate de-

margination of polymorphonuclear cells in other circumstances, rises substantially during pregnancy and is the substance presumed to be most responsible for neutrophilia in pregnancy. When a modest elevation in neutrophils is discovered during pregnancy, a diagnostic evaluation is rarely necessary. A normal physical examination in an afebrile and asymptomatic woman is usually sufficient to rule out infection. Leukocyte Döhle bodies (blue cytoplasmic inclusions consisting of rough endoplasmic reticulum) and metamyelocytes frequently are seen in sepsis as well as pregnancy, and their presence alone is not an indication for additional blood tests or cultures.

Differential Diagnosis

Distinguishing the neutrophilia of pregnancy from leukemia usually is not a difficult problem. Bone-marrow biopsy and aspirate, histochemical stains, chromosome analysis, and peripheral blood flow cytometric analysis of white blood cells help identify the rare pregnancy complicated by leukemia. When leukemia does occur during pregnancy, difficult decisions are presented by the anticipated toxic effects of chemotherapy on mother and fetus (the most active stage of fetal organogenesis is during the first trimester) as well as the long-term prospects for survival. Although a number of case reports detail successful, uncomplicated births following chemotherapy for acute leukemia, the most common outcomes are abortion and fetal loss. Leukapheresis may serve as an effective stopgap measure to control leukocyte counts in chronic leukemia until after delivery and thus delay the use of drugs that are potentially immunosuppressive and teratogenic.

THROMBOCYTOPENIA

Although the subject is somewhat controversial, there is now a large body of literature to suggest that during late pregnancy, many healthy women become thrombocytopenic, defined by a platelet count below 150,000/μL. The reasons for the development of mild thrombocytopenia during normal pregnancy are complex. Alterations in plasma volume probably result in a "dilutional thrombocytopenia." Increased platelet consumption related to low-grade disseminated intravascular coagulation (DIC) within the uteroplacental circulation also has been proposed as a physiologic adaptation allowing preservation of the uteroplacental interface. Following delivery, mild thrombocytopenia resolves spontaneously.

In a large prospective study of more than 6000 pregnant women in Hamilton, Ontario by Burrows and Kelton, approximately 8% had mild thrombocytopenia at term, yet no adverse results were experienced by the women or their infants. Because a platelet count in the range of 100,000–150,000/µL in an otherwise uncomplicated pregnancy rarely causes problems, several authors have suggested restraint in evaluating and treating patients with this finding. The cause of thrombocytopenia should not be overlooked, however, when platelet counts are less than 100,000/µL or when other medical problems supervene. Finding and eliminating the cause has special significance, because bleeding complications can threaten both mother and fetus and may have important implications vis-à-vis determining the method of delivery and defining the infant's needs for postnatal care.

IMMUNE THROMBOCYTOPENIC PURPURA

Immune thrombocytopenia purpura (ITP) is characterized by a decreased platelet count caused by splenic sequestration mediated by antiplatelet antibodies. It is relatively common during pregnancy, occurring once or twice in 1000 deliveries. Although pregnancy has not been thought to have a significant impact on the development or severity of ITP, this assertion recently has been challenged by McCrae.

ITP can be classified based on its chronicity. The acute form typically affects children more often than adults and occurs following a viral illness. Thrombocytopenia and purpura usually develop within 1–2 weeks of a viral prodrome, affect males and females with equal frequency, and are self-limiting. Chronic ITP is more likely to affect young women and, as suggested by its designation, is longer lasting. Platelet counts usually remain low; remission refers to absence of purpura rather than normality of the platelet count. When platelet counts fall below 50,000–70,000/µL, therapy with glucocorticoids or other methods is considered. In pregnancy-associated ITP, maternal death is rare, and morbidity correlates with the severity of thrombocytopenia. Postpartum hemorrhage caused by cervical or vaginal laceration is the most common complication of a low platelet count. The aspect of ITP that is unique to pregnant patients is that the fetus may be affected by the disorder. Although maternal platelet-associated IgG antibodies can cross the uteroplacental barrier and affect fetal platelets, significant fetal thrombocytopenia at or following delivery (50,000/µL) occurs in only 10–15% of instances and is rarely associated with significant morbidity.

Clinical Findings & Diagnosis

If thrombocytopenia develops in the first half of pregnancy, it is unlikely to be pregnancy-associated and more likely to be ITP. A healthy woman who is found on the basis of routine laboratory studies to have isolated thrombocytopenia, normal-appearing or mildly enlarged platelets on peripheral blood smear, and a bone marrow containing normal or increased numbers of megakaryocytes presumably has ITP. Most patients with platelet counts less than 30,000–50,000/µL offer a history of easy bruising and findings of petechia, epistaxis, or gingival oozing. Overt hemorrhage is uncommon, however, unless the platelet count is below 20,000/µL. Physical examination is otherwise unremarkable, and the presence of significant lymphadenopathy or splenomegaly should call into question the diagnosis of ITP. Assays for platelet-associated antibody rarely are helpful in establishing the diagnosis; the antibody is not always present and may not correlate with clinical findings.

Differential Diagnosis

Other causes of thrombocytopenia, such as infection with the human immunodeficiency virus (HIV) or other viruses, neoplasms, aplastic anemia, vitamin deficiency, eclampsia, DIC, and autoimmune disorders, must be excluded by laboratory or clinical evaluation. A careful drug history should be elicited; a number of drugs used commonly during pregnancy may cause thrombocytopenia (Table 40–2). Two drug-induced syndromes relatively unique to pregnancy deserve mention: (1) acute cocaine ingestion has been associated with the transient development of a syndrome resembling severe preeclampsia and may be accompanied by profound thrombocytopenia;

Table 40–2. Drugs occasionally associated with thrombocytopenia in pregnancy.

Class	Drug
Cytotoxic agents	Nitrogen mustard
	Cyclophosphamide
	5-Fluorouracil
	Methotrexate
Antacids	Cimetidine
	Ranitidine (Zantac)
	Nizatidine
	Omeprazole (Prilosec)
Diuretics	Chlorothiazide
Antihypertensives	Hydralazine
Antibiotics	Penicillin
	Sulfa-containing drugs
Oral hypoglycemics	Sulfonamides
	Tolbutamide
	Glyburide
Anticonvulsants/hypnotics/ antiemetics	Chlorpropamide
	Diazepam
	Diphenylhydantoin
	Chlorpromazine
Pain modulators	Acetaminophen
Miscellaneous	Gold salts
	Heparin
	Heroin
	Cocaine
	Alcohol

*Many other agents used in cancer chemotherapy could be listed.

and (2) neonatal thrombocytopenia may occur in the infants of women who have taken thiazide diuretics or hydralazine, which are used occasionally to manage pregnancy-induced hypertension.

Treatment

Treatment for ITP during pregnancy typically is initiated once platelet counts fall below 50,000/μL. Prednisone at a dose of 1–1.5 mg/kg/d is the treatment of choice. Eighty percent of women respond to this regimen with a rise in platelet counts within 10–14 days. If the patient does not respond within 2–4 weeks or if there are relative contraindications to use of steroids (eg, poorly controlled diabetes, active psychiatric problems, or labile hypertension), high-dose intravenous immunoglobulins (IVIGs) are infused to raise maternal platelet counts. IVIGs presumably impart a beneficial effect on platelet counts by blocking the maternal reticuloendothelial receptor uptake of IgG-coated platelets. The usual total dose is 2 g/kg divided into daily dosages given over 1–5 days. Although a response is seen within days, platelet increases are usually short-lived, and therapy may need to be repeated every 3 weeks.

Although splenectomy can be performed safely in the second trimester of pregnancy, it usually can be avoided because of the ready availability and success of steroids and IVIGs. Other drugs that are used occasionally for non-pregnancy-associated ITP, such as cyclophosphamide, vincristine, and azathioprine, usually are held in reserve because of concerns regarding their immunosuppressive or teratogenic potential. Danazol, 200 mg orally 3 times daily, is prescribed occasionally; however, platelet count increases are not consistent, and concern for possible hepatotoxicity mandates blood draws to detect liver enzyme elevations. Platelet transfusions are of questionable benefit also because of their rapid elimination from the circulation. As a result, they are used only in the setting of life-threatening or difficult-to-control hemorrhage. Drugs that inhibit platelet aggregation such as aspirin and other nonsteroidal anti-inflammatory drugs (NSAIDs) should be avoided; women should not receive intramuscular injections of any drugs, because they can lead to painful hematomas. Patients should be instructed not to use hard toothbrushes, dental floss, or metal razors.

A major area of controversy among those who care for patients with maternal thrombocytopenia is how best to manage the fetus. In theory, head trauma associated with the passage of the fetus through the birth canal during labor and delivery could precipitate a devastating intracranial hemorrhage. Efforts to predict or influence fetal platelet counts by looking at the maternal platelet count, assaying for platelet-associated IgG, and providing the mother with corticosteroids have proved to be unreliable. In the absence of a simple, accurate method to determine or influence fetal platelet counts, cesarean section often has been recommended, in the hope of protecting the fetus from bleeding during labor and delivery.

More recently, scalp blood sampling has been employed to assess fetal platelet counts directly. The value of this test is compromised by the need for adequate cervical dilatation before the procedure is performed and the possibility of inaccuracy owing to dilution with amniotic fluid or clotting of the sample. Cordocentesis (umbilical vein sampling) may be a more accurate means of assessing fetal platelet counts and can be performed before the onset of labor.

There is disagreement as to what risk maternal ITP poses to the fetus. It appears that severe thrombocytopenia (platelet level below 20,000/μL) rarely occurs; the incidence may be in the range of 4%. Furthermore, in a retrospective study by Samuels et al of 90 cases of fetal ITP over a 20-year period, no antenatal or neonatal intracranial hemorrhage occurred. In another study, an incidence of 1–2% of fetal or neonatal intracranial hemorrhage was seen. The low probability of encountering severe thrombocytopenia and the small risk of serious hemorrhage have led some investigators to conclude that the risks of cordocentesis, which vary widely according to the experience of the treating physician, are unwarranted.

Although there is still support for giving steroids and IVIGs to ITP-affected mothers during the 3 weeks before delivery for their effect on the fetus, no studies have shown convincingly a reliable benefit to the fetus. Despite lack of evidence to substantiate that cordocentesis is helpful, many practitioners are reluctant to allow vaginal delivery with a maternal or fetal platelet count below 50,000/μL, and a single cordocentesis is performed at term at many institutions.

PREECLAMPSIA- & ECLAMPSIA-RELATED HEMATOLOGIC ABNORMALITIES

Preeclampsia is a frequent complication occurring in as many as 5–13% of pregnancies. Most commonly, these patients are primigravidas in their third trimester. The pathogenesis of preeclampsia-associated thrombocytopenia is uncertain. Patients with preeclampsia and thrombocytopenia have large mean platelet volumes and increased megakaryocytes on bone-marrow sampling. Suggested reasons for low platelet counts include increased consumption of platelets owing to damaged or activated endothelium, alterations in thrombin generation, and enhanced sequestration of platelets caused by the deposition of IgG or circulating immune complexes on their cell surface. Between 15 and 50% of patients with preeclampsia develop thrombocytopenia at some point during their illness, making preeclampsia a common cause of significant thrombocytopenia during the third trimester.

Clinical Findings & Diagnosis

The diagnosis of preeclampsia is established by an increase in blood pressure to at least 140/90 mmHg, accompanied by edema, proteinuria greater than 0.3 g/24 h or 10 mg/dL in at least two random specimens collected 6 hours apart, or both. For unknown reasons, preeclampsia is observed most often in women who are younger than 20 or older than 30 years.

In severe preeclampsia, a reduction in plasma volume may be reflected by a rapid increase in the HCT over 5–10 days. In mild preeclampsia, alterations in HCT usually are not seen. In more than 20% of patients with severe preeclampsia, consumption of procoagulants takes place. DIC also may contribute to this process, with low levels of antithrombin III and elevated dimers of fibrin split products found in DIC screening assays.

Differential Diagnosis

When thrombocytopenia is noted in a patient in whom classic signs of preeclampsia (edema, followed by hypertension and proteinuria) or eclampsia (seizures/coma) are developing, the cause of the thrombocytopenia is usually easy to identify. Thrombocytopenia also may accompany hepatic forms of toxemia in which the usual signs of preeclampsia are absent. Acute fatty liver of pregnancy is one of these variants; clinical attention is drawn to liver abnormalities including profound elevations in transaminases along with less impressive rises in bilirubin and alkaline phosphatase. The hematologic alterations in pregnancy may extend to encompass the HELLP (hemolysis, liver dysfunction, low platelets) syndrome. Criteria for diagnosis include (1) microangiopathic hemolytic anemia with schistocytes on the peripheral blood film; (2) bilirubin above 1.2 g/dL, lactate dehydrogenase (LDH) above 600 u/L, and serum glutamic oxaloacetic transaminase (SGOT) at least 70 u/L; and (3) platelet count less than 100,000/µL. Because many patients with HELLP also manifest hypertension and proteinuria, the clinical overlap with eclampsia is evident.

Thrombotic thrombocytopenic purpura and the hemolytic uremic syndrome are additional disorders characterized by microangiopathic hemolytic anemia and severe thrombocytopenia. Although both diseases are rare in pregnancy, they should be considered when evaluating a pregnant patient with thrombocytopenia. All pregnant women with platelet counts less than 75,000/µL should be evaluated by a hematologist.

Treatment

Management of toxemia and its variants involves medical stabilization of the patient followed by delivery of the fetus as soon as possible. A few case reports suggest a benefit to a trial of aspirin in the rare instance when thrombocytopenia occurs in the mid to late second trimester. The beneficial effect of NSAIDs suggests a causal relationship of prostaglandin and arachidonic acid metabolism in eclampsia.

Although significant bleeding usually does not occur in patients with preeclampsia, minor bleeding and postoperative oozing are common. Occasionally, bleeding is the result of a coagulopathy such as DIC. Because heparin may enhance the bleeding tendency, its use should be avoided. Rather, platelet transfusions are ordered just before delivery in an effort to maintain platelet numbers greater than 20,000–50,000/µL, especially if cesarean section is contemplated. The benefits of platelet transfusions in this instance are unclear given their rapid consumption shortly after they have been infused. Steroid administration just before delivery may increase platelet counts.

DISSEMINATED INTRAVASCULAR COAGULATION

DIC is an acquired syndrome of laboratory and clinical findings in which proteins important in coagulation are consumed and the fibrinolytic system is activated. It is a frequent cause of abnormal bleeding in obstetric patients. Activation of the coagulation system has been associated with abruptio placentae, sepsis, retained intrauterine fetal death, and amniotic fluid embolus. Other causes of DIC include liver disease, trauma, and hypovolemic shock. Common to many of these conditions is the release of a thromboplastin or endotoxin-like substance into the circulation, resulting in intravascular clotting and fibrin formation in the microvasculature (Fig 40–1).

The coagulation factors most readily consumed in DIC include platelets, prothrombin, factor V, and factor VIII. The body has a finite capacity to replace these factors, which are critical to clot formation. When procoagulants are consumed, a bleeding diathesis may ensue. Activation of the fibrinolytic system produces fibrin-fibrinogen degradation products (FDP), which interfere with normal clotting mechanisms. Systemic manifestations include endothelial damage with increased vascular permeability, hemorrhage, and end-organ ischemia.

Laros has divided the obstetric diseases associated with DIC into three major groups based on the mechanisms by which the primary disease initiates vascular clotting. DIC is triggered in the first group by the intravascular infusion of tissue thromboplastins. Abruptio placentae and the dead fetus syndrome fall into this grouping. In the dead fetus syndrome, consumption occurs slowly over a period of days to weeks. With abruptio placentae, consumption is

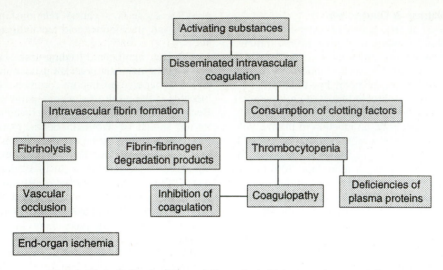

Figure 40–1. Pathophysiology of disseminated intravascular coagulation.

rapid and fulminant, and the chief complication is hemorrhage.

A second group of pathologic conditions causing DIC includes those associated with endothelial damage. An example already reviewed is eclampsia or preeclampsia.

A third group of conditions associated with DIC encompasses nonspecific or indirect effects of certain diseases. This group includes amniotic fluid embolus, gram-negative sepsis, and saline abortion. Amniotic fluid embolism is usually fatal (85% mortality rate), more as a result of cardiovascular collapse than of its hemorrhagic complications. This life-threatening entity occurs most frequently during difficult deliveries in multiparous women. Hypoxemia, shock, and hemorrhage in this setting should suggest the diagnosis. The prototype for sepsis causing DIC is clostridial infection. This aftermath of septic abortions also is characterized by severe intravascular hemolysis attributed to the direct bacterial by-product attack of lecithinase on the RBC membrane.

Clinical Findings & Diagnosis

The signs and symptoms of DIC are those of the underlying disease with the addition of hemorrhage, thrombosis, or both. Acute DIC most often is associated with bleeding, and chronic DIC, with thrombotic complications. Acute DIC poses a great risk to the mother, with intracranial hemorrhage the most worrisome complication. Thrombotic presentations may be neurologic, with seizures, delirium, or coma, or they may be dermatologic, with focal ischemia and superficial gangrene. Thrombosis of the renal vasculature can cause cortical necrosis and renal failure. Infarcts and emboli represent pulmonary vascular obstruction, whereas phlebitis and extremity gangrene

are the result of thrombosis of peripheral blood vessels.

DIC must be considered a possibility in any obstetric patient presenting with risk factors as noted or who has unexplained bleeding or thrombosis. The laboratory diagnosis of acute DIC is usually clear (Table 40–3). As RBCs are forced through the obstructed microvasculature, they are sheared. The fragmented forms are referred to as schistocytes and helmet cells and are seen on peripheral blood smear. Thrombocytopenia is invariably present. Fibrinogen, which usually is elevated to supranormal levels in uncomplicated pregnancy, is low or low-normal (less than 250 mg/dL), and circulating FDPs are elevated. The prothrombin time (PT) and partial thromboplastin time (PTT) are prolonged in most cases. If intravascular hemolysis is sufficiently brisk, hemoglobinuria occurs, and serum haptoglobin levels decline to absent or barely detectable levels. Like fibrinogen, serum haptoglobin is an acute-phase reactant and is elevated in uncomplicated pregnancies. The laboratory diagnosis of chronic DIC may prove more subtle

Table 40–3. Typical laboratory findings in acute disseminated intravascular coagulation.

Laboratory Test	Result
Platelet count	Decreased
Fibrinogen	Decreased
Antithrombin III	Decreased
Prothrombin time	Usually prolonged
Activated partial thromboplastin time	Usually prolonged
Fibrinogen-fibrin degradation products	Increased
Schistocytes on peripheral blood smear	Present

and require the expertise of a hematologist to interpret.

Treatment

Of major importance in the management of a patient with DIC is recognizing and treating the underlying cause. In the obstetric arena, in particular, treating the underlying cause produces profound improvement in hematologic and clinical parameters. Chronic DIC is now infrequently a problem because its principal cause, fetal death in utero, is recognized easily by oxytocin induction of delivery with blood component support.

Treatment of acute DIC triggered by abruptio placentae consists of delivery of the infant under the coverage of the appropriate blood components—platelets, cryoprecipitate, and fresh frozen plasma. Guidelines for the replacement of blood products include maintenance of a HCT of 20–25%, normovolemia reflected by a urine output of greater than 30 mL/h, a platelet count in excess of 20,000/μL, and a fibrinogen level of greater than 100 mg/mL.

Treatment of amniotic fluid embolism is focused on vigorous supportive therapy directed toward gas exchange with mechanical respiratory assistance and intravascular fluid and pressor infusions to maintain adequate cardiac output. In patients in whom continued entry of amniotic debris may be contributing to intravascular clotting, heparin may be a reasonable adjunct to therapy. Because heparin may exacerbate bleeding and possibly thrombocytopenia, it should be employed in the coagulopathic patient under direction of the consulting hematologist.

During the second trimester, saline-induced abortions often result in mild DIC. Most of these patients do not have clinical signs of bleeding, although brisk oozing is sometimes seen at delivery. This complication is short-lived and disappears after the fetus is delivered. In the rare instance in which bleeding persists and fibrinogen or platelet counts are low, the patient should be treated appropriately with cryoprecipitate and platelet transfusions to correct the deficiency. If vaginal bleeding occurs in the face of normal hemostatic factors, however, the bleeding may be due to retention of fetal products rather than a systemic hemostatic defect.

VON WILLEBRAND'S DISEASE

von Willebrand's disease (vWD) is an inherited qualitative or quantitative abnormality of von Willebrand factor (vWF). vWF functions in two ways: (1) as an adhesive protein that permits efficient binding of platelets to the endothelium and (2) as a carrier molecule for factor VIII. vWD is the most common coagulopathy that causes problems during pregnancy and delivery. Abnormalities in vWF most commonly are inherited in an autosomal dominant or autosomal recessive fashion with variable penetrance, although they may be acquired also.

Structurally, vWF consists of a series of multimers. Cross-immunoelectrophoretic experiments reveal variable mobility of the multimers, with the smallest multimers having the most rapid mobility. The clinical relevance of these multimer fractions is the apparent relationship between size and hemostatic efficacy. Larger multimeric fractions are the most functionally active, and deficiencies of these factors frequently result in bleeding-time abnormalities.

Clinical Findings & Diagnosis

The clinical symptoms among patients with vWD vary greatly. In the usual heterozygous form, defects of primary hemostasis are seen including bruising, epistaxis, gingival oozing, and gastrointestinal blood loss. In female patients, the only clue to this condition may be a history of menorrhagia, and frequently, postextraction and posttraumatic bleeding is moderately prolonged. Homozygous or doubly heterozygous patients may experience severe bleeding such as postsurgical bleeding, hemarthrosis, or, more rarely, uncontrollable gastrointestinal hemorrhage. Many persons with vWD are not diagnosed until adulthood. Bleeding symptoms show considerable variability within a family as well as in an individual on different occasions.

Inherited vWD is classified into three major subtypes depending on laboratory findings (Table 40–4). Type I has a mild reduction in quantity of apparently normal vWF, with a normal multimeric profile; type II and its subgroups have qualitative abnormalities in vWF, either in function or in electrophoretic multimer distribution; and type III is characterized by absent or low levels of vWF. Clinical severity varies by group, with type III the most severe.

The laboratory diagnosis of vWD is complex and expensive and should be undertaken only under the direction of a hematologist or coagulation technician. The criteria for the laboratory diagnosis of vWD include quantitative and qualitative abnormalities of vWF. Because several of the clinical and laboratory findings mimic those of hemophilia (eg, easy bruisability, postprocedure hemorrhage, prolonged PTT, and reduced factor VIII levels), it may be necessary to perform tests for vWD in persons with decreased factor VIII levels and no clear evidence of sex-linked bleeding history. A prolonged bleeding time is characteristic of vWD; in hemophilia, bleeding is a function of reduced factor VIII or factor IX levels, but platelet function (in the absence of recent NSAID use) is normal. A complete discussion of the available tests is beyond the scope of this chapter; there are several excellent reviews of this topic.

Table 40–4. Classification of von Willebrand's disease based on laboratory abnormalities.

Factor	Type I	Type IIA	Type IIB	Type III
Genetic transmission	Autosomal dominant	Autosomal dominant	Autosomal dominant	Autosomal recessive
Bleeding time	Prolonged	Prolonged	Prolonged	Prolonged
Factor 8 coagulant	Decreased	Decreased or normal	Decreased or normal	Markedly decreased
von Willebrand factor antigen	Decreased	Decreased or normal	Decreased or normal	Minute amounts or absent
Ristocetin cofactor	Decreased	Markedly decreased	Decreased or normal	Absent
von Willebrand factor function	Decreased or normal	Absent or markedly decreased	Increased	Absent
Multimeric structure	Normal in plasma and platelets	Absence of large and intermediate multimers from plasma and platelets	Absence of only large multimers from plasma; normal in platelets	Variable
Treatment	Desmopressin ± cryoprecipitate	Desmopressin ± cryoprecipitate	Cryoprecipitate; desmopressin is contraindicated	Cryoprecipitate

Prolongation of the bleeding time is not specific for vWD; it can be observed in a myriad of platelet and vessel wall abnormalities. In vWD, the bleeding time is abnormal because platelet adherence to subendothelium is compromised, thus preventing a normal hemostatic plug. Rarely, bleeding times in vWD remain normal; further testing is recommended if there is a personal or family history of hemorrhage. In the type I variant, in particular, there is an increase in factor VIII coagulant and antigen levels during pregnancy. The PTT and thrombin time are usually normal, although modest elevations in PTT are seen when factor VIII is decreased secondary to the decline in vWF.

Patients with type I vWD may be partially protected during pregnancy because factor VIII and vWF levels increase, often to near-normal levels; therefore, immediate postpartum hemorrhage is an infrequent occurrence. There remains a risk of bleeding after delivery in these women because of the rapid return of the coagulant levels to a nonpregnant, deficient state. In type II vWD, in which a qualitative defect in vWF exists, increased levels of vWF during pregnancy may not translate into normalization of the bleeding time. Thrombocytopenia may occur in type IIB disease, presumably because of the increased concentration of more reactive, high-molecular-weight multimers of vWF.

Treatment

Cryoprecipitate infusion remains the treatment of choice for patients with all subtypes of vWD who are actively hemorrhaging. Single-donor cryoprecipitate has all the fractions of vWF found in normal plasma. Bleeding usually is arrested once factor VIII procoagulant activity and vWF levels of 50% of normal are achieved. Because the therapeutic effects last ap-

proximately 4 hours, cryoprecipitate must be reinfused to maintain normal hemostatic control.

Although cryoprecipitate infusion has been the standard therapy for nonemergent vWD in the past, because of the risks of infection, desmopressin (a synthetic analog of vasopressin) has been used recently. Desmopressin provides temporary benefit to patients with type I vWD by inducing release of vWF from endothelial stores. Its use is limited by the development of tachyphylaxis after repeated administration. In persons with type II vWD, response to desmopressin is limited and unpredictable. In persons with type IIB vWD, administration of desmopressin can accentuate thrombocytopenia, further aggravating the bleeding problem. Persons with type III vWD do not respond to desmopressin.

SUMMARY

In evaluating pregnant women, it is important to be aware of the physiologic changes in pregnancy that affect the HCT and other laboratory parameters. Although the treatment and obstetric management of most hematologic disorders is well established, controversy exists concerning conditions such as ITP, DIC, and sickle cell disease. To ensure optimal health of the pregnant woman and fetus, a hematologist should be consulted in the evaluation of patients with moderate-to-severe thrombocytopenia, anemia that is not responsive to iron supplementation, or a prior history of moderate-to-severe bleeding after surgical procedures.

REFERENCES

Alderot LM: Treatment of von Willebrand's disease. Mayo Clin Proc 1991;66:841.

Aster RH: "Gestational" thrombocytopenia: A plea for conservative management. N Engl J Med 1990;323:264.

Bloom AL: von Willebrand factor: Clinical features of inherited and acquired disorders. Mayo Clin Proc 1991;66:743.

Browning J, James DK: Immune thrombocytopenia in pregnancy. Fetal Med Rev 1990;2:143.

Burrows RF, Kelton JG: Fetal thrombocytopenia and its relation to maternal thrombocytopenia. N Engl J Med 1990;329:1463.

Burrows RF, Kelton JG: Thrombocytopenia at delivery: A prospective study of 6715 deliveries. Am J Obstct Gynecol 1990;162:731.

Cook RL et al: Immune thrombocytopenic purpura in pregnancy: A reappraisal of management. Obstet Gynecol 1991;78:578.

Duffy TP: Hematologic aspects of pregnancy. In: *Hematology: Basic Principles and Practice*. Hoffman R et al (editors). Churchill Livingstone, 1991.

Fisher J, Dietl J, Goelz R: Fetal and maternal thrombocytopenia. (Letter.) N Engl J Med 1994;330:940.

Ginsburg D, Bowie EJ: Molecular genetics of von Willebrand disease. Blood 1992;79:2507.

Horn E: Iron and folate supplements during pregnancy: Supplementing everyone treats those at risk and is cost effective. Br Med J 1988;297:1325.

Koshy M et al: Prophylactic red-cell transfusions in pregnant patients with sickle cell disease: A randomized, prospective study. N Engl J Med 1988;319:1147.

Laros RK Jr: Acquired coagulation disorders. In: *Blood Disorders in Pregnancy*. Laros RK Jr (editor). Lea & Febiger, 1986.

Marder VJ et al: Consumptive thrombohemorrhagic disorders. In: *Hemostasis and Thrombosis: Basic Principles and Clinical Practice,* 3rd ed. Colman RW et al (editors). Lippincott, 1994.

Martin JN, Stedman CW: Imitators of preeclampsia and HELLP syndrome. Obstet Gynecol Clin North Am 1991;18:181.

McCrae KR, Samuels P, Schreiber AD: Pregnancy associated thrombocytopenia: Pathogenesis and management. Blood 1992;80:2697.

Perry KG, Morrison JC: Hematologic disorders in pregnancy. Obstet Gynecol Clin North Am 1992;19:783.

Pollack CV Jr: Emergencies in sickle cell disease. Emerg Med Clin North Am 1993;11:365.

Rosenberg IH: Folic acid and neural-tube defects: Time for action. N Engl J Med 1992;327:1875.

Samuels P et al: Estimation of the risk of thrombocytopenia in the offspring of pregnant women with presumed immune thrombocytopenia purpura. N Engl J Med 1990;323:299.

Stein ML, Gunston KD, May RM: Iron dextran in the treatment of iron deficiency anaemia of pregnancy. S Afr Med J 1991;79:195.

Suharno D et al: Supplementation with vitamin A and iron for nutritional anaemia in pregnant women in West Java, Indonesia. Lancet 1993;342:1335.

United States Preventive Services Task Force: Routine iron supplementation during pregnancy: Policy statement. JAMA 1993;270:2846.

Warkentin TE, Kelton JG: Current concepts in the treatment of immune thrombocytopenia. Drugs 1990;40:531.

Williams MD, Whelby MS: Anemia in pregnancy. Med Clin North Am 1991;76:631.

41

Chronic Fatigue Syndrome

Dedra Buchwald, MD

Definition
Incidence
Pathophysiology
Signs & Symptoms
Clinical Findings
Differential Diagnosis & Cormorbid
   Conditions
Diagnosis
Treatment
Prognosis

Fatigue is a common experience. Large surveys in the developed world have found that between 10 and 50% of people report current fatigue, usually of an unspecified severity and limited duration. Fatigue is also a common complaint in primary care settings. Among patients seeking medical care, for example, the prevalence of fatigue is at least 20%. In most cases, fatigue is transient, explained by prevailing circumstances, relieved by rest, and little cause for concern. In both community and clinical settings, the prevalence of fatigue often has been observed to be greater in women than in men.

Fatigue can be both chronic and debilitating, however. In some cases, it may be the result of a medical or psychological condition such as thyroid disease or depression. Less commonly, chronic fatigue may be the hallmark of chronic fatigue syndrome (CFS), an illness characterized by profound fatigue often accompanied by sleep disturbances, myalgias, pharyngitis, and depression. CFS has been reported worldwide. In the United States, a formal case definition has been developed by the Centers for Disease Control and Prevention (CDC) (see next section).

Definition

Although diagnostic criteria for CFS have been formulated only recently, the condition is not new. Several clinical syndromes, both sporadic and epidemic, described previously by clinicians and researchers in retrospect appear to share some of the features of CFS. These disorders include neurasthenia, myalgic encephalomyelitis, and chronic Epstein-Barr virus (EBV) infection. The current definition of CFS used in the USA originated in the controversies concerning reports in the medical literature and lay press of an epidemic initially attributed to chronic EBV infection in the Lake Tahoe, Nevada, area. In 1987, a group of public health epidemiologists, academic researchers, and clinicians was convened by the CDC to develop a consensus statement on the salient clinical characteristics of the syndrome. This group proposed a working case definition designed to improve the comparability and reproducibility of clinical research and epidemiologic studies and to provide a rational basis for evaluating patients with chronic fatigue of unknown cause. Furthermore, the group proposed that chronic EBV infection be re-

named CFS, thus removing the implication that EBV is the causal agent and emphasizing the syndrome's most dominant feature.

The original CDC case definition published in 1988 consisted of two major and fourteen minor criteria; the minor criteria included 11 symptoms and 3 physical criteria. A revised case definition has recently been published (Table 41–1). A case of CFS is defined by the presence of clinically evaluated, unexplained, persistent or relapsing fatigue that has been present for longer than 6 months. It also mush be of definite onset, not alleviated by rest, and result in substantial reduction in occupational, educational, social, or personal activities. The new case definition requires the concurrent occurrence of at least four of eight symptoms, all of which must have persisted or recurred during 6 or more consecutive months and must not have predated the onset of fatigue. No abnormalities on physical examination or laboratory studies are required to make the diagnosis of CFS. The CDC criteria for CFS are not empirically based and have never been subjected to rigorous scrutiny.

Among the first problems encountered by researchers in attempting to use the CDC criteria was distinguishing CFS from psychiatric disorders. This difficulty results from the enormous overlap between the symptoms of CFS and those of affective, anxiety, and somatization disorders. For example, a patient who reports fatigue, clearly a prerequisite for CFS, is simultaneously describing a symptom of major depression. In fact, the similarity of CFS symptoms to those of major depression and the apparently high rate of preexisting psychiatric disorders in patients

Table 41–1. The Centers for Disease Control and Prevention working case definition of chronic fatigue syndrome.

Both fatigue criteria and four of eight symptom criteria must be present to fulfill the case definition.

Fatigue

1. Persistent or relapsing fatigue that:
   a. has been clinically evaluated
   b. is of definite onset
   c. is not the result of exertion
   d. results in substantial reduction in activity
2. Other conditions that explain the fatigue have been excluded including:
   a. active medical conditions, eg, untreated hypothyroidism
   b. previously diagnosed medical condition whose resolution has not been clinically documented (eg, treated malignancies)
   c. past or present psychotic or melancholic depression, bipolar disorder, schizophrenia, delusional disorders, dementia, anorexia nervosa, bulimia
   d. alcohol or substance abuse within 2 years of the onset of fatigue or anytime thereafter.

Symptom criteria

Persistent or recurrent symptoms lasting more than 6 consecutive months:

1. Self-reported impairment in short-term memory or concentration, which causes substantial reduction of occupational, educational, social, or personal activities.
2. Sore throat
3. Tender posterior cervical, anterior cervical, or axillary lymphnode pain
4. Muscle pain
5. Multijoint noninflammatory arthralgias
6. New or different headaches
7. Unrefreshing sleep
8. Prolonged (at least 24 hours) generalized fatigue following previously tolerable levels of exercise

---

with CFS have led to the suggestion that CFS is simply depression or the modern version of neurasthenia.

There also has been confusion regarding the psychiatric exclusion criterion imposed by the CDC case definition. The 1988 criteria was not explicit and does not identify clearly which patients and which disorders should be excluded. The revised case definition published in 1994 does not exclude patients with major depression, panic, generalized anxiety, and somatization disorder. Psychiatric diagnoses that are grounds for exclusion are schizophrenia, bipolar disorder, psychotic depression, and substance abuse. It is recommended that patients with CFS be screened for psychological distress and psychiatric disorders.

Incidence

A. Prevalence in Clinical Settings: There have been several studies of CFS (or CFS-like illnesses) among patients in general medical settings. In a study conducted before the development of the CFS case definition using much less stringent criteria, chronic fatigue associated with headache, sore throat, and myalgias was reported approximately 20% of patients seeking primary care. However, many of the symptoms in the CDC case definition were not elicited, the severity of fatigue was not quantified, and comorbid illnesses that could have produced fatigue were not systematically pursued. In another survey of 611 British ambulatory patients, it was found that only one patient had a CFS-like illness with at least 6 months of significant fatigue. In a subsequent investigation in which patients underwent a comprehensive medical and psychological evaluation, 17 cases of CFS were detected among 686 patients attending a primary care practice. Finally, a recent prospective study in a primary care practice in the USA identified three cases of CFS among 1000 patients seeking care. In these investigations, the point prevalence of CFS ranged from 164 to 2500 per 100,000 persons among general medical patients.

B. Prevalence in the Community: Many previous population-based studies have examined the frequency of complaints of fatigue, but few have attempted to evaluate the prevalence of CFS in the community. Three studies in the USA, Australia, and Great Britain indirectly estimated the prevalence of CFS in the community by identifying patients seeking care for fatigue through sentinel physicians. These investigators have reported the prevalence of CFS to range from 3.4 to 130 per 100,000 persons. Other approximations of the prevalence of CFS have used data from an epidemiologic study of psychiatric illness or information from viral serology request forms neither of which contained all the items required to assess whether the CFS case definition was met. In the only true population-based study to date, a large random sample of enrollees in a health maintenance organization, selected irrespective of whether they sought medical care, were surveyed by mail for the presence of chronic fatigue. Those who reported chronic fatigue underwent a thorough medical and psychological evaluation. It was found that unexplained, debilitating chronic fatigue of at least 6 months duration (not necessarily meeting the CDC case definition) had a point prevalence of 2316 to 6321 per 100,000 persons. CFS was considerably less common, with an estimated point prevalence of 98 to 267 per 100,000 persons. Persons with CFS as well as chronic fatigue had greater psychological distress and poorer functional status than healthy control participants. An interesting finding was that the population-based nature of this study (ie, persons not seeking medical care) resulted in the representation of a broader spectrum of illness. For example, only 14% of the participants in this community study who reported chronic fatigue and none of those with CFS were unemployed, in contrast to 35–45% in consultative practices of CFS patients.

C. Gender, Race, and Ethnicity: Early reports in the lay press about the so-called yuppie flu and findings published in the medical literature suggested that chronic fatigue alone (but not CFS) and CFS primarily affected young, successful, white women. An inspection of 30 studies on CFS-like illnesses, published between 1985 and 1993, found among the five studies reporting incidence in ethnic and racial groups race, three had no minority-group participants (in one instance, 50% of the practice was composed of blacks), and the remaining two reported a striking preponderance of whites. However, a growing body of evidence suggests that chronic fatigue and CFS affect persons from all socioeconomic classes, all racial and ethnic groups, and both genders. A clinic-based study found that the spectrum of illness, including the demographic, clinical, laboratory, functional, and psychosocial features, is similar in white and nonwhite patients. In one community study, nonwhites were underrepresented and blacks were overrepresented, compared with the local and national population.

It seems likely, therefore, that the paucity of minority-group patients with chronic fatigue or CFS seen in referral settings is in part a function of health care seeking. Other factors may be equally important, however, such as the affordability and accessibility of medical care; cultural factors affecting the perceived need for, acceptability of, and desirability of mainstream medical services; and cultural dynamics that dictate the degree to which symptoms are perceived as problems.

Pathophysiology

Although there have been many theories of the cause of CFS, strong evidence to support any of them is lacking. Most investigators believe that no single agent will prove to be the cause in all—or even in most—cases. Nonetheless, the fact that CFS frequently is reported to be precipitated by an acute viral illness may be important. Previous work has shown that viruses have the ability to alter neuroendocrine function, as well as to reset sleep mechanisms, either directly or through intermediary factors such as cytokines. These observations have led to speculation that a triggering event, usually a viral infection, leads to the persistent production of cytokines in CFS patients, such as those elaborated as part of the acute phase response (Fig 41–1). These cytokines, in turn, disrupt sleep both directly and indirectly through their effects on the normal functioning of the hypothalamic-pituitary-adrenal (HPA) axis. Dysregulation of the HPA axis also may result from the infection itself or through the effects of cytokines. In any case, a disruption of sleep is manifested, and a syndrome characterized by chronic fatigue eventually results. It is of interest that cytokines are known to cause the flulike symptoms associated with many acute infections and have been shown to induce a CFS-like syndrome when administered for therapeutic purposes. As in any chronic illness,

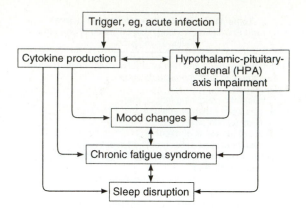

Figure 41–1. Postulated pathophysiologic mechanism for chronic fatigue syndrome.

symptoms lead to disability, which is both due to, and results in psychological dysfunction.

Signs & Symptoms

A. Symptoms: A compelling piece of evidence that CFS is an "organic" illness is its sudden onset in up to 85% of patients. Many state that their illness began on a particular day, with a flulike syndrome characterized by fever, pharyngitis, adenopathy, myalgias, and related symptoms. Unlike the usual experience with the flu, however, these patients never fully recovered. Several points require emphasis: (1) these symptoms are present most of the time; (2) many cases are sufficiently severe to substantially impair normal functioning; and (3) in response to explicit questioning, most patients state that these symptoms were not a problem before their illness began.

The hallmark of CFS is fatigue. Approximately 25% of CFS patients describe themselves as regularly bedridden or shut-in and unable to work, and one-third can work only part-time. Patients typically were physically active before the illness began; since becoming ill, however, even modest physical exertion results in an exacerbation of many of their symptoms. Although the exertion itself may be tolerated reasonably well, most patients report a marked worsening of their fatigue, cognitive function, adenopathy, pharyngitis, and fever 6–24 hours later. After fatigue, sleep and neurocognitive disturbances are the most prominent symptoms. Disturbed sleep may be the most frequent complaint in CFS, reported by up to 95% of patients. Sleep complaints in CFS take many forms including hypersomnia, inability to fall or stay asleep, inadequate sleep time, and feeling unrested on rising. In addition, symptoms suggestive of sleep disorder, such as sleepiness, drowsiness, snoring with apnea, and sleep attacks, are surprisingly common among CFS patients and should trigger the search for a comorbid sleep disorder. Neuropsychiatric symptoms such as word groping, decreased concentrating ability, and impaired short-term memory are common, and one-third of adults report at least one episode of extreme confusion or disorientation. One study found subtle information-processing deficits on neuropsychological testing in patients with CFS.

In addition to the symptoms that define CFS, other commonly reported chronic symptoms include muscle weakness, weight gain, daily napping, and shortness of breath (Table 41–2).

B. Physical Examination Findings: Abnormalities in the physical examination are unusual (Table 41–3). Fevers, posterior and anterior cervical adenopathy, and organomegaly have been described. The presence of "tender points" is the most common physical finding. The three physical examination findings included in the original CDC case definition have little diagnostic value and have been removed from the revised criteria.

C. Psychiatric Disorders: Many investigators have found considerable psychiatric comorbidity in CFS, especially major depression (Table 41–4). Current and lifetime major depression have been reported in 15–54% and 40–76% of patients, respectively. Studies that examined the temporal sequence of CFS and psychiatric disorder found that the psychiatric disorder often preceded the onset of fatigue. In fact, the apparently high rate of preexisting psychiatric disorders and the overlap of symptoms of CFS with those of major depression have led to suggestions that CFS is a form of depression or neurasthenia. This explanation is insufficient, however, because at least 25% of CFS patients have no current or lifetime psychiatric illness, and among those who do have major depression the classic biologic accompaniments appear to be absent.

There are several lines of evidence that argue against the contention that CFS is a form of depres-

sion and suggest a different mechanism for the associated affective symptoms. For example, the polysomnographic findings characteristic of major depression, such as increases in sleep latency, number of awakenings, and rapid eye movement (REM) density, as well as decreases in REM sleep latency and slow-wave sleep, are not observed in CFS. Another piece of evidence is the fact that the pattern of HPA axis dysregulation in CFS differs dramatically from the classic neuroendocrine findings of major depression. In the latter, resistance to pituitary-adrenal suppression has been used clinically in the form of the dexamethasone suppression test. In contrast to the nonsuppression or "hypercortisolemia" seen in many severely depressed patients, nonsuppression is rare in CFS. Similarly, the changes in monoamine metabolism characteristic of major depression are not observed in CFS. Finally, the pattern of event-related brain potentials in CFS patients does not resemble that seen in major depression. Taken together, these studies, particularly those of neuroendocrine function and sleep, raise the possibility that different mechanisms are responsible for the depressive symptoms of major depression and CFS.

Clinical Findings

Many laboratory abnormalities have been reported in patients with CFS. However, these findings are diverse, sometimes conflicting, and frequently modest in degree. In addition, these findings have not been shown to explain the symptoms of CFS, nor to correlate with changes in symptoms over time.

Table 41–3. Physical findings in chronic fatigue syndrome.

Finding	Frequency
Tender points	33–70
Inflamed pharynx	40–60
Posterior cervical adenopathy	20–40
Macular rash	10–20
Temperature above 37.5 °C*	10–20
Hepatomegaly	5–10
Splenomegaly	5–10
Axillary adenopathy	5–15

*Detected at a single visit.

Table 41–2. Commonly reported symptoms in chronic fatigue syndrome.

Symptom	Frequency (%)
Muscle weakness	91
Feel worse under stress	89
Weight gain	78
Need for daily nap	76
Shortness of breath	72
Unsteadiness	69
Morning stiffness	69
Blurred vision	66
Dizziness	64
Dry throat or mouth	63
Frequent nausea	62
Decreased sexual function	61
Rapid heartbeat	55
Tinnitus	54

Table 41–4. Frequency of psychiatric diagnoses in chronic fatigue syndrome.

Diagnosis	Frequency (%) Current	Frequency (%) Lifetime
Major depression	15–54	40–76
Generalized anxiety disorder	2–17	0–31
Panic disorder	6–13	5–30
Somatization disorder		2–46
Any current diagnosis	21–72	
Any lifetime diagnosis		26–86

A. Routine Studies: Standard serum hematologic tests are generally normal. Atypical lymphocytes have been reported in up to 30% of selected patients. Slightly elevated erythrocyte sedimentation rates (ESRs) are an occasional finding; however, values greater than 50 mm/hr should alert clinicians to other causes of fatigue. Standard serum chemistry tests also are generally unremarkable. In a study comparing routine laboratory test results obtained in approximately 600 patients with a chronically fatiguing illness with those of 150 control subjects, the patients were significantly more likely to have increased levels of cholesterol (54% versus 33%) decreased levels of and alkaline phosphatase (18% versus 5%). In addition, approximately 20% of patients have modestly elevated transaminases.

B. Immunologic Tests: Patients with CFS may be more likely than healthy individuals to have circulating autoantibodies. In particular, antinuclear antibodies are found in as many as 20% and rheumatoid factor in up to 10% of patients, typically in low concentrations without other evidence for lupus or rheumatoid arthritis. Antibodies to thyroid gland and other tissues are found occasionally. A recent report suggested that rheumatoid factor, antinuclear antibodies of at least 1:80, and anti-Ro (or SS-A, an autoantibody associated with Sjögren's syndrome) may be present in some patients with CFS and a Sjögren's syndrome-like clinical presentation.

A large number of studies that have examined humoral immunity in CFS have reported conflicting results. Most commonly, immunoglobulin levels have been normal or mildly diminished. IgG subclass deficiencies, usually IgG_1 or IgG_3, also have been reported by some investigators. Several investigators have found low levels of circulating immune complexes in up to one-third of CFS patients. Despite this abnormality, few patients have depressed complement, and none have clinical manifestations of immune-complex-mediated disease.

The symptoms of CFS have been postulated to result, at least in part, from the inappropriate production of cytokines. Among the first observations lending support to this theory were two reports of increased activity of the interferon-induced enzyme, 2'5'-oligoadenylate synthetase in the leukocytes of a small number of CFS patients. A subsequent, ongoing search for objective evidence of increased cytokine production in CFS has yielded mixed results, however. Although the assays used may have been insensitive, the combined data from many studies have suggested that circulating interferons are infrequently present. Other markers of immune activation, including interleukin-1, interleukin-4, soluble interleukin-2 receptor, tumor necrosis factor, and β_2-microglobulin, have not been detected in CFS. In contrast, compared with control subjects, higher levels of circulating interleukin-2, transforming growth factor-β, neopterin, and interleukin-6 have been reported in some patients with CFS. These abnormalities have not been found consistently or replicated reliably, however. In one study using functional assays of cytokine production, mitogen-stimulated release of interleukin-1-β and tumor necrosis factor-α from peripheral lymphocytes was shown to be significantly greater, and release of transforming growth factor-β lower, in patients with CFS than in healthy individuals.

The numbers of CD4+ and CD8+ T lymphocytes and the CD4:CD8 ratio are usually normal in CFS, although both increases and decreases have been reported. However, deranged T-cell function has been demonstrated more consistently. Some patients have been reported to be anergic; two studies found significantly decreased delayed hypersensitivity to multiple antigens in patients compared with matched healthy and depressed control subjects. Several investigators also have reported decreased responsiveness to standard mitogen-stimulation assays.

More recently, extensive analyses of lymphocyte cell surface markers among patients with CFS-like illnesses have demonstrated an increase in the expression of activation markers, lending support to the theory of underlying immune dysregulation. The most striking findings have been elevated numbers of CD2 cells expressing the CDw26 activation marker and increases in the CD8+, CD38+, and CD8+ HLA-DR subsets. The latter two abnormalities were not observed in a subsequent study, however. Replicated findings have included a significant reduction in the suppressor subset, CD8+ CD11b−; a decrease in the CD4 CD45RA+ suppressor-inducer subset; and increases in the expression or density of the ICAM (CD54) on CD4 cells.

Finally, although abnormalities of natural killer-cell number and function have been demonstrated in a number of independent laboratories, findings have been inconsistent. Most studies have found a diminution in the absolute number, percentage, or both, of natural killer cells. Similarly, natural killer-cell function has been found to be increased, decreased, and normal as measured by cytolytic activity against several different target cell lines. These findings are interesting given the important role of these cells in the host defense against viral infections.

C. Virologic Assays: CFS-like illnesses have been attributed, either directly or indirectly, to a variety of infectious agents. The viruses that have been the object of the greatest scientific inquiry are the herpes viruses, including Epstein-Barr virus (EBV) and human herpes virus 6 (HHV-6); the enteroviruses; and a putative novel retrovirus. Despite the often acute onset of CFS following an infectious illness, however, the demonstration of elevated antibody titers and other objective evidence of viral involvement in CFS has been inconsistent.

Early studies in the USA found elevated levels of antibodies to Epstein-Barr viral capsid antigen IgG and early antigen in patients with a CFS-like illness. However, subsequent investigations did not detect other markers of EBV infection in blood and throat cultures or in EBV in situ hybridization studies of lymphocytes. A substantial overlap in antibody titers between patients and healthy individuals also was documented, indicating that EBV is unlikely to be the causative agent in most cases.

In one outbreak of a chronically fatiguing illness, significantly higher titers of Epstein-Barr viral capsid antigen IgG and antibodies to early antigens were noted in cases compared with control subjects. Evidence also was found of active replication of HHV-6 in stimulated primary lymphocyte cell cultures from 70% of patients compared with 20% of control subjects. These observations underscore that, at least in the case of HHV-6, antibody titers may not accurately reflect active viral replication or reactivation. In another study of 10 viruses, higher titers of antibodies to the early antigens of EBV, HHV-6, and coxsackievirus B4 and lower titers of antibodies to EBV nuclear antigens were found among patients with CFS than control subjects. These findings were interpreted by the authors to reflect an underlying defect in T-cell function rather than a primary viral infection or clinically significant viral reactivation.

Several serologic surveys in the United Kingdom found abnormal coxsackie B virus test results among individuals with "myalgic encephalomyelitis." Two studies reported circulating complexes of coxsackievirus antigen and IgM in the majority of patients, with isolation of enterovirus from stool in 22%, findings that were not replicated by another group. Additional support for the presence of an enteroviral infection came from work showing that enteroviral nucleic acid was found in muscle cells of chronically fatigued patients more often than in those of control subjects. These techniques did not detect virus in many patients, however, and are not available routinely in most clinical settings. Moreover, attempts at replication have not been successful.

A report presenting indirect evidence of a novel retrovirus in CFS patients that shares some nucleic acid sequence homology with human T lymphotropic virus II has not been replicated by others. In addition, infection with human T lymphotropic virus I or II is unlikely to be associated with CFS. Finally, CFS has not been found to be caused by many other infectious agents including hepatitis C virus, *Chlamydia, Toxoplasma,* and the Lyme disease spirochete, although it has been known to develop subsequent to acute infection with the latter.

D. Allergy Testing: It has been speculated that individuals who respond with unusual vigor to infectious antigens also may have a heightened reactivity to allergens. In fact, up to 60% of patients with CFS have worsening of preexisting or development of new allergies. Several investigators have explored this association and found increased cutaneous reactivity to allergens, increased levels of circulating IgE and IgE-bearing T and B cells, and greater lymphocyte responsiveness to allergens. The mechanisms linking allergy and CFS remain unknown.

E. Neuroendocrine Abnormalities: Recent investigations have highlighted the importance of factors other than the immune system, such as neuroendocrine function, in CFS. In the first study to document neuroendocrine changes, the activity of the HPA axis was assessed in patients and healthy participants using both basal and functional measurements. A novel pattern of HPA axis dysfunction was described, characterized by a significant reduction in plasma and urinary glucocorticoid levels, elevated basal evening adrenocorticotropin hormone (ACTH) concentrations, enhanced adrenocortical sensitivity to ACTH with a reduced maximal response, and normal cerebrospinal corticotropin-releasing hormone levels. The mild glucocorticoid deficiency, enhanced adrenocortical sensitivity to exogenous ACTH, and blunted response to corticotropin-releasing hormone were interpreted to be incompatible with primary adrenal insufficiency and most consistent with a central failure of corticotropin-releasing hormone production or release by the hypothalamus.

Patients with CFS also show a significant reduction in basal plasma levels of 3-methoxy-4-hydroxyphenylglycol and an increase in 5-hydroxyindoleacetic acid—a pattern contrasting with that seen in depression. Additional evidence of perturbation of neuroendocrine function comes from studies demonstrating low baseline levels and erratic secretion of arginine vasopressin and possible upregulation (ie, increase in number of receptors) of hypothalamic 5-hydroxytryptamine receptors as assessed by buspirone challenge and measurement of basal and peak prolactin levels.

Although some of the preceding laboratory findings have been reported consistently, others await confirmation. Most of the abnormalities observed in CFS are found in laboratory tests performed only in research settings. Systematic, blind studies using healthy controls have failed to confirm many of the abnormalities initially thought to be characteristic of CFS, and new evidence of dysfunction in immunologic and neuroendocrinologic domains has surfaced. It remains to be demonstrated whether these findings reliably distinguish CFS patients from those with illnesses that can present with a similar clinical picture, particularly depression.

Differential Diagnosis & Cormorbid Conditions

Although it is uncommon for systemic disorders to present solely with fatigue, many medical conditions are associated with fatigue, including anemia, hypothyroidism, multiple sclerosis, inflammatory bowel disease, connective tissue diseases, neoplasms, and infectious processes such as sinusitis or hepatitis. All patients should be evaluated to exclude these possibilities. In addition to the well-known causes of chronic fatigue, several other conditions appear to coexist often with CFS such as fibromyalgia, sleep disorders, and Sjögren's syndrome. Although these conditions have many demographic and clinical features in common with CFS and may represent overlapping clinical syndromes, their exact relationship to CFS is not clear.

A. Fibromyalgia: Fibromyalgia is a common rheumatologic condition characterized by chronic myalgias, fatigue, and disrupted sleep; it often is associated with headache, irritable bowel syndrome, paresthesias, Raynaud's syndrome, and a variety of other signs and symptoms. It occurs most commonly in women and may follow a viral illness or trauma. The American College of Rheumatology has proposed criteria for fibromyalgia that require widespread musculoskeletal pain in conjunction with tenderness at a minimum of 11 of 18 specified tender points. Up to 70% of patients with CFS simultaneously meet criteria for fibromyalgia. The presence of fibromyalgia does not preclude a diagnosis of CFS.

Although a variety of laboratory abnormalities have been described, no diagnostic tests exist, and the cause of fibromyalgia remains unknown. Polysomnography consistently has demonstrated a non-rapid eye movement (non-REM) sleep anomaly, ie, the spontaneous appearance of an alpha EEG frequency during non-REM sleep. These alpha-wave intrusions are considered an objective index of arousal during sleep and may be experienced by the patient as unrefreshing sleep.

B. Disturbances of Sleep: Well-documented sleep disorders are surprisingly common in CFS. Between 33 and 80% of chronically fatigued patients have sleep disorders such as sleep apnea, nocturnal myoclonus, periodic limb movements, and narcolepsy. It is not surprising that investigators screening CFS patients for subjective drowsiness or sleepiness have found higher rates of sleep disorders than those testing unselected patients. Of note is the fact that in studies using measures of depression, sleep disorders occurred with at least equal frequency in depressed and nondepressed patients with CFS.

Perturbations in sleep duration and architecture in the absence of overt sleep disorders also may be important in CFS. Compared with healthy participants, patients with CFS have significantly decreased sleep efficiency and diminished proportion of time spent in REM sleep; increased onset latency to stage 2 sleep and stage 4 sleep; and increased time spent in delta sleep.

At the present time, it is not known whether sleep disorders are causative or comorbid conditions in CFS. However, direct and indirect support for the hypothesis that sleep disruption is a manifestation of CFS comes from several observations. First, many patients who meet strict criteria for CFS do not have a primary sleep disorder on polysomnography. Second, there is a striking disparity between the objective severity of the sleep disorder (usually mild) and the degree of fatigue reported by patients. Third, treatment meets with only limited success. Unlike the striking improvement typical of patients treated for well-documented sleep disorders not associated with CFS, those with CFS infrequently recover entirely, and most report only moderate improvement. In summary, although an underlying sleep disorder may masquerade as CFS, in most cases, sleep disorders and CFS are likely to be separate, although potentially overlapping, conditions.

C. Sjögren's Syndrome: Many patients with CFS report sicca symptoms compatible with Sjögren's syndrome, as well as overwhelming fatigue and other symptoms typical of CFS. Moreover, approximately up to 60% of such patients have a positive Schirmer's test. On laboratory testing, antinuclear antibodies (ANA) is found in more than 50%, for rheumatoid factor in 14%, and for anti-Ro in 5%. In comparing CFS patients who have a Sjögren's syndrome-like condition with those who have only CFS, the former were significantly more likely to have recurrent fever and a positive ANA but less likely to have an acute onset. Currently, it is unclear whether this subset of patients has unrecognized Sjögren's syndrome or a Sjögren's syndrome-like comorbid condition. The relatively low prevalence of autoantibodies, particularly anti-Ro, suggests that this condition occurs concurrently with CFS. It also is not known whether the natural history of Sjögren's syndrome in the context of CFS differs from that of CFS alone.

Diagnosis

A detailed history, physical examination, and selected laboratory tests are indicated in individuals with chronic fatigue that significantly affects daily activity. Equal emphasis must be placed on the psychosocial evaluation, in particular evaluating patients for anxiety and depression. Although no laboratory tests are diagnostic of CFS, an initial laboratory test battery in evaluating patients with possible CFS should consist of the following: a complete blood cell count (CBC), with manually performed differential white blood cell count; ESR; chemistry panel, including liver function tests; thyroid-stimulating hormone level; and a urinanalysis. Other tests such as antinuclear antibodies, immune complexes, immunoglobulin levels, and lymphocyte subsets may be appropriate in some patients or settings. Taken together, these tests may be helpful in supporting a diagnosis of CFS or in ruling out other diseases that can produce fatigue.

Treatment

There is no specific treatment for CFS. Treatment should be directed at relief of specific symptoms and reintegration into the patient's social network. Symptomatic therapy may include antipyretic and non-steroidal anti-inflammatory agents. There have been anecdotal reports of successful treatment using antiviral and immunomodulating drugs, vitamins, holistic remedies, dietary modifications, and rest. In adults, low dosages of antidepressants such as fluoxetine in the morning or amitriptyline, nortriptyline, or doxepin at bedtime may be beneficial. The role of therapeutic dosages of antidepressant medications remains unknown. Several agents, including acyclovir, a liver extract–B_{12}-folate preparation, antifungal agents, and intramuscular magnesium have undergone a vigorous evaluation and do not appear to be more effective than placebo.

A supportive approach aimed at enhancing self-efficacy and reconditioning is effective in many cases. Emphasis should be placed on attainment of regular sleep patterns, with avoidance of napping and significant changes in the sleep cycle. Diet should be well balanced with meals appropriately spaced throughout the day. Physical activities previously enjoyed should be increased gradually in a structured manner, often with the assistance of a physical therapist, because complete inactivity appears to promote fatigue. Continuity of care, education, instruction in coping skills, and counseling often are neglected, but they are important aspects of treatment for CFS. Reassurance that gradual improvement will occur with time is a powerful aspect of any treatment program. Reassessment for organic and psychiatric disorders should be performed at regular intervals; however, extensive laboratory testing without additional indications is not indicated.

Prognosis

CFS is not a progressive disease. Symptoms usually are most severe during the first 6 months of the illness, plateau relatively early, and recur with varying degrees of severity. Although detailed longitudinal studies are lacking, it appears most patients report a gradual recovery, usually punctuated with relapses precipitated by overexertion, stress, or infection. Moderate to complete recovery has been found in 26–57% of patients with CFS-like illnesses over varying periods of follow-up. Predictors of return to work and clinical improvement may include absence of affective disorders and shorter duration of illness. With the exception of suicide, death resulting directly from CFS has not been reported.

REFERENCES

Buchwald D, Komaroff AL: Laboratory findings in chronic fatigue syndrome. Rev Infect Dis 1991;13:S12.

Buchwald D et al: A chronic illness characterized by fatigue, neurologic and immunologic disorders, and active human herpes type 6 infection. Ann Intern Med 1992;116:103.

Buchwald D et al: Sleep disorders in patients with chronic fatigue. Clin Infect Dis 1994;18(Suppl 1):S68.

Demitrack MA et al: Evidence for impaired activation of the hypothalamic-pituitary-adrenal axis in patients with chronic fatigue syndrome. J Clin Endocrinol Metab 1991;73:1224.

Fukuda K and the International Chronic Fatigue Syndrome Study Group. The Chronic Fatigue Syndrome: A comprehensive approach to its definition and study. Ann Int Med 1994;121:943.

Goldenberg DL et al: High frequency of fibromyalgia in patients with chronic fatigue seen in a primary care practice. Arthritis Rheum 1990;33:381.

Holmes GP et al: Chronic fatigue syndrome: A working case definition. Ann Intern Med 1988;108:387.

Katon WJ et al: Psychiatric illness in patients with chronic fatigue and rheumatoid arthritis. J Gen Intern Med 1991;6:277.

Komaroff AK, Buchwald D: Symptoms and signs of chronic fatigue syndrome. Rev Infect Dis 1991;13:S8.

Landay AL et al: Chronic fatigue syndrome: Clinical condition associated with immune activation. Lancet 1991;338:707.

Schluederberg A et al: Chronic fatigue syndrome research: Definition and medical outcome assessment. Ann Intern Med 1992;117:325.

Shafran SD: The chronic fatigue syndrome. Am J Med. 1991;90:730.

Straus SE et al: Lymphocyte phenotype and function in the chronic fatigue syndrome. J Clin Immunol 1992;13:30.

Ware N, Kleinman A: Culture and somatic experience: The social course of illness in neurasthenia and chronic fatigue syndrome. Psychosom Med 1992;54:546.

42

Headache

Laird G. Patterson, MD

MIGRAINE

Migraine (MG) is a ubiquitous disorder whose cause is obscure. There is no universally accepted definition of the condition. In 1988 the International Headache Society published criteria that are useful for gathering data and assessing treatment; however, the criteria are too complex for everyday use.

Migraine can be defined generally as paroxysmal or periodic recurrent attacks of headache, frequently unilateral, and often preceded by or associated with widespread premonitory systemic or neurologic symptoms. Migraine is no longer classified as common or classic but rather as MG without aura and MG with aura (see the section following, Migrainous Aura).

Essentials of Diagnosis
- Strong family history.
- Pattern altered by hormonal factors including menses, pregnancy, menopause, ingestion of oral contraceptives, and hormone replacement therapy.
- Existence of endogenous and exogenous triggering factors.
- Consisting of a prodrome, aura (15–20% of patients), headache, associated symptoms, and postdrome.
- Headache responds to medications that have agonist and antagonist actions at the serotonin (5-HT) receptor site.

Incidence & Risk Factors
Although the heterogeneity makes prevalence difficult to estimate, studies suggest that MG occurs in 18% of women and 6% of men. Peak onset is in the third and fourth decades. Prevalence of MG seems to increase steadily from childhood until approximately age 40 and then decrease beginning in the fifth decade. Although MG tends to resolve with age, in fully 25% of patients, it continues into old age. Migraineurs have a strong family history of MG; 50–60% identify first-degree relatives as affected. The risk of developing MG is especially high if the condition is present in both parents.

Migraine prevalence is inversely related to household income and is not related to intelligence test

---

Migraine
  Essentials of Diagnosis
  Incidence & Risk Factors
  Pathogenesis
  Signs & Symptoms
  Clinical Findings
  Treatment
  Prognosis
  Variations & Complications of Migraine
  Psychosocial Issues
Pseudotumor Cerebri (PTC)
  Essentials of Diagnosis
  Incidence
  Pathophysiology
  Associated Conditions
  Signs & Symptoms
  Clinical Findings
  Treatment
  Prognosis
  Pregnancy & PTC
Coital Headache
  Essentials of Diagnosis
  Signs & Symptoms
  Treatment
  Prognosis
Chronic Paroxysmal Hemicrania
  Essentials of Diagnosis
  Incidence
  Signs & Symptoms
  Clinical Findings
  Treatment

---

scores or socioeconomic class. Migraineurs with higher intelligence test scores and in higher socioeconomic groups, however, are more likely to consult a physician.

Pathogenesis
Any attempt to explain the cause of MG must encompass all of its features including trigger factors, prodrome, aura, headache, associated systemic and neurologic symptoms, and the aftermath, or postdrome. Earlier, vasomotor theories did not explain adequately this conflation of events. Although an exact cause remains elusive, reproducible changes in

brain biochemistry and physiology have been documented repeatedly.

Serotonin has been recognized for a long time to be a neurotransmitter of interest in MG. Platelet serotonin levels fall dramatically prior to an attack and rise later. A variety of serotonin (5-HT) receptors populate the intra- and extracranial vasculature, and their activation produces both vasoconstriction and vasodilatation. Serotonin acts as a regulatory neurotransmitter in the endogenous pain control pathway and stimulates peripheral nociceptive nerve terminals. It is important in the regulation of mood, appetite, and sleep. Several drugs affecting serotonin release and uptake may cause headache, and anti-MG drugs have an agonist or antagonist function at the 5-HT receptors.

Brain stem areas such as the locus ceruleus and dorsal raphe nuclei innervate intracranial vasculature and may influence its reactivity. Stimulation of these centers may initiate some of the hemodynamic and vascular changes that occur during MG; however, the factors that initially activate neurons in these nuclei are unknown.

A corollary to the brain stem neural hypothesis of MG is the observation that the aura is associated with spread of a transient depolarizing wave beginning posteriorly and propagating anteriorly across the cortical surface. During this event, neurons are depolarized; repolarization is delayed; and transient, reversible fluxes in potassium, sodium, and calcium can be measured. An increase in blood flow accompanies the initial wave, followed by prolonged hypoperfusion. The inciting event is not known, although projections from the brain stem nuclei may stimulate the cortex and cortical vessels and disrupt normal neurophysiologic and vasomotor function.

Headache is another feature of MG that is not explained easily, but there is evidence that the trigeminovascular system may be an integral component in the genesis of MG cephalgia. Unknown triggers stimulate trigeminal afferents in vessel walls and generate nociceptive impulses. Neuropeptides, eg, substance P and bradykinin, are released within the vascular endothelium causing plasma extravasation, inflammation, and persistent pain. The frontal and occipitocervical distribution of the trigeminal nerve is coincidentally the distribution of MG pain.

Although no single theory accounts for all of the phases of MG, it appears certain that neural and vascular components both are necessary and that serotonin is an important mediator of the neurovascular events that culminate as the MG phenomenon.

Signs & Symptoms

The heterogeneity of MG symptoms implies a widespread disruption of normal physiologic function that is not confined to the brain and cerebral vessels. Migraine with aura constitutes only 15–20% of all MG. Many migraineurs who experience aura have attacks that are aura-free. In addition, the aura can occur without headache. Whether or not the various forms of MG are the same disorder, they share many of the same clinical, biochemical, and electrophysiologic characteristics.

A. The Prodrome: Migraineurs may have vague premonitory or prodromal experiences preceding their headache by 24–48 hours. These include insidious changes in mood, behavior, and appetite; fatigue; gastrointestinal disturbances; and fluid retention. Mild confusion, irritability, elation, depression, or anxiety can also can be part of the prodrome.

B. Triggers or Precipitants: A multiplicity of exogenous triggering factors are recognized by MG patients (Table 42–1). Endogenous genetic and biologic factors also may initiate an attack. Foods con-

Table 42–1. Triggering factors for migraine.

Diet
  Processed, fermented, preserved foods
  Bioactive amines
    Phenylmethylamine—chocolate
    Tyramine—red wine, cheese
    Octopamine—citrus fruits
  Additives
    Monosodium glutemate (MSG)
    Nitrites, nitrates
    Aspartame
    Excess salt
  Beverages
    Alcohol
    Caffeine (withdrawal)
Physical/environmental factors
  Exertion
  Heat, cold
  Visual stimulus—glare, flashing lights
  Noise
  Odors, fumes
    Solvents
    Hydrocarbons
    Perfumes
    Smoke
  Barometric pressure
    Weather change
    High altitude
  Head trauma
Psychologic factors
  Stress, stress letdown
  Depression
  Anxiety
Biorhythm disturbances
  Sleep disruption, deprivation
  Weekends, holidays
  Fasting, overeating
  Time-zone changes
Hormonal changes
  Menses, ovulation
  Pregnancy
  Menopause
Medications (see Table 42–2)
Other systemic symptoms
  Fever
  Dehydration
  Dialysis
  Anemia

taining biogenic amines or additives such as monosodium glutamate, nitrites, or aspartame are major precipitants. Biogenic amines are concentrated principally in cheese, dairy products, chocolate, seafood, and citrus fruits. Alcohol (in particular, red wine) may contain impurities or biogenic amines. Physical factors such as exertion, glare, or bright or flashing lights may evoke headache. Many patients are sensitive to loud noises, odors, or changes in barometric pressure. Disruption of eating and sleeping routines, stress, and letdown from stress are all disturbances of biologic rhythm that can initiate attack. Head trauma, especially in young patients with familial MG, may trigger a series of attacks. Medications are often responsible for the onset or perpetuation of an episode (Table 42–2).

Migraineurs often cannot identfy a consistent relationship between a triggering factor and the development of headache. In addition, with the passage of time and changes in the MG pattern, patients become sensitive to factors to which they previously were resistant. Precipitants may induce changes in vascular reactivity, neurotransmitter function, or receptor sensitivity that eventuate in the MG attack.

C. Migrainous Aura: An aura is a well-defined neurologic symptom that is often, but not always, followed by headache. The most common aura is either a negative or a scintillating scotoma marching slowly across the visual field. Unilateral face and arm paresthesias, lateralized mild weakness or clumsiness, language and cognitive impairment, alterations in consciousness such as dreamlike states, de-

Table 42–2. Medication triggers.

Illicit drugs
  Cocaine
  Amphetamines
Antibiotics
  Griseofulvin
  Trimethoprim
Antihypertensives
  Captopril
  Minoxidil
  Nifedipine
  Reserpine
Nitrates
  Isosorbide dinitrate
  Trinitroglycerine
Hormones
  Estrogen
  Oral contraceptives
  Danazol
  Medroxy progesterone acetate (Depo-Provera)
Nonsteroidal anti-inflammatory drugs (NSAIDs)
  Indomethacin
  Ibuprofen
H_2-receptor antagonists
  Cimetidine
  Ranitidine
Miscellaneous
  Vitamin A derivatives
  Abuse or overuse of over-the-counter drugs

personalization, and distortions of the visual environment all have been reported. Vertigo; olfactory or gustatory sensations, and nonspecific intracranial, visceral, or abdominal sensations occur independently or accompany other, better-defined symptoms. Auras persist for minutes to as long as an hour and may vary in intensity and duration from one attack to another.

Complicated migraine is a term reserved for episodes of headache with an aura of severe unilateral paralysis, aphasia, and sensory or visual loss. Deficits may be prolonged or persistent. An unusual entity that occurs in young persons, **basilar migraine** includes a variety of brain stem and cerebellar symptoms, viz, dramatic changes in the visual fields, diplopia, dysarthria or anarthria, vertigo, ataxia, and weakness or numbness. Transient unresponsiveness, syncope, or a confusional state may accompany basilar MG.

D. Headache Characteristics: Headache that follows an aura may occur as the aura is resolving or any time 1–2 hours later. Migrainous head pain is often unilateral, although strictly so in only 50% of adult patients. Headache typically begins unilaterally in the occipitocervical region and radiates anteriorly, but it is frequently holocranial from the onset. Pain frequently radiates to the orbit or retroorbital area and face, particularly the cheek or jaw, or even to shoulders and arms. Headaches are usually contralateral to the aura. Head pain is sometimes sharply localized and accompanied by focal scalp tenderness. Cervical paraspinous and trapezius soreness or tenderness may precede a full headache.

MG pain may be throbbing and pulsatile or simply dull and aching in character. At times, an intense, pounding headache is relieved by vomiting. Pain may be incapacitating and only partially attenuated by lying quietly in a dark room. Physical activity, jolting, or Valsalva maneuver intensifies the pain. Headache may last from a few minutes to as long as several days; a nagging, dull, cephalgia or scalp tenderness may persist even after the primary headache has resolved. Discrete jabbing, sharp, ice pick-like pains may be superimposed on the headache or continue after it has resolved.

E. Associated Symptoms: Although headache is the salient feature of an MG attack, other associated symptoms may be even more disabling. Patients experience sonophobia and photophobia of varying severity, and they may have an aversion to smells that are normally pleasurable. Nausea or vomiting complicate the headache in more than 50% of cases. Vomiting may intensify the headache or may provide relief. If vomiting is severe and prolonged, it causes dehydration and electrolyte depletion, further aggravating the condition. Diarrhea and bowel hyperactivity can be prodromal symptoms but often occur during the headache. Gastric emptying is usually slowed. Light-headedness, severe orthostatic dizziness, or even syncope may accompany attacks. Patients can experience a vague sense of disequilibrium or even have true vertigo.

During an attack, it is common for patients to feel mildly disoriented or confused, and concentration is poor. Mood changes overwhelm many patients; they may become agitated, tearful, irritable, hostile, and easily angered, or they may withdraw and desire seclusion or isolation. Lassitude, enervation, drowsiness, and an overwhelming sleepiness appear during and after the peak of the headache. In severe cases, there may be extreme disorganization of thought processes, depersonalization, and impaired memory or even amnesia.

Other ictal changes include signs of vasomotor instability such as flushing, pallor, diaphoresis, and unilateral swelling of the face, periorbital tissues, or scalp. Although more commonly seen in cluster headaches, unilateral ptosis, miosis, conjunctival injection, and nasal congestion may be evident with strongly unilateral migraine. Temperature dysregulation and elevation of blood pressure may be recorded during the episode. Many female patients experience fluid retention prior to the attack and later undergo a diuresis.

F. Postdromal Symptoms: Premonitory and ictal symptoms often obscure the postdromal or postictal phase. Some patients note that sleep restores a feeling of well-being; however, many continue to feel mentally dull and slightly dazed, with mild head discomfort, for 24–48 hours afterward. For 1–2 days or even a week, patients may note listlessness, fatigue, somnolence, and a subdued or depressed mood. Cognitive function, including concentration and memory, may remain impaired, although some patients emerge from an attack feeling refreshed, elated, and energetic. Enhanced appetite can occur, but nausea, often in association with the smell of certain foods, can persist for several days.

G. Headache Patterns: Migraine peaks between the ages of 20 and 40. In many patients, MG develops in early childhood, becomes latent, and reemerges in early or mid adulthood. The frequency of attacks varies considerably. There may be lengthy periods without headaches, followed by a clustering or grouping of headaches. Some patients have predictable episodic cephalgia, eg, during the menstrual cycle. Others have headache only when they fail to avoid a known trigger factor. Migraineurs may go for months or years without experiencing an attack, but when they do have one, it can be severe and prolonged. Headache duration averages 12–72 hours, but it can be briefer, and headaches can persist for a week or more. Headache-free intervals are the norm between attacks, but ice pick pains or dull, chronic daily headache may complicate the interictal period. Discrete MG attacks with interposed chronic daily headache often result from overuse of ergotamines or over-the-counter (OTC) medications. The migraine

pattern may change during the childbearing years and perimenopausally.

Episodes often occur at or near the same time of day, week, or month. Some patients are awakened with headache in the middle of the night or in early morning, possibly during rapid eye movement (REM) sleep. Others note attacks at the end or beginning of a work week. Vacations or holidays are other likely periods of risk, and a clustering of attacks may disrupt major holiday periods. Migraineurs who travel frequently and cross multiple time zones may experience headache because of a change in their usual diurnal pattern.

Clinical Findings

The diagnosis of MG relies almost exclusively on historical information, because there are no tests that support the diagnosis. A careful search for the typical features previously mentioned aids in characterizing a syndrome that may have seemed vague to the patient or other examiners and allows for appropriate therapy. Essential aspects of the headache evaluation are listed in Table 42–3.

A. History: Many patients mistakenly believe that they have several different varieties of headache

Table 42–3. Headache/migraine history.

Chronology
  Age and circumstances of onset
  Frequency and duration
  Timing (day, week, month, season)
Pain descriptors
  Location and radiation
  Course and severity
  Character of pain
Precipitating factors
  Exogenous
  Endogenous
Aggravating factors
  Exertion
  Position, movement
  Valsalva maneuver
Associated systemic and neurologic features
  Prodrome
  Aura
  Headache
  Postdrome
Past and present therapy
  Nonpharmacologic
  Pharmacologic
    Drug, dose, duration
    Combinations
  Response to therapy
  Abuse or overuse
Other illnesses
Personal history
  Occupation
  Family situation
  Habits
  Emotional state
  Biorhythms
    Sleep
    Eating habits
  Family history of migraine or other headaches

when they experience occipitocervical pain on one occasion, sharp stabbing pains on another, and intense, throbbing hemicranial pain on a third. In fact, these headaches are all part of the MG syndrome. The misattribution of allergy as a cause of headache is due to the mistaken impression that foods cause headache through allergic rather than biochemical mechanisms. Sinus disease, ophthalmologic and dental conditions, and temporomandibular joint (TMJ) syndrome often mistakenly are considered causes of headaches that are of migrainous origin.

The circumstances of the first recognized attack, premonitory symptoms, aura (if any), and temporal profile of the headache itself with its associated features are all important in identifying a headache as migrainous or not. Pain location, quality, and severity should be determined. The episodic nature and associated features of the MG syndrome best define it, and these symptoms should be sought in detail. The patient's memory of the attacks may be inaccurate, and only specific questioning may elicit the necessary information.

It is important to know the particulars of past headache treatments. Medications and combinations of medications, doses, duration of therapeutic trials, and treatment response all should be detailed, because patients may have been taking subtherapeutic doses for inappropriately short periods. Presumed side effects that prevented the use of effective drugs may turn out to have been insignificant, and another trial may be initiated. Prior nonpharmacologic interventions and their benefits are also important to know about before a new treatment strategy is designed.

The patient's occupation, with its stresses or exposure to triggering factors, may contribute to the MG syndrome. Family difficulties; poor health habits, particularly smoking and excessive drinking; overuse of caffeine; sleep disruptions; and situations that produce wide emotional swings all provoke MG.

Other illnesses often have an impact on MG either because of medications required for their treatment or because of the illness itself. Head injuries can precipitate or aggravate migrainous headache. Use of medications that are not prescribed for headache or illicit drugs can cause headache or may contain impurities that contribute to it.

A search for familial MG should consist of more than an inquiry as to whether or not other family members have headaches. Patients often mistakenly attribute familial headaches to sinus disease, allergy, or head injury, or may state that a relative with headaches was told that the problem was not MG. Further questioning often discloses that family members who were thought to have nonmigrainous headache may have had MG syndrome.

B. Physical Examination: The interictal physical examination usually is normal. If patients are examined during the attack, they are pale and diaphoretic, appear acutely ill, are sitting or lying in a darkened room when the examiner enters, and may vomit during the course of the evaluation. Blood pressure elevation and tachycardia are often present. Facial flushing, tearing, conjunctival injection, nasal stuffiness, and even unilateral ptosis and miosis may be encountered. Patients who have mentioned focal swelling of the scalp, periorbital tissues, or face may demonstrate that finding. Some patients appear reluctant to answer questions, may seem dazed or confused, or may even have a hemiparesis, hemisensory abnormalities, aphasia, or brain stem signs such as disconjugate gaze, nystagmus, dysarthria, ataxia, paresis, or sensory loss.

C. Diagnostic Tests: Blood tests are unnecessary in the investigation of typical MG, but they can be important in evaluating alternative causes of headache such as temporal arteritis or a systemic illness. Occasionally, patients have a dramatic aura accompanying their headache that is suggestive of a seizure disorder; such patients need an EEG to help differentiate MG aura from the aura of a seizure disorder. Lumbar puncture (LP) usually is reserved for patients in whom subarachnoid hemorrhage or infection is suspected. It is necessary if a previously asymptomatic patient experiences a fulminating headache even though it may have some of the features of MG.

Imaging studies are appropriate only if there is confusion about the diagnosis. Computed tomography (CT) with and without contrast or magnetic resonance imaging (MRI) and magnetic resonance angiography may be useful depending on the situation. When MG is clearly the cause of a patient's symptoms, imaging studies are not needed. Percutaneous angiography is performed rarely now that MR angiography is available. Some patients cannot be dissuaded from pursuing testing, because they want to know the cause of their headaches. Neuropsychiatric testing may be helpful in validating complaints of persistent cognitive dysfunction.

Treatment

A. General Principles: The goal of MG therapy, whether aimed at alleviating the acute attack or preventing recurrent attacks, is the reduction in headache frequency, severity, and duration, and in associated symptoms. Complete success is not always achieved, however, and symptom reduction rather than absolute relief may be the best that can be accomplished. Many migraineurs have tried numerous OTC and prescription medications and had numerous physician interactions and remain discouraged. They need to be made aware that headache therapy is a long-term process. A good doctor-patient relationship is critical to the success of any treatment program.

The foundation of any treatment plan is nonpharmacologic management. This aspect includes alterations in adverse life-style practices; identification and elimination of triggering factors; and a review of the social, familial, and occupational situation of the patient to determine what changes will enhance the success of a headache management program.

Pharmacologic treatment strategy depends on a variety of considerations such as the frequency and severity of the MG syndrome. Infrequent headache, even though severe, may not warrant preventive therapy if it can be managed with abortive and symptomatic medications. Patients with fewer than 2–4 hedaches a month usually do not require prophylactic medication. However, frequent headaches or headaches that are infrequent but severe and disruptive require the addition of prophylactic therapy. Patients who have an identifiable prodrome or aura often respond well to abortive medication, because they can take it early in the course of the episode before symptoms are fully developed. Delayed use of abortive medications is generally ineffective and may even contribute to the headache.

The route of administration for acute therapy must be chosen on the basis of convenience, suitability, and patient acceptability. Because gastric emptying time often is delayed or vomiting intervenes, oral administration frequently is impossible. Use of an antiemetic such as metoclopramide prior to other medication may improve tolerance of the oral route, however. Rectal administration gives the best absorption of medication and avoids the problem of vomiting. Nasal and inhalant forms of medication are either available or being developed. Self-administered subcutaneous injection of various medications is an option for patients willing to learn self-injection techniques.

The physician must be aware of such contraindications to medications as pregnancy, concomitant diseases, or interactions with other medications. Most drugs should not be used by pregnant patients. Cardiovascular, gastrointestinal, hepatic, renal, or pulmonary disease precludes the use of many anti-MG drugs. Potential adverse interactions with drugs used to treat systemic illnesses may limit treatment choices.

Prophylactic therapy is reserved for patients with frequent or severe disruptive headache or for those in whom acute therapy has failed or is contraindicated. It is important for patients taking prophylactic medications to record treatment effects to guide changes in medication in complicated or resistant cases. It should be emphasized to patients that prophylactic therapy is not a cure; it is considered effective if it reduces the frequency, severity, and duration of the MG episode or enhances the benefits of symptomatic therapy. Preventive therapy is selected with careful attention to drug safety and is used at the lowest effective dose.

Minor side effects may emerge with administration of prophylactic drugs; in many cases, however, patients adapt with continued use. If side effects remit, patients should be encouraged to continue.

Cost is a consideration when devising a treatment plan. Although many medications are generic and inexpensive, visits to the emergency room, newer medications, and some prophylactic medications are expensive.

B. Nonpharmacologic Treatment: Life-style changes may be difficult to enact, but they should be pursued. Stress reduction may be accomplished through counseling. Job changes and family therapy may eliminate some obstacles to headache improvement without resorting to medication.

Personal habits are important to explore. Smoking or other forms of tobacco use not only are potential triggering factors for MG, but also negate the effects of symptomatic and prophylactic therapy. These habits must be discontinued before therapy can succeed.

Dietary factors often are known and avoided, but it may take further questioning to identify obscure items in the diet that also trigger headache. So-called elimination diets, which attempt to eliminate all foods that might potentially cause headache, are generally not effective.

Management of biorhythm disturbances, such as unconventional eating habits, sleep disruption, and frequent time zone changes, improves many MG patients. An aerobic exercise program may aid in eliminating symptoms of MG (if they are not precipitated or aggravated by exercise).

Other techniques such as biofeedback, manipulative therapy, physical therapy, massage, acupuncture, and acupressure have been tried, but adequate studies validating their use are not available; anecdotal and testimonial evidence of success can be found.

C. Treatment of the Acute Attack: Treatment of the acute attack has two phases. If there is any warning prior to the headache, abortive therapy is employed. If headache occurs without warning and is the only harbinger of the attack, abortive therapy may be less useful, and purely symptomatic therapy in an attempt to suppress the headache is the treatment employed.

Medications used for the abortive treatment of acute MG (Table 42–4) share the characteristic of agonist activity at 5-HT_1-receptor sites. To be effective, abortive therapy mustas possible after a warning, and the dosage must be adequate to suppress the headache. Frequently, patients either are misinstructed or are reluctant to take an adequate dose of medication and lose the opportunity to abort the attack. The ergotamines (with or without caffeine) are effective abortive medications in patients who tolerate them. The oral route is used frequently, but absorption may be poor, and ergotamine may contribute to nausea and vomiting. Rapid and higher drug levels are achieved with the rectal route.

A combination of a vasoconstrictor (isomethep-

Table 42–4. Abortive therapy for migraine.

Drug	Route	Dosage
Ergotamine and caffeine, 1 mg	PO	2 mg at onset; repeat 1–2 mg $q\frac{1}{2}$–1h; limit: 4 mg/d, 6 mg/wk
Ergotamine and caffeine, 2 mg	PR	1–2 mg at onset; repeat in $\frac{1}{2}$–1 h; limit: 4 mg/d, 6 mg/wk
Ergotamine, 2 mg	SL	2 mg at onset; repeat in 1 h; limit: 4 mg/d, 6 mg/wk
Isometheptene and acetaminophen	PO	2 caps at onset; repeat $q\frac{1}{2}$–1h × 2
Dichloralphenazone, acetyl salicylic acid, and caffeine	PO	2–3 tabs at onset; repeat q3–4h
Naproxen sodium, 550 mg	PO	550–775 mg at onset; repeat 550 mg q4h × 2
Ibuprofen, 400 mg	PO	400–1200 mg at onset; repeat 400–800 mg q3–4h
Metoclopramide, 10 mg	PO	10 mg at onset; repeat 10 mg q4–6h
Butorphanol, 1 mg	NS	1 mg (one spray) at onset; repeat q1–2h × 4
Sumatriptan, 6 mg	SQ	6 mg at onset; repeat × 1 in 1–2 h
Dihydroergotamine, 1 mg	SQ	0.5–1 mg 1h × 3

tene), a mild sedative (dichloralphenazone), and acetaminophen is also a reliable abortive medication and produces less nausea than the ergotamine-caffeine combination (Table 42–5). Subcutaneous or intranasal dihydroergotamine mesylate (DHE) prevents headache and is not associated with significant rebound or nausea. It can be given later in the cycle and still suppress symptoms.

Sumatriptan, a medication specifically developed as a 5-HT$_1$-receptor agonist, is a new abortive drug that is given subcutaneously by self-injection. Although generally well regarded, its drawbacks are expense, unacceptable side effects in some patients, and a tendency for the headache to rebound after initial suppression. In addition, recent labeling changes have been issued, reflecting the need for proper diagnosis before use; describing rarely reported adverse events, including drug-associated fatalities; and reporting the effects of interaction with monoamine oxidase inhibitors (MAOIs), which produces increased systemic exposure to sumatriptan. Thorough familiarity with the drugis recommended before use. Sumatriptan has been an excellent medication for many patients who previously did not respond to other therapy. Any of the medications discussed in this section may need to be administered with an antinauseant.

Symptomatic therapy is used if patients experience no warning prior to the headache or as an adjunct to abortive therapy. Simple measures should be given an adequate trial before more complicated and expensive medications, with a greater potential for side effects, are prescribed. Aspirin and nonsteroidal antiinflammatory drugs (NSAIDS) such as ibuprofen and naproxen sodium are simple but effective symptomatic drugs.

Combination prescription medications such as aspirin or acetaminophen with butabarbital and caffeine seem to be more effective than single analgesics in many patients. They need to be carefully monitored, however, because of the potential for abuse. Patients who experience frequent headaches may overuse these medications and may develop rebound headaches as a complication. Restricted use of opioids is appropriate for patients who have no more than two or three headaches per month. Some patients respond well to low-dose propranolol taken at the time of the headache. Twenty milligrams every 4 hours in combination with a simple analgesic may eliminate the headache completely.

Patients who fail to respond to self-administered abortive and symptomatic measures may have intractable headache with vomiting and dehydration and must be treated in the office or emergency department. Patients can receive DHE intramuscularly or intravenously in combination with a parenteral

Table 42–5. Symptomatic therapy for migraine.

Drug	Route	Dosage
Naproxen sodium	PO	550–775 mg q4–6h
Ibuprofen	PO	600–800 mg q4–6h
Ketorolac	PO	10 mg qid
	IM	60 mg q4h × 2
Acetylsalicylic acid, acetaminophen, caffeine, butalbital	PO	1–2 tabs q4–6h
Analgesic-narcotic combination	PO	Use as directed for acute headache; monitor use
Promethazine	PO, PR, IM	50–100 mg q4–6h
Hydroxyzine	PO, IM	50 mg q4–6h
Prochlorperazine	PO, PR, IM	10–25 mg q4–6h
Dihydrotryotamine	IV, SQ, IM	0.5–1 mg q6–8h
Meperidine	IM	75–125 mg q3–4h × 2; use with antiemetic; limit 2–4 injections/m; monitor use
Dexamethasone	IV	10–16 mg; may repeat q6–8h × 1

antiemetic. Ketorolac, 60 mg intramuscularly, relieves headache in some patients. No more than two sumatriptan injections should be administered within a 24-hour period; patients should be asked whether they have self-injected at home, and if so, at what time. Parenteral antiemetics and opioids relieve headache in many patients, although there may be rebound. Opioids should be given in adequate doses but used selectively and monitored rigorously because of their potential for abuse. Meperidine, 75–125 mg, and an antiemetic such as promethazine or prochlorperazine can be given concomitantly. If patients experience repeated headache and initial emergency department therapy does not control symptoms, intravenous dexamethasone, 10–20 mg, eventually may terminate the attack.

D. Prophylactic Therapy: Prophylactic treatment aims to decrease the frequency and severity of attacks that occur more than 2–4 times per month or are severe enough to be disruptive. It also may improve the effectiveness of symptomatic therapy if headaches break through the protective barrier of a prophylactic regimen. The prophylactic medications have a variety of biologic effects, making it impossible to attribute their success to any one mechanism. Most of the effective prophylactic drugs appear to have antagonist activity at the 5 HT_2–receptor site. There are no definitive guidelines for the selection of one medication over another, but side effects, patient tolerance, effective dosage, and cost are considerations that make it important to individualize treatment. Preventive therapy is considered successful if it reduces the frequency, duration, and intensity of the attacks by 50% or more. If stabilization and control are established after a period of treatment of 6 months to 1 year, medications can be discontinued slowly, and there may be a prolonged remission.

The most successful of the drugs available for prophylactic therapy (Table 42–6) include beta-blockers, calcium channel blockers, and tricyclic antidepressants (TCA). They are effective in 50–70% of patients, either alone or in combination.

1. Beta-blockers–Beta-blockers are perhaps the most widely used agents. Propranolol, nadolol, and atenolol are all effective. The nonselective beta-blockers are more highly regarded than the selective group, but they may have more side effects. Low-dose regular-acting or long-acting treatment is preferred, and the dosage should be increased gradually until an effect is apparent or side effects intervene. If there is no significant response after 6–8 weeks of treatment at the maximal dosage, a different beta-blocker may be tried. Caution must be used so that hypotension and bradycardia do not occur. Some patients note lassitude, depression, poor endurance, and weight gain, although the medications are well tolerated by most patients, especially at lower doses. The beta-blockers should be avoided in patients with asthma, insulin-dependent diabetes, and heart failure,

Table 42–6. Prophylactic therapy for migraine.

Drug	Daily Dosages
Beta-blockers	
Propranolol	60–160 mg
Nadolol	40–180 mg
Atenolol	50–100 mg
Calcium channel blockers	
Verapamil	120–480 mg
Nifedipine	20–80 mg
Tricyclic antidepressants	
Amitriptyline	10–100 mg
Imipramine	25–100 mg
Nortriptyline	25–100 mg
Protriptyline	10–40 mg
Doxepin	25–100 mg
Other antidepressants	
Trazodone	50–100 mg
Fluoxetine	20–40 mg
Phenelzine	15–45 mg
5-HT-receptor-influencing drugs	
Methysergide	4–8 mg
Cyproheptadine	4–12 mg
Ergotamine, belladonna, phenobarbital	1–2 tab
Nonsteroidal anti-inflammatory drugs	
Naproxen	250–750 mg
Ketoprofen	50–150 mg
Indomethacin	50–150 mg
Miscellaneous drugs	
Divalproex sodium	500–1500 mg
Lithium	300–900 mg

and should not be used in combination with other antihypertensive agents.

2. Calcium channel blockers–Verapamil is the most effective of the calcium channel blockers. Dosages ranging from 40 to 240 mg twice daily can be effective. The long-acting preparation is quite effective, although the dosage may need to be split because 24-hour prophylaxis may not be achieved with single-dose therapy. For the response to verapamil to be evaluated thoroughly, patients need to take the maximal dosage for at least 4–6 weeks. Although initial aggravation of headache may occur, the verapamil should be continued if the headaches are not disabling, because improvement often follows. Prolonged aura or complicated MG may be treated more effectively by calcium channel blockers than other agents. In addition to hypotension, side effects of verapamil include constipation and fluid retention. Although other calcium channel blockers may be useful at times, they may cause or aggravate headaches.

3. Tricyclic antidepressants–The prophylactic effect of the TCAs is independent of any antidepressant activity. The best medications for headache are amitriptyline, doxepin, and imipramine, which inhibit serotonin reuptake and block the 5-HT_2 receptor. The more adrenergic TCAs such as nortriptyline and desipramine are used if the other TCAs fail. The newer serotonin reuptake inhibitors such as fluoxetine have not fulfilled their initial promise as prophylactic agents and in some cases seem to cause or intensify headache. As with the beta-blockers, lack of effectiveness of one TCA does not preclude switching to another. Side effects that limit the use of TCAs include drowsiness, dry mouth, constipation, urinary dysfunction, and weight gain. They are contraindicated in patients with hypertension or significant cardiovascular disease. Some of the less bothersome side effects often disappear with continued use; if the drug is started at a low dosage and gradually increased, some of the side effects can be avoided altogether. TCAs are effective at lower dosages than used for depression, nd dosages above 75–100 mg of amitriptyline or its equivalent provide little added benefit. When given once a day before bedtime, TCAs are particularly effective against headache that awakens patients from sleep.

4. Other 5-HT$_2$-receptor antagonists–Methysergide, cyproheptadine, and the ergotamines may be tried if drugs in the major three categories for prophylaxis have failed. Methysergide is one of the oldest anti-MG preparations, but its use has been limited because of fear of tissue fibrosis. It is considered safe when administered with periods of discontinuation of 4 weeks every 5–6 months. Minor gastrointestinal symptoms, drowsiness, and changes in cognitive function are initial side effects that may be avoided if the drug is started at a low dosage and gradually increased. The most potentially dangerous side effect is intense vasoconstriction causing arterial insufficiency and anginal pain. It can occur as an idiosyncratic response after use of only small doses of the medication. Many of the minor side effects are temporary, however, and the drug is useful in patients whose headaches are refractory to other medications.

Cyproheptadine is a relatively safe drug with drowsiness and weight gain as its only major side effects. It is more useful as an adjunctive drug than a primary therapeutic agent. The ergotamines are not only effective for abortive therapy; taken once daily in low doses, they act as prophylactic agents.

5. Nonsteroidal anti-inflammatory drugs (NSAIDs)–NSAIDS can be given alone or in combination with other classes of drugs for MG prophylaxis. Their usefulness may be limited by gastrointestinal or renal side effects. Naproxen, ketoprofen, fenoprofen, and indomethacin are all effective. It has been noted that 325 mg of aspirin at bedtime sometimes has a prophylactic effect.

6. Anticonvulsants–Phenytoin and carbamazepine rarely are prescribed as first-line or add-on therapy; however, sodium valproate recently has found use as a primary agent. It is an effective single prophylactic medication, but it also can be combined with some of the other primary drugs. Drug levels between 75 and 100 μg/mL should be achieved before the drug is considered ineffective, although many patients respond at lower levels. Side effects such as sedation and ataxia can occur, but they are generally not a serious problem. Hepatic dysfunction is reported, and enzymes should be monitored. The drug should not be given in patients with hepatic disease.

7. Other drugs–Several other medications are reserved for prophylaxis in refractory cases. Lithium, 300 mg 2–3 times daily, sometimes prevents cyclic MG. Lithium levels require careful monitoring, and the drug should not be used in patients with renal or cardiac disease.

Phenelzine, an MAOI, also may be tried when other medications fail. With MAOIs, the diet must be restricted to prevent exogenous vasoactive amine ingestion. Sympathomimetics should be avoided. Narcotics, particularly meperidine, should never be administered to patients taking MAOIs because death has been reported. Other drugs to be avoided when MAOIs are taken include fluoxetine, beta-blockers, and calcium channel blockers because of the potential for severe hypotension. Patients with hypertension or hepatic, cardiovascular, or renal disease should not be treated with MAOIs.

Drugs that are likely to cause dependency, including the opiates and the benzodiazepines, should not be used on a chronic basis. Many of these medications as well as OTC analgesics are overused by patients who experience frequent MG attacks and cause rebound headache or the failure of prophylactic therapy.

8. Combination therapy–In cases refractory to single drug therapy, combination therapy provides added treatment flexibility. The best combinations are a beta-blocker or calcium channel blocker and a TCA or valproate. Cyproheptadine, an NSAID, or lithium also can be used as a second-line drug in combination with any of the aforementioned medications. When combination therapy is used, lower dosages of both medications are generally preferable. Adding a third drug rarely provides additional benefit.

Prognosis

Forty percent of children in whom MG develops between ages 7 and 15 may be in remission by age 30; after prolonged MG-free intervals, however, some experience recurrence. At least one-third of such children have no remission at any time. The prognosis for remission tends to be better in boys than in girls. There is controversy about the mortality rate of MG patients compared with the general population. Some studies have suggested a higher and others a lower rate.

Variations & Complications of Migraine

A. Chronic Daily Headache (CDH): This condition occurs often in patients with prior attacks of MG in whom there has been transformation from episodic headache with headache-free intervals to daily headache with superimposed attacks of MG. In this group, there usually is a strong family history of

MG, and hormonal changes are a triggering factor; many patients report associated gastrointestinal and neurologic symptoms. Transformation of MG to CDH is common in mid-life or during the perimenopausal years. Tobacco use may contribute to CDH of this and other types.

A second group of patients with CDH have had episodic tension-type headache, which may have been associated with cervical and pericranial tenderness. The headaches may be intermittent initially and transform gradually into CDH, although some patients have headaches that are daily in occurrence from the onset. Associated features are rare, but photophobia and nausea can occur. Patients with chronic tension-type headache do not have a history of episodic MG-type headache with clear-cut attacks and associated migrainous features.

A third group of patients with CDH have symptoms related to viral infections, particularly Epstein-Barr. Following the onset of headaches, prolonged CDH, often self-limited, occurs. Symptoms may continue for months.

There are several distinctive clinical features of CDH. There is an increased incidence of depression. Medication overuse is common and includes excessive ingestion of OTC medications such as aspirin, acetaminophen, and headache preparations containing caffeine. Medications may be overprescribed, contributing to dependency and analgesic rebound. In particular, ergotamine overuse or abuse can lead to CDH. It must be remembered that some medications used for prophylactic therapy can produce headache that resembles CDH as a side effect.

The headache caused by analgesic rebound or medication overuse varies in location and severity. It often is precipitated by minimal activity or stress, and many patients become irritable, cannot concentrate, complain of sleep-related difficulties, awaken in the morning with severe headache, and become physically inactive and socially withdrawn.

Among the consequences of continued medication overuse are reduction or nullification of the effectiveness of other symptomatic and prophylactic therapies. The headache is perpetuated by the continued use of medication, and short periods of withdrawal or partial reduction in the frequency or dosage of medication does not result in significant improvement.

Management of CDH can be difficult and requires a multidisciplinary or multimodal approach. Complete discontinuation of the offending medications is mandatory if the headache cycle is to be interrupted. Judicious and temporary use of benzodiazepines to help patients taper and discontinue the offending drugs may be necessary. Stress management, biofeedback, other forms of counseling, and a vigorous exercise program should be instituted if appropriate. Patients should be instructed clearly on the deleterious effects of medication overuse. Prophylactic treatment can begin with a reasonable chance for effec-

tiveness once patients have been withdrawn successfully from their medications. These patients need close follow-up care and continued monitoring of their medication use.

The prognosis of CDH is somewhat discouraging. Despite attempts to withdraw medication, initiate changes in life-style, and institute effective prophylaxis, at least one-third of patients continue to experience headache. There is a discouraging relapse rate if patients are not carefully followed. Some authors believe these patients get little or no relief despite all the changes that are made and resume their previous habits of medication overuse. In refractory cases, there may be some advantage in enrolling patients in a pain clinic or a specialized headache clinic for intense outpatient or inpatient therapy.

B. Status Migrainosus (SM): Status migrainosus is defined as a continuous severe headache lasting longer than 72 hours with less than 4 hours during that period (not counting sleep) of headache-free time with or without treatment. In addition to the usual triggering factors, viral or other febrile illness or a minor head injury may precede the develoment of SM. Even when the inciting event remits, the headache may continue. Changes in hormonal status such as menopause or changes in the menstrual cycle may be associated with SM in susceptible persons.

Features of SM in addition to intractability and long duration include sleep deprivation (which undoubtedly aggravates the headache), nausea, vomiting, dehydration, and behavioral changes such as irritability, agitation, and withdrawal. Often multiple attempts to control the headache have failed, and patients may have complicated the situation by self-medication with other drugs or alcohol in an attempt to control the headache. When a patient has SM, a careful search should be made for other causes of severe unremitting headache, such as infection, subarachnoid hemorrhage, or a space-occupying lesion, although these conditions often are clinically apparent.

Treatment of SM often requires hospitalization for rehydration and intravenous medication. DHE (0.5 mg) and metoclopramide (10 mg) can be administered intravenously over a 2–3 minute period, and repeated every 8 hours if the initial dose provides temporary relief of the headache. Higher doses of DHE (0.75–1 mg) may be given if the lower dose is not effective and nausea is not a limiting side effect. This schedule of DHE and metoclopramide may be continued until the headache is relieved completely, but should not exceed 3 days. Treatment of other complications, such as electrolyte disturbances and dehydration, and the addition of intravenous methylprednisolone or dexamethasone may help to terminate SM.

C. Cerebrovascular Complications: Persistence of neurologic deficits and abnormal imaging studies that suggest cerebral ischemia occur in some patients with MG. It has been estimated that approximately 10% of cases of stroke seen in patients under age 40 are related to an attack of MG. The incidence is significantly higher in women by a factor of 3 or 4. Strokes occur more often in patients who have a discrete, intense aura associated with their headache. Smoking and hypertension increase the risk of MG-related stroke. It is not clear whether oral contraceptives are associated with an increased incidence of migrainous stroke, because study results are conflicting.

The pathophysiology of MG stroke is not completely understood. Cerebral imaging and blood flow studies demonstrate persistent hypoperfusion and ischemia, but whether these are caused by vasospasm or whether neural activity influences the perfusion abnormalities is yet to be determined. There may be an increase in platelet aggregation, and a hypercoagulable state may contribute to the ischemic process.

The clinical features of the stroke often resemble the symptoms of a previous aura. Stroke often occurs during the course of an MG attack or may begin with the aura. Other causes of stroke must be excluded even in young patients who have MG. Medications that intensify vasoconstriction are among the factors thought to precipitate MG stroke. The ergotamines have been of concern, although no direct evidence exists that they cause stroke. Trauma and arteriography sometimes are identified as precipitating causes of stroke in migraineurs.

Stroke is most common in the posterior cerebral circulation, although middle cerebral artery branch ischemia is seen also. Patients may have monocular symptoms caused by retinal infarction. A variety of visual, somatosensory, motor, and cognitive changes have been reported with MG stroke. Fortunately, recovery is often good, although it may be incomplete.

Patients who have severe aura and in whom stroke is a concern should avoid vasoconstrictor therapy and undergo long-term treatment with verapamil and aspirin. They should be encouraged strongly to discontinue any adverse life-style habits such as smoking and any medications that may be harmful such as oral contraceptives. If stroke occurs, hospitalization, evaluation for other causes of stroke, and treatment with heparin followed by warfarin (Coumadin) and verapamil are the measures to be taken.

D. Migraine and the Hormonal Cycle:

1. Catamenial migraine–Menstrual MG affects approximately 60% of female MG sufferers, in whom some or all of their headaches are related to the menstrual cycle. Most attacks occur during the first 2–3 days preceding the onset of menstruation or during the first or second day of the menses. The timing is consistent for individual patients. Headaches are frequently severe; are somewhat longer lasting than other forms of MG, persisting for 2–3 days; and are accompanied by nausea and vomiting. Most of the attacks occur without aura, although patients who have MG with aura at other times often experience aura with catamenial MG. Catamenial MG may be absent for several cycles only to occur repetitively for several subsequent cycles before remitting again. In women whose menstrual cycle is irregular, headaches are unpredictable. Other women may have headache only during ovulation at mid cycle, although both mid- and end-of-cycle headaches can coexist in the same patient. The onset of catamenial MG often coincides with menarche. The age of onset seems to be slightly younger than that of MG that is not related to the menstrual cycle.

The role of hormones in the genesis of catamenial MG is not fully understood; however, it is clear that headache is associated with a rapid fall in plasma estradiol levels. Progesterone fluctuations do not play a significant role. Absolute estrogen levels are not as important as the rate and degree of their fall. Artificially maintaining a high estrogen level during the menstrual period may delay headaches until the estrogen level falls. Other hormones that have been studied include prostaglandins, prolactin, and the endorphins, but their roles in the genesis of catamenial MG are unclear.

Treatment of catamenial MG depends on the patient's history. If an attack of MG is similar to other attacks occurring during the month, the timing represents menstrual worsening of the underlying MG, and treatment is no different than for other forms of MG. MG that is purely catamenial can be resistant to therapy. If headache is predictable, prophylactic therapy begun 1 week before onset of menses and continued for the week afterward allows for intermittent rather than daily therapy. At times, however, daily therapy may be necessary. Effective medications include NSAIDS, beta-blockers, TCAs, and the ergotamines. Calcium channel blockers, which often require considerable time to exert their effect, are less likely to be successful. Although diuretics might seem useful because the premenstrual period often is associated with fluid retention, they generally are not helpful.

Because of the relationship between headache and the drop in estrogen levels, hormonal manipulation has been attempted to prevent menstrual MG; however, there has not been a consistent response. Although oral estrogen replacement is usually ineffective, the use of transdermal estradiol may suppress symptoms. Estrogen therapy usually delays the onset of headache rather than eliminating it. Androgens, tamoxifen, and bromocriptine mesylate all have been tried, but reports of success have been anecdotal only.

Overall, the best approach to therapy is restricted prophylaxis in patients who have predictable menses and headaches. A combination of naproxen and ergotamine tartrate begun 3–4 days prior to the predicted onset of an attack is often best, and more complicated regimens may be unnecessary.

2. Oral contraceptive use—An increased incidence of headache in previously headache-free women and aggravation of existing MG are reported by 20–50% of patients taking oral contraceptives. As might be expected, the attacks tend to occur during the period when medication is not taken, when estrogen levels are falling. One-third of patients taking oral contraceptives report improvement in their headache syndromes, but most patients experience no change. If onset of MG occurs with oral contraceptive use, it is generally during the earlier cycles, but it can emerge after months or even years of use. On occasion, headaches may be related to a change in the type of oral contraceptive. A family history of MG is absent in up to 60% of women who develop symptoms with oral contraceptive use, making it difficult to predict who might be at risk.

Guidelines for the use of oral contraceptives are not formally established, and many contraindications are relative. Family history, as noted, is not a good predictor of risk, but a strong family history of MG may be a relative contraindication. If new-onset MG that develops early in the course of oral contraceptive use is severe, disruptive, or associated with significant neurologic dysfunction, the patient should discontinue the drug. Patients with preexisting MG who have marked aggravation of their symptoms may respond best to a lower dose oral contraceptive or to withdrawal rather than an attempt to treat the headache and continue the oral contraceptive. Stroke risk is difficult to assess; however, there is some suggestion that patients with severe and prolonged aura or neurologic symptoms should discontinue oral contraceptives, because stroke sometimes occurs in this group. Change in the pattern of MG from headache without aura to headache with aura may define another subgroup of patients who should discontinue oral contraceptives. The rate of migrainous infarction is greater in patients with risk factors such as smoking, hypertension, or lipid disorders, and these factors are strong contraindications to use of oral contraceptives.

Treatment of patients with oral contraceptive-related MG clearly involves withdrawal of the offending agent. If the headache persists, taking 6 months to a year to resolve, routine symptomatic or prophylactic MG therapy is employed.

3. Pregnancy and the postpartum period—Pregnancy usually has a beneficial effect on MG, and suppression or resolution of the attacks is seen in 50–90% of cases. Improvement often begins during the last two trimesters. It is much less likely that a patient will have worsening of attacks during pregnancy. In 10–15% of cases, MG makes its initial appearance in the first trimester of pregnancy. Uncommonly, MG may mark the onset of preeclampsia or eclampsia. Some patients with MG have a less well-defined headache at the onset of their pregnancy, which later resolves. Nonspecific, limited peripartum headache is also frequent in migraineurs. Elevated hormone levels may play a role in the genesis of pregnancy-related MG, and the rapid fall associated with delivery may be the cause of postpartum headaches.

Treatment of MG during pregnancy rarely requires prophylaxis or significant amounts of abortive or symptomatic medication, because patients often are able to cope with the pain. If medication must be used, small doses of acetaminophen or codeine are relatively safe. Nondrug therapies should be emphasized. If prophylaxis is required, beta-blockers and amitriptyline are acceptable. For acute, severe headache, injections of meperidine and antinauseants such as metoclopramide, if used infrequently, are deemed safe. Intravenous dexamethasone given on rare occasions for persistent headache also is not associated with complications.

Other causes of headache during pregnancy besides MG should be considered. Hypertension, pseudotumor, subarachnoid hemorrhage caused by aneurysm or arteriovenous malformation (AVM), expanding tumors (particularly of the pituitary gland or meningiomas), and *Listeria* meningitis all are possible causes of headache during pregnancy and should be excluded by appropriate studies before MG therapy is instituted.

If headaches requiring treatment recur during the postpartum period in a nursing mother, consideration must be given to concentrations of anti-MG drugs in breast milk. Aspirin and the ergotamines are likely to be present at high levels. Medications that are considered safe include acetaminophen, most of the NSAIDS, beta-blockers and calcium channel blockers, and codeine. Headache in some patients may be refractory to treatment because of life-style changes, such as sleep disruption or deprivation, that occur with mothering an infant. It may be necessary to discontinue nursing if the mother is incapacitated by headache.

4. Menopause—Although MG may disappear during menopause, in some patients it makes its initial appearance, changes character, or worsens. A change in MG may precede menopause by 5 or more years, possibly because of hormonal changes that ultimately lead to cessation of the menses.

The course of MG often is altered by the need for hormone replacement therapy (HRT). Although it may be associated with improvement in the MG syndrome, HRT often produces no change or even a marked worsening of MG, and it may be responsible for a dramatic alteration in the character of the headache. Excessive use of OTC medications may be largely responsible for the changing character of the headache.

Treatment of menopausal and postmenopausal MG relies on the medications previously outlined. Attempts to manipulate the hormonal status of the patient by HRT or by more drastic measures such as hysterectomy generally have failed. Occasionally, a shift in the dosage and type of HRT or a change to a continuous from a cyclic regimen may be of benefit. Discontinuing oral HRT and using the transdermal delivery route may improve symptoms in some patients. The lowest possible dosage of estrogen necessary to maintain the desired effect or a change in the type of estrogen may diminish or eliminate the headaches. If hormonal manipulation is not effective, routine anti-MG prophylaxis or symptomatic therapy can be employed.

Psychosocial Issues

Migraine is responsible for considerable social, personal, and economic disruption. Women, who now constitute a major part of the work force and in addition are responsible for the majority of home care, are disproportionately affected. Patients from lower income groups may go undiagnosed and untreated. The monetary cost to society is enormous. Headache is one of the 10 most common reasons for visits to a physician and is expensive to diagnose and treat. An average of 10 working days a year are lost either totally or partially because of reduced worker effectiveness. Indirect costs of MG in the United States are conservatively estimated to be nearly $5 billion each year.

Associated depression may require therapy, and patients are often withdrawn or pathologically anxious. The mood and personality changes induced by acute headache or by the stress of dealing with chronic pain produce substantial personal and social dysfunction leading to disruption of family or social ties. The economic cost to a family when a member of the household suffers severe MG is potentially disastrous. Job stability may be affected, and some patients with refractory MG are incapable of holding a regular job. Self-employed persons may be overwhelmed by severe MG to the point that their business suffers drastically.

PSEUDOTUMOR CEREBRI (PTC)

Pseudotumor cerebri (PTC) is a condition of elevated intracranial pressure documented by lumbar puncture (LP). Neurologic examination is unremarkable with the exception of papilledema and possible sixth-nerve oculomotor dysfunction. Imaging studies show no evidence of ventricular enlargement, meningeal thickening, inflammation, or a space-occupying lesion.

Essentials of Diagnosis

• Increased cerebrospinal fluid (CSF) pressure documented by LP.
• Papilledema.
• Negative imaging studies.
• Female sex (female:male ratio, 8:1).

• Associated obesity and endocrine disturbances.
• Headache and visual disturbances (often the only symptoms).

Incidence

PTC has an overall prevalence of 1 in 100,000. In obese women between the ages of 20 and 44 who weigh more than 20% above their ideal weight, the incidence rises dramatically to nearly 20 in 100,000. The female:male ratio in the general as well as the overweight population is 8:1.

Pathophysiology

The cause of PTC is not known, although several mechanisms have been proposed. These include increased outflow resistance leading to a decrease in CSF absorption via the arachnoid villi, excess brain water content, and elevated intracranial blood volume. None of these mechanisms have been confirmed in all cases of PTC.

Associated Conditions

Patients with PTC often have endocrine disturbances, and menstrual irregularities are common. Corticosteroid abnormalities, thyroid disease, disorders of the hypothalamic-pituitary axis, and hypoparathyroidism or pseudohypoparathyroidism all have been reported. The incidence is high in obese young women, and recent weight gain and obesity are common in the year prior to the onset of symptoms. Use of numerous medications, drugs, and supplements has been reported in association with PTC, including tetracycline, nitrofurantoin, indomethacin, oral contraceptives, vitamin A, isotretinoin, and corticosteroids.

Signs & Symptoms

Headache is the symptom that usually provokes patients to seek medical evaluation. The headache is nondescript and can be either throbbing or nonthrobbing in character; it may be holocranial and worse in the reclining position. Visual disturbances are frequent and may include fixed visual field defects, transient visual obscurations, or even visual loss. Diplopia, if present, usually is due to a sixth-nerve paresis. Patients often complain of tinnitus or other intracranial noises. Focal neurologic symptoms generally are not reported; if they are, they raise the possibility of a different cause of headache.

Clinical Findings

A. Physical Examination: Papilledema is almost always present in PTC, although it can be subtle with blurring only of the upper and lower disk margins or absence of spontaneous venous pulsations. Long-standing papilledema may be associated with optic atrophy. Sixth-nerve dysfunction, although uncommon, is the only oculomotor abnormality. Visual field defects such as enlarged blind spots or diminished peripheral vision presumably are due to disk edema.

B. Diagnostic Tests: Laboratory studies are usually normal, although endocrine or calcium metabolism abnormalities may be detected. Lumbar puncture should document a pressure of at least 250; however, lower levels, particularly in thinner patients, may indicate disease. Pressures above 180 but below 250 are in the equivocal range. All CSF studies should be negative.

Imaging studies disclose no abnormalities except for possible decrease in ventricular size. Transependymal absorption can be evident on both CT and MRI. Increased pressure on the suprasellar leptomeninges may be associated with the empty-sella syndrome.

Treatment

Because many patients with PTC are obese or have experienced recent weight gain, weight loss and maintenance of ideal body weight often reverse the process. A diagnostic LP can be permanently therapeutic, but repeat LPs may be needed to manage recurrent pressure elevation. Carbonic anhydrase inhibitors or loop diuretics may relieve cerebral edema, although carefully controlled studies documenting their effectiveness are not available. Steroid pulse therapy sometimes controls severe symptoms temporarily.

Surgery is a last resort; lumboperitoneal or ventriculoperitoneal shunt restores normal CSF pressure. Fenestration of the optic nerve sheath also is advocated as a method of surgically lowering the CSF pressure.

Prognosis

PTC is a self-limiting condition in many patients; once it remits, however, there is a recurrence rate of approximately 10%. Some patients enter a phase of chronic PTC with gradual worsening of vision and may be unaware of gradual visual field deterioration unless formal evaluation is performed. It is estimated that permanent visual disturbances occur in 25% of patients with PTC. Blindness, formerly seen in 10% of patients, is now a rare complication.

Pregnancy & PTC

Onset of PTC during pregnancy is usually in the first trimester. Nonpharmacologic treatment of PTC during pregnancy is similar to management of PTC in nongravid patients. If medication is absolutely necessary because weight control and serial LPs have not controlled the pressure, acetazolamide or steroids can be used after 20 weeks of gestation. Therapeutic abortion almost never is indicated. Visual fields should be monitored carefully during pregnancy if there are visual complaints. The recurrence rate in subsequent pregnancies is low.

COITAL HEADACHE

Essentials of Diagnosis

- Precipitated by sexual activity or exertion.
- May recur with repeated sexual activity or other exertion if not treated, but is usually self-limited.

Signs & Symptoms

This headache is precipitated by sexual activity, including arousal, intercourse, and masturbation. It seems to occur more frequently in patients with an MG diathesis. Onset can be sudden or may be gradual, with the headache building in severity. It often resolves after release of tension; however, it may persist in the occipitonuchal area and be accompanied by tenderness of the cervical muscles. Although the headache can recur subsequently, it frequently remits spontaneously. Diagnosis is usually not difficult in typical cases; however, other causes of explosive headaches, such as subarachnoid hemorrhage or sudden increase in intracranial pressure resulting from ventricular occlusion, may need to be ruled out.

Treatment

Medication is sometimes effective in preventing recurrent coital headache. Anti-inflammatory medications such as indomethacin or naproxen taken during a 24- to 48-hour period before anticipated sexual activity or exertion may prevent the headache. Beta-blockers and verapamil are useful prophylactic medications in patients who suffer frequent, recurrent attacks.

Prognosis

Headache accompanying sexual activity or exertion usually spontaneously remits. Such headaches are almost never due to underlying disease and are self-limited.

CHRONIC PAROXYSMAL HEMICRANIA

Essentials of Diagnosis

- Hemicranial, frequent, and brief but often severe headaches.
- Absolute response to indomethacin.

Incidence

Chronic paroxysmal hemicrania (CPH) is a rare disorder with a predominance in women; the female:male ratio is 7:1. Mean onset is in the third and fourth decades.

Signs & Symptoms

The headache of CPH is unilateral and almost always is confined to the same side. Pain is throbbing or pulsatile, but it can be sharp and localized to the periorbital region. Multiple attacks occur in the course of a 24-hour period, lasting from a few minutes to as long as an hour. Nocturnal attacks are uncommon in this type of headache. The menstrual cycle has a variable effect on the occurrence of the CPH; the fact that the headache almost invariably diminishes during pregnancy, however, indicates some hormonal relationship. Whereas its counterpart, cluster headache, occurs more frequently in smokers, patients with CPH have no increased incidence of smoking. Also, cluster headache has a male predominance. Other differences from cluster headaches include the higher attack frequency and shorter duration of CPH. Patients with cluster headaches tend to have little pain between attacks, whereas CPH often is associated with a lingering discomfort in the affected area between attacks.

Clinical Findings

Findings during a period of headache are similar to those in cluster headache. Patients have lacrimation, miosis, ptosis, conjunctival injection, unilateral nasal congestion, and rhinorrhea. Unilateral periorbital edema on the symptomatic side may occur.

Treatment

CPH may be defined by its absolute response to indomethacin. Dosages of 150 mg/d for several days suppress the headache, but continued treatment is often necessary at a lower dose (25–100 mg/d). After 2–4 weeks of therapy, long-lasting remission may occur. Other medications are not likely to provide relief.

REFERENCES

Davidoff RA: *Migraine: Manifestations, Pathogenesis, and Management.* Contemporary Neurology Series. Davis, 1994.

Lange JW (supplement editor): Advances in biology and pharmacology of headaches. Neurology 1993;43(Suppl 3).

Lipton RB, Stewart WF (supplement editors): The impact of migraine. Neurology 1994;44(Suppl 4).

Olesen J, Tfelt-Hansen P, Welch KMA (editors): *The Headaches.* Raven Press, 1993.

Radhakrishnan K et al: Idiopathic intracranial hypertension. Mayo Clin Proc 1994;69:169.

Rapoport AM (supplement editor): Severe headache: Focus on migraine. Neurology 1994;44(Suppl 3):43.

Raskin NH: Serotonin receptors and headache. N Engl J Med 1993;329:1476.

Rothrock J et al: Migraine and migrainous stroke. Neurology 1993;43:2473.

Sheftell FD: Chronic daily headache. Neurology 1992;42(Suppl 2):32.

Silberstein SD, Merriam GR: Estrogens, progestins, and headache. Neurology 1991;41:786.

Welch KMA: Drug therapy of migraine. N Engl J Med 1993;329:1476.

Asthma

43

Joyce Lammert, MD, PhD

Essentials of Diagnosis
- Inflammation of the lungs with bronchial hyperreactivity and variably reversible air flow obstruction
- Frequently, normal pulmonary function tests and chest x-ray
- Variable triggers, including allergens, viral infections, sinus infections, exercise, and nonspecific irritants

Incidence & Risk Factors

There are approximately 10 million people in the United States who have asthma. Asthma is most common in childhood, declines in the late teens, and then increases steadily into the 70s. Asthma rates are higher in males than in females below the age of 20. For older age groups, rates are higher in females than males. Asthma prevalence, rates of hospitalization, and mortality rates appear to be on the rise in many countries. Results from the National Health Interview Survey (NHIS) showed an increase in asthma prevalence in the USA of 29% from 1980 to 1987. In persons younger than 20, rates increased by 42% for the whole group and 69% for females. Prevalence rates are greater in blacks than whites and greater in urban than rural areas. Air pollution, exposure to tobacco smoke, and allergen exposure all are believed to increase the risk of asthma.

Low income has been found to be a strong independent predictor of asthma prevalence and outcome. A variety of complex social factors may explain this finding, including increased exposure to allergens and to irritants such as tobacco smoke, a less nutritional diet, and lack of medical care.

Genetic factors are also important in the development of asthma. Studies of twins have shown an increased prevalence in monozygotic compared with dizygotic twins both in children and in adults. Allergic disease also has a strong genetic component, and multiple studies have shown an increased prevalence of allergic disease in individuals with asthma.

Pathophysiology

In 1892 William Osler described asthma as a special form of inflammation of the airways. Recent bronchoscopy studies looking at lavage fluid and biopsies in patients with mild asthma have confirmed

> Essentials of Diagnosis
> Incidence & Risk Factors
> Pathophysiology
> Signs & Symptoms
> Clinical Findings & Diagnosis
> Treatment
> Prognosis
> Referral to a Specialist
> Issues of Pregnancy & Asthma
> Psychosocial Concerns

Osler's impression of the disease. Bronchoalveolar lavage fluid from these patients contains increased inflammatory cells including eosinophils, macrophages, and activated T cells. The activated T cells produce increased amounts of a variety of lymphokines including interleukin-3 (IL-3), IL-4, IL-5, and granulocyte macrophage—colony stimulating factor (GM-CSF). These lymphokines are important for recruitment of eosinophils and mast cells and for IgE production. Recent studies have suggested an association between increased numbers of activated T cells and lymphokines and clinical parameters including pulmonary function tests, bronchial hyperreactivity as measured by challenge testing, and symptom scores. Treatment of asthma now focuses on therapy for the underlying inflammation (see "Treatment" section).

Signs & Symptoms

Major symptoms of asthma include dyspnea, wheezing, chest tightness, and cough. The history is the most important aspect in arriving at the correct diagnosis. Although wheezing is common, not everyone with asthma wheezes. Patients may complain of difficulty taking a deep breath and exhaling completely, of not getting enough air in, or of having to concentrate when breathing. An isolated cough has been shown to be associated with bronchial hyperreactivity in about one-third of cases. The history should include questions about exposures or activities that make symptoms better or worse. Factors that influence symptoms of asthma may include allergen exposure, respiratory tract infections, physical activity, weather, the menstrual cycle, aeroirritants, medications, and emotions.

Physical signs of asthma depend on the degree of obstruction present. The examination may be unremarkable, or findings may include tachypnea, tachycardia, pulsus paradoxus, diaphoresis, use of accessory muscles, prolongation of the expiratory phase, and wheezing or rhonchi on auscultation. The physical examination should include examination of the ears and posterior pharynx, a speculum examination of the nose, and a careful cardiac examination.

Clinical Findings & Diagnosis

Not all wheezing represents asthma. It is important to document the diagnosis because asthma is a chronic disease, and the medications used in treatment are expensive. Pulmonary function tests can help establish the diagnosis, give an idea of severity, and be used to monitor the course. An improvement of the forced expiratory volume in 1 second (FEV_1) of 15% following beta-agonist treatment is generally accepted as diagnostic. The finding of normal pulmonary function tests does not rule out asthma, however; a challenge test with a stimulus such as methacholine or histamine may be necessary.

A selected allergy evaluation should be done in all patients with asthma who require regular medication use. Sinus x-rays should be obtained if (1) the patient has symptoms, (2) gives a history of chronic sinusitis, or (3) has a persistent exacerbation of the asthma that is otherwise unexplained. Chest x-rays are usually normal in uncomplicated asthma. An eosinophil count and total IgE level are useful if there is concern about allergic bronchopulmonary aspergillosis.

Treatment

The goals of the treatment of asthma are to control symptoms, including nocturnal symptoms; maintain normal activity levels, including exercise; and prevent acute exacerbations.

A. General Approach: Although inflammation of the airways is the common mechanism in asthma, the clinical disease is complex, and treatment needs to be individualized. Education is the first step. The patient needs to understand the nature of the disease, the role of triggers, and the purpose of medications. Meter dose inhalers should be used with spacers to improve deposition of the drug into the lungs. Inhaler and spacer technique should be taught and periodically reevaluated. Avoidance of clinically significant triggers is important in improving control. Peak flow meters and symptom diaries help with early recognition of an asthma exacerbation. Early recognition combined with a written treatment plan allows for prompt treatment of flares. The chronic treatment plan needs to be simple to ensure long-term compliance. Influenza and pneumococcal vaccines should be prescribed at appropriate intervals.

B. Medications: Beta-adrenergic agonists re-

lax smooth muscle in the airway and may modulate mediator release from mast cells and basophils. They are the primary medications for treatment of acute bronchospasm. Inhaled therapy is preferred over oral therapy because it has a more rapid onset of action, achieves a similar therapeutic effect, and has fewer systemic side effects. Most of the currently available agents (albuterol, terbutaline, pirbuterol) have a 4- to 6-hour duration of action. Salmeterol was released recently and has an extended duration of action (10–12 hours); it should provide better control for patients who have nocturnal asthma. Beta-adrenergic agents typically are used on an as-needed basis; for occasional asthma or exercise-induced asthma, these products can be the sole medication. If a beta-adrenergic agent is being used on a regular basis once a day, it has been suggested that an anti-inflammatory medication be started.

There has been some controversy with regard to the safety of routine use of inhaled bronchodilators as maintenance medications. Separate reports by Sears et al and Spitzer et al have suggested that regular use of fenoterol, a potent, long-acting beta-agonist, is associated with increased asthma deaths. A more recent study by Suissa et al found that the increased mortality was confined primarily to the use of these drugs in excess of recommended limits (1.4 canisters per month).

Anti-inflammatory agents interrupt the development of bronchial inflammation and have a preventive action. It has been suggested that anti-inflammatory medications be initiated if a beta-adrenergic agent is being used on a daily basis for symptom control. Corticosteroids are the most effective available anti-inflammatory drugs. The inhaled medications are safe and have been shown to reduce significantly bronchial hyperreactivity. Bronchial biopsies of patients with asthma who use inhaled corticosteroids have demonstrated a marked reduction in the number of mast cells and eosinophils and a clearing of epithelial desquamation. Preparations available in the USA include beclomethasone dipropionate, triamcinolone acetonide, and flunisolide. Local adverse side effects include oropharyngeal candidiasis, dysphonia, and cough. These effects can be reduced or prevented with use of a spacer and rinsing out of the mouth after use. Cromolyn sodium and nedocromil sodium are the two nonsteroidal anti-inflammatory drugs available for inhalation. These drugs also may reduce nonspecific bronchial hyperreactivity. The primary advantage of these medications is the minimal incidence of side effects. They are would be appropriate as the first-line anti-inflammatory drug in patients with mild disease.

Oral corticosteroids should be used to treat acute episodes of asthma that do not respond to inhaled corticosteroids and bronchodilators. Dose and length of treatment need to be individualized based on clinical response. The goal is to use the lowest dose for the shortest length of time to ensure adequate treatment of the underlying inflammation. Immunotherapy might be indicated in a patient who has tested positively on skin tests, but the asthma is not controlled by avoidance of allergens and use of inhaled anti-inflammatory and bronchodilator medications.

Prognosis

Most studies that have looked at the natural history of asthma were performed before inhaled corticosteroids were available. Because these medications reduce bronchial hyperreactivity and the inflammatory infiltrate normally seen in asthma, they might have the potential to alter the course of the disease. Remission rates are high only during adolescence. At any point in time, the remission rate is about 20%. The remission rate is lowest in those with severe disease in whom fixed obstruction develops.

Asthma mortality appears to be increasing in the USA. From 1980 to 1987, total asthma deaths rose from 2891 to 4360 or from 1.3 to 1.7 per 100,000. Rates increased twofold in women relative to men. Mortality is high in children, the elderly, urban dwellers, blacks, and those in lower socioeconomic groups. These increases remain after taking into account changes in coding. The causes for this apparent increase in morbidity and mortality are not clear.

Referral to a Specialist

Referral to a specialist is indicated when (1) a patient has symptoms of asthma, but examination and pulmonary function tests are unremarkable and a therapeutic trial of medication is not helpful; (2) multiple emergency room visits or hospitalizations have taken place; (3) the patient has lost significant time from work, has ongoing nocturnal symptoms, or has been unable to return to her usual activity level despite apparently appropriate treatment; (4) there is question of a possible allergic component; (5) the family or patient needs ongoing education or close follow-up; or (6) the patient requires frequent use of systemic corticosteroids.

Issues of Pregnancy & Asthma

Up to 10% of women of childbearing age have bronchial asthma, and studies suggest that up to 4% of pregnancies are complicated by asthma. The asthma symptoms can be affected by pregnancy; exact numbers vary, but approximately one-third of the time the asthma improves, one-third of the time it stays the same, and one-third of the time it worsens during pregnancy. This phenomenon appears to reflect more than the natural history of asthma, because the disease tends to revert to the prepregnancy level 3 months postpartum. Although only a few women have been studied, the course appears to be consistent with each pregnancy. The peak incidence of episodes during pregnancy appears to be between the

twenty-fourth and thirty-sixth weeks of pregnancy. During weeks 37–40, women experience fewer episodes, and most asthma is under control during labor and delivery.

Most studies of the outcome of pregnancy in women with asthma have found that the major variable predicting outcome is how well the asthma is controlled. Both maternal and fetal complications can occur in patients with uncontrolled asthma. Undertreatment of asthma because of fears about the effects of medication use is a major problem in the management of asthma in pregnancy. Goals for the treatment of asthma during pregnancy are exactly the same as for nonpregnant women.

A. Nonpharmacologic Management: Pregnant women with asthma should avoid exposure to both allergens and nonspecific irritants. Exposure to tobacco smoke should be eliminated. Smoking has been shown to cause low-birth-weight infants, and this effect may be additive if maternal asthma flares secondary to smoke exposure. Immunotherapy can be continued at the dose achieved before pregnancy unless the patient has experienced frequent reactions. It is recommended that immunotherapy not be started during pregnancy. Influenza vaccine is recommended for pregnant patients with moderate or severe asthma.

Women with asthma should be followed regularly during pregnancy. They should have regular objective measurements of pulmonary function and facilitated access to the health care provider for increased symptoms. Many women experience some dyspnea during pregnancy, which is believed to be associated with the progressive increase in progesterone. Pulmonary function tests help sort out dyspnea of pregnancy from true asthma flares. These tests also allow the health care provider to identify patients with minimal symptoms but significant obstruction that might have an impact on the pregnancy.

B. Pharmacologic Management: Most retrospective studies of the adverse outcomes associated with the use of asthma medications during pregnancy have had negative or inconclusive results. In contrast, there are well-performed studies that have shown adverse outcomes of hypoxemia on the fetus. Patients need to be reassured that asthma medications not only are safe and necessary but also help to ensure a healthy outcome of the pregnancy. The choice of medications for use in pregnancy is based on a variety of considerations including human and animal data. Other considerations when deciding which medication to recommend include whether or not the medication has a track record for effectiveness and whether the medication is topical or systemic. Table 43–1 lists medications recommended by the National Asthma Education Program Working Group on Asthma and Pregnancy. It is important also to control associated conditions, including allergic rhinitis and

Table 43–1. Drugs used for asthma and rhinitis in pregnant women.*

Asthma

Class	Drug	Dose
Anti-inflammatory	Cromolyn	2 puffs qid
	Beclomethasone	2–5 puffs bid–qid
	Prednisone	Burst for active symptoms
Bronchodilator	Inhaled beta-agonist	2 puffs prn

Rhinitis

Class	Drug	Dose
Anti-inflammatory	Cromolyn	2 sprays each nostril bid
	Beclomethasone	2 sprays each nostril bid
Antihistamine	Chlorpheniramine	4 mg up to qid
	Tripelennamine	25–50 mg up to qid
		100 mg sustained-release
Decongestant	Pseudoephedrine	60 mg up to qid
	Oxymetazoline	Spray up to 5 d

*National Heart, Lung, and Blood Institute, National Institutes of Health: *Management of Asthma During Pregnancy.* National Asthma Education Program Working Group on Asthma and Pregnancy. NIH Publication No. 93–3279 A, 1993.

rhinosinusitis. Amoxicillin is the initial antibiotic of choice; others include erythromycin and, for persistent disease, cephalosporins. Tetracycline and the sulfonamides should be avoided during pregnancy.

Psychosocial Concerns

Asthma is a chronic disease that can be disruptive to the patient both at home and at work. Some asthmatics deal with their disease with denial of symptoms and noncompliance with medications. The results can be frequent emergency care, the need for treatment with systemic corticosteroids, and possible fatality. Asthma can be used for secondary gain such as avoidance of school or work activities. Occasionally, asthmatics develop manipulative behaviors that have an impact on their friends and family. Although emotional stress does not cause asthma, it can make poorly controlled asthma worse. Depression and anxiety or panic disorders can intensify asthma, as can associated behaviors such as hyperventilation.

Side effects of the medications also can have an impact on the patient's psychologic well-being. Systemic corticosteroids can cause a variety of side effects that can be devastating to the patient's body image. These include marked weight gain with central obesity, fluid retention, ecchymoses, striae, increase in lanugo hairs, and growth suppression in younger patients. Systemic corticosteroids also can cause or worsen affective disorders such as depression.

It is important for the health care provider to be sensitive to these issues and to discuss them with the patient. Appropriate referrals to a psychologist or psychiatrist can be helpful in some cases.

REFERENCES

Beasley R et al: Cellular events in the bronchi in mild asthma after bronchial provocation. Am Rev Respir Dis 1989;139:806.

Evans R: Epidemiology and natural history of asthma, allergic rhinitis, and atopic dermatitis. In: *Allergy Principles and Practice,* 4th ed. Middleton E et al (editors). Mosby, 1993.

Greenberger PA: Asthma. In: *Allergic Diseases: Diagnosis and Management,* 4th ed. Patterson R et al (editors). Lippincott, 1993.

Haahtela T et al: Comparison of a B$_2$-agonist, terbutaline, with an inhaled corticosteroid, budesonide, in newly detected asthma. N Engl J Med 1991;325:388.

Laitinen LA, Laitinen A, Haahtela T: Airway mucosal inflammation even in patients with newly diagnosed asthma. Am Rev Respir Dis 1993;147:697.

Mathison DA: Asthma in adults: Diagnosis and treatment. In: *Allergy Principles and Practice,* 4th ed. Middleton E et al (editors). Mosby, 1993.

National Heart, Lung, and Blood Institute, National Institutes of Health: *Guidelines for the Diagnosis and Management of Asthma.* National Asthma Education Program Expert Panel Report. NIH Publication No. 91–3042, 1991.

National Heart, Lung, and Blood Institute, National Institutes of Health: *Management of Asthma During Pregnancy.* National Asthma Education Program Working Group on Asthma and Pregnancy. NIH Publication No. 93–3279 A, 1993.

Robinson DS et al: Relationships among numbers of bronchoalveolar lavage cells expressing messenger ribonucleic acid for cytokines, asthma symptoms, and airway methacholine responsiveness in atopic asthma. J Allergy Clin Immunol 1993;92:397.

Schatz M: Asthma during pregnancy: Interrelationships and management. Ann Allergy 1992;68:123.

Sears MR et al: Regular inhaled beta-agonist treatment in bronchial asthma. Lancet 1990;336:1391.

Spitzer WO et al: The use of beta-agonists and the risk of death from asthma. N Engl J Med 1992:326:501.

Sporik R et al: Exposure to house-dust mite allergen and the development of asthma in children. N Engl J Med 1990;323:502.

Suissa S et al: A cohort analysis of excess mortality in asthma and the use of inhaled beta-agonists. Am J Respir Crit Care Med 1994;149:604.

Section XII.
Gynecologic Disorders

44

Premenstrual Syndromes

Leslie Hartley Gise, MD

The widespread belief that premenstrual syndrome (PMS) does not exist and that it is "all in a woman's head," combined with lack of clear diagnostic criteria, has complicated the evaluation and treatment of the premenstrual syndromes. These conditions range from mild, normal changes to severe symptoms that interfere with functioning. Despite these difficulties, premenstrual syndromes can be diagnosed in the primary care setting and can be treated effectively.

Evaluation
Etiology
Incidence & Risk Factors
Clinical Findings
Differential Diagnosis
Treatment
Prognosis & Course
Referral to a Specialist
Issues Related to Sex & Reproduction
Psychosocial Concerns
Controversies & Unresolved Issues

Evaluation

Four kinds of premenstrual symptoms must be differentiated:

1. Premenstrual symptoms or premenstrual changes– Women in this category have one or more symptoms (Table 44–1) that are mild to moderate in severity but not severe enough to interfere with functioning. These changes may be normal, typically do not warrant consultation with a physician, and occur in up to 95% of women.

2. Premenstrual syndrome–Approximately one-third of women have two or more symptoms, such as fatigue and irritability, which may be problematic but are not severe enough to interfere with daily living and are not classified as a mental disorder. Patients often complain about such symptoms during routine evaluations, but they rarely seek consultation specifically for them. Women with premenstrual syndrome often medicate themselves with over-the-counter preparations. This is the population of women with premenstrual symptoms who are most commonly seen by primary care providers.

3. Premenstrual disorder–These women have a mood symptom (eg, depression, anxiety, irritability, lability) plus four or more other symptoms (eg, decreased interest, fatigue, difficulty concentrating, change in appetite, change in sleep pattern, physical symptoms such as breast or abdominal swelling or musculoskeletal pain); the symptoms are severe enough to impair daily functioning. This condition corresponds to the late premenstrual dysphoric disorder (PDD) described in the *Diagnostic and Statistical Manual of the American Psychiatric Association (DSM-IV)* and is classified as a "depression disorder

not otherwise specified." Less than 4% of women have this disorder and are likely to seek treatment specifically for it. Such patients may be misdiagnosed easily with other psychiatric disorders because they have mood and behavior symptoms. In a primarily biomedical environment with little psychosocial orientation, these patients often get the impression that they are not being taken seriously.

4. Premenstrual exacerbation–Some medical and psychiatric disorders get worse premenstrually. Such medical disorders include migraine headaches, asthma, allergy, endometriosis, and seizure disorders. Psychiatric disorders that are exacerbated premenstrually include mood disorders, anxiety disorders, eating disorders, personality disorders, and substance use disorders. Premenstrual exacerbation may be difficult to distinguish from true premenstrual disorder. Hallmarks of premenstrual exacerbation include the lack of a symptom-free period and presence of symptoms during the week after menses.

Symptoms of the premenstrual syndromes typically occur during the week before menstruation and stop within a day or two after the onset of menses. It is the **timing** of the symptoms, not their nature, that is critical to the diagnosis. In some cases symptoms may last longer than one week, and symptoms may occur for 1–2 days at the time of ovulation (Fig 44–1). Many women experience **mittelschmerz**, or ovulatory pain at about day 14 of the menstrual cy-

Table 44–1. Common signs and symptoms of PMS.*

Cognitive
Loss of interest
Indecision
Difficulty concentrating
Memory impairment
Obsessional thinking
Confusion
Feel unreal, like in a dream
Poor judgment

Mood
Mood swings
Irritability
Anxiety
Depression
Can't cope
Feel insecure
Suicidal thoughts
Guilty thoughts
Feel empty

Behavioral
Increased drug and alcohol
    use
Increased sensitivity to
    alcohol
Smoke more
Impulsive
Increased appetite
Social withdrawal
Accident prone
Clumsiness
Restlessness (fidgeting,
    hand-wringing, can't sit
    still)
Lack of self-control, violent
    behavior
Crying
Self-indulgent
Change in interest in sex

Energy level
Fatigue
Malaise
Sleep changes
    (hypersomnia, insomnia)
Weakness
Frequent naps

Autonomic
Fainting, dizziness, vertigo
Sweating
Nausea
Vomiting
Ringing in ears
Numbness
Tingling of skin
Trembling
Lightheadedness
Palpitations
Headaches, migraines

Gastrointestinal
Increased appetite
Food cravings
Thirst
Nausea
Vomiting
Abdominal bloating,
    discomfort
Constipation

Fluid retention
Edema
Abdominal bloating,
    discomfort
Puffy hands
Breast tenderness, pain, or
    swelling
Leg heaviness
Weight gain

Allergic
Asthma
Breathing difficulties
Watery nose, nasal conges-
    tion
Red eyes
Urticaria
Pruritus

Miscellaneous
Urinary frequency or
    retention
Acne
Joint and muscle pain
Backache
Stiffness

*Reproduced, with permission, from Gise LH: Premenstrual syndrome: Which treatments help? Medical Aspects of Human Sexuality 1991:62.

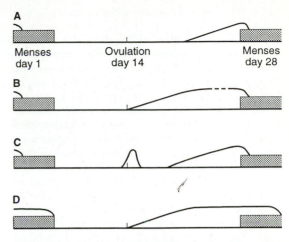

Figure 44–1. Patterns of premenstrual symptoms. (Reproduced, with permission, from Reid RL, Yen SSC: Premenstrual syndrome. Clin Obstet Gynecol 1983;26:710.)

The patient participates actively in the evaluation process by charting her symptoms daily for 2 months. This **longitudinal** approach differs from the traditional approach to medical diagnosis (history, physical examination, laboratory tests), which is **cross-sectional**. Overdiagnosis occurs when the diagnosis is made on the basis of the history, ie, on the basis of **retrospective** rather than **prospective** reporting. In specialized premenstrual treatment programs, only two of ten women seeking treatment for PMS meet the criteria for a premenstrual disorder, and in research studies, up to 100 patients must be screened for each subject admitted.

There is considerable discrepancy among the history, the clinical examination, and the woman's daily reporting of her symptom pattern. Typically, the history sounds like that of a premenstrual disorder, eg, "I look forward to getting my period because I feel dramatically better within a day or two of getting it and I feel entirely well for 2 weeks after I get it." The clinical examination may reveal a major depression, and the daily ratings may show no relationship between the symptoms and the cycle. This lack of concordance between subjective and objective data is a characteristic of premenstrual symptoms. For example, chronic job, relationship problems, or both may be confused with premenstrual worsening. A woman may have problems throughout the month but focus on the week before her period. Despite these discrepancies, women report that keeping daily ratings is helpful to them; they learn exactly what their symptoms are and how the symptoms relate to their menstrual cycle. Women also report that record-keeping helps them to anticipate, plan for, and manage their symptoms. This process appears to work in a similar way to biofeedback, in which becoming aware of a

cle. (Day 1 of the cycle is the first day of bleeding.) Mittelschmerz is usually not severe and simply indicates to the woman that she is ovulating. It is usually the associated premenstrual-like symptoms that are distressing rather than the pain.

A symptom-free period is a hallmark of the premenstrual syndromes. A woman who reports that she does not have an asymptomatic period during which she feels entirely well and symptom-free is likely to have a premenstrual exacerbation of a medical or psychiatric disorder rather than a true premenstrual disorder.

bodily function is associated with the ability to control it.

After 2 months of record-keeping, most women are considerably improved; they often state that although they still have "PMS," the symptoms are less severe and do not last as long. They also typically report that now they can cope with their symptoms, which no longer interfere with their functioning, and that they do not feel that they need medication. Most women with significant premenstrual symptoms are willing or even eager to chart their symptoms for 2 months. If a woman is unwilling to give a few minutes a day to record-keeping, she may not have severe symptoms. Rarely, women get angry when they are asked to record their symptoms, stating that they already know they have PMS, "self-diagnosed PMS," that is. The practitioner should explain patiently that the diagnostic procedure is standard practice, nationally and internationally, and that it will help her to gain a better understanding of her symptoms. These women may have personality disorders or may be reacting to past experiences in which they felt they were not being taking seriously and that their symptoms were being dismissed.

The Daily Rating Form (DRF) (Appendix G) provides a convenient way to record symptoms. Figure 44–2 shows the second of five pages of a filled-in form, the page that contains references to mood symptoms. The date is indicated on the left; menstruation is indicated as a yes or a no. Each symptom is rated daily on a scale from 1 to 6. It is clear from this record that symptoms are severe before menses and disappear shortly after the onset of menses. Ratings for each month must include the week before and the week after menses. Thus, if a woman starts keeping records during her menstrual period or right after, it may take more than 2 calendar months to complete the records for two consecutive menstrual cycles.

Women are asked to do the ratings each night before they go to bed, a task that should take only a few minutes. Women should be encouraged not to obsess but to record the first rating that comes to mind. They should be reassured that the form is designed with so many ratings that if the scores are off by one number, it will not affect the overall rating. If patients forget to do the ratings at night, they should do them first thing in the morning. If they forget until the next night, they should leave the space for that day blank. It is too hard to reconstruct symptoms after a day has gone by, and missing a day or two may not interfere with the characterization of a whole month. If a patient misses more than a few days, it may not be possible to evaluate the ratings for that month.

When evaluating daily rating forms, the physician looks for a 30% change between the week before menstruation and the week after menstruation. For example, if the symptom reaches a severity level of 6 premenstrually, it should not reach a level greater than 4 during the week after menses. If a symptom

reaches a severity level of 5 premenstrually, it should not be higher than 3 during the week after menses. If there is not a week during which all the symptoms are rated 1 or 2, the diagnosis may be premenstrual exacerbation, not premenstrual disorder. If the symptom reaches a severity level of only 3 or 4, it is not severe and may represent a **premenstrual syndrome** rather than a premenstrual disorder. It should be noted that five or more symptoms with a clear premenstrual pattern are required to make a diagnosis of a **premenstrual disorder**. To meet this criterion, the week before the menstrual period must be significantly different from the week after the menstrual period.

Eight of ten women seeking treatment for premenstrual symptoms produce records like those shown in Figure 44–3. Clearly there are symptoms during the week after menses and there is no symptom-free period. Physical symptoms such as abdominal bloating or breast pain typically show a clear premenstrual pattern, but generally these symptoms are not as troublesome as mood and behavior symptoms, particularly irritability and depressed mood.

The Premenstrual Assessment Form (Appendix H) is a 95-item inventory of mood, behavior, and physical symptoms that takes a few minutes to complete and can be used on a monthly basis as a measure of severity. Each symptom is rated in terms of its change from the patient's usual level of functioning. Ratings range from 1 (no change from usual level) to 6 (extreme change, eg, even people who do not know you might notice). At the beginning of treatment, women typically have about 35 severe (level 5) or extreme (level 6) symptoms; the number is reduced to 10 or fewer such symptoms after treatment.

Etiology

Many causes for premenstrual symptoms have been proposed, but none explains the whole picture. The strongest evidence that premenstrual syndromes are linked to the ovarian sex steroids, estrogen and progesterone, comes from the dramatic disappearance of symptoms with gonadotropin-releasing hormone (GnRH) agonists such as leuprolide. To date, hormone levels in women with premenstrual disorder have not been found to differ from those of controls. Serotonergic abnormalities have been reported and coincide with the dramatic response to serotonergic medications. Serotonin is one of the neurotransmitters in the brain involved in the causation of mood disorders and other psychiatric conditions. Because physicians see primarily mood and behavior symptoms in the premenstrual syndromes, they assume brain chemistry is involved. It is presumed that the brains of some women are more susceptible to changing hormone levels, because all women who menstruate have changing hormones but not all women have premenstrual symptoms. Abnormalities

Date	Menstru-ating?	Active, restless	Mood swings	Depressed, sad, low, blue, lonely	Anxious, jittery, nervous
2/26	N	1 (2) 3 4 5 6	(1) 2 3 4 5 6	1 2 (3) 4 5 6	(1) 2 3 4 5 6
2/27	N	(1) 2 3 4 5 6	(1) 2 3 4 5 6	(1) 2 3 4 5 6	(1) 2 3 4 5 6
2/28	N	1 2 (3) 4 5 6	(1) 2 3 4 5 6	(1) 2 3 4 5 6	(1) 2 3 4 5 6
2/29	N	1 (2) 3 4 5 6	(1) 2 3 4 5 6	(1) 2 3 4 5 6	(1) 2 3 4 5 6
3/01	N	1 (2) 3 4 5 6	1 2 (3) 4 5 6	1 (2) 3 4 5 6	1 (2) 3 4 5 6
3/02	N	1 2 3 (4) 5 6	1 2 3 (4) 5 6	1 2 3 (4) 5 6	1 2 3 (4) 5 6
3/03	N	1 2 3 (4) 5 6	1 2 3 4 5 (6)	1 2 3 4 5 (6)	1 2 3 4 5 (6)
3/04	N	1 2 3 (4) 5 6	1 2 3 4 5 (6)	1 2 3 4 5 (6)	1 2 3 4 5 (6)
3/05	N	1 2 3 (4) 5 6	1 2 3 4 5 (6)	1 2 3 4 5 (6)	1 2 3 4 5 (6)
3/06	N	1 2 3 (4) 5 6	1 2 3 4 5 (6)	1 2 3 4 5 (6)	1 2 3 4 5 (6)
3/07	N	1 2 3 4 (5) 6	1 2 3 4 5 (6)	1 2 3 4 5 (6)	1 2 3 4 5 (6)
3/08	Y	1 2 (3) 4 5 6	1 (2) 3 4 5 6	(1) 2 3 4 5 6	(1) 2 3 4 5 6
3/09	Y	(1) 2 3 4 5 6	(1) 2 3 4 5 6	(1) 2 3 4 5 6	(1) 2 3 4 5 6
3/10	Y	(1) 2 3 4 5 6	(1) 2 3 4 5 6	(1) 2 3 4 5 6	(1) 2 3 4 5 6
3/11	Y	(1) 2 3 4 5 6	(1) 2 3 4 5 6	(1) 2 3 4 5 6	(1) 2 3 4 5 6
3/12	Y	(1) 2 3 4 5 6	(1) 2 3 4 5 6	(1) 2 3 4 5 6	(1) 2 3 4 5 6
3/13	Y	(1) 2 3 4 5 6	(1) 2 3 4 5 6	(1) 2 3 4 5 6	(1) 2 3 4 5 6
3/14	Y	(1) 2 3 4 5 6	(1) 2 3 4 5 6	(1) 2 3 4 5 6	(1) 2 3 4 5 6
3/15	N	(1) 2 3 4 5 6	(1) 2 3 4 5 6	(1) 2 3 4 5 6	(1) 2 3 4 5 6
3/16	N	(1) 2 3 4 5 6	(1) 2 3 4 5 6	(1) 2 3 4 5 6	(1) 2 3 4 5 6
3/17	N	(1) 2 3 4 5 6	(1) 2 3 4 5 6	(1) 2 3 4 5 6	(1) 2 3 4 5 6
3/18	N	(1) 2 3 4 5 6	(1) 2 3 4 5 6	(1) 2 3 4 5 6	(1) 2 3 4 5 6
3/19	N	(1) 2 3 4 5 6	(1) 2 3 4 5 6	(1) 2 3 4 5 6	(1) 2 3 4 5 6
3/20	N	(1) 2 3 4 5 6	(1) 2 3 4 5 6	(1) 2 3 4 5 6	(1) 2 3 4 5 6
3/21	N	(1) 2 3 4 5 6	(1) 2 3 4 5 6	(1) 2 3 4 5 6	(1) 2 3 4 5 6
3/22	N	(1) 2 3 4 5 6	(1) 2 3 4 5 6	(1) 2 3 4 5 6	(1) 2 3 4 5 6
3/23	N	(1) 2 3 4 5 6	(1) 2 3 4 5 6	(1) 2 3 4 5 6	(1) 2 3 4 5 6
3/24	N	(1) 2 3 4 5 6	(1) 2 3 4 5 6	(1) 2 3 4 5 6	(1) 2 3 4 5 6
3/25	N	1 (2) 3 4 5 6	1 (2) 3 4 5 6	(1) 2 3 4 5 6	(1) 2 3 4 5 6
3/26	N	(1) 2 3 4 5 6	1 (2) 3 4 5 6	1 (2) 3 4 5 6	1 (2) 3 4 5 6
3/27	N	(1) 2 3 4 5 6	(1) 2 3 4 5 6	(1) 2 3 4 5 6	(1) 2 3 4 5 6
3/28	N	1 2 3 (4) 5 6	1 2 3 4 (5) 6	1 2 3 4 (5) 6	1 2 3 (4) 5 6
3/29	N	(1) 2 3 4 5 6	1 2 3 4 (5) 6	1 2 3 4 5 (6)	1 2 3 4 5 (6)
3/30	N	1 2 3 (4) 5 6	1 2 3 4 (5) 6	1 2 3 4 5 (6)	1 2 3 4 5 (6)
3/31	N	1 2 3 (4) 5 6	1 2 3 4 (5) 6	1 2 3 4 5 (6)	1 2 3 4 5 (6)
4/01	N	1 2 3 (4) 5 6	1 2 3 4 (5) 6	1 2 3 4 5 (6)	1 2 3 4 5 (6)
4/02	N	1 2 (3) 4 5 6	1 2 3 4 (5) 6	1 2 3 4 5 (6)	1 2 3 4 5 (6)
4/03	N	1 2 (3) 4 5 6	1 2 3 4 (5) 6	1 2 3 (4) 5 6	1 2 3 (4) 5 6

(handwritten margin note: Premenstrual disorder)

Figure 44–2. Daily Rating Form: Clear premenstrual pattern. (Reproduced, with permission, from Gise LH: Premenstrual syndrome: Which treatments help? Med Aspects Hum Sex 1991:66.)

PM Syndrome

Date	Menstru-ating?	Headaches	Back, joint, or muscle pain	Abdominal pain	Breast pain
6/22·	N	1 2 3 (4) 5 6	1 2 3 4 5 (6)	1 2 (3) 4 5 6	1 2 3 4 (5) 6
6/23	N	1 2 3 4 (5) 6	1 2 (3) 4 5 6	1 2 3 (4) 5 6	1 2 3 4 (5) 6
6/24	N	1 2 3 4 5 (6)	1 2 (3) 4 5 6	1 2 3 (4) 5 6	1 2 3 4 5 (6)
6/25	N	1 2 3 4 5 (6)	(1) 2 3 4 5 6	1 2 3 4 (5) 6	1 2 3 4 5 (6)
6/26	N	1 2 3 4 5 (6)	(1) 2 3 4 5 6	(1) 2 3 4 5 6	1 (2) 3 4 5 6
6/27	N	1 2 3 (4) 5 6	1 2 (3) 4 5 6	1 2 3 (4) 5 6	1 2 3 (4) 5 6
6/28	N	1 2 (3) 4 5 6	1 2 3 (4) 5 6	1 (2) 3 4 5 6	1 2 3 4 (5) 6
6/29	N	1 2 3 4 5 6	1 2 3 4 5 6	1 2 3 4 5 6	1 2 3 4 5 6
6/30	N	1 2 3 4 5 6	1 2 3 4 5 6	1 2 3 4 5 6	1 2 3 4 5 6
7/01	N	1 2 3 (4) 5 6	1 2 3 4 (5) 6	1 2 3 (4) 5 6	1 2 3 4 (5) 6
7/02	N	1 2 3 4 (5) 6	1 2 3 (4) 5 6	1 2 3 4 (5) 6	1 2 3 4 5 (6)
7/03	N	1 2 3 4 5 (6)	1 2 3 4 5 (6)	1 2 3 4 5 (6)	1 2 3 4 5 (6)
7/04	N	1 2 3 (4) 5 6	1 2 3 4 (5) 6	1 2 3 4 5 (6)	1 2 3 4 5 (6)
7/05	N	1 (2) 3 4 5 6	1 2 (3) 4 5 6	1 2 3 (4) 5 6	1 2 3 4 (5) 6
7/06	N	1 2 (3) 4 5 6	1 2 3 4 (5) 6	1 2 3 4 (5) 6	1 2 3 4 5 (6)
7/07	N	1 (2) 3 4 5 6	1 2 3 4 (5) 6	1 2 3 4 (5) 6	1 2 3 4 5 (6)
7/08	N	(1) 2 3 4 5 6	1 2 3 4 (5) 6	1 2 3 4 (5) 6	1 2 3 4 5 (6)
7/09	Y	(1) 2 3 4 5 6	1 2 3 4 5 (6)	1 2 3 4 5 (6)	1 2 3 4 5 (6)
7/10	Y	1 2 3 4 5 (6)	1 2 3 4 5 (6)	1 2 3 4 5 (6)	1 2 3 4 5 (6)
7/11	Y	1 2 (3) 4 5 6	1 2 3 4 5 (6)	1 2 3 4 5 (6)	1 2 3 4 5 (6)
7/12	Y	1 2 (3) 4 5 6	1 2 3 (4) 5 6	1 2 3 (4) 5 6	1 2 3 (4) 5 6
7/13	N	1 2 3 4 5 6	1 2 3 4 5 6	1 2 3 4 5 6	1 2 3 4 5 6
7/14	N	1 2 3 4 (5) 6	1 2 3 4 (5) 6	1 2 (3) 4 5 6	1 2 3 4 (5) 6
7/15	N	1 2 (3) 4 5 6	1 2 3 (4) 5 6	1 2 3 (4) 5 6	1 2 3 4 (5) 6
7/16	N	1 2 3 4 5 (6)	1 2 3 4 5 (6)	1 2 3 4 5 (6)	1 2 3 4 5 (6)
7/17	N	1 2 3 4 5 (6)	1 2 3 4 5 (6)	1 2 3 4 5 (6)	1 2 3 4 5 (6)
7/18	N	(1) 2 3 4 5 6	(1) 2 3 4 5 6	1 2 3 4 5 (6)	1 2 3 4 5 (6)

Premenstrual exacerbation

Figure 44–3. Daily Rating Form: No association between symptoms and cycle. Four items from the patient's full 21-item form are shown. Severity ratings: 1 = not at all; 2 = minimal; 3 = mild; 4 = moderate; 5 = severe; 6 = extreme. (Reproduced, with permission, from Gise LH: Premenstrual syndrome: Which treatments help? Med Aspects Hum Sex 1991:67. Daily Rating Forms reproduced with permission from Jean Endicott, PhD.)

in melatonin, sleep and temperature regulation have been described.

There may be predisposing, precipitating, and sustaining causes of premenstrual syndromes. Past and family history of mood instability may be predisposing causes including a history of significant postpartum and mood changes. Precipitating causes may be stress, childbirth, cessation of birth control pills, bilateral tubal ligation, and other surgical and diagnostic procedures. Once a woman has a premenstrual

disorder, health behaviors (such as those related to diet, exercise, alcohol, nicotine, caffeine, and stress) may function as sustaining causes to make the symptoms worse and enduring.

Incidence & Risk Factors

Although premenstrual symptoms or changes and premenstrual syndrome are common, true premenstrual disorders are rare. Up to 95% of women have at least one premenstrual **symptom**, which may be mild. Premenstrual **syndrome** occurs in about one-third of women. Although the onset may be in the teens or twenties, women seeking treatment for premenstrual symptoms are usually in their thirties and symptoms commonly worsen until they cease at menopause. A true premenstrual **disorder** with symptoms severe enough to interfere with functioning occurs in less than 4% of women. Of women with mood disorders, 60% have premenstrual **exacerbations** with dysphoric mood.

Women with a past history or a family history of mood instability, mood disorders, anxiety disorders, or substance use disorders may be at increased risk for premenstrual syndromes. Women who have had significant adjustment problems in the past also may be at increased risk. Family history is considered to increase risk if a first-degree relative is affected, ie, parent, sibling, or child. Finally, a past history of sexual abuse also may place a woman at risk.

Clinical Findings

A. Signs and Symptoms: Common signs and symptoms of premenstrual syndrome are shown in Table 44–1. Unusual symptoms may occur, however; for example, some professional singers report voice changes with difficulty hitting certain notes premenstrually, presumably caused by edema of the vocal cords. Professional athletes may complain of subtle changes in coordination.

Women with premenstrual symptoms often are anxious. They frequently feel misunderstood by their friends and relatives and also by their physicians. They get the message from others that it is "all in their head," and because they are having mood and behavior symptoms, they typically feel that they are going crazy. Anxiety heightens the awareness of any symptom, and the symptom is intensified.

Although musculoskeletal aches and pains are among the most typical premenstrual symptoms, abdominal and pelvic pain are not. Abdominal and pelvic pain are **common during** menstruation (dysmenorrhea), but they are **not typical before** menses. Women who have abdominal or pelvic pain during the week before the menstrual period or at other times (chronic pelvic pain) should have a gynecologic evaluation, possibly with laparoscopy, to rule out endometriosis or another gynecologic cause.

About 15% of women report that they feel **better** premenstrually, according to Stewart. Women have talked in the past of experiencing bursts of energy before menstruation, leading them to clean out the closets; other women, particularly artists, sometimes say they have increased access to their creative potential at this time. Increased libido is common premenstrually, but for women who are extremely irritable, this may result in masturbation rather than sexual activity with a partner.

Although women often report cognitive symptoms premenstrually, studies of high-level cognitive func-tioning have failed to demonstrate significant differences on psychophysiologic testing across phases of the menstrual cycle. Here, again, there is a discrepancy between subjective and objective data. It appears to be the perception of cognitive functioning that is impaired rather than the functioning itself. Although cognitive symptoms such as difficulty thinking, indecision, difficulty concentrating, memory problems, obsessional thinking, depersonalization, derealization, and poor judgment are typical premenstrual symptoms, they are also common symptoms of major depression. This fact should be kept in mind when one must differentiate a mood or personality disorder from a premenstrual disorder.

B. Screening: Premenstrual syndromes not only are overdiagnosed, they are underdiagnosed as well. Many women have fluctuating symptoms for years without making the connection between their symptoms and their menstrual cycle phase. It is rewarding to make this connection, make a diagnosis, and help these women get concrete help. In a routine evaluation, an appropriate screening question might be as follows: "Have you ever had difficulty with your periods, with pain, or with moodiness?" Women with significant premenstrual symptoms typically respond to such a question positively. This inquiry also should be made of women who are no longer menstruating to elicit a past history of mood reactivity. These women may be at risk for mood symptoms from other hormonal changes, such as menopause, or from medications, such as corticosteroids.

Differential Diagnosis

It may be difficult to differentiate a premenstrual syndrome from a mood disorder or a personality disorder. In addition to obtaining daily ratings, it is important to see the patient at two different times of the month. For example, a woman who is suicidal and appears to require admission to a psychiatric unit may come back the next week and appear completely normal.

Treatment

Treatment of the premenstrual syndromes starts with the evaluation, which is therapeutic in many cases. This situation is fortunate for clinicians but unfortunate for researchers. Physicians are best advised to delay prescription of medication for two menstrual cycles until daily ratings are completed. Most women—even those with the most severe symptoms—have had symptoms for years before seeking help; therefore, waiting 2 more months is rarely unbearable. Of course, if the patient has extremely severe symptoms or suicidal ideation, pharmacologic treatment may be instituted at the first visit. The physician should keep in mind that the placebo response is as high as 80% and that symptoms may remit for 3–4 months before they return to their original level after about 6 months.

Treatment of the premenstrual syndromes is an on-going process, not a one-time visit in which a prescription is written. Ideally, women should be monitored on a weekly basis; if this is not possible, one should monitor monthly until the diagnosis is established. In a premenstrual program in which group follow-up sessions are held weekly, women offer great support to one another, which is helpful in alleviating symptoms.

A. Nondrug Treatment—Modification of Health Behaviors: During the 2 months that the woman is keeping track of her symptoms, she may be encouraged to think about one of six specified health behaviors. Only one health behavior is selected because each of the six is hard to change; by selecting just one, the physician maximizes the chances of the patient making changes. The six health behaviors involve the areas of exercise, diet, caffeine, nicotine, alcohol, and stress. The health behavior selected should be one that is problematic and the one the woman is most likely to be able to modify over a 2-month period. For example, if a woman has been smoking three packs of cigarettes a day for 20 years, which may be contributing to irritability and moodiness, she is unlikely to quit smoking in 2 months. Frequently, exercise is selected as the area most conducive to change within this time frame.

1. Increasing exercise—For women who have never exercised, a program of walking may be the most realistic goal. Many women have a past history of establishing an aerobic exercise routine, which they abandoned after changes in their work schedule or family status. If the physician tells the patient what to do, eg, to return to her previous exercise routine, she may feel angry and misunderstood, saying she does not have the time, and may not comply. Instead, if physicians encourage these busy women to think about their exercise needs, the women are more likely to assume responsibility for their health and to comply.

The ideal exercise program is 20–30 minutes or more each day, 6 days a week. Some women have difficulty starting and should receive encouragement for any positive behavior in this direction, such as joining a gym, buying an exercise tape, or even exercising once a week. Exercise reduces tension and may elevate beta-endorphins in the brain. Studies such as those by Prior et al have shown that regular aerobic exercise reduces the severity of premenstrual symptoms. Furthermore, women report that they feel better when they exercise.

Women know of the benefits of exercise, and if they are not exercising, they often feel guilty and become self-critical. They also may become rebellious toward the physician, who is an authority figure and thus may activate old conflicts. Women often are better at taking care of others than of themselves.

2. Modifying diet—Many diets have been recommended for the treatment of premenstrual syn-drome, but there are no data to support their efficacy. A diet low in fat and high in complex carbohydrates, with plenty of fresh fruits and vegetables, is advised. Some women feel that a regimen of six small meals a day is helpful, but no association between hypoglycemia and premenstrual syndromes has been found. There is some evidence that a carbohydrate meal with no protein raises serotonin levels in the brain, improves mood, and reduces food cravings for several hours. Clinically, this suggestion has been useful for women who overeat at certain times of the day, eg, between lunch and dinner or after dinner. Eating a carbohydrate meal with no protein at these times may be helpful. Whether or not the change in diet is helpful, the feeling of being out of control is disturbing to many women. Feeling that one is in control of eating has a beneficial effect.

Because symptoms of fluid retention are common, salt restriction is reasonable. Craving of carbohydrates such as potato chips may be associated with excessive salt intake, which may aggravate bloating and swelling. Magnesium supplements have been advocated as helpful by some, but their usefulness is disputed by others. Plasma magnesium has not been found to differ between women with premenstrual syndrome and controls, and there are no good studies of magnesium supplements used as a single treatment method.

3. Eliminating use of caffeine—Caffeine abuse is common in our society and socially acceptable. Many women with premenstrual irritability are unusually sensitive to caffeine without knowing it, and anxious people tend to be more sensitive to caffeine. Although many women are reluctant to eliminate caffeine for fear of lowering their energy level, after the typical withdrawal symptom of severe headache is gone, most women find that their energy level is the same as before. It is best to eliminate caffeine every day of the month, not just premenstrually, because the goal is to stabilize mood throughout the month.

4. Eliminating use of nicotine—Many women report an improvement in premenstrual symptoms when they stop smoking; nicotine is known to cause irritability. Women seeking treatment for premenstrual symptoms often stop smoking at this time without being advised to. It may be that women seek treatment for premenstrual symptoms at a time when they are ready to make significant changes in their lives. Most of these women have had symptoms for years before making a commitment to change. It is highly rewarding to treat a woman who says, at first, "Doctor, it's my hormones," but proceeds to participate actively in her treatment and recovery. Stopping smoking is one example of such active involvement.

5. Eliminating alcohol abuse—Alcohol abuse is not uncommon among women complaining of premenstrual symptoms, but it is hard to diagnose (see Chapter 11). Denial is a characteristic feature of alcohol abuse. It may take from 6 months to a year for a woman to admit that she has an alcohol problem and agree to treatment. It is rewarding, however, to see a woman accept her problem and begin to address it. The physician should be aware also that seeking treatment for premenstrual symptoms may be a convenient way to avoid confronting other issues such as alcohol abuse and marital problems. Some women report that alcohol has an increased effect premenstrually, ie, one drink will have the same effect as two. Many women who do not abuse alcohol find that eliminating alcohol helps to stabilize mood and reduce premenstrual symptoms.

6. Reducing stress–Stress aggravates premenstrual symptoms as it does other medical symptoms. Women who have been in psychotherapy or have accumulated self-knowledge through other means know the sources of stress in their lives and know how to reduce stress. Others may first consider psychotherapy or behavioral treatments to reduce stress when they are seeking treatment for premenstrual syndromes. Psychotherapy is an individual matter, and a woman must be motivated to invest time and energy in learning how to increase her control over her life. Physicians cannot force patients into psychotherapy because they think it will help. One must respect individual preferences and timing and note that some women will find psychotherapy unacceptable.

B. Drug Treatment: Vitamin B_6, diuretics, oral contraceptive agents, and progesterone are the four agents gynecologists most commonly prescribe for PMS. They all have been condemned in the gynecologic literature as both ineffective and dangerous.

1. Antianxiety medication–Even women with five or more premenstrual symptoms (including a mood symptom) confirmed by 2 months of daily ratings may be significantly better after 2 months of nondrug treatment. If symptoms persist, alprazolam $\frac{1}{4}$ or $\frac{1}{8}$ mg orally every 4 hours as needed during the premenstrual cycle phase may help. Some women feel more comfortable taking this medication on a set schedule, eg, three times daily. Women with a past history of substance use disorders should not be given medications that have the potential for abuse. The nonaddicting antianxiety agent buspirone (ie, 15–40 mg orally daily) can be substituted. Benzodiazepine dependence has not been seen in women with premenstrual syndromes when the medication is taken for only a few days out of the month, however. Typically women take less and less medication over time; after about 6 months, they often report that they are carrying the medication with them for security and do not take it anymore.

For women with a past history of substance use problems combined with brief psychotic episodes or significant impulse control problems, including features of borderline personality disorder, a small dose of a low-potency neuroleptic such as thioridazine,

10–25 mg orally every 4 hours as needed, may be helpful.

2. Antidepressant medication–When symptoms persist after a trial of antianxiety medication, the selective serotonin reuptake inhibitors (SSRIs) often produce a dramatic improvement. These drugs currently include fluoxetine, 10–20 mg orally daily; sertraline, 50–200 mg orally daily; and paroxetine, 20 mg orally daily. Fluoxetine is best taken in the morning; sertraline and paroxetine are best taken at night. Similar results were obtained in the past with tricyclic antidepressants, but side effects were more problematic. Women typically have a dramatic response to serotonergic medications even when they do not meet *DSM-IV* criteria for major depression, ie, they do not have depressed mood or loss of interest for 2 weeks or more. Women may have symptoms for as short a time as one day, but if the symptoms are severe and disruptive, such as suicidal ideation, they require treatment. For some women, irritability and anxiety may mask underlying depressive symptoms, which may emerge after treatment with antianxiety medication and respond to antidepressant medication. Treatment studies have looked only at antidepressants used daily. There is one case report of 10 patients treated by increasing the antidepressant dosage for 7–10 days premenstrually to maximize effectiveness and minimize side effects. There have been anecdotal reports of antidepressant therapy given premenstrually only, but no studies have been reported.

3. Vitamin B_6–Vitamin B_6 may improve mood, but there is no evidence of a specific premenstrual effect. A dosage of 25 mg daily is adequate, and the dosage should not exceed 100 mg. Above a dosage of 200 mg daily, peripheral neuropathy with numbness and tingling in the hands has been reported. Some PMS vitamin preparations contain toxic levels of vitamin B_6, and the physician is best advised to check for this.

4. Diuretics–Diuretics such as spironolactone, 25 mg orally 4 times daily, may alleviate fluid retention symptoms but do not affect the mood and behavior symptoms, which are usually the most troubling. The dangers of electrolyte imbalance from the chronic use of diuretics are well-known.

5. Oral contraceptive agents–One-third of women who take oral contraceptive agents for premenstrual symptoms improve, one-third are unchanged, and one-third get worse. Birth control pills may improve mood and reduce symptoms in women with mild premenstrual symptoms, but they often cause severe symptoms to worsen and may precipitate a clinical depression.

6. Progesterone–In the past, premenstrual syndrome was said to be caused by progesterone deficiency, and there was anecdotal evidence of successful treatment with progesterone. There is no clear evidence of progesterone deficiency in women who have premenstrual syndrome, however, and well-designed studies have shown progesterone to be no more effective than placebo. Progesterone may produce improvement by a placebo effect for up to 3–4 months, but after about 6 months, the original symptoms tend to return. Progesterone, especially synthetic progestogens such as medroxyprogesterone acetate, may produce symptoms or side effects such as sedation, dysphoria, and even clinical depression. It is largely progesterone that is responsible for the mood symptoms found with use of oral contraceptive agents and hormone therapy for menopause. Natural progesterone has been advocated in preference to synthetic progestogens because of its fewer side effects; natural progesterone is available from two pharmacies in Madison, Wisconsin: Madison Pharmacy (800-558-7046) and Women's International Pharmacy (800-792-3505).

7. Bromocriptine–Bromocriptine is effective in relieving severe, painful mastalgia, but this is rarely a major symptom of premenstrual syndrome. Bromocriptine is a dopamine agonist that suppresses the secretion of prolactin; however, there is no evidence that prolactin causes premenstrual syndromes. Prolactin is under inhibitory control of the hypothalamus, mediated by dopamine; it is stimulated by estrogen and causes salt and water retention. But bromocriptine has a high incidence of adverse side effects, and most women complaining of severe breast tenderness reject such a medication.

8. Gonadotropin-releasing hormone agonists–Gonadotropin-releasing hormone analogs are administered subcutaneously or nasally on a daily basis or by monthly injection (leuprolide acetate). This reversible, chemical menopause, or "medical ovariectomy," causes loss of menstrual cycles and abolishes premenstrual symptoms; however, it is a drastic treatment that precipitates all the short- and long-term symptoms of menopause, including the risk of osteoporosis. Supplementation with estrogen and progesterone, originally conceived of as an experimental model of premenstrual syndrome, prevents menopausal symptoms and does not precipitate a recurrence of premenstrual symptoms. But GnRH analogs are very costly and have not been covered by medical insurance. Because of the cost, this treatment is used rarely. Most patients whose symptoms are severe enough to warrant such drastic treatment are eventually treated with hysterectomy, including ovariectomy.

Prognosis & Course

The prognosis of the premenstrual syndromes is excellent. Most women with premenstrual symptoms have one of the milder forms—premenstrual changes or premenstrual syndrome—which readily respond to behavioral treatment and rarely require medication. True premenstrual disorders, which are severe

enough to interfere with functioning, are rare but also respond to treatment.

Premenstrual symptoms may get worse over time (see Fig 44–1), initially lasting 3–4 days (A) and progressing to a week to 10 days (B) or even 2–3 weeks (D) and symptoms may occur with ovulation (C). Thus a woman may report that she has only one good week (D), or only a few good days each month. From an endocrinologic point of view, symptoms cannot last longer than 2 weeks, the duration of the luteal phase of the menstrual cycle, days 14–28. But when a significant upset in mood and behavior occurs regularly, on a monthly basis, the patient can find it harder to bounce back, and recovery may take longer. This secondary disability may pose a diagnostic problem in differentiating premenstrual disorder from premenstrual exacerbation. The differentiation can be accomplished by using daily ratings. With premenstrual exacerbation, there are symptoms during the week following menses and a more inconsistent pattern (see Fig 44–3). With premenstrual disorder, there is a much clearer premenstrual pattern (see Fig 44–2). This worsening premenstrual syndrome with symptoms lasting longer than 2 weeks overlaps with major depression. Indeed, a course characterized by worsening premenstrual symptoms is a risk factor for a full-blown major depressive episode and may herald its onset.

Although premenstrual symptoms appear in adolescence and young adulthood, women seeking treatment for premenstrual symptoms are usually about 35 years old and have had symptoms for about 5 years. Symptoms usually get worse until menopause, when they cease. During perimenopause, women may go through a period of relative estrogen excess caused by anovulatory periods. Without ovulation, there is no rise of progesterone during the second half of the menstrual cycle (luteal phase); although estrogen levels are lower, the effect of estrogen is unopposed by progesterone. Thus a relative estrogen excess syndrome may occur, with increased moodiness and fluid retention, followed by lowering of estrogen levels after menopause.

Referral to a Specialist

Rarely, a woman has suicidal ideation during her premenstrual cycle phase; although the episode may last for as little as one day and is likely to be benign, the patient should be evaluated by a mental health specialist. Women who have a true premenstrual disorder and do not respond to simple behavioral or pharmacologic treatment also should be referred to a specialist. Finally, women with premenstrual exacerbations of a medical or psychiatric illness who do not respond to increased treatment for the underlying disorder should be referred simultaneously to two specialists, one for the underlying disorder and the other for premenstrual syndrome. Women who have abdominal or pelvic pain before menstruation should be evaluated for endometriosis.

Issues Related to Sex & Reproduction

Increased interest in sex or increased libido is a common premenstrual change that usually is not reported as a symptom. Childbirth is one of the precipitating causes of premenstrual syndromes; symptoms often first appear or worsen after childbirth. Significant mood changes postpartum are a risk factor for the development of premenstrual symptoms and may predispose women to these problems. Many women eagerly await menopause for the cessation of menstrual periods and premenstrual symptoms; however, symptoms may recur after menopause in the context of cyclic estrogen and progesterone therapy. Progesterone seems to be the offending agent; some women become dysphoric during the days they take progesterone. As mentioned previously, substitution of natural progesterone for synthetic progestogens may alleviate symptoms for some.

Psychosocial Concerns

One conceptualization of premenstrual symptoms is that women are socialized in this society to avoid the expression of anger, so that these feelings are suppressed for 3 weeks out of the month; with the lessening of inhibitions and increased irritability premenstrually, however, women express the feelings that bother them, even if they do it in a maladaptive way.

In addition, midlife psychosocial concerns and stress-related events interact with premenstrual symptoms. Symptoms typically continue until menopause, often worsening during the patient's 40s.

Stress aggravates premenstrual symptoms as it does most other medical illnesses. Women who have delayed childbearing may become anxious about establishing a relationship before it is too late to have a child. With menopause talked about readily, women in their 20s and 30s are now beginning to worry about hormonal changes decades in advance and to focus on their menstrual cycles. Midlife issues such as difficulties with adolescent and young adult children appear at this time, as do losses, relationship problems, and responsibilities for caring for elderly parents.

Controversies & Unresolved Issues

Clearly there is an overlap between premenstrual syndromes and mood disorders, but many women have severe, clear-cut premenstrual disorder without any current or past history of mental illness. Premenstrual dysphoric disorder is classified as a depressive disorder not otherwise specified in the *DSM-IV* although the criteria remain in the appendix indicating the need for further study. Furthermore, premenstrual tension appears in the *ICDM-9-CM* as a medical diagnosis. Some have suggested that premenstrual syndrome be classified as an organic mood disorder because there is "a specific organic factor judged to be etiologically related to the disturbance" (American Psychiatric Association, 1987).

The cause of the premenstrual syndromes remains an enigma. Multiple causes have been proposed, but for each, there is some experimental evidence that does not fit the hypothesis. It is presently believed that the premenstrual syndromes are the result of the interaction of a multitude of factors.

REFERENCES

American Psychiatric Association: *Diagnostic and Statistical Manual of Mental Disorders,* 4/e. American Psychiatric Association, 1994.

Gise LH: Group approaches to the diagnosis and treatment of the premenstrual syndromes. In: *Group Psychodynamics: New Paradigms and New Perspectives.* Halperin DA (editor). Yearbook Medical, 1989.

Gise LH: Premenstrual syndrome: Which treatments help? Medical Aspects of Human Sexuality 1991:62.

Gise LH (editor): *Premenstrual Syndromes: New Findings and Controversies.* Churchill Livingstone, 1988.

Gise LH: Reproductive endocrinology. In: *Medical-Psychiatric Practice,* vol 2. Stoudemire A, Fogel BS (editors). American Psychiatric Press, 1993.

Muse KN et al: The premenstrual syndrome: Effects of "medical ovariectomy." N Engl J Med 1984;311:1345.

Paddison PL et al: Sexual abuse and premenstrual syndrome: Comparison between a lower and higher socioeconomic group. Psychosomatics 1990;31:265.

Prior JC et al: Conditioning exercise decreases premenstrual symptoms: A prospective, controlled six-month trial. Fertil Steril 1987;47:402.

Severino SK, Moline ML: *Premenstrual Syndrome: A Clinician's Guide.* Guilford, 1989.

Smith S, Schiff I: The premenstrual syndrome: Diagnosis and management. Fertil Steril 1989;52:527.

Stewart DE: Positive changes in the premenstrual period. Acta Psychiatr Scand 1989;79:400.

Wurtman JJ et al: Effect of nutrient intake on premenstrual depression. Am J Obstet Gynecol 1989;161:1228.

45

Dysmenorrhea, Endometriosis, & Pelvic Pain

Michael M. Klotz, MD

DYSMENORRHEA

Essentials of Diagnosis

- Primary dysmenorrhea arises from the normal release of prostaglandins with menses and usually presents with the onset of ovulatory cycles within the first few years after menarche.
- Secondary dysmenorrhea is caused by disease of the uterus or pelvis and generally presents later in a woman's reproductive life.

Incidence & Risk Factors

The incidence of primary dysmenorrhea in women of reproductive age is approximately 50–75%. It is greatest in women in their late teens to early twenties and declines with age. Parity has a variable effect. The degree of discomfort is related directly to the duration of flow but not to the cycle length. Use of oral contraceptives and exercise can reduce the severity of dysmenorrhea. Intrauterine devices can worsen it. The incidence of secondary dysmenorrhea is unknown; the condition generally occurs in women older than 25 years.

Symptoms

Patients who present with primary dysmenorrhea typically complain of painful cramping in the central lower abdomen or pelvis beginning just before or at the onset of menses and usually lasting for the first 1–3 days of flow. The pain can be severe and may radiate to the back or down the medial thighs. Symptoms related to prostaglandin excess may be present, such as diaphoresis, tachycardia, headache, nausea, vomiting, and diarrhea.

The symptoms of secondary dysmenorrhea can be similar to those of primary dysmenorrhea, but they usually begin after the teenage years and progress with age. The symptoms can be suggestive, but they are not diagnostic, of an underlying pathologic condition. These symptoms include pelvic heaviness or bloating, menorrhagia, deep dyspareunia, and more generalized pelvic pain.

Clinical Findings & Diagnosis

The history should include a description of the pa-

Dysmenorrhea
  Essentials of Diagnosis
  Incidence & Risk Factors
  Symptoms
  Clinical Findings & Diagnosis
  Treatment
  Prognosis
  Referral to a Specialist
  Psychosocial Issues
  Controversies & Unresolved Issues
Acute Pelvic Pain
  Essentials of Diagnosis
  Incidence & Risk Factors
  Symptoms
  Clinical Findings
  Referral to a Specialist
  Issues of Pregnancy & Acute Pelvic Pain
  Psychosocial Issues
  Controversies & Unresolved Issues
Endometriosis
  Essentials of Diagnosis
  Incidence & Risk Factors
  Symptoms
  Clinical Findings & Diagnosis
  Treatment & Prognosis
  Referral to a Specialist
  Issues of Pregnancy & Endometriosis
  Psychosocial Issues
  Controversies & Unresolved Issues
Chronic Pelvic Pain
  Essentials of Diagnosis
  Incidence & Risk Factors
  Symptoms
  Clinical Findings & Diagnosis
  Differential Diagnosis & Treatment
  Surgical Treatment
  Long-term Management
  Referral to a Specialist
  Controversies & Unresolved Issues

420

tient's symptoms, the time of onset in relation to the first day of the menses, the severity of symptoms, and whether they have been progressive or stable. The patient should be asked about her current and past menstrual pattern, presence of dyspareunia, history of a gynecologic procedure, history of endometriosis, and contraceptive method. Her use of analgesics and their effectiveness should be detailed.

Primary dysmenorrhea is diagnosed by a history of pain with the onset of regular or ovulatory cycles. The pelvic examination may reveal mild uterine tenderness at the time of menses, but it is otherwise normal.

Possible causes of secondary dysmenorrhea include adenomyosis, cervical stenosis, endometriosis, intrauterine device (IUD), submucosal fibroid tumors, uterine polyps, and congenital anomalies of the reproductive tract. These causes may be suggested by the patient's history or physical examination, but frequently hysteroscopy or laparoscopy is required to confirm the diagnosis. Adenomyosis typically presents in a multiparous woman between 35 and 50 years old. In adenomyosis, dysmenorrhea increases in severity and is associated with menorrhagia and midline deep dyspareunia. The uterus is enlarged, globular, and tender at the time of menses. Cervical stenosis may be suspected when there is a history of scant menstrual flow with severe cramps, or of cervical ablation or conization, or when a small probe or dilator cannot be passed through the cervix. The presence of an IUD should be confirmed by visualization of the string or by ultrasonography if the string is not visible.

Regardless of the category of dysmenorrhea, the patient's impression of the severity of the pain, the degree of dysfunction it imposes on her life, and her concern regarding the cause should determine the extent of the initial diagnostic evaluation.

Treatment

The treatment of primary dysmenorrhea is aimed at decreasing prostaglandin production and release in the endometrium. Nonsteroidal anti-inflammatory drugs (NSAIDs) are an effective first-line approach (Table 45–1). The patient should begin taking the medication at the onset of menses or just before her expected menses. The medication should be continued for the first 2–3 days of flow. For patients desiring contraception or who have contraindications or an intolerance to NSAIDs, combination oral contraceptives are also an excellent first-line management choice. They can diminish the amount and duration of flow and may decrease the frequency of menses in women with a short menstrual interval. Patients who have not obtained sufficient relief may benefit from the use of continuous oral contraceptives (without the usual 7-day hiatus) for 3 months at a time to reduce menstrual frequency significantly. The use of other hormonal contraceptive methods such as implantable or injectable progestins is not well documented in the treatment of dysmenorrhea; these methods could be expected to provide relief through ovulation suppression and possible amenorrhea.

It is best to avoid the use of narcotic analgesics unless all other options have been exhausted and their use can be monitored closely. If the patient requires narcotics for more than 1–3 days of her cycle or if she requires increasing doses, the diagnosis of primary dysmenorrhea should be questioned.

If the patient presenting with secondary dysmenorrhea has an obvious underlying cause, such as cervical stenosis or an IUD, early treatment should address the cause. IUD-associated dysmenorrhea may respond to NSAID therapy. In most cases, however, the examination is normal, and the cause is unclear. If the symptoms are not severe and the patient is willing, a trial of NSAIDs or oral contraceptives should be attempted. This treatment may provide adequate relief and avoid the expense and risk of invasive procedures.

If the patient is unwilling to undertake symptomatic treatment or it does not provide sufficient relief, a definitive diagnosis is warranted. When intrauterine disease such as submucosal fibroids or uterine polyps is suspected, the next step in evaluation is hysteroscopy. Not only is this procedure diagnostic, but it is also therapeutic because it allows excision of fibroids and large polyps or can be followed

Table 45–1. Nonsteroidal anti-inflammatory drugs (NSAIDs) for the treatment of dysmenorrhea.

Drug	Dose	Frequency	Maximum Daily Dosage
Etodolac*	200–400 mg PO	q6–8h	1200 mg
Ibuprofen**	400–800 mg PO	q6 or 8h	3200 mg
Ketoprofen	25–50 mg PO	q6–8h	300 mg
Meclofenamate	100 mg PO	q8h	400 mg
Mefenamic acid	500, then 250 mg PO	q6h	Unavailable
Naproxen sodium**	550, then 275 mg PO	q6–8h	1375 mg
Ketorolac*	30 mg IM	q6h	120 mg

*Not approved for use in dysmenorrhea.
** Available over the counter in lower doses.

by a dilation and curettage (D&C) to remove multiple small polyps. D&C sometimes can be performed in the office setting, but anesthesia may be required for more extensive procedures. When endometriosis is suspected or hysteroscopy fails to confirm the diagnosis, laparoscopy is performed. Hysteroscopy and laparoscopy can be done as combined procedures in the operating room when office hysteroscopy is not available or the patient cannot tolerate the procedure without anesthesia. Treatment of endometriosis can be initiated at the time of laparoscopy.

Adenomyosis can be diagnosed definitively only from pathologic evaluation of the hysterectomy specimen, and this should be undertaken only in severe cases of dysmenorrhea refractory to conservative management and only in women who do not wish to preserve their fertility. Hysterectomy also is used in the management of severe endometriosis. Patients with severe dysmenorrhea whose major symptom is central pain, whether from endometriosis, suspected adenomyosis, or unknown causes, may benefit from laparoscopic presacral neurectomy or laser uterosacral nerve ablation (LUNA), although the success has been variable. Endometrial ablation has been used successfully in the treatment of menorrhagia; it may reduce or alleviate dysmenorrhea in patients with menorrhagia and no other treatable cause for pain.

Prognosis

The majority of patients with primary dysmenorrhea respond to medical treatment, and those who do not should be reevaluated for the causes of secondary dysmenorrhea. Medical treatment for secondary dysmenorrhea is less successful; however, an underlying cause usually can be identified and treated. Hysterectomy is the definitive treatment, but it should be reserved for severe and refractory cases.

Referral to a Specialist

When medical management of dysmenorrhea fails or symptoms are too severe to allow time for a trial of medications, the patient should be referred to a gynecologist capable of performing hysteroscopy, D&C, and laparoscopy for diagnosis and treatment of the underlying cause. Presacral neurectomy, LUNA, endometrial ablation, and hysterectomy should be performed only by those who are experienced with the techniques and are capable of managing potential complications of the procedures.

Psychosocial Issues

Dysmenorrhea has a significant impact on patients' ability to function at work, in their families, and in their recreational pursuits. Because it is a condition with poor social acceptance as a source of physical impairment, it can be embarrassing for the patient to disclose.

Secondary dysmenorrhea often develops in otherwise healthy women who may fear that their symptoms are secondary to cancer or other serious disease or are worried about the effect of the problem on their fertility. When hysterectomy is a treatment option, the surgery may have an impact on the woman's self-image and sexuality. Dysmenorrhea can be a manifestation of chronic pelvic pain and, therefore, a clue to underlying psychological problems that require treatment for a successful outcome.

Controversies & Unresolved Issues

The effects of treating the symptoms of secondary dysmenorrhea without diagnosing their cause, particularly in the case of endometriosis, are unknown. There could be an adverse effect on the patient's future fertility; however, given the risk of recurrence and the morbidity of treatment, symptomatic treatment may be a safe approach in some circumstances.

ACUTE PELVIC PAIN

Essentials of Diagnosis

- Duration is less than 6 months.
- Source may be gynecologic, pregnancy-related, gastrointestinal, or urologic (Table 45–2).

Incidence & Risk Factors

Acute pelvic pain is a common reason that women seek urgent gynecologic evaluation. The great majority of these patients are in the reproductive age

---

Table 45–2. Causes of acute pelvic pain.

Gynecologic
  Adnexal torsion
  Endometriosis
  Infection
    Pelvic inflammatory disease
    Tuboovarian abscess
  Ovarian
    Corpus luteum cyst
    Endometrioma
    Mittelschmerz
    Neoplasm
    Ruptured cyst
  Uterine
    Fibroids: degeneration, torsion
    Dysmenorrhea
Pregnancy-related
  Abortion: septic, spontaneous
  Ectopic pregnancy
Gastrointestinal
  Appendicitis
  Constipation
  Diverticulitis
  Gastroenteritis
  Inflammatory bowel disease
Urologic
  Acute cystitis
  Renal calculi

group, because acute pelvic pain results most commonly from sexual activity or ovarian ovulatory function. Approximately 1 million women are diagnosed with pelvic inflammatory disease (PID) each year, and about one-fourth of these women require hospitalization.

Symptoms

Although the presenting symptoms are variable, the patient typically complains of pain in the lower abdomen and pelvis. However, midabdominal pain or pain in the upper aspects of the lower quadrants may lead the patient to seek evaluation for perceived pelvic pain. Her pain may be mild and described as a discomfort or severe enough to cause guarding and immobility. Cyclic pain may occur at midcycle or with the onset of menses. Severe pain is usually of recent onset, and in some cases, it may have diminished or resolved by the time of the evaluation. Nausea and deep dyspareunia are common complaints regardless of the cause of the pain. Anorexia, vomiting, and fever, however, are more specific to the underlying problem. Proctitis or dysuria can arise from peritoneal irritation; they are not necessarily indicative of a primary rectal or bladder process. A thorough history often helps to narrow the differential diagnosis; pertinent aspects are outlined in Table 45–3.

Clinical Findings

The physical examination should begin with vital signs, including postural changes, and observation of the patient's posture and mobility. She should be asked to point to the location of the pain. The abdominal examination includes observation for bowel tones, distention, guarding, rigidity, rebound (generalized, local, and referred), and masses. If the pain can be localized by the examination, repeat palpation should be done to confirm this finding. During the pelvic examination, the presence of vaginal discharge and evidence of cervicitis should be noted. On bimanual examination, cervical motion tenderness, either bilateral or unilateral, and uterine motion tenderness reflect peritoneal irritation and are clues to the extent of the painful process. Cervical or uterine motion tenderness does not necessarily localize the source of pain to the pelvis. If a source of pain can be isolated to the uterus or adnexa, the patient should be asked if the pain is the same as her complaint. If there is significant abdominal guarding, the patient may tolerate manipulation more easily with the vaginal hand over the abdominal one in evaluating for the presence of a pelvic mass. A rectovaginal examination should be done to evaluate the posterior pelvis. Common causes of acute pelvic pain related to findings from the history and physical examination are shown in Table 45–4.

A. Ectopic Pregnancy:

1. Incidence–Ectopic pregnancy has an overall incidence of about 15 in 1000 reported pregnancies and is the second leading cause of pregnancy-related mortality. The incidence increases with age, peaking at 35–44 years, and is higher in black than in white women. Risk factors include IUD use, a history of PID, tubal surgery, or prior ectopic pregnancy.

2. Symptoms–The spectrum of presentations ranges from vague, mild, unilateral pelvic discomfort to severe generalized pain in a hemodynamically unstable patient. The most common presentation is unilateral sharp pain of recent and progressive onset. The patient may have had a missed menses or experienced irregular bleeding. Generalized pain can result from a hemoperitoneum that may cause diaphragmatic irritation and the complaint of posterior shoulder or neck pain.

Examination may reveal a normal size or appropri-

Table 45–3. Patient history for pelvic pain.

Menstrual: frequency, duration, dysmenorrhea, association with pain, changes since onset of pain
Sexual: orientation, contraception, age at first coitus, number of partners, most recent coitus, dyspareunia
Psychosocial: rape, incest, sexual or physical abuse, depression, alcohol or drug abuse
Infection: pelvic inflammatory disease, sexually transmitted disease (in self or partner)
Surgical: abdominal or pelvic surgery, documented endometriosis
Obstetric: parity, abortions (spontaneous, induced), ectopic pregnancy, desire for current pregnancy if applicable, desire for fertility
Current pain complaint:
  Description: location, quality, intensity, duration, frequency, radiation, changes since onset, factors that ameliorate and exacerbate, association with menstrual cycle
  Associated symptoms: breast tenderness, fever, nausea, vomiting, change in bowel habits, dysuria, vaginal bleeding
Use of pain medications
Patient's concerns and fears regarding the cause

Table 45–4. Causes of acute pelvic pain related to history and physical examination findings.

Cyclic pain
  Dysmenorrhea
  Endometriosis
  Mittelschmerz
Painful mass
  Adnexal torsion
  Corpus luteum cyst
  Ectopic pregnancy
  Endometrioma
  Functional cyst
  Ovarian neoplasm
  Tuboovarian abscess
Unilateral or diffuse pain without a mass
  Appendicitis
  Ectopic pregnancy
  Endometriosis
  Pelvic inflammatory disease
  Ruptured ovarian cyst

ately enlarged uterus. Typically, there is adnexal tenderness in the region of pain, but a palpable mass is frequently absent, and its presence is not diagnostic. The other pelvic structures may be mildly tender, and cervical motion tenderness can be present with stretch of the involved adnexa.

3. Diagnosis and treatment–The diagnosis of ectopic pregnancy is rarely obvious on initial presentation, and the consequences of missing it can be fatal for the patient; therefore, the clinician must maintain a high index of suspicion. Any woman in the reproductive age group presenting with acute pelvic pain must have a pregnancy test regardless of her menstrual or contraceptive history. A recent normal menstrual period or the absence of pregnancy-related symptoms cannot exclude the diagnosis. In the setting of pelvic pain, a positive pregnancy test is considered an ectopic pregnancy until proved otherwise.

The diagnosis of ectopic pregnancy has been revolutionized by the availability of sensitive urine tests (human chorionic gonadotropin [HCG]), serum HCG titers, and ultrasonography (U/S), especially endovaginal scans. The differential diagnosis includes an intrauterine pregnancy (IUP) with an adnexal mass, most commonly a corpus luteum cyst, which, with rupture, can produce pain and hemorrhage identical to those of an ectopic pregnancy, PID or abscess after a miscarriage or abortion, septic abortion, and causes unrelated to pregnancy such as appendicitis. The time allotted for confirmation of the diagnosis varies with the severity of the symptoms. The keys to making the diagnosis are the combination of HCG levels and U/S findings (see Chapter 56).

Contemporary treatment of ectopic tubal pregnancy is discussed in Chapter 56. Although newer, alternative methods of treatment may involve medical management, immediate referral to a gynecologic surgeon is necessary to optimize the outcome.

B. Pelvic Inflammatory Disease: PID is found most commonly in women between 15 and 25 years, with the greatest incidence between ages 15 and 19. Risk factors for PID include a history of sexually transmitted diseases, sexual activity with a male partner, and IUD use.

1. Diagnosis–Patients presenting with PID encompass such a broad spectrum of severity, symptoms, and signs that making the diagnosis is difficult. The goals of diagnosis are to hospitalize patients when appropriate, to avoid leaving mild cases undiagnosed, and to avoid misdiagnosing cases of appendicitis or ruptured ectopic pregnancy. The only uniform complaint is lower abdominal or pelvic pain that is of several days to weeks in duration and is progressive.

Because of this variable presentation, the threshold for diagnosis should be low; the Centers for Disease Control and Prevention (CDC) recommends making the diagnosis based on minimal criteria from the physical examination. If the patient has lower abdominal tenderness, cervical motion tenderness, and adnexal tenderness and there is no competing diagnosis, she should be treated for PID. Her pregnancy test should be negative, and an IUD, if present, should be removed after initiation of antibiotics. All patients must be reevaluated in 48–72 hours and hospitalized if they are not improved. In all cases of PID, the patient's partner should have a culture taken, if possible, and should be treated whether or not symptoms or signs are present.

If the presenting symptoms and signs are severe, additional criteria should be used to aid in the differential diagnosis: a temperature greater than 38°C, leukocytosis, positive test for cervical *Chlamydia trachomatis* or *Neisseria gonorrhea,* elevated C-reactive protein, elevated erythrocyte sedimentation rate (ESR), or presence of inflammation on endometrial biopsy. The latter three tests are much more sensitive and specific than the others for the diagnosis of PID. The finding of an adnexal mass or an examination limited by guarding should be followed by pelvic ultrasonography to evaluate for a tubo-ovarian abscess (TOA). If the diagnosis remains unclear, a laparoscopy should be performed.

2. Treatment–Inpatient therapy should be initiated for the patient with moderate or severe findings, a tubo-ovarian abscess, failed response to outpatient therapy, or one in whom compliance is questionable. Inpatient treatment should lead to improvement in 3–5 days and should be continued for 48 hours after significant clinical improvement is seen. Patients in whom treatment fails require laparoscopy to confirm the diagnosis and evacuate abscesses.

3. Prognosis–The prognosis for immediate cure in PID, when diagnosed and treated early, is excellent; however, there is a long-term risk of infertility. In advanced cases, there is a high risk of subsequent development of infertility, ectopic pregnancies, and chronic pelvic pain.

C. Ovarian Neoplasm: When the examination of a woman with pelvic pain reveals a tender adnexal mass, the management depends on the severity of the pain and the U/S findings. Functional ovarian cysts are believed to result from ovarian follicles that failed to rupture with ovulation and usually present in the last 2 weeks of the menstrual cycle or with a history of delayed or missed menses. The U/S finding is of a unilocular, thin-walled cyst. If the cyst diameter is greater than 8 cm, spontaneous resolution is unlikely and surgery is indicated. Cysts of smaller diameter generally resolve in 4–8 weeks and are best managed by observation. Ovarian suppression with oral contraceptives is used commonly in management, but there is evidence that this treatment has little benefit over observation for resolution of the cyst. Persistence of the cyst requires surgical intervention. Painful solid ovarian tumors in the reproductive age group are usually benign but rarely resolve and are best managed by surgery as well.

1. Differential diagnosis—The U/S finding of a cystic-solid or complex ovarian mass in a woman of reproductive age may represent a hemorrhagic corpus luteum cyst or a unilateral endometrioma. Bilaterality indicates the diagnosis of endometrioma. If the symptoms allow and strong support for the diagnosis of endometriosis is lacking, it is best to follow the patient for spontaneous resolution, which occurs with most corpus luteum cysts. Corpus luteum cysts can rupture spontaneously or after trauma from a pelvic examination, coitus, or exercise. Rupture can cause severe pain and possible intraperitoneal hemorrhage, necessitating serial hematocrits or surgery. The differential diagnosis for a painful adnexal mass and negative pregnancy test includes appendiceal abscess, TOA, endometrioma, adnexal torsion, or torsion of a pedunculated fibroid.

2. Diagnosis—A common diagnosis made in the evaluation of acute pelvic pain when no mass is detected is that of a ruptured ovarian cyst. This diagnosis rarely is confirmed; it is presumed by excluding other possibilities. The patient typically presents in the last 2 weeks of her cycle or with delayed menses. She complains of acute onset of unilateral or generalized moderate-to-severe pelvic pain that often is receding or even resolved at the time of her evaluation. The examination may reveal unilateral or generalized pelvic tenderness of mild-to-moderate intensity, but it is otherwise normal. Her pain resolves in 24–48 hours and may require analgesics. This presentation differs from PID by its rapid onset and resolution.

3. Treatment—The surgical approach in these patients is to perform laparoscopy and, ideally, cystectomy to preserve ovarian function and fertility. Laparotomy is necessary for very large masses, cases in which the procedure cannot be completed with the laparoscope, or cases of a malignant mass. A postmenopausal patient presenting with a painful adnexal mass requires surgical evaluation, because these masses rarely resolve and carry an increased risk of malignancy.

D. Adnexal Torsion:
1. Signs and symptoms—Adnexal torsion can occur with normal ovaries, an ovarian mass, or a parovarian cyst; it involves the right side more often than the left. The patient usually presents with the acute onset of severe, progressive, unilateral pain that may have been preceded by mild intermittent pain for days or weeks. In advanced cases, there may be generalized pain with guarding and rebound, and nausea and vomiting are often present. Examination reveals a tender mass that on U/S is complex and may have engorged blood vessels. Adnexal torsion occurs in younger women, with an average age of onset of 20. It is most common when an adnexal mass is present or during the second trimester and early postpartum periods of pregnancy.

2. Diagnosis and treatment—In the early stages, the diagnosis may remain unclear, but the pain eventually becomes so severe that surgery is required for confirmation of the diagnosis and treatment. In the past, the standard treatment was laparotomy with adnexectomy, because there was the fear that detorsion of the mass would lead to emboli of blood clot and necrotic tissue. Recent studies have shown that detorsion, usually with a laparoscopic approach, is a safe procedure. Unilateral salpingo-oophorectomy is reserved for nonviable tissue.

E. Mittelschmerz: Mittelschmerz is a mild, unilateral, midcycle pain that some women feel with follicular rupture during normal ovulation. It is usually intermittent and may be associated with vaginal spotting. Treatment is simply reassurance or, if the patient desires, ovulation suppression.

F. Appendicitis: Appendicitis most commonly occurs in women between 20 and 40 years.
1. Signs and symptoms—The classic presentation is of poorly localized umbilical pain that in 1–12 hours localizes to the right lower quadrant; in many cases, however, the right lower quadrant is the first site of pain. The pain location can vary with the location of the appendix, and the occurrence in a long appendix may suggest an adnexal source. The pain is typically moderate to severe and constant, and it increases with movement. The classic complaint on directed questioning is anorexia, which precedes the onset of pain. Although anorexia can occur with other sources of pain, its absence makes appendicitis unlikely. Vomiting frequently follows the onset of pain, but it is rarely prolonged and is not necessary for the diagnosis. Other gastrointestinal symptoms such as constipation or diarrhea are variable in occurrence.

The patient presenting with acute appendicitis is often afebrile but may have a low-grade fever. A temperature of greater than 38°C may represent perforation if the abdominal findings are confirmatory. The abdominal examination classically reveals tenderness at McBurney's point (located one-third of the distance above the anterior iliac spine on a line between that spine and the umbilicus), but as noted, the site varies with the location of the appendix. Rebound tenderness is often present at the site of pain, as is in voluntary guarding. The white blood cell count (WBC) usually shows a mild-to-moderate elevation with an increased percentage of polymorphonucleocytes and band cells. Values greater than 20,000 cells/μL are consistent with perforation.

2. Diagnosis and treatment—The traditional treatment for appendicitis is laparotomy with appendectomy; however, many cases are now treated with the laparoscope. If the diagnosis is unclear but appendicitis is suspected strongly, diagnostic laparoscopy is the procedure of choice. The differential diagnosis includes ectopic pregnancy, PID, and ruptured ovarian cyst.

3. Prognosis—The prognosis is excellent for an uncomplicated recovery if appendicitis is treated prior to rupture. A ruptured appendix is a serious condition that can lead to abscess and extensive adhesion formation with subsequent chronic pain and infertility. The consequences of rupture warrant a low threshold for diagnosis and a willingness to err on the side of removing normal appendixes.

Referral to a Specialist

Most patients presenting with acute pelvic pain can be managed by a primary health care professional. If the patient is severely ill and the diagnosis is unclear, however, an appropriate consultation is imperative. Any diagnosis with the potential need for surgery requires a consultation; the need for surgery may develop on an emergent basis. The availability of a gynecologic or general surgeon is crucial for cases of ectopic pregnancy, adnexal torsion, and appendicitis; the surgeon should be notified as soon as the diagnosis is considered.

Issues of Pregnancy & Acute Pelvic Pain

Pregnant women with pelvic pain deserve special consideration. The causes of acute pelvic pain discussed previously occur most frequently in the reproductive age group and therefore can occur in pregnant patients. The confusion with normal pregnancy-related symptoms, alterations in abdominal anatomy, and the reluctance to perform invasive or other potentially risky procedures all can lead to a delay in diagnosis and the risk of pregnancy loss.

Adnexal torsion can present in the second trimester and early postpartum period when the uterus undergoes a rapid change in size. As pregnancy advances, the appendix may rotate into the right upper quadrant, confusing the diagnosis of appendicitis. PID rarely occurs in early pregnancy; it usually requires termination of pregnancy for adequate treatment. Pregnant patients with unusual abdominal or pelvic pain should be evaluated by a provider who has a firm understanding of the alterations the condition may impose on the patient's presentation.

Psychosocial Issues

As mentioned in the discussion of dysmenorrhea, many women presenting with acute pelvic pain have an underlying concern about fertility and cancer. Many of these patients are young, and hospitalization for PID or an ectopic pregnancy may require disclosure of their sexual activity to unaware parents. PID usually is caused by a sexually transmitted disease (STD), which raises the issue of exposure to other STDs including the human immunodeficiency virus (HIV). The relative youth of PID patients makes compliance for them, as well as their partners, a major factor in treatment.

Controversies & Unresolved Issues

Studies on the long-term effects of outpatient treatment for PID on fertility are lacking. The early mild symptoms and difficulty in making the diagnosis frequently lead to inadequate treatment. Until outpatient therapy is proved to be effective, the provider should choose inpatient management if fertility is a major concern.

ENDOMETRIOSIS

Essentials of Diagnosis

- Endometrial glands and stroma are located outside the uterus.
- Dysmenorrhea, acute pain, or chronic pain is present.
- Asymptomatic endometriosis in patients with infertility is well documented.

Incidence & Risk Factors

Endometriosis has an estimated incidence of 7% in the general female population of reproductive age. In infertility patients the incidence is 30%, and a similar value (28%) has been found for patients with chronic pelvic pain. Approximately 5% of cases are diagnosed in postmenopausal patients, most of whom are undergoing estrogen replacement therapy. The typical presentation of endometriosis is in a nulliparous woman in her mid 30s with infertility; however, dysmenorrhea or acute and chronic pelvic pain are also common presentations. Patients may relate a family history of the disease.

Symptoms

The patient with endometriosis may complain of worsening primary dysmenorrhea or secondary dysmenorrhea; often the pain begins 1–2 days prior to her menses and lasts throughout her flow. She may present with central, unilateral, or generalized pelvic pain that can range in intensity from a dull ache to severe pain. Other complaints include premenstrual deep dyspareunia, low back pain, pelvic heaviness or bloating, radiation of pain to the legs, and dyschezia at the time of menses. The symptoms are usually chronic, but they may be acute and severe in the case of a ruptured endometrioma. In advanced cases, the patient may complain of persistent dyspareunia and continuous pelvic pain that is worse with her menses.

Clinical Findings & Diagnosis

Findings on pelvic examination vary with the extent of the disease; however, there is a poor correlation between the disease extent and the patient's pain. An examination performed near the time of menses may be entirely normal or may reveal only mild tenderness. Tender uterosacral ligaments or tender nodules in the posterior cul-de-sac are suggestive of the disease. In advanced cases, the uterus may be retroverted and fixed, the ovaries fixed, and the posterior vaginal fornix narrowed. Unilateral or bilateral enlarged, tender ovaries may represent endometriomas; U/S shows cysts with low-level homogeneous internal echoes. CA-125 levels often are elevated in endometriosis, but this test is neither specific nor sensitive enough to aid in diagnosis.

Neither the history nor the physical examination findings are pathognomonic for endometriosis; the diagnosis can be confirmed only by laparoscopic observation and biopsy of implants.

Treatment & Prognosis

If endometriosis is suspected and the symptoms are cyclic, the patient can be offered symptomatic treatment as described for primary dysmenorrhea. If the patient is unable or unwilling to take that approach, the diagnosis should be confirmed before specific treatment is initiated. The patient who presents with recurrence of documented endometriosis can be offered medical therapy directly, but she may benefit from laparoscopy if her symptoms are severe. The role of laparoscopy is threefold: to confirm the diagnosis, to stage the extent of disease (the American Fertility Society classification system is used most commonly), and to treat visible disease with surgery, laser, or electrocautery.

Most patients benefit from long-term postoperative treatment, which acts to suppress residual disease by either decreasing estrogen production or decreasing the endometrial response to estrogen. The medical treatment options and their costs are shown in Table 45–5.

Gonadotropin releasing hormone (GnRH) agonists act, after an initial transient stimulation, to suppress pituitary gonadotropin secretion. The various agents are equally effective among themselves and in comparison to danazol. Although these agents are the most expensive of the treatment options, they are the most frequently used because of better patient compliance. The common side effects are those related to the hypoestrogenic state such as hot flushes, insom-

nia, decreased libido, vaginal dryness, and headache, all of which are reversible. A decrease in bone-mineral density has been shown with the use of these agents, which may be reversible only partially. Amenorrhea usually occurs in 4–6 weeks, and treatment is continued for 6 months; however, recent reports suggest 3 months may be adequate. There are also studies showing that the addition of norethindrone and conjugated estrogens, the so-called "add-back" therapy, may be able to reduce the side effects without compromising treatment.

Danazol is an androgen derivative that causes an inhibition of endometrial growth. The side effects reflect the hypoestrogenic state as well as the androgenic and anabolic effects of the medication. Hot flushes, vaginal dryness, emotional lability, weight gain, fluid retention, and acne are the more common side effects; there is a lower incidence of hirsutism, decreased breast size, and deepening of the voice. The drug may cause a mild elevation of liver function tests and a decrease in high-density lipoprotein levels. These side effects generally are reversible, although there are a few cases of permanent voice changes. The fear of these effects has led to decreased patient acceptance of danazol as the GnRH agonists have become available.

Medroxyprogesterone acetate is as effective as danazol in the treatment of endometriosis, but it is used less often as other agents have gained favor. The most common side effect is breakthrough bleeding; others include weight gain, bloating, edema, and irritability. Depomedroxyprogesterone acetate should be considered as a cost-effective long-term therapy.

Combination oral contraceptives given in a continuous (noncyclic) fashion are also effective; however, the daily dosage may have to be increased to 2–3 pills to maintain amenorrhea. The side effects of breast tenderness, nausea, edema, and breakthrough bleeding, especially at higher doses, have led to a high discontinuation rate. Cyclic therapy with oral contraceptives may diminish the patient's symptoms but is not effective as treatment. The medical management of endometriosis leads to symptomatic im-

Table 45–5. Medical therapies for endometriosis.

Agent	Dose	Route	Frequency	Duration	Price*
GnRH† agonists					
Depot leuprolide	3.75 mg	IM	qmo		$370
Nafarelin acetate	200 µg	Intranasal	bid	3–6 mo	$323
Goserelin acetate	3.75 mg	IM implant	q28d	3–6 mo	$345
Danazol	200–400 mg	PO	bid	3–6 mo	$210 (400 mg)
Progestins					
Medroxyprogesterone acetate	30–50 mg	PO	qd	4–6 mo	$24
Megestrol acetate	40 mg	PO	qd	4–6 mo	$12
Depomedroxyprogesterone acetate	150 mg	IM	q3mo	6 mo +	$12
Oral contraceptives					
Ethinyl estradiol + levonorgestrel	30 µg + 0.15 mg	PO	qd	6 mo	$25

*Average wholesale price, USA, 1994, for 30 days of treatment.
†Gn-RH = gonadotropin releasing hormone.

provement in approximately 80% of patients; however, the 5-year recurrence rate is 30–50%.

The definitive treatment for endometriosis, total abdominal hysterectomy with bilateral salpingo-oophorectomy, is reserved for severe cases in women who do not desire fertility. Estrogen replacement therapy can be initiated postoperatively, but a delay of 3–6 months may decrease the small chance of recurrent disease. Laparoscopic presacral neurectomy may benefit those suffering from refractory central pain, but it has shown limited success, as has LUNA. Involvement of other organs with endometriosis such as the bladder, ureter, or bowel requires surgical treatment.

Referral to a Specialist

Because women who are suspected of having endometriosis should not be treated without a laparoscopic diagnosis, referral to a gynecologist is necessary for the initial diagnosis and for recommendations for continued treatment. The gynecologist should have expertise in complicated operative endoscopy to maximize the chances of thorough laparoscopic treatment.

When future pregnancy is an issue and the endometriosis is recurrent or severe, consultation with a reproductive endocrinologist should be arranged to increase the patient's chances of achieving a pregnancy.

Issues of Pregnancy & Endometriosis

Women with moderate or severe endometriosis (stage III or IV) have decreased fertility, probably through distortion of anatomy and possibly because of factors secreted into the peritoneal fluid that affect various steps in reproduction. Data do not show conclusively that minimal or mild (stage I or II) endometriosis has an impact on fertility. Endometriosis does not increase the risk for spontaneous abortion or impact in any other way on a pregnancy.

It is a common misconception that pregnancy cures endometriosis. The elevated progestins and amenorrhea may have a positive impact on endometriosis, but pregnancy also may have no effect on the progression of disease.

Psychosocial Issues

The recurrent nature of endometriosis means that women with the disorder may have repeated surgeries or medical treatments. Some women undergo a hysterectomy and associated sterility at a young age. Others must deal with the psychosocial issues associated with infertility (see Chapter 52); with severe endometriosis, pregnancy is sometimes possible only with assisted reproductive technologies.

Even though a clear physical problem exists for women with endometriosis, the chronicity of their pain puts them at risk for a chronic pain syndrome.

Controversies & Unresolved Issues

Many of the treatments for endometriosis are expensive and no more effective than less expensive options. As the control of health care costs becomes a primary treatment concern, the less expensive alternative may become the first-line therapy, with the expensive regimens reserved for treatment failures. The long-term effects of the loss of bone mineral seen with GnRH agonists are unknown. Decreasing the duration of treatment to 3 months or adding estrogen may prevent this loss, but the effect of these modifications on treatment success is not well studied. The addition of etidronate to prevent bone-mineral loss currently is being evaluated.

CHRONIC PELVIC PAIN

Essentials of Diagnosis

- Noncyclic pelvic or lower abdominal pain greater than 6 months in duration
- Underlying disease processes that are somatic psychologic, or combined

This section discusses the approach to the patient with chronic pelvic pain (CPP) and the evaluation and treatment of common somatic causes. Chapter 46 gives an overview of long-term management strategies regarding the psychologic component of the problem.

Incidence & Risk Factors

Approximately 10% of outpatient gynecologic visits, 25–40% of diagnostic laparoscopies, and 13% of hysterectomies are for chronic pelvic pain. CPP usually affects women between the ages of 25 and 35 years. Patients often use prescription medications. Frequently, there is a history of childhood sexual abuse (20–64%), substance abuse, marital discord, sexual dysfunction, depression, somatization, or other chronic pain syndromes. Not infrequently, the patient has had multiple evaluations and surgical procedures for her complaint.

The causes diagnosed by laparoscopy are endometriosis and adhesions. Adhesions are found in 25–50% of CPP patients, although some studies have shown an equal incidence in pain-free controls. Risks for the formation of intra-abdominal adhesions include PID, endometriosis, ruptured appendix, and abdominal surgery. Patients with PID have approximately a 20% risk of developing CPP.

Symptoms

With the variety of causes of CPP, there is no one pattern of pain. The pain may be well localized and constant; more commonly, it covers a broad area of the pelvis and lower abdomen. It also typically varies in intensity and location. A patient who describes a current severe pain may not display any associated behavior changes. Dyspareunia, protracted dysmenorrhea (beginning well before and lasting long after the menses), and menorrhagia are other common complaints. There is a high incidence of somatic symptoms such as headache, low back pain, dizziness, shortness of breath, fatigue, and weakness.

Clinical Findings & Diagnosis

The psychologic component of CPP only recently is becoming understood. It is not clear whether this component is the result of a psychologic disorder preceding the onset of pain and exacerbated by it, or the result of the patient's response to her chronic pain. Differentiation is unnecessary; the psychologic component of the patient's condition needs to be addressed for an adequate chance of treatment success.

Multiple studies have shown a poor correlation between the location and extent of disease and the patient's pain. The treatment of an organic cause has a variable effect on relief of pain; frequently, no disease is discovered.

At presentation the patient often is frustrated from the impact her condition has had on her life, from the past failure to obtain a diagnosis, and from being told her pain is "all in her head." Providers may have a poor understanding of the chronic pain process and, for fear of alienating the patient, are reluctant to address the psychologic issues. This attitude can lead to an abuse of treatments the provider is comfortable with, such as antibiotics, narcotics, and surgery.

It is imperative to begin an integrated approach to the patient at the onset of evaluation. This approach decreases the risk of somatic fixation on the part of the patient and decreases the pursuit of inappropriate treatment such as "definitive surgery." The patient should be advised that in many cases of CPP an underlying cause is found; regardless of the presence or absence of an organic cause, however, she needs to be aware of the role the psychologic component plays. The clinician should explain the role of stress—past, present, or secondary to pain—in one's ability to cope with pain. It is best to mention at the first visit that the diagnostic workup may involve a psychiatrist, psychologist, social worker, physical therapist, and nutritionist, among others.

The guidelines for the patient history outlined in Table 45–3 apply for both acute and chronic pain. Most patients have significant psychosocial problems and have the chronic pelvic pain syndrome (CPS) as defined by Steege and Stout. This definition requires, in addition to pain for greater than 6 months, at least three of the following criteria: inadequate relief attained through prior treatments, impaired physical function, at least one vegetative sign of depression, and altered family role. During the history, emphasis should be placed on eliciting these factors. The effect of the pain on the patient's work, activity, relationships, sexual function, and family responsibilities, as

well as any change in the behavior of others toward her, reveals the impact of the condition on her life and may uncover pain-reinforcing behaviors. Also important are perceptions the patient and her family have concerning the cause of her pain.

In light of the frequent somatic complaints associated with CPP, a complete physical examination should be performed. A detailed back, abdominal, and pelvic examination is needed to focus on the pain symptom and reveal possible somatic causes. Palpation of the abdominal wall with the patient in a half sitting position tenses the rectus muscle and helps to differentiate pain within the wall from that of a deeper source. If the patient complains of vaginal pain or dyspareunia, palpation with a cotton swab may reveal trigger points. The pelvic floor muscles (levators and piriformis) should be examined for tenderness, and an attempt to duplicate deep dyspareunia should be made with the bimanual examination. It should be kept in mind that the physical examination results rarely correlate with the presence or absence of disease or the patient's pain symptoms.

Laboratory tests include a WBC, fecal occult blood test, tests for cervical infection with N gonorrhea and C trachomatis, and a urinalysis. In the presence of an adequate examination with normal findings, U/S is rarely helpful. More invasive tests such as computed tomography (CT), magnetic resonance imaging (MRI), barium enema, and intravenous pyelography are appropriate only when strongly indicated.

Laparoscopy has been considered the ultimate diagnostic test for CPP. In light of the recent understanding of the disease, however, this assumption is incorrect. Laparoscopy remains an excellent diagnostic tool if the history is suggestive of endometriosis or adhesions, examination suggests pelvic disease, or the pain is well localized and reproducible. However, it should be used judiciously, not routinely. Studies have shown that approximately 28% of CPP patients have endometriosis, and 25% have adhesions at the time of laparoscopy. How these factors relate to the patient's pain is not well understood, because many asymptomatic patients also have these findings. The location and extent of disease in CPP patients rarely explains their pain, and treatment of the pathologic condition alone has limited success Other studies have shown a 47% incidence of occult somatic disease (eg, urethral syndrome, irritable bowel syndrome, abdominal wall trigger points) in patients with CPP and a negative laparoscopic evaluation. Overall, it is estimated that about 39% of patients have no abnormal findings with laparoscopy. It is important to be aware that the patient who was told her laparoscopic findings were normal and never returned was not cured but was treated inadequately and probably sought care elsewhere. The patient who presents with a recent laparoscopy should not be sub-

jected to a repeat procedure. Videotaping laparoscopic findings helps to prevent repeat procedures.

Differential Diagnosis & Treatment

Table 45–6 lists many of the known causes of
CPP. The underlying mechanisms for many of these
causes are poorly understood; they may, in part, be
somatic manifestations of the psychological disorder
in these patients.

A. Psychopathology: This is the only diagnosis found in up to 50% of patients with CPP and is a
cofactor in up to 30% of cases in which organic disease is found. As emphasized previously, this component cannot be overlooked even when other diagnoses are present.

B. Abdominal Wall Trigger Points: These are
diagnosed by eliciting reproducible pain during
palpation of the abdominal wall. The pain distribution is usually within a dermatome and can be localized further with a needle. The underlying mechanism is unknown, because no pathologic tissue has
been detected. Treatment is by injection of a local
anesthetic agent such as 0.25% bupivicaine. Repeat
injections usually are required.

C. Myofascial Pain: This condition is diagnosed by finding irritable areas within a tight band of
muscle or fascia often associated with a prior incision. There may be muscle twitching and distant pain
radiation with palpation. Methods of treatment have
included transcutaneous electrical nerve stimulation
(TENS), local anesthetic injection, acupuncture, and
scar revision.

D. Vaginal Wall Trigger Points: An underlying cause is rarely found, but there may be improvement after local anesthetic injection.

E. Vulvar Vestibulitis: This condition is diagnosed by the finding of erythema and exquisite ten-

Table 45–6. Causes of chronic pelvic pain.

Gynecologic
  Adhesions
  Chronic pelvic inflammatory disease
  Endometriosis
  Ovarian remnant
  Pelvic floor myalgia
  Pelvic congestion
  Retained ovary syndrome
  Vaginal wall trigger points
  Vulvar vestibulitis
Psychopathologic
Abdominal wall factors
  Myofascial pain
  Trigger points
Gastrointestinal
  Constipation
  Diverticulitis
  Inflammatory bowel disease
  Irritable bowel syndrome
Urologic
  Interstitial cystitis
  Urethral syndrome

derness in the vestibular region. The most common
complaint is severe vaginal entrance dyspareunia.
There has been a recent association with human papillomavirus infection, and alpha-interferon injections or 5-fluorouracil cream has been used with limited success. Other treatments that have had variable
success include local steroid or anesthetic injections
and surgery (perineoplasty).

F. Pelvic Floor Myalgia: Spasm and tenderness of the levator plate musculature can result from
prior surgery or trauma, but usually no underlying
mechanism is detected. The patient generally complains of dyspareunia, and treatment includes physical therapy with biofeedback techniques.

G. Pelvic Congestion: Engorgement of the
pelvic vasculature is a well-known finding, but its
role in pelvic pain is unclear. It is believed to cause a
dull, aching pelvic pain that is worse premenstrually
and with prolonged standing. Venography and U/S
have been used in the diagnosis, but there are no controlled trials evaluating this condition as a cause of
CPP. Treatment usually has been hysterectomy, but
venous ligation also has been performed.

H. Residual Ovary Syndrome: Between 1 and
3% of posthysterectomy patients require surgical
evaluation for pain from a retained ovary. Adhesions
of the ovary or the development of functional cysts,
endometriomas, or other neoplasms is the usual
cause. Scarring of the ovary to the vaginal cuff may
lead to symptoms of dyspareunia. The ovary often
can be palpated and the patient's pain duplicated, but
if the diagnosis is uncertain, U/S or MRI is helpful.
Treatment is usually oophorectomy, which can be
done laparoscopically in many cases.

I. Ovarian Remnant Syndrome: Women
presenting with pain and a small (3–4 cm) pelvic
mass after a hysterectomy and bilateral salpingo-
oophorectomy may be suffering from the effects of a
retained portion of an ovary. These are often fixed to
the pelvic sidewall. The pain is associated with normal ovarian function that can be confirmed by the
finding of premenopausal follicle-stimulating hormone (FSH) levels if the patient stops her estrogen
replacement. Although laparoscopic treatment can be
attempted, the dense scarring, poor tissue planes, and
frequent intimate association with the ureter make laparotomy a safer approach.

J. Intra-abdominal Adhesions: The risk factors for the formation of adhesions were discussed
previously. The patient with CPP may be presenting
years after the appearance of such a risk factor. It is
unlikely that the location of adhesions has changed.
Rather, the chronicity most likely has led to a chronic
pelvic pain syndrome. As reviewed previously, the
role of adhesions as a cause of CPP is unclear. In one
study, an improvement in pain at 1 year following lysis of adhesions was found in 75% of patients without the chronic pain syndrome and in only 40% of
those with it. The patients who benefit most from ad-

hesiolysis are those with a concurrent history of a risk factor for adhesions and the onset of pain as well as localized pain. Laparoscopic adhesiolysis is preferred because it is associated with a shorter recovery time, and the procedure itself may induce less adhesion formation than a laparotomy. If laparoscopy is performed in patients with chronic pain syndrome, the treatment of adhesions found is unlikely to provide prolonged relief. Patients relating a history of surgery for their pain without relief may have adhesions that are unrelated to their pain.

K. Endometriosis: Endometriosis can be a cause of chronic pain or it may be present but unrelated to a chronic pain syndrome. Because it also presents with acute pain and dysmenorrhea, it is discussed in the previous section.

Surgical Treatment

The role of laparoscopy has been discussed in the section preceding, "Clinical Findings & Diagnosis." Presacral neurectomy and LUNA have been used in the treatment of CPP. There are no controlled trials, and long-term follow-up is lacking. Hysterectomy with or without bilateral salpingo-oophorectomy has often been employed as "definitive" therapy for CPP. Long-term follow-up results are rarely available, and most studies do not support this treatment. In one study of hysterectomies done for pelvic pain with a presumed uterine source, no pathologic condition was found in 66% of specimens. There was no correlation between relief of pain at 1-year follow-up and the presence of disease. Given these results and the risk of psychologic morbidity from hysterectomy, this procedure should be contraindicated in CPP except in rare circumstances.

Long-term Management

Most patients with CPP require more than diagnosis and treatment of underlying disease. Addressing the psychologic component from the beginning may help the patient to understand the depth of the problem and the lack of an immediate cure. Reassurance that her physical findings are not life-threatening and that definitive surgery will not cure her pain may help her to accept a treatment plan. Frequently scheduled visits for emotional support and to monitor treatment may decrease the pain-reinforcing behavior of emergency visits. Psychological and sometimes musculoskeletal considerations are key to a long term treatment plan and are described in more detail in Chapter 46.

Referral to a Specialist

The primary care provider is in an excellent position to treat patients with CPP. These patients require extensive education and counseling as well as coordination of specialty consultations with psychologists, gynecologists, or physical therapists. A physical therapy consultation should be considered when musculoskeletal components are suspected or identified or when biofeedback is a consideration for treatment. CPP is a complex, poorly understood process that in many cases requires skilled, long-term treatment. Severely dysfunctional patients are best managed in multispecialty pain clinics or by providers who have appropriate resources available.

Controversies & Unresolved Issues

The mechanisms of chronic pain perception are poorly understood. There are many theories about pain perception, and future research may influence the appropriate treatment of chronic pain. Psychologic tests also are limited in their ability to guide the management of these patients. As improvement in this area occurs, the large role that psychosocial issues play may become even more obvious.

REFERENCES

Barbieri RL: Gonadotropin-releasing hormone agonists: Treatment of endometriosis. Clin Obstet Gynecol 1993;36:636.

Dawood MY: Dysmenorrhea. Clin Obstet Gynecol 1990; 33:168.

Gambone JC, Reiter RC: Nonsurgical management of chronic pelvic pain: A multidisciplinary approach. Clin Obstet Gynecol 1990;33:205.

Howard FM: The role of laparoscopy in chronic pelvic pain: Promise and pitfalls. Obstet Gynecol Surv 1993;48:357.

Olive DL, Schwartz LB:Endometriosis. N Engl J Med 1993;328:1759.

Peters AAW et al: A randomized clinical trial to compare two different approaches in women with chronic pelvic pain. Obstet Gynecol 1991;77:740.

Reiter RC: A profile of women with chronic pelvic pain. Clin Obstet Gynecol 1990;33:130.

Rock JA et al: Zoladex (gosarelin acetate implant) in the treatment of endometriosis: A randomized comparison with danazol. Obstet Gynecol 1993;82:198.

Schwartz SI: Appendicitis. In: *Principles of Surgery,* 6th ed. Schwartz SI, Shires GT, Spencer FC (editors). McGraw-Hill, 1994.

Shalev E, Peleg D: Laparoscopic treatment of adnexal torsion. Surg Gynecol Obstet 1993;176:448.

Slocumb JC: Chronic somatic, myofascial, and neurogenic abdominal pelvic pain. Clin Obstet Gynecol 1990;33:145.

Slocumb JC: Operative management of chronic abdominal pelvic pain. Clin Obstet Gynecol 1990;33:196.

Steege JF, Stout AL: Resolution of chronic pelvic pain after laparoscopic lysis of adhesions. Am J Obstet Gynecol 1991;165:278.

Stovall TG, Ling FW, Crawford DA: Hysterectomy for chronic pelvic pain of presumed uterine etiology. Obstet Gynecol 1990;75:676.

Stovall TG et al: Nonsurgical diagnosis and treatment of tubal pregnancy. Fertil Steril 1990;54:537.

Surrey ES et al: The effects of combining norethindrone with a gonadotropin-releasing hormone agonist in the treatment of symptomatic endometriosis. Fertil Steril 1990;53:620.

Vercellini P et al: A gonadotropin-releasing hormone ago-nist versus a low-dose oral contraceptive for pelvic pain associated with endometriosis. Fertil Steril 1993;60:75.

Wheeler JM, Knittle JD, Miller JD: Depot leuprolide ac-etate versus danazol in the treatment of women with symptomatic endometriosis: A multicenter, double-blind randomized clinical trial. II. Assessment of safety. Am J Obstet Gynecol 1993;169:26.

Wheeler JM, Knittle JD, Miller JD: Depot leuprolide versus danazol in treatment of women with symptomatic en-dometriosis: I. Efficacy results. Am J Obstet Gynecol 1992;167:1367.

Management of Chronic Pelvic Pain: Musculoskeletal & Phsychological Considerations

46

Edward A. Walker, MD, & Kathe Wallace, PT

In the management of women with chronic pelvic pain, care must be taken to consider both organic and functional causes. Although it may appear at first that organic disease is absent or minimal, it could be discovered later that there is an occult or prodromal pathologic condition. Conversely, some patients who are found to have organic disease, such as endometriosis, eventually develop comorbid chronic pelvic pain syndrome (Chapter 45).

Several factors that modify the course of chronic pelvic pain need to be understood. Not all women who experience chronic pelvic pain feel it is severe enough to seek medical help; some live productive lives with persistent, low-level pain. Some patients who find their discomfort severe enough to warrant treatment become disabled by their pain, whereas others do not. The development of disability appears to be an important factor in the establishment and maintenance of chronic pelvic pain and is predictive of both high levels of use of medical care and poor treatment outcome.

Musculoskeletal factors have been overlooked frequently in a traditional biopsychological model of chronic pelvic pain. The musculoskeletal origin of chronic pelvic pain must be considered in a comprehensive evaluation of and treatment plan for patients with chronic pelvic pain. In addition, physical therapy addresses the physical changes brought on by the vicious cycle of chronic pain (Fig 46–1).

MUSCULOSKELETAL CONSIDERATIONS

In patients with chronic pelvic pain, identification of any musculoskeletal dysfunction is important. A chronic pain-tension cycle can develop from orthopedic malalignment, postural abnormalities, pelvic floor muscle dysfunction, urogynecologic and colorectal disease, or psychological dysfunction.

Specifically, lumbar, sacroiliac, or hip joint malalignment or disease can affect the pelvic muscles, causing limitations in range of motion, strength, muscle length, posture, and functional activities. Myofascial pain and dysfunction have been identified in specific muscles of the pelvic region by Travell and

> Musculoskeletal Considerations
>   Clinical Findings & Diagnosis
>   Treatment
> Psychological Considerations
>   Clinical Findings
>   Disability
>   Evaluation
>   Treatment

Simons. The coccygeus, levator ani, obturator internus, adductor magnus, piriformis, and oblique abdominal muscles can have trigger points that refer pain to the pelvic region.

Psychological causes of pain can lead to changes in posture as well as chronic muscle tension. Although psychological causes of pain frequently are difficult to separate from musculoskeletal causes, patients often consider musculoskeletal causes of pain more tangible and acceptable.

Painful medical conditions such as endometriosis or interstitial cystitis can cause tension to be held in the pelvic floor musculature. Chronic tension in these muscles can lead to pain in the pelvic region. This condition is called a **hypertonus dysfunction of the pelvic floor.** Frequently, such a dysfunction may be caused by any of the following factors:

- Pelvic inflammation, infection, or disease
- Postural dysfunction
- Surgeries with urogenital or rectal approaches and episiotomy
- Sexual abuse
- Psychogenic factors
- Muscle tension in pelvic floor and abdomen caused by stress
- Abnormal use of pelvic floor muscles such as chronic holding patterns
- Habitual poor posture
- Point or soft-tissue restrictions of the musculoskeletal system

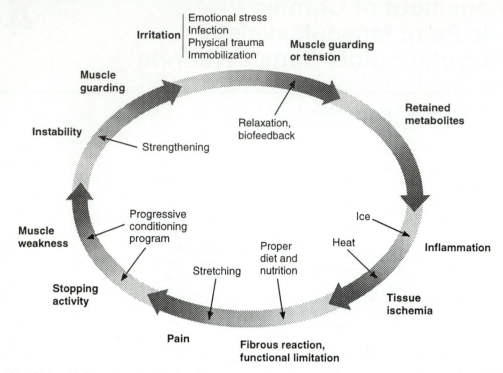

Figure 46–1. Typical pain cycle. (Reproduced from Sanders P: Breaking the chronic pain cycle. Clinical Management 1991;11(4):76, with the permission of the American Physical Therapy Association.)

Clinical Findings & Diagnosis

Pelvic floor tension myalgia is a diagnostic term used to describe a wide variety of syndromes of pelvic floor muscle hypertonus. These syndromes include levator ani syndrome, levator spasm syndrome, coccygodynia, vaginismus, and piriformis syndrome. Often, pelvic floor hypertonus problems are labeled **levator ani syndrome.** The primary symptom is pain that is usually poorly localized in the perivaginal area, perirectal region, lower abdominal quadrants, or pelvis. In addition, suprapubic, coccygeal, posterior thigh, vulvar, or clitoral localization of pain is sometimes present.

Other conditions that may have a component of pelvic floor hypertonus dysfunction include chronic low back pain, urethral syndrome, vulvodynia, sphincter dyssynergia, and fibromyalgia.

A. Screening Examination: A musculoskeletal screening examination is indicated in patients who present with pelvic and abdominal pain, suprapubic pressure, or urogenital symptoms. Key factors in a patient's history include symptom alteration caused by stress, activity, or position changes. It is important to screen for a history of spinal or lower extremity trauma, injury, or pathologic condition. Musculoskeletal examinations include a postural assessment, range of motion and strength testing, and pelvic floor muscle examination.

Pelvic floor muscle examinations should be a routine part of the screening evaluation. In a pelvic examination, the speculum covers the pelvic floor musculature, and its examination frequently is overlooked. Internal and external palpation of the pelvic floor can locate and isolate specific muscle problems including increased tone (pelvic floor hypertonus), tenderness, or trigger points. One component of this examination is the specific palpation of the pelvic musculature. When performed externally, it is called the **pelvic clock examination,** which is illustrated in Figure 46–2. With the patient in a lithotomy position, an external palpation examination is performed to assess muscle tone, tenderness, or trigger points of the perineum. The individual muscles of the perineum can be assessed clockwise, starting from the symphysis pubis and moving to the ischial spines, the ischial tuberosities, and the perineal body. Each number on an imaginary clock is palpated to identify the muscle that may be contributing to the pain or hypertonus dysfunction. The urogenital triangle is represented by the 1, 2, 3, 9, 10, 11, and 12 o'clock positions. The deeper levator ani muscles in the anal triangle are represented by the 4, 5, 7, and 8 o'clock positions. The 1 and 11 o'clock positions represent the ischiocavernosus muscle. The 2 and 10 o'clock positions represent the bulbocavernosus muscle. The 3 and 9 o'clock positions represent the superficial

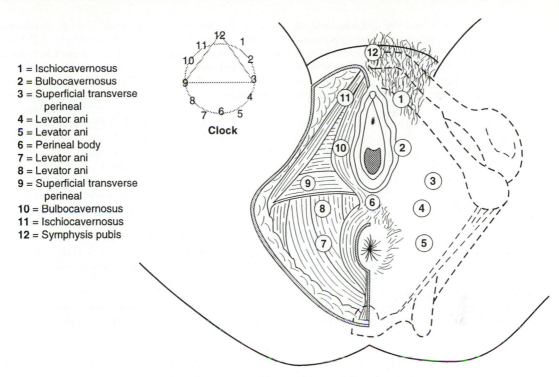

1 = Ischiocavernosus
2 = Bulbocavernosus
3 = Superficial transverse perineal
4 = Levator ani
5 = Levator ani
6 = Perineal body
7 = Levator ani
8 = Levator ani
9 = Superficial transverse perineal
10 = Bulbocavernosus
11 = Ischiocavernosus
12 = Symphysis pubis

Clock

Figure 46–2. Pelvic clock examination. Muscles of perineum are palpated in order, according to corresponding numbers of superimposed clock face. (Reproduced, with permission, from Herman H, Wallace K: *The APTA Section on Obstetrics and Gynecology, Pelvic Floor Seminar Manual.* American Physical Therapy Association, 1993.)

transverse perineal muscle. The 4, 5, 7, and 8 o'clock positions represent the levator ani muscles. The 6 o'clock position represents the perineal body.

B. Comprehensive Evaluation: Positive findings in the initial screening examination warrant a comprehensive musculoskeletal evaluation by a physical therapist. Physical therapists routinely perform musculoskeletal evaluations and treat acute and chronic pain problems. Some physical therapists specialize in obstetric and gynecologic conditions.

A comprehensive physical therapy evaluation should include a patient interview and a review of the patient's medical history. During the interview, the patient's functional limitations are outlined, and a list is made of the patient's present pain-management techniques. The physical examination includes a neurologic scan examination and an assessment of muscle strength, active and passive range of motion, joint mobility, and myofascial and scar tissue restrictions. Static and dynamic postural alignment in standing, sitting, and walking also is assessed. In addition, specific muscle palpation in the pelvic floor (the pelvic clock examination), trunk, and hip musculature can identify the muscles that may be referring pain to the pelvic region.

Surface electromyography (SEMG) evaluation with biofeedback can objectify muscle activity and monitor skeletal muscle tension of the pelvic floor and the related musculature.

Treatment

The physical therapy evaluation identifies musculoskeletal problems requiring treatment. Goals of the treatment include management and reduction of musculoskeletal factors that could contribute to or cause chronic pelvic pain.

Orthopedic malalignment should be treated with manual therapy techniques. Functional and postural limitations should be treated with specific exercise programs. Chronic pain and muscle guarding require patient education in the physiology of pain and instruction on muscle relaxation techniques. Therapeutic interventions include specific pelvic floor exercises, scar mobilization, myofascial release, and trigger point treatment. Physical therapy modalities such as heat, cold, and electrotherapy may provide pain relief and physiologic quieting. The emphasis should be on introducing treatment that is aimed at reducing the musculoskeletal factors of chronic pelvic pain and breaking the chronic pain cycle using physical therapy interventions and biofeedback. An additional home program of relaxation and key exercises is also beneficial.

Biofeedback: Biofeedback can be used to facilitate self-regulation of pain and to assist with the diagnosis of hypertonus dysfunction and treatment of chronic pelvic pain. It works by shaping a self-management response to pain. The goal of biofeedback is to learn control of typical physiologic responses to pain and dysfunction through the use of SEMG, electrodermal response, respiration, and skin temperature.

Computer-assisted equipment is available to enhance the quality of the feedback provided. Visual and audio signals assist the patient in learning self-regulation of pain. Typical relaxation training such as diaphragmatic breathing, Jacobson relaxation techniques, imagery, and autogenic training all are enhanced by the use of biofeedback.

SEMG biofeedback is helpful in the demonstration of the difference between a contracted and a relaxed muscle. This training helps the patient identify chronic muscle tension holding patterns and assists with pelvic floor exercises. Patients learn to detect changes in muscle tension that can occur from increased pain. They also learn how to perform pelvic floor exercises. Specific vaginal and rectal electrodes are available to treat pelvic floor muscles with SEMG; they are particularly useful because the pelvic floor muscles are frequently difficult to identify and exercise properly. Specific treatment of the pelvic floor muscles includes re-education of normal muscle use through pelvic floor strengthening and relaxation training. Frequently, when there is prolonged pain and muscle tension, the patient is unaware of the muscle function.

The goals of biofeedback treatment are to encourage behavioral changes in pain management and to learn and practice normal use of the pelvic floor muscles. As part of a comprehensive treatment program using a biopsychosocial model, biofeedback treatment can provide a nonpharmacologic approach to relaxation and pain management.

PSYCHOLOGICAL CONSIDERATIONS

Clinical Findings

Although the physiologic factors that maintain chronic pelvic pain remain obscure, in the last decade several studies of chronic pelvic pain have highlighted important psychosocial associations. These include current and lifetime psychiatric disorders, somatization, and prior emotional, sexual, and physical trauma.

When compared with women undergoing laparoscopy for tubal ligation and infertility, women with chronic pelvic pain are significantly more likely to have current and lifetime episodes of major depression, somatization disorder, sexual dysfunction, and medically unexplained physical symptoms in several organ systems, despite the lack of significant difference in objective laparoscopic findings.

Chronic pelvic pain also is found frequently in patients presenting with irritable bowel syndrome (IBS). Nearly 40% of women in one study of IBS reported prior or current pelvic pain, distinct from their gastrointestinal discomfort. Women with histories of both IBS and chronic pelvic pain were more distressed than women with IBS alone or pain-free controls. Patients with both disorders showed the highest rates of current and lifetime psychiatric disorders, somatization, dissociation, and gynecologic disorders including dysmenorrhea and dyspareunia; they also had higher rates of hysterectomy.

Several studies have found significantly higher rates of sexual, physical, and emotional abuse in patients with chronic pelvic pain compared with women who did not report pelvic pain. Prevalence rates for childhood rape or incest as well as adult sexual victimization are 2–3 times higher than for women without pain. Physical and emotional abuse are also significantly more common in these patients. Indeed, psychological distress, early and recent sexual and physical abuse, and lifetime psychiatric disorders may be better predictors than physical diagnostic techniques of whether pelvic pain is functional or organic. These factors also may be important predictors of which patients will go on to develop chronicity through disability.

Disability

Recent studies have investigated the relationship of chronic pain to functional disability. Studies of other chronic abdominal pain disorders such as inflammatory bowel disease (IBD) have shown that most patients continue to function remarkably well despite the stress of repeated surgeries, parenteral nutrition, and recurrent episodes of diarrhea and pain. Despite the long-term medical and surgical distress endured by IBD patients, they do not display psychiatric disorder or abuse prevalence rates that are much higher than comparable medical clinic patients. On the other hand, patients with chronic abdominal pain syndromes such as chronic pelvic pain and IBS experience a much more benign course of illness and do not undergo such extreme treatments but show far greater levels of distress.

One of the important differences appears to be disability. People who are not disabled perceive themselves to be primarily healthy with occasional periods of illness. People with disability, on the other hand, perceive themselves as ill, with occasional periods of health. The view of oneself as disabled often is found in people with somatization, and both somatization and disability can occur in patients with early experiences of abuse or neglect. It is not surprising, therefore, that patients with chronic pelvic pain, with their higher prevalence rates of psychiatric disorders and developmental stressors, should have an increased risk for disability. Once disability has been established firmly, it is very difficult to return the patient to the prior, nondisabled state.

Although abdominal disease frequently is associated with acute pelvic pain, the relationship of physical findings to chronic pelvic pain recently has been called into question (see Chapter 45). Several controlled studies have shown no association between laparoscopic findings and severity of pain. Laparoscopies of women with chronic pelvic pain are frequently negative, whereas abnormal findings often are discovered unexpectedly in pain-free women undergoing laparoscopy for tubal ligation or infertility.

Chronic pain syndrome and its associated disability can develop in patients with known organic pelvic disease. This comorbidity can occur because the relatively benign pathophysiologic findings of chronic pelvic pain are likely to be distinct from the more severe organic disease.

Evaluation

A patient with chronic pelvic pain frequently endures a long biomedical workup only to hear her doctor announce that no explanation can be found for her incessant pain. Not only is this finding unbelievable intellectually, it is unsatisfying emotionally. Fears of abandonment, of a lifetime of pain, and of overlooked disease such as cancer can engender a range of emotions from hopelessness to rage. The serial process of performing a systematic biomedical evaluation before pursuing psychosocial factors may be problematic.

Several techniques can help maintain a therapeutic liaison with the patient. It is imperative for the clinician to make the patient aware that he or she believes the pain to be real regardless of cause. The clinician should insist on an integrated biopsychosocial model that considers the interaction of physical and psychosocial factors from the beginning of the evaluation to demonstrate the importance of considering all aspects of her pain. This task can be carried out by alternating between biomedical and psychosocial emphases in the evaluation and using the term **stress** as a common explanatory model for the pain.

Hearing the cause of her problem described as stress may assist the patient who is ambivalent about making links between her pain and depression, anxiety, and psychosocial vulnerabilities. Education about a "vicious cycle of pain" (ie, pain leads to stress, which leads to worsening pain) may help the patient see that stress is a factor in the worsening of all forms of pain. Many patients have discovered that narcotic analgesics are of minimal value; helping patients to understand the differences between functional and nociceptively derived pain may be useful.

Treatment

The treatment plan focuses on the reframing of pain as a stress symptom. Techniques aimed at changing pain behavior rather than understanding it may be more effective than those requiring insight. The provider should focus on coping and should not promise a cure. Reduction of disability by restoration of adaptive coping skills is a far better goal than the possibly unreachable outcome of elimination of pain.

A. Biopsychosocial Model: It is useful to employ the biopsychosocial model as a guide to care. This model can be divided conveniently into biomedical, psychological, and social components. Each of these components has a separate diagnostic and treatment formulation. Careful alternation between a graded, judicious biomedical investigation, including musculoskeletal factors, and a rational, progressive psychosocial evaluation should result in a treatment plan that is efficient, cost-conscious, and effective.

In many patients who have chronic pain, these biologic, social, and developmental forces form interlocking, mutually reinforcing maladaptive patterns that need to be modified together. Interventions that do not address all of these areas are likely to have limited effectiveness. Multidisciplinary pain treatment centers that emphasize integrated, multimodal treatment strategies have been successful. Their goal is to break the chronic pain cycle and return the patient to a functional level.

Although many patients resist the biopsychosocial model as an explanation of their pain, most readily accept that their physical illness causes them stress, which worsens their pain. Although these stress factors may be causal in the development of pain, it is better not to press this point at the beginning. The acceptance that stress is an object of treatment in pain reduction is enough. Open communication between a mental health provider and the primary care clinician is essential in gradually moving the patient away from a disease-oriented model to one that includes treatment of disability and psychological factors as primary goals. The patient should consider both providers to be working together actively and should have strong therapeutic bonds to both.

B. Treatment Strategies: Although a thorough biomedical evaluation may have been accomplished previously with few positive findings, several biologically based strategies can be employed. Patients who have developed a narcotic dependence require careful withdrawal. Antidepressants have demonstrated efficacy in patients with other forms of chronic pain. Many women with chronic pelvic pain respond to antidepressants although they are not believed to be clinically depressed. A trial of antidepressant medication may be an important initial therapeutic step that can provide benefit while other physical and psychosocial strategies are being started.

Physical therapy interventions including biofeedback should be considered. These interventions may provide a nonpharmacologic alternative to the management of chronic pain. They should be considered even when the primary cause of pain is believed to be psychological. In addition, patients often find biofeedback and physical therapy interventions more acceptable than therapy to address a psychological cause directly. Beginning with the more easily understandable physical conditions can open a pathway to the patient's final understanding of the mind-body connection. This approach may allow for an introduction of the psychological component of chronic pelvic pain into the treatment plan.

Patients may live in situations that reinforce or maintain their pain. Attention to support structures and family and work dynamics may suggest social and life-style interventions that provide benefits similar to those attained by using pain behaviors. For example, a woman who is in a physically abusive relationship may experience less abuse when her partner perceives her chronic illness. Many pain behaviors are reinforced by financial, emotional, or situational factors that provide essential benefits to the patient while the pain is present but disappear when the pain subsides. Learning to "live despite the pain" is often the first step in restructuring the world of the patient with chronic pain.

Inquiring about early family experiences of abuse or neglect may raise issues that need to be dealt with in psychotherapy. Many women need to understand that experiences of early sexual or physical victimization as well as emotional abuse or neglect can have long-lasting emotional and medical sequelae and may be important factors in maintaining their pain. This understanding should be reached in the context of psychotherapy. If psychotherapy is unavailable, the clinician can recognize and empathically support the patient as she struggles with these memories.

Collaborative interaction between the mental health and primary care providers leads to earlier psychosocial evaluation and treatment as well as better outcomes for these highly distressed patients.

REFERENCES

Baker PK: Musculoskeletal origins of chronic pelvic pain: Diagnosis and treatment. Obstet Gynecol Clin North Am 1993;20:719.

Kasman G: Use of integrated electromyography for the assessment and treatment of musculoskeletal pain: Guidelines for physical medicine practitioners. In: *Surface EMG for Clinical Recordings.* Vol 2. Cram JR (editor). Clinical Resources, 1990.

Sinaki M, Merrit J, Stillwell GK: Tension myalgia of the pelvic floor. Mayo Clin Proc 1977;52:717.

Steege JF, Stout AL, Somkutu SG: Chronic pelvic pain in women: Toward an integrative model. J Psychosom Obstet Gynecol 1991;12(Suppl):3.

Travell J, Simons D: *Myofascial Pain and Dysfunction: The Trigger Point Manual.* Williams & Wilkins, 1983.

Travell J, Simons D: *Myofascial Pain and Dysfunction: The Trigger Point Manual.* Vol 2: *The Lower Extremity.* Williams & Wilkins, 1992.

Walker EA, Stenchever M: Sexual victimization and chronic pelvic pain: Clinical and research issues. Obstet Gynecol Clin North Am 1993;20:795.

Walker EA, Sullivan MD, Stenchever M: Use of antidepressants in the management of women with chronic pelvic pain. Obstet Gynecol Clin North Am 1993;20:743.

Walker EA et al: Chronic pelvic pain: The relationship to psychiatric diagnoses and childhood sexual abuse. Am J Psychiatry 1988;145:75.

Walker EA et al: Medical and psychiatric symptoms in women with childhood sexual abuse. Psychosom Med 1992;54:658.

Walker EA et al: The prevalence of chronic pelvic pain and irritable bowel syndrome in two university clinics. J Psychosom Obstet Gynecol 1991;12(Suppl):65.

Walker EA et al: Psychiatric diagnoses and childhood sexual abuse in women with chronic pelvic pain. Psychosomatics. [In press.]

Wallace K: Female pelvic floor function, dysfunction and behavioral approaches to treatment. Clin Sports Med 1994;13:459.

Approach to Abnormal Vaginal Bleeding

47

Beth Skrypzak, MD

Menstruation is the physiologic shedding of the endometrium that occurs at approximately monthly intervals from menarche to menopause. Menarche generally occurs between 11 and 14 years of age, with a mean of 13 years. Menopause generally occurs between 45 and 55 years of age, with a mean of 51 years. The cycle interval is usually 28 (±7) days. Most cycle interval irregularities occur during the first 2 years after menarche and the 3 years before menopause, when anovulatory cycles are more frequent. Average length of flow is 4 (±2) days, with longer than 7 days considered menorrhagia. It is more difficult to determine what constitutes a normal amount of flow. One definition of excessive flow is frequently passing quarter-sized or larger clots or the need to change a saturated tampon or sanitary pad more than 6 times daily.

The normal phases of the menstrual cycle have been defined by the endometrial and ovarian changes (Fig 47–1). The preovulatory part of the cycle is called **proliferative** (referring to the endometrium) or **follicular** (referring to the ovary). The postovulatory part of the cycle is called **secretory** (referring to the endometrium) or **luteal** (referring to the ovary). The secretory, or luteal, phase is followed by the menstrual phase of the cycle. The luteal phase is fairly consistently 14 days, based on the normal life span of the corpus luteum. The proliferative and menstrual phases contribute the variability of cycle length (Fig 47–1).

Complicated neuroendocrine changes occur each month to ensure the regularity of the cycle. The interaction between the hypothalamus, pituitary, ovary, and endometrium is complex, but it can be summarized in the following manner (Figs 47–1 and 47–2): The low estradiol level during menstruation stimulates pulsatile gonadotropin-releasing hormone (GnRH) production in the hypothalamus. GnRH stimulates follicle-stimulating hormone (FSH) and luteinizing hormone (LH) release from the pituitary. FSH and LH cause folliculogenesis in the ovary. The ovary primarily produces estradiol in the follicular phase, which stimulates the development of the endometrium in preparation for the fertilized ovum. An estradiol peak followed by an LH surge midcycle provides the stimulation for ovulation. The corpus lu-

Secondary Amenorrhea & Oligomenorrhea
    Essentials of Diagnosis
    Incidence & Risk Factors
    Signs & Symptoms
    Clinical Findings & Diagnosis
    Treatment
    Prognosis
    Referral to a Specialist
    Controversies & Unresolved Issues
Menorrhagia & Metrorrhagia
    Essentials of Diagnosis
    Incidence & Risk Factors
    Signs & Symptoms
    Clinical Findings & Diagnosis
    Treatment
    Prognosis
    Referral to a Specialist
    Issues of Pregnancy & Excessive Vaginal
        Bleeding
    Controversies & Unresolved Issues

teum, which develops from the site on the ovary where the egg was released, now produces both estradiol and progesterone to maintain the endometrial lining. Without the appearance of human chorionic gonadotropin (HCG) from the developing placenta, the corpus luteum degenerates after 14 days and progesterone levels fall rapidly. Within 1–2 days, this drop in progesterone causes the organized shedding of the endometrium. If all these events do not occur in a sequential fashion, abnormal vaginal bleeding can occur (Fig 47–2).

SECONDARY AMENORRHEA & OLIGOMENORRHEA

Essentials of Diagnosis

- Pregnancy must be excluded early in the evaluation.
- Hypothalamic amenorrhea, such as from anorexia, vigorous exercise, or emotional stress, is a diagnosis of exclusion. The other causes must be searched for before hypothalamic amenorrhea is assumed.

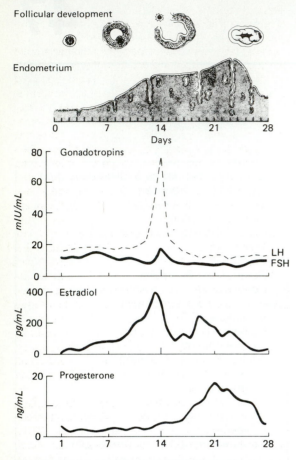

Figure 47–1. The menstrual cycle, showing pituitary and ovarian hormones and histologic changes in the endometrium. (Reproduced, with permission, from Katzung BG (editor): *Basic and Clinical Pharmacology*, 2/e. Lange, 1984.

- Premature ovarian failure is rare.
- Primary amenorrhea: lack of secondary sexual characterictics and no menses before age 14 or no menses before age 16 regardless of development of secondary sexual characteristics.
- Oligomenorrhea: infrequent menses (interval greater than 35 days).

Incidence & Risk Factors

Amenorrhea can occur in up to 5% of the general population, excluding pregnant women. In an unselected adolescent population, the figure may be as high as 8.5%. Between 10 and 20% of vigorously exercising women and perhaps as many as 40–50% of long distance runners and professional ballet dancers are amenorrheic.

Absent or infrequent menses may be a sign of an illness, or it may be a sign of emotional or physical stress. Hypothyroidism can be associated with menstrual irregularities. A history of autoimmune disorders could suggest possible premature ovarian fail-

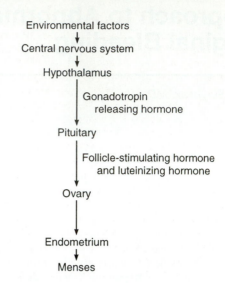

Figure 47–2. Endocrinologic factors of normal menstruation.

ure. A prior uterine curettage in the setting of pregnancy or infection can lead to Asherman's syndrome. Eating disorders such as anorexia or bulimia can lead to rare or absent menses.

Signs & Symptoms

Amenorrhea means absence of menses and can be categorized as primary or secondary. **Primary amenorrhea** refers to lack of menses before 14 years of age in the absence of growth and development of secondary sexual characteristics or the lack of menses before 16 years of age regardless of the presence of normal growth and development of secondary sexual characteristics. In a previously menstruating woman, **secondary amenorrhea** is defined as 6 months or longer without menses or lack of menses for a length of time equivalent to a total of at least three of her previous cycles. For example, if the woman normally has a 30-day cycle, absent menses for longer than 3 months would establish the diagnosis of secondary amenorrhea.

Oligomenorrhea means infrequent menses occurring at intervals greater than 35 days. Although these intervals can represent a woman's normal pattern, several abnormalities should be excluded before that assumption is made. Because there is a great deal of overlap in the causes and treatment of secondary amenorrhea and oligomenorrhea, these two conditions are dealt with together in the following sections.

In taking the patient's history, several issues can be addressed that may help direct the evaluation. The possibility of pregnancy should be considered. If the woman is in a heterosexual relationship, it is important to determine whether she is using a reliable method of birth control. Symptoms of hypothyroidism such as weight gain or hair changes should be sought. Any history of galactorrhea, headaches, or visual field defects may suggest a pituitary microadenoma. Long-standing hirsutism suggests polycystic ovarian syndrome, but an androgen-secreting tumor should be considered if hirsutism suddenly appeared or worsened (see Chapter 19). Any history of hot flashes, night sweats, vaginal dryness, or sleep disturbances could identify the rare patient with premature ovarian failure. Recent emotional or physical stresses can be contributing factors. A history of vigorous exercise or eating disorders should be elicited.

When evaluating patients for amenorrhea or oligomenorrhea, it is important to exclude several other possible causes: (1) pregnancy, (2) hypothyroidism, (3) prolactin-secreting pituitary tumor, (4) hyperprolactinemia without tumor (medications, breast trauma, damaged pituitary stalk), (5) pituitary tumor with normal prolactin (PRL) level (rare), (6) chronic anovulation, (7) polycystic ovarian syndrome, (8) hypothalamic dysfunction, (9) Asherman's syndrome, and (10) ovarian failure.

Clinical Findings & Diagnosis

A careful physical examination should be performed. General appearance may suggest an eating disorder. Height and weight should be measured. Percentage of body fat can be estimated or measured with calipers. The distribution and amount of hirsutism present at the time of examination should be noted as well as other signs of androgen excess such as acne or temporal balding. The neck examination should exclude thyromegaly. At the time of the breast examination, the nipples should be squeezed gently to demonstrate galactorrhea. If secretions are present, they should be examined microscopically to confirm the presence of fat globules. On pelvic examination, attention should be focused on excluding atrophic vaginitis, adnexal masses, and signs of early pregnancy. Visual field testing may help in the evaluation of possible pituitary microadenoma.

Initial laboratory evaluation should include a urine pregnancy test (HCG) and levels of thyroid-stimulating hormone (TSH), PRL, and FSH. There is no need to obtain a level of LH, because it will not be cost-effective. Some textbooks on gynecology do not recommend checking FSH as part of the initial laboratory evaluation; however, in most situations, obtaining the FSH at this time expedites the evaluation, saves the patient time and repeat venipuncture, and avoids missing the diagnosis of premature ovarian failure. Figure 47–3 contains an algorithm that combines laboratory testing and treatments for amenorrhea.

A sensitive urine pregnancy test can detect low levels of HCG in the range of 25–50 mIU/mL, which correspond to a pregnancy approximately 12–14 days from ovulation. Thus, most pregnancies may be detected by this method at or just before the missed menses. The urine test is less expensive than serum HCG levels. If the patient has a positive pregnancy test and is having abnormal bleeding, the possibility of a spontaneous abortion, ectopic pregnancy, or gestational trophoblastic disease should be considered. Quantitative HCG levels and gynecologic consultation are recommended.

Hypothyroidism can be associated with a modest elevation of the PRL level, ie, 20–40 ng/mL. The elevated level of thyrotropin releasing hormone (TRH) associated with hypothyroidism also stimulates PRL release from the pituitary. Generally, treatment of hypothyroidism normalizes the PRL, and any concern over a pituitary microadenoma is resolved. The combination of an elevated PRL level (above 20 ng/mL)

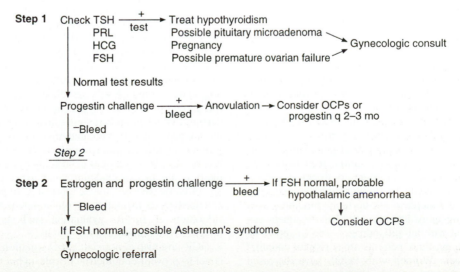

Figure 47–3. Algorithm for the evaluation and treatment of secondary amenorrhea. TSH = thyroid-stimulating hormone; PRL = prolactin; HCG = human chorionic gonadotropin; FSH = follicle-stimulating hormone; OCPs = oral contraceptives.

and a normal TSH level warrants a repeat PRL in midmorning and gynecologic consultation.

The interpretation of the FSH level can be confusing. If the woman has amenorrhea and an elevated FSH, it is helpful to recheck this level 2 weeks later if she fails to have a menses within 2 weeks. The FSH level is increased mid cycle and can mimic menopause if tested on only one occasion (see Fig 47–1). If the woman has oligomenorrhea and is perimenopausal, the FSH may be elevated on some occasions but normal at other times.

If there has been recent-onset or rapidly progressive hirsutism, levels of serum testosterone and dehydroepiandrosterone sulfate (DHAS) should be drawn to exclude an androgen-producing tumor. If the level of testosterone is greater than 200 mg/dL or DHAS is greater than 700 μg/dL, a tumor should be suspected and a referral initiated (See Chapter 19).

The diagnosis of polycystic ovarian syndrome (PCOS) usually can be established by history and physical examination. PCOS has been associated classically with the Stein-Leventhal syndrome, which has the clinical picture of obesity, hirsutism, oligomenorrhea, and enlarged ovaries with multiple tiny cysts in the cortex. Previously, this diagnosis was made by discovery of an LH:FSH ratio greater than 3. Currently, any woman with chronic anovulation and hyperandrogenemia (by clinical or laboratory findings) satisfies the criteria for PCOS. Not all patients with PCOS have the classic clinical manifestations. Some patients with PCOS are slim, although most are overweight. Some women with markedly elevated androgen levels are amenorrheic, although most are oligomenorrheic. There is wide variation in the appearance of the ovaries; many are normal in size. There are many theories about the pathogenesis of PCOS: whether the basic defect is adrenal, ovarian, or hypothalamic is debated. However, the final result is noncyclic gonadotropin and androgen production and chronic anovulation.

Treatment

If a specific disorder such as hypothyroidism is diagnosed, the appropriate therapy should be initiated, as outlined in Chapter 20. Treatment of hyperprolactinemia should be determined by the consultant; it can include bromocriptine.

Treatment of the patient with PCOS depends on the specific manifestations. If fertility is desired, clomiphene citrate or menopausal gonadotropins often are required to induce ovulation (see Chapter 52). When hirsutism is a problem, oral contraceptives (OCPs) can be given to suppress ovarian androgen production and increase sex hormone binding globulin, inhibiting more hair growth. This treatment can be combined with an antiandrogen (see Chapter 19). Most important, these patients are at risk for endometrial neoplasia. Women with PCOS have increased estrone levels from peripheral conversion of androgens to estrogen, and the chronic anovulation results in low or absent progesterone production. Both of these problems contribute to excessive estrogenic stimulation of the endometrium. Use of OCPs or of medroxyprogesterone acetate (MPA), 10 mg daily for 10 days at least every 2–3 months, should prevent endometrial neoplasia.

If the FSH is persistently elevated (greater than 30 mIU/mL), a gynecologic consultation is in order. Premature ovarian failure is defined as menopause before age 40 and can be associated with organ-specific autoimmune diseases. Hormone replacement therapy (HRT) should be initiated to prevent osteoporosis and cardiovascular disease. Continuous HRT with conjugated estrogens, 0.625 mg, or 17-β-estradiol, 1 mg daily, and MPA, 2.5 mg daily, usually works well. These patients also can be treated with OCPs. If pregnancy is desired, referral to a reproductive endocrinologist is indicated to discuss options.

There are two steps in treating amenorrhea and oligomenorrhea (Fig 47–3):

Step 1: If the TSH, PRL, and FSH levels are normal and the HCG is negative, a progestin challenge test is given. MPA, 10 mg, given for 10 days should induce a withdrawal bleed within 2–7 days of completing the course if there are adequate levels of endogenous estrogen to stimulate the development of an endometrial lining.

If a withdrawal bleed occurs, amenorrhea is most likely a result of anovulation, and no other studies are necessary; however, medical therapy should be considered to prevent endometrial neoplasia. The patient should be offered OCPs or MPA every 2–3 months if the amenorrhea continues. Although the appropriate frequency of progestin administration is unknown, this regimen will most likely protect against neoplasia.

Step 2: If the progestin challenge does not produce a withdrawal bleed, a trial using estrogens followed by progestin may be initiated. This therapy supplements an inadequate production of endogenous estrogen. OCPs for 1 month or conjugated estrogens, 2.5 mg daily for 21 days, with MPA, 10 mg for the final 10 days, (days 12–21) should be given.

If a withdrawal bleed occurs this time, the cause of the amenorrhea probably is related to the low endogenous estrogen levels associated with hypothalamic-pituitary dysfunction. It is necessary to try to understand why the endogenous estrogen production is not adequate, because the endometrium required this supplementation to induce a bleed. If serum FSH is low or normal, the absent or infrequent menses most likely is due to hypothalamic amenorrhea. If there is no obvious reason for a patient's hypothalamic amenorrhea, consultation is recommended for consideration of further evaluation such as pituitary imaging with computed tomography.

OCPs are also beneficial in this situation. The goal is not to prevent endometrial neoplasia but to provide estrogen replacement to prevent the increased risk of osteoporosis and lipid changes associated with hypoestrogenism. Occasionally, bone-mineral density studies show early osteoporosis, and the results may help convince a patient to use OCPs.

If the patient fails to have a withdrawal bleed to the estrogen and progestin challenge and if the FSH level is normal, there may be an end-organ problem with the uterus, such as Asherman's syndrome. This condition is associated with intrauterine scarring usually related to a prior endometrial curettage. Gynecologic consultation is recommended, especially if the patient is interested in pregnancy.

Once the cause of amenorrhea is determined, most patients benefit from some therapy, not just to induce a menses but to prevent other medical complications.

Prognosis

If the cause of the amenorrhea or oligomenorrhea is identified and the patient receives the appropriate long-term therapy, the condition should be alleviated. It is important to identify the patient with premature ovarian failure, normal menopause, or hypothalamic amenorrhea so that hormonal therapy can be initiated early to prevent osteoporosis. The risk of endometrial neoplasia in patients with chronic anovulation is increased throughout their life span. Any excessive vaginal bleeding in these women, even when they are younger than 40 years, needs to be evaluated with an endometrial biopsy.

Patients with PCOS have associated increased risks of cardiovascular disease, hypertension, and diabetes, and they should be monitored appropriately. Preventive health changes such as diet and exercise modifications may be especially beneficial in these patients, because they often are identified at a young age.

Referral to a Specialist

Appropriate timing of referrals was mentioned throughout the preceding section but is summarized here. An adolescent with primary amenorrhea should be referred to a pediatrician with an interest in this area, a pediatric endocrinologist, a general gynecologist with an interest in adolescent gynecology, or a reproductive endocrinologist. A woman with hyperprolactinemia, possible premature ovarian failure, elevated androgens, possible Asherman's syndrome, or possible pregnancy should be referred to a gynecologist with an interest in the specific disorder or to a reproductive endocrinologist. If the patient has PCOS or premature ovarian failure and desires pregnancy, referral to a reproductive endocrinologist is appropriate.

Controversies & Unresolved Issues

The timing of the initiation of HRT in the perimenopausal patient with intermittently elevated FSH levels is controversial. Usually, therapy is initiated when the patient is experiencing symptoms of estrogen deficiency, even if some menstrual bleeding continues.

The use of hormonal therapy such as OCPs in the adolescent with primary or secondary amenorrhea is also controversial. If laboratory and diagnostic tests do not reveal any significant disease, expectant management may be appropriate. However, recent data about bone deposition and growth may prompt more aggressive use of hormonal therapy in the future.

Pituitary microadenomas are generally slow growing and do not always require bromocriptine therapy; therapy is required if the patient has significant galactorrhea, has visual field changes, or wishes to conceive. Menstrual abnormalities associated with hyperprolactinemia usually can be treated with OCPs.

Many studies have established the recommended doses of estrogen replacement therapy to prevent osteoporosis in the postmenopausal woman, but few studies have been performed in the premenopausal woman with hypothalamic amenorrhea. It is not known whether these patients need higher dosing to prevent osteoporosis.

MENORRHAGIA & METRORRHAGIA

Essentials of Diagnosis

- Pregnancy must be excluded with any abnormal vaginal bleeding.
- Menorrhagia: menstrual bleeding for longer than 7 days or excessive flow (greater than 80 mL) at regular intervals.
- Metrorrhagia: bleeding at irregular intervals or intermenstrual bleeding.
- Presence of neoplasia, hormonal abnormalities, or anatomic abnormalities should be evaluated.

The term **dysfunctional uterine bleeding** is a diagnosis of exclusion. It suggests that no neoplastic or anatomic cause has been found for excessive bleeding, and thus it should not be used until these conditions have been ruled out.

Incidence & Risk Factors

The exact incidence of menorrhagia or metrorrhagia is not known. Excessive bleeding is a common problem, but it can be confusing because of the many causes, which can overlap. The multiple causes are sometimes only partially understood by clinicians, and the treatments may not be optimal.

Medical risk factors include a history of coagulation disorders or liver disease, such as von Willebrand's disease, idiopathic thrombocytopenia, and cirrhosis. It is estimated that about 20% of adolescents with menorrhagia have a coagulation disorder. Anovulatory cycles are more common just after menarche and just before menopause. Women taking anticoagulants or undergoing chemotherapy can develop excessive bleeding that can be challenging to treat. Also, thyroid disorders can present with abnormal bleeding.

Gynecologic risk factors include possible pregnancy, neoplasia, and uterine abnormalities. If there has been a long interval since the patient's last Papanicolaou (Pap) smear, suspicion of cervical neoplasia is increased. Only 1% of endometrial polyps are neoplastic. If the patient has a history of diabetes, hypertension, obesity, or chronic anovulation, she could be at increased risk for endometrial neoplasia. About one-third of women with leiomyoma complain of menorrhagia. Leiomyoma can cluster in families; leiomyoma occurs in about 1 in 4–5 white women and in about 1 in 3 black women. Less than 0.1% of leiomyomas are malignant. Endometriosis also can have familial tendencies, and about 20% of women with laparoscopically proven endometriosis can have adenomyosis. Adenomyosis can cause menorrhagia in 40–50% and dysmenorrhea in 25–30% of patients.

Signs & Symptoms

Menorrhagia, or **hypermenorrhea,** is defined as menstrual bleeding for longer than 7 days or with excessive flow (greater than 80 mL) but at regular intervals. More than 80 mL per menses is equivalent to more than six saturated pads or tampons per day. The mean loss for normal menses is 35 mL. Ninety-five percent of women bleed less than 60 mL, which corresponds to 10–15 pads or tampons per menses.

Metrorrhagia is defined as light or heavy bleeding at irregular intervals or intermenstrual bleeding. **Menometrorrhagia** is excessive prolonged flow without any predictable pattern. It can be normal for a woman in her 40s to develop a shortened cycle interval as a result of a physiologic shortened luteal phase.

Metrorrhagia suggests neoplasia, hormonal abnormalities, or polyps and menorrhagia often suggests uterine abnormalities such as leiomyoma or adenomyosis. The distinction is more significant in the later stages of diagnosis and treatment after gynecologic referral.

When taking the woman's history, eliciting the amount and pattern of bleeding is important. Is the frequency regular or irregular, and what is the exact amount of flow? Women have different perceptions of heavy bleeding. What may seem excessive to one patient may be within an acceptable range when compared with other women. Often a "bleeding calendar" is helpful to define the pattern and to record the number of pads or tampons used each day. Postcoital bleeding suggests a cervical problem such as an endocervical polyp or cervical neoplasia. Midcycle spotting is usually normal and is related to the physiologic drop in estradiol levels at the time of ovulation. Screening for symptoms of iron deficiency anemia, such as fatigue, dizziness, or headaches, is also important. Pregnancy should be considered.

Any history of uterine leiomyomas or uterine or endocervical polyps can indicate recurrent problems from these anatomic abnormalities. Prior or current endocervical polyps can be associated with endometrial polyps.

Clinical Findings & Diagnosis

A careful pelvic examination is the first step in defining the cause of excessive bleeding. Possible causes for excessive vaginal bleeding include (1) pregnancy, (2) thyroid disorder, (3) coagulopathy, (4) chronic anovulation, (5) cervicitis or endometritis, (6) endometrial or endocervical polyps, (7) leiomyoma, (8) adenomyosis, (9) endometrial hyperplasia or carcinoma, and (10) cervical dysplasia or carcinoma. The bleeding also may be idiopathic. A cytobrush Pap smear should be done. Care should be taken to inspect the cervix for any lesions or polyps. Assessing the amount of flow from the cervical os, if there is any, may be important in deciding on appropriate acute therapy. Bimanual examination should attempt to exclude any obvious leiomyoma or pregnancy or the soft, enlarged, "boggy" uterus associated with adenomyosis.

Pap smears can result in diagnosis of endometrial carcinoma in only about 20% of women with carcinoma. It is not an adequate test for endometrial carcinoma; endometrial biopsy should be used if appropriate. Endometrial cells sometimes can be seen in a premenopausal patient, but their presence in a postmenopausal woman carries a 10% risk of endometrial hyperplasia or carcinoma.

Laboratory evaluation should include a hematocrit and a urine pregnancy test, if pregnancy is suspected. Rarely, thyroid disorders can be associated with menorrhagia or metrorrhagia, and the TSH should be checked if the patient manifests other symptoms or signs. Generally, cervical cultures are not helpful, but they should be obtained if purulence is seen on cervical examination. Coagulation tests, such as prothrombin time (PT), partial thromboplastin time (PTT), and bleeding time, should be checked in the adolescent with menorrhagia.

An ultrasonographic scan should be obtained if the provider is unable to perform an adequate pelvic examination because of obesity or patient discomfort. If leiomyomas are suspected by bimanual examination, ultrasonography is useful to establish a "baseline" examination and to exclude adnexal masses. Any provider can be fooled by a pelvic mass that is presumed to be a leiomyoma but is actually an adnexal mass distorting the pelvic anatomy. The ultrasonographic scan also may help distinguish the location of the leiomyoma. A submucosal location (just below the endometrium) is associated with menorrhagia or sometimes intermenstrual bleeding and often can be resected hysteroscopically. However, if the leiomyomas are primarily intramyometrial, resection is not as effective. Leiomyomas can cause menorrhagia, even in an intramural location, probably by inhibiting the contractility of the spiral arterioles in the basalis layer of the endometrium.

Transvaginal ultrasonography has been introduced over the past several years and has become helpful in determining endometrial thickness, especially after menopause. There have not been extensive studies on its use in premenopausal women. The hyperechoic endometrium is measured in two layers from one adjacent inner myometrium to the other adjacent inner myometrium. It is normal for there to be a small fluid collection in a premenopausal woman. Biopsy of an asymptomatic *premenopausal* patient based on the thickness measurement is still unclear, but a thickness of more than 15 mm is grounds to suspect neoplasm. This test can be especially helpful in the evaluation of women in whom the office endometrial sampling cannot be accomplished easily. A thin lining (less than 6mm) may spare this patient a dilation and curettage (D&C) procedure.

Office endometrial biopsy (EMB) is performed by many primary care providers. Its use has eliminated the need for many outpatient D&C procedures. The following describes the technique for obtaining an endometrial biopsy:

1. Premedicate the patient with 600 mg ibuprofen 1 hour before the procedure.
2. Perform a bimanual examination to determine the size and direction of the uterus.
3. Insert the speculum and clean the cervix with antibacterial solution.
4. Provide a paracervical block if needed for patient comfort, especially if the cervix is stenotic. Ten milliliters of 1% lidocaine is administered using a 22-gauge spinal needle.
5. Place a single-tooth tenaculum on the anterior lip of the cervix.
6. Using sterile technique, gently insert the endometrial suction curette into the cervical os while placing traction on the tenaculum. A "release" should be felt on entering the endometrial cavity and some resistance should be felt at the top of the fundus. If there is no release, the curette may still be within the cervical canal. If there is no fundal resistance, perforation may have occurred; suction should not be applied, and the curette should be removed. The depth of the uterus should be noted; in a premenopausal woman, it is unlikely the cavity has been entered if the depth of the sound is less than 5 cm.
7. If the cavity is not clearly entered, make a single attempt to dilate the cervix gently with the smallest available dilator. A paracervical block can be placed at this time.
8. Apply suction with the curette, and while maintaining traction on the tenaculum, obtain circumferential sampling of the endometrium from the fundus to the internal os for 15 seconds.
9. After confirming hemostasis of the anterior

cervix, remove all instruments from the vagina and place the specimen in formalin. Bleeding points on the cervix usually can be controlled with silver nitrate applicator sticks.

Most patients can undergo the procedure successfully in the office and tolerate it well with premedication with nonsteroidal anti-inflammatory drugs (NSAIDs). The sensitivity of the test for diagnosis of endometrial carcinomas is in the range of 95–97%. Thus, this is a useful screening test. If the EMB is abnormal or inadequate or if the result is normal but the bleeding continues, gynecologic referral for hysteroscopy and D&C should be considered. A report of "inadequate tissue" can be reassuring in a postmenopausal woman, if the biopsy curette clearly entered the uterus and atrophic endometrium is strongly suspected. However, inadequate tissue is not an acceptable diagnosis in the pre- or perimenopausal woman with excessive bleeding, and further diagnostic procedures are warranted.

EMB should be performed to exclude neoplasia in any woman over age 40 who is experiencing abnormal excessive vaginal bleeding. Even if the patient has a leiomyoma, she could also have endometrial hyperplasia or carcinoma; one should not assume that the bleeding is related to the leiomyoma without excluding neoplasia first. If the patient has had a normal biopsy within the past year, a repeat test is probably not necessary. If the patient has risk factors such as diabetes, obesity, chronic anovulation, or a family history of endometrial neoplasia, EMB should be performed even if she is in her 30s.

The diagnosis of adenomyosis can be established only by histologic examination of endometrial glands and stroma within the myometrial layer of the uterus. Hysterectomy is the only known cure and the only way to establish the diagnosis histologically. Generally, this is a presumptive diagnosis made preoperatively when a patient has intractable menorrhagia and dysmenorrhea unresponsive to medical management, and no leiomyomas, polyps, or neoplasia is found.

Treatment

Figure 47–4 presents an organized approach to treating excessive bleeding. Any patient with iron deficiency anemia should be treated with iron therapy.

If the patient does not require an EMB, initial therapy includes MPA, 10 mg daily for 10 days each month (days 19–28 of the cycle); monophasic OCPs; or NSAIDs. The OCPs promote atrophy of the endometrial lining to decrease menorrhagia and provide the progestin lacking when anovulation is the cause of metrorrhagia. NSAIDs also have been shown to decrease the endometrial blood flow by their antiprostaglandin effect. Alone, they may reduce blood loss by 30%.

If the patient is having an acute hemorrhage and is not pregnant, estrogens are often helpful initially.

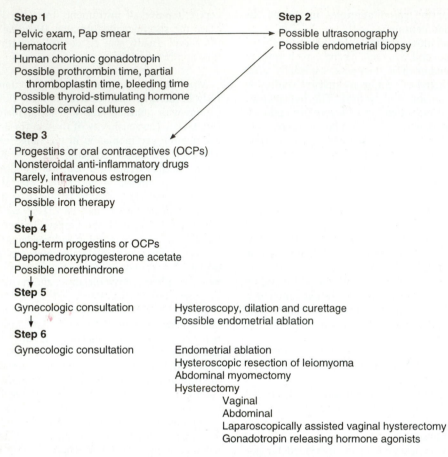

Step 1

Pelvic exam, Pap smear ────────────→
Hematocrit
Human chorionic gonadotropin
Possible prothrombin time, partial
   thromboplastin time, bleeding time
Possible thyroid-stimulating hormone
Possible cervical cultures

Step 2

Possible ultrasonography
Possible endometrial biopsy

Step 3

Progestins or oral contraceptives (OCPs)
Nonsteroidal anti-inflammatory drugs
Rarely, intravenous estrogen
Possible antibiotics
Possible iron therapy

Step 4

Long-term progestins or OCPs
Depomedroxyprogesterone acetate
Possible norethindrone

Step 5

Gynecologic consultation

Hysteroscopy, dilation and curettage
Possible endometrial ablation

Step 6

Gynecologic consultation

Endometrial ablation
Hysteroscopic resection of leiomyoma
Abdominal myomectomy
Hysterectomy
    Vaginal
    Abdominal
    Laparoscopically assisted vaginal hysterectomy
    Gonadotropin releasing hormone agonists

Figure 47–4. Algorithm for diagnosis and treatment of excessive vaginal bleeding.

With hemorrhage, much of the endometrium is thought to have been shed, and rebuilding it initially with estrogen halts the bleed from the denuded spiral arterioles of the basalis layer. OCPs are given twice daily for 1 week, then once daily for the next 2 weeks. Conjugated estrogens, 1.25 mg twice daily for 1 week, then once daily with MPA, 10 mg for another 2 weeks, also can be used. Rarely, if this regimen is not successful, intravenous estrogens may be needed along with a gynecologic consultation. After the acute hemorrhage is controlled, further diagnostic studies can be performed and a long-term plan formulated.

Treatment can be directed by the results of the EMB. Not only can the biopsy exclude neoplasia, but it also provides some information on the present hormonal status of the endometrium and what therapy is appropriate. If the biopsy is insufficient for diagnosis, a repeat may be necessary. The diagnoses of menstrual or secretory endometrium are helpful only in excluding neoplasia and any obvious hormonal imbalance. Such patients often can benefit from monophasic OCPs. Proliferative endometrium in the presumed secretory phase of the cycle or disordered

proliferative endometrium often responds to progestin supplementation in the last 10 days of the cycle (days 19–28).

Acute or chronic endometritis is an easily treated cause of abnormal bleeding in a premenopausal patient. Antibiotic therapy with doxycycline, 100 mg twice daily for 7 days, should be successful. In a postmenopausal patient, there can be hyperplasia or carcinoma underneath the endometritis, and the biopsy only samples the surface. Postmenopausal patients should be given antibiotic therapy, and repeat biopsy should be performed within 1–3 months to exclude any neoplasia.

Simple or cystic hyperplasia can be treated with MPA, 10 mg daily 10 days each month for 3 months; repeat biopsy is needed 3 months later to assess the efficacy of treatment. Atypical adenomatous hyperplasia, which is considered premalignant, requires higher progestin dosing, D&C, or both, so that gynecologic consultation is necessary. Carcinoma needs immediate consultation.

Long-term hormonal therapy for dysfunctional uterine bleeding includes monophasic OCPs, monthly luteal-phase MPA, or possibly, depot MPA,

150 mg intramuscularly every 3 months. Initially, some patients taking depot MPA have abnormal bleeding, but approximately 50% achieve amenorrhea after 1 year of use. This treatment may be a satisfactory nonsurgical option for women who can be patient with the lack of results in the initial months of therapy. Women who have side efects of depression, headache, or nausea from the MPA may do better with norethindrone, 0.35–0.7 mg daily.

Patients who do not respond to any of these hormonal therapies require hysteroscopy to exclude endometrial polyps, submucosal leiomyoma, or occult endometrial neoplasia. D&C usually is done at the time of the hysteroscopy.

Endometrial ablation with a "roller-ball" attachment or a resectoscope may be performed if future fertility is not desired. These patients require contraception postoperatively, because this procedure is not always associated with infertility. Additionally, endometrial ablation is a fairly new procedure that destroys the endometrial lining with electrosurgical techniques under hysteroscopic guidance.

If the patient has no leiomyoma and no adenomyosis, this procedure results in amenorrhea in about 50% and hypomenorrhea in another 30–40% of women. This procedure is performed as outpatient surgery and may prevent a future hysterectomy and the need for hospitalization.

If the patient has leiomyomas, many treatment alternatives exist. For leiomyomas that are larger than 12 weeks in size (ie, the uterus is greater than 15 cm), rapidly enlarging leiomyomas, or significant anemia (hematocrit less than 30), gynecologic consultation is recommended. Hydronephrosis can occur with larger leiomyomas. If the patient is not having any of these problems, expectant management is best initially. If the patient is older than 40 and having abnormal bleeding, endometrial biopsy should be performed to exclude neoplasia. One should not assume leiomyomas are the cause of the abnormal bleeding without further investigation. If the patient has menorrhagia caused by the leiomyoma, progestins or OCPs may promote atrophy of the endometrial lining and improve the bleeding pattern. There is a theoretic concern regarding estrogenic stimulation of leiomyomas with combination OCPs, but this is not often a problem. The risk of this stimulation needs to be weighed against that of continued menorrhagia if progestins alone are not helpful.

If the woman does not respond to hormonal therapy, some leiomyomas can be resected hysteroscopically, especially if in a submucosal location. Ablation procedures can be done at the same time and may augment the resection, if future fertility is not desired. An abdominal myomectomy procedure can be considered by the consulting gynecologist if future fertility is desired. These patients sometimes are treated with GnRH agonists preoperatively to decrease the size of the leiomyomas and reduce intra-

operative blood loss. GnRH therapy is associated with bone loss if continued longer than 6 months; therefore, it is generally used preoperatively and not for long-term therapy.

As a final treatment option, hysterectomy can be considered for the patient who fails to respond to hormonal therapy. Less invasive options, if appropriate, may be considered in conjunction with this procedure. If the patient has large leiomyomas or significant anemia and does not desire future fertility, hysterectomy may be the best option. Vaginal hysterectomy is preferred, if feasible, because hospitalization and recovery time are usually shorter and less pain medication is required than with an abdominal approach. Sometimes abdominal hysterectomy is the best surgical approach, depending on the uterine size or lack of descensus. Laparoscopically assisted vaginal hysterectomy is a newer procedure that may convert an abdominal approach to a vaginal approach, again with a faster recovery. Sometimes GnRH therapy is used to reduce the size of the leiomyoma to make a vaginal approach possible. As stated earlier, adenomyosis is diagnosed and cured only with a hysterectomy.

Prognosis

Many women can be treated successfully without a hysterectomy. Atypical endometrial hyperplasia, if left untreated, has a 20–30% risk of progressing to carcinoma. Early endometrial carcinomas usually can be treated successfully with total abdominal hysterectomy and bilateral salpingo-oophorectomy without adjuvant therapy. Polyps have a tendency to recur. Many leiomyomas are quiescent, but they may increase in size, especially during pregnancy with the added estrogenic stimulation. Any woman who chooses a conservative procedure for the treatment of leiomyomas, such as a myomectomy, should understand that the risk of recurrence is unknown. Endometrial ablation is successful in creating amenorrhea or hypomenorrhea in about 90% of patients, with failures usually associated with multiple leiomyomas or undiagnosed adenomyosis.

Referral to a Specialist

When a woman's bleeding affects her life-style and the interventions by the primary care provider are not effective, gynecologic consultation is recommended. If the patient has normal results on EMB and fails to respond to hormonal therapy, a referral to a gynecologist for hysteroscopy to exclude polyps or submucosal leiomyomas is appropriate. If the EMB shows atypical hyperplasia or carcinoma, a referral to a gynecologist or gynecologic oncologist is needed. If the patient is pregnant and is having abnormal bleeding, obstetric consultation may be helpful. If the patient is having an acute hemorrhage and is hemodynamically compromised, acute interventions by a gynecologist may be lifesaving. If the woman has symptomatic leiomyomas and has infertility or recurrent pregnancy losses, she should see a gynecologist or reproductive endocrinologist for possible myomectomy.

Issues of Pregnancy & Excessive Vaginal Bleeding

It is important to exclude pregnancy if the patient is heterosexual, especially if the abnormal bleeding is a first-time event. The possibility of a spontaneous abortion, gestational trophoblastic disease, or ectopic pregnancy always should be considered. Even if the woman has had a tubal ligation, she could have an ectopic or intrauterine pregnancy because of the 1 in 300 failure rate of the sterilization procedure. If the patient is pregnant, her blood type should be determined; if she is Rh-negative, Rh immune globulin

should be given (see Chapter 56). Gynecologic consultation should be obtained.

Controversies & Unresolved Issues

At present, some theoretic concern exists that endometrial ablation may hide endometrial glands that can develop later into cancer without obvious early bleeding as a symptom. After more than 10 years of experience, few cases of carcinoma have been reported. Long-term studies will not be available for several years.

The use of ultrasonography, rather than histologic evaluation to exclude endometrial neoplasia is still in a preliminary phase, but increasing data support its use as an alternative to biopsy in selected circumstances, especially in postmenopausal women.

REFERENCES

Benson RC: *Current Obstetric and Gynecologic Diagnosis and Treatment,* 5th ed. Lange, 1984.
Herbst AL et al: *Comprehensive Gynecology,* 2nd ed. Mosby, 1992.
Lin MC et al: Endometrial thickness after menopause: Effect of hormone therapy. Radiology 1991;180:427.

Marshall LA: Clinical evaluation of amenorrhea in active and athletic women. Clin Sports Med 1994;13:371.
Speroff L, Glass RH, Kase NG: *Clinical Gynecologic Endocrinology and Infertility,* 5th ed. Williams & Wilkins, 1994.

Diseases of the Vulva & Vagina

48

Raymond H. Kaufman, MD

Before any attempt at therapy is undertaken in the management of the patient with disease involving the vulva or vagina, it is imperative that a correct diagnosis be made. One of the major problems associated with conditions affecting these areas is the fact that often the patient has received multiple treatments prior to the establishment of an accurate diagnosis, making it difficult for the clinician to evaluate and manage the patient. This is often the case in patients complaining of vaginal discharge or vulvar pruritus and pain. Often therapy is prescribed over the phone on the basis of an initial diagnosis made years before.

VULVAR DISEASES

Examination of the Vulva

In the majority of cases, visual examination of the vulva allows the clinician to define clearly the changes that are present. Often, the use of a handheld magnifying glass allows the physician to inspect the vulva in greater detail. The use of a colposcope also may be of value, especially in defining possible changes related to human papillomavirus (HPV) infection. Frequently, washing the vulva and vestibule with 3–5% acetic acid highlights lesions, especially those related to HPV infection and those representing intraepithelial neoplasia, particularly on the mucosal surfaces of the vulva, ie, inner labia minora and vestibule.

It is also advisable to inquire about and inspect other areas of the body in the patient presenting with vulvar disease to look for the presence of dermatologic problems that may involve the glabrous skin as well as the vulva. For example, the individual with erosive lichen planus of the vulva often has lesions involving the buccal mucosa. The changes of psoriasis that may be classical elsewhere on the body may be present in an atypical fashion on the vulva because of the local environment of warmth and moisture. Thus, a clue to the cause of the vulvar disease may be found by careful inspection of the skin and mucosal surfaces elsewhere on the body.

> Vulvar Diseases
>   Examination of the Vulva
>   Technique of Vulvar Biopsy
>   Clinical Findings & Treatment
>   Vulvodynia
> Vaginitis
>   Clinical Findings & Treatment

In evaluating the patient presenting with complaints relative to the vulva, it is also advisable to evaluate the vagina and cervix for the presence of vaginitis or cervicitis. Often, the individual with a candidal infection of the vagina has secondary manifestations present on the vulva or may have an associated cutaneous candidiasis involving the vulva. The irritating discharge associated with trichomoniasis frequently results in secondary changes on the vulva. The diagnosis of vaginal infection often is made easily in the office on the basis of saline and potassium hydroxide (KOH) wet mount preparations obtained from vaginal secretions. This laboratory test, associated with establishment of the vaginal pH using pH "strips," allows the clinician to make an accurate diagnosis in the majority of cases. When the vaginal pH is normal, it is highly unlikely that the patient has a bacterial vaginosis or trichomonal infection of the vagina. Cultures are rarely necessary to establish a diagnosis; when they are necessary, the laboratory should be advised specifically concerning the organism suspected so that the appropriate culture media can be used. Cultures for *Candida* are worthwhile performing in most instances in patients with vulvar complaints, however, because a positive culture often is obtained in the presence of a negative wet mount preparation. The use of Sabouraud's medium is recommended. Numerous patients presenting with a complaint of recurrent candidal infection of the vagina do not in fact have such an infection. Verification by appropriate culturing of the vulva and vagina avoids incorrect treatment and overtreatment.

Technique of Vulvar Biopsy

Biopsy of the vulva should be liberally performed in the office because adequate therapy is based on a correct diagnosis. This simple office procedure is virtually free from complications and is essentially painless when performed using local anesthesia. Small, discrete lesions are best handled by excisional biopsy. Larger lesions or widespread skin lesions can be biopsied easily using the Keye's cutaneous dermal punch biopsy instrument. A sharp, disposable cutaneous biopsy instrument is also available and has the advantage of not requiring periodic sharpening as is necessary with the Keye's punch (Fig 48–1). In most instances, a 4-mm instrument is sufficient to obtain the biopsy.

The area from which the specimen will be obtained is infiltrated with 1% lidocaine solution using a small-gauge (30-mm) needle. The sharp edges of the dermal punch are then twisted up and back into the site of the biopsy. After the epithelium and dermis have been cut through, the circular portion of tissue is lifted with small tissue forceps, and the base of the specimen is severed with small scissors. The small area of the biopsy site obviates the need for sutures. Hemostasis is easily accomplished by the application of Monsel's solution (ferric subsulfate) or by cautery with a silver nitrate applicator. The tissue specimen should be placed on a small piece of filter paper or paper towel with the epithelial surface on top. This allows for proper orientation of the tissue when sections are cut. Poorly oriented tissue specimens often result in tangential cutting, which occasionally can lead to an erroneous diagnosis. Washing the vulva with 3–5% acetic acid highlights mucosal lesions such as intraepithelial neoplasia, which often turn acetowhite after the application of this solution. Similar changes are seen in the presence of an HPV infection.

One percent toluidine blue has been used to help define the biopsy site. The vulva is covered with this stain, and after it dries, the tissues are washed with 1% acetic acid. In the absence of significant cellular atypia, this process should result in the removal of the toluidine blue. Because nuclei retain toluidine blue, lesions such as invasive and intraepithelial carcinoma retain the dye after they are washed with acetic acid. The dye, however, is retained on any ulcerated site whether benign or malignant. Frequently, when a thick keratin layer covers the surface of intraepithelial or invasive carcinoma, the dye is not retained. Thus, this method is not highly sensitive or specific for selecting a biopsy site.

When multifocal or diffuse lesions are present, it is advisable to obtain biopsy specimens from several different locations. When an erosive lesion involves the vulva, the differential diagnosis is often confusing.

Immunofluorescent staining often is valuable in establishing the diagnosis. Direct immunofluorescent testing using the patient's own tissue is most often employed. This type of study is of value in distinguishing among the different chronic "vesiculobullous" diseases such as pemphigus, pemphigoid, lupus erythematosus, and leukocytic vasculitis. If immunofluorescent staining is to be performed, it is important that the biopsy specimen not be taken directly from the lesion but rather from the normal-appearing tissue adjacent to it. The specimen must be examined in the "fresh" state and should be kept in either a special "holding" solution or transported in phosphate-buffered normal saline. The location of various immunoglobulins, as well as various antigens such as carcinoembryonic antigen (CEA), S-100 protein, and HMB 45, often is valuable in clarifying the diagnosis.

Clinical Findings & Treatment

There are various approaches that the clinician can take in establishing a differential diagnosis of the diseases that involve the vulva. These lesions are classified in this chapter as they present to the clinician, ie, red lesions, white lesions, pigmented lesions, erosive and ulcerated lesions, and tumors. There are several disease processes that can present with different appearances, eg, vulvar intraepithelial neoplasia (VIN) may be seen as a white, red, or pigmented lesion or as all of the preceding.

A. White Lesions:

1. Nonneoplastic epithelial disorders–The International Society for the Study of Vulvar Disease has established a classification for the nonneoplastic epithelial disorders. Unlike the prior classification, which was based purely on histopathologic findings, the current classification is based on a combination of gross appearance and histopathologic changes. The classification is as follows:

Squamous cell hyperplasia (formerly hyperplastic dystrophy)

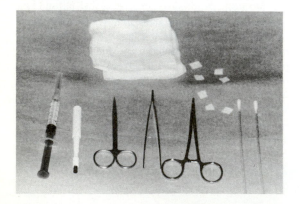

Figure 48–1. Vulvar biopsy with disposable 4-mm cutaneous punch instrument.

Lichen sclerosus

Other dermatoses (eg, psoriasis, eczematoid dermatitis, lichen planus)

Squamous cell hyperplasia represents changes for which no specific cause has been established and in which significant squamous cell hyperplasia is noted in the biopsy specimen. These changes probably represent lichen simplex chronicus and are related to persistent rubbing or scratching of the vulva as a result of pruritus from any cause. Lichen sclerosus is a specific dermatologic problem that may involve other areas of the body in addition to the vulva. It was formerly classified as a mixed dystrophy when associated with squamous cell hyperplasia. When these two changes are associated, the current recommendation is to report both lichen sclerosus and squamous cell hyperplasia. The other specific dermatoses, such as psoriasis and lichen planus, should be diagnosed specifically. Lesions with associated squamous cellular atypia should be classified under VIN. When intraepithelial neoplasia is associated with a nonneoplastic epithelial disorder, both diagnoses should be listed separately.

a. Squamous cell hyperplasia–As already indicated, most examples of squamous cell hyperplasia probably represent lichen simplex chronicus. Hyperplastic lesions are usually associated with epithelial thickening and hyperkeratosis. Moisture, scratching, and rubbing, as well as the application of medications, may cause variation in the appearance of lesions in the same patient.

Squamous cell hyperplasia may be localized, elevated, well demarcated, or poorly demarcated (Fig 48–2). The vulvar tissues may appear red, or if a thick keratin layer is seen on the surface, they appear white. Lichenification, an accentuation of the skin markings, frequently occurs. Fissures and excoriations may result from chronic scratching. The latter

requires careful evaluation, because a carcinoma may appear first as a minute ulcer.

The microscopic findings consist of a variable degree of acanthosis with associated elongation and blunting of the epithelial folds. The granular layer is frequently prominent, and a thick keratin layer is often seen on the surface. An inflammatory infiltrate consisting primarily of lymphocytes and plasma cells is often seen in the upper dermis.

b. Lichen sclerosus–The vulva is a common site of lichen sclerosus (Fig 48–3). Occasionally, however, lichen sclerosus is found exclusively in nongenital areas. It may involve any or all areas of the vulva, including the perineal skin, the skin folds adjacent to the thighs, and the inner buttocks. Often, the changes extend around the anus in a figure-of-eight or keyhole fashion. The hood of the clitoris is frequently involved as well. Hart et al observed extragenital lesions in 5% of a group of patients they followed.

In lichen sclerosus, the skin frequently has a crinkled or parchmentlike appearance. At times, edema of the clitoral foreskin completely hides the clitoris. Phimosis of the clitoris may be seen late in the

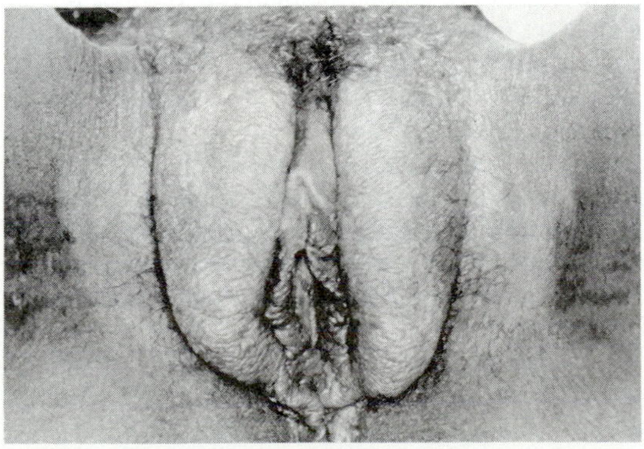

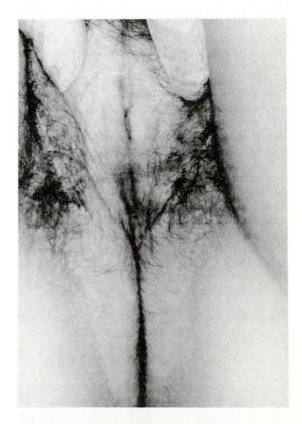

Figure 48–2. Squamous cell hyperplasia. Marked lichenification of the labia majora is evident.

Figure 48–3. Lichen sclerosus. The tissues have a crinkled white appearance. Phimosis is evident.

course of the disease. Often, the labia minora fuse to the labia majora and are not seen as distinct entities. Fissures often develop in the natural folds of the skin and in the posterior fourchette. The introitus may become stenotic and preclude sexual relations. Small areas of ecchymosis and telangiectasia are often noted.

The microscopic features of lichen sclerosus consist of epithelial thinning with flattening of the pegs, hyperkeratosis, cytoplasmic vacuolation of basal cells, and follicular plugging. Beneath the epidermis, a characteristic homogeneous pink-staining, relatively acellular zone is seen. An inflammatory infiltrate of lymphocytes and plasma cells is often seen deep to this acellular zone. Not uncommonly, areas of squamous cell hyperplasia are seen in association with lichen sclerosus. These changes probably represent a secondary response of the epithelium to chronic scratching of the tissues.

Occasionally, lichen sclerosus may be seen in a child. It has the same gross and microscopic features as noted in the adult.

Pruritus is the primary complaint of most individuals with squamous cell hyperplasia and lichen sclerosus. Occasionally, vulvar pain is the primary complaint. In individuals with introital stenosis, dyspareunia may be an associated complaint as well.

The likelihood of invasive squamous cell carcinoma developing in an individual with pure squamous cell hyperplasia is quite low. In the presence of lichen sclerosus, this probability increases to between 3 and 5% over a prolonged period of time. Cancer is seen most commonly in individuals with persistent pruritus with associated scratching who develop squamous cell hyperplasia along with the lichen sclerosus. Although the likelihood that vulvar squamous cell carcinoma will develop in a patient with squamous cell hyperplasia or lichen sclerosus is low, the risk is higher than that in the general population. Thus, these patients require careful management and follow-up.

Prior to undertaking therapy, a correct diagnosis should be established. This can best be accomplished by biopsy. Any aggravating factors such as candidiasis or other vaginitis, allergy, or contact irritants should be looked for and, if found, treated accordingly. Attention subsequently can be directed to specific control of the patient's symptoms, primarily pruritus.

The hyperplastic lesions are best treated with topical corticosteroids. The use of 0.025 or 0.01% fluocinolone acetonide, 0.01% triamcinolone acetonide, 1% or 2.5% hydrocortisone cream, or similar preparations 2–3 times daily usually relieves pruritus. One of the newer superpotent steroids, clobetasol 0.05%, may be successful in relieving pruritus when the preceding preparations are not successful. Long-term topical use of the mid- and high-potency steroids

should be with caution, because atrophy of the treated tissue may result.

Once pruritus is brought under control, these potent steroids should be discontinued and replaced with a medication containing hydrocortisone. Warm sitz baths 2–3 times daily offer temporary relief of pruritus. Lichen sclerosus can be treated with an ointment of testosterone in petrolatum. Testosterone propionate in sesame oil, 100 mg/mL, is mixed in petrolatum to obtain a 2% ointment. In the presence of significant pruritus, it is often of value to mix the testosterone in 1% hytone ointment—the latter containing a petrolatum base. This medication is applied 2–3 times daily for at least 3–6 months or until pruritus has subsided. Thereafter, the frequency of application is gradually reduced over 1–2 years until a maintenance level of application once or twice weekly is reached.

Clobetasol (0.05%) has been reported to be extremely effective in the management of lichen sclerosus. Bracco et al compared the efficacy of topical testosterone and topical progesterone with clobetasol. Clobetasol proved to be the most effective drug for relief of symptoms and improvement of objective and histopathologic findings. Clobetasol should be applied twice daily for 1 month, once daily for 2 months, and twice weekly for an additional 3 months.

On occasion, vulvar pruritus may persist despite medical therapy. Under these circumstances, the subcutaneous injection of triamcinolone may be used. Five milligrams of triamcinolone suspension is diluted in 2 mL of saline. A 3-inch spinal needle is inserted just below the mons pubis and passed subcutaneously through the labium majus to the perineum. As the needle is slowly withdrawn, the suspension is fanned out into the subcutaneous tissue. This process is repeated on the opposite side. The tissue should be gently massaged to disperse the suspension. If this approach does not offer lasting relief from pruritus, the subcutaneous injection of absolute alcohol may relieve the symptoms. This treatment requires hospitalization and anesthesia. Aliquots of 0.1–0.2 mL of alcohol are injected subcutaneously at 1-cm intervals over the vulva. After injection of the alcohol, the vulva should be gently massaged to disperse the alcohol.

The treatment of lichen sclerosus in a child is directed toward the relief of pruritus. This can often be accomplished with intermittent use of topical corticosteroids. Occasionally, a mixture of progesterone (100 mg in oil) mixed in 1 ounce of petrolatum may be effective.

c. Dermatoses–The characteristic findings of many dermatoses on the glabrous skin often are not observed when these changes involve the vulva. The local environment of moisture and warmth often alters the gross appearance of these lesions. For this reason, whenever changes are observed on the vulva that are not easily diagnosable, the remaining skin of the body should be carefully examined, looking for lesions that may give a clue to the changes seen on the vulva. The characteristic papular hyperemic scaly lesions of psoriasis may present as diffuse, well-demarcated, hyperemic areas on the vulva. Likewise, the violaceous papular lesions often associated with lichen planus are rarely seen involving the vulva. The most common manifestation of lichen planus involving the vulva is that of erosive lichen planus. Under these circumstances, the changes seen on the vulva consist of hyperemic eroded areas primarily involving the inner labia minora and vestibule. The lacy, white Wickham's striae also may be seen adjacent to these changes. Well-demarcated, hyperemic, eroded areas also are often seen within the vagina in such individuals. Approximately two-thirds of patients with erosive lichen planus involving the vulva have or eventually develop similar erosive lesions involving the gums. The management of the various dermatoses involving the vulva is complex and in most cases should be left to an experienced dermatologist.

2. Vulvar intraepithelial neoplasia–The International Society for the Study of Vulvar Disease has proposed a classification for intraepithelial neoplasia involving the vulva; the diseases of squamous cell type have been grouped under a single heading. Paget's disease and melanoma also may present as intraepithelial lesions, but they have distinctly different histopathologic appearances, histochemical characteristics, and natural history. Therefore, they have been listed separately in this classification. The classification is as follows:

Vulvar Intraepithelial Neoplasia (VIN)

1. Squamous cell (may include HPV change)
    a. VIN I (mild dysplasia)
    b. VIN II (moderate dysplasia)
    c. VIN III (severe dysplasia, carcinoma in situ)
2. Other
    a. Paget's disease (intraepithelial)
    b. Melanoma in situ (level 1)

a. VIN I and II–The appearance of these lesions is often quite distinct; they can be distinguished from hyperplastic lesions that do not show cellular atypia. The majority of lesions are well delineated, white, slightly elevated, and irregular. Occasionally, pigmented and red areas may be noted. Microscopic examination demonstrates mild cellular atypia beginning in the deeper portion of the epithelium with cell maturation occurring as the cells move toward the surface. The size and shape of the nuclei vary, and they are often hyperchromatic. Scattered atypical mitoses may be seen. The microscopic changes noted in VIN I and II must be distinguished from those observed in a "flat condyloma." In the latter, the nuclei may be hyperchromatic, large, and irregular, and multinucleated cells often are observed. Koilocytosis

is a prominent feature of the flat condyloma, but it also may be seen in association with VIN. The lack of significant pleomorphism and atypical mitotic figures distinguishes the flat condyloma from VIN.

b. VIN III (squamous carcinoma in situ)–No specific gross or microscopic feature is characteristic of VIN III. The changes seen grossly may vary from a localized, white, slightly raised lesion (Fig 48–4) to one that is diffuse (Fig 48–5) and involves labia majora, hood of the clitoris, labia minora, and perineum and may extend into the anal canal, vagina, and distal urethra. Lesions may at times appear red, moist, and crusted, and on other occasions, hyperpigmentation is the predominant finding. Not uncommonly, lesions may have a white, red, and pigmented appearance. Areas of ulceration, induration, and granularity should arouse suspicion of invasive carcinoma. Biopsy provides a definitive diagnosis.

Multifocal lesions are quite common, especially in individuals under 40 years of age. Bornstein et al, as well as Barbero et al, observed that at least one-third of the patients studied with VIN III had multifocal lesions.

The histopathologic features associated with VIN III include the presence of hyperchromatic, irregular nuclei arranged in a disorderly fashion. Multinucleated epidermal cells are occasionally present, and periodically, cytoplasmic vacuoles may be seen. Atypical mitoses are seen scattered throughout the epithelium. These changes may extend through the full thickness of the epithelium, or there may be a few layers of a superficial granular or hyperkeratotic layer. Occasionally, a well-differentiated form of VIN III may be seen. These lesions are believed to be unusually aggressive with a high propensity to progress to invasive squamous cell carcinoma.

c. Paget's disease–Extramammary Paget's disease is a slowly progressive intraepithelial carcinoma containing typical vacuolated Paget cells. The overwhelming majority of cases are intraepithelial in

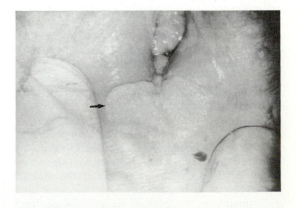

Figure 48–4. Vulvar intraepithelial neoplasia (VIN) III. A sharply demarcated, white lesion is noted *(arrow)*.

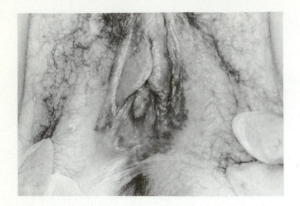

Figure 48–5. Vulvar intraepithelial neoplasia (VIN) III. Diffuse, confluent, pigmented lesions are seen.

location, and when recurrences occurs, they are usually intraepithelial. Rarely does primarily intraepithelial Paget's disease progress to invasive Paget's disease. However, it may be seen primarily as invasive disease and may, in a small percentage of instances, be associated with underlying sweat gland adenocarcinoma. Paget's disease also may be associated with a primary carcinoma of the anus or rectum, urethra, or bladder, especially when it involves the perianal region.

The typical appearance of Paget's disease is that of an erythematous, eczematoid lesion with scales and crusts scattered over the surface. It may also present as a white lesion or as a hyperemic lesion with scattered white plaques. The histopathologic changes are typical but occasionally can be confused with squamous cell carcinoma in situ and melanoma. Large, irregular Paget's cells containing clear vacuolated cytoplasm are characteristic. The nuclei are vesicular, vary in size and shape, and may exhibit hyperchromatosis. The Paget's cells often are seen in clusters in the deeper portions of the epithelial folds, and scattered cells may be distributed throughout the epithelium above. Occasionally, Paget's cells may be seen in the underlying skin appendages; this does not represent invasive carcinoma or a primary underlying adnexal carcinoma. The intraepidermal migration of Paget's cells is common, and often these cells extend well beyond the grossly visible disease. The latter accounts for incomplete excision and so-called recurrence of the tumor.

Histochemical staining should confirm the diagnosis of Paget's disease and rule out such lesions as melanoma and squamous cell carcinoma in situ. The finding of acid or neutral mucopolysaccharides within the cells is pathognomonic of the disease. Various monoclonal antibodies also have been used in distinguishing the cells of Paget's disease from those of intraepithelial squamous cell carcinoma and melanoma. The monoclonal antibodies KA-4 and GCDFP-15 can be used to distinguish the cells of Paget's disease from other intraepithelial disorders. In addition, Paget's cells almost invariably are positive with immunohistochemical staining for CEA.

The most commonly used treatment for intraepithelial neoplasia of the vulva is that of wide local excision of the lesion. This is easily accomplished in the presence of unifocal lesions; however, when multifocal disease is present, the wide local excision may consist of a "skinning" vulvectomy. The latter allows for the preservation of the normal anatomy of the vulva yet permits removal of extensive lesions. On occasion, the surgical defect must be covered with a skin graft. The carbon dioxide laser also has been found to be extremely effective in treating intraepithelial neoplasia of the vulva, especially for unifocal disease. Some clinicians avoid use of laser therapy when disease involves hair-bearing areas of the vulva. The intraepithelial neoplasia often extends down into the hair shafts, making it necessary to carry the laser destruction down to a depth of approximately 3 mm if all potential disease is to be eradicated. This often results in a prolonged, painful period of healing and resulting scarring.

In the presence of disease involving the clitoris, the vulvar lesions can be excised by wide local excision, and disease involving the clitoris can be eradicated using the carbon dioxide laser. This method allows for preservation of the clitoris. When local excision is used, it is advisable to obtain frozen sections of the excised margins of tissue to be sure that the disease has been adequately excised. If margins are positive, additional tissue should be excised.

Paget's disease of the vulva should be treated somewhat more aggressively because of the occasional association of an underlying skin-appendage adenocarcinoma. In addition, the intraepidermal migration of Paget's cells requires that a wide margin of normal tissue be removed when the primary lesion is excised. Even in the latter instance, recurrence of disease is not uncommon.

3. Vitiligo–Vitiligo is an autoimmune disease resulting in lack of pigmentation of the skin. The overwhelming majority of patients with vitiligo involving the vulva also demonstrate areas of vitiligo elsewhere on the body. Thus, the remaining glabrous skin should be carefully examined when these changes are noted on the vulva. In the presence of vitiligo, the tissues have a white, "nonpigmented" appearance. The skin appears perfectly normal in all other respects (Fig 48–6). Because of the white appearance of the skin associated with vitiligo, the condition may be confused with other white lesions involving the vulva. No effective therapy is available for the treatment of this condition.

B. Red Lesions:

1. Contact irritant dermatitis–One of the more common, yet often unrecognized, problems involving the vulva is that of contact irritant dermatitis.

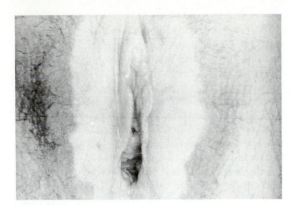

Figure 48–6. Vitiligo. Lack of pigmentation of the vulvar tissue is noted. In contrast to lichen sclerosus, the texture of the skin is normal.

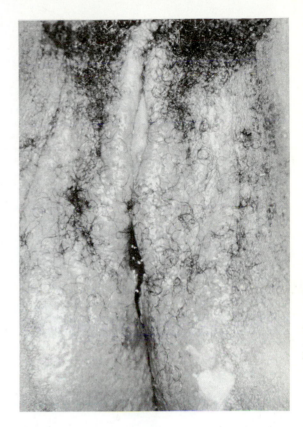

Figure 48–7. Severe contact irritant vulvitis. Long-term vulvitis secondary to topical use of various medications. (Reproduced, with permission, from Kaufman RH, Faro S: *Benign Diseases of the Vulva and Vagina.* Mosby-Yearbook, 1994.)

Often patients present with clinical symptoms related to a specific disease process such as candidiasis. Treatment of these conditions may result in a contact irritant or contact allergic dermatitis. Unfortunately, with the exacerbation of symptoms, it is assumed that the patient is not responding adequately to the treatment of the originally diagnosed disease. Other medications are prescribed, which often exacerbate the symptoms.

On inspection of the vulva, the tissues often have an erythematous, edematous appearance (Fig 48–7). Occasionally, vesiculation may occur with rupturing of the vesicles being accompanied by a moist "weeping" appearance. It is important that the clinician recognize the underlying cause of the patient's complaints, because the most appropriate treatment is to discontinue all local therapy and allow the tissues to undergo healing spontaneously. Warm sitz baths are of value in alleviating symptoms, and occasionally, the use of a topical 1% hydrocortisone cream helps alleviate the pruritus. An oral antihistamine may be of some value in reducing symptoms.

2. Candidiasis—Erythema of the vulvar vestibule and inner labia minora is common in association with vaginal candidiasis. Not uncommonly, however, patients also have a cutaneous candidiasis, which is associated with significant, diffuse hyperemia of the outer labia minora, the labia majora, and often the inner aspect of the thighs (Fig 48–8). Peripheral pustules also are often seen in the presence of cutaneous candidiasis. These patients usually complain of severe pruritus. The diagnosis is easily established by obtaining a scraping from the lesion, which is placed on a slide with 15% potassium hydroxide. The slide should be gently heated over a flame to help dissolve the keratinized cells, and the specimen is examined under the microscope. The presence of typical spores and mycelia establishes the diagnosis.

Cutaneous lesions can be treated effectively with

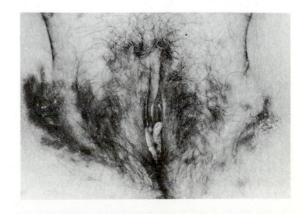

Figure 48–8. Cutaneous candidiasis. Diffuse erythema involving the labia majora and crural folds is seen.

topical 1% clotrimazole or 2% ketoconazole cream. Any one of a variety of antifungal medications can be used intravaginally to treat any vaginal infection present.

3. Invasive squamous cell carcinoma–Invasive squamous cell carcinoma most often presents as a raised, red, granular lesion (Fig 48–9). When seen early, these lesions may vary from 0.5 to 1 cm in diameter. In long-standing cases, however, the entire vulva may be replaced by an ulcerated, necrotic, indurated mass. Biopsy of the lesion confirms the diagnosis of invasive squamous cell carcinoma.

The treatment of invasive squamous cell carcinoma consists of wide local excision of the lesion. In the presence of large lesions, an extensive deep vulvectomy should be performed on the side of the lesion. If the carcinoma involves the midline or both sides of the vulva, bilateral inguinal femoral groin dissection should be carried out. If nodes are positive on the side of the neoplasm, the nodes on the opposite side should be surgically removed followed by radiotherapy to the deep pelvic lymph nodes.

4. Dermatophytoses–The dermatophytoses

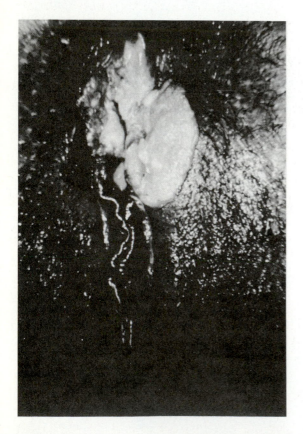

Figure 48–9. Invasive squamous cell carcinoma. A raised, red granular lesion is apparent involving the upper labia majora, labia minora, and clitoris.

are superficial fungal infections that involve the skin and its appendages. The fungi thrive best on softened skin such as that found in the groin area, where the environment of warmth and moisture predisposes to the growth of these organisms.

Tinea cruris is a fungal infection of the genitocrural area. The etiologic agents are *Epidermophyton floccosum, Trichophyton mentagrophytes,* and *T rubrum.* These organisms do not invade the tissue, and thus the lesions remain superficial and limited to the stratum corneum of the epidermis.

Infection begins as a small, erythematous patch with crusting or scale formation. The lesions spread peripherally and coalesce as they enlarge, with clearing occurring at the center of the lesion. The infection usually occurs on the upper, inner aspects of the thighs and may spread to the groin, perineum, and buttocks. The lesions are well circumscribed and have sharply defined margins that are erythematous and slightly elevated. They may vary in color from slightly pigmented to fiery red. Pruritus is the chief complaint.

The gross appearance of these lesions is characteristic enough to suggest the diagnosis strongly. Final diagnosis, however, depends on confirmation by smear or culture. The hyphae of the fungus can be found in marginal scrapings suspended in 10–20% KOH solution. On gentle heating over a lightbulb for 15–20 seconds, the keratinized, cellular debris dissolves, and the organisms are easier to find. The fungi also can be cultured on Sabouraud's medium.

The identification of hyphae alone on KOH smear helps distinguish tinea cruris from cutaneous candidiasis. Both hyphae and spores are formed in the presence of the latter infection.

Erythrasma is similar to tinea cruris in appearance, although it lacks an active border. It is associated with minimal or no itching and is fluorescent under Wood's light.

Miconazole nitrate cream, clotrimazole liquid or cream, and ketoconazole cream are specific therapeutic agents for most of the fungi causing the superficial mycoses. Any of these creams can be applied twice daily for a period of 2–3 weeks.

Erythrasma is effectively treated with oral erythromycin, 200 mg 4 times daily for 7 days. Scrubbing the affected area twice daily with an antibacterial soap also results in a cure in most patients.

5. Seborrheic dermatitis–Seborrheic dermatitis most commonly involves the scalp, mid portion of the face, and presternal and interscapular regions. However, the pubic, genital, and perianal regions also may become involved. The diagnosis of seborrheic dermatitis of the vulva is usually confirmed following identification of seborrheic dermatitis involving other areas of the body. The typical lesions of seborrheic dermatitis are pale to yellowish red and may be covered with dull, greasy, nonadherent scales and crusts. They are usually superficial and poorly defined. The lesions often take on an eczematoid appearance in the vulvar area because of the local environment of moisture and friction. The primary complaint is of mild-to-moderate pruritus.

Seborrheic dermatitis must be differentiated from psoriasis, cutaneous candidiasis, tinea cruris, and squamous cell hyperplasia (lichen simplex chronicus). Examination of scrapings from the lesion mixed in 10–20% KOH usually helps distinguish seborrheic dermatitis from candidiasis and tinea cruris.

Treatment of seborrheic dermatitis consists of the local application of a corticosteroid lotion or cream.

C. Pigmented Lesions:

1. Nevus–Nevi may be found on the vulva as well as other areas of the body. Their chief significance lies in their distinction from and possible development into melanoma. More than 50% of melanomas arise from preexisting nevi. Certain types of nevi carry a greater risk for the development of melanoma than others; these types are the dysplastic nevus and the congenital nevus. Individuals with dysplastic nevi usually have many lesions in contrast to the solitary or occasional lesion of the common nevus. The common nevus usually appears in young adulthood, whereas the dysplastic nevus appears in adolescence and may continue to appear in adulthood. Nevi are usually described as flat, slightly elevated, papillomatous, dome-shaped, and pedunculated. The flat nevus is usually junctional, whereas the other types are usually compound or intradermal.

The pigmented nevi vary in color from light tan to dark brown and vary considerably in size from 1 to 2 cm. The diagnosis is established by biopsy of the lesion.

Treatment of vulvar nevi consists of local excision. All pigmented lesions of the vulva should undergo biopsy, which can be accomplished easily by local excision.

2. Melanosis–Melanosis of the vulva is often confused with junctional nevi and melanoma. It usually presents as a pigmented patch that is flat and smooth (Fig 48–10). It may be focal or may present as a large, diffuse, macular, pigmented area. Biopsy of the area reveals the presence of increased numbers of typical melanocytes arranged in solitary units at the dermoepidermal junction of a hyperpigmented epidermis. These lesions are asymptomatic, and their significance lies in their confusion with other pigmented vulvar lesions such as VIN III or melanoma. Once the diagnosis is established, no therapy is required.

3. Melanoma–Approximately 1% of deaths from neoplasia are from melanomas. One to three percent of all malignant vulvar neoplasms are melanomas. Prevalence and associated mortality of melanoma make the early diagnosis extremely important. Any pigmented lesion demonstrating an increase in size, deepening of color, ulceration, or pigment incontinence along the edges should arouse

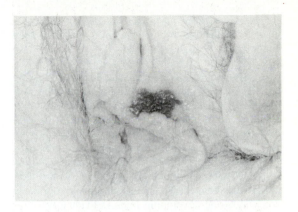

Figure 48–10. Melanosis. A sharply demarcated, pigmented area is seen on the outer aspect of the labium minus extending to the inner labium majus. (Reproduced, with permission, from Kaufman RH, Faro S: *Benign Diseases of the Vulva and Vagina.* Mosby-Yearbook, 1994.)

suspicion of melanoma. Melanomas may be seen as superficial spreading or nodular lesions. The superficial type usually has a better prognosis than the nodular melanoma. Biopsy is necessary to confirm the diagnosis. The prognosis is directly related to the depth of invasion of the melanoma. Disease limited to the epithelium or dermal papillae has an excellent prognosis, whereas melanoma cells that extend to the reticular dermis or subcutaneous fat have an extremely poor prognosis.

Treatment for melanoma consists of wide, deep excision of the lesion (partial deep vulvectomy) with removal of the ipsilateral inguinal and femoral lymph nodes. In the presence of metastasis to the regional lymph nodes, supplemental radiation therapy to the inguinal and femoral areas on both sides, as well as the deep pelvic lymph nodes should be carried out.

4. Seborrheic keratosis–Seborrheic keratosis is most commonly found on the trunk, face, neck, and arms of postmenopausal women. On occasion, however, lesions may appear on the vulva either as a solitary tumor or in association with similar growths elsewhere in the body.

Seborrheic keratoses are sharply demarcated, raised lesions that are usually papular but may appear flat. They vary in diameter from one to several centimeters and may appear singly or in groups. Most often, they are flesh-colored to brown, but they may appear black. The lesions often have a scaly appearance.

Treatment of seborrheic keratosis involves local excision. The lesion is limited in its growth potential and does not become malignant.

5. VIN III–VIN may present as a pigmented lesion or lesions. Often, multiple pigmented papules may be seen covering the labia majora and perineum.

The term **bowenoid papulosis** has been used to designate such lesions; morphologically, however, they demonstrate the changes of VIN III.

D. Erosive and Ulcerated Lesions:

1. Herpes simplex viral infections (HSV)–The majority of individuals infected with the herpes simplex virus never develop clinical manifestations of this infection. It is a sexually transmitted disease, and most infections involving the vulva are caused by HSV II. Herpes simplex viral infections of the lips are usually caused by HSV I. When clinical manifestations develop, they present as an initial primary, nonprimary, or recurrent infection. An initial primary infection is one developing in an individual who has never been exposed and developed antibodies to herpes simplex virus I or II. An initial nonprimary infection is defined as the first occurrence of clinical symptoms in an individual who already has antibodies to HSV I or II. Recurrent infection is defined as clinical manifestation in an individual with prior documented clinical manifestations of infection.

Herpes genitalis infection is acquired through sexual contact. The symptoms of a primary infection occur within 3–7 days after exposure. Mild paresthesia and burning may be experienced before lesions become visible. Occasionally, the patient may complain of a neuralgic pain radiating to the back or hips or down the legs. When lesions develop, the patient reports severe pain and tenderness in the affected tissues. She also may complain of dysuria, as well as inguinal and pelvic pain. The lesions seen in primary infections are often extensive and may involve the entire vulva, perineal skin, vestibule, vagina, and ectocervix. Initially, multiple vesicles may be seen, but these rupture rapidly and leave shallow, pink, ulcerated areas (Fig 48–11). Lesions may coalesce to form bullae that ultimately lead to large ulcerations. Superficial ulcerations may be seen on the ectocervix and within the vagina. Occasionally, a fungating necrotic mass may cover the entire ectocervix and be confused with invasive carcinoma of the cervix. The lesions seen in primary infection may persist for 2–6 weeks. After healing, no residual scarring or induration is noted.

Occasionally, meningitis and encephalitis may be associated with a primary infection. The recovery rate following meningitis is excellent; however, the mortality associated with HSV II encephalitis is quite high.

The symptoms associated with recurrent genital herpes viral infections are milder than those associated with primary infections. Frequently, prodromal symptoms of burning and tingling occur. These are followed by the formation of vesicles, which quickly rupture, leaving superficial ulcerated lesions (Fig 48–12). Healing usually occurs within 7–10 days after the onset of recurrences and leaves the vulva completely normal in appearance. Pain with recurrent infection may last from 5–7 days.

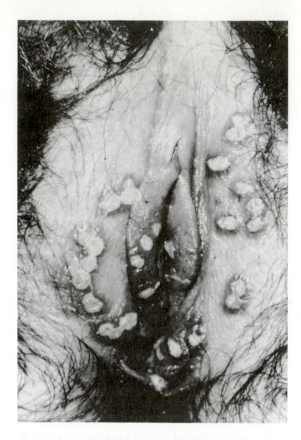

Figure 48–11. Primary herpes. Multiple ulcerated areas are scattered over the labia majora, labia minora, and perineum. A red area is noted around many of the ulcerations. (Reproduced, with permission, from Kaufman RH, Faro S: *Benign Diseases of the Vulva and Vagina.* Mosby-Yearbook, 1994.)

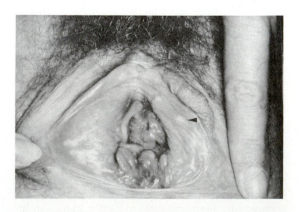

Figure 48–12. Recurrent herpes. Several superficial ulcers following rupture of the vesicles are noted *(arrow).*

Before any patient is labeled as having genital herpes, the diagnosis should be confirmed by both clinical and laboratory evaluation. This task is best accomplished by viral culture. The virus can be readily isolated from sterile cotton-tipped swab specimens taken from ulcers or recently ruptured vesicles. The swab should be placed in Eagle's medium containing 2% fetal bovine serum and antibiotics. The specimen should be transported rapidly to the virology laboratory. If rapid transport is not possible, the culture tube should be kept in a refrigerator at 4 °C until it can be sent to the laboratory. A positive culture can be established within 48–72 hours after inoculation of the culture medium. Viral cultures should be obtained as soon as possible after the onset of clinical symptoms, because viral titers quickly begin to diminish 48 hours after the onset of lesions.

Acyclovir is currently the most effective treatment for genital herpes simplex virus infections. For primary lesions, treatment should be instituted as soon as possible with 200 mg taken 5 times daily by mouth. This regimen should be continued until symptoms have disappeared (7–10 days). In the presence of severe primary infection, meningitis, or encephalitis, intravenous acyclovir should be instituted. Five milligrams per kilogram should be administered every 8 hours. In the presence of central nervous system involvement, 10–15 mg/kg every 8 hours should be given.

Treatment of recurrent infection should be instituted as soon as prodromal symptoms begin. Acyclovir, 200 mg 5 times daily, should be given orally for a period of 5 days or until the lesions regress. In the individual with frequently recurring episodes, long-term suppressive therapy with acyclovir is effective in preventing recurrences. In a recent completed study, 389 patients who completed 5 years of continuous suppressive treatment (400 mg twice daily) had a progressive decline in recurrences. Prior to institution of therapy, these individuals had an average of 12 recurrences per year. During the fifth year of therapy, an average of 0.8 recurrences for the year was noted.

The side effects from long-term suppressive therapy are minimal, and laboratory studies including complete blood cell count (CBC), liver enzymes, blood urea nitrogen (BUN), and urea remain consistently normal.

Valacyclovir will soon be available for the treatment of herpes viral infections. This drug converts to acyclovir following ingestion and has an oral potency equivalent to acyclovir administered intravenously.

2. Chancroid–The annual incidence of chancroid has increased in the United States over the last 40 years. However, its occurrence among women in the USA is still uncommon. Chancroid is responsible for 25–60% of genital ulcers in Asia and Africa, making it an important consideration when evaluating patients from these areas with a genital ulcer.

The lesion usually begins as a tender papule surrounded by erythema. Within 48 hours, it develops a pustular center that rapidly erodes and becomes ulcerated. The ulcer is extremely tender in contrast to the chancre of syphilis. Approximately one-third of the patients have multiple lesions, and closely approximated ulcers may fuse to form large ulcers. Inguinal lymphadenopathy is a common characteristic of this infection and occurs in approximately 50% of cases.

Diagnosis is based on history, clinical findings, symptoms, and the exclusion of other ulcerative diseases of the vulva. A Gram-stained smear is often diagnostic; diagnosis is based on the morphologic features and the arrangement of the bacilli causing this infection. The bacterium is a short, plump, coccobacillus and is gram-negative. Organisms may be seen intracellularly, but more often they are found in clusters outside polymorphonuclear leukocytes and arranged in groups often referred to as a "school of fish" arrangement. Obtaining a culture from the base of the ulcer or following aspiration of a suppurative bubo often confirms this infection. However, selective media must be used for culturing this organism, and the laboratory should be informed of the clinical diagnosis that is suspected.

Systemic antibiotic therapy with trimethoprim-sulfamethoxazole is effective in eradicating the causative organism, *Haemophilus ducreyi*. The recommended dose is one tablet (160 mg trimethoprim and 800 mg sulfamethoxazole) every 12 hours for 7–10 days. Erythromycin, 500 mg every 6 hours for 7–10 days, is also effective, as is azithromycin, 1 g orally in a single dose.

3. Syphilis–Both the primary and secondary lesions of syphilis may present as ulcerative vulvar lesions. If this infection is undiagnosed and left untreated, the long-term consequences are devastating. The causative agent, *Treponema pallidum,* is transmitted by intimate contact of an infected individual with another. The chancre, the lesion of primary syphilis, usually appears approximately 3 weeks after inoculation, although it may not appear for up to 3 months. It usually begins as an erythematous macule, following which a papule develops, which erodes in the center forming an ulcer. The ulcer has a clean, smooth base with a well-defined border (Fig 48–13). The chancre is painless unless it becomes secondarily infected. Approximately 1 week after the appearance of the chancre, unilateral or bilateral regional lymphadenopathy may occur. The chancre lasts for 2–8 weeks and then spontaneously disappears.

The diagnosis of primary syphilis is made by darkfield examination. The specimen should be obtained from the clean surface of a chancre by gentle rubbing of the ulcer. The serous exudate, free of red blood cells and cellular debris, is then examined using darkfield microscopy to identify the motile *T pallidum.* Lesions of secondary syphilis begin to appear

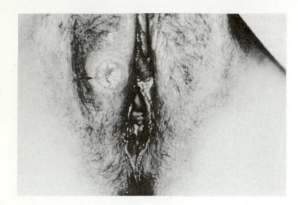

Figure 48–13. Chancre of primary syphilis **(arrow).** Darkfield examination revealed motile *Treponema pallidum.*

approximately 6 weeks after the chancre first appears. Vulvar manifestations include the development of papulosquamous, macular, and maculopapular lesions. These may coalesce to form large plaques and often are seen as moist, slightly raised, eroded, nontender areas. Inguinal lymphadenopathy is frequently seen.

The diagnosis of secondary syphilis commonly is missed, because the physician fails to consider syphilis in the differential diagnosis. The diagnosis can be confirmed on darkfield examination. At this stage of the disease, serologic tests also are positive. Benzathine penicillin, 1.2 million units intramuscularly into each buttock, is the usual treatment with both primary and secondary syphilis.

4. Granuloma inguinale—Granuloma inguinale is a chronic, progressively destructive infection if left untreated. The initial lesion is a papule that undergoes central necrosis to form a clean, granulomatous, sharply defined ulcer. The lesions have a beefy red base of granulation tissue and bleed easily on contact. The ulcers often are multiple because of autoinoculation, and these eventually may become confluent. The infection is caused by the organism *Calymmatobacterium granulomatis.* Secondary infection of the regional lymph nodes results in the development of bubos. The diagnosis of this infection is easily established by the demonstration of Donovan bodies in scrapings, tissue smears, or histopathologic specimens. Smears can be performed easily by taking a scraping from the lesion or by placing a small piece of tissue from the base of the lesion on a slide, crushing it between two slides, allowing it to air dry, and staining with Wright's or Giemsa stain. The Donovan bodies are seen as dark organisms that resemble a safety pin. They are frequently found within the numerous histocytes seen within the tissue.

Treatment of this infection is usually effective; it consists of tetracycline, 500 mg orally every 6 hours for 3 weeks or until the lesion has disappeared completely. Trimethoprim-sulfamethoxazole, two tablets twice daily for 14–21 days, is also effective therapy.

5. Erosive lichen planus, pemphigus, pemphigoid, and Behçet's disease—A number of autoimmune-related diseases may affect the vulva. These also are frequently associated with oral lesions, and in Behçet's disease, there are ocular manifestations. Erosive lichen planus may present as diffuse, eroded areas involving the inner labia minora, vulvar vestibule, and vagina. When the vagina is involved, a profuse seropurulent exudate may be present. In approximately two-thirds of patients, similar oral lesions are found or ultimately develop. Biopsy of the edge of an eroded area frequently demonstrates a characteristic bandlike infiltrate of lymphocytes approximating the epithelium or the eroded surface. The use of intravaginal hydrocortisone suppositories (one-half of a 25-mg suppository) inserted into the vagina twice daily has proved to be the most effective therapy for the vulvovaginal lesions.

Pemphigus vulgaris is a rare autoimmune blistering disease that usually affects older people. The mouth is often the first site to be affected, and the vulva is involved in approximately 10% of women with the disease. The changes are noted most often on the inner labia minora and vulvar vestibule. Bullae quickly rupture and present as shallow, red ulcerations with serpiginous borders. Immunofluorescent staining of a biopsy taken from the border of an eroded area (to include normal-appearing tissue) distinguishes this lesion from other erosive lesions. Pemphigoid is similar to pemphigus in that it is autoimmune in nature and is characterized by the formation of bullae with subsequent ulceration. Once again, immunofluorescent staining of a biopsy taken adjacent to a lesion allows for a specific diagnosis to be made. Both pemphigus and pemphigoid are treated most effectively using systemic steroids.

Behçet's disease is characterized by genital and oral ulceration, as well as ocular inflammation. In the more severe form of this disease, systemic manifestations involving the central nervous system, intestines, and kidneys are noted. The vulvar ulcers begin as small vesicles or papules that ulcerate and become craterlike. These ulcers tend to heal and recur at irregular intervals. Biopsy of a lesion often demonstrates findings that are suggestive but not diagnostic of Behçet's disease. No specific treatment has been successful; the best results have been obtained using 40 mg of triamcinolone injected intramuscularly 2 or 3 times at 10- to 14-day intervals.

Occasionally, vulvar manifestations may be seen in association with Crohn's disease. These may include perineal and vulvar abscesses, rectoperineal and rectovaginal fistulas, sinus tracts, and characteristic "knife cut" ulcers in the inguinal, genitocrural, and inner labial folds. Management is aimed at treatment of the intestinal disorder, although Millar has suggested the use of a local injection of triamcinolone suspension into the affected vulvar areas.

6. Basal cell carcinoma–Approximately 2–4% of the neoplasms involving the vulva are basal cell carcinomas. Typically, the vulvar tumors are slightly raised, slowly growing nodules with central ulceration and pearly rolled borders (Fig 48–14). The base of the ulcer may be covered with small amounts of necrotic debris or small crusts. If left untreated, the tumor may erode deeply into the underlying tissues and even into the bone of the symphysis pubis. These are locally destructive tumors that rarely metastasize. Biopsy confirms the diagnosis. Treatment is directed toward wide, local excision of the lesion.

E. Benign Tumors: A wide variety of benign cystic and solid tumors may involve the vulva. They may be classified as shown in Table 48–1. The majority of these tumors can be diagnosed easily on

Table 48–1. Classification of benign solid and cystic tumors.

Solid tumors
  Epidermal origin
    Condyloma acuminatum
    Molluscum contagiosum
    Acrochordon
    Seborrheic keratosis
    Nevus
    Keratoacanthoma
  Epidermal appendage origin
    Hidradenoma
    Sebaceous adenoma
    Basal cell carcinoma
  Mesodermal origin
    Fibroma
    Lipoma
    Neurofibroma
    Leiomyoma
    Granular cell tumor (myoblastoma)
    Hemangioma
    Pyogenic
    Lymphangioma
    Vulvovaginal polyp
  Bartholin's and vestibular gland origin
    Adenofibroma
    Mucous adenoma
  Urethral origin
    Caruncle
    Prolapse of urethral mucosa
Cystic tumors
  Epidermal origin
    Epidermal inclusion cysts
    Pilonidal cysts
  Epidermal appendage origin
    Sebaceous cysts
    Hidradenoma
    Fox-Fordyce disease
    Syringoma
  Embryonic remnant origin
    Mesonephric (Gartner's) cysts
    Paramesonephric (müllerian) cysts
    Urogenital sinus cysts
    Cysts of canal of Nuck (hydrocele)
    Adenosis
    Cysts of supernumerary mammary glands
    Dermoid cysts
  Bartholin's gland origin
    Duct cysts
    Abscesses
  Urethral and paraurethral origin
    Paraurethral (Skene's duct) cysts
    Urethral diverticula
  Miscellaneous origins
    Endometriosis
    Cystic lymphangioma
    Liquefied hematoma
    Vaginitis emphysematosa

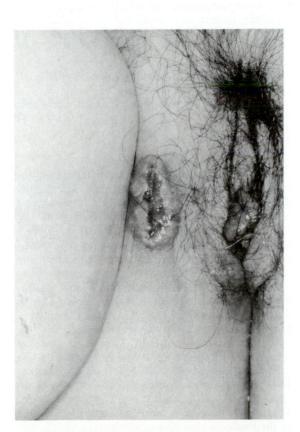

Figure 48–14. Basal cell carcinoma. Raised border and central ulceration are noted. (Reproduced, with permission, from Kaufman RH, Faro S: *Benign Diseases of the Vulva and Vagina.* Mosby-Yearbook, 1994. Courtesy of Dwayne Townsend, MD.)

gross inspection. The most important factors to consider are whether or not the lesion appears to be malignant and whether or not it is symptomatic. If even the slightest doubt exists concerning the correct diagnosis or potential malignancy of such a tumor, it should be either removed or biopsied.

Vulvodynia

One of the most perplexing problems faced by the clinician is that of persistent vulvar burning. The International Society for the Study of Vulvar Disease defines vulvodynia as "chronic vulvar discomfort, especially that characterized by the patient's complaint of burning, stinging, irritation, or rawness." This symptom must be distinguished from the complaint of pruritus. In some instances, there are no, or minimal, physical findings associated with the burning.

A. Approach to the Patient with Vulvodynia: In many instances, vulvar burning is associated with specific gross changes; therefore, it is important that, in addition to a careful history regarding the intensity of burning, cyclicity of symptoms, and relationship to contact with medications, a careful physical examination of the vulva and vagina should be carried out. It is also important to define specifically in what areas of the vulva the burning occurs. Does it involve primarily the labia majora and mons pubis, the region of the vulvar vestibule, or both? The following list shows several of the problems that may be associated with vulvodynia:

Dermatoses (erosive lichen planus or lichen sclerosus)
Behçet's syndrome, bullous dermatoses (ie, pemphigus vulgaris)
Contact irritant dermatitis (periorificial dermatitis)
Cyclic candidiasis
Herpes genitalis (postherpetic neuralgia)
Vulvar vestibulitis (HPV infection)
Referred nerve root pain
Pudendal neuralgia
"Essential or dysesthetic vulvodynia"

A careful history and physical examination often demonstrate obvious gross findings that give a clue to the correct diagnosis. The following steps should be carried out during the course of the examination:

1. Culture of vulva and vagina for candidal organisms.
2. Biopsy of any abnormalities noted.
3. Washing the vulva with 4–5% acetic acid looking for acetowhite change. Special attention should be directed toward the vestibule.
4. Wet mount preparation of vaginal secretions.
5. In the presence of erosive or bullous disease, biopsy with appropriate immunofluorescent staining (IgG, IgA, IgM, CIII) of biopsy.
6. Colposcopy.

The following steps should be followed in managing the patient with vulvodynia:

1. A correct diagnosis must be made.

2. Prior treatment must be stopped, especially if it is not relevant to the clinical impression or findings.
3. Steroids may be used for specific processes.
4. Long-term candidal therapy may be prescribed for individuals with chronic or cyclic candidiasis.
5. Acyclovir is given to the patient with herpes genitalis or possible postherpetic neuralgia.
6. Antidepressants, eg, amitriptyline or desipramine, may be helpful.
7. Emotional support is important.

B. Vulvar Vestibulitis: One of the most perplexing problems related to vulvodynia is vulvar vestibulitis. The largest subset of patients with vulvar pain is composed of patients suffering from this problem. Vestibulitis is associated with an exquisitely painful inflammatory process involving the vulvar vestibule.

Woodruff and Parmley reported a group of cases with vestibular pain and speculated that the disease represented infection of the minor vestibular glands. Friedrich termed this disorder "vulvar vestibulitis syndrome" and defined the diagnostic criteria as follows:

1. Severe pain on vestibular touch or attempted vaginal entry.
2. Tenderness to pressure localized within the vulvar vestibule.
3. Gross physical findings limited to vestibular erythema.

Most patients have had symptoms lasting for months to years and have seen many physicians in an attempt to obtain relief. Many patients report an absence of sexual lubrication, with a feeling that the vulvar tissues are being rubbed with sandpaper during intercourse. Many also have a history of recurrent vaginal candidiasis and condylomata acuminata. Turner and Marinoff reported an association of vulvar vestibulitis with HPV infection. More recently, Umpierre et al reported a subset of patients with vulvar vestibulitis in whom HPV DNA was identified in biopsy specimens taken from the vestibule.

Vestibulitis is best identified by careful history and careful inspection of the vulvar vestibule and vagina. Palpation of the vestibule with a moist cotton-tipped applicator usually elicits a sensation of severe pain. Not infrequently, areas of hyperemia are seen in the vestibule, especially around the openings of the Bartholin's and Skene's ducts (Fig 48–15). After the vestibule is washed with 5% acetic acid, an acetowhite change often is demonstrated covering either large areas of the vestibule or focal areas where tenderness is most pronounced.

Traditional therapy for vestibulitis has been peri-

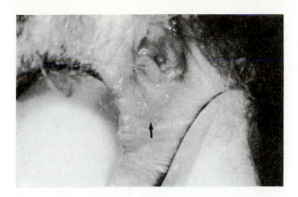

Figure 48–15. Vulvar vestibulitis. Hyperemic areas are noted in the posterior vestibule *(arrow)*. (Reproduced, with permission, from Kaufman RH, Faro S: *Benign Diseases of the Vulva and Vagina.* Mosby-Yearbook, 1994.)

neoplasty. This procedure encompasses surgically removing the vulvar vestibule and undermining the vaginal mucosa, which is brought down to cover the defect. Perineoplasty results in relief of symptoms in approximately 70–75% of cases. More recently, the intralesional injection of interferon has proved effective in treating these patients. One million units of recombinant alpha-interferon II is injected submucosally at a different location in the vestibule 3 times weekly for a total of 12 injections until the entire vestibule is injected with interferon in a clockwise fashion. The therapeutic success using this form of treatment has been reported as 50% or higher. One advantage is the fact that it is a noninvasive approach to management. Solomons et al have studied the use of a low-oxalate diet along with the ingestion of calcium citrate tablets in relieving the symptoms of vestibulitis. They have reported success using this approach to treatment, although success with this treatment has not been impressive.

VAGINITIS

The symptoms of leukorrhea, vulvar pruritus, irritation, and burning frequently are associated with one of several vaginal infections. The three most common types of vaginitis encountered by the clinician include candidiasis, bacterial vaginosis, and trichomoniasis. Although other, less common vaginal infections also can be associated with symptoms, this chapter is concerned primarily with these three infections.

In the presence of a mucopurulent discharge coming from the cervix or a hyperemic friable-appearing cervix, cultures should be taken from this area for *Chlamydia* and *Neisseria gonorrhoeae*. Both of these organisms can cause infections resulting in a profuse discharge coming from the cervix, which presents to the patient as a vaginal discharge.

Clinical Findings & Treatment

Careful inspection of the vulva and vagina often leads to a presumptive diagnosis; however, treatment should not be instituted until laboratory confirmation of the cause of the infection has been established. In the presence of a candidal infection, the vestibule often appears hyperemic. The characteristic white, cheesy, thrushlike patches are seen uncommonly in association with this infection; more often, a white, cheesy, or even creamy discharge is present. In the presence of trichomoniasis, the vulvar inner labia majora, labia minora, and vestibule frequently appear hyperemic, and a tan, creamy discharge that is occasionally frothy is noted. The discharge associated with bacterial vaginosis often has a disagreeable odor and appears grayish-tan. Rarely are there any irritative signs noted in association with bacterial vaginosis.

In the overwhelming majority of instances, a specific diagnosis is made on the basis of wet mount preparations and examination of the vaginal pH. The vaginal pH probably provides the best objective evidence regarding the vaginal ecosystem. The normal vaginal pH varies between 3.8 and 4.4. In the presence of a pH in this range, it is almost certain that trichomoniasis or bacterial vaginosis is not present. Candidal vaginitis, however, may be found when the vaginal pH is within the normal range. Bacterial vaginosis usually is associated with a pH of 5.0–6. Trichomoniasis is seen in the presence of a vaginal pH that is often 6.0 or higher. The saline and KOH wet mounts allow one to make a specific diagnosis of the cause of the vaginitis in most instances. A small amount of vaginal secretion is obtained on a cotton-tipped applicator and mixed with several drops of normal saline on a glass slide. A coverslip is added, and the secretion is examined under the microscope at both low and high powers. The presence of motile trichomonads, "clue" cells, or the hyphae and spores of *Candida* allow for a correct diagnosis. It is usually not necessary to perform cultures to establish a diagnosis. Furthermore, the finding of a predominant organism in a vaginal culture does not necessarily mean that this organism is the cause of the patient's symptoms. However, obtaining cultures from the vagina for *Candida* is often of value, because in a significant number of cases, the saline and KOH wet mount preparations are negative in the presence of a positive culture for *Candida*. If cultures are taken, it is of extreme importance for the clinician to inform the laboratory of the type of infection suspected so that the appropriate culture medium can be used.

A. Vaginal Candidiasis: *Candida albicans* is the species that is most often associated with this infection. Other species of *Candida* that occasionally result in clinical vaginitis include *C glabrata* and *C* *tropicalis.* Other species are occasionally recovered from the vagina, but these only rarely give rise to vaginitis.

1. Signs and symptoms–Vulvar pruritus is the main symptom of candidiasis. The itching may vary from slight to severe and may interfere with the individual's normal activities and rest. Patients often complain of a burning sensation, especially on urination. Dyspareunia is not uncommon. Leukorrhea is not a predominant symptom of candidiasis, although the majority of women with this infection complain of a slight discharge at some stage of the infection. Examination often reveals an abnormal redness of the vagina, although it is unmistakably present in only a small percentage of infected women. Typical thrushlike patches are not often seen, but when present, they consist of loosely adherent white or yellow curdy-appearing material (Fig 48–16). The vaginal secretions in most nonpregnant women with candidiasis are essentially normal in consistency, color, volume, and odor.

2. Diagnosis–Diagnosis depends on a demonstration of the *Candida* species and the presence of clinical symptoms compatible with the disease. As indicated, the vaginal pH usually remains within the normal range. Microscopic examination of vaginal material mixed with physiologic saline often reveals the spores and hyphae of the candidal organisms (Fig 48–17). Often, it is easier to identify the candidal organisms using 20% KOH rather than saline, because the former usually causes dissolution of the epithelial cells present in the smear. In the absence of identification of the organisms on KOH preparations, a culture should be taken using Sabouraud's medium.

3. Treatment–The most commonly used medications for treating candidal vaginitis include the various imidazole compounds. These act by interfering with the demethylation steps in ergosterol synthe-

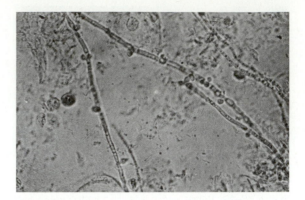

Figure 48–17. Candidiasis. Hyphae and conidia are seen using saline wet mount preparation.

sis, which is found within the yeast membrane wall, thus preventing the formation of normal yeast cell walls. Dosage recommendations vary from drug to drug; however, clotrimazole, miconazole, butaconazole, tioconazole, and ketoconazole intravaginally all appear to be equally effective. Depending on the medication and dosage used, treatment lasts from 3 to 7 days.

B. Trichomoniasis: Trichomoniasis is caused by infection with the organism *Trichomonas vaginalis.* It is a unicellular protozoan flagellate that usually can be identified easily by morphologic findings and movement characteristics in a saline wet mount preparation.

1. Signs and symptoms–Trichomoniasis exhibits a wide variety of clinical patterns. The symptoms associated with acute infection differ significantly from those seen in the individual with long-standing infection. The typical manifestations are a copious vaginal discharge, pruritus, and burning. Although the characteristics of this discharge are variable, usually there is a profuse, frothy discharge that is greenish in color and foul smelling. In the presence of a chronic infection, the discharge is usually moderately profuse, may be slight gray to tan in appearance, and is homogeneous. Generalized erythema is the only gross change noted within the vagina of some patients with acute infection. Pruritus of the vulva is found frequently in association with trichomoniasis. Erythema of the vulvar vestibule and inner labia minora are not uncommon. The diagnosis is established following identification of the motile trichomonad on a saline wet mount preparation (Fig 48–18). A culture is rarely necessary to identify the organism.

2. Treatment–Metronidazole is currently the standard for the treatment of this infection. A single dose, of 2 g of the medication may be used. Other approaches to therapy include a regimen of 250 mg, 3 times daily for 7 days, or 500 mg, twice daily for 5

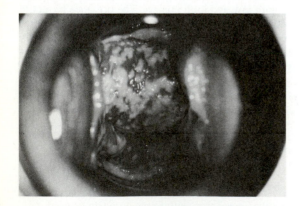

Figure 48–16. Candidiasis. "Thrush" patches are seen adherent to the vaginal wall. (Reproduced, with permission, from Kaufman RH, Faro S: *Benign Diseases of the Vulva and Vagina.* Mosby-Yearbook, 1994.)

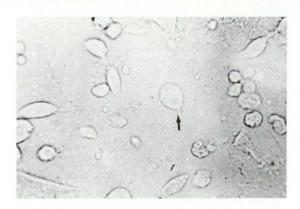

Figure 48–18. Trichomoniasis. Wet mount preparation with physiologic saline reveals multiple trichomonads *(arrow)*.

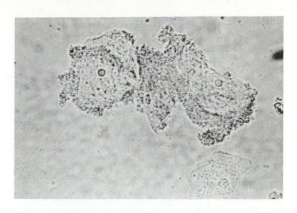

Figure 48–20. Bacterial vaginosis. Clue cells are evident. (Reproduced, with permission, from Kaufman RH, Faro S: *Benign Diseases of the Vulva and Vagina.* Mosby-Yearbook, 1994.)

days. However, the single 2-g oral dose appears to be as effective as the other approaches to treatment. The sexual partner of the patient also should be treated.

C. Bacterial Vaginosis: Bacterial vaginosis is a polymicrobial syndrome occurring as the result of a synergism between *Gardnerella vaginalis* and anaerobic bacteria, including mobiluncus species and *Bacteroides*. Bacterial vaginosis is regarded as a sexually transmitted disease by many individuals, but there is some disagreement on this issue.

1. Signs and symptoms–The predominant symptom is a profuse, foul-smelling vaginal discharge. Examination reveals a normal-appearing vulva with a slate-gray, homogeneous discharge present within the vagina (Fig 48–19). The vaginal mucosa appears normal, and there is none of the inflammatory response noted with candidal or trichomonal infections. The vaginal discharge usually has an offensive, foul odor.

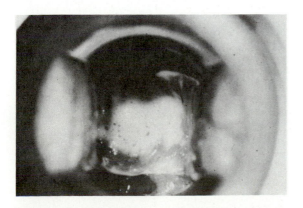

Figure 48–19. Bacterial vaginosis. A thin, creamy discharge is noted within the vagina. (Reproduced, with permission, from Kaufman RH, Faro S: *Benign Diseases of the Vulva and Vagina.* Mosby-Yearbook, 1994.)

2. Diagnosis–The diagnosis usually can be readily established on careful examination of the patient, measurement of vaginal pH, and examination of a wet mount preparation. The vaginal pH is elevated above 5. As already indicated, the discharge has a foul odor, but if this is not readily noticeable, the addition of a few drops of 20% KOH to some of this discharge results in an offensive odor (whiff test). Wet mount preparation demonstrates the presence of characteristic "clue" cells (Fig 48–20). These are squamous epithelial cells covered by adherent, rodlike bacteria. In addition to the clue cells, the absence of lactobacilli is another essential feature seen in association with this infection.

3. Treatment–Metronidazole is still the first-line therapy for this infection. Five hundred milligrams twice daily for 7 days is effective in eliminating the symptoms. As indicated, there is some dispute as to whether the male consort should be treated. If resolution of symptoms after treatment is followed by a recurrence, certainly both the female and male partner should be treated at that time.

Several topical agents have been found to be extremely effective in treating bacterial vaginosis. Clindamycin 2% cream used once daily for 7 days and metronidazole gel applied twice daily for 5 days have proved to be effective agents in eradicating the infection.

REFERENCES

Barbero M et al: Vulvar intraepithelial neoplasia: A clinical pathologic study of 60 cases. J Reprod Med 1990; 35:1023.

Bornstein J et al: Multicentric intraepithelial neoplasia involving the vulva. Cancer 1988;62:1601.

Bracco GL et al: A critical evaluation of clinical and histologic effects of topical treatment of lichen sclerosus with 2% testosterone, 2% progesterone, and 0.05% clobetasol and cream base. Proceedings of The International Society for the Study of Vulvar Disease, September 1991.

Friedrich EG Jr: Vulvar vestibulitis syndrome. J Reprod Med 1987;32:110.

Goldberg LH et al: Long term suppression of recurrent genital herpes with acyclovir. Arch Dermatol 1993;120:582.

Hart WR, Norris, HJ, Helwig EB: Relation of lichen sclerosus and atrophicus of the vulva to the development of carcinoma. Obstet Gynecol 1975;45:369.

Internal Society for the Study of Vulvar Disease: ISSVD committee report on vulvodynia, vulvar vestibulitis, and vestibular papillomatosis. J Reprod Med 1991;36:413.

Kaufman RH, Faro S: *Benign Diseases of the Vulva and Vagina,* 4th ed. Mosby-Yearbook, 1994.

Lever WF, Schaumburg-Lever G: *Histopathology of the Skin,* 7th ed. Lippincott, 1990.

Mann MS, Kaufman RH: Erosive lichen planus of the vulva. Clin Obstet Gynecol 1991;34:605.

Mann MS et al: Vulvar vestibulitis: Significant variables in treatment outcome. Obstet Gynecol 1992;79:122.

Millar D: Crohn's disease of the vulva. J R Soc Med 1992;85:305.

Solomons CC, Melmed MH, Heitler SM: Calcium citrate for vulvar vestibulitis. J Reprod Med 1991;36:879.

Turner MLC, Marinoff SC: Association of human papillomavirus with vulvodynia and the vulvar vestibulitis syndrome. J Reprod Med 1988;33:533.

Umpierre SA et al: Human papillomavirus DNA in tissue biopsy specimens of vulvar vestibulitis patients treated with interferon. Obstet Gynecol 1991;78:693.

Woodruff JD, Parmley TH: Infection of the minor vestibular gland. Obstet Gynecol 1983;62:609.

Woodruff JD, Thompson B: Local alcohol injection in the treatment of vulvar pruritus. Obstet Gynecol 1972; 40:18.

Cervical Cancer Screening & Management of the Abnormal Papanicolaou Smear

49

Howard G. Muntz, MD

Essentials of Diagnosis

- Most women with abnormal Papanicolaou smears are asymptomatic.
- Early cytologic detection of preinvasive lesions or minimally invasive cancers in asymptomatic women allows effective treatment without significant morbidity and usually with preservation of fertility.
- Colposcopy is essential to the diagnosis and management of preinvasive and microinvasive cervical neoplasia because it shows the changes in color, vascular pattern, and surface contour that identify neoplastic regions on the cervix.
- Women with deeply invasive cervical cancer usually report abnormal vaginal bleeding or discharge, and a gross cervical tumor is seen on pelvic examination.
- Signs of advanced cervical cancer include replacement of the cervix and upper vagina by a large friable tumor mass, erosion into the bladder or rectum, ureteral obstruction, and metastatic spread to the liver, lungs, and retroperitoneal lymph nodes.

Incidence

In developed countries with Papanicolaou (Pap) smear cytologic screening programs, there has been a dramatic fall in cervical cancer incidence and mortality rates and an increase in the incidence of cervical carcinoma in situ (CIS). In the United States in 1994, there were an estimated 50,000 cases of CIS, but only 15,000 cases of invasive cervical cancer, resulting in 4600 deaths. These favorable ratios are related to the high proportion of patients with preinvasive or early-stage cervical neoplasia detected by Pap smear screening. Overall, cervical cancer ranks as only the seventh cause of cancer mortality among women in the USA. In underdeveloped countries with inadequate Pap smear screening programs, cervical cancer is still the leading cause of cancer deaths among women.

The age-specific incidence of cervical CIS and invasive cancer (Fig 49–1) affects the rational approach to Pap smear screening. The incidence of cer-

> Essentials of Diagnosis
> Incidence
> Risk Factors
> Screening
> Pap Smear Classification Systems
> Evaluation
> Treatment of Cervical Dysplasia
> Referral to a Specialist
> Issues of Pregnancy & an Abnormal Pap Smear
> Psychosocial Concerns
> Controversies & Unresolved Issues

vical CIS peaks between ages 25 and 35, whereas invasive cervical cancer rates increase with age. In some populations, preinvasive cervical lesions occur at a very early age, perhaps related to sexual practices among young teenagers. At the opposite end of the age spectrum, epidemiologic data indicate a problem with controlling cervical cancer in elderly women.

The overall incidence of Pap smear abnormalities has risen rapidly over the last 2 decades. Currently, in a typical screening program, up to 5% of all Pap smears may be interpreted as abnormal, although the exact proportion varies widely. A major challenge in women's health care is to provide cost-effective yet reliable evaluation of a large number of abnormal smears.

Risk Factors

Epidemiologic and other circumstantial evidence suggests that cervical neoplasia is initiated by sexually transmitted carcinogens. Strong evidence has emerged linking human papillomavirus (HPV) infection with cervical neoplasia. HPV types 16 and 18 are associated most often with cervical cancer and higher grades of dysplasia (Table 49–1). Research has shown recently that the E6 and E7 gene products of HPV types 16 and 18 interact with the retinoblastoma and p53 factors, resulting in deregulation of cell

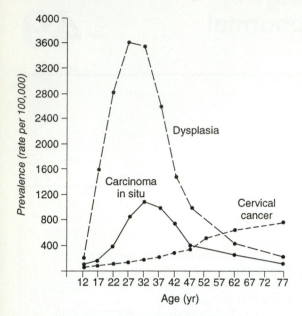

Figure 49–1. Age-specific incidence of cervical dysplasia, carcinoma in situ (CIS), and invasive cancer. The incidence of cervical dysplasia and CIS rises sharply at approximately age 20 and peaks between ages 25 and 35. Invasive cervical cancer rates have a more gradual rise, with the highest incidence from age 50 through senescence. (Reproduced, with permission, from Reid R, Fu YU: In: *Banbury Report 21: Viral Etiology of Cervical Cancer.* Peto R (editor). Cold Spring Harbor Laboratory Press, 1986.)

proliferation. Although HPV-mediated effects appear important in the process of malignant transformation, they are not sufficient to cause cervical cancer. Presence of cofactors, such as exposure to carcinogens in cigarette smoke, may be as important as infection with a high-risk HPV type.

Most of the well-known epidemiologic risk factors for cervical cancer (Table 49–2) can be accounted for by such a multistep theory of carcinogenesis. Unfortunately, many of these factors, such as early age at first intercourse and exposure to a "high-risk" male partner, are beyond the province of the health care provider. Also, HPV is highly infectious, and dis-

Table 49–1. Common types of human papillomavirus (HPV) and association with different clinical conditions.

HPV Type	Association
1–4	Common skin wart
6, 11	Benign condylomata of lower genital tract
16, 18	Invasive cancers and high-grade dysplasia of the cervix
31, 33	Intermediate risk for cervical dysplasia and cancer

Table 49–2. Risk factors associated with cervical cancer.

Early age at first intercourse
Multiple sex partners
"High-risk" male consort
Low socioeconomic status
Black race
Early age at childbearing
Intrauterine diethylstilbestrol (DES) exposure
Human papillomavirus (HPV) infection
Herpes simplex virus (HSV II) infection
Compromised immunity, including HIV infection
Deficiency in vitamins A and C
Cigarette smoking

semination in a sexually active population is probably not preventable. Although the use of condoms and other safe sex practices should be encouraged on general principles, they are ineffective against transmission of HPV, which has a large reservoir in genital tract skin and mucous membranes. Clinicians must be aware that, based on epidemiologic data, almost all women in the USA are at risk for cervical cancer.

Screening

A. Guidelines: There is universal agreement that an effective Pap smear screening program can dramatically reduce cervical cancer incidence and mortality. However, the optimal interval for obtaining smears remains controversial. The theoretic benefit of annual screening is supported by a number of case-control studies that demonstrate progressively decreasing cervical cancer incidence and mortality rates as screening intervals are shortened. However, most of the benefit from Pap smear screening can be achieved with intervals of 2–3 years, which is more cost-effective than shorter intervals, as emphasized by the original 1976 Canadian Walton Report. A consensus was reached in 1988 among the American Cancer Society, American College of Obstetricians and Gynecologists, American Medical Association, National Cancer Institute, and other organizations (Table 49–3). The 1988 guidelines endorse annual

Table 49–3. Recommendation for cervical cancer screening.*

Papanicolaou (Pap) smear screening should begin when a woman becomes sexually active or reaches age 18.
Screening should be performed every year until three or more annual Pap smears have been normal; thereafter, it can be performed less frequently if recommended by a physician.
There is no upper age limit on testing.

*American Cancer Society, 1988 (with consensus of American Medical Association, National Cancer Institute, American Nurses' Association, American Academy of Family Physicians, American Medical Women's Association, and American College of Obstetricians and Gynecologists).

screening, but they recommend that the clinician lengthen screening intervals after three consecutive negative smears for individual patients who are at low risk for cervical cancer.

Whether elderly women require Pap smear screening is also controversial. The 1988 consensus guidelines have no upper age limit for Pap smear screening. Other organizations (including the Canadian and US Preventive Services Task Forces) have recommended that Pap smear screening cease at age 60, on the assumption that a woman with serial normal smears in her younger and middle-aged years will have a negligible risk of developing cancer as an older woman. As noted previously, however, the incidence and mortality rates in the USA for cervical cancer are highest among older women, which is evidence that this population is currently underscreened. Primary care practitioners must ensure that their older patients have had several documented normal smears before Pap smear screening is halted solely on the basis of age. After that time, annual inspection of the female genital tract to screen for pelvic tumors and gynecologic problems should continue.

A related issue is vaginal apex Pap smear screening of posthysterectomy patients. Any woman who underwent a supracervical hysterectomy still has a cervix and thus needs to have Pap smears. Fortunately, almost all hysterectomies performed in the last 2 decades involved complete resection of the cervix (total abdominal hysterectomy or any vaginal hysterectomy). Because vaginal cancer is so rare, vaginal apex Pap smear screening after a hysterectomy is probably not necessary for most women. However, the risk of vaginal cancer is significant for women previously treated for lower genital tract dysplasia or cancer or who were exposed to diethylstilbestrol (DES) in utero; Pap smear screening should continue indefinitely for those two groups of women. Women who have had a hysterectomy for endometrial cancer also should have vaginal apex Pap smears indefinitely.

B. Pap Smear Technique: Most cervical dysplasias arise in the transformation zone. This region is usually located at or near the cervical os and represents the junction between the squamous epithelium of the vagina and exocervix and the columnar epithelium of the endocervix and endometrium (Figs 49–2 and 49–3).

Most false-negative Pap smears are due to sampling error by the clinician rather than faulty interpretation by the cytologist. The specimen should not be contaminated by lubricant and should be obtained before samples are acquired for cervical cultures. Large amounts of vaginal discharge, if present, should be removed gently. With care taken to avoid excessive bleeding, the clinician scrapes a wooden or plastic spatula circumferentially over the exocervix; this step is followed by a gentle, partial rotation of an endocervical brush within the cervical canal. An ad-

ditional circumferential smear of the upper two-thirds of the vagina should be obtained in DES-exposed women. The material obtained should be smeared on a glass slide and fixative rapidly applied. Air drying, which can occur within a few seconds, renders the sample uninterpretable.

The adequacy of the specimen should be described in the report from the cytologic laboratory. Smears should be repeated when considered unsatisfactory for evaluation because of too few endocervical cells, excessive blood, or inflammation. In the latter situation, a repeat smear can be delayed until after treatment for any infectious cause of cervicitis or vaginitis. The clinician should recognize that the intense inflammation and bloody discharge associated with an occult cancer could be the underlying reason for the inadequate smear.

Pap Smear Classification Systems

A. Background: The cytologic assessment of cervicovaginal smears, as originally proposed by Papanicolaou and Traut in 1941, was intended specifically for the early detection of invasive cervical cancers. It was not until the 1960s that preinvasive disease of the cervix was appreciated fully, leading to changes in both cytologic and histologic terminology. Figure 49–2 illustrates the spectrum of cervical disease, ranging from normal squamous epithelium to microinvasive squamous carcinoma. Progressive replacement of the epithelium by dysplastic cells defines the worsening degrees of dysplasia. The cervical intraepithelial neoplasia (CIN) nomenclature, introduced in the 1970s, closely parallels the dysplasia system (Table 49–4).

B. The Bethesda System: Although together the dysplasia and CIN nomenclatures have been used for several decades, variability in reporting results from different laboratories has hampered effective clinical management. A national interdisciplinary group was convened, therefore, in 1988 to standardize the interpretation of cervical Pap smears and biopsies, leading to the Bethesda system (Table 49–5, which includes minor 1991 revisions). The most sweeping change was the use of only two terms, low-grade squamous intraepithelial lesion (LSIL) and high-grade squamous intraepithelial lesion (HSIL), to encompass the entire spectrum of squamous cell carcinoma precursors. The LSIL category includes CIN I (mild dysplasia) as well as HPV-associated changes (koilocytosis). Although it is controversial, the Bethesda system thereby recognizes both the linkage of HPV infection with cervical neoplasia and the practical difficulty in distinguishing koilocytosis from mild dysplasia by cytologic or histologic criteria. The HSIL category includes CIN II and III (moderate dysplasia, severe dysplasia, and carcinoma in situ). Because the management of CIN II and CIN III is so similar, clinicians have welcomed this change.

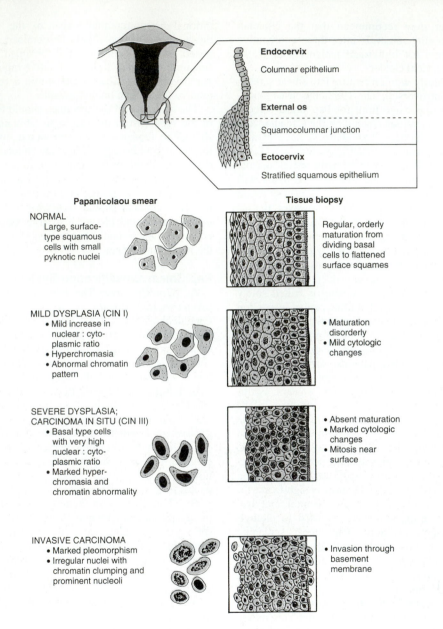

Papanicolaou smear

Tissue biopsy

NORMAL
  Large, surface-
  type squamous
  cells with small
  pyknotic nuclei

Regular, orderly
maturation from
dividing basal
cells to flattened
surface squames

MILD DYSPLASIA (CIN I)
  • Mild increase in
    nuclear : cyto-
    plasmic ratio
  • Hyperchromasia
  • Abnormal chromatin
    pattern

• Maturation
  disorderly
• Mild cytologic
  changes

SEVERE DYSPLASIA;
CARCINOMA IN SITU (CIN III)
  • Basal type cells
    with very high
    nuclear : cyto-
    plasmic ratio
  • Marked hyper-
    chromasia and
    chromatin abnormality

• Absent maturation
• Marked cytologic
  changes
• Mitosis near
  surface

INVASIVE CARCINOMA
  • Marked pleomorphism
  • Irregular nuclei with
    chromatin clumping and
    prominent nucleoli

• Invasion through
  basement
  membrane

Figure 49–2. Squamous epithelial dysplasia and carcinoma of the cervix, showing criteria used to grade dysplasia. (Reproduced, with permission, from Chandrasoma P, Taylor CR: *Concise Pathology.* Appleton & Lange, 1991.)

Another important change is the requirement that adequacy of the cytologic specimen be described. The Bethesda system also sought to define more precisely the term **atypia,** which in the past had become so overused it was clinically meaningless. The new category **atypical squamous cells of undetermined significance (ASCUS)** should be applied to relatively few cases. Glandular cell abnormalities also are reported more precisely in the Bethesda system. However, the accurate diagnosis of cervical adenocarcinoma precursors by cytologic testing can be dif-

ficult, and such cases should be reviewed by an experienced gynecologic cytopathologist.

Evaluation

A. Indications for Colposcopy: An abnormal Pap smear report merely identifies a patient who needs additional evaluation. The severity of the cervical lesion and its precise topographic location can be determined best by colposcopically directed cervical biopsies. Any woman with a Pap smear diagnosis

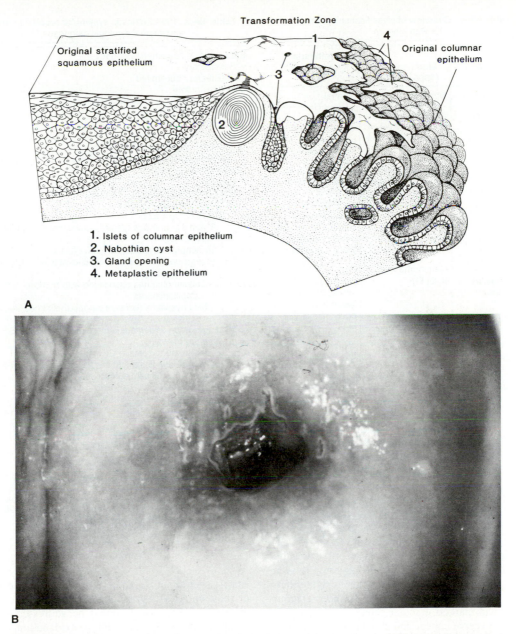

1. Islets of columnar epithelium
2. Nabothian cyst
3. Gland opening
4. Metaplastic epithelium

A

B

Figure 49–3. The transformation zone and the physiologic squamocolumnar junction. At birth, the squamocolumnar junction usually is located on the exocervix. Beginning in adolescence, it gradually migrates into the cervical canal as columnar epithelium, undergoes metaplasia, and matures into squamous epithelium. **A:** Schematic diagram. **B:** Colpophotograph of normal transformation zone. Note the squamocolumnar junction and gland openings. (Reproduced, with permission, from Burke L, Antonioli DA, Ducatman BS: *Colposcopy: Text and Atlas.* Appleton & Lange, 1991.)

of SIL (either low- or high-grade) should undergo colposcopic evaluation promptly.

Significant controversy exists concerning the evaluation of the atypical Pap smear, however. Earlier series have identified dysplasia in 15–77% of patients with persistently atypical smears. This wide disparity can be attributed to variable definitions of atypia and to dissimilar patient populations. Under the Bethesda system, there should be a low rate of occult dysplasia among smears classified in the new ASCUS category. Official recommendations for management of these ASCUS smears are still lacking, however, because of interlaboratory variability and limited long-term experience with the Bethesda system. Table 49–6 lists acceptable management options.

B. Technique of Colposcopy: Colposcopic

Table 49–4. Overview of classification systems for Pap smears.*

Original "class" system	Modifications (1960s, 1970s)	Bethesda system† (1988, 1991)
Class I–normal	Normal	Normal
Class II–slightly suspicious for malignancy	Atypical cells, but below the level of cervical neoplasia	Atypical squamous cells of undetermined significance (ASCUS)
Class III–moderately suspicious for malignancy	Dysplastic cells present consistent with intraepithelial neoplasia; often graded as cervical intraepithelial neoplasia (CIN) I–III	Low-grade squamous intraepithelial lesion (LSIL); equivalent to changes associated with human papillomavirus (HPV) and CIN I
Class IV–highly suspicious for malignancy	Carcinoma in situ (CIN III)	High-grade squamous intraepithelial lesion (HSIL); equivalent to CIN II–III
Class V–diagnostic for malignancy	Invasive cancer	Invasive cancer

*These systems are not directly interchangeable.
†Table 49–5 contains additional details of the Bethesda system.

Table 49–5. 1988 Bethesda system for reporting cervical and vaginal cytologic diagnoses.*

Statement on specimen adequacy
  Satisfactory
  Satisfactory but limited
  Unsatisfactory
  (Specify reason for nonsatisfactory smears)
General categorization
  Within normal limits
  Benign cellular changes
  Epithelial cell abnormality
  (See descriptive diagnosis for details)
Descriptive diagnoses
  Infection
  Reactive and reparative changes
  Epithelial cell abnormalities
    SQUAMOUS CELL
      Atypical squamous cells of undetermined significance (ASCUS)
      Squamous intraepithelial lesion (SIL)
      Low-grade squamous intraepithelial lesion (LSIL) encompassing:
        Cellular changes associated with human papillomavirus
        Mild dysplasia (cervical intraepithelial neoplasia [CIN]–I)
      High-grade squamous intraepithelial lesion (HSIL) encompassing:
        Moderate dysplasia (CIN-II)
        Severe dysplasia and carcinoma in situ (CIN-III)
      Squamous cell carcinoma
    GLANDULAR CELL
      Presence of unexpected endometrial cells
      Atypical glandular cells of undetermined significance (AGCUS)
      Endocervical adenocarcinoma
      Endometrial adenocarcinoma
      Other adenocarcinoma
Nonepithelial malignant neoplasm: specify
Hormonal evaluation (applies to vaginal smears only)
Recommended action

*Complete Bethesda system is reported in JAMA 1989;262: 931 and in J Reprod Med 1992;37:383.

evaluation relies on stereoscopic magnification to visualize the changes in color, vascular pattern, and surface contour that identify neoplastic regions on the cervix (Fig 49–4). The vagina and vulva also should be evaluated carefully, because vulvovaginal dysplasias and cancers may coexist with cervical lesions. The application of 3% acetic acid causes neoplastic regions to appear white as the result of transient dehydration. Abnormal vascularity, usually recognized as mosaic or punctate patterns, is seen more easily when viewed with a green light filter. Dense acetowhitening, unusual surface contour changes, and marked vascular changes are hallmarks of occult invasive cancer and should be recognizable by any clinician performing colposcopic examinations.

A careful description of the extent of the dysplastic lesions is necessary in planning subsequent therapy. Colposcopy is considered satisfactory when the entire transformation zone and any associated abnormalities can be visualized fully. An unsatisfactory colposcopic examination is dangerously inaccurate, because occult carcinoma may escape detection. Use of an endocervical speculum converts to satisfactory many examinations initially considered unsatisfactory. Areas demonstrating colposcopic changes consistent with neoplasia can then be biopsied with minimal discomfort (Fig 49–5). In general, an endocervical curettage (ECC) also should be performed. HSIL Pap smears should not be ignored if biopsies are negative or show only LSIL. Although possible "over-call" of the original Pap smear should be addressed by the cytopathologist, the more likely explanation of this discrepancy is an error by the colposcopist. Repeat colposcopy should be performed promptly. A diagnostic cervical conization may be necessary.

C. Cervical Conization: As a diagnostic procedure, cone biopsy of the cervix (Fig 49–6) should be performed when any of the following four clinical situations is present: (1) the colposcopic examination is unsatisfactory; (2) the endocervical curettage is positive for neoplasia; (3) the cytologic diagnosis is significantly more severe than shown by the colposcopically directed biopsies; or (4) biopsies suggest a microinvasive cancer or adenocarcinoma in situ. The wide adoption of colposcopic technique has reduced the number of diagnostic cone biopsies performed in the USA.

Table 49–6. Management options* for the diagnosis of atypical squamous cells of uncertain significance (ASCUS) on Pap smear.†

Immediate referral for colposcopy
Patients at significant risk of occult dysplasia or cancer
Persistently atypical smears
Prior treatment for dysplasia
Epidemiologic high risk (see Table 49–2)
AIDS or HIV-seropositive
Patient considered unreliable for long-term monitoring
Antibiotic therapy for cervicitis,‡ followed by repeat Pap in 6–12 wk
Yeast, *Chlamydia,* or *Trichomonas* infections
Treatment of nonspecific inflammatory changes with metronidazole
Estrogen therapy for atrophy, followed by repeat Pap in 3 mo
Postmenopausal women with lower genital tract atrophy
Repeat Pap smear in 3–4 mo
All other patients§

*Accurate information about the patient's clinical history and close dialogue between the primary practitioner and laboratory are essential for optimal management of patients in this Pap smear category.
†Patients with atypical glandular cells detected on Pap smears should be referred to an experienced colposcopist for evaluation.
‡Inflammation can be associated with normal metaplasia, so in the absence of cytologic atypia is not necessarily abnormal; severe inflammation may mask invasive cancer.
§Persistent ASCUS requires colposcopy.

Treatment of Cervical Dysplasia

A. Role of Expectant Management: Women with HSIL should undergo prompt treatment because of the risk of progression to invasive cancer. Although progression is not a certainty and it may take several years, there is a subset of patients who rapidly develop cancer. Furthermore, early treatment of preinvasive neoplasia can be accomplished by any of several office procedures outlined in the following section, with preservation of fertility. The only reason to delay treatment of HSIL is a concurrent pregnancy.

On the other hand, the observation that over 50% of all mildly dysplastic lesions may resolve spontaneously has prompted some practitioners to defer therapy for these lesions. Surveillance is most appropriate for a young woman found to have koilocytotic atypia bordering on mild dysplasia who agrees to at least semiannual Pap smears and colposcopic examinations. Certainly, many women classified in the new Bethesda system with LSIL have only HPV-associated changes, and most experts currently recommend that such patients not be treated.

B. Treatment Methods: A variety of techniques may be used to treat preinvasive neoplasia of the cervix. These include ablative therapy (electrocoagulation diathermy, cryocautery, carbon dioxide laser vaporization) and excisional procedures (scalpel or laser conization, loop excision). The choice of therapy depends on the severity, size, and distribu-

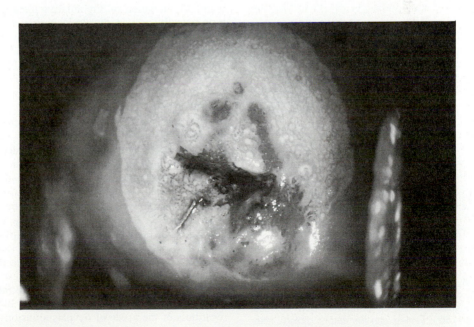

Figure 49–4. Colpophotograph after application of 3% acetic acid demonstrating acetowhitening and a mosaic vascular pattern. Biopsies revealed high-grade squamous intraepithelial lesions (HSIL). The broad area of dysplasia in this case is best treated with carbon dioxide laser vaporization rather than cryocautery. (Reproduced, with permission, from Burke L, Antonioli DA, Ducatman BS: *Colposcopy: Text and Atlas.* Appleton & Lange, 1991.)

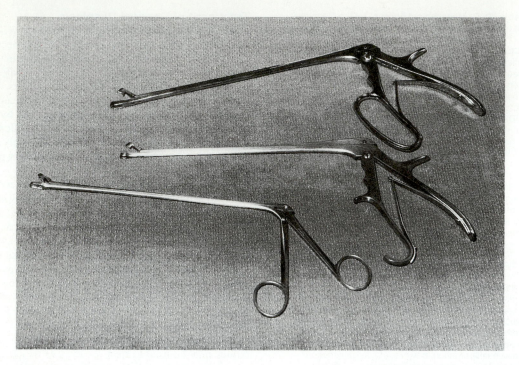

Figure 49–5. Biopsy instruments used during colposcopy. From top to bottom: Tischler, Burke, and Eppendorfer biopsy forceps. (Reproduced, with permission, from Burke L, Antonioli DA, Ducatman BS: *Colposcopy: Text and Atlas.* Appleton & Lange, 1991.)

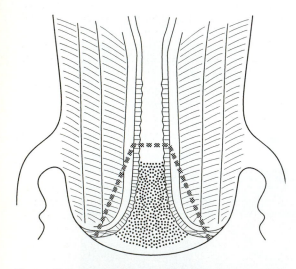

Figure 49–6. Schematic of traditional broad, deep cervical conization. Smaller, more precise conizations under colposcopic guidance can be performed now for most women in an office setting with the carbon dioxide laser or the loop electrosurgical excision procedure (LEEP). (Reproduced, with permission, from Berek JS, Hacker NF: *Practical Gynecologic Oncology,* 2nd ed. Williams & Wilkins, 1994.)

tion of the lesion. It is of paramount importance that, before the initiation of any ablative therapy, there is histologically proven dysplasia consistent with the cytologic diagnosis and no evidence of endocervical involvement or occult invasion. Up to one-half of invasive cervical cancers occurring after ablative therapy for dysplasia are due to errors by the colposcopist, usually because an indication for excisional conization was not recognized.

Cryocautery with a liquid nitrogen or carbon dioxide–cooled probe is effective therapy for small, low-grade lesions of the exocervix. It is a readily learned, inexpensive technique with a low complication rate. Cryocautery is most effective when applied in two 3-minute freezings with a 5-minute period for thaw between applications. Using the double-freeze technique, 94–97% of mild or moderately dysplastic lesions occupying less than 25% of the surface of the portio are treated effectively.

There are a number of disadvantages to the use of cryocautery in all cases. First, its success rate depends on the degree of dysplasia. Failure rates in the treatment of CIS range from 18 to 39%. In addition, regardless of the grade of dysplasia, lesions occupying more than half of the cervical portio (see Fig 49–4) or involving endocervical glands may have a 20–50% failure rate. Another disadvantage to cryocautery is that it may cause migration of the squamocolumnar junction into the endocervical canal, rendering all subsequent colposcopic examinations unsatisfactory.

Vaporization of the abnormal cervical epithelium to a depth of 7–8 mm with a carbon dioxide laser has significant advantages over cryocautery. Over 90% of women can be treated successfully with laser therapy, and unlike cryocautery, cure rates are not related to lesion size or degree of dysplasia. In addition, healing is rapid, with less posttreatment vaginal discharge. When this treatment is performed properly, the transformation zone remains visible.

The major disadvantages of laser vaporization are its cost and technical complexity. The complication rate is somewhat higher than that of cryosurgery, with minor bleeding episodes reported in up to 15% of patients. The rate of cervical stenosis is approximately 4% for both cryotherapy and laser ablation.

Although primarily a diagnostic procedure, scalpel conization may be therapeutic if the lesion is excised completely with negative margins. A high power density carbon dioxide laser also can be used by a skilled surgeon to perform excisional conizations. If the lesion is resected completely, the recurrence rate following conization of squamous lesions is 2% or less. Management of the less common, adenocarcinoma in situ lesions is more controversial, although carefully selected young women can be managed safely by conization alone.

The **loop electrosurgical excision procedure (LEEP)** is an office technique growing in popularity for the treatment of cervical dysplasia (Fig 49–7). It has the benefit of histologic evaluation without the associated cost and complication rate of a formal cervical conization. Removal of the entire transformation zone to a depth of 7–8 mm is termed **large loop excision of the transformation zone (LLETZ)** and is equivalent to laser vaporization of the exocervix. Several specimens can be removed sequentially, or one larger loop can be used to perform office cone biopsies. However, crucial histologic detail can be destroyed by an inexperienced surgeon because of thermal artifact.

Hysterectomy has little role in the treatment of women with cervical SIL. In general, hysterectomy is advised only for women who have completed childbearing and have dysplasia at the endocervical margin of an adequate cone biopsy. Occasionally, it is appropriate for the patient who will not adhere to long-term surveillance. When fertility is important and dysplasia involves a cone margin, a careful colposcopic examination, Pap smear, and ECC should be repeated after 3 months. If dysplasia is detected again, reconization can be considered before a hysterectomy is recommended.

C. Posttreatment Surveillance: After treatment for cervical dysplasia, the first follow-up Pap smear should be done in 3–4 months; repeat colposcopy and endocervical curettage are generally ad-

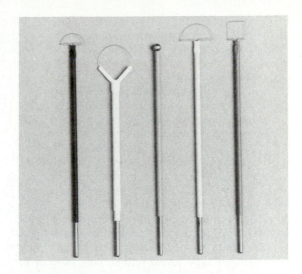

Figure 49–7. Selection of electrodes used for loop electrosurgical excision procedures (LEEP). Large loop excision of the transformation zone (LLETZ) usually can be done in a single pass with a loop that is 15 mm wide and 7 mm deep. Narrow loops can excise portions of the endocervical canal, and large loops are useful for office conizations. Ball electrodes are used for hemostasis. (Courtesy of Virginia Mason Medical Center Medical Art and Photography.)

vised when monitoring patients after treatment for HSIL or endocervical dysplasia. Patients should be followed subsequently with Pap smears and selective colposcopic examinations every 3–4 months for the first year and every 4–6 months for the second year. Almost all recurrences (or treatment failures) are detected within the first 2 years. Long-term annual follow-up is required, nonetheless, because recurrences can occur years later and involve any portion of the lower genital tract. The future risk of invasive cancer is low (less than 3%) after appropriate management of preinvasive lesions, but it must be guarded against.

Referral to a Specialist

Gynecologic oncologists and obstetrician-gynecologists who have received specialized training currently perform most colposcopic examinations in the USA. Considering the increasing number of women with abnormal Pap smears, it is appropriate for primary care clinicians with an interest in women's health care to become proficient in colposcopy. Similarly, although most patients who require treatment are referred to a specialist, some primary care providers may choose to learn techniques of cryotherapy, laser therapy, or loop excision. This circumstance is most appropriate in rural or other areas underserved by gynecologic specialists. Some clinical situations that may require consultation with a specialist in obstetrics and gynecology, gynecologic oncology, or gynecologic cytopathology are listed in Table 49–7.

Issues of Pregnancy & an Abnormal Pap Smear

Only experienced physicians with specialty training should manage pregnant women with abnormal Pap smears. Increased vascularity and other morphologic changes of the cervix make diagnostic biopsies and colposcopic examinations more difficult. The primary goal is protection of the mother's health; detection of invasive cancer must prompt immediate referral to a gynecologic oncologist. If only dysplasia is present, therapy can be postponed until after delivery. Cervical biopsies and conizations can be performed with a reasonable degree of safety during pregnancy, but they should be done only when invasive cancer is suspected.

Psychosocial Concerns

Psychological surveys consistently rank an abnormal Pap smear report as one of the most stressful situations a woman may face. She must confront the possibility of a potentially fatal malignancy while at the same time dealing with a disease process and necessary treatments that together threaten core elements of her sexual, reproductive, and gender identities.

It is imperative that the patient be provided with complete and accurate information about her Pap smear abnormality. Women often complain that they were notified of their abnormal Pap result by inexperienced office staff. Additionally, every effort should be made to avoid stigmatizing cervical cancer as a sexually transmitted disease.

Controversies & Unresolved Issues

The practicing clinician can expect to encounter

Table 49–7. Evaluation of the abnormal Pap smear: Indications for specialty referral.

A. Suspicion of cancer, based on one or more of the following:
1. Malignant cells on Pap smear
2. Colposcopically directed biopsies
3. Colposcopy suggestive of cancer, even if not confirmed by biopsy
B. Unsatisfactory colposcopy or other situation requiring cervical conization
C. Unexplained discrepancy between cytologic and histologic findings*
D. Pregnancy complicated by abnormal Pap smear
E. Nonsquamous lesions, including atypical glandular cells of undetermined significance (AGCUS); cytologic findings consistent with endocervical, endometrial, or other adeno-carcinoma; and unusual diagnoses (lymphoma, sarcoma)*

*Review by a gynecologic pathologist may be required in addition to referral to a clinical specialist.

the following problems and trends during the next 10 years:

1. Inadequate screening of poor women will continue.
2. The controversy between a 1- and a 3-year screening interval will be a factor in the national health care debate.
3. More colposcopic examinations will be done in primary care settings as clinicians struggle with an increasing number of mildly abnormal smears.
4. The pathogenesis of cervical cancer will be better understood, especially with respect to HPV and other cofactors.

REFERENCES

Alvarez RD et al: Prospective randomized trial of LLETZ versus laser ablation in patients with cervical intraepithelial neoplasia. Gynecol Oncol 1994;52:175.

Burke L, Antonioli DA, Ducatman BS: *Colposcopy Text and Atlas.* Appleton & Lange, 1991.

Goff BA et al: Human papillomavirus typing in patients with Papanicolaou smears showing squamous atypia. Gynecol Oncol 1993;48:384.

Johnson N et al: Decision analysis for best management of mildly dyskaryotic smear. Lancet 1993;342:91.

Kurman RJ et al: From Papanicolaou to Bethesda: The rationale for a new cervical cytologic classification. Obstet Gynecol 1991;77:779.

Morrow CP, Curtin JP, Townsend DE: Premalignant and related diseases of the lower genital tract. In: *Synopsis of*

Gynecologic Oncology, 4th ed. Churchill Livingstone, 1993.

Muntz HG et al: Adenocarcinoma in situ of the uterine cervix. Obstet Gynecol 1992;80:935.

Reid R: Preinvasive disease. In: *Practical Gynecologic Oncology,* 2nd ed. Berek JS, Hacker NF (editors). Williams & Wilkins, 1994.

Shy K: Concepts in the application of cervical cytology. In: *Gynecologic Oncology: Treatment Rationale and Techniques.* Greer BE, Berek JS (editors). Elsevier, 1991.

Wright TC Jr, Richart RM: Pathogenesis and diagnosis of preinvasive lesions of the lower genital tract. In: *Principles and Practice of Gynecologic Oncology.* Hoskins WJ, Perez CA, Young RC (editors). Lippincott, 1992.

Evaluation of Pelvic Masses & Screening for Ovarian Cancer

50

Joseph L. Yon, Jr., MD

Essentials of Diagnosis

- Pelvic masses are usually benign and are often found in the asymptomatic patient. The goal of the primary care provider is to differentiate between patients who require surgery and those who do not.
- Disorders of the urinary and gastrointestinal tracts and of other intra-abdominal organs can present as pelvic masses (Table 50–1).
- Gynecologic causes of pelvic masses may be uterine or adnexal (Tables 50–2 and 50–3). The differential diagnosis varies depending on whether the patient is pre- or postmenopausal and pregnant or not pregnant. Acute symptoms suggest an urgent event such as infection, rupture, bleeding, or infarction.
- There is currently no effective screening test for ovarian cancer.

Incidence

Ovarian cysts are the fourth most common cause for female admissions to the hospital in the United States. Sixty-five percent of women in the USA younger than 40 operated on for an ovarian enlargement ultimately prove to have a functional, ie, corpus luteum or follicular, cyst.

Ovarian cancer is the most malignant of the gynecologic tumors; it is the fifth most common cancer in women and the third most common cause of cancer death in women. It is projected that there will be 23,000 cases and 13,600 deaths in 1994. This figure exceeds the number of deaths in the USA from cervical and endometrial cancer combined. Eighty percent of ovarian tumors are epithelial in origin and as such have a cystic component. Therefore, evaluation of ovarian cysts is an important component of detecting early ovarian tumors.

Risk Factors

Although the cause of ovarian cancer is unknown, several potential risk factors have been identified. This cancer tends to be a disease of Western industrialized countries and of nulliparous white women. Associated but unproven risk factors include a history of severe mumps, increased fat in the diet, increased

| Essentials of Diagnosis |
| Incidence |
| Risk Factors |
| Screening for Ovarian Cancer |
| Signs & Symptoms |
| Clinical Findings & Diagnosis |
| Management of Specific Disorders |
| Prognosis of Ovarian Cancer |
| Referral to a Specialist |
| Issues of Pregnancy & Adnexal Masses |
| Psychosocial Issues |
| Unresolved Issues |

coffee or caffeine intake, exposure to talc or asbestos, and infertility.

The lifetime risk of a woman developing ovarian cancer is quoted to be 1 in 70, or a % risk of 1.4 (this varies in different studies). The risk varies with age groups: in the 20- to 29-year-old group, the risk is 4 in 100,000, which increases to 15 in 100,000 in the 40- to 44-year-old group and to 54 in 100,000 in the 75- to 79-year-old group. Ovarian cancer is a disease of older women; it predominantly affects women of the age group that tends not to present for routine examinations.

Multiparity, breast-feeding, and the use of oral contraceptives seem to be protective, possibly by decreasing the number of lifetime ovulatory events. A recent study has shown a decrease in the incidence of ovarian cancer in patients with a history of tubal ligation, although the reason is unknown. The protection provided by oral contraceptives appears to be real and increases as the duration of pill use increases. A reduction in risk of up to 60% may occur when oral contraceptives are used for longer than 5 years. Oral contraceptive use and prophylactic oophorectomy are at the present time the only established preventive measures available.

Familial Ovarian Cancer: The most significant risk factor for the development of ovarian cancer is a family history. Although a strong family history on the maternal side has been recognized for a number

Table 50–1. Nongynecologic sources of pelvic masses.

Organ or System	Disorder
Urinary tract	Distended bladder (urinary retention)
	Bladder diverticulum
	Pelvic kidney
	Polycystic kidney disease
	Urachal cyst
	Carcinoma of the bladder
Gastrointestinal tract	Cecum, redundant
	Sigmoid, redundant
	Appendiceal abscesses or tumors
	Diverticular disease
	Mesenteric cysts
	Carcinoma of the colon or small bowel
Spleen	Splenic cysts
	Enlarged spleen or malaria
	Accessory spleen
Others	Abnormal, asymmetric, or hypertrophic pelvic musculature
	Aneurysms of the pelvic vessels

Table 50–3. Nonuterine gynecologic causes of pelvic masses.

Nonovarian
  Nonovarian endometriosis
  Salpingitis: tuboovarian abscesses
  Hydrosalpinx
  Paraovarian cysts
  Leiomyoma of the round ligament
  Tubal pregnancy
  Actinomycosis
  Malignant disease of the tubes
Ovarian—benign
  Follicular cysts
  Corpus luteum cysts
  Endometrioma
  Benign neoplasms
    Fibroma
    Cystadenoma
    Cystic teratoma
Ovarian—malignant neoplasms
  Epithelial
  Germ cell
  Stromal
  Metastatic

of years as being important, recent data have shown that paternal history may be equally important. The risk of developing the disease increases as the number of family members affected increases. Having one first-degree family relative affected, eg, a mother, increases a woman's lifetime risk from 1.4% to as high as 3.0–3.5%. Having two or more first-degree relatives affected may increase the risk to as high as 50%, consistent with the current theory that this is an autosomal dominant gene with variable penetrance.

Three different syndromes fall under the heading of familial ovarian cancer. First, there is the site-specific, **hereditary ovarian cancer (HOC) syndrome,** in which only ovarian cancer is recorded. More common is the **hereditary breast-ovarian cancer (HBOC) syndrome,** in which there is a mixture of both diseases, both often occurring in the same patient. Last, there is the **Lynch II syndrome,** in which there are breast, ovarian, colon, endometrial, and other cancers presenting throughout the pedigree.

One of the characteristics of these familial syn-

Table 50–2. Uterine causes of pelvic masses.

Pregnancy
  Uterine
  Cornual
Leiomyomas
Hematometra
  Congenital anomaly
  Acquired
Pyometra
Adenomyosis
Malignant tumor
  Fundal
  Cervical

dromes is that the ovarian cancers tend to occur at a younger age in successive generations, and it is recommended that prophylactic oophorectomy be considered in women in these families between the ages of 30 and 35. These families also have a significantly increased incidence of benign neoplasms of the ovary, such as cystadenomas. The malignant potential of these processes is unknown at this time, although there is evidence that at least some of these may be premalignant. The prophylactic effect of oral contraceptives in these families is unknown. It should be recognized that less than 5% of all ovarian cancers occur in families with these histories.

Screening for Ovarian Cancer

A screening test should be inexpensive, safe, widely available, accurate, noninvasive, and useful in asymptomatic patients who are potentially curable. A screening test does not necessarily have to detect the disease in question, but it should detect patients who require more sophisticated testing. To develop such a screening test would require that the natural history of the disease be well known, that there be a preinvasive or curable early stage, and that false-positive results could be minimized. Unfortunately, there are no such tests or combination of tests available for ovarian cancer. Recent evidence suggests that there may be a preinvasive form of ovarian cancer, but detection of this condition is problematic at best.

The pelvic examination is unreliable as a screening test. There is a greater than 30% inaccuracy level in the physical assessment of pelvic disease compared with that found with ultrasonography, laparoscopy, or laparotomy. Masses as large as 8–10 cm are missed by experienced examiners. It has been estimated that it would take approximately 10,000 pelvic examinations to detect one case of ovarian cancer in the general female population.

Ultrasonography, particularly transvaginal, is being investigated as a screening tool for ovarian disease. The newer, more powerful 5- to 7.5-mHz transducers are accurate but have a short depth of penetration. These transducers can be used without a full bladder, but the depth of field is limited. Unfortunately, there are currently no standards that can be used as a basis of screening. Premenopausal ovaries are constantly changing with the ovarian cycle. Even in the postmenopausal patient, there are ethnic and racial differences in normal ovarian size. Because ultrasonography can detect changes in the ovary, it may be more useful in longitudinal studies with serial examinations. Color Doppler flow can increase the accuracy of diagnosing a potentially neoplastic problem, but the complexity of the equipment and the expense are unacceptable. In the future, a type of transvaginal ultrasonography may become part of the "routine" annual examination of women. The machines need to become much less expensive and more available in offices, however, and all practitioners performing pelvic examinations need to have adequate training in ultrasonography. Ultrasonographic evaluation is most useful when results are negative, ie, excluding an abnormality. An additional advantage of the use of routine ultrasonography is its ability to evaluate uterine and endometrial disease.

Screening has other limitations. There is strong evidence that at least some cases of so-called advanced ovarian cancer are not ovarian in origin but multifocal, arising de novo on peritoneal surfaces. These cases may represent as many as 9–10% of "ovarian" cancers and have been reported to occur in patients who have had their ovaries removed prophylactically or for other reasons. Clearly, screening the pelvis for ovarian disease has no effect on the early detection of cancer in these patients.

In April 1994, the Consensus Development Conference on Ovarian Cancer recommended against routine screening in the general population. They found that using the three most available tests, ie, pelvic examination, CA-125 (see the section, Laboratory Tests), and ultrasonography, 65 laparotomies would have to be performed for the detection of one case of early ovarian cancer. There is no evidence that the use of routine screening has had any impact on the mortality and morbidity of ovarian cancer. In addition, significant morbidity has been caused by unnecessary operations performed. A positive laparotomy rate of approximately 1 in 10, similar to that for appendicitis, would be considered acceptable, but 1 in 65 is not acceptable. Using these tests to screen the general population at age 45 would increase the life expectancy of the cohort by 8 hours; to screen at age 65 would increase the life expectancy of the cohort by 18 hours. Therefore, screening procedures should be limited to patients considered to be at high risk, ie, women with a family history of ovarian cancer.

Screening of high-risk patients, either before the age that prophylactic oophorectomy is advised or as an alternative, may be cost-effective considering the high incidence of disease in this population. The frequency of screening, however, remains to be determined. The biology of the disease is not understood well enough to determine the progression rate from preinvasive to invasive cancer. As more is learned about the biology of the disease, both in high-risk families and in the general population, the necessary information may be forthcoming. Use of gene markers such as BRCA-1 might prove to be helpful in the future.

Signs & Symptoms

A careful history often can lead the clinician to the correct ancillary tests. A change in bowel habits might suggest gastrointestinal origin, particularly if the patient is older than 40 years of age, and evaluation of the colon might be worthwhile. Colonoscopy or barium enema combined with flexible sigmoidoscopy can rule out diverticular disease or cancer. Barium enemas are not particularly useful for the last few centimeters of the rectosigmoid, however, so that a digital examination and flexible sigmoidoscopy are essential if colonoscopy is not to be done.

Endometriosis is suspected by a history of infertility, increasing dysmenorrhea, and premenstrual spotting. Adenomyosis is a diagnosis that can be made only in retrospect by the pathologist, but it is suggested by increasing dysmenorrhea and menorrhagia in a woman older than 35.

Acute salpingitis usually has associated with it fever, peritoneal signs, and adnexal tenderness. There may be a history of prior episodes, but the clinician should not be lulled into making a diagnosis of pelvic inflammatory disease (PID) just because the patient has had that diagnosis in the past. The prior diagnosis may have been in error.

Leiomyomas (fibroids) are particularly common in black women, less common in Asians, and tend to run in families. In premenopausal patients, a menstrual history may raise the suspicion of a complication of pregnancy, although it is predicted that in the future less than 50% of patients with ectopic pregnancies will have a palpable mass. Any bleeding in a postmenopausal patient is significant, and any change in urinary habits needs to be investigated.

In a patient with ascites, a history of ethanol intake plus the proper diagnostic studies can save a cirrhotic patient from an unnecessary and potentially life-threatening operation.

Most women with ovarian cancer present with ascites, abdominal distention, vague gastrointestinal symptoms, and pelvic or abdominal masses; the earlier stages usually are found serendipitously while the clinician is looking for something else. The older woman with ovarian cancer is likely to have vague, nondescript gastrointestinal symptoms of other causes and to attribute her abdominal distention to weight gain. It is not unusual for ovarian cancer to be detected in women undergoing laparoscopy as part of an infertility evaluation. Therefore, some sort of effective screening program that is readily available to detect early disease is desirable.

Clinical Findings & Diagnosis

The following is a list of factors to consider in the workup of a patient with a pelvic mass:

Age
Acuteness of onset
Location
Size
Consistency (solid versus cystic)
Mobility (mobile versus fixed)
Tenderness
Bilaterality
Contours (smooth versus irregular)
Associated symptoms
Ascites or pleural effusion

A. Physical Examination: On physical examination, the clinician needs to consider such findings as the location and consistency of the mass, tenderness, associated fever, and peritoneal signs.

When evaluating the gastrointestinal tract, it is important to know that diverticulosis tends to be left-sided, although right-sided disease can occur. This condition can be confused with appendicitis, which tends to be right-sided, except in very young girls. In PID both adnexa are almost always tender, and the disorder is associated with an elevated white cell count and temperature. Although unilateral tuboovarian abscesses can occur in patients with a history of intrauterine device (IUD) use, these abscesses tend to be bilateral. Chlamydial disease is known for its protean signs and symptoms, however, and should always be suspected in cases of pelvic infection.

Ascites in the presence of a pelvic mass should suggest malignant disease until proved otherwise. **Meigs' syndrome,** a benign solid ovarian fibroma associated with ascites and a right-sided pleural effusion, is rare. However, alcoholic patients with cirrhosis can present with ascites and pelvic masses of almost any cause and even an elevated CA-125 level, causing confusion and sometimes unnecessary and life-threatening surgical interventions.

B. Laboratory Tests: A complete blood cell count (CBC) with differential can be useful in sorting out inflammatory processes. A mildly elevated white cell count with a slight shift can be found in low-grade or chlamydial salpingitis, diverticulitis, or torsion of the ovary. Sedimentation rates are seldom helpful, but C-reactive protein determination might be useful if the process is less than 3–5 days old. A

normal white cell count, however, does not exclude any of these disease processes; many patients with significant inflammatory processes including peritonitis and even sepsis can present with normal counts.

In a premenopausal patient, a serum or urinary qualitative HCG determination can be useful. If an ectopic pregnancy or abnormal intrauterine pregnancy is suspected, a quantitative HCG level should be obtained in anticipation of following its increase (see Chapter 56). An elevated platelet count in excess of 400,000–500,000 has been associated with many cases of ovarian cancer but is not consistent enough to be used as a screening test or even a marker.

In prepubertal girls with an ovarian cyst, thyroid function should be checked, because the cysts may be the only sign of subtle thyroid abnormalities.

Alpha-fetoprotein (AFP) and carcinoembryonic antigen (CEA) are fairly tumor-specific, are elevated in germ cell tumors of the ovary, and tend to occur in younger women. They should be determined postoperatively if the histologic findings show a tumor for which these markers might be helpful. They are not useful as screening tests for pelvic masses.

C. CA-125: CA-125, first described by Bast in 1983, is a high-molecular-weight surface glycoprotein expressed by coelomic epithelium. This antibody was found to be elevated in some cases of epithelial ovarian cancer, and when elevated, its level is somewhat proportional to the amount of tumor present. Therefore, in patients with epithelial tumors that react to CA-125, the test can be used to follow the progress of the disease under treatment or in remission.

Ninety-nine percent of normal women have a level of CA-125 below 35, and 99.8% have a level below 65. Therefore, 35 is considered the upper limits of normal. The antibody is elevated in a large number of both benign and malignant processes, however (Table 50–4). In ovarian malignant disease, it tends to be elevated mainly in serous tumors.

An effective marker would differentiate patients who do not need further investigation or surgical in-

Table 50–4. Elevations of CA-125.

Benign	Malignant
Normal variation with menstrual cycle	Ovarian cancer
Endometriosis	Endometrial cancer
Adenomyosis	Cervical cancer
Pelvic inflammatory disease	Tubal cancer
Pancreatitis	Biliary tract cancer
Renal failure	Liver cancer
Leiomyomas	Pancreatic cancer
Early pregnancy	Breast cancer
Liver disease	Lung cancer
Cirrhosis	Colon cancer
Peritonitis	
History of abdominal or pelvic radiation	

tervention. Although CA-125 has been approved by the United States Food and Drug Administration (FDA) for use only as a marker in the treatment of ovarian cancer and as an alternative to second-look operations in patients previously diagnosed, four million tests were run in the USA in 1993 at a cost of approximately $100 million dollars. This test is not, and was never intended to be, a screening test. The sensitivity and specificity, especially in premenopausal women, are too poor to use for detection of early disease. Indeed, less than 40% of stage I and II ovarian cancers of any cell type have an elevated CA-125 level above 35, and some reports place this level at 25%. Conversely, 1% of the normal female population have a CA-125 level above 35, and only 0.3% of asymptomatic women with a normal examination and an elevated CA-125 greater than 35 have ovarian cancer. In the postmenopausal patient with an adnexal mass, determination of a CA-125 level may be more useful, because the incidence of false-positive results in this group is significantly less.

In an attempt to improve the accuracy of the serologic screening, other tumor-associated markers have been combined in "panels." Many of these panels are commercially available, but their usefulness remains to be proved. These include CA-15-3, TAG 75, CA-19-9, CA-15, NB/70K, CA-195, CST-1, and others. To date, no combination of tests has proved to be an accurate, consistent screening tool.

D. Imaging Studies: Once a pelvic mass has been found on examination, the next step is to select one or more of the available imaging studies to help formulate a diagnosis and a treatment plan. Currently available are magnetic resonance imaging (MRI), computed tomography (CT), and ultrasonography (both abdominal and vaginal, with or without Doppler flow studies), as well as the more conventional intravenous pyelography (IVP), barium enema, upper gastrointestinal (GI) series, and cystography.

CT generally is less helpful in diagnosing diseases of the pelvis than ultrasonography or MRI, although CT scans are probably a more cost-effective procedure for diseases of the upper abdomen. MRI is particularly useful in differentiating leiomyomas, dermoids, and endometriomas from other pelvic masses. Ultrasonography, especially transvaginal, however, is the method of choice for most adnexal and uterine diseases, particularly in the asymptomatic patient. The newer, more powerful vaginal probes give better definition at the expense of a shorter depth of field; however, their results are quite accurate and reproducible. These tests are most useful when the study shows normal anatomy and saves the patient from further investigation. However, Doppler flow is expensive, somewhat complicated to use, and not universally available.

The availability and possible overuse of some tests has led to some dilemmas. This is especially evident in postmenopausal women in whom it appears that ovarian cysts are far more common than was previously known. At one time, it was clinical dogma that any enlargement in an ovary in a postmenopausal patient was an indication for surgical removal. Although this is still true for solid enlargement, increased use of pelvic ultrasonography and CT has taught clinicians that small unilocular cysts in postmenopausal patients come and go. Although these cysts cannot be called functional, they are undoubtedly physiologic.

In patients who present with a pelvic mass but do not have any upper tract symptoms, there is no reason to do an upper GI series or a small-bowel follow-through study. When gastrointestinal symptoms are present, an evaluation of the colon may be worthwhile. In addition, patients with proven endometrial or ovarian cancer should have a barium enema and flexible sigmoidoscopy to rule out synchronous or metastatic tumors.

Management of Specific Disorders

A. Leiomyomas: Until recently, it was common gynecologic practice to recommend hysterectomy in patients with leiomyomas when the aggregate uterine size was greater than 10–12 weeks gestational size. The rationale was that at this size, the uterus filled the pelvis, precluding adequate physical examination of other pelvic structures, particularly the ovaries. With the use of modern ultrasonographic instruments, it is almost always possible to visualize ovaries and to document accurately the change in size of the uterus. Therefore, size alone is no longer an indication for hysterectomy. Patients who are symptomatic from their fibroids can be treated with myomectomy or, if they desire, hysterectomy. Treatment with gonadotropin releasing hormone (GnRH) agonists is also an option in selected patients either alone or in conjunction with surgery. Although expensive to use, these medications sometimes can replace surgery or lower its morbidity.

B. Endometriosis: Laparoscopy is still the "gold standard" for diagnosing endometriosis, although the diagnosis can be suspected from the history, physical examination, and ultrasonographic findings suggestive of an endometrioma. There may be a mildly elevated CA-125 level up to 200. Quite often, endometriomas and endometriosis can be removed adequately and safely with the laparoscope using newer operative techniques.

C. Ovarian Cysts: Ninety percent of ovarian growths are benign. The most common is the ovarian cyst. Most ovarian cysts are functional, ie, corpus luteum or follicular cysts, and most are no more than 8 cm in diameter. Ultrasonography is helpful in determining which cysts can be followed and which cannot. In the premenopausal patient, cysts of less than 8 cm can be followed for one or two cycles with the expectation that they are functional and will resolve. Clinicians can expect about 25–35% of these to persist. Cysts greater than 8 cm, even if considered functional, usually do not resolve spontaneously and are subject to rupture, bleeding, or torsion and infarction. Also, cysts less than 8 cm that persist beyond one to two menstrual cycles tend not to be functional and might need to be investigated surgically, especially if they are multilocular or septate. Hemorrhagic cysts such as corpora lutea are expected to resolve, whereas endometriomas do not.

It is common practice to "suppress" women with suspected functional cysts by using oral contraceptives for 2–3 months. Currently, there are no data that support the contention that oral contraceptives accelerate the resolution of functional ovarian cysts.

In the postmenopausal patient, the guidelines are different. Any solid enlargement of an ovary must be investigated and considered to be cancer until proved otherwise. However, numerous studies have demonstrated that unilocular cysts less than 5 cm in diameter may be observed. This is true only if there are no other, associated risk factors such as ascites; in this situation, a CA-125 serum test might be useful, because false-positive results are less common in the postmenopausal patient. If the cyst is followed, it should be restudied by ultrasonography after 6 weeks, 3 months, and 6 months. Many of these cysts resolve under observation. In one study of unilocular cysts, 40% were in postmenopausal women. If there is any increase in size during follow-up, the ovary needs to be removed expeditiously and its histologic structure examined.

Once it has been determined that an ovarian cyst is not likely to be functional, surgical intervention via laparoscopy is a viable option, particularly in the premenopausal patient. The use of this method in postmenopausal patients remains somewhat controversial, although there are reliable studies available that indicate its safety when correctly applied. Further studies need to be done to determine the safety and indications of this technique.

Prognosis of Ovarian Cancer

The prognosis of ovarian cancer is related directly to the stage of the disease at the time of diagnosis. Although there is at least a 95% 5-year survival rate in patients who have a low-grade ovarian cancer confined to one ovary, this situation is seldom encountered except by accident while investigating the patient for something else. Generally speaking, patients with stage I and II carcinomas of the ovary have a 5-year-plus survival rate of greater than 75%; however, the rate for stage III and IV ovarian cancer is in the 15% range. Unfortunately, because of the insidious nature of the disease, most tumors are stage III or IV when first detected. Hence, the ongoing search for effective screening tests.

Referral to a Specialist

When and to whom to refer the patient once the evaluation of an adnexal mass has begun can be a difficult decision. If the studies outlined in this chapter suggest that the mass is benign or a complication of pregnancy, referral to a general gynecologist, particularly one with expertise in laparoscopy, is appropriate. If there is any question that the mass may be malignant, early referral to a gynecologic oncologist may avoid unnecessary testing and can provide the patient with the best possible surgical intervention. Often a phone call to a specialist can guide the practitioner along the proper route of investigation and possibly save the patient from the expense and stress of unnecessary invasive procedures.

Issues of Pregnancy & Adnexal Masses

When a patient presents in early pregnancy with an adnexal mass, the first step is to make sure that the mass is not a complication of pregnancy such as ectopic pregnancy. This is done most easily with an ultrasonographic examination, particularly transvaginal ultrasonography. A fetal sac should be seen at an HCG level of 6500 IU with an abdominal probe and of approximately 2000 IU with a vaginal probe. Once it has been established that the mass is not a complication of pregnancy, particularly if the mass is ovarian, further evaluation, including surgery, is best delayed until the patient is at 14–16 weeks of gestation. Intervention at that time does not risk disruption of the corpus luteum and loss of the pregnancy.

Psychosocial Issues

Indiscriminate use of screening tests can have a devastating effect on the patient. False-positive findings using CA-125 and other ill-advised procedures such as "routine" ultrasonography have led to numerous unnecessary invasive procedures, some with considerable morbidity. Strict adherence to established, scientifically valid procedures avoids unnecessary anxiety and suffering. It is worthwhile to note that in England, the rate of surgical investigation of adnexal masses is less than 50% of that in the USA and that the morbidity and mortality from ovarian cancer are equivalent to that in the USA.

Unresolved Issues

The increased and often unjustified use of screening tests in the USA has failed to produce any effect on the morbidity and mortality of ovarian cancer. It is important that researchers continue to search for more cost-effective methods of screening that do not subject low-risk patients to invasive procedures.

At the present time, the use of laparoscopy and endoscopic techniques to diagnose and treat adnexal masses, particularly in the postmenopausal patient, remains controversial. However, reliable data are emerging gradually that in the proper setting, such as with a gynecologic oncologist attending the case, some of the newer, minimally invasive procedures are acceptable.

REFERENCES

Boente MP, Goodwin AK, Hogan WM: Screening, imaging, and early diagnosis of ovarian cancer. Clin Obstet Gynecol 1994;37:377.

Carter J et al: How accurate is the pelvic exam compared to transvaginal sonography? J Reprod Med 1994;39:32.

Daly MB, Lerman C: Ovarian cancer risk counseling: A guide for the practitioner. Oncology 1993;7:27.

Kerlikwski K, Brown JS, Grady D: Should women with a family history of ovarian cancer undergo prophylactic oophorectomy? Obstet Gynecol 1992;80:700.

Lynch HT et al: Hereditary ovarian cancer. Hematol Oncol Ann 1994;2:107.

Mann WJ, Reich H: Laparoscopic adnexectomy in postmenopausal women. J Reprod Med 1994;37:121.

Rulin MC (guest editor): Controversies in the management of adnexal masses. Clin Obstet Gynecol 1993;36:361.

Schwartz PE: Ovarian masses: Serological markers. Clin Obstet Gynecol 1991;34:423.

Seltzer V (chairman): Consensus Development Conference on Ovarian Cancer at the National Institutes of Health, 1994. See JAMA 1994;271:1305; Oncology Times 1994;XVI:1; and Cancer Control (May) 1994;286.

Squatrito RC, Buller RE: Use of CA-125 for monitoring and prognosticating outcome in patients with epithelial ovarian cancer. Female Patient 1994;19:13.

Steege JF: Laparoscopic approach to the adnexal mass. Clin Obstet Gynecol 1994;37:392.

Vreeland L: Ovarian cancer: Should you be tested? Lears, February 1994.

Section XIII.
Reproductive Health Issues

51

Contraception

Gerard S. Letterie, MD, & Romy Royce, MS, ARNP

The contemporary birth control movement can be traced to the efforts of two women on either side of the Atlantic. The early efforts of Margaret Sanger (1879–1965), an American nurse, led to the establishment of the Birth Control League and its successor, Planned Parenthood Federation of America (Fig 51–1). Marie Stopes (1880–1958), a British paleontologist, established the first birth control clinic for contraceptive counseling, dissemination of information, and distribution of contraceptive devices. The publications by Sanger, *The Woman Rebel* and *Family Limitations,* and by Stopes, *Married Love,* gave the public its first informative description of contraception and female sexuality.

A period of dormancy characterized contraceptive research and development from the 1920s to the 1950s. A disinterest in contraceptive development was partly influenced by a less than receptive social climate. Primarily through the efforts of Margaret Sanger, sufficient funds were finally raised in the 1950s for formal investigations of contraceptive techniques. These studies came approximately 50 years after the initial description of hormonal contraceptives was made by Halverstadt in Vienna.

In 1959, after clinical trials demonstrated efficacy and effectiveness, the Searle Company planned on marketing an oral contraceptive (Enovid E). The systematic investigations into oral contraception and the eventual marketing of the products represent landmark achievements in the cooperation between commercial and scientific endeavors in response to a clear-cut social need. However, the need continues unabated as the world population growth continues. Alternative forms of contraception are needed, and wider dissemination to both male and female populations appears to be crucial.

CONTRACEPTION COUNSELING

The widespread availability of contraceptive techniques has not been matched by widespread dissemination of accurate information about these techniques. Misunderstandings among patients persist and, in some circumstances, contribute to a failure to use contraception. According to a 1993 survey of females from 15 to 45 years, only 73% of those who

Contraception Counseling
Contraceptive Techniques
   Hormonal Contraception
   Intrauterine Devices
   Barrier Methods
   Vaginal Spermicides
   Natural Family Planning
Emergency Contraception (Postcoital
   Contraception)
   Background
   Mechanism of Action
   Clinical Management
Female Sterilization
   Background
   Mechanism of Action
   Clinical Management
Referral to a Specialist
Pregnancy & Failed Contraception
Unresolved Issues
   RU486
   Gonadotropin Releasing Hormone:
     Agonists & Antagonists

wished to avoid pregnancy used contraception. The remainder, primarily adolescents and women older than 40 years, stated that they did not use any contraception because of fears regarding side effects and health risks. Fears concerning oral contraceptives included a suspicion of increased cardiovascular disease and various types of cancer. These misconceptions have changed little since a 1985 Gallup Poll found that 75% of women thought oral contraception caused cancer.

It is essential for clinicians to dispel such fears and concerns. This goal is most appropriately achieved through an adequate counseling session regarding contraceptive options. In discussing options, each technique should be described in detail and an individual's needs matched to a technique.

Every patient has contraceptive needs that are unique not only for herself but also for particular times in her life. These needs may change depending on age, relationship status, and fertility plans. Discussions should be undertaken describing the various

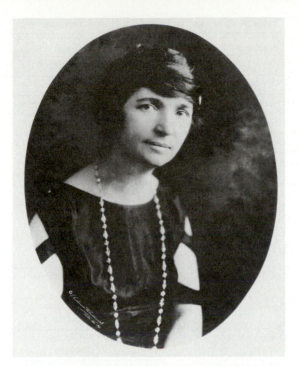

Figure 51–1. Portrait of Margaret Sanger (1879–1965).

both the lowest possible number and an expected number may be cited.

Once a contraceptive method has been chosen, recommendations for that method must be accompanied by detailed explanations of how the technique works; the risks, benefits, contraindications, and alternatives of the method; the amount of follow-up and the timing of follow-up visits; the signs of potential complications; and the need for condom use in some circumstances. The last factor is particularly important when discussing protection from sexually transmitted diseases (STDs). To prevent transmission of the human immunodeficiency virus (HIV) and other STDs, patients should be counseled that oral contraceptives, implantable and injectable contraceptives, intrauterine devices (IUDs), and natural membrane condoms do not protect against STDs. Use of a latex condom should be advised when appropriate.

All patients, regardless of contraceptive choice, should be informed of emergency contraceptive measures in case a primary method fails.

CONTRACEPTIVE TECHNIQUES

Hormonal Contraception

A. Combination Oral Contraceptives:

1. Background—Oral contraceptives (OCPs) are the most commonly used reversible form of contraception. Currently, approximately 12 million women in the United States use OCPs. These steroid preparations consist of a combination of a synthetic estrogen and a progestin. The estrogenic component is either ethinyl estradiol or mestranol. First-generation progestins include norethindrone, norethindrone

methods of contraception and the effectiveness of each method. In discussing contraceptive effectiveness, the best estimate of efficacy for a particular contraceptive method (method effectiveness) can be compared with the usual field experience for a particular contraceptive method (use effectiveness) (Table 51–1). A range of effectiveness that incorporates

Table 51–1. Failure rates for contraceptive methods.

Method	Percentage of Women with Pregnancy	
	Lowest (Method Effectiveness)	Typical (Use Effectiveness)
Combination pill	0.1	3.0
Progestin-only pill	0.5	3.0
Intrauterine device (IUD)		
Progesterone IUD	2.0	< 2.0
Copper T 380A	0.8	< 1.0
Implantable agents	0.2	0.2
Female sterilization	0.2	0.4
Male sterilization	0.1	0.15
Depot medroxyprogesterone	0.3	0.3
Spermicides only	3.0	21.0
Withdrawal	4.0	18.0
Cervical cap	6.0	18.0
Sponge		
Parous women	9.0	28.0
Nulliparous women	6.0	18.0
Diaphragm and spermicides	6.0	18.0
Condom and spermicides	2.0	12.0

*Failure rates are the lowest expected and typical pregnancy rates for first year of use.

acetate, norethynodrel, ethynodiol diacetate, and norgestrel. These progestins are 19-nortestosterone derivatives and maintain a small and variable aspect of their androgenic heritage. Androgenic actions may be manifested at times by adverse side effects such as mild acne and unfavorable changes in lipoprotein profiles. A second generation of progestational agents has become available recently, including desogestrel, gestodene, and norgestimate. This group of compounds has a marked reduction in androgenicity. Such a favorable profile has positive implications for both long-term use and use in patients older than 40 years.

The improved safety profile for OCPs may be traced to a reduction in the estrogen and progestin content of the pills and the introduction of the newer progestin compounds. The 1960s saw the introduction of OCPs with estrogen concentrations more than 3–4 times those of the currently available agents. Initial efforts at improved formulations in the 1970s and 1980s focused on a gradual reduction in the estrogen concentration to as low as 20 μg/tablet. Current formulations have estrogen concentrations that range from 20–50 μg of ethinyl estradiol (Table 51–2). The 1980s and 1990s have seen marked changes in the type and concentration of the progestins. The introduction of bi- and triphasic combination pills and the second-generation progestational agents has led to a marked improvement in the profile of the currently available pills (Table 51–3).

2. Mechanism of action—Oral contraceptives exert their contraceptive effect primarily at the level of the hypothalamic-pituitary axis. The estrogenic component suppresses follicle-stimulating hormone (FSH) and the progestational component suppresses luteinizing hormone (LH). Secondary effects are changes in tubal motility and ovum transport, sperm penetration and implantation, and cervical mucus, all significant factors contributing to contraceptive efficacy.

3. Clinical management—Oral contraceptives are extremely well tolerated and safe medications. OCPs may be prescribed to patients without absolute contraindications or risk factors (Table 51–4). Absolute contraindications preclude pill use. Relative contraindications are guidelines under which oral contraceptives may be prescribed cautiously, with close follow-up.

An initial evaluation should include a general examination with blood pressure determination and cervical cytologic study. In patients at risk, the initial evaluation also may include screening for lipoprotein profiles, fasting serum glucose level, and liver function. Follow-up visits may be scheduled at 12-month intervals and should include, at a minimum, blood pressure determination, pelvic examination, and cervical cytologic study. For some patients, a follow-up visit at 3 or 6 months may be advantageous for further discussion to answer any questions about trou-

Table 51–2. Monophasic combination oral contraceptives.

Commercial Name	Estrogen (μg)	Progestin (mg)
Norinyl 1+50	mestranol, 50	norethindrone, 1
Ortho-Novum 1/50	mestranol, 50	norethindrone, 1
Ovcon-50	ethinyl estradiol, 50	norethindrone, 1
Norinyl 1+35	ethinyl estradiol, 35	norethindrone, 1
Ortho-Novum 1/35	ethinyl estradiol, 35	norethindrone, 1
Brevicon	ethinyl estradiol, 35	norethindrone, 1
Modicon	ethinyl estradiol, 35	norethindrone, 0.5
Ovcon 35	ethinyl estradiol, 35	norethindrone, 0.4
Loestrin (Fe) 1/20	ethinyl estradiol, 20	norethindrone acetate, 1
Loestrin (Fe) 1.5/30	ethinyl estradiol, 30	norethindrone acetate, 1.5
Demulen 1/50	ethinyl estradiol, 50	ethynodiol diacetate, 1
Demulen 1/35	ethinyl estradiol, 35	ethynodiol diacetate, 1
Ovral	ethinyl estradiol, 50	norgestrel, 0.5
Lo/Ovral	ethinyl estradiol, 30	norgestrel, 0.3
Levlen	ethinyl estradiol, 30	levonorgestrel, 0.15
Nordette	ethinyl estradiol, 30	levonorgestrel, 0.15
Ortho-Cyclen	ethinyl estradiol, 35	norgestimate, 0.25
Desogen	ethinyl estradiol, 30	desogestrel, 0.15
Ortho-Cept	ethinyl estradiol, 30	desogestrel, 0.15

Table 51–3. Bi- and tri-phasic combination oral contraceptives.

Commercial Name	Estrogen (μg) Ethinyl Estradiol	Progestin (mg) Norethindrone
Ortho-Novum 10/11*	35/35	0.5/1
Tri-Norinyl*	35/35/35	0.5/1/0.5
Ortho-Novum 7/7/7*	35/35/35	0.5/0.75/1
Jenest 28*	35/35/35	0.5/1/1
		Norgestimate
Ortho Tricyclin*	35/35/35	0.18/0.215/0.25
		Levonorgestrel
Triphasil*	30/40/30	.05/.075/.125
Tri-Levlen*	30/40/30	.05/.075/.125

*Variable dose of progestin only.
*Variable dose of both estrogen and progestin.

Table 51–4. Relative and absolute contraindications to combination oral contraceptive use.

Relative	Absolute
Migraine headaches	Thromboembolic disease or thrombophlebitis, cerebral vascular disease, coronary artery disease, or history of these conditions
Hypertension	Known or suspected carcinoma of the breast
Uterine leiomyoma	Known or suspected estrogen-dependent neoplasia
Epilepsy	Undiagnosed abnormal genital bleeding
Varicose veins	Known or suspected pregnancy
Gestational diabetes	
Elective surgery	

blesome side effects or worries and to ensure compliance.

The oral contraceptive that provides adequate contraception with the fewest side effects at the lowest possible dose should be used. Multiphasic preparations usually fulfill these criteria, but any low-dose pill may be used. Several commercial brands are available, and none has a distinct advantage over another.

Compliance is essential for successful use of OCPs. Adequate counseling has been shown to improve compliance, especially in adolescents. Patients should be carefully counseled regarding when to start. Pills may be initiated on either the first day of the menstrual cycle or as a "Sunday start." Effective contraception is ensured when the medications are taken on the first day of the menstrual cycle; should the patient elect to initiate a Sunday start, the effectiveness of the oral contraceptives for that cycle may be questioned if the Sunday start is not within a day or two of the first day of the patient's menstrual cycle. If this scenario applies, the first pill cycle should be considered at risk, and a reliable alternative method should be used for 1 month.

In the postpartum setting, oral contraceptives should be prescribed within 3 weeks after delivery, because ovulation may occur as early as the third week post partum. Low-dose preparations may be used in breast-feeding patients with little influence on either the quantity or quality of the milk or the growth of the infant. After an elective termination of pregnancy, oral contraceptives may be started on the day of the procedure.

Some guidelines should be given to patients when OCPs are first prescribed. If one pill is missed, the dose should be doubled for the next day. If two pills are missed, two pills on two successive days should be taken until the patient is back in phase with her package. If more than two pills are missed, the patient should be considered at risk for pregnancy, and an alternative form of contraception should be used

until the onset of menses. Repeated compliance problems suggest an alternative form of contraception should be discussed.

In counseling patients regarding the use of OCPs, adequate emphasis must be placed on the risks, benefits, alternatives, and potential beneficial side effects of oral contraceptive use. Oral contraception is an extremely safe method of birth control, but bothersome side effects do exist. Side effects commonly experienced are breakthrough bleeding, weight gain, and mild acne and oily skin. Breakthrough bleeding appears to be the most troublesome and may be managed with the use of supplemental estrogen, either 1.25 mg of conjugated estrogens or 20 μg of ethinyl estradiol at the time of the irregular bleeding.

Benefits of OCPs include a reduction in the risk for iron deficiency anemia, pelvic inflammatory disease, ovarian cysts, ovarian cancer, and endometrial cancer.

Contraceptive choices for women over the age of 35 were few until recently. Data evaluating oral contraceptives have shown that these agents may be used safely throughout reproductive years. If no contraindications exist, such as smoking or hypertension, oral contraceptives may be used until menopause for excellent contraceptive efficacy with good tolerance and virtual lack of side effects. Prior reports suggested increased episodes of cardiovascular side effects, primarily as a result of the high estrogen concentration and possibly the type of progestin. The use of these agents in this age group has the added benefit of cycle control with no apparent pill-related changes in lipoprotein patterns or coagulation parameters. Frequency of surveillance remains yearly. Screening may also include lipoprotein profiles (for possible age-related changes) and mammography.

B. Progestin-Only Pills (Minipills): Compared with combination OCPs, progestin-only tablets account for a small portion of oral contraceptive use (0.2% in the USA). These pills consist of the progestin norethindrone or norgestrel (Table 51–5). They are used continuously, ie, one tablet daily without the 7-day pill-free interval characteristic of combination OCPs. These agents are associated with more irregular bleeding than the combination pills; hence, their acceptability to patients is considerably less. Breakthrough bleeding is experienced by 20–30% of patients who use progestin-only pills. This incidence decreases with continued use. The nonmenstrual side effects from the use of these pills are few. Progestin-only pills have a slightly increased pregnancy rate, possibly secondary to a failure of the method itself but possibly secondary to poor compliance because of the side effects. Failure rates appears to be higher in heavier women, as is the case with most other progestin-containing contraceptives. Progestin-only pills were initially prescribed in patients who had a contraindication to estrogen use, such as breast-feeding or age greater than 35. Their

Table 51–5. Progestin-only (minipill) contraceptives.

Commercial Name	Estrogen (μg) Ethinyl estradiol	Progestin (mg) Norethindrone
Nor QD	0	0.35
Micronor	0	0.35
		Norgestrel
Ovrette	0	0.075

role has been markedly decreased in view of the safety of combination OCPs in both of these clinical circumstances.

C. Long-Acting Implantable Contraceptive Agents:

1. Background–Contraception with an implantable device was initially described in the mid-1960s. These early studies sought to devise a means of passive hormonal contraception with a prolonged duration of action. Implementation, however, awaited the availability of safe and reliable subcutaneous Silastic capsules. A delivery system for the progestin, norgestrel, became available in 1967. Over 500,000 women worldwide have used this method of contraception successfully. The Norplant system was approved by the US Food and Drug Administration (FDA) for use in the USA in December 1990.

Since the initial demonstration of contraceptive efficacy with the Norplant system, these implantable contraceptive agents have undergone a number of revisions and refinements, making them better able to meet the demands of clinical practice. Newer delivery systems under investigation may contain fewer implants, shorter-acting systems, biodegradable capsules, and different progestins. These changes are intended to improve the ease of insertion and removal, as well as to increase safety and compliance. None are available for use in the USA.

2. Mechanism of action–The Norplant system delivers a constant serum level of norgestrel. The mechanism of action of the norgestrel is identical to that of all progestin-only contraceptive techniques. These agents act primarily by altering ovulation, cervical mucus, and endometrial receptivity. Suppression of ovulation occurs in approximately 50% of cycles, and current data suggest that when ovulation does occur, the endometrium is sufficiently hostile to prevent implantation.

3. Clinical management–Norplant consists of six Silastic capsules that are placed subcutaneously. Six capsules are essential to maintain constant serum concentrations of norgestrel over a 5-year period. These capsules are easily placed under local anesthesia using a trocar supplied by the manufacturer (Fig 51–2). Removal has been more problematic; in a recent series, the time required to remove the capsules ranged from 4 to 215 minutes, with approximately 50% of the removals completed in less than 30 min-

utes and approximately 20% requiring longer than 1 hour. The data further describe "significant" pain associated with removal in approximately one-fourth of the patients. The capsules provide constant contraception for a 5-year period, and because of this and their passive nature, they have been well accepted in a variety of circumstances.

The 1-year removal rate in the USA has been 13%, with the rate in other countries ranging from 1.25–10%. A patient's experience with previous methods of contraception does not predict satisfaction or dissatisfaction with implantable agents. The side effects of Norplant include changes in bleeding patterns (60%) and pain at the site of insertion (32%). A desire for pregnancy or reaction to the bleeding pattern were the most common reasons for removal. Caution should be exercised in counseling women who anticipate a change in their marital status or who desire more children in the near future.

Implantable contraceptives should be inserted within 7 days of a menstrual cycle, after an abortion, or after establishing two negative pregnancy tests (either urine or serum) 10 days apart with reliable contraception in the interval between tests. In a recent study it was found that 6 of 10 pregnancies reported with Norplant were diagnosed shortly after insertion, and the patients were in fact pregnant at the time of insertion. Hence, if a patient cannot fulfill the first two criteria for insertion, obtaining two sensitive pregnancy tests and ensuring their negativity 10 days apart provides further assurance that the patient is not pregnant at the time of insertion.

Key aspects to the use of implantable contraception appear to be patient selection and provision of adequate counseling. The patient's ability to tolerate the two most significant side effects, ie, irregular bleeding and weight gain, appears to be related to the adequacy of counseling of patients prior to insertion. If contraception is for spacing of pregnancies, a shorter acting agent should be considered. Most important, pregnancy should be excluded at the time of insertion. Furthermore, because it is a long-acting contraceptive, the follow-up in annual examinations has been less than ideal. Hence, appropriately timed reminders for routine annual care are recommended.

D. Long-Acting Injectable Contraceptive Agents–The concept of an injectable progestational contraceptive was initially introduced in 1950. Long-acting injectable progestational agents provide a passive means of contraception that must be renewed at 3-month intervals. These agents have the advantage of requiring little daily involvement by the user and are ideal for patients with problems in compliance.

Depot medroxyprogesterone acetate (DMPA) is the most commonly used injectable contraceptive; it has been in use in more than 90 countries. Its use has attracted considerable controversy because initial studies in beagle dogs suggested an association between long-acting progestational agents and breast

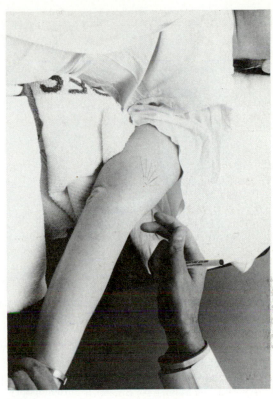

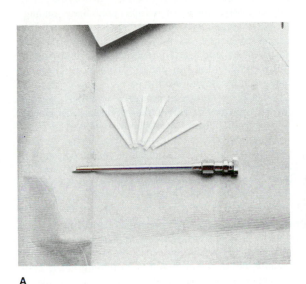

A   B

Figure 51–2. Norplant system *(A)* and outline of pattern of insertion on the medial aspect of the brachium *(B)*.

cancer. Subsequent studies did not confirm this finding, and the agent was recently approved by the Food and Drug Administration as a contraceptive agent. The controversy continues, however, because long-term follow-up studies are lacking.

DMPA is used as a single 150-mg dose repeated at 3-month intervals. The most common side effects of these long-acting drugs are irregular bleeding and weight gain. After a 150-mg injection of DMPA, the mean interval for return of ovulation is 4–5 months. There is no correlation between the number of injections and the length of time for return of ovulatory function. Seventy percent of DMPA users conceive within the first 12 months following discontinuation and 90% within 24 months. The efficacy rate of DMPA is similar to that cited for oral contraceptives.

Intrauterine Devices

Through the late 1960s and early 1970s, IUDs were used by 10% of women as contraceptive devices. However, the initial descriptions of severe pelvic inflammatory disease and maternal death when pregnancy occurred with the Dalkon shield (Fig 51–3) in situ led to an expanding investigation of the Dalkon shield and of intrauterine devices in general regarding their safety and efficacy.

In an increasingly litigious atmosphere, concerns regarding product liability led to a dramatic decrease in IUD use. When the public was polled regarding the safety of IUDs, no distinction was made by respondents between Dalkon shields and other IUDs. All IUDs were withdrawn from the market in the early 1980s, which left a substantial gap in choices of passive types of contraception. The debate persists regarding the exact association between infertility and pelvic inflammatory disease and IUD use. It is only in the case of the Dalkon shield that this association appears unquestionable. With further scrutiny of the data in the contemporary literature, it may be possible to expand the population for whom the IUD offers a viable contraceptive method. A new generation of IUDs is now available that are distinct from their predecessors. These devices offer contraception that appears to be as safe as other contraceptive methods. However, despite a favorable profile, IUD use accounts for only 1% of contraception in the USA.

There are currently two IUDs available for insertion in the USA: a copper-containing device, the T380, marketed as the Paragard and the Progestasert, and a progesterone-containing intrauterine device. The copper-containing T380 has a longer placement

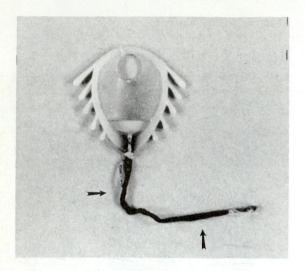

Figure 51–3. Dalkon shield intrauterine device (IUD). Note multifilament tail (arrow).

life than the original copper-containing IUDs, 4–8 years as opposed to 3 years.

A. Mechanism of Action: Copper-containing IUDs act by the induction of a sterile inflammatory reaction within the uterine cavity. This reaction fosters a milieu unsuitable for implantation; data suggest there is also interference with fertilization. The copper in the devices may contribute to the interference by increasing the inflammatory reaction, decreasing the viability of sperm, and limiting the transport of ovum.

Progesterone-containing intrauterine devices combine the potential advantages of an intrauterine device as a passive means of contraception and hormonal contraceptives known to decrease the risk of pelvic inflammatory disease. These devices are designed to release a fixed amount of a progestin per day. Their primary activity appears to be at the level of the endometrium and cervix. Progestasert is the only progesterone-containing IUD marketed in the USA at this time. This device releases progesterone from the long stem of the T-shaped device. The effectiveness of this device decreases markedly after 1 year, and annual replacement is essential. Data suggest that in addition to its efficacy as a contraceptive agent, the local effect of the progesterone results in less blood loss during menstruation and a decrease in the incidence of dysmenorrhea. Levonorgestrel-containing IUDs are available in Europe; they have been shown to be effective contraceptive agents in addition to reducing the incidence of pelvic inflammatory disease, probably secondary to a local progesterone effect.

Additional IUDs are available in other countries and are under investigation. Data from two of these studies show a favorable profile for user safety. The most significant aspect of these IUDs is the low rate of pelvic inflammatory disease associated with each model; although incidence may be no different in user versus non-user populations, PID presents a problem regardless of IUD use.

B. Clinical Management: The cornerstone to safe IUD use is patient selection. Patients are not candidates for IUD use if there is a history of pelvic inflammatory disease or ectopic pregnancy, undiagnosed dysfunctional uterine bleeding, or multiple sexual partners or if they are is unable to assess string placement. Careful consideration and caution should be exercised in patients who have structural abnormalities of the uterine cavity, such as fibroids or a history of in utero exposure to diethylstilbestrol (DES); a history of valvular heart disease; an allergy to copper; or a history of impaired fertility.

Placement may occur at any time in the cycle if the woman is reliably using other contraception or if two sensitive pregnancy tests are negative at least 10 days apart. Data suggest that infection and expulsion rates are lower if the placement occurs on a nonmenstruating day in the cycle. In the immediate postpartum period, placement is associated with higher expulsion rates and is best avoided. The IUD should be placed 6 weeks post partum if the woman is breastfeeding, is not sexually active, is reliably using contraception, or has had negative pregnancy testing as just described.

The patient must be well informed regarding the signs and symptoms of infection, perforation, ectopic pregnancy, and expulsion. She should be instructed in the means of access to care in such instances. Past unfavorable publicity on the topic of IUDs has created an emotionally charged atmosphere for a decision concerning this method. It is essential that adequate counseling take place before IUD insertion. Preplacement counseling to minimize the fears and complications of this method cannot be over-emphasized. Informed-consent materials are distributed with the IUDs and provide an opportunity for discussion. It is essential for the physician or clinic representative to review and sign these documents with each patient.

Menorrhagia may occur during the first 2–3 months after placement of an IUD. If this symptom persists, the patient should undergo further evaluation to rule out infection or pregnancy. Nonsteroidal anti-inflammatory agents may be used in an attempt to decrease the amount of monthly bleeding; dysmenorrhea also may be managed with these drugs. Should the pain become severe, culture and appropriate treatment for possible STDs or pelvic infection should be considered.

Barrier Methods
A. Male Condoms:
1. Background—The demonstration that the

transmission of the virus responsible for AIDS could be prevented with the use of appropriate barrier contraceptive techniques brought condom use to the forefront of contraceptive technology after some period of dormancy. The importance of condom and spermicidal use cannot be overemphasized. These agents may be viewed not only as a technique of contraception, but also as a necessary adjunct to the use of other contraceptive techniques that do not prevent the spread of STDs.

Male condoms may be lubricated, textured, tinted, contoured, or equipped with a spermicidal jelly or a reservoir tip. Regardless of options, male condoms are all basically of the same design, measuring 19 cm in length and 2.5 cm in width. The types available depend on locale and market and the number available ranges from one to several dozen. The importance of condom use regardless of choice of contraceptive must be discussed in all counseling sessions. The effectiveness of condoms is enhanced when combined with the use of spermicidal agents, which have the additional benefit of activity against a variety of viruses, *Chlamydia,* and gonorrhea, and efficacy in the reduction of pelvic inflammatory disease in the female partner. The combination of the mechanical barrier with spermicidal jelly presents an attractive choice for the couple who are engaging in behaviors that may place them at increased risk for STDs or HIV infection.

2. Mechanism of action–Placement of a condom is intended to prevent sperm from entering the female reproductive tract. The use of a spermicidal gel or foam may increase effectiveness by reducing viable sperm and is recommended routinely. The use of these agents also improves protection against AIDS and STDs. Spermicidal condoms became available in the early 1980s. This addition has been shown to reduce the motile sperm detected 60 seconds after ejaculation from 50% without spermicide to 4% with spermicide.

3. Clinical management–The male condom is used by 15% of couples. Its widespread availability is a distinct advantage over some of the other methods. The rate of breakage varies widely depending on the study population. The average rate per act of intercourse is approximately 1 in 100. It is part of routine counseling to encourage all couples in the early phases of a new relationship to employ condoms and spermicide until there is certainty that neither partner is HIV-positive. Latex condoms, as opposed to those made of natural products, seem to offer the greatest protection against HIV; those that are impregnated with spermicide appear to be particularly protective.

Regular use of male condoms presents unique social aspects not found with other techniques. Both men and women may report some degree of dissatisfaction with this method, owing to decreased sensation during intercourse, lack of spontaneity, and irritation. Although most users prefer a prelubricated condom, any additional lubricants should be water-based. Mineral-based lubricants may weaken the latex at body temperature and predispose to breakage when used. Surgical jelly such as K-Y lubricant jelly is preferred. Mineral and vegetable oil, cold cream, and petroleum jelly are to be avoided.

Condoms and spermicidal agents may be recommended to any person at high risk for HIV infection and to couples with an intolerance for any other method of contraception. It is essential that patients be adequately counseled regarding the need for effective use of condoms. This counseling should include women who plan to use them as their method of contraception. Such counseling includes proper placement and the need to use the method reliably with each coital episode.

B. Female Condoms:

1. Background–Recent approval by the FDA has brought the female condom to the marketplace. This device offers women for the first time the opportunity to be autonomous in condom use; no participation from a male partner is required. This aspect may be important when the male partner refuses to use a condom. The female condom is a long polyurethane pouch that is designed to line the vagina. It is designed with two rings: an inner ring fitted over the cervix (similar to a diaphragm) and an outer ring to anchor the pouch outside the vagina (Fig 51–4). Although not yet widely used, the female condom is available through agencies such as Planned Parenthood. Data on effectiveness are limited. The use effectiveness failure rate at 1 year has been estimated at 15%.

2. Clinical management–The female condom is considered an over-the-counter method that is a reasonable alternative to the male version. Because it is relatively new in use, the ability to describe the "ideal" user is difficult. Physical sensation does not appear to be compromised for either the male and female partners. In one study, male users described the sensation of the female condom to be more acceptable than that of the male condom. Disadvantages described include the fact that it is more cumbersome to use than other barrier methods. Specifically, it can be pushed entirely into the vagina or fall completely out of the vagina. The outer ring can irritate the external genitalia of both the male and female partner. It is also a concern that vaginal penetration may occur outside of the condom (between the pouch and the vaginal wall).

C. Diaphragm:

1. Background–Margaret Sanger established the first diaphragm manufacturing firm in 1925, thus bringing contemporary contraceptive techniques to the USA. With FDA approval as a medical device, the diaphragm received an early initial endorsement and widespread use among the public. This early endorsement and approval by the FDA led to a distinct

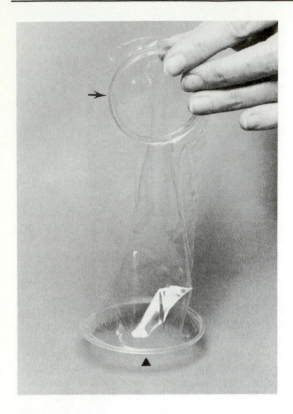

Figure 51–4. Female condom demonstrating the inner cervical ring (arrow) and outer vaginal ring (arrowhead).

The diaphragm needs to be fitted to each woman. Diaphragms should be fitted to accommodate the largest diameter possible for a patient without any discomfort. Diaphragms are available in a variety of sizes and are numbered according to the diameter of the rim. The rims may be made of a flat spring, a coil spring, an arching spring, or a wide-seal rim. The diaphragm may be inserted by folding it in half after placement of the spermicidal jelly and sliding it into the vagina. Adequate positioning should be verified after placement. For patients who have difficulty with the vaginal insertion of the diaphragm, a plastic introducer is available that may facilitate placement.

Diaphragms may be considered in patients who are unable to use alternative methods. Because diaphragms are available by prescription only, the cost of an office visit must be considered. The inconvenience of insertion in advance of sex, although not different from other over-the-counter methods, has been cited as altering the spontaneity of the sex act. Education in its proper use is essential to maximize its effectiveness. The woman who uses this method has to be motivated and informed. The continuation rate for 1 year is between 50 and 80%. The patient should demonstrate to a provider her ability to use it properly. To maximize effectiveness, the patient should be instructed in the use of both a diaphragm and spermicidal jelly. A diaphragm should not be fitted within 6 weeks of delivery and should not be used in patients with a history of toxic shock syndrome.

A common complaint is recurrent candidal infection. Switching to a different spermicidal preparation may be of some benefit. Consideration of a serum glucose concentration in the woman with frequent recurrence may be worthwhile, because candidal infection can be a heralding symptom of diabetes. Continued irritation may be managed by consideration of other methods of contraception. In some cases, a change to the cervical cap may reduce the irritation, because there is significantly less spermicide used for this method.

D. Cervical Cap:

1. Background–The cervical cap is a barrier method similar to the diaphragm. It is snugly fitted over the cervix, unlike the arching dome of the diaphragm, which covers the anterior portion of the vagina and includes the cervix (Fig 51–5). The only approved cervical cap in the USA is the Prentif Cavity Rim Cervical Cap. Other caps in use in other parts of the world offer some advantages in certain situations. The cap, perhaps more than any other barrier method, requires a highly motivated woman to learn the appropriate method of use. This subset of women report high satisfaction with this method, especially when there have been problems with other methods in the past. The cap must be inserted prior to intercourse.

2. Mechanism of action–The mechanism of

advantage over the cervical cap, which received no such endorsement until 1988.

2. Mechanism of action–The diaphragm provides a vaginal barrier method to prevent viable sperm from entering the upper female reproductive tract. In addition to providing a physical barrier, the diaphragm also provides a vehicle for the administration of spermicidal jelly. The use of these agents has been shown to increase markedly the use effectiveness of the diaphragm.

3. Clinical management–The diaphragm is a soft dome of latex on a flexible rim, allowing for its insertion in the vagina and expansion to cover the cervix. It may be used in conjunction with spermicidal jelly to maximize its contraceptive effectiveness and as a further guard against infectious disease. The diaphragm must be inserted prior to intercourse and left in place for at least 6 hours after intercourse. It should be taken out at least every 24 hours, but it should not be removed if doing so would cut short the 6 hours required after intercourse. If the couple has intercourse more than once or if the diaphragm is inserted more than 6 hours in advance of intercourse, it is suggested that the woman insert an extra applicator of spermicide without removing the diaphragm.

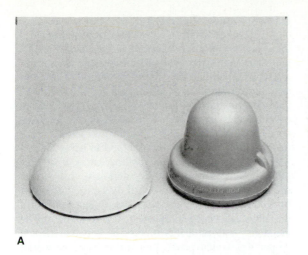 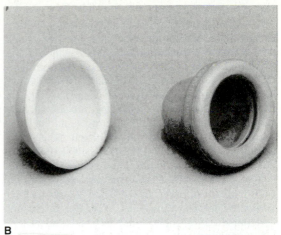

Figure 51–5. Prentif and Dumas cervical caps, vaginal side **(A)** and cervical side **(B).**

action of the cap is multifold and is somewhat different from other barrier forms. First, it is a barrier between sperm and egg. When the cap is inserted, it is filled approximately one-third full with spermicide, thus providing the second mechanism of action. It is theorized that the most significant mechanism of action has to do with the fact that the cervical secretions are sequestered within the cap. In this fashion, vaginal secretions predominate and create an acidic environment. This alteration of the pH creates an environment that is naturally spermicidal. The woman has to wear the cap for at least 8 hours after intercourse to maintain this environment and ensure the maximal effectiveness.

3. Clinical management–The cap is available by prescription only. The supplier of the cervical cap sells the caps for dispensing only to a person or institution that has been "certified" in the fitting of caps. The fitter should describe to the wearer techniques of use and insertion. An initial and follow-up visits are required; in addition, the FDA requires a repeat Papanicolaou (Pap) smear after 3 months of use and routine cytologic study thereafter.

The cervical cap may be considered an alternative barrier technique for couples who find that condoms, the diaphragm, or spermicidal agents inhibit sexual responsiveness. Literature suggests that sexual responsiveness may be more favorable with the cap. The fact that the cervix is within the cap may heighten the awareness of the uterine contractions at climax. Male partners, who may be able to feel the cap, have described its use both positively and negatively. Because the cap may be placed hours to a day or more in advance of intercourse, it does not have to interfere with the spontaneity of sex. It is significantly less cumbersome than the diaphragm, because the required amount of spermicide is much less, and the spermicide is contained within the vessel of the cap. The contraindications for the use of the cap include a history of DES exposure, a history of toxic shock syndrome, and untreated cervical dysplasia.

The cap is approved for use for 48 hours. It should be removed for a few hours every other day. However, the wearer should always err on the side of protecting against pregnancy. The fact that the cap may stay in place for 48 hours is more convenient than the 24-hour limit of the diaphragm. Extra spermicide should not be inserted if intercourse occurs more than once when the cap is in place or if the cap is inserted hours in advance of intercourse. To insert extra jelly or cream may alter the manner in which the cap is secured onto the cervix.

It is essential that the placement of the cap be checked both before and after intercourse because of the possibility of dislodgment during intercourse. The placement is checked by running a finger around the top edge of the cap to make sure that the cervix is fully contained within the cap. Although this aspect is perhaps the most difficult part of using the cap, with coaching, nearly all women can manage this check. The person who is not able to do this check is probably not a candidate for the cap. The fitter and the patient have to feel confident that the patient can identify both appropriate and inappropriate placement. Cervical caps must be used by patients who are highly motivated both in the placement and in the subsequent checking for accurate insertion.

It is recommended that the new cap wearer use a backup method for the first month while she is gaining proficiency in the use of the cap. If the woman has been taking oral contraceptives, she should continue for 1 month. A routine follow-up appointment is recommended at that time to ensure proper fit and technique.

Vaginal Spermicides

A. Background: Spermicidal preparations have been available for use for some time. The two agents most commonly used are nonoxynol 9, which is the active ingredient in most spermicidal jellies, and octoxynol 9. Their relative ease of use and affordability make them an important over-the-counter method of contraception. Benefits of the spermicides include activity against a wide range of viruses and bacteria, which appears to provide an additional measure of protection against STDs. They are available in a variety of forms, such as foams, jellies, and creams. The contraceptive sponge is now available and is impregnated with 1 g of nonoxynol 9. These agents may be considered for use in patients who have infrequent intercourse and in whom compliance is not an issue.

B. Mechanism of Action: Spermicidal preparations are surface active agents that destroy the sperm cell membrane. This is the most important mechanism of action of nonoxynol 9 and octoxynol 9. Other spermicidal agents with surface active properties include menfegol and benzalkonium chloride, which are available in other parts of the world. Enzymatic inhibition is a second mechanism of action in these agents. In addition to their inhibitory action on sperm, these agents are active also in preventing STDs. Data suggest that there is significant protection against gonorrhea and *Chlamydia* when nonoxynol 9 products are used. This agent also has been shown to be effective against the herpes virus, *Trichomonas*, syphilis, and HIV. The protection against STDs and HIV appears to be enhanced when the spermicidal agents are used in conjunction with a barrier method.

C. Clinical Management: The failure rate for the first year of use for the spermicidal agents as sole contraceptive agents is extremely high at 21%, probably because of nonuse. When used reliably, however, vaginal spermicides provide an effective means of contraception, with failure rates of 3%. Their greatest disadvantage is the need for absolute compliance. There are no data to suggest that the use of one agent over the other is more effective. Each product appears to offer comparable contraception. If foams, films, or suppositories are used, adequate time must be factored into the use of these agents to permit dissolution and dispersion of the agent within the vagina. The use of a barrier method in conjunction with the spermicide markedly increases the effectiveness. In the absence of a barrier method, reliable and consistent use is absolutely essential. Accurate placement high in the vagina is required; spermicidal applicators can assist in placement. The use of spermicides for vaginal douching after intercourse is not acceptable. If an individual wishes to douche following vaginal intercourse and is reliably using a vaginal spermicidal jelly, she should wait 6–8 hours after intercourse.

Natural Family Planning

A. Background: Natural family planning (also known as the rhythm method) is based on the fact that there are observable and measurable changes in a woman's body at the time of ovulation. These observable changes serve as signals to the couple to avoid intercourse or "intimate genital contact" during the times that are considered to be high risk for pregnancy. The World Health Organization (WHO) estimates worldwide use of this method to be as high as 11%. Women choose this method because of religious preferences, availability and low cost, or the desire to have a sense of control over their body. The method requires a significant commitment to identify the physical changes specific for ovulation. The pregnancy rate with this method is between 10 and 25 per 100 woman years. In some areas of the world, the method, used correctly, has a nearly perfect effectiveness rate.

B. Mechanism of Action: Natural family planning has as its underpinning the definition of a "fertile zone." The exact definition of this interval is essential in determining both the earliest and latest possible times of fertility. Implicit in this method is abstinence or other contraceptive use during the fertile interval.

C. Clinical Management: Detailed instruction in temperature charting, definition of time of ovulation, and awareness of events of the menstrual cycle are essential prerequisites for natural family planning. The woman who participates in this technique, sometimes referred to as the Billings method, is instructed in the distinct features of the cervical secretions during each phase of the cycle. The critical phases suggesting fertility are identified, and intercourse is avoided during these phases. Fertile days are those in which the secretion is changing from watery to a consistency resembling raw egg white and for 3 days thereafter.

Data suggest that the cervical mucus method alone is not as effective as a combined use of temperature charting, menstrual calendar tracking, and monitoring other symptoms of ovulation. Basal body measurements that are taken and charted correctly provide useful visual data for the prediction of ovulation. To maximize the accuracy of this method, the woman measures her temperature each day on awakening and before engaging in any activity. The reading is plotted on a graph so that the marked increase in temperature that occurs with ovulation is apparent. Intercourse should be avoided 3 days prior to ovulation and the 3–4 days following ovulation, although cycle variation may occur.

Patients who are candidates for use of natural family planning are highly motivated women with an understanding of the menstrual cycle and the subtleties of the cyclic changes in their body. Irregular cycles or any menstrual disorder seriously limits the applicability of this technique. Essential to natural family planning is a skilled instructor who is readily available to the user. The fact that this method is free and within the control of most women makes it attractive worldwide. It is consistent with teachings of the Catholic religion on family planning and thereby appeals to the large segment of the world population that strictly follows these teachings. The most obvious shortcomings are a high failure rate, particularly among women who are not motivated or do not fully understand the method, and the need for intensive instruction sessions and instructors available for consultation.

EMERGENCY CONTRACEPTION
(Postcoital Contraception)

Background

What has come to be known as a "morning after" pill should be labeled "emergency contraception." It is essential that patients understand that this form of contraception may be used after an interval greater than 1 day after unprotected intercourse. Different forms of emergency contraception may be reliably implemented for up to five days after an episode of unprotected intercourse. Patients frequently have the impression that even if they were evaluated in the late afternoon or evening on the day after an episode of unprotected coitus, that any of these methods of emergency contraception would be ineffective. The data simply do not support this. Emergency contraceptive techniques may be used effectively as late as 72 hours for hormonal emergency contraception and as late as 5 days for IUD insertion to avoid an unwanted pregnancy. Hence, the term morning after pill is an unfortunate misnomer and should be avoided in most circumstances.

Mechanism of Action

Postcoital hormonal contraception appears to act primarily through an alteration in the endometrial receptivity. The mechanism of action for the IUD appears to be the inhibition of implantation by the sterile reaction initiated by the IUD and the cytotoxic effects of the copper in the IUD.

Clinical Management

Emergency contraception should be part of any counseling session regardless of the primary contraceptive technique chosen. Hormonal therapy as emergency contraception may be instituted using a variety of agents. Most commonly, 50 µg of ethinyl estradiol and 0.5 mg of norgestrel, two tablets twice a day, 12 hours apart, for a total of two doses (four tablets), should be initiated within 72 hours after an episode of unprotected intercourse. These agents may be used any time within 72 hours, and there are no data to suggest that if used earlier or later they are more or less efficacious. After administration of

these agents, it is prudent to wait 2–3 weeks for the onset of menses and, if no bleeding occurs, to order a pregnancy test. During this interval, the patient must either abstain from intercourse or use a barrier method of contraception such as condoms or foam to avoid the possibility of a second episode of unprotected intercourse. Should the patient have a second episode of unprotected intercourse, this regimen should be repeated. The failure rate is approximately 3% for this method. Should the patient become pregnant secondary to failed emergency contraception, there is no evidence to suggest that the pregnancies are in any way affected adversely. Danozol (Danocrine) and the combination of of ethinyl estradiol and norgestrel (Ovral) tablets are the most commonly used agents; danazol, 400–600 mg 12 hours apart, appears to be slightly more effective than the Ovral regimen. Other hormonal regimens may be applied, depending on the availability of the different agents (Table 51–6).

Contraindications to these regimens are identical to those for oral contraceptives. The indications for emergency contraception include unprotected intercourse during the critical midcycle window in patients with regular monthly menses or at any time in patients with an uncertain first day of last menstrual period or irregular cycles; in patients who have missed two pills and did not use an alternative contraceptive technique; when a diaphragm becomes dislodged earlier than expected; and when the interval since depot medroxyprogesterone (Depo-Provera) injection exceeds 15 weeks.

Insertion of a copper-containing IUD may be considered emergency contraception in multiparous patients in the following circumstances: if there have been multiple unprotected exposures during the critical time of ovulation; if the patient wants to opt for an IUD as her method of contraception; and if the patient presents for evaluation and therapy at a time after intercourse that exceeds the 72-hour time limit for hormonal emergency contraception.

Table 51–6. Emergency contraceptives: hormonal regimens.

Hormonal Agent	Method of Administration
Ovral	2 tablets PO stat, then 2 more tablets 12 hr later
Nordette, Levlen, or Lo/Ovral	4 tablets stat, then 4 more tablets 12 hr later
Triphasil or Tri-Levlen	4 yellow tablets stat, then 4 more tablets 12 hr later
Ethinyl estradiol (Estinyl)	2.5 mg PO bid or 5 mg PO daily for 5 d
Conjugated estrogens (Premarin)	30 mg PO daily for 5 d, 10 mg PO for 5 days, or 25 mg IV stat and 25 mg IV 24 hr later
Estrone sulfate (Ogen)	5 mg PO bid for 5 d
Danazol (Danocrine)	400–600 mg PO stat, then repeated 12 hr later
Mifepristone (RU486)	600 mg PO as a single dose

FEMALE STERILIZATION

Background

There has been a three- to fourfold increase since the early 1970s in the number of women who annually undergo sterilization. The original descriptions of the procedure involved a transabdominal approach with ligation and resection of the tube in what is commonly referred to as a **Pomeroy tubal ligation.** The advent of sophisticated endoscopic equipment in the early 1970s made possible the performance of tubal ligations through the laparoscope. This approach was facilitated by the widespread use of safe electrical generators for electrocoagulation in the early 1970s and the subsequent development of spring-loaded clips and Silastic rings in the mid-1970s. The availability of an operating laparoscope has enabled this procedure to be performed through a single infraumbilical incision. Postpartum tubal ligations had been described as early as 1903. This procedure has remained relatively unchanged. and involves an infra-umbilical incision and Pomeroy tubal ligation.

Mechanism of Action

Tubal ligations interrupt the fallopian tube and exert their contraceptive effect simply by mechanical interruption of tubal continuity. There has been a suggestion that a tubal ligation is associated with compromise to ovarian function and may result in irregular bleeding after the procedure, but this has not been proven conclusively and is currently being debated.

Clinical Management

The cornerstone for management of patients requesting a tubal ligation is adequate counseling. Concomitant with the increase in tubal ligations has been a definition of the legal rights of individuals seeking sterilization and the legal responsibilities of the practitioners performing them. Contemporary legal doctrine is explicit in describing the expectations that patients may have and the duties that are incumbent on the practitioner performing the tubal ligation. It is essential that the patient be informed of the nature of the procedure, whether the approach is laparoscopy or laparotomy, the type of tubal ligation, the risks and benefits, potential complications, and alternative methods of contraception available to the patient in a manner intelligible to her. It is essential that patients be aware that, although the procedure is considered permanent, there are failure rates inherent to the procedure. Adequate counseling of patients regarding these points of management will reduce the likelihood of litigation should a pregnancy occur in the future. Average failure rates for all types of tubal ligations may be quoted to patients in the range of 1 in 250 to 1 in 500. Although the procedure is considered safe, there is a case fatality rate of 4 in 100,000 procedures. This extremely low rate makes deaths attributable to sterilization a rare event, secondary to anesthetic complications, technical complications, or concomitant medical illnesses.

Preoperative laboratory screening should be kept to a minimum, but a hematocrit and urinary pregnancy test are essential. Other tests should be ordered only as indicated by history; there is no suggestion that extensive preoperative laboratory screening is beneficial or cost-effective in this setting. Patients should be counseled to continue their method of reversible contraception until the time of the procedure. For patients using oral contraceptives, the procedure may be performed at any time. In these circumstances, the patients should be counseled to continue their oral contraceptives until they have completed a full cycle. Continued OCP use will minimize the likelihood of irregular bleeding after the tubal ligation. For patients using an IUD, the device may be removed at the time of the tubal ligation. For patients who are not using a reliable form of contraception, the tubal ligation may be performed either at the time of menses or after two negative urinary pregnancy tests obtained 10 days apart while the patient uses reliable contraception in the interim. The majority of tubal ligations performed are by the laparoscopic approach, because this method seems to minimize complications and hospitalization and is more cost-effective.

Patients frequently inquire regarding the reversibility of a tubal ligation. The procedure should not be performed on any patient who even remotely is considering a reversal. If the patient does harbor such hopes, a reversible form of contraception is a better choice.

REFERRAL TO A SPECIALIST

The majority of complications from the use of any contraceptive agent can usually be managed by simple intervention. Techniques for managing these complications are outlined for each type of contraception in this chapter. However, there are unusual circumstances that may require further evaluation and referral to a specialist.

Patients with irregular and persistent bleeding while taking low-dose OCPs that does not respond to supplemental estrogen therapy should be referred to a specialist for evaluation to rule out anatomic abnormalities such as endometrial polyps. This evaluation may be done through hysteroscopy on an outpatient basis or by detailed transvaginal and transabdominal pelvic ultrasonography.

Patients with medical problems such as diabetes or migraine headaches may take OCPs; however, should their medical problems become exacerbated in association with OCPs, they should be evaluated further by a specialist prior to discontinuing the use of the OCPs. If a patient is pleased with the reliability of an oral contraceptive, the patient should be evaluated to make sure that there are not other factors contributing to the symptoms.

Patients who use implantable devices should be referred to a specialist if there is extreme difficulty in removing the implants or if not all the implants can be retrieved. Patients who have used long-acting, injectable contraceptive agents should be referred for evaluation if their menses have not begun after a 12-month interval.

If intrauterine devices cannot be removed easily or if the string is not immediately evident, patients should be referred for evaluation. In select circumstances, an IUD may be retrieved during pregnancy by hysteroscopic means without interrupting the pregnancy.

PREGNANCY & FAILED CONTRACEPTION

Contemporary contraceptive techniques, in spite of their high reliability, are occasionally associated with failure. When a patient becomes pregnant while using any contraceptive, the immediate priority should be to verify the location of the pregnancy. There is a clear increase in the incidence of ectopic pregnancies in patients who use either a progestin-only contraceptive or an IUD or who have had a tubal ligation. There is no evidence to suggest that there is a higher incidence of ectopic pregnancies in oral contraceptive or barrier method users. In these circumstances, early transvaginal ultrasonography to verify an intrauterine location of the pregnancy is warranted.

There is no evidence to suggest that conception while taking a hormonal contraceptive has a higher incidence of birth defects. The original suspicion that pregnancies occurring while patients were using OCPs resulted in more birth defects—specifically limb bud defects—has not been verified by larger studies. Patients who continue to term in whom emergency hormonal contraceptive measures failed similarly do not have a higher incidence of birth defects. Data published in 1981 suggested a potential association between spermicide use at the time of conception and a broad range of congenital anomalies. Subsequent studies failed to confirm this association.

Special circumstances apply when a patient becomes pregnant and an IUD is in place. This situation requires careful management. Approximately 30% of IUD-related pregnancies are associated with inadvertent expulsion of the IUD. The management of a pregnancy complicated with an IUD in place is dictated by the patient's interest in maintaining or aborting the pregnancy. If the patient requests termination, the IUD should be removed at the time of the abortion. However, it is essential prior to performing the abortion, to attempt to locate the IUD by ultrasonography, because it may have been expelled or may have perforated the uterus. If the patient wishes to maintain the pregnancy and the IUD string is visible, the IUD should be removed and an early transvaginal ultrasonographic examination performed to determine the location of the pregnancy. If the patient is interested in maintaining the pregnancy and the IUD string is not visible, management depends on the presence or absence of signs and symptoms of infection. Any suggestion of an infection necessitates evacuation of the uterus and appropriate treatment of the infection using aggressive intravenous antibiotic therapy. Aggressive treatment of serious pelvic infections cannot be overemphasized. If there are no signs of infection, the patient should be informed of her options and managed conservatively. A transvaginal ultrasonographic scan should be performed to exclude an ectopic pregnancy and to verify the position of the IUD. Since the discontinuation of Dalkon shields and the recommendation to remove IUDs in the event of pregnancy, no deaths have been reported among pregnant women with an IUD in situ.

Five percent of women who are pregnant with an IUD in place have an ectopic pregnancy. Data further suggest that progesterone-containing IUDs are associated with a 6- to 10-fold increase in the ectopic rate over other IUDs. When an event of pregnancy has been verified, early testing for serum HCG concentrations and a transvaginal ultrasonographic examination should be performed.

UNRESOLVED ISSUES

RU486

RU486 (mifepristone) is an antiprogesterone steroid initially described in 1982 when the understanding of the mechanism of action of steroid hormones and steroid receptors evolved. The use of this agent in early pregnancy interruption and as an emergency contraceptive was based on the hypothesis that the interruption of progesterone action would frustrate implantation by irreversibly altering the endometrial environment (see Chapter 54). When RU486 is administered during the menstrual cycle, it exerts a luteolytic effect and induction of menses. When given in critically timed doses, RU486 may have a role as an effective contraceptive agent. Its use as an emergency contraceptive agent is predicated on similar principles; it may be effective when used within 48 hours of the LH surge.

Gonadotropin Releasing Hormone: Agonists & Antagonists

The definition of the gonadotropin releasing hormone (GnRH) led to the subsequent development of two analogs, the agonist and the antagonist. The agonist is currently available as a depot injection or nasal spray, but antagonists are not yet clinically available. Both agents exert a profound blockade on the pituitary gland with subsequent hypogonadism. When used chronically in males and females, the GnRH agonist has led to anovulation and azoospermia, respectively. These effects are reversible on discontinuation of the agent. The difficulty with this approach is in the induction of a hypogonadal state and subsequent decrease in sex steroids. In one pilot trial, this prob-

lem has been overcome with the addition of an estrogen and progestin regimen without compromise to the efficacy of these agents as a contraceptive. The GnRH antagonist may be used as an emergency contraceptive agent and has been effective in blocking the midcycle LH surge when given as late as the day of the surge. The exact role of these agents in the future development of contraceptives remains speculative.

REFERENCES

Alvarez F: New insights on the mode of action of intrauterine contraceptive devices in women. Fertil Steril 1988;49:768.

Baird DT, Glasier AF: Hormonal contraception. N Engl J Med 1993;328:1543.

Bucksbee K: Phase three clinical trial with Norplant 2: Report on five years of use. Contraception 1993;48:120.

Couzinet B et al: Termination of early pregnancy by the progesterone antagonist RU486. N Engl J Med 1986; 315:1565.

Derman R: Oral contraceptives: A reassessment. Obstet Gynecol Surv 1989;44:662.

Dixon GW et al: Ethinyl estradiol and conjugated estrogens as postcoital contraceptives. JAMA 1980;244:1336.

Dubois C, Ulmann A, Baulieu EE: Contraception with late luteal administration of RU-486. Fertil Steril 1988;50: 593.

Farley TN: Intrauterine devices and pelvic inflammatory disease: An international perspective. Lancet 1992;339: 785.

Frank ML: One year experience with subdermal contraception implants in the US. Contraception 1993;48:229.

Glasier A et al: Mifepristone (RU-486) compared with high-dose estrogen and progesterone for emergency postcoital contraception. N Engl J Med 1992;327:1041.

Hatcher RA, Warner DL: New condoms for men and women, diaphragms, cervical caps, and spermicides: Overcoming barriers to barriers and spermicides. Obstet Gynecol 1992;4:513.

Howie PW: The progestin only pill. Br J Obstet Gynecol 1985;982:1001.

Kuhl H et al: The effect of a biphasic desogestrel-containing oral contraceptive on carbohydrate metabolism in various hormone parameters. Contraception 1993;47:55.

Paul C, Skeegg DC, Spears GFS: Depomedroxyprogesterone and risk of breast cancer. Br Med J 1989;299:759.

Rubin GL, Ory HW, Layde PM: Oral contraceptives and pelvic inflammatory disease. Am J Obstet Gynecol 1982;144:630.

Shoupe E, Mishell DR, Bopp BL: Significance of bleeding patterns in Norplant users. Obstet Gynecol 1991;77:256.

Sivin I, Schmidt F: Effectiveness of IUDs: A review. Contraception 1987;36:55.

Toivonen J, Luukkrainen T, Allonen H: Protective effect of intrauterine release of levonorgestrel on pelvic infection. Obstet Gynecol 1991;77:261.

Trussel J, Grommer-Strawn L: Further analysis of contraceptive failures of ovulation method. Am J Obstet Gynecol 1991;165:2054.

VanStaten MR, Haspels AA: Postcoital low dose estrogens and norgestrel combination: For interception. Contraception 1985;31:275.

Volpe A et al: Contraception in older women. Contraception 1993;47:229.

Webb A, Russell J, Elstein M: Comparison of Yuzpe regimen, Danazol and mifepristone (RU-486) as oral postcoital contraception. Br Med J 1992;305:927.

Yum K: Fertility awareness in the 1990s: the Billing ovulation method of natural family planning. its scientific basis, practical application and effectiveness. Adv Contracept 1991;7:301.

Zeken GL: Barrier contraceptive use and HIV infection among high risk women in Cameroon. AIDS 1993; 1:725.

Infertility

52

Lorna A. Marshall, MD

Essentials of Diagnosis
- Failure to conceive after unprotected intercourse for 12 months.
- Female factors: Ovulatory dysfunction, tubal disease, advanced age (over 34 years old), endometriosis, cervical abnormalities.
- Male factors: Varicocele, obstruction, infections, hormonal abnormalities, idiopathic.
- Fifteen percent of couples have unexplained infertility.

Essentials of Diagnosis
Incidence & Risk Factors
Etiology
Clinical Findings & Diagnosis
Treatment
Prevention
Prognosis
Referral to a Specialist
Psychosocial Issues
Controversies & Unresolved Issues

Incidence & Risk Factors

Since the 1980s, infertility has become an increasingly visible problem. There are greater numbers of women in the reproductive age group. Career demands and contraceptive availability have resulted in delayed conception, increasing the incidence of age-related infertility. Couples are anxious to build their families in a shorter period of time, increasing the use of the health care profession for assistance. The media have focused on the availability of the reproductive technologies and on dramatic procedures such as micromanipulation of sperm and embryos. Finally, alternative routes to parenting such as adoption have become more difficult. Fewer infants are available for adoption, possibly because of legalization of abortion and a greater acceptance of single parents.

Surveys to determine the prevalence of infertility have been taken of married women and sometimes of married couples. However, surveys do not include such groups as single women desiring childbirth. These surveys estimate that 8–15% of married couples in the United States are infertile.

The older the age of the female partner, the greater is the risk for infertility. The risk for infertility is doubled for women ages 35–44 compared to women 30–34. It is estimated that one-third of women who delay pregnancy until their mid to late 30s have an infertility problem. This finding is believed to be related to the effect of aging on egg quality and ovulatory function as well as to an increased chance of disorders such as endometriosis. In addition, the risk of pregnancy loss increases substantially with age, to greater than 30% in women in their early 40s.

Other risk factors for infertility include a history of menstrual abnormalities, sexually transmitted diseases or pelvic inflammatory disease (PID), ruptured appendix, in utero diethylstilbestrol (DES) exposure to male or female partner, and mumps orchitis in the male partner.

Etiology

It is a common misconception that infertility is a woman's problem; in fact, a male factor is involved in 40–50% of cases. Table 52–1 lists an estimated distribution of the causes for infertility. The total adds up to more than 100% because multiple factors may be present, involving both the female and male partners. Male factors include abnormalities recognized in the semen analysis, as well as functional abnormalities in sperm such as antisperm antibodies, poor penetration of the zona pellucida, or failed in vitro fertilization. Ovulatory dysfunction includes amenorrhea or oligomenorrhea from a variety of causes, as well as more subtle defects in ovulation such as a luteal phase defect. The term **unexplained infertility** refers to the couple who has tried for more than 2 years to conceive and who has undergone an entire evaluation, including laparoscopy and sperm penetration assay, with no abnormalities uncovered. Unexplained infertility is more common when the female partner is in her late 30s or early 40s; it may be termed **age-related infertility** in this group of women.

Clinical Findings & Diagnosis

When possible, the male and female partner should present together for the initial interview. A careful menstrual history should be taken, with attention to the recent pattern of menstrual flow and dys-

Table 52–1. Causes of infertility.

Cause	Percentage
Male factor	40–50
Tubal disease	15
Ovulatory disorders	20
Endometriosis	5
Other female factor	5
Unexplained	15

Table 52–2. Normal values for semen analysis.

Factor	Values
Volume	≥ 2mL
Viscosity	Liquefaction in 1 h
pH	7–8
Count	≥ 20 million/mL
Motility	≥ 50%
Morphologic factors	≥ 60% forms normal
White blood cell count	< 1 million/mL

menorrhea. A history of contraceptive practices, sexually transmitted diseases, pelvic surgery, and pregnancies should be taken. The possibility of in utero DES exposure and any family history of reproductive problems should be reviewed. For the male partner, the history should include any testicular injury or surgery, mumps orchitis, heat exposures, environmental exposures, smoking, alcohol use, recreational drug use including anabolic steroids, and in utero exposure to DES.

An initial evaluation for infertility gives the provider a chance to provide preconception counseling (see Chapter 55). Medical, genetic, and medication histories should be reviewed; appropriate laboratory testing should be performed; and vaccinations should be given if indicated.

Physical examination of the female partner should include attention to lean body mass, abnormal hair growth, and galactorrhea as well as a careful pelvic examination. A fixed, retroverted uterus or tender nodularity in the cul-de-sac could suggest endometriosis and should be evaluated before the infertility evaluation progresses further.

The male partner can be examined at the initial visit or later if semen abnormalities are present. A semen analysis should be the first test conducted in the infertility evaluation. Neither a history of past paternity nor a normal postcoital test replaces the semen analysis. The specimen should be collected by masturbation into a clean container after 2–3 days of abstinence. If the specimen is collected at home, it should be brought to the laboratory within 1 hour, preferably within 30 minutes, of collection. The male partner may use a silicone condom if masturbation to obtain a specimen is unsuccessful or too stressful. Normal semen parameters are listed in Table 52–2.

A clinician should not designate a male as infertile based on a single semen analysis, because there may be variation from sample to sample. The time for spermatogenesis is about 72 days, so that a second specimen should be requested after 2–3 months has elapsed. If the second specimen is abnormal, further diagnostic procedures in the female partner should be delayed until decisions are reached concerning the male partner. The semen analysis is so crucial to the evaluation of an infertile couple that many physicians believe the workup should not proceed further without this information. Certainly, no treatment such as

ovulatory medications should be prescribed without these results.

If the semen analysis is normal, the couple should be reassured. However, it should be made clear that this test is only a screening test for male factor fertility and that abnormalities of sperm function may be identified later. The couple should be discouraged from assigning responsibility to the female partner at this point in the evaluation.

The basal body temperature (BBT) chart is a useful tool that may give indirect evidence of ovulation. Temperature is taken immediately on awakening with either a BBT or digital thermometer. This constant vigilance of the menstrual cycle can cause significant stress to the couple. Usually, 2–3 cycles should be sufficient to establish whether or not and when ovulation occurs. For women with cycle intervals consistently greater than 35 days, BBTs are not recommended. Such patients are oligo- or anovulatory and should be offered ovulation induction. It is important to recognize that ovulation usually occurs before the first temperature elevation; therefore, a rise in the BBT should not be used by the infertile couple as a signal to have intercourse.

It is important to avoid overreading of BBT charts. The intent is to screen for anovulation and to help the patient identify the approximate day of ovulation. There is no evidence, for example, that a gradual rather than an abrupt rise in temperature indicates the presence of an ovulatory abnormality.

Ovulation predictor tests are readily available and are accurate means to detect the luteinizing hormone (LH) surge, which begins about 36 hours before ovulation. These tests are useful in timing intercourse for couples with busy schedules and infrequent intercourse. Careful recording of the day of onset of a menstrual cycle, the day of the LH surge, and the first day of the subsequent cycle gives the clinician as much information as BBT charts do and may be less stressful for the patient.

Women who have normal menstrual cycles can have a progesterone level drawn on approximately day 21 of a 28-day cycle to document ovulation. A level less than 5 ng/mL suggests anovulation; ovulation induction medications should be offered to patients with such levels. A level over 10 ng/mL is reassuring, and other aspects of the evaluation should be pursued in patients with those results. If the level is intermediate (5–10 ng/mL), the test should be repeated. Further testing such as a luteal phase endometrial biopsy may be considered if levels continue to be less than 10 ng/mL.

Women who have irregular menses should have prolactin, thyroid-stimulating hormone (TSH), and follicle-stimulating hormone (FSH) levels drawn. FSH levels are most useful when drawn on day 3 of the menstrual cycle. Levels higher than 15 mIU/mL are predictive of poor results with assisted reproductive technologies, and probably also with other fertility treatments. Even if menstrual cycles are regular, a day 3 FSH level may be obtained in women over 35 years of age to provide information about the expected success of various treatment options.

Postcoital testing can be offered easily in the office. Usually, sperm is destroyed in the vagina within 5 minutes of ejaculation into the vagina. However, just prior to ovulation, sperm may survive in cervical mucus for up to 72 hours. A postcoital test measures the ability of the sperm to reach and survive in the cervical mucus. The test usually is performed 2–8 hours after the couple has had intercourse, after 48 hours of abstinence. The "sex on demand" aspect of this technique is difficult for some couples, and the physician and office staff need to be sensitive to this issue. A specimen of mucus is obtained with a nasal polyp forcep or a tuberculin syringe and examined grossly and microscopically. The cervical mucus should be clear and hypocellular, with 6–10 cm of elasticity (spinnbarkeit). Most important, at least five motile sperm with forward progression should be seen for the test results to be considered acceptable.

A normal postcoital test is reassuring, but a test may be abnormal (less than 5 motile sperm/high power field) for many reasons, including poor timing. Once ovulation has occurred, the mucus is no longer receptive to sperm. Abnormal tests should be repeated at least once before treatment is recommended, with careful attention to proper timing. If the test result is abnormal and excessive numbers of white blood cells (WBCs) are seen, cervical cultures should be obtained for *Chlamydia* and gonorrhea, and antibiotic treatment should be initiated, if indicated.

Hysterosalpingography (HSG) should be offered early in the evaluation. If a patient has undergone several cycles of treatment before learning that her fallopian tubes are blocked, she may be frustrated that the testing was not discussed earlier. Several studies suggest that pregnancy rates may be enhanced in the subsequent months when the results are normal. In addition to determining tubal patency, the HSG is an excellent screening tool for uterine abnormalities, for the evaluation of both infertility and recurrent pregnancy losses (Fig 52–1). Many fertility specialists prefer to perform hysterosalpingogram injections and evaluate the results themselves. In some centers, the radiologist performs the procedure, including the injection of dye, and the test can be ordered by any physician. It should be recognized that there are significant false-negative and false-positive rates for this test. It cannot detect pelvic adhesions or endometriosis. The risk of serious PID after HSG in women with a history of previous PID is 3%; therefore, some specialists recommend laparoscopy instead of HSG in these women. No studies support the ability of prophylactic antibiotics to prevent these infections. However, clinicians generally administer prophylactic doxycycline to women with a possible history of pelvic inflammatory disease, and to treat after the procedure if findings are consistent with tubal disease.

If these initial tests are normal, a younger couple usually is advised to continue timed intercourse for an additional 6 months before further testing or treatment is initiated. However, a luteal phase (10–12 days after ovulation) endometrial biopsy can be performed at this time if there is a suspicion of an ovulatory abnormality, eg, borderline progesterone levels, shortened or lengthened menstrual interval, or mild elevation in level of prolactin. Other tests that are often useful in the evaluation of infertile couples include sperm antibody testing, sperm penetration assay, ultrasonography, laparoscopy, and hysteroscopy. These tests add considerable expense to the evaluation, and their use should be considered carefully. Often, it is more cost-effective to refer the patient to a specialist at this time so that the remainder of the evaluation can be integrated into the overall treatment plan.

Treatment

Some treatments are offered before a complete evaluation has been performed in an effort to allow the couple to conceive in the most cost-effective manner. However, it should be kept in mind that many couples have several factors preventing conception. If one problem has been corrected, but pregnancy does not occur, other problems should be considered.

If the female partner is anovulatory or oligomenorrheic (cycle interval greater than 35 days), treatment with clomiphene citrate is usually the first step. It is essential that other causes for anovulation such as hyperprolactinemia and ovarian failure be excluded before ovulation induction is initiated. Clomiphene citrate is a nonsteroidal medication that binds to the estrogen receptor and can initiate ovulation in women who have some endogenous estrogen. Generally, it is given orally in doses of 50–100 mg for 5 days, beginning on day 3, 4, or 5 of a menstrual cycle. It also can be given after a menstrual bleed has been induced with 10 mg of medroxyprogesterone acetate for 5–10 days. Ovulation usually occurs 5–10 days after the last day of medication. BBT charts provide the most useful method for monitoring of ovulation in a patient taking clomiphene citrate.

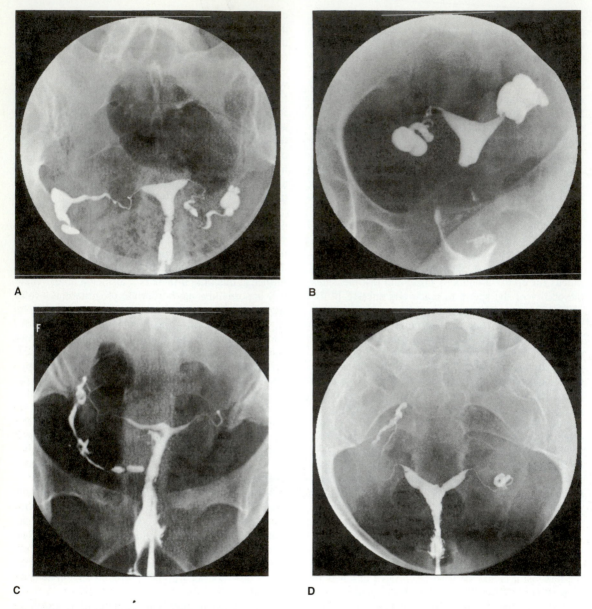

Figure 52–1. *A:* Normal hysterosalpingogram demonstrates a normal cavity and oil droplets seen exiting from patent tubes. ***B:*** Fallopian tubes markedly dilated from bilateral hydrosalpinges. ***C:*** Filling defect in uterine cavity caused by Asherman's syndrome. ***D:*** Abnormal uterine cavity, found at hysteroscopy/laparoscopy to be a midline septum.

Clomiphene should be started at a dose of 50 mg and increased to 100 mg if ovulation does not occur or occurs later than 10 days after the last dose of the medication. If ovulation occurs but pregnancy does not, there is no reason to increase the dose of clomiphene citrate. After the first cycle of treatment, and about every 2 months thereafter if pregnancy does not occur, the woman should have her BBT chart reviewed and her ovaries examined to exclude persistent ovarian cysts. If large ovarian cysts are present, no more clomiphene should be administered until the cysts resolve.

There is little evidence that clomiphene is beneficial to women who have normal menstrual cycles; in some cases, its antiestrogenic effect on cervical mucus and the endometrial lining may prevent conception. Therefore, the practice of administering clomiphene to ovulatory women is not recommended.

About 80% of anovulatory women ovulate after taking clomiphene, and approximately 40% conceive. A referral should be initiated if ovulation does not occur on a regimen of 100 mg of clomiphene or if pregnancy does not occur after 3–6 months of treatment. Ultrasonographic monitoring generally is recommended if doses greater than 100 mg are used. The multiple pregnancy rate is about 5%; the multiple births are almost entirely twins. No increased risk of birth defects has been reported. Side effects of clomiphene include vasomotor symptoms, mood changes, and, less commonly, headache, visual symptoms, and ovarian enlargement. Recent reports have raised the question of an increased risk of ovarian cancer in infertile women who have taken fertility drugs, but small numbers and questionable controls make it difficult to draw any conclusions from these reports.

If the postcoital test is persistently abnormal (less than 5 sperm/high power field) and the semen analysis normal, intrauterine inseminations of processed sperm of the male partner are indicated. Couples with this profile are the best candidates for intrauterine inseminations. If inseminations are not an available option, conjugated estrogens, 0.625–1.25 mg, may be given for 8–10 days before ovulation in an attempt to improve the cervical mucus.

Intrauterine inseminations often are advised for a limited period of time for male factor infertility, but they have not been shown to benefit couples with unexplained infertility. They are generally more successful than intravaginal inseminations when donor sperm is used. Usually, inseminations are performed best at an office that has access to a laboratory for the preparation of sperm and can perform inseminations 7 days of the week. Inseminations usually are performed 1 day after the LH surge is detected. A variety of catheters can be used, including the sheath of an 18-gauge intravenous catheter. A tenaculum may be used if intrauterine placement of the catheter is difficult.

Other treatments offered depend on the problems identified, the age of the female partner, and the couple's emotional and financial resources. Most reproductive surgery, including microsurgical tubal repair, is performed using the laparoscope or hysteroscope. Proximal tubal obstruction often can be treated with cannulation of the tube under fluoroscopic or hysteroscopic guidance. Menopausal gonadotropins are used with or without inseminations for the treatment of most ovulatory disorders that are unresponsive to clomiphene and also are useful for the treatment of unexplained infertility. Bromocriptine, progesterone, and pulsatile gonadotropin releasing hormone are useful in the treatment of selected ovulatory disorders. Varicocele repairs can improve semen quality and function in carefully selected men.

The primary care provider can play a significant role in patient education, even after a referral to a specialist has occurred. Myths abound in this area, and the provider should dispel them whenever appropriate. For example, couples who adopt do not conceive at an increased rate, and relaxation has not been shown to be therapeutic in the treatment of infertility.

Many couples who are infertile want to be as informed as possible about the treatment process, and the primary care provider can complement the educational services provided by the specialist. Patient brochures about the evaluation and treatment of infertility are available from the American College of Obstetricians and Gynecologists (ACOG), the American Society for Reproductive Medicine, and pharmaceutical companies that make infertility medications. Most chapters of RESOLVE, a support organization for infertile couples, keep libraries with patient educational material.

1. Assisted Reproductive Technologies: Since the birth of the first child resulting from in vitro fertilization (IVF) in 1978, the reproductive technologies have evolved into important and efficient treatments for tubal disease, male factor infertility, endometriosis-related infertility, and unexplained infertility. More than 35,000 egg retrievals were performed in the USA in 1992, resulting in over 7000 births. Unfortunately, these procedures are not available to most couples who could benefit from them, primarily because of their cost ($6,000–10,000/cycle) and the failure of most insurance plans in this country to cover even a limited number of cycles.

It is important that the primary care provider understand the options available and their approximate success rates. In 1992, about 17% of egg retrievals performed for IVF in the USA and Canada resulted in a delivery. Each reproductive technology program is required by the Society for Assisted Reproductive Technology to maintain outcome data. This information, as well as patient satisfaction, may help guide appropriate referrals.

IVF is the most commonly performed assisted reproductive procedure today. It was developed initially to bypass the function of the fallopian tube for women with severe tubal disease. After stimulation of oocyte development with menopausal gonadotropins, the eggs are retrieved under transvaginal ultrasonographic guidance. Insemination with the partner's sperm occurs in the laboratory, and the fertilized and cleaving embryo is transferred transcervically into the uterus about 2 days after the retrieval. The availability of embryo cryopreservation allows embryos to be saved for future transfer after the initial placement of a limited number of embryos in the uterus.

Variants of IVF, gamete intrafallopian transfer (GIFT) and zygote intrafallopian transfer (ZIFT), are more successful than IVF in some clinics for the treatment of unexplained infertility and some cases of male factor infertility. Normal fallopian tubes are usually necessary for both GIFT and ZIFT. In GIFT, the eggs are retrieved and, during the course of the procedure, placed into a catheter with sperm and transferred into the ampullary portion of the fallopian tube. This transfer usually is done laparoscopically, although it also can be performed transcervically with less success. In ZIFT, egg retrieval occurs as with IVF; when fertilization is documented, zygotes rather than gametes are transferred into the tubes.

Recent advances have allowed some couples to have more available options. Women with ovarian failure, even those with primary ovarian failure from Turner's syndrome, can conceive with donated eggs, fertilized in vitro with the husband's sperm. Ovum donation is frequently the best option for couples when the female partner is older than 40. Clinical pregnancy rates are low, and rates of pregnancy loss are high in women over 40 with all other reproductive technologies. Microinjection techniques have allowed couples with sperm counts too low for conventional IVF to reconsider the option. With intracytoplasmic sperm injection (ICSI), a single sperm is placed into the cytoplasm of the egg. In some states, surrogate arrangements are used to allow a couple in which the female partner lacks a normal uterus to use a "host uterus" to carry their genetic child. The complex ethical and legal issues are addressed continually through professional societies such as the American Society for Reproductive Medicine.

Prevention

The primary care provider is in an excellent position to take steps toward the prevention of infertility. To lower the risk of sexually transmitted diseases, condoms should be advised for contraception, and limitation of the number of sexual partners should be encouraged strongly. Sexually transmitted diseases should be treated promptly to prevent pelvic inflammatory disease and subsequent tubal infertility. Intrauterine devices should not be placed in nulliparous women who may desire a future pregnancy because of a possible increased risk of tubal infertility. Patients with progressive dysmenorrhea and pelvic pain should be evaluated aggressively to exclude endometriosis.

Couples should be encouraged to conceive before the female partner reaches her late 30s. Older women have an increased chance of infertility as well as a shorter period of time during which conception can occur.

When a couple is considering conception, they should be counseled about life-style factors that may diminish their chances of conception. Smoking and recreational drug use may diminish the fertility of either partner. The female partner should scale down a vigorous exercise program, especially if her menstrual periods are abnormal.

The male reproductive system is probably more sensitive to environmental influences than the female system. Nevertheless, both partners should be encouraged to minimize occupational exposures. The male partner should avoid prolonged exposure to heat, such as in hot tubs or saunas or in wearing tight briefs. Anabolic steroids can act as a contraceptive in men. Many lubricants are spermicidal; if a lubricant is necessary, vegetable oil is advised.

Preconception counseling should include a discussion of the menstrual cycle and of the appropriate frequency and timing of intercourse. In general, the optimal frequency of intercourse is every 36–48 hours from 3–4 days before until 2 days after ovulation. Few couples have intercourse too frequently for conception to occur. The couple should be reassured that it is safe and even encouraged to have intercourse on consecutive days in the periovulatory period. Ovulation usually occurs about 14 days before the subsequent menses, or on about day 14 of a 28-day cycle. Normal sperm can fertilize eggs for 24–48 hours after ejaculation, but an egg can be fertilized for only about 6–12 hours after ovulation. Couples need to understand that it is important for sperm to be available before ovulation. When the BBT has begun to climb, ovulation usually has already occurred. Rigorous attention to timing of intercourse should not be encouraged when a couple first attempts pregnancy, however, because of the potential for adversely affecting a couple's sexual relationship.

Finally, couples who are at high risk for infertility should be identified, and an evaluation or referral should be initiated earlier than the 1-year mark. Examples include women with a history of endometriosis or PID or of menstrual cycles that are more than 35 days apart; men with a history of mumps orchitis; and men or women in whom infertility has occurred in a previous relationship. In addition, clinicians may evaluate couples in whom the female partner is older than 37 years after 6 months of unprotected intercourse.

Prognosis

It is often difficult to evaluate the success of each treatment because of a significant spontaneous conception rate. It is estimated that half of couples who present for evaluation after 1 year of infertility and have a normal evaluation will achieve pregnancy in the next year without treatment. There are few randomized, controlled trials that are large enough to give accurate chances of conception for most infertility treatments. In general, most treatments other than some assisted reproductive technologies do not exceed the monthly conception rate in normal couples, which is about 20%. All treatments become significantly less successful when the female partner is older than 40.

When treatments are not successful, the provider can help the patient to understand the limitations of treatment. In addition, decisions about adoption or living without children should be reinforced when appropriate.

Referral to a Specialist

The primary provider for male and female partners is in a position to treat infertile couples. The provider may play a vital role in the prevention of infertility, including preconception counseling to maximize a couple's chance of conception. Providers choose variable involvement in infertility evaluations and treatments. It is important to have a general understanding of the available treatments and processes involved so that appropriate referrals can be made and emotional support given.

The timing of referral depends on the provider's training, interest, and office organization, as well as on the availability of infertility specialists in the area. Infertility is a rapidly changing field, with reproductive technology services becoming more available and successful. Patients are increasingly aware of the services available and often seek out a specialist to initiate an evaluation.

The best option for referral of the female partner is a board certified reproductive endocrinologist, who can guide a couple from a basic evaluation to consideration of the assisted reproductive technologies. Many gynecologists who have a special interest in infertility can perform a basic evaluation and initiate treatments other than the reproductive technologies.

If semen abnormalities are identified on two specimens, a referral to a urologist is recommended to evaluate the male partner further, treat any pyospermia, and recommend therapy. A urologist also should be seen if impotence may be affecting fertility. If a varicocele is present, repair may improve sperm parameters and increase the chance of pregnancy. The decision whether or not to fix a varicocele is sometimes difficult and requires input from both the urologist and the provider who is managing the female partner's evaluation.

Many couples, especially those with an older female partner, express frustration that referrals were not made soon enough. It is important for the provider to identify couples who require an early referral and to leave that option open for them from the onset of their complaint.

Psychosocial Issues

Emotional issues surrounding the evaluation and treatment of infertility are numerous and important for the primary care provider to understand. These are discussed extensively in Chapter 53. Ethical issues involve the many options available to build a family and are discussed briefly in Chapter 6.

Controversies & Unresolved Issues

There are many medical controversies in the field of infertility that center on the most appropriate and cost-effective approach to help a couple or woman to achieve pregnancy. Rigorous studies are lacking in this area because of lack of federal funding for many years and the difficulties in assigning patients to "no-treatment" arms of studies when they are hoping to conceive.

When to apply the available reproductive technologies to a particular couple is generally a medical and economic issue. However, possible restrictions on research in the field and on the application of the technologies is a source of legal and ethical controversy.

REFERENCES

Barnea ER, Holford TR, McInnes DRA: Long-term prognosis of infertile couples with normal basic investigations: A life-table analysis. Obstet Gynecol 1985;66:24.

Hammond MG, Halme JK, Talbert LM: Factors affecting the pregnancy rate in clomiphene citrate induction of ovulation. Obstet Gynecol 1983;62:196.

Lutjen P et al: The establishment and maintenance of pregnancy using in vitro fertilization and embryo donation in a patient with primary ovarian failure. Nature 1984; 307:174.

Menken J, Trussell J, Larsen U: Age and infertility. Science 1986;23:1389.

Rossing MA et al: Ovarian tumors in a cohort of infertile women. NEJM 1994;331:771.

Schwabe MG, Shapiro SS, Haning RV Jr: Hysterosalpingography with oil contrast medium enhances fertility in patients with infertility of unknown etiology. Fertil Steril 1983;40:604.

Scott RT et al: Follicle-stimulating hormone levels on cycle day 3 are predictive of in vitro fertilization outcome. Fertil Steril 1989;51:651.

Society for Assisted Reproductive Technology (SART), The American Fertility Society: Assisted reproductive technology in the United States and Canada: 1992 results generated from the Society for Assisted Reproductive Technology Registry. Fertil Steril 1994;62:1121.

Speroff L, Glass RH, Kase NG: *Clinical Gynecologic Endocrinology and Infertility,* 5th ed. Williams & Wilkins, 1994.

Steptoe PC, Edwards RG: Birth after implantation of a human embryo. Lancet 1978;2:366.

Whittemore A et al: Characteristics related to ovarian cancer risk: Collaborative analysis of twelve U.S. case-control studies. II. Invasive epithelial cancer in white women. Am J Epidemiology 1992;135:1184.

53
Emotional Aspects of Infertility

Mary Ann Draye, ARNP, MPH, FNP

Infertility has been described as a developmental crisis; as such, it has the potential to disrupt the progression of adult development. According to Erickson's theory of development, **generativity,** or guiding the next generation, is a major developmental task of adulthood. Most often in society, the task of generativity is translated into bearing and raising children. Failure to achieve generativity can lead to stagnation and self-absorption.

One theory of family development notes that couples think of themselves as potential parents long before children arrive. Infertility may result in a developmental crisis by defying the cultural norm (despite some support for child-free living) and the individual's own goal of parenthood. If parenthood is viewed as the primary means of role fulfillment, the threat of failure is significant, resulting in a sense of despair and loneliness. Components of generativity include creativity and productivity as well as nurturing. Parenting is one way—not the only way—of accomplishing these tasks.

The chronicity of infertility has an impact that needs consideration. Infertility brings one crisis after another (eg, negative pregnancy tests and monthly disappointments as new treatments are tried and failed). As time goes on, certain events such as birthdays or holidays may mark the attempts and failures at becoming pregnant.

Unruh and Mcgrath have pointed out that the steps of resolution employed in crisis and grief models do not always hold for infertility. Rather, the ongoing nature of infertility contributes to a chronic sorrow. The emotional pain is cyclic; it is experienced periodically as one is reminded of one's losses. In addition, the sorrow that accompanies infertility is not only for what is perceived as lost, but also for the current distress.

Common Responses to Infertility

Infertility is exhausting for all those involved. Extensive treatment and testing over time, the experience of hopes rising only to be shattered, and the expenditure of resources exact an emotional toll. Increasingly, the emotional aspects of infertility have been acknowledged in the literature. Common feelings associated with infertility are anger, denial, guilt, depression, isolation, grief, and decreased self-

Common Responses to Infertility
Gender Differences
Assisted Reproductive Technologies
Strategies for Helping

esteem. In addition, a patient may feel profoundly out of control. The feeling of lack of control, coupled with decreased self-esteem, leads to feelings of inadequacy.

A. Anger and Frustration: The patient's anger results primarily from feeling out of control and from the perceived unfairness of infertility. Many patients feel angry when they encounter parents who seem unfit, children who are abused, or news accounts of unwanted pregnancies. Frustration accompanies anger, because the demands and sacrifice associated with treatment are upsetting but must be tolerated to increase the chance of achieving pregnancy. Also, the inability to comfort one's partner is a source of extreme frustration for some (see the section following, "Gender Differences").

Anger can be rational, if it is directed at the situation, or irrational. Anger may be projected onto providers, one's partner, family and friends, or a stranger who has children. Anger also can be turned inward resulting in depression.

B. Denial: Denial is one of the early feelings associated with infertility. Most individuals assume they are fertile, especially when they are healthy. Reluctance to participate in certain procedures or refusal to accept a negative result may indicate some denial on the part of patient. Denial serves as a protective mechanism until a person can comprehend the magnitude of the crisis. However, denial is appropriate and effective only as a short-term coping mechanism.

C. Guilt: In trying to explain infertility, cause and effect relationships often are sought. Past thoughts and actions are reviewed as possible causes of infertility. Issues that commonly produce guilt include premarital sex, masturbation, previous abortion, contraceptive use, sexually transmitted diseases, divorce, and even ambivalence about parenting. Self-

506

blame over these events leads to feelings of guilt or of being punished.

D. Anxiety: Feelings of impending doom, worry, and uncertainty about the future all contribute to anxiety. In addition, treatment procedures may contribute to anxious feelings. Waiting for tests, worrying about how the partner will react, financial worries, and deciding how to tell others what is happening are dominant concerns.

E. Isolation: Often, infertile patients experience the loss of friends who become parents. For some, the pain of being around friends with children is too much to bear. If information regarding infertility is not shared, the person may be the recipient of pressure, well-meaning advice, and worse—bad jokes. If the information is shared with others, even more advice may be forthcoming along with stories of cures, others' successes, unwelcome sympathy, and uncomfortable silence. Whether or not the information is shared, the result may be that gatherings with family and friends become so painful that the infertile couple withdraws. Many infertile couples report feeling alone in a fertile world. They often turn to each other for their support, which can put further strain on a relationship that is already stressed. Although frequent communication is necessary, a common complaint of couples is that infertility is all they ever talk about anymore.

F. Grief: The grief associated with infertility has some unique characteristics. **Grief** is defined as a response to loss. For infertile couples, the grief process is different because they feel a potential loss rather than the concrete loss experienced with the death of a child. There is nothing tangible to mourn, and there are no rituals of support to help bear this loss. Moreover, the loss may be trivialized by well-meaning people who point out the benefits of being free of parenting responsibilities.

Simultaneously, couples experience grief over painful and costly treatments, strained relationships, and an uncertain future. The pain and loss are not forgotten but experienced repeatedly.

G. Depression: Feelings of sadness, despair, pessimism, and fatigue accompany infertility. Apathy and loss of pleasure also can characterize the normal depression of infertility. Usually, however, patients with mild depression are able to continue to function and do not use maladaptive coping strategies for extended periods of time. Patients with more severe depression have intense symptoms that significantly affect their functioning over time.

Worsening persistent sadness (depression), extreme changes in sleep and eating patterns, anxiety, increased use of alcohol and drugs, feeling out of control, persistent thoughts of suicide and death, and obsessive behavior all indicate more than the normal depression associated with infertility; referral to a mental health professional is indicated for patients with these symptoms.

H. Decreased Self-Esteem: Infertile patients are at risk for decreased self-esteem. Both women and men report feeling that their sexuality has been attacked by infertility. Women report feeling incomplete, less feminine, or a failure as a woman. Men report feeling defective and less virile. Consequently, both men and women may feel less desirable sexually or less confident about their sexuality. In addition, some medications used in fertility treatment may decrease sexual desire and pleasure.

Loss of self-confidence may occur in other areas of life as well. Pursuing treatment and working through the feelings involved take precedence over other activities. Competence in other areas of life such as career and partner relationships is minimized. Olshansky found that for infertile couples, infertility can become the central focus of their lives. When one's central view of oneself is associated with failure, as in the inability to achieve pregnancy, one's self-esteem suffers.

Gender Differences

Infertility and its treatment affect women and men differently. Initially, women seem to be more vulnerable to the infertility crisis than their male partners. Women appear to experience more distress, regardless of the medical cause. They report disruption in their personal lives, worries over role failure, decreased self-esteem, and a significant sense of loss. Women may increase medical and mental health-seeking behavior, whereas men may be less inclined to use such services. Commonly, the woman is the initiator of all types of treatment and has the most interactions with the health care system.

When the cause for infertility is a male medical factor, men report more feelings of loss and decreased self-esteem than men without a medical factor. However, these men do not report the same degree of disruption as their female counterparts. Women without a medical factor feel the loss of childbearing as strongly as those with such a factor. Men without a medical factor feel loss because of their inability to help their partner.

A. Coping Patterns: Women and men cope differently in response to infertility (Table 53–1). Women typically use a greater variety of coping methods. Social coping includes talking, seeking support, reading, and attending lectures. Emotion-focused coping, eg, wishing and hoping, also is employed although not to the exclusion of problem-solving coping.

Men are less likely to use social coping. Rather they employ a more private, problem-solving style of coping. Problem-focused coping implies developing and following an action plan. Men often substitute other activities for those lost, and they are more likely than women to continue to find pleasure in those other activities.

B. Communication Patterns: It has been sug-

Table 53–1. Common responses to infertility by gender.

Area	Male Response	Female Response
Communication	Less need or desire to discuss infertility	Needs and desires to discuss repeatedly
	Use of conversation primarily to problem-solve or compete	Use of conversation primarily to connect, relax, and discuss feelings
Coping	Private coping	Social coping
	Primarily problem-focused	Primarily emotion-focused, variety of strategies
Isolation	Some; generally able to compartmentalize infertility	Often significant; infertility pervades all areas of life; feels separate from other women
Frustration	Major source of frustration is feeling helpless to comfort partner; cannot seem to "make it better"	Major source of frustration is childlessness; lack of "success"
Options for parenting	Often able to consider child-free life earlier	Usually strong drive for motherhood

gested that if women and men talked through interpreters, they might have a better chance of staying together. Differing communication styles present a challenge to all couples, but they are of greater magnitude for partners facing infertility. During the course of treatment, many decisions need to be made including those concerning options for parenthood and expenditure of resources. These decisions require effective communication between partners. Furthermore, the emotions associated with infertility need to be shared with the partner.

Couples need to be open and honest in their communication and avoid making assumptions about their partner. To assume one knows what the partner thinks about an issue or feels in response to a loss is dangerous. These assumptions can be wrong and lead to resentment and hurt feelings.

Another danger in communication is to judge the value of a communication style. For example, women tend to cope with infertility by verbalizing. It is helpful for them to talk about how they feel and review the dilemma of infertility. The male partner, on the other hand, may tire of hearing the same words over and over. To him, to communicate is to problem-solve and sometimes to be assertive and show what he knows. Therefore, he offers a solution to her verbalizing when a solution is not what she desires. She simply wants to express herself and be listened to empathically. The deleterious effect occurs when value judgments are ascribed to the styles. He thinks she is overemotional, compulsive, and obsessive. She thinks he is uninterested, less caring, and detached. He tends to withdraw and feel nagged. She feels alone and unsupported. In truth, they are merely using different styles of communications.

Studies indicate that when communication becomes difficult or upsetting, men feel threatened and less equipped to handle their partner's expressions of negative emotions. This reaction contributes to frustration. He may express himself as follows: "I try to help her but nothing seems to work, so I just quit and wait it out, but it's getting tiring." "I wish I could be more in touch with my feelings like she is, but I'm not—that's just the way I am." Repeatedly and

poignantly, men have shared their profound sense of frustration at (1) not being recognized for trying to communicate and (2) inability to comfort their partner no matter how hard they try.

The existence of these differing styles does not mean that women and men do not communicate successfully concerning infertility or that women never problem-solve and men never support. Rather, these are some of the prevailing patterns and pitfalls that can be difficult for some partners.

Assisted Reproductive Technologies

The advancing technologies of assisted reproduction (see Chapter 52) bring new hope to couples who previously had none. Although changes occur in technology, the emotional aspects of infertility are not changed. When patients consider the wide range of treatment options, however, additional dynamics related to the "high tech" nature of treatments are added to the emotional aspects of infertility. It is worth considering the blessings as well as the burdens of these new technologies.

The assisted reproductive technologies (ART) offer patients more hope than ever before, sometimes making it hard for patients to stop treatment. Many patients report that they feel compelled to try ART to "close the door" on infertility treatment. For some patients, ART represents the next logical step in treatment. ART often is viewed as the last chance for a biologic child, and chances for success may be overestimated. Taking advantage of the reproductive technologies usually requires significant expenditure of resources, not only financial but emotional and physical as well. In addition, a significant amount of time is required for clinic appointments and procedures. Life is rearranged around the demands of the treatment protocols.

Issues common to ART patients include expenditure of resources, confidentiality, ethics and values, handling loss, informed consent, and coping with the intrusion of technology into their lives. Balancing hope with realism proves to be a significant task for most patients. Worry for the welfare of the woman and normalcy of a child conceived through ART is also present (despite data showing that these pregnancies and outcomes are no different from spontaneous pregnancies). The rigors of ART treatment can have significant impact on patients. Daily monitoring and complex physical procedures can be stressful. Moreover, patients undergo these treatments with the knowledge that the chances for success are relatively low. This can contribute to worry and anxiety. For some couples the strain of waiting can be more difficult than the physical aspects of treatment (eg, "Did the eggs fertilize?" "Did pregnancy occur?"). When ART fails, the feelings of loss and sadness are profound. Although most couples eventually work through their grief, the emotional stress surrounding a failed ART cycle is significant.

Strategies for Helping

Primary care providers can play a valuable role in helping infertility patients. It may be the primary care provider who first discovers or hears about fertility problems. The relationship with the patient that has already been established can be helpful even as specialty care is being considered.

The primary care provider should inform patients of various options and services available and facilitate an appropriate referral. This includes a transfer of records and assistance as patients move from a familiar provider to the care of a specialist. Even while patients are being seen by specialists, the primary care provider may play a role in ongoing support. Obtaining feedback from specialists is important also, especially if the provider continues to see these patients for support, counseling, and other areas of primary care. Being accessible to provide information or discuss feelings in the office or by phone is important.

A. Empathy: The principal component of each interaction with patients should be empathy. **Empathy** is defined as an emotional sensitivity; it implies understanding of the other person's thoughts and feelings. Empathic listening involves sincerely hearing what the patient is saying in a nonjudgmental way. Sometimes merely interacting with an empathic provider is immensely helpful to patients.

B. Empowerment: A second role of the provider is to facilitate the empowerment of infertility patients. Clinicians do not directly empower patients, because that connotes a hierarchy of power. Rather, clinicians provide information and choices and support patients in their decision making. When recommendations are made by the health care team, patients are encouraged to weigh them in light of their life goals, values, and resources. For example, the recommendation may be to undertake another cycle of in vitro fertilization (IVF) when the patient's present goal is to stop treatment and reevaluate.

Another part of facilitating empowerment is helping patients to redefine the concepts of success and failure. Surely, taking home a baby is defined as success. Although facing adversity with courage, redefining life goals, and planning for the future are components of successful maturity, such qualities are rarely affirmed or acknowledged in the course of infertility treatment. Providers should use every opportunity to acknowledge the significant emotional work being done by infertility patients.

C. Anticipatory Guidance: Providing information is another way to facilitate empowerment in patients. When patients understand the treatment protocol, they usually feel more in control. Potentially serious errors can be avoided, and patient anxiety can be reduced. Anticipatory guidance helps to prepare patients for the future stages of treatment. For example, outlining the steps for obtaining a hysterosalpingogram helps the patient to know what to expect (eg, length of procedure, medications, side effects). Providing such guidance usually reduces fear of the unknown.

A part of anticipatory guidance includes information regarding community resources. Perhaps patient support groups, relaxation training, or a RESOLVE chapter is available. (RESOLVE is a national, nonprofit organization that offers information and support for infertile patients.) Crisis phones and professional therapists may be needed for a small percentage of patients. Primary care providers need to be aware of and develop effective referral networks.

REFERENCES

Abbey A, Andrews FM, Halman LJ: Gender's role in responses to infertility. Psychol Women Q 1991;15:295.

Domar A, Seibel M, Benson H: The mind/body program for infertility: A new behavioral treatment approach for women with infertility. Fertil Steril 1990;53:246.

Draye MA: Telephone counseling: The infertility patient. Obstet Gynecol Nurs Forum (Sept 3) 1991:3.

Draye MA, Woods NF, Mitchell E: Coping with infertility in couples: Gender differences. Health Care Women Int 1988;9:163.

Erickson E: *Childhood and Society.* Norton, 1950.

Greenfield DA (editor): *Infertility and Reproductive Medicine Clinics of North America: Psychosocial Issues in Infertility.* Vol 4. Saunders, 1993.

Klock SC, Maier D: Guidelines for the provision of psychological evaluations for infertile patients at the University of Connecticut Health Center. Fertil Steril 1991;56:489.

Olshansky E: Redefining the concepts of success and failure in infertility treatment. NAACOG's Clinical Issues in Perinatal & Women's Health Nursing 1992;3:343.

Unruh A, Mcgrath P: The psychology of female infertility: Toward a new perspective. Health Care Women Int 1985;6:369.

Woods NF, Olshansky E, Draye MA: Infertility: Women's experiences. Health Care Women Int 1991;12:179.

Wright J et al: Psychological distress and infertility: Men and women respond differently. Fertil Steril 1991;55: 100.

Pregnancy Termination

54

Kathy Preciado-Partida, MD

Since the 1973 United States Supreme Court decision of *Roe v Wade,* a woman may elect to terminate her pregnancy during the first trimester for her own reasons. During the second and third trimesters, each state may regulate the abortion procedures in ways that are reasonably related to maternal health.

Elective abortion, or voluntary termination of pregnancy, is the interruption of pregnancy before fetal viability at the woman's request. **Therapeutic abortion** is the termination of pregnancy before viability to protect maternal health or because the fetus is affected by disease or deformity. Certainly, the vast majority of abortions currently performed in the USA are elective.

Incidence

It is estimated that approximately 25% of pregnancies worldwide are terminated by induced abortion, rendering this perhaps the most common method of birth control. The number of legal abortions performed in the USA has risen steadily since 1973 and leveled off in 1980 (Fig 54–1). In 1989, there were 1.4 million abortions in the USA, or 346 induced abortions per 1000 live births.

The ratio of abortions to live births was highest for members of ethnic minority groups and women younger than 15 years of age. In 1988, there were 860,000 pregnancies in teenagers, with recent statistics indicating an almost 10% annual teenage pregnancy rate. In 1988, 23,000 women under 15 years of age terminated their pregnancies.

Generally, women obtaining abortions were young, white, and unmarried (25% were married), had no previous live births, and were having the procedure for the first time. Approximately 50% of abortions in 1989 were performed at 8 weeks or less gestational age, and 87% before the thirteenth week. Four percent of abortions were performed at 16–20 weeks of gestation, and 1% at greater than 21 weeks.

Clinical Findings

As in any procedure, it is essential to obtain informed consent. The nature, risks, alternatives, benefits, and indications for the proposed procedure or treatment need to be discussed in detail with the patient. All of her questions should be answered satisfactorily. The clinician should feel certain that the

---

Incidence
Clinical Findings
Technique
Complications
Referral to a Specialist
Psychosocial Issues
Current Controversies

---

patient requests this procedure of her own volition. It is prudent to mention other options for unplanned pregnancies such as adoption but important to respect the woman's right to self-determination.

A. History: The preoperative evaluation should include a medical history with particular attention paid to previous surgical problems, gynecologic disease, allergies, possible coagulopathy, and perceived pain tolerance. All of these factors may influence the planning and performance of the procedure.

B. Physical Examination: Physical examination should include heart, lung, abdominal, and pelvic examinations. It is essential to establish gestational age, because this generally determines the type of procedure to be performed. If the patient is uncertain of gestational age or if there is discordance between reliable dates and pelvic examination, it is wise to obtain an ultrasonographic scan to guide therapy decisions. Ultrasonography also may be appropriate if there has been abnormal bleeding to identify the occasional molar or ectopic pregnancy.

C. Laboratory Tests: Routine laboratory tests include a pregnancy test, hematocrit, and Rh typing and antibody screen. Controversy exists over the need for screening for sexually transmitted diseases (STD) and cervical neoplasia (see Chapter 37). Rho (D) immune globulin should be administered to women who are Rho (D) negative without Rh antibodies. Fifty grams should be given when the gestational age is 12 weeks or less, and 300 g should be given when the gestational age is greater than 12 weeks.

D. Counseling: Contraceptive counseling is a crucial part of a visit to terminate a pregnancy. Oral contraceptives can be started on the day of the procedure.

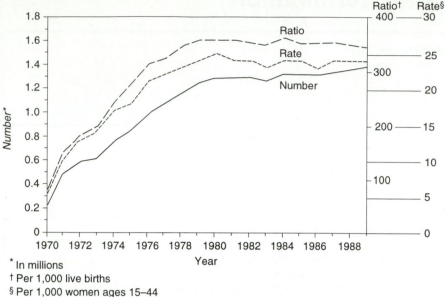

Figure 54–1. Number (in millions), ratio (per 1000 live births), and rate (per 1000 women ages 15–44) of legal abortions in the United States between 1970 and 1988. (Reproduced, with permission, from Koonin et al: Abortion Surveillance. Centers for Disease Control/U.S. Department of Health and Human Services 1989;41:55.)

Technique

There are three main methods for performing an abortion: instrumental evacuation vaginally, stimulation of uterine contractions, and major surgical procedures. Generally speaking, gestational age determines the technique.

A. Menstrual Extraction: Menstrual aspiration or extraction is early suction curettage of the endometrium; it may be performed up to 50 days after the last menstrual period. A flexible plastic cannula is used, 4–6 mm in diameter, with a self-locking syringe to provide suction. Menstrual aspiration has the advantage that anesthesia and cervical dilation often are not required. If a chosen cannula cannot be passed, a smaller one of the set might serve as a dilator. After the appropriate size cannula is inserted, the syringe is attached and the pinch valve released to begin suction. Uterine contents flow into the syringe. The procedure is done by radial passes starting at the fundus and moving to the lower uterine segment, covering all of the uterine cavity until the gritty feel of the endometrium is present and bubbles appear in the syringe. Two cautions should be emphasized: (1) the cannula must not be removed while a vacuum exists in the syringe and (2) the plunger of the syringe should not be advanced while the cannula is connected within the uterus because an air embolism could result.

Because this procedure is performed so early in pregnancy, it could be done unnecessarily on a nonpregnant woman. It should not be performed unless a positive result on a pregnancy test is obtained. There exists a higher failure rate in terminating a pregnancy before 6 weeks of gestation, perhaps because the target is so small. Microscopic examination of the products of conception, plus careful follow-up, can reduce the likelihood of a persistent pregnancy going unrecognized.

B. Suction Curettage: This procedure has proved to be the most effective surgical technique for pregnancy termination during the first trimester. Its advantages over sharp curettage include less blood loss, shorter procedure time, and lower incidence of uterine perforation. The use of a strong vacuum (50–60 mmHg) quickly shears the products of conception away from the uterine wall, evacuates them from the uterine cavity, and induces uterine contractions. This process minimizes blood loss.

Preoperatively, the patient is instructed to consume only a clear liquid diet. Preoperative medications include a nonsteroidal anti-inflammatory agent such as ibuprofen, 600 mg (for cramps); diazepam 10 mg (for anxiety); and tetracycline 250 mg, all taken 1 hour before the procedure begins.

After the procedure, ibuprofen is continued every 6 hours as needed. The patient is instructed to call the physician if she experiences fever, chills, vaginal bleeding heavier than a normal menses, severe abdominal or pelvic pain, or persistent nausea and vomiting.

Patients report less discomfort when preoperative cervical laminaria tents are used. This procedure also facilitates use of local anesthesia, which decreases the surgical risk and total cost. Laminaria are hygroscopic, long, thin aggregates of desiccated, sterilized seaweed. Although the mechanism of action may be multifactorial, the principal mechanism seems to be desiccation of the cervix, causing it to soften and dilate. Most dilation occurs in the first 4–6 hours, with some additional dilation occurring throughout 24 hours. Synthetic laminaria work more quickly, often in the course of 2 hours. The use of laminaria greatly reduces cervical trauma and laceration, as well as the incidence of uterine perforation.

Placement of laminaria is straightforward. The cervix is cleaned antiseptically. The cervical lip is grasped with a Jacobs tenaculum (which tears the pregnant cervix less than a single tooth) to render the endocervical canal parallel to the vagina. The anterior lip is grasped on an anteflexed uterus and the posterior lip on a retroflexed uterus (Fig 54–2). Care is taken to judge the length of the canal either by gentle, minimal sounding or by digital examination. Steady traction to stabilize the cervix is applied, the appropriate width tent is selected, and with ring or packing forceps, the laminaria tent is placed gently through the cervix just past the level of the internal os (Fig 54–3). Its position is maintained with soft vaginal tamponading by one or two 4- × 4-in gauze sponges.

At the time of the evacuation procedure, the vagi-

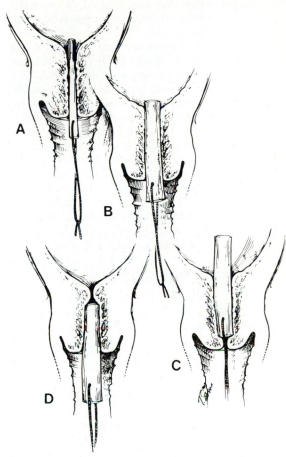

Figure 54–3. Insertion of laminaria. **A:** Laminaria immediately after being placed appropriately with its upper end just through the internal os. **B:** The swollen laminaria and dilated, softened cervix about 18 hours later. **C:** Laminaria inserted too far through the internal os; the laminaria may rupture the membranes. **D:** Laminaria not inserted far enough to dilate the internal os. (Reproduced, with permission, from Cunningham FG et al (editors): Abortion. In: *Williams Obstetrics,* 19/e. Appleton & Lange, 1993.)

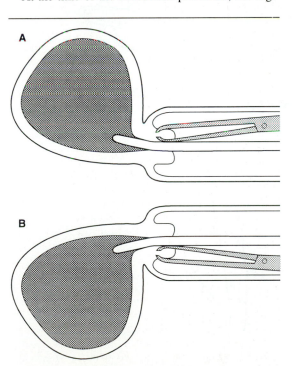

Figure 54–2. Traction on cervix during dilation. **A:** The tenaculum is placed vertically on the anterior lip. **B:** The tenaculum is placed vertically on the posterior lip for a retroverted uterus. (Reproduced, with permission, from Thompson JD, Beck JA: *Te Linde's Operative Gynecology,* 7/e. Lippincott, 1992.)

nal sponges and laminaria are removed and a bimanual examination is performed again to guide the physician in determining the cannula size and direction of its passage. Exposure of the upper vagina and cervix is obtained with a bivalve speculum, generally the Graves. Some physicians prefer the Moore modification, in which the blades are 1 inch shorter, which allows the cervix to be drawn closer to the introitus. The cervix and upper vagina are cleansed antiseptically.

In the USA, most abortions are done with local anesthesia, which is quicker, cheaper, and safer than general anesthesia. However, its use is predicated on patient cooperation and relaxation. If these criteria cannot be met or if the informed patient requests it, general anesthesia is used.

The paracervical block is effective in decreasing pain, but the patient should be informed that the placement itself may be uncomfortable. Most physicians use 1% lidocaine because it is effective and inexpensive. Chloroprocaine is considerably less toxic than lidocaine and has a faster onset of action, but it is more expensive. To minimize the discomfort of placing this submucosal anesthetic, the needle tip can be placed on the mucosa over the chosen site and the patient asked to cough. The clinician should anesthetize the tenaculum site similarly. It is important to wait 1 minute (chloroprocaine) to 3 minutes (lidocaine) after injection for the block to be most effective.

Like the laminaria tent, the tenaculum is placed on the cervix, with traction applied, thereby aligning the cervical canal parallel to the vagina (Fig 54–4). Tapered mechanical dilators, eg, Pratt, are associated with easier dilation and a lower perforation rate than nontapered dilators, eg, Hegar. Tenaculum traction is applied.The fourth and fifth fingers of the dilating hand are maintained against the patient's buttocks and perineum to minimize excessive force and perforation (Fig 54–4). The cervix is dilated until the appropriate-size cannula can be placed.

Should the clinician find the cervix difficult to dilate to the desired width, two options are available: (1) using a smaller cannula or (2) packing the os with laminaria and returning to complete the operation several hours later.

Next the cannula is inserted into the uterus. Rigid

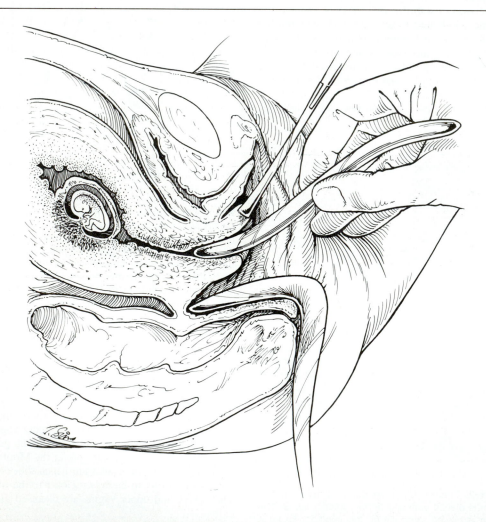

Figure 54–4. Dilation of cervix. Note that the fourth and fifth fingers rest against the perineum and buttocks, lateral to the vagina, to lower the risk of perforation of the uterus. (Reproduced, with permission, from Cunningham FG et al (editors): Abortion. In: *Williams Obstetrics,* 19/e. Appleton & Lange, 1993.)

cannulas are best. The cannula size generally is one less than the gestational age in weeks from the last menses. If the slightly angled type of cannula is used, the cannula is placed just above the internal os at the level of the lower uterine segment. If the straight type of cannula is selected, it is placed gently just below the level of the fundus. In either case, suction of 50–60 mmHg is generated, and the cannula is rotated 360 degrees slowly, multiple times, until bubbles are seen in the cannula. A gentle, sharp curettage can confirm that the cavity is empty, and a subsequent quick pass with the suction removes any clots or tissue that might promote excessive postoperative bleeding. The tenaculum is removed and direct pressure applied for a few minutes to stop any bleeding from the puncture sites.

It is critical to examine the aspirated tissue to confirm completion of the procedure, to identify a molar pregnancy, and to exclude the possibility of an ectopic pregnancy. If the uterus seems empty after the procedure but the tissue appears insufficient or atypical, the specimen should be submitted for pathologic examination, and gynecologic consultation should be sought.

C. Dilation and Evacuation (D&E): From 1975 to 1989, the percentage of second-trimester (greater than 13 weeks) abortions performed by D&E increased from 33% to 92%, whereas the percentage performed by intrauterine instillation decreased from 57% to 6%. The increasing use of D&E may have resulted from the improved technology, especially ultrasonographic guidance, and the lower risk of complications associated with the procedure. The patient's age is inversely correlated with the gestational age at which abortion is sought, ie, younger women account for a higher percentage of these advanced procedures.

D&E differs from suction curettage in two ways: (1) D&E requires greater cervical dilatation, usually accomplished by placing multiple laminaria the afternoon before the procedure, and (2) forceps are needed to evacuate the more advanced pregnancies. From 13–16 weeks, vacuum aspiration alone is sufficient; thereafter, specialized forceps extraction is needed. Confirmation of completeness of uterine evacuation is accomplished with gentle, sharp curettage or ultrasonography. In D&E, the skill and expertise of the surgeon determines in large part the safety of the procedure.

D. Stimulation of Uterine Contractions: This technique is used predominantly for more advanced pregnancies, usually over 16–17 weeks of gestation. In 1989, less than 1% of legal abortions were accomplished by intrauterine saline or prostaglandin instillation, with the latter technique being more prevalent. Intrauterine saline or urea generally results in fetal death, with labor following thereafter. The prostaglandin directly activates myometrial fibers, inducing labor. In the United Kingdom and Sweden, use of

the antiprogesterone mifepristone (RU486) with vaginal and intracervical prostaglandins has resulted in a shorter time from induction to abortion.

E. Hysterotomy and Hysterectomy: These methods should not be considered primary methods for abortion. They carry undue risk, expense, and pain when compared with the aforementioned techniques. Indeed, less than 0.02% of abortions were performed by these methods in 1989. Hysterectomy should be performed only as dictated by preexisting disease.

Complications

Morbidity is determined largely by gestational age and abortion method. The safest interval has been reported to be 7–10 weeks of gestation (Table 54–1). Suction curettage appears to be the safest method available (Table 54–2).

Immediate complications of suction abortion include hemorrhage (0.05–4.9%), cervical laceration (0.01–1.6%), uterine perforation (0.2%), and acute hematometra (0.2–1%). The latter condition is characterized by severe cramping within 2 hours of the procedure; less than expected vaginal bleeding; weakness; perspiration; and a tender, enlarged uterus. Treatment involves prompt reevacuation. Often neither anesthesia nor dilation is necessary. Removal of the liquid and clotted blood gives prompt relief.

Retained tissue often is expelled with vaginal bleeding. Otherwise, it manifests itself by cramping and bleeding several days after the procedure in less than 1% of abortions. Reevacuation is indicated if symptom severity persists, ultrasonographic findings demonstrate persistent tissue, or a fever occurs.

Postabortal infection occurs in less than 1% of suction D&Cs and in 1.5% of D&E procedures. The organisms usually responsible are group B β-hemolytic streptococci, *Bacteroides* species, *Neisseria gonorrhoeae, Escherichia coli,* and *Staphylococcus aureus.* Treatment consists of appropriate antibiotics

Table 54–1. Serious complication rates for legal abortion by gestational age, United States, 1975–1978.*

Gestational Age (wk)	Rate[†]
≤ 6	0.4
7–8	0.2
9–10	0.1
11–12	0.3
13–14	0.6
15–16	1.3
17–20	1.9

*For women with follow-up and without concurrent sterilization or preexisting conditions; serious complications include fever of 38 °C or higher for 3 d or more, hemorrhage requiring blood transfusion, and any complication requiring unintended surgery (excluding curettage). (Reproduced, with permission, from Thompson JD, Beck JA: *Te Linde's Operative Gynecology,* 7/e. Lippincott, 1992.)
[†]Per 100 abortions.

Table 54–2. Serious complication rates for legal abortion by method, United States, 1975–1978.*

Method	Rate†
Suction curettage	0.2
Dilation and evacuation	0.7
Saline instillation	2.1
Prostaglandin instillation	2.5
Urea and prostaglandin instillation	1.3

*For women with follow-up and without concurrent sterilization or preexisting conditions; serious complications include fever of 38 °C or higher for 3 d or more, hemorrhage requiring blood transfusion, and any complication requiring unintended surgery (excluding curettage). (Reproduced, with permission, from Thompson JD, Beck *JA: Te Linde's Operative Gynecology*, 7/e. Lippincott, 1992.)
†Per 100 abortions.

and careful follow-up. Curettage is indicated if the infection is associated with retained tissue.

The incidence of Rho sensitization should be minuscule if the health care provider follows standard care guidelines for Rho (D) immune globulin administration.

More than 1 million abortion procedures were performed in 1987, with six maternal deaths, which is equivalent to a case-fatality rate of 0.4 in 100,000. Deaths from legal abortion declined fivefold between 1973 and 1985 (from 3.3 to 0.4 deaths per 100,000 procedures), reflecting increased physician education and skills, improvements in medical technology, and earlier termination of pregnancy. Risk factors include ethnic minority group membership, age greater than 35 years, and increasing gestational age. The mortality rate for legal abortions between 1979 and 1985 was 0.6, more than 10 times lower than the 9.1 maternal deaths per 100,000 live births for that time interval.

There is no evidence that a single vacuum aspiration procedure increases the risk of subsequent infertility, ectopic pregnancy, or other complications of pregnancy. Insufficient data are available for women who have had multiple or second-trimester procedures.

Referral to a Specialist

Many primary care providers choose to refer all patients desiring an abortion to providers or clinics that perform large numbers of these procedures. Most providers who are comfortable with endometrial biopsies and D&C procedures can perform first-trimester abortions safely in their office.

Patients requesting second-trimester abortions should be referred to providers who perform large enough numbers of them to demonstrate a low complication rate. Not all gynecologists who perform first-trimester abortions fall into this category.

When the products of conception are absent or abnormal at the time of suction curettage, a gynecologist should be consulted. In addition, any indication of an ectopic, molar, or cornual pregnancy at the time of preprocedure ultrasonography should prompt a referral. Women with significant medical problems such as von Willebrand's disease, unstable cardiovascular disease, or pulmonary hypertension should be referred for medical consultation, and the abortion usually should be performed in the operating room with an anesthesiologist present.

Psychosocial Issues

The decision to terminate a pregnancy can be difficult. Many women anguish over the possibility of future infertility or unhealthy children. The provider may reassure the patient that the data refute these worries. Studies on the emotional impact of abortion show that severe adverse emotional reactions are rare. Most women experience relief and reduced distress after an abortion. Sadness, regret, anxiety, and guilt are mild when they occur. Negative emotions are much more common when the procedure is performed for medical or genetic indications, when second-trimester abortion is performed, or when ambivalence about the decision is present.

The legal, ethical, religious, political, and societal issues that surround abortion in the USA are complex and beyond the scope of this chapter (see Chapter 6). The impact of some of these issues on access to abortion procedures is significant; restricted access is most likely to affect disproportionately adolescents, low-income women, and women from rural areas.

Current Controversies

Mifepristone (RU486) is an antiprogesterone steroid initially described in 1982. This medication was developed for pregnancy interruption on the hypothesis that the interruption of progesterone action would alter the endometrial environment and prevent implantation. Early studies in France and Switzerland demonstrated its effectiveness.

Terminations are successful in 95% of pregnancies up to 10 weeks of gestation when given in conjunction with an intramuscular prostaglandin. Recently, the combination of RU486 and an oral prostaglandin (misoprostol) has been shown to be equally effective. The latter technique has the added advantage that no visit to a physician's office is required.

Mifepristone is available in many countries throughout the world, including China, France, and Great Britain. In the USA, the political influence of the "right to life" groups has delayed its development. It may be many years before this alternative is clinically available.

REFERENCES

Blumenthal PD: Abortion: Epidemiology, safety, and technique. Curr Opin Obstet Gynecol 1992;4:505.

Bonavoglia A (editor): *The Choices We Made: 25 Women and Men Speak Out About Abortion.* Random House, 1991.

Centers for Disease Control: *Abortion Surveillance— United States, 1989.* US Government, 1992.

Council on Scientific Affairs, American Medical Association: Induced termination of pregnancy before and after Roe v. Wade. Trends in the mortality and morbidity of women. JAMA 1992;268:3231.

Cunningham et al: Abortion. In: *Williams Obstetrics.* Appleton & Lange, 1993.

Droegenmueller W et al: Abortion. In: *Comprehensive Gynecology.* Mosby, 1992.

Grimes DA: Surgical management of abortion. In: *TeLinde's Operative Gynecology.* Thompson, Rock (editors). Lippincott, 1992.

Grimes DA et al: Local vs. general anesthesia: Which is safer for performing suction curettage abortions? Am J Obstet Gynecol 1979;135:1030.

Laufe LE: The menstrual regulation procedure. Stud Fam Plann 1977;8:253.

Thong KJ, Baird DT: Induction of abortion with mifepristone and misoprostol in early pregnancy. Br J Gynecol 1992;99:1004.

Thong KJ, Baird DT: Induction of second-trimester abortion with mifepristone and gemeprost. Br J Obstet Gynecol 1993;100:758.

55

Preconception Counseling & Care of Common Medical Disorders in Pregnancy

Susan K. Hendricks, MD, MaryAnn Von Eschen, MS, & Margo C. Grady, MS

GENETIC COUNSELING & RISK ASSESSMENT

A vital segment of the preconception counseling visit is genetic risk assessment. Identification of factors that place the pregnancy at increased risk is important for preconception as well as pregnancy management. Identifying risk factors prior to pregnancy allows time for reduction or elimination of risk as well as consideration of alternative pregnancy choices. Genetic counselors help women to understand difficult obstetric issues so that they can make informed decisions about pregnancy. The American Society of Human Genetics has adopted the following definition of genetic counseling:

Genetic counseling is a communication process which deals with human problems associated with the occurrence, or risk of occurrence, of a genetic disorder in a family. This process involves an attempt by one or more appropriately trained person(s) to help the individual or family

1. Comprehend the medical facts, including the diagnosis, probable course of the disorder, and the available management
2. Appreciate the way heredity contributes to the disorder and the risk of recurrence in specified relatives
3. Understand the options for dealing with the risk of recurrence
4. Choose the course of action which seems appropriate to them in view of their risk, and the family goals, and act in accordance with that decision
5. Make the best possible adjustment to the disorder in an affected member and/or to the risk of recurrence of that disorder

---

Genetic Counseling & Risk Assessment
Risk Identification
    Advanced Maternal Age
    Previous Child With a Chromosomal
        Abnormality
    Structural Chromosomal Rearrangement
    Previous Child With an Isolated or Multiple
        Congenital Anomalies
    Previous Stillborn
    Family History of Mendelian Disorder
    Ethnic Background
    History of Multiple Miscarriages
Types of Prenatal Diagnosis
    Chorionic Villus Sampling
    Amniocentesis
    Ultrasonography
    Triple Screen
Maternal Medical Disorders: Preconception
    Counseling
Teratogen Exposure
Common Medical Disorders in Pregnancy
    Diabetes
    Urinary Tract Disorders
    Thyroid Disease
    Hypertensive Disorders of Pregnancy
    Cardiac Disease

RISK IDENTIFICATION

Part of the preconception intake should include a preliminary family and personal history as shown in Figure 55–1. Positive responses to any of these questions indicate an increased risk; such families should see a geneticist, genetic counselor, or maternal-fetal medicine subspecialist. These professionals are able to give nondirective information regarding individual risks, carrier screening, and options for prenatal diagnosis as well as to counsel and support these families.

Yes   No

○   ○   1. Will you be 35 years or older when the baby is born?
Age when due_____.

○   ○   2. Have you or the baby's father had two or more pregnancies that ended in miscarriages?

○   ○   3. Have you or the baby's father had a stillborn baby?

○   ○   4. Do you or the baby's father have a birth defect, handicapping condition, or disorder that may be hereditary?

○   ○   5. Do you or the baby's father have any children with birth defects, handicaps, mental or growth retardation, learning disabilities, or genetic disorders?

○   ○   6. Do you or baby's father have brothers, sisters, uncles, aunts, cousins, nieces, nephews, or grandparents with any birth defects, handicaps, mental or growth retardation, or genetic disorders?

○   ○   7. Are you or the baby's father from any of the following ethnic or racial groups?
Jewish ○   Black ○   Asian ○
Mediterranean (Greek, Italian) ○

○   ○   8. Are you currently taking any drugs or medications such as seizure medications, alcohol (more than two drinks or glasses daily), anticancer drugs, anticoagulants (blood thinners), lithium, or isoretinoin?

○   ○   9. Are you and the baby's father related to each other (eg, cousins)?

Figure 55–1. Questionnaire detailing personal and family history for the preconception counseling visit.

An essential part of prenatal risk assessment is the development of a family pedigree. The pedigree should contain at least three generations and should include all the children of a sibship, whether abnormal or normal, living or dead. A multigenerational pedigree is mandatory in the assessment of the inheritance pattern of a disorder in a particular family. This is important because of the possibility of generation skipping in disorders such as X-linked recessive or autosomal dominant disorders in which reduced penetrance is present. Basic information should include age and cause of death. Specific questions should be asked about congenital malformations, mental retardation, genetic conditions, infant deaths, stillbirths, and pregnancy losses. If accurate information is unobtainable, such as the age or cause of death of an individual, this ambiguity should be included in the pedigree. It is imperative to obtain medical records for confirmation of diagnosis as well as clarification of unclear or inaccurate information. For example, if a patient reports a family history of hemophilia and prenatal diagnosis is offered for that condition, an incorrect diagnosis of the fetus may be given if it was hemophilia B, and not hemophilia A,

that was present in this family. Pedigree terminology is reviewed in Figure 55–2.

Advanced Maternal Age

It is considered the standard of care in this country and is the recommendation of the American College of Obstetrics and Gynecology to inform women age 35 or older of the availability of prenatal counseling and testing. Genetic counseling for discussion of age-related chromosomal abnormalities such as Down syndrome and other nondisjunctional events resulting in fetal aneuploidy should precede any testing. The relevant prenatal diagnostic procedures should be explained, and the possible risks should be detailed. The maternal age of 35 years has been established as the cutoff point at which pregnant women are referred for prenatal diagnosis for fetal aneuploidy. When the criteria for prenatal diagnosis were established in the 1970s, the risk of having an aneuploid fetus outweighed the risk of procedure-related miscarriage at the maternal age of 35 years. Studies of complications from amniocentesis indicated that 35 was the age when the risk of having an aneuploid fetus equaled or was greater than the risk of losing the

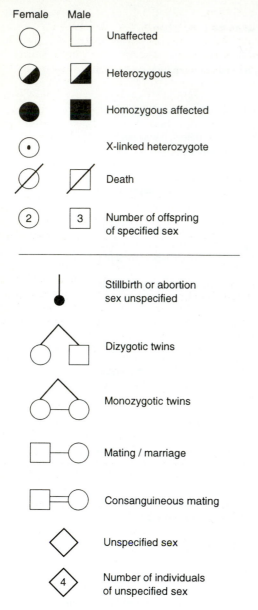

Female   Male

○   □   Unaffected

◑   ◪   Heterozygous

●   ■   Homozygous affected

⊙   X-linked heterozygote

⊘   ⊘   Death

②   ③   Number of offspring
of specified sex

Stillbirth or abortion
sex unspecified

Dizygotic twins

Monozygotic twins

Mating / marriage

Consanguineous mating

Unspecified sex

④   Number of individuals
of unspecified sex

Figure 55–2. Terms and symbols used in family pedigrees.

investigators have suggested that the cutoff age for amniocentesis should be lowered so that it is offered to all women over the age of 30. Table 55–1 lists age-related risks for Down syndrome and all chromosomal abnormalities.

Previous Child With a Chromosomal Abnormality

Parents who have had a child with an extra chromosome (aneuploidy) such as trisomy 21 (Down syndrome), trisomy 13, or trisomy 18, have an empirical recurrence risk of 1–2%. When a child has a chromosomal translocation, deletion, or duplication, the parental chromosomes should be tested to determine whether the parents are balanced translocation carriers. If one of the parents is found to be a balanced translocation carrier, there is an increased risk to future pregnancies, and prenatal diagnosis should be offered in all subsequent pregnancies. Elevated risks to future pregnancies include delivery of a live-born child with an unbalanced translocation as well as stillbirth, spontaneous abortion, and infertility. However, if neither parent carries a chromosomal translocation, the couple can be reassured that there is not

Table 55–1. Age-related risks of chromosomal abnormalities (live births).*

Maternal Age	Down Syndrome	All Chromosomal Abnormalities
20	1/1667	1/526†
21	1/1667	1/526
22	1/1429	1/500
23	1/1429	1/500
24	1/1250	1/476
25	1/1250	1/476
26	1/1176	1/476
27	1/1111	1/455
28	1/1053	1/435
29	1/1000	1/417
30	1/952	1/384
31	1/909	1/384
32	1/769	1/322
33	1/635	1/317
34	1/500	1/260
35	1/385	1/204
36	1/294	1/164
37	1/227	1/130
38	1/175	1/103
39	1/137	1/82
40	1/106	1/65
41	1/82	1/51
42	1/64	1/40
43	1/50	1/32
44	1/38	1/25
45	1/30	1/20
46	1/23	1/15
47	1/18	1/12
48	1/14	1/10

*Reproduced with the permission of the American College of Obstetrics and Gynecology from Hook EB: Rates of chromosome abnormalities at different maternal ages. Obstet Gynecol 1981;58:282.
†47, XXX excluded for ages 20 to 32 (Data not available).

pregnancy as the result of complications from the procedure (approximately 0.5%). This reference base has been applied to chorionic villus sampling (CVS), although the risk of pregnancy loss from this procedure appears to be slightly higher (approximately 1%). It has been suggested that a maternal serum test called the triple screen or AFP+ (see the section following, "Types of Prenatal Diagnosis") be offered as an alternative to all women over the age of 35. This is not a current recommendation in the United States, because the screening test has neither the sensitivity nor the specificity of fetal karyotype analysis. Some an increased risk for having another child with a chromosomal abnormality.

Structural Chromosomal Rearrangement

Although parents who are carriers of balanced chromosomal rearrangements do not have any medical or physical problems related to this rearrangement, they are at increased risk for having a child with an unbalanced rearrangement. The risk of having a child with an unbalanced chromosomal rearrangement varies with the type of parental balanced translocation as well as the gender of the parent carrying the translocation. The overall risk is 10–12%. Robertsonian translocations (the fusion of two acrocentric chromosomes, such as 14 and 21) carry a transmission risk of 15% if the mother carries the translocation and 2–4% if the translocation is paternal. The risk of having an offspring with unbalanced translocation to a couple who carries a reciprocal translocation (the transference of chromosomal material between two nonhomologous chromosomes) depends on the ascertainment of the abnormality. The risk to a carrier couple ascertained by delivery of an affected child or identification in a relative is 20%; if the abnormality is ascertained by a history of multiple miscarriages, the risk falls to 2–5%.

Genetic counseling for individual risk assessment and prenatal diagnosis, such as CVS or amniocentesis, to determine fetal karyotype should be offered to the couple at risk.

Previous Child With an Isolated or Multiple Congenital Anomalies

The delivery of a child with a birth defect, such as a congenital heart defect, increases the risk that siblings may be born with a similar problem. Recurrence risk counseling depends on the mode of inheritance as well as the relationship of the affected individual to the couple. For example, the parents of a child with a congenital heart defect would have a recurrence risk of 1–4%, but a second degree relative would have a risk of approximately 1% that their child would also be affected. Many birth defects follow a multifactorial pattern of inheritance. In these cases, a collection of factors, some known, most unknown, have to combine to reach a threshold before a child is affected. Common isolated defects have known empirical risks of recurrence based on large population studies. However, children with multiple congenital anomalies should be evaluated by a geneticist for a pattern of defects that might lead to a diagnosis. If a definitive diagnosis is made, it could alter the risk for the parents of having a second affected child (Table 55–2). If there is a known environmental agent that increases the risk of having a child with a particular birth defect, this agent can be avoided in future pregnancies. Also, some agents have been discovered that can be protective. For example, couples who have had a previous child with a neural-tube defect, eg, spina bifida or anencephaly, have a 3–5% risk of recurrence. Recent studies have shown, however, that if folic acid supplementation is given to the mother prior to neural-tube closure (21–28 days postconception), the risk for a second affected child may be reduced by as much as 70%.

Previous Stillborn

Parents with a previous pregnancy resulting in a stillbirth of unknown cause may be at increased risk for a second stillbirth. Proper evaluation of a stillbirth may determine the cause of fetal death and therefore help to assess risks to future pregnancies. Maternal evaluation also is indicated to establish maternal causes of pregnancy loss. If no cause for stillbirth is found, couples who have experienced one stillbirth have an empirical recurrence risk of 3%; in families with two previous stillbirths, the overall risk to subsequent pregnancies is about 15%.

Table 55–2. Common congenital abnormalities.

Type	Incidence in Newborns	Recurrence Risks
Congenital heart disease	8/1000, 0.8%	1–4%
VSD: Ventricular Septal Defect	1/532, 0.19%	1.7–4.2%
ASD: Atrial Septal Defect	1/1548, 0.6%	0.7–2.9%
PDA: Patent Ductus Arteriosis	1/1340, 0.75%	1–3.5%
Neural-tube defects	1–2/1000	3–5%
Clubfoot	3/1000	3%
Diaphragmatic hernia	1/2000–1/3000	0–2%
Cleft lip and palate	1/1000	4%
Dislocation of hip	1/1400	6%
Tracheoesophageal fistula	1/3000	1%
Gastroschisis	1/10, 000	1/10,000
Omphalocele	1/4000	1/4000, some inherited
Duodenal atresia	1/10,000	
Nonimmune hydrops	1/1500–1/4000	
Down syndrome	1/700	1% (all aneuploidies)

Family History of Mendelian Disorder

A family history of a Mendelian disorder may put a couple at risk for having a child with that disorder. Risks to the pregnancy vary depending on both the type of inheritance of the condition in the family as well as which members of the family are affected. Carrier screening before pregnancy may reassure a couple that they are not at increased risk of having a child with a specific genetic disorder. If an increased risk is identified preconceptionally, however, more time is available for the couple to discuss options in pregnancy such as prenatal diagnosis. Early risk identification also gives the couple sufficient time to discuss pregnancy management with their physician. Couples who are identified prenatally as at an increased risk for having a child with a Mendelian disorder also have the option to discuss and choose alternatives to conventional pregnancy including in vitro fertilization (IVF), preimplantation screening, artificial insemination by donor, surrogacy, or adoption.

Ethnic Background

Each ethnic group has genetic disorders that are more common within the ethnic group than in the general population (Table 55–3). For example, cystic fibrosis and phenylketonuria (PKU) are more common in the Northern European population and Tay-Sachs disease is more common in the Ashkenasi Jewish and French Canadian populations.

By determining the disorders for which the couple

Table 55–3. Ethnic distribution of mendelian disorders.

Ethnic Group	Disorder
Northern European	Phenylketonuria (PKU) Cystic fibrosis
African	Sickle cell anemia Alpha-thalassemia Glucose-6-phosphatase dehydrogenase deficiency
Mediterranean	Beta-thalassemia Glucose-6-phosphatase dehydrogenase deficiency
Southeast Asian	Alpha-thalassemia Glucose-6-phosphatase dehydrogenase deficiency
Ashkenasi Jewish	Tay-Sachs disease Gaucher's disease Familial dysautonomia
Quebec French	Tay-Sachs disease Morquio's syndrome Agenesis of the corpus callosum
Sephardic Jewish	Congenital adrenal hyperplasia Cystinosis

is at risk, carrier screening, if available, can be performed before conception. Some screening tests, such as for Tay-Sachs and hemophilia, are more accurate prior to conception than during pregnancy.

At this time, population screening for identification of heterozygote carriers is offered to individuals of Jewish ancestry for Tay-Sachs disease; to blacks for sickle cell anemia and alpha-thalassemia; and to individuals of Mediterranean or Southeast Asian descent for the thalassemias. Although the gene for cystic fibrosis has been identified, screening for cystic fibrosis usually is not performed unless there is a positive family history or congenital absence of the vas deferens in the male partner. Heterozygote carrier testing is indicated for families with a history of cystic fibrosis, because testing is nearly 100% informative in these families if there is an identifiable mutation. If a DNA sample is available from an affected individual, linkage analysis can be performed if the affected individual carries an unidentifiable mutation. However, cystic fibrosis screening is not indicated if there is a negative family history. The current cystic fibrosis mutation detection rate is 85%; therefore, 15% of mutations are not identifiable by screening, and carriers of these mutations would have false-negative results. Because the current cystic fibrosis mutation rate is not 100%, both the American Society of Human Genetics and the National Institutes of Health Workshop on Population Screening have issued statements that population-based carrier testing is not recommended at this time.

History of Multiple Miscarriages

It is estimated that approximately one-half of all recognized pregnancies that result in miscarriage involve chromosomal abnormalities. Recurrent miscarriages occur in approximately 2% of pregnant women. Couples who have recurrent miscarriages have a 6% risk that one partner has a balanced chromosomal rearrangement. Karyotype analysis of parental blood determines whether or not this couple is at an increased risk for having a child with an unbalanced karyotype. If a balanced rearrangement is identified in one of the parents, a probable cause of the spontaneous abortion has been identified. However, if the parental chromosomes are normal, further investigation into the cause of the miscarriages is indicated (see Chapter 56).

TYPES OF PRENATAL DIAGNOSIS

Chorionic Villus Sampling

CVS is performed early in pregnancy, typically at 9–12 weeks of gestation. CVS involves a placental biopsy of the chorionic villi to obtain tissue for chromosomal analysis. Depending on the placement of the placenta, which is determined by ultrasonography, villi are obtained either transcervically or transabdominally. Approximately 10–20 mg of tissue is obtained during the procedure. This tissue is suitable also for enzyme or molecular analysis if the family is known to be at risk for a specific genetic disorder. The major complication from CVS is spontaneous abortion, which occurs less than 1% of the time. This risk is in addition to the 3–10% loss rate at this stage of pregnancy. Results of the chromosomal analysis are available in 10–14 days.

Two types of chorionic villus cell types can be used for cytogenetic analysis. The rapidly dividing cytotrophoblasts, which are derived from extraembryonic trophectoderm, often are used for direct chromosomal analysis, and the results are available within 24–48 hours. The final results of the chromosomal analysis are derived from slowly dividing mesenchymal core cells, whose origins are from both extraembryonic and embryonic mesenchyme. Final results are usually available in 7–10 days. The result of the direct analysis should be considered preliminary, with the final results considered conclusive. It is more common to have discrepancies in findings such as mosaicism or chromosomal rearrangements between the karyotype results of the direct analysis and the actual karyotype of the fetus than between the final results and the actual fetal karyotype.

There has been some controversy concerning the safety of the CVS procedure. Two reports have suggested that CVS was responsible for a sixfold increase in the rate of limb reduction defects over the general population rate. The safety of CVS early in pregnancy (7–8 weeks) is being debated. However, the CVS registry indicates that fetal defects of all anatomic locations are similar in frequency to those of the base population and that CVS is safe if performed by an experienced clinician within a program and done after the ninth week of gestation.

Amniocentesis

Amniocentesis is a procedure used to obtain a sample of amniotic fluid for karyotypic and alpha-fetoprotein (AFP) analysis. Amniocentesis for prenatal diagnosis is performed in the second trimester of pregnancy (between 15 and 20 weeks of gestation). After the fetus and the placenta are located by ultrasonography, approximately 20 mL of amniotic fluid is aspirated directly. Depending on the preference of the physician, local anesthesia may be used. The risk of miscarriage is estimated to be between 1 in 200 and 1 in 500. The results of the AFP screen are ready in approximately 1 week, and the chromosome results are typically available in 10–14 days.

Some programs have used early amniocentesis, which is performed prior to 15 weeks of gestation, as an alternative form of prenatal diagnosis. The technique for early amniocentesis is similar to that of traditional amniocentesis except that less fluid is aspirated, usually 1 mL for each completed week of gestation. Because early amniocentesis is a relatively new procedure and no prospective controlled studies have been conducted, the effectiveness and safety are still unknown.

Ultrasonography

Ultrasonography can visualize fetal anatomy during pregnancy and can help rule out some congenital anomalies that cannot be detected by CVS or amniocentesis. The best time during pregnancy to obtain a complete scan of the fetal anatomy is at 18–20 weeks of gestation. After numerous studies, there has been no documentation of ultrasonic waves damaging fetal hearing. The incidence of karyotypic abnormalities in a population of fetuses ascertained by ultrasonography to have a single structural abnormality is 15–22%; in fetuses ascertained to have multiple anomalies, the incidence is approximately 33%. The frequency of chromosomal abnormalities is greater with certain anatomic abnormalities, such as cardiovascular anomalies (approximately 35%), CNS anomalies (approximately 22%), and omphalocele (30–55%) (Table 55–4).

It is important to emphasize to patients that even if CVS or amniocentesis and ultrasonographic findings are reported as normal, a perfect infant cannot be guaranteed. For example, a fetus may be found to have normal chromosomes and a normal ultrasonographic scan and still be born with a genetic disorder such as beta-thalassemia.

Triple Screen

Triple marker screening (TMS) is a relatively new test that uses alpha-fetoprotein (AFP), human chorionic gonadotropin (HCG), and unconjugated estriol (uE_3) levels in maternal serum at 15–20 weeks of gestation to screen for trisomy 21 (Down syndrome) and neural-tube defects. Recent studies have reported that low AFP, elevated HCG, and low uE_3 levels are associated with an increased risk of trisomy 21 in the fetus. The TMS test combines the results of these three determinations along with maternal age at delivery to calculate individual risks. Calculated risks also are adjusted for maternal race, weight, diabetes, and smoking habits. For women under age 35, the TMS detects approximately 60% of pregnancies with trisomy 21, with a false-positive rate of approximately 5%.

The TMS should be offered to pregnant women under 35 at 15–20 weeks of gestation; optimal timing is at 15–17 weeks of gestation. Although the risk of having a fetus with trisomy 21 does increase with age, the majority (80%) of babies with trisomy 21 are born to women under the age of 35. If a woman's TMS result indicates an increased risk for aneuploidy, genetic counseling and prenatal testing should be offered. It is not recommended that the TMS be used as a substitute for prenatal diagnosis for women over the age of the 35. However, it may

Table 55–4. Risk of abnormalities related to ultrasonographic findings.*

Ultrasonographic Finding	Risk of aneuploidy	Risk of other abnormalities
Omphalocele	30–55%	50%
Gastroschisis	0–3%	4–25%
Duodenal atresia	33%	48–78%
Nonimmune hydrops	34%	64%
Nuchal folds	33%	—
Cystic hygroma	50%	—
IUGR-Intrauterine growth retardation	2–5%	10–30%
Congenital heart disease	22%	5.2%
ASD-Atrial Septal Defect	14%	
VSD-Ventricular Septal Defect	8%	4.7%
Renal abnormalities		
Urethrovesical junction	23%	—
Urethropelvic junction	4%	—
Central nervous system		
Neural-tube defects	8–33%	—
Holoprosencephaly	40–60%	37% intracranial
Hydrocephalus	3–9%	63% extracranial
Agenesis of the corpus callosum	14%	—
Choroid plexus cysts	1%	—
Diaphragmatic hernia	6–25%	50–57%
Single umbilical artery	0–5%	21%
Cleft lip or palate	0.15%	13%
Clubfoot	25–31%	77%
Esophageal atresia	19%	50–70%

be offered to help define the risk for fetal aneuploidy if amniocentesis or CVS is declined.

A recent study by Haddow et al investigated the effectiveness of the TMS as an alternative to amniocentesis in women age 35 or older. Using a risk cutoff of 1 in 200 and a false-positive rate of 25%, 89% of fetuses with Down syndrome would have been identified. However, only 47% of other autosomal trisomies and 44% of gender aneuploidies were identified using these criteria. Haddow concluded that TMS can provide a basis for decision making in the cases of women older than 35 as well as younger women.

MATERNAL MEDICAL DISORDERS: PRECONCEPTION COUNSELING

Ideally, any woman considering pregnancy would have preconception counseling. In addition to a family history, an extensive maternal medical history should be obtained at all preconception intake interviews. Clinicians should pose specific questions regarding maternal illnesses that may cause increased risks. Use of an extensive medical history checklist helps to ensure that all potential risks are identified. Nutrition; exercise; adverse habits such as smoking, drinking, and drug abuse; and physical disorders should be discussed. The patient should be encouraged to eliminate all avoidable hazards to a pregnancy with the appropriate social and medical support, eg, nutritional counseling for weight loss, referral to social services and referral to programs for

substance abuse. Occupational hazards should be eliminated, and any preexisting medical condition should be controlled with appropriate therapy, including a review of all medications and treatments that may have an impact on the pregnancy, ie, potential teratogens. Appropriate laboratory tests may include the following:

Rubella titers
Varicella titers
Toxoplasmosis
Cytomegalovirus
Hepatitis screening
HIV (for high-risk patients)
Glucose testing
Rh testing
Hemoglobin electrophoresis (Asian and black patients)
Tuberculosis testing

Patients who require vaccinations (rubella or varicella nonimmune, tetanus toxoid) should receive them preconception; those who are susceptible to high-risk perinatal infections (cytomegalovirus, toxoplasmosis) should be counseled regarding prophylaxis and avoidance of high-risk situations.

Women older than 35 are prone to the development of chronic disease. Medical illnesses that are more prevalent in these women include diabetes, hypertension, renal disease, and heart disease. The incidence of (superimposed) preeclampsia increases with age as does the severity of the condition. Gestational diabetes is threefold more common in older women, as is overt diabetes. Other complications of pregnancy that develop with increasing frequency include miscarriage (two- to threefold increase), preterm labor and premature rupture of membranes (twofold increase), fetal macrosomia (related to the increase in gestational diabetes and postterm pregnancies), fetal intrauterine growth retardation (related to the increase in vascular disease), placental abruption and previa, and ectopic pregnancy. These issues should be discussed thoroughly.

The following is a list of signs that should alert the primary physician to high-risk pregnancies:

Advanced maternal age (older than 35)
Grand multiparity (greater than four)
Small stature (less than 5 feet tall)
Low maternal weight (less than 55 kg)
Obesity (more than 20% over ideal weight)
Preexisting medical disorders
Abnormal uterine bleeding
Infertility
Sexually transmitted disease (increased risk of ectopic pregnancy)
Prior poor pregnancy outcome (fetal or neonatal loss, prematurity)

Table 55–5 lists high-risk medical conditions that could affect the mother and fetus.

TERATOGEN EXPOSURE

A **teratogen** is an agent that produces abnormality or anomaly in a fetus that is exposed to it during organogenesis. There are three defined developmental periods in the fetus. The first is commonly known as the "all or none" period, which exists from the day of conception to day 9–13. During this period, the

Table 55–5. High-risk medical conditions.

Diabetes mellitus
  Type 2, diet-controlled
  Type 1 or 2, insulin-dependent*
Malignant disease
Hypertension
  Chronic*
  Pregnancy-induced hypertension
    Mild
    Severe
Heart disease
  Class 1*
  Class 2, 3, 4†
Pulmonary disease
  Asthma, well-controlled
  Unstable asthma†
Gastrointestinal problems
Hepatitis

*Consultation with subspecialty physician in maternal-fetal medicine is advised.
†Care by maternal-fetal medicine subspecialist is advised.

pregnancy is either lost because of the exposure or it is unaffected. The next period extends to approximately day 70 and is considered the period of **organogenesis** or **embryogenesis.** During this period, exposure to a teratogen affects individual organ systems. The period of fetal growth is from day 70 to term. During this time, teratogens can impact on fetal growth and development and can affect the organs that are still in the process of development, specifically the eyes, ears, and central nervous system. The major teratogenic agents are listed in Table 55–6.

COMMON MEDICAL DISORDERS IN PREGNANCY

Diabetes

Diabetes affects 3–5% of all pregnant women, making it one of the most common medical complications of pregnancy. Diabetes is a heterogeneous disorder with a wide spectrum of manifestations ranging from insulin-dependent diabetes mellitus (IDDM) to gestational diabetes. Glucose intolerance detected in pregnancy is called **gestational diabetes mellitus (GDM).** GDM is one of the most frequent and significant risks for adverse maternal and fetal outcome in pregnancy; it accounts for 90% of cases of diabetes in pregnant women, whereas IDDM and noninsulin-dependent diabetes mellitus (NIDDM)

Table 55–6. Major teratogenic agents.

Class	Agent
Drugs and chemicals	Angiotensin converting enzyme (ACE) inhibitors
	Alcohol
	Androgens
	Antibiotics (tetracycline, streptomycin, chloramphenicol)
	Anticoagulants (warfarin, dicumarol)
	Anticonvulsants (phenytoin, trimethadione, paramethadione)
	Valproic acid
	Tricyclic antidepressants (amitriptyline, imipramine, desipramine)
	Antifungals (amphotericin B, griseofulvin, nystatin, clotrimazole, miconazole, flucytosine)
	Antithyroid drugs (propylthiouracil, iodide, methimazole)
	Chemotherapeutic drugs
	Diethylstilbestrol
	Isoretinoin
	Lead
	Lithium
	Organic mercury
	Thalidomide
Infections	Cytomegalovirus
	Rubella
	Syphilis
	Toxoplasmosis
	Varicella
Radiation	X-ray therapy

(type I and type II diabetes) account for the remainder. Gestational diabetes is considered a marker for the development of future diabetes, but the exact risk is unknown. Controversy exists regarding implications for mother and child both during pregnancy and following delivery. It is unclear which diagnostic criterion is most accurate in the diagnosis of gestational diabetes; even more controversy surrounds methods of treatment.

The metabolic adaptations that occur in pregnancy increase the risk of glucose intolerance. Whether or not this is a true pathologic condition is debatable. It is clear that the effects of maternal hyperglycemia include fetal hyperinsulinemia, which results in fetal macrosomia, fetal metabolic disorders, neonatal complications, and possible long-term complications for both fetus and mother. Neonatal morbidity and mortality in well-controlled gestational diabetes is equivalent to that of nondiabetic pregnancies, lending credence to the belief that gestational diabetes may be a metabolic adaptation to pregnancy.

A. Periconceptional Counseling: Genetic counseling concerning diabetes mellitus is complex. Identical twin studies have investigated the genetic inheritance of insulin dependent diabetes mellitus (IDDM) and noninsulin-dependent diabetes mellitus (NIDDM). In NIDDM, identical twins approach 100% concordance in the development of the disorder. The concordance rate in IDDM is much less, with the average study reporting between 25 and 35%. In their review of diabetes mellitus in pregnancy and periconceptional genetic counseling, Reece and Hagay review the information regarding HLA linkage. IDDM is an HLA-linked disorder; it appears that NIDDM is not. Because of the uncertainty regarding the extent of genetic contribution in both disorders, the exact mechanism of inheritance cannot be elucidated.

B. Recurrence Risks of IDDM: Medical preconception counseling with intensive diabetic management has resulted in a reduction in the incidence of congenital malformations. The most frequent fetal malformations are found in the cardiovascular system and the central nervous system. The correlation between long-term control and malformations has been confirmed by multiple investigators. High levels of glycosylated hemoglobin in the first trimester during the critical period for organogenesis have been correlated with an increased number of malformations. Recent studies in the USA using programs that have developed preconception counseling and strict metabolic control in the first trimester of pregnancy have shown a reduction in the incidence of congenital malformations in infants of diabetic mothers.

A glycosylated hemoglobin level of less than 6.9% is considered consistent with good control. The risk of early abortion has been shown to diminish with tight control prior to and in the first month of pregnancy. Congenital malformations seem to increase the risk of miscarriage following 8–10 weeks; preconception counseling with tight metabolic control reduces the incidence of spontaneous abortion during this time. The vascular complications of pregnancy (including the manifestations of hypertension, proliferative retinopathy, renal disease, and neuropathy) should be assessed and treated. A thorough ophthalmologic examination with treatment of proliferative retinopathy should be performed prior to pregnancy. The medical management of the woman with IDDM or GDM is complex. A major key is the involvement of an entire team with the woman and her partner including a diabetes nurse educator, nutritionist, endocrinologist, obstetrician, ultrasonographer, and pediatrician. Optimal management includes normal glycemia prior to conception with maintenance throughout the pregnancy and throughout the antepartum and intrapartum periods.

Management of normal glycemia during pregnancy involves cooperation between the medical team and the nutritionist. Strict dietary management and self-monitoring of capillary blood glucose should be thoroughly explained to the patient prior to conception with frequent reviews. Glycosylated hemoglobin values below 6.9% should be the ultimate goal, preferably prior to conception. The majority of investigators use a fasting blood glucose level of below 100 and a 2-hour postprandial level of below 120 mm%. Gestational diabetes often can be managed by dietary control alone. However, some investigators have reported a decrease in the incidence of macrosomia and neonatal metabolic disturbances, the most common complications of gestational diabetes, with the use of prophylactic insulin.

C. Obstetric Management of Diabetes: The intense medical management and strict metabolic control have decreased both the maternal and perinatal morbidity and mortality in the pregnancies of women with IDDM over the last decade. Complications such as polyhydramnios, macrosomia, intrauterine growth retardation, hypertensive disorders, and intrauterine fetal demise occur with much less frequency, but they are present in women with type I diabetes with inadequate glycemic control. In the first trimester, spontaneous abortion or fetal embryopathy are the most frequent complications. Fetal malformations can be detected by a combination of second-trimester surveillance techniques such as the triple screen (inclusive of alpha-fetoprotein to detect neural-tube defects), genetic amniocentesis (for alpha-fetoprotein and acetylcholinesterase), and ultrasonographic evaluation with fetal echocardiography at 16–20 weeks of gestation. Sonography is also the method of choice for detection of polyhydramnios and growth abnormalities in the fetus and should be performed every 6–8 weeks in the diabetic.

Urinary Tract Disorders

A. Asymptomatic Bacteriuria: Asymptomatic bacteriuria (ASB) occurs in as many as 10% of all pregnant patients; its presence increases the risk to the gravida of acute urinary tract infection and pyelonephritis. The incidence of these acute infections following ASB is approximately 10-fold greater than those whose bacteriuria is treated. Diagnosis is made from culture of a midstream clean catch with a count of greater than 10^5 per milliliter of urine.

Diabetes mellitus and sickle cell trait increase the risk of asymptomatic bacteriuria. Patients with increased parity and black patients have a higher risk than patients who are white or of low parity.

Asymptomatic bacteriuria requires therapy with a sensitive agent (see the section following, Acute Pyelonephritis). After drug treatment is complete, a repeat culture should be performed to confirm the effectiveness of the treatment.

B. Cystitis: Cystitis is a symptomatic urinary tract infection. Inflammation or infection of the bladder or bladder wall is common in pregnancy. Symptoms include abdominal discomfort, dysuria, frequency, and urgency. The diagnosis is made in the same manner as for asymptomatic bacteria. More than 10^5 bacteria on a midstream clean catch specimen confirms the diagnosis. Escherichia coli is present in more than 75% of patients diagnosed with cystitis with variable sensitivities to ampicillin. *Chlamydia trachomatis* and *Staphylococcus saprophyticus* are other common pathogens. Sensitivities of the organism should be examined. The patient can be treated effectively with the appropriate oral medications. A "test of cure" culture should be performed after completion of therapy.

C. Acute Pyelonephritis: The presence of fever, chills, costovertebral angle tenderness, and low abdominal pain in combination with frequency, dysuria, and urgency is consistent with the diagnosis of acute pyelonephritis. The diagnosis is confirmed when a symptomatic patient has a midstream clean catch urine with greater than 10^5 bacteria per milliliter of urine, with the presence of numerous white blood cells. E coli is the most frequent organism. Other organisms that can be seen include enterococci, staphylococci, *Proteus,* and *Klebsiella.* The distinction between lower and upper tract disease is largely clinical. Acute infection of the lower urinary tract should not be associated with systemic symptoms, such as costovertebral angle tenderness, suprapubic pain, fever, or chills. There is no consistent laboratory technique to differentiate between the two.

The treatment of pyelonephritis is hospitalization and intravenous antibiotics until the patient has been afebrile for 24–48 hours, followed by oral antibiotics for 10–14 days. As in both asymptomatic bacteriuria and cystitis, antibiotic therapy is aimed at sensitivities. Ampicillin has been the traditional drug of first choice; however, the increase in resistance of E coli

to ampicillin may dictate the use of an aminoglycoside or cephalosporin in conjunction with or in place of ampicillin. Oral medications for the renal infectious disorders include the sulfonamides, ampicillin, amoxicillin plus clavulanate, and trimethoprim-sulfamethoxazole. If a patient has a history of pyelonephritis or recurrent urinary tract infections, suppression therapy using nitrofurantoin can be maintained at a dosage of 100 mg/d.

It is important to remember that appropriate therapy of pyelonephritis is critical. Reports over the last 5–7 years have indicated that inadequately treated pyelonephritis may result in adult respiratory distress syndrome (ARDS). This extremely serious complication can be avoided by appropriate and timely therapy.

D. Urolithiasis: Urolithiasis, or urinary calculus, is an infrequent occurrence in pregnancy. Smooth-muscle relaxation caused by increases in progesterone concentration and the mechanical obstruction of the uterus caused by its increasing size predispose pregnant women to both infection secondary to urinary stasis and the formation of renal calculi.

Urolithiasis, which occurs in 0.02–0.05% of pregnancies, has potentially disastrous implications for the fetus and mother. Because urolithiasis can be confused with other abdominal or pelvic disorders during pregnancy, serious consideration must be given to this diagnosis in pregnant women with abdominal or flank pain, hematuria, or unresolved bacteriuria. Urinary tract infection is the most common presentation of this disorder in pregnancy. When antibiotic therapy is unsuccessful in resolving urinary tract infection or pyelonephritis in the patient in whom culture reveals a susceptible organism, the diagnosis of urolithiasis should be suspected.

The diagnosis of urolithiasis is critical. Ultrasonography can be surprisingly useful. Diagnosis of urinary tract calculi may be made in greater than 70% of patients with urolithiasis, even in the third trimester. Noninvasive testing always should be attempted initially. In the presence of complications that may require invasive intervention, pregnancy should not deter appropriate roentgenographic evaluation. When the diagnosis is uncertain, modified excretory urography may be definitive. A routine four- to six-film examination results in an exposure of 0.4–1 rad. The minimal risk of this low-level radiation exposure is outweighed by the possible complications of mismanagement. A suggested algorithm for the management of urolithiasis is illustrated in Figure 55–3.

Thyroid Disease

A. Hypothyroidism: Symptomatic hypothyroidism in pregnancy is an uncommon phenomenon. Many cases are subclinical and difficult to detect. Symptoms include obesity or hypometabolism; dry,

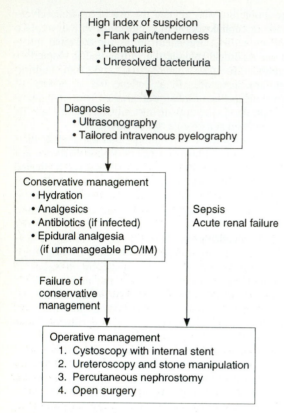

Figure 55–3. Algorithm for management of urolithiasis in pregnant women.

coarse hair and skin; cold intolerance; and gastrointestinal dysfunction. It is diagnosed by an increase in thyroid-stimulating hormone (TSH) with or without below normal levels of T_4 and T_3.

Complications of hypothyroidism include infertility, which serves as a partial explanation for the decreased incidence in pregnancy. In patients who become pregnant, hypothyroidism is associated with an increased risk of intrauterine growth retardation, stillbirth, placental abruption, and preeclampsia. There is also a four- to fivefold increase in miscarriage.

Patients who are diagnosed with hypothyroidism should be treated with levothyroxine. The initial dosage is 50 μg daily. The dosage should be increased every 3–4 weeks based on the impact of the therapy on TSH levels (normal levels: below 6 μU/mL). Most patients can be maintained adequately in pregnancy on dosages of 100–150 μg daily.

B. Hyperthyroidism: Hyperthyroidism is relatively common in pregnancy, occurring in approximately 1–2 pregnancies per thousand. The most common cause is Graves' disease, although Hashimoto's thyroiditis, hyperemesis, and trophoblastic disease also occur in association with this condition.

Symptoms of hyperthyroidism include hyperdynamic cardiovascular function (tachycardia, palpitations, tremor), increased appetite with weight loss, heat intolerance, nervousness, weakness, fatigability, and insomnia. There may be diffuse enlargement of the thyroid or, in the presence of a tumor, a thyroid nodule. A bruit may be heard over the organ.

The diagnosis of hyperthyroidism is made clinically and by laboratory tests. An elevation of T_4, T_3, or both, and an increased free thyroxine index are generally present. Treatment of hyperthyroidism in pregnancy is described in Chapter 20.

Hypertensive Disorders of Pregnancy

Hypertension associated with pregnancy is a common complication of primigravid pregnancies in the USA, occurring in 6–8% of the population. The pathophysiologic mechanism of this condition has yet to be defined. Chesley showed an increased incidence of the disorder in the daughters of women who had a history of pregnancy-induced hypertension (PIH) that was consistent with an autosomal recessive mode of inheritance. Other investigators have postulated an autoimmune cause, suggested by the preponderance of primiparous women who acquire the disease. An increased vasoreactivity has been reported by Gant et al; pregnant women in whom PIH developed had a greater reaction to infused angiotensinogen, which persisted until delivery. Although vasoconstriction is thought to be the final common pathway, recent studies by Easterly suggest that patients at risk for PIH can be identified in the second trimester by a significant increase in cardiac output over pregnancy baseline. This hyperdynamic model suggests that the subsequent increase in renal perfusion causes microvascular damage in the renal vasculature, resulting in albuminuria and positive feedback in the renin-angiotensin system.

The following classification of hypertension in pregnancy has been generally accepted:

1. Hypertension
   a. Without proteinuria or edema (pregnancy-induced hypertension)
   b. With proteinuria, edema, or both (mild or severe preeclampsia)
   c. With proteinuria, edema, or both, and convulsions (eclampsia)
2. Chronic hypertension alone
3. Chronic hypertension with superimposed preeclampsia or eclampsia

The presence of preexisting hypertension, any intrinsic vascular or autoimmune disease, diabetes, multiple gestation, trophoblastic disease, or a hydropic fetus increases the risk of PIH.

The diagnosis of preeclampsia is defined by the

College of Obstetricians and Gynecologists as follows:

1. Systolic blood pressure greater than 140 mmHg
2. Diastolic blood pressure greater than 90 mmHg OR an increase in systolic pressure of more than 30 mmHg or of diastolic pressure more than 15 mmHg on two separate occasions greater than 6 hours apart
3. Proteinuria greater than 300 mg per 24 hours OR 1 g/L in two random collections
4. Weight gain greater than 5 pounds/wk, edema, or both (especially facial or hands)

Severe preeclampsia is defined as follows:

1. Blood pressure greater than 160/110 on two separate occasions more than 6 hours apart
2. Proteinuria of 3–4+ on dipstick testing or greater than 5 g in a 24-hour specimen
3. Oliguria
4. Cerebral or visual disturbances
5. Pulmonary edema or cyanosis
6. Fetal intrauterine growth retardation
7. Epigastric or right upper quadrant pain
8. Abnormal laboratory values (elevated liver function tests, increased serum creatinine or uric acid, thrombocytopenia, hemolysis)

The management of PIH is defined by the severity of the disorder. Ultimately, only delivery of the fetus cures the disease. However, fetal well-being and maternal well-being both must be considered. In the case of extreme prematurity, conservative therapy may be indicated.

In a near-term pregnancy, delivery may be the best option. The fetal maturity is a vital piece of information. If maternal condition does not dictate immediate delivery, amniocentesis for lung maturity may be indicated. If the lungs are immature, steroids and conservative management for the mother are appropriate. Bed rest (at home if patient is compliant and stable) is vital. Hospitalization is necessary for patients who cannot remain on bed rest at home or whose blood pressure is sustained above 140/90 despite rest.

Cardiac Disease

Maternal cardiac disease is a serious complication of pregnancy and can lead to increased morbidity and mortality in both the mother and fetus. The incidence of these disorders is relatively low in pregnancy. However, the physiologic changes that occur in pregnancy may exacerbate an underlying cardiac abnormality or may make the diagnosis difficult.

An increase in cardiac output occurs early and maximizes at 30–50% of normal values by the beginning of the third trimester. It is recognized that the red blood cell mass does not increase to the same extent that plasma volume expands, creating the so-called physiologic anemia that is seen in the gravid female. Excessive iron utilization may result in iron deficiency anemia. Cardiac output increases 30–40% above nonpregnant values by mid pregnancy. The increase begins as early as 6–8 weeks and reaches its peak at 26–28 weeks. Stroke volume is increased 15–20%, and the maternal heart rate is increased 10–15 beats in the average pregnant woman.

Other physiologic parameters and hemodynamic changes in pregnancy can make the diagnosis of a pathologic condition difficult. Physical examination of a pregnant woman often reveals a systolic flow murmur (greater than 90%), a venous hum, S_3 90%, S_4 (less than 10%), tachycardia, cardiomegaly, prominent jugular veins, and peripheral edema. Changes may occur in the electrocardiogram. The average pregnant female evidences a shift of the main QRS, with minor ST depression and T-wave flattening or inversion often seen in leads 3 and aVF. Small Q waves also are sometimes present. Tachycardia is seen in more than 90% of pregnant women and is atrial in origin; extrasystoles and premature ventricular contractions (PVCs) are also common.

Preconception Counseling: It is vital that a woman with a history of cardiac disease discuss the ramifications of the disease and pregnancy with her physician prior to pregnancy. The risk to the mother during pregnancy varies with the type of preexisting disease. Functional status traditionally has been measured by the New York Heart Association classification as follows:

- Class I—asymptomatic
- Class II—symptoms with greater than normal activity
- Class III—symptoms with normal activity
- Class IV—symptoms at bed rest

In patients with preexisting heart disease, a careful search for diagnosis and a thorough evaluation of cardiac function should be performed before the risks of pregnancy are discussed. Cardiac condition is evaluated by the traditional methods of physical examination, echocardiography, and ECG; the more invasive procedures such as cardiac catheterization and evaluation of pulmonary pressure are performed only in more serious cases. The information gathered by appropriate diagnosis and definition of functional status is useful in counseling the patient regarding risks of pregnancy to herself and her fetus.

Specific risk factors for maternal mortality resulting from a pregnancy with preexisting maternal congenital heart disease (CHD) are listed Table 55–7. This table can be used to approximate the risk to a woman with known CHD. The risk level of the first category is acceptable to most pregnant women, and these patients may be followed by a generalist in obstetrics and gynecology. Women in group 2 require

Table 55–7. Maternal mortality associated with pregnancy.*

Group 1—mortality < 1%
  Atrial septal defect[†]
  Ventricular septal defect[†]
  Patent ductus arteriosus[†]
  Pulmonic or tricuspid disease
  Tetralogy of Fallot, corrected
  Porcine valve
  Mitral stenosis, NYHA class I and II
Group 2—mortality 5–15%
  Mitral stenosis, NYHA class III and IV
  Mitral stenosis with atrial fibrillation
  Artificial valve
  Aortic stenosis
  Coarctation of aorta[†]
  Tetralogy of Fallot, uncorrected
  Previous myocardial infarction
  Marfan syndrome with normal aorta
Group 3—mortality 25–50%
  Pulmonary hypertension
  Coarctation of aorta, with valvular involvement
  Marfan syndrome with aortic involvement

*Reproduced, with permission, from Clark SL et al (editors): *Critical Care Obstetrics,* 2nd ed. Blackwell Scientific Publications, 1991.
[†]Uncomplicated.

specific counseling by a specialist familiar with cardiac disease (preferably a subspecialist in maternal-fetal medicine) and appropriate follow-through in the event of pregnancy. Patients in group 3 should be counseled by a subspecialist in maternal-fetal medicine; the high risk to the mother requires discussion of pregnancy termination.

Counseling must include discussion of the risk to the fetus. The incidence of congenital cardiac defects in the fetus of an affected mother ranges from 5 to 10%; the defect is concordant in less than 50%. The perinatal outcome of affected pregnancies depends on the severity of the maternal disease. In general, maternal hypoxemia (pO_2 below 70%) and hyperemia (hematocrit greater than 65%) are associated with poor perinatal outcome. Increased risks of intrauterine growth retardation; preterm labor; and birth, stillbirth, and miscarriage are seen in affected pregnancies.

REFERENCES

American College of Obstetrics and Gynecology: Cardiac disease in pregnancy. Tech Bull No. 92, 1992.

American College of Obstetrics and Gynecology: Management of diabetes mellitus in pregnancy. Tech Bull No. 92, 1986.

American College of Obstetrics and Gynecology: Thyroid disease in pregnancy. Tech Bull No. 181, 1993.

Burton BK et al: Limb anomalies associated with chorionic villus sampling. Obstet Gynecol 1992;79:726.

Chesley LC: History and epidemiology of preeclampsia/eclampsia. Clin Obstet Gynecol 1984;27:801.

Clark SL et al (editors): *Critical Care Obstetrics,* 2nd ed. Blackwell Scientific Publications, 1991.

Creasy RK, Resnik R (editors): *Maternal-Fetal Medicine: Principles and Practice,* 3rd ed. Saunders, 1994.

Easterly TR, Benedetti TJ: Preeclampsia: A hyperdynamic disease model. Am J Obstet Gynecol 1989;160:1447.

Evans MI et al (editors): *Fetal Diagnosis and Therapy.* Lippincott, 1989.

Firth HV et al: Severe limb abnormalities after chorion villus sampling at 56-66 days gestation. Lancet 1991;337:762.

Gant NF et al: A study of angiotensin II pressor response throughout primigravid pregnancy. J Clin Invest 1973; 52:2682.

Haddow JE et al: Reducing the need for amniocentesis in women 35 years of age or older with serum markers for screening. N Engl J Med 1994;330:1114.

Hendricks SK, Ross SO, Krieger JN: An algorithm for diagnosis and therapy of management and complications of urolithiasis during pregnancy. Surg Gynecol Obstet 1991;172:49.

Tulchinsky D, Little AB (editors): *Maternal-Fetal Endocrinology,* 2nd ed. Saunders, 1994.

Pregnancy Losses

56

Laura R. Stone, MD

A **spontaneous abortion** is an intrauterine pregnancy that ends before the twentieth week of gestation. It is complete (Fig 56–1) if the placenta and fetus have been passed and incomplete (Fig 56–2) if some fetal or placental tissue remains in the uterus. A **missed abortion** is defined by lack of fetal cardiac activity after 7 weeks in the absence of bleeding or cramping. A **threatened abortion** occurs when there is vaginal bleeding or cramping and the cervical os is not dilated. **Inevitable abortion** is diagnosed when bleeding and cramping occur and either the cervical os is dilated or tissue is present in the cervical canal. An **ectopic pregnancy** is a pregnancy that is not located in the endometrial cavity. Ectopic pregnancies can be located in the fallopian tube, cervix, uterine cornu, ovary, or peritoneal cavity (see Fig 56–3).

Incidence & Risk Factors

The incidence of ectopic pregnancy (expressed as ectopic pregnancies per live births) has been rising dramatically over the last 30 years. The Centers for Disease Control and Prevention (CDC) reports that between 1970 and 1986, the rate of ectopic pregnancies increased from 4.5 in 1000 to 14.3 in 1000. In 1986, ectopic pregnancies represented only 1.4% of all pregnancies but accounted for 13.2% of all maternal deaths. At present, 1 in 60 pregnancies is ectopic. Multiple explanations are given for the increase in incidence of ectopic pregnancy: earlier and more accurate diagnosis, better treatment of pelvic inflammatory disease (thus preserving fertility), use of intrauterine devices (IUDs), and increased availability of abortion (fewer live births).

Risk factors for ectopic pregnancy include the following:

History of sexually transmitted diseases or pelvic
  inflammatory disease (PID)
Multiple sexual partners
Tubal ligation
Use of IUD
Progestin-only oral contraceptive or implant
Previous ectopic pregnancy
History of appendicitis
History of infertility and infertility treatments

Incidence & Risk Factors
Signs & Symptoms
Clinical Findings & Diagnosis
Treatment
Prognosis
Referral to a Specialist
Psychosocial Concerns
Unresolved Issues

Infection after delivery or gynecologic procedure
History of tubal surgery

A history of multiple partners, sexually transmitted diseases, PID, tubal surgery, or a ruptured appendix can increase the risk of tubal damage. Progestin-only birth control pills and subcutaneous progestin implants are believed to increase the risk of ectopic pregnancy because of decreased tubal motility. IUDs are thought to increase ectopic pregnancy risk through decreased tubal motility or increased intrauterine inflammation; they are also risk factors for PID and subsequent tubal scarring. Most pregnancies in women who have had tubal ligations are ectopic. Any patient who has been infertile is at higher risk for ectopic pregnancy, even if tubal disease has not been diagnosed. Use of clomiphene citrate for ovulation induction or one of the reproductive technologies carries a higher risk of ectopic pregnancy than that of the general population. Any such treatment that results in multiple ovulations increases the risk of multiple pregnancy and is one of the few circumstances in which heterotopic (intrauterine plus extrauterine) pregnancies can occur. Endometritis or pelvic infections following previous delivery or gynecologic procedure also can cause tubal injury. Finally, any woman with a history of previous ectopic pregnancy should be assumed to have another until proved otherwise.

The incidence of miscarriage (spontaneous abortion) is unknown. One half of all conceptions are not recognized clinically. Of those that are recognized

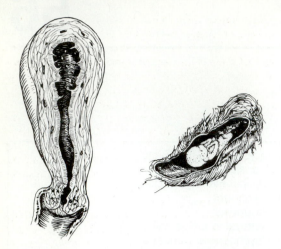

Figure 56–1. Complete abortion. *At right:* Product of complete abortion. (Reproduced, with permission, from Benson RC: *Handbook of Obstetrics & Gynecology,* 8th ed. Lange, 1983.)

clinically, 15–30% are lost in the first trimester, and another 2–3% are lost later during the pregnancy. The incidence of miscarriage increases after age 40, along with the incidence of genetic abnormalities.

Signs & Symptoms

The most common signs and symptoms of early pregnancy are missed menstrual period, nausea,

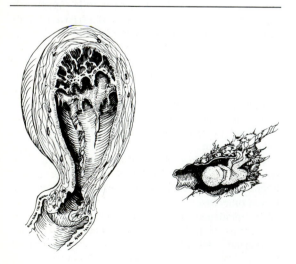

Figure 56–2. Incomplete abortion. *At right:* Product of incomplete abortion. (Reproduced, with permission, from Benson RC: *Handbook of Obstetrics & Gynecology,* 8th ed. Lange, 1983.)

breast tenderness, fatigue, occasional irregular uterine cramping, and intermittent adnexal pain caused by tension and strain of the round ligaments or a corpus luteum cyst. Occasionally, mild spotting can occur 1 week before the expected and missed period, at the time of embryonic implantation.

Symptoms that should alert clinicians to potential problems are sharp, unilateral, lower quadrant pain that recurs and increases in intensity; persistent spotting or bleeding; rectal pain; shoulder pain; lightheadedness or syncope; increasing "menstrual" cramps; and pain with intercourse. Decreasing or suddenly absent symptoms of breast tenderness, nausea, and fatigue are also clues that the pregnancy may not be progressing normally.

There is a great deal of overlap between symptoms of normal and abnormal pregnancies. Some women with normal intrauterine pregnancies deny any symptoms at all, and some women with ectopic pregnancies describe symptoms consistent with normal pregnancy. It is essential for clinicians to remember that ectopic pregnancies can be life-threatening. Any pregnancy with abnormal bleeding or pain must be considered ectopic until proved otherwise.

Clinical Findings & Diagnosis

When a woman presents with vaginal bleeding or pelvic pain and may be pregnant, the history should focus on a description of symptoms, risk factors for ectopic pregnancy (see the section preceding, Incidence & Risk Factors), and the exclusion of diseases in the differential diagnosis for ectopic pregnancy, which include the following (numbers 3 through 10 can occur concurrently with ectopic pregnancy or spontaneous abortion):

1. Spontaneous abortion
2. Anovulatory cycle
3. Ruptured corpus luteum
4. Ruptured ovarian cyst
5. Torsion of ovary
6. Endometriosis
7. Acute salpingitis
8. Appendicitis
9. Degenerating fibroids
10. Trauma

A. Pain Location and Severity: Midline or suprapubic pain associated with menstrual-like cramps is more common with possible miscarriage. Pain that is persistently one-sided or radiating to the midline is suggestive of ectopic pregnancy. Ninety-nine percent of ectopic pregnancies are located in the fallopian tube, usually the ampullary portion (Fig 56–3).

B. Last Menstrual Period: The date of the last normal menstrual period (LMP) should be recorded, as well as the date of onset of abnormal bleeding. Ectopic pregnancies frequently present at approximately 6–8 weeks past the LMP, whereas miscarriages often present 8–10 weeks past the LMP, although there is considerable overlap.

C. Other Symptoms: Presence of fever or chills and color of vaginal discharge may or may not be related to the pregnancy. Infected and septic abortions should be included in the differential as well as gastroenteritis or appendicitis concurrent with pregnancy.

D. Physical Examination: Rapid pulse and orthostatic hypotension indicate possible internal hemorrhage, which can result from ruptured ectopic pregnancy or ruptured corpus luteum cyst. A "surgical abdomen" with rebound and guarding should be regarded as such. If immediate ultrasonography is not available in this situation, culdocentesis should be considered as part of the pelvic examination (see the section following, Culdocentesis). If the patient remains unstable, evaluation for surgery is required. A surgical abdomen is extremely rare with miscarriage, although it may be present with a ruptured corpus luteum.

On pelvic examination, an attempt should be made to locate the pain over either the uterus or the adnexa. Approximately 50% of ectopic pregnancies present with an adnexal mass. Cervical motion tenderness is nonspecific and can be associated with ectopic pregnancy, miscarriage, or other pelvic disease. The amount of bleeding should be assessed. Large clots in the vagina and brisk bleeding usually are associated with threatened or incomplete abortion. Brownish spotting or bleeding consistent with menses could be either miscarriage or ectopic pregnancy. Any tissue seen at the cervical os should be removed carefully with ring forceps and sent for pathologic study for further identification. Any clots or tissue passed into the vagina should be sent as well. If closed ring forceps can be passed easily through the internal os, the cervix is "open," and the diagnosis is almost always inevitable or incomplete abortion.

E. Laboratory Tests:

1. β-Human chorionic gonadotropin (βHCG)– βHCG is produced by placental villi. The α subunit is common to pituitary hormones, whereas the β subunits of these molecules are unique. βHCG can be measured in both serum and urine. For serum, most laboratories use the First International Standard Preparation (FSIP), which is a radioimmunoassay. Values are expressed in IU/L with the lower limits of detection being 5–10 IU/L. A "qualitative" serum pregnancy test determines the presence or absence of pregnancy. A "quantitative" serum pregnancy test provides the amount of βHCG that is present. Urine pregnancy tests are available that measure a minimum of 25–50 IU/L. The urine tests available are various combinations of monoclonal and polyclonal immunoassays and enzymatic assays.

During the first 6 weeks of gestation, the βHCG fraction doubles approximately every 48 hours, but there can be wide variations from this pattern with both normal and abnormal pregnancies. A 66% rise every 48 hours is considered acceptable. Pregnancies that do not maintain this doubling curve may be abnormal, ie, ectopic pregnancies or pregnancies that will miscarry. βHCG increases more rapidly in multiple gestations and molar pregnancies.

2. Progesterone–Same-day progesterone levels are not widely available, and their value in differentiating normal and abnormal pregnancies is controversial. A value less than 5 ng/mL may suggest ectopic gestation, whereas levels greater than 25 ng/mL generally are associated with intrauterine pregnancy. There is wide overlap with intermediate values.

3. Other laboratory tests–Hematocrit, blood type and screen (to determine whether the patient needs Rh immune globulin (RhoGAM), as well as βHCG level should be ordered. Cross-match is indicated when suspicion of ruptured ectopic is high. Cultures of the cervix for gonorrhea and *Chlamydia trachomatis* can be considered, but the cultures are not valid when there is significant bleeding.

F. Imaging Studies:

1. Ultrasonography–The primary use of ultrasonography is to locate an intrauterine sac. When the sac has been clearly located, an ectopic gestation al-

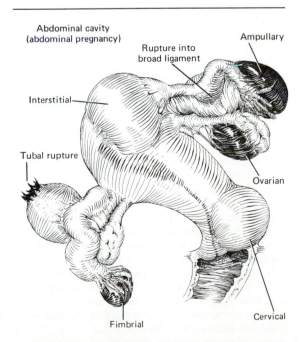

Figure 56–3. Sites of ectopic pregnancies. (Reproduced, with permission from Benson RC: *Handbook of Obstetrics & Gynecology,* 8th ed. Lange, 1983.)

most always is ruled out. Occasionally, an irregular or "pseudogestational" sac is associated with an ectopic gestation. It is rare to have concurrent intrauterine and ectopic (heterotopic) pregnancies, but this situation can occur when there have been multiple ovulations.

Most ultrasonography departments and laboratories work together to establish "discriminatory zones." These zones define the level of βHCG required to visualize the pregnancy with ultrasonography. When the FSIP is used, a gestational sac should be visualized by transabdominal ultrasonography when the βHCG is 6000–6500 IU/L. Transvaginal transducers are able to visualize an intrauterine sac at approximately 2000 IU/L. It is important to know which preparation is used and how βHCG levels correlate with available ultrasonographic examinations. The discriminatory zone may vary between institutions. When an intrauterine gestation is not seen, the sonographer views the adnexa carefully for any apparent masses. The pelvis also is checked for free fluid (blood in the case of ectopic pregnancy). The fetal pole and fetal cardiac activity should be seen by 7 weeks of gestation (menstrual dating) by transabdominal scan. Transvaginal scan often identifies the fetal pole and cardiac activity by 6 weeks.

2. Doppler ultrasonography–Color Doppler is now being evaluated in diagnosing ectopic gestations. Color Doppler works by noting the direction of blood flow relative to the transducer. It is hoped that visualization of abnormal blood flow patterns in the adnexa may help to define ectopic gestation further.

Differentiating between ectopic pregnancies and early threatened abortions can be difficult. Abnormal bleeding and pain associated with pregnancy should be considered an ectopic pregnancy until proved otherwise. Any female patient of childbearing age with unexplained pelvic or abdominal pain should have a serum pregnancy test. When the diagnosis is not clear initially, the patient should be sent home to follow "ectopic versus miscarriage precautions." These precautions are as follows:

- Avoid intercourse and tampons
- Save and bring in tissue passed
- Notify the provider in case of worsening pain, bleeding that requires more than one pad per hour, a temperature above 100.5 °F, or lightheadedness, syncope, or shoulder pain.

If she passes tissue, she should put a plastic bag over her hand, pick up the tissue, turn the bag inside out, and bring the tissue to the office or emergency room. Tissue should be sent to the pathology laboratory for further identification. The patient should have the phone number of the emergency department. The process of losing a pregnancy can be frightening; specific instructions on how to obtain help can be reassuring.

3. Culdocentesis–Culdocentesis can provide indirect evidence of ruptured ectopic pregnancy by demonstrating the presence of nonclotting intraperitoneal blood (Fig 56–4). It is performed less frequently than in the past because of the availability of ultrasonography to detect intraperitoneal bleeding. A speculum is placed in the patient's vagina, and the cervix and upper vagina are swabbed with antiseptic. The posterior lip of the cervix is grasped with a tenaculum and retracted downward and anteriorly. An 18-gauge spinal needle attached to a 20-mL syringe is inserted through the vagina posterior to the cervix and between the uterosacral ligaments into the posterior cul-de-sac. Traditionally, these steps have been done without local anesthetic. However, 1–2 mL of 1% lidocaine injected into the posterior lip of the cervix and 1–2 mL injected into the vaginal wall covering the cul-de-sac decrease discomfort.

In ruptured ectopic pregnancies, nonclotting blood usually is obtained. The blood does not clot because of fibrinolysis of a previously formed clot in the peritoneum. A hematocrit of nonclotting blood greater than 15% is consistent with ectopic gestation. However, clotting also can occur if bleeding into the abdominal cavity is brisk or if an artery is entered with the needle. No blood indicates that either the cul-de-sac has not been entered or there is no internal bleeding. A large amount of straw-colored fluid indicates possible ovarian cyst rupture or ascites.

G. Diagnosis of Ectopic Pregnancy: Ectopic pregnancies, like appendicitis, can be "great foolers." The differential diagnosis should be kept in mind as the evaluation progresses (see the section preceding, "Clinical Findings & Diagnosis"). Figure 56–5 describes one approach to the diagnosis of ectopic pregnancy. If the diagnosis is suspected and the serum pregnancy test is positive, an ultrasonographic scan should be obtained. If an intrauterine sac is clearly seen, an ectopic pregnancy is excluded. If an intrauterine sac is not seen, and the βHCG is greater than the discriminatory zone, the patient should be referred immediately for treatment of a probable ectopic pregnancy. If the βHCG is less than the discriminatory zone and the patient is stable, another quantitative βHCG should be obtained in 48 hours. If the values double normally, another ultrasonographic scan should be performed when the value reaches the discriminatory zone.

If the βHCG values rise slowly (ie, less than 66% in 48 hours) or plateau, another ultrasonographic scan should be obtained. If no adnexal mass is seen, the patient requires a suction dilation and curettage (D&C) to examine the contents of the uterus. If villi are not identified, further diagnosis of ectopic pregnancy should be pursued. Decidual tissue or an Arias-Stella reaction is suggestive of ectopic preg-

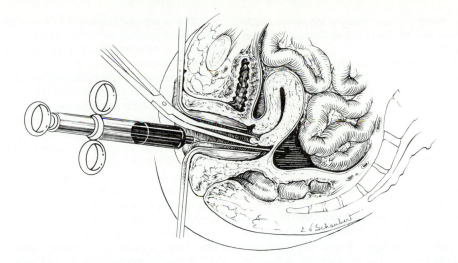

Figure 56–4. Culdocentesis. (Reproduced, with permission, from DeCherney AH, Pernoll ML: *Current Obstetric & Gynecologic Diagnosis & Treatment,* 8/e. Appleton & Lange, 1994.)

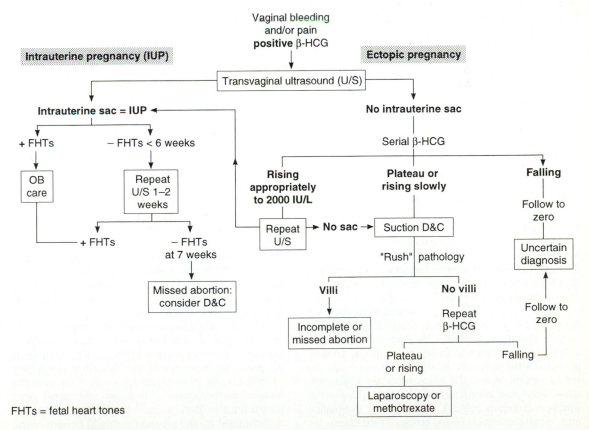

FHTs = fetal heart tones

Figure 56–5. Algorithm for diagnosis and treatment of spontaneous abortion and ectopic pregnancy.

nancy. The patient needs surgery or methotrexate therapy unless βHCG levels fall dramatically immediately after the D&C.

In some asymptomatic stable patients with a βHCG less than 2000 IU/L that continues to fall and an empty uterus, observation and continued serial βHCGs can be relied on. A small intrauterine pregnancy may have been missed by the D&C. In addition, some small degenerating ectopic pregnancies may resolve spontaneously. The patient must be reliable, and the βHCGs should be followed until the findings are negative.

Treatment

A. Prevention of Isoimmunization: Isoimmunization of the mother can occur with both ectopic pregnancies and miscarriages if fetal red cells enter the maternal system. Red blood cells are present in the developing embryo at approximately 6 weeks. All women who are Rh-negative and who have been treated for ectopic pregnancy or spontaneous or therapeutic abortion up to and including 12 weeks should be given 50 µg Rh immune globulin (MICRhoGAM). This dose is designed to suppress the immune response to 2.5 mL or less of blood. Losses occurring after 13 weeks should receive the full 300-µg dose of immune globulin (RhoGAM), which covers 15 mL or less. Patients who have bleeding episodes with threatened abortions also should be given immune globulin. Maternal side effects are extremely rare, but treatment should be avoided in anyone known to have had an anaphylactic reaction to any immune globulin.

Some centers advocate the use of the 300-µg dose in all cases, because the amount of blood transfused is difficult to estimate with certainty, the cost differential is small, the side effects to the mother are rare, and the potential consequences to future pregnancies are great if isoimmunization should occur. The full dose offers protection against future bleeds for 2–4 months.

B. Ectopic Pregnancy: The details of surgical treatment are beyond the scope of this book. Conservation of the affected tube is attempted in all cases in which a woman wants to preserve her fertility. Most surgery is done laparoscopically to minimize patient discomfort and hospital stay. Linear salpingostomy is the procedure of choice for unruptured ampullary ectopic pregnancies less than 3 cm in diameter. Postoperatively, serial βHCGs are followed until they are negative. Levels should be checked 48 hours after surgery and then weekly, if they are falling. Larger ectopic pregnancies and those located in the isthmic portion of the tube are treated by excising the affected portion of the tube. Microsurgical reanastomosis is done at a later date after healing is complete. The less common cornual, or interstitial, pregnancy may require resection of the cornua of the uterus or, if ruptured, a hysterectomy. The patency of the opposite tube is not evaluated at the time of initial surgery because of possible infection and edema. If fertility is desired, a hysterosalpingogram can be obtained 3 months postoperatively.

Methotrexate inhibits dihydrofolic acid reductase and blocks DNA synthesis, causing rapid involution of villi. It has been used extensively as a chemotherapeutic agent in treating choriocarcinoma or trophoblastic disease. This agent is being used to treat selected ectopic pregnancies and persistent elevations of βHCG after surgery. Persistent elevations of βHCG in the low range (below 2000 IU/L) also have been treated with methotrexate when the exact location of the pregnancy cannot be determined and laparoscopic surgery seems too invasive in a stable patient. Various regimens for methotrexate therapy have been devised with intramuscular, intravenous, and intratubal administration, with single- or multiple-dose therapy. One approach is a single intramuscular injection of 40 mg/m^2 or 1 mg/kg, to be repeated weekly if βHCG levels fall less than 10% per week. Complete blood cell count (CBC), serum glutamic-oxaloacetic transaminase (SGOT), and clinical symptoms need to be monitored carefully. The prospect of a nonsurgical approach for these patients is promising. Side effects are usually minimal and include nausea and fatigue. However, few long-term studies have been done in these patients to assess residual tubal damage from the ectopic tissue and future fertility.

C. Miscarriage: When an abortion is threatened, bleeding is present, cramping may be present, and the internal os of the cervix is closed. No tissue has been passed, and an ultrasonographic scan may have identified a sac or even a viable fetus. The pregnancy continues in greater than 50% of cases. Rh-negative women should receive Rh immune globulin.

There are no studies showing that restriction in activity alters the outcome. However, many women feel reassured by reducing activity for 1–2 days. If bleeding and cramping decrease or disappear, ultrasonography should be repeated in 1–2 weeks to verify continuation of the pregnancy. At times, serial βHCGs may provide reassurance if appropriate increases can be shown.

Supplemental progesterone has not been proved to alter the outcome of a threatened abortion. Its value may be only to make the patient feel she is doing something to help, and its use after the diagnosis of threatened abortion is discouraged.

When the abortion is incomplete, cramping is variable, the internal os of the cervix is open, and bleeding can be profuse. Suction D&C usually is required; the procedure is similar to that described in Chapter 54. Usually, the placenta or a portion of the placenta remains in the uterus. All tissue and blood clots passed prior to D&C as well as products of conception obtained by the procedure should be sent to the pathology laboratory. In early losses, the fetus may not be easily identified, but villi should be seen. If villi are not found, serial βHCGs should be followed until they are negative. If values plateau or continue to rise, an ectopic pregnancy or gestational trophoblastic disease needs to be excluded. Rh-negative women should receive Rh immune globulin. Doxycycline or erythromycin usually is given for 7–10 days following D&C as prophylaxis against *Chlamydia trachomatis,* which may have been introduced into the upper genital tract from the procedure.

When the abortion is complete, cramps decrease or stop. Bleeding ceases or is slight. The cervix may be open. All products of conception are passed. If tissue is available, it should be sent to the pathology laboratory for identification of villi. If no tissue is available or no villi are seen, βHCG levels should be followed until they are negative.

Sometimes it is difficult to distinguish between incomplete and complete abortions. Some practitioners perform a D&C in all situations to ensure that the uterus is empty. Alternatively, ultrasonography may be performed. An endometrial thickness of 10 mm or less is consistent with a complete abortion, and D&C is not required.

A missed abortion has been defined in the past as retention of fetus and placenta for 8 weeks beyond the time of fetal death. With widespread availability of ultrasonography, it is now defined by the lack of fetal cardiac activity after 7 weeks gestation. The outlook is also poor if no fetal pole is seen by 6 weeks gestation. Accurate dating of the pregnancy is essential. If dates are not known for certain, repeat ultrasonography in about 1 week will show no further progression of the pregnancy if it is not viable. Serial βHCGs that are level or falling also help confirm the diagnosis. In these situations, therapy can be individualized. Many women elect to proceed with D&C. Others choose to allow a spontaneous abortion to occur and undergo a D&C if medically necessary. Complete abortion (not requiring a D&C) occurs most often when the gestation is early (ie, at 7 weeks or less) or when no fetal pole has been identified. Most pregnancies 8 weeks or greater require D&C because of increased bleeding.

Missed abortions in the second trimester require dilation and evacuation (D&E) or prostaglandin induction of uterine contractions. The options available depend on the comfort level and skill of the practitioner. It is important to find skilled surgeons with low complication rates and warm, supportive staffs to whom to make referrals. The uterus is soft and easy to perforate in the second trimester with D&E. Prostaglandin inductions are usually done in an inpatient setting. Patients with missed abortions late in the second trimester that have been retained in utero for a month or longer since fetal demise are at risk for coagulation abnormalities caused by necrotic tissue. The uterus needs to be evaluated promptly.

Evidence of an infected or septic abortion is an indication for hospital admission, broad-spectrum intravenous antibiotic treatment (gentamicin and clindamycin), and D&C or D&E to evacuate the uterus after the first dose of all antibiotics has been administered. Evidence of maternal sepsis requires the addition of penicillin G. Intravenous antibiotics should be administered until the patient has been afebrile for 48 hours. Oral antibiotics should be administered to complete treatment of pelvic inflammatory disease. If the pregnancy is too far advanced for D&E, induction of uterine contractions with oxytocin or prostaglandins is indicated.

D. Counseling After a Pregnancy Loss: Frequent questions asked by patients include "What did I do wrong?" "When can we have sex?" and "When can we try to conceive again?"

It is important to dispel the concept that the pregnancy loss was caused by anything the patient did either before or during the pregnancy. It is useful to find out what the couple thinks may have caused the loss and address these issues.

After ectopic pregnancies and early uncomplicated miscarriages, the cervix is generally closed. Vaginal bleeding can continue for several weeks afterward. Many practitioners advise patients not to have intercourse until after bleeding ceases. Most advise at least 3 days abstinence after D&C to allow the cervix to close completely to avoid possible infection.

Traditionally, a 3-month waiting period has been advised before attempting conception. This time period is intended to allow the couple time to grieve, to let the woman's cycles become regular, and to allow the endometrial cavity or fallopian tube to heal. However, pregnancies that begin in the month following a miscarriage have a similar outcome to those that are delayed by 3 months or more. Some couples want to attempt conception right away, whereas others decide to wait a longer time. Couples postponing pregnancy should be counseled about contraception.

Prognosis

Any woman treated for an ectopic pregnancy should be considered at increased risk for subsequent ectopic pregnancy. Approximately 50% of women have an intrauterine pregnancy with the next attempt, but 20% have a repeat ectopic pregnancy. Therefore, serial βHCGs and early ultrasonography are indicated with all subsequent pregnancies. The remaining 30% of patients are unable to conceive without in vitro fertilization.

The chance of a couple conceiving after a miscarriage is excellent. Ninety-five percent of women conceive and carry a pregnancy to term within the next 2 years (Table 56–1). No evaluation is advised after one miscarriage.

Traditionally, women were not classified as "habitual aborters" until after three miscarriages. However, it is now generally recommended that a consultation and some testing be performed after two

Table 56–1. Recurrence risks for spontaneous abortions.*

	Prior Abortions	Risk (%)
Women with liveborn infants	0	12
	1	24
	2	26
	3	32
	4	26
Women without liveborn infants	2 or more	40–45

*Gabbe SO, Niebyl JV, Simpson JL: *Obstetrics: Normal & Problem Pregnancies.* Churchill Livingstone, 1991.

spontaneous abortions in the first trimester. Losses in the second trimester should prompt immediate referral.

First-trimester losses frequently have genetic causes. The incidence of genetic anomalies in spontaneously aborted fetuses is approximately 50%, compared with the 6% rate in elective abortions. Karyotyping of tissue obtained from D&C of a second loss can help determine whether the couple should be screened for balanced translocation or mosaicism; however, the screening is expensive. Less than 6% of couples with recurrent pregnancy losses.

Up to 15% of recurrent spontaneous abortions are caused by structural anomalies of the upper genital tract such as a uterine septum. These anomalies can be identified by hysterosalpingography. The remainder of the evaluation is controversial, but it often includes testing for antiphospholipid antibodies and an endometrial biopsy to exclude a luteal phase defect.

Approximately 70% of the time, recurrent pregnancy losses remain unexplained. The lack of an identifiable cause should be presented to the patient as reassuring. Currently, there are no data that support the use of other interventions such as leukocyte immunization or immunoglobulin infusions, and these treatments should be offered only as part of experimental protocols.

Second-trimester losses frequently are attributed to maternal causes, but they also can be caused by genetic anomalies. Rapidly enlarging leiomyomas or other structural anomalies can lead to expulsion of the fetus. An "incompetent cervix" (painless dilation of the cervix) should be followed carefully during a subsequent pregnancy with possible cerclage placement. Systemic maternal disease such as diabetes, systemic lupus erythematosus, or chronic renal disease should be managed by a medical specialist and an obstetrician prior to conception of the next pregnancy.

Referral to a Specialist

The skill level and knowledge base of the provider are the most important determinants of referral for specialty care. Resources for referral vary widely in communities and geographic areas.

The diagnosis of ruptured ectopic pregnancy should prompt immediate referral to a gynecologic surgeon for emergency surgery. The diagnosis of possible unruptured ectopic pregnancy requires referral to a gynecologic surgeon for either surgery or methotrexate therapy. Rupture can occur at any time with ectopic pregnancy, but it usually occurs within the first 2 weeks following methotrexate injection. Methotrexate should be administered under the guidance of a gynecologic surgeon.

Women who are found to have pelvic adhesions or other abnormalities at the time of surgery for ectopic pregnancy or who have recurrent ectopic pregnancies should be referred to a reproductive endocrinologist for consultation if fertility is desired.

D&C for incomplete or missed abortions in the first trimester should be performed only by providers comfortable with the procedure and management of complications. All women with molar pregnancies should be referred to a gynecologist. Not all gynecologists are skilled in second-trimester abortions; therefore, patients needing a D&E in the second trimester should be referred to gynecologists who perform the procedure regularly and have low complication rates.

Women experiencing two spontaneous abortions in the first trimester or one spontaneous abortion after 13 weeks of gestation should be referred to an obstetrician or reproductive endocrinologist for further evaluation.

All couples should be offered emotional support at each visit. If further counseling is needed, patients should be referred to mental health workers experienced in dealing with grief and loss. If suicidal ideation is elicited, immediate psychiatric evaluation is indicated.

Psychosocial Concerns

Stress following miscarriage and ectopic pregnancy can be enormous. When women learn they are pregnant, they often anticipate the next 9 months and beyond and are crushed to find out they are no longer pregnant. Many women have surgery for the first time in their life. However, the outcome is clearly negative—no baby to hold, no new family.

Women and their partners should be told to expect that the pregnancy loss will have a strong emotional impact. The woman may cry easily or for no apparent reason. She may have a difficult time on her projected due date. Much like infertile women and their partners (see Chapter 52), the couple may not want to see friends who have children or who are pregnant. This is normal grieving for what might have been, and the reaction will diminish with time.

Frequently, women and their partners deal differently with a pregnancy loss. Clinicians can encourage partners to comfort each other and communicate, but it is important to realize they may not be recovering at the same rate.

The psychological impact of miscarriage only recently has been examined by controlled observational study. Women who experienced miscarriage had a 3.4–4.3-fold greater chance of having depressive symptoms than women who were pregnant or women in a community control group. Women who were childless and lost a wanted pregnancy were 11 times more likely to be significantly depressed than childless community women. The more children a woman had at the time of the loss, the better she was able to cope. Women with recurrent losses were not more symptomatic than women experiencing their first loss. Women who viewed the pregnancy as a "fetus" felt the impact much less than those who viewed the pregnancy as a "baby." The researchers found also that women were the most symptomatic in the first few weeks following a loss. Six months after miscarriage, women were 3 times as likely to be depressed as women in the community.

Another ongoing study found that 10% of women reported having seriously considered suicide following miscarriage. Most significantly, the researchers determined that the interviews themselves were helpful in alleviating depressive symptoms.

Patients need to be given adequate counseling time so that the provider can review their emotional status and offer support. Many women feel much better knowing that the provider is aware of their feelings. If symptoms are significant, suicidal ideation should be elicited. It is important to be aware of the resources in the community, especially counselors and therapists who are experienced in grief and loss therapy. The organization RESOLVE provides support to couples with pregnancy losses as well to infertile couples (see Chapter 53).

Unresolved Issues

Long-term follow-up studies of methotrexate therapy for ectopic pregnancy currently are underway. Tubal patency, future fertility, and cost-effectiveness as compared with traditional surgical techniques are being examined. The ideal dose and route of administration of methotrexate continue to be evaluated.

The causes of recurrent spontaneous abortion are still poorly understood. Advances in the fields of genetics, immunology, embryo research, reproductive technology, infectious disease, and systemic medical illness all will contribute to future advances in therapy.

REFERENCES

American College of Obstetricians and Gynecologists: *Ectopic Pregnancy.* Technical Bulletin No. 150. ACOG, 1990.

American College of Obstetricians and Gynecologists: *Ultrasonography in Pregnancy.* Technical Bulletin No. 187. ACOG, 1990.

DeFrain J: Learning about grief from normal families: SIDS, stillbirth and miscarriage. J Mar Fam Ther 1991;17:215.

Gabbe SG, Niebyl JR, Simpson JL: *Obstetrics: Normal and Problem Pregnancies.* Churchill Livingstone, 1991.

Neugebauer R et al: Depressive symptoms in women in the six months after miscarriage. Am J Obstet Gynecol 1992;166:104.

Ory SJ: New options for diagnosis and treatment of ectopic pregnancy. JAMA 1992;267:534.

Plouffe L et al: Etiologic factors of recurrent abortion and subsequent reproductive performance of couples: Have we made any progress in the past 10 years? Am J Obstet Gynecol 1992;167:313.

Steinkampf MP, Nichols JE: Ectopic pregnancy: The deadly gestation. Emerg Med 1990;7:17.

Stovall TG, Ling FW, Gray LA: Single-dose methotrexate for treatment of ectopic pregnancy. Obstet Gynecol 1991;77:754.

57

Psychological Aspects of Perinatal Loss

Irving G. Leon, PhD

Perinatal loss is the outcome of approximately 1.5% of all pregnancies beyond 20 weeks. Some causative factors such as congenital abnormalities and cord entanglements are unlikely to recur. To the degree that poor prenatal care persists (eg, untreated acute and chronic diseases poor nutrition, and poor health habits such as drinking and smoking), which contributes to prematurity and perinatal loss, subsequent pregnancies have a higher than average mortality rate.

Few areas in medical practice have undergone as radical a revision and as great an improvement as the professional response to perinatal loss has in the past 20 years. Before the mid-1970s, medical practitioners usually tried to inhibit parental mourning of a perinatal death by preventing parental contact with the dead baby, disposing of the body unceremoniously and anonymously, prescribing tranquilizers for the parents to dull any expression of shock or grief, advising the parents to forget the experience, and often suggesting another pregnancy as soon as possible. Today, the opposite approach is recommended. Parents are encouraged to see, touch, hold, name, and bury their stillborn or dead infant to make the child's life and death more real. They are discouraged from taking tranquilizers; instead, parents are encouraged to share their feelings about the loss with each other. They are advised not to attempt another pregnancy for 6 months to a year, the period generally considered necessary to mourn a child's death.

Historical Perspectives

Early studies of perinatal loss during the 1970s documented, often in rich, descriptive detail, the unique aspects of this family death that made effective coping especially challenging. It is difficult to mourn a person whose social identity has not been established clearly and whose image is so heavily laden with fantasies as opposed to memories of interaction. Grief is complicated further by the incomplete separation of the baby from the physical and psychological selves of the parents, often resulting in profound disorientation, disappointment, and lowered self-esteem. By denying that a baby was lost,

> Historical Perspectives
> The Meanings of Perinatal Loss
> Implications for Practice
> Future Directions

clinicians did not provide the necessary assistance to parents grieving from perinatal loss.

Quantitative investigations during the 1980s made it clear that perinatal loss in the Western, industrialized world was a major loss of a family member. Studies in the United States, Canada, Great Britain, Sweden, and Australia demonstrated a similar pattern of intense grieving following this loss. Methodologic weaknesses such as using measures nonspecific to perinatal loss and failing to track the trajectory of this grief made it difficult to understand clearly what is unique about this death at the inception of life. Both the clinical richness of earlier anecdotal reports and an appreciation of the unique aspects of this death occurring during pregnancy were lost in most of this empirical research. However, this decade marked a dramatic advance in hospitals, in which protocols and perinatal bereavement programs were developed to help parents grieve over the death of their child.

During the late 1980s and early 1990s, more sophisticated measures of perinatal loss were applied to track long-term outcome longitudinally. Theut et al reported that resolution of pregnancy loss, including miscarriage, often was facilitated by a successful subsequent pregnancy. Lasker and Toedter's Perinatal Grief Scale, a 33-item questionnaire, demonstrated that three different components of this grief (ie, active grieving, difficulty coping, and despair) were associated differentially with long-term outcome. Although earlier research often suggested that a more intense grief reaction predicted poorer outcome (contrary to the growing clinical wisdom of facilitating grief), Lasker and Toedter indicated that it was not the intensity of grief but prepregnancy mental health that seemed to have the greatest influence on continued difficulties in coping and depression for couples 2 years after the loss. The three-factor structure of this scale allowed for a more comprehensive understanding of perinatal loss involving not only grieving over the loss of a baby, ie, active grieving, but managing the damage to the self represented by lowered self-esteem, psychosomatic symptoms, and a sense of emptiness ("despair").

As theoretic models for understanding perinatal loss have become available, it has been possible to embed significant findings in a clearer conceptual framework, which can advance clinical practice as well. For example, as it is discovered that "active grieving" follows a painful but ultimately benign course, it is important to consider ways of clinically addressing variables (eg, premorbid level of self-esteem, vulnerability to depression, and earlier conflicts) that may portend chronic problems and are less visible than overt grief.

The Meanings of Perinatal Loss

The context in which perinatal loss occurs—pregnancy—critically determines the experience of this loss, making it significantly different from other family deaths. Several additional factors can make perinatal loss especially challenging and complicated.

A. Developmental Issues: When perinatal losses prevent the couple from attaining parenthood, the potentially powerful interference in the normal course of adult development needs to be considered. Couples are deprived of a crucial milestone and organizer of meaning in life. Increased stagnation as well as isolation from other couples and families contribute to psychosocial alienation. These issues are not addressed through grieving over the death of a baby, but they may be amenable to the therapeutic effects of support groups, which an provide a sense of belonging and fitting in with others.

B. Prior Psychological Conflicts: In pregnancy, earlier stages of psychological development with their salient problems typically are revisited. This phenomenon may lead to the bereaved mother constructing distorted understandings of her perinatal loss based on these earlier issues. For example, a perinatal loss may be experienced unconsciously as a punishment for unresolved sexual or aggressive feelings. Such a loss also may exacerbate difficulties in the process of separation-individuation typically revived in pregnancy. Although long-term psychoanalytic psychotherapy is usually not the treatment of choice following recent perinatal loss, increased integration of these dynamics is often possible in short-term psychodynamic therapy for bereaved parents who seek professional help.

C. Mourning the Lost Person: By the last trimester of pregnancy or earlier, parents usually develop an intense attachment to the unborn child as a separate, distinct person. Based on this understanding, most research and practice recommendations view perinatal loss as synonymous with grieving over the death of a baby. This fact explains the great importance placed on encouraging a couple to see, touch, and hold their dead baby—to consolidate bonding with that child—to facilitate the concurrent process of mourning. It also needs to be recognized that depression associated with earlier, unresolved grief, especially for a mother or parental figure who died when the patient was a child, sometimes is precipitated by perinatal loss. Because pregnancy often resurrects the feelings surrounding important parental relationships, mourning perinatal loss sometimes requires resolving the legacy of past images of others conferred on that child along with grieving over the baby who has died.

D. Injuries to the Self: Procreation enhances self-esteem and enriches identity by (1) fostering a sense of omnipotence, both in the act of creation and in becoming a parent (who is imbued with much power in the mind of a young child); (2) affirming one's gender through reproduction; and (3) defusing death anxiety by ensuring a biologic continuity in the next generation. Perinatal loss, therefore, results in multiple blows to self-worth and self-image. Especially for a woman, there is usually a powerful feeling that her body has failed and that, ultimately, she has failed. This feeling can help explain why for many women a significant recovery coincides with the achievement of a successful pregnancy following their loss. Having a baby allows them not only to parent but also to achieve some repair of a damaged self.

Implications for Practice

A. Long-Term Outcomes: Perinatal grief normally subsides over the first year, although as many as 25% of women experience psychological difficulties 2 years after the loss, typically in the form of prolonged depression. Quantitative studies have been notoriously unsuccessful in predicting later adjustment based on early reactions to the loss. Prior mental health problems and poor social support appear to be the two most important factors associated with later psychological difficulties. Both clinical and quantitative studies indicate that a close, supportive marital relationship provides a crucial buffer to distress and facilitates resolution of grief. Owing to the increased attachment to the fetus as a baby with the advance of pregnancy, later term losses are associated with a more intense, although not necessarily more problematic, grief reaction. A clinical study of women seeking psychotherapy following perinatal loss suggests that a crucial risk factor leading to psychological difficulty is the awakening of unresolved childhood loss, disappointment, or deprivation, especially concerning her own mother.

Following perinatal loss, women tend to experience significantly more guilt, more intense grief and depression, and a greater blow to their self-esteem than their partners. However, male responses to perinatal loss rarely have been systematically explored and may be less accessible to investigation because of societal prohibitions of masculine expression of feelings. Men may grieve less, but they also may be saying less about their grief. Even when grief is substantially resolved and functioning resumes, it is normal for parents to experience a less intense, transient grief evoked by anniversaries of the death and due dates as well as experiences touching their memories about the loss (eg, seeing a child the same age as their child would have been). Although perinatal loss can increase marital stress, most couples who weather the storm together, sharing their feelings, report an improved marital relationship.

Too often, surviving and subsequent children experience this death as an invisible loss; they are denied the opportunity to grieve for a brother or sister and are deeply affected by the psychological loss of parents consumed by grief. It is vital that they are provided both an explanation of the circumstances of the loss at their cognitive level and continuity of parenting to prevent the development of later emotional disturbance.

B. Hospital Management: The cornerstone of current psychological management of perinatal loss is the facilitation of the resolution of grief by creating multiple opportunities for the parents to get to know the baby as a person. Seeing, touching, and holding the baby are encouraged. Pictures are taken routinely. Memorabilia such as locks of hair and foot and handprints are given. Naming the child along with having a funeral or memorial service helps to establish a social identity. Parents are advised to share their feelings, hopes for, and memories of this child to continue the process of grieving begun in the hospital.

Parents cherish the memories of their child created in the hospital and clearly are helped by these guidelines. Yet medical practitioners need to be careful about how these recommendations are put into practice. Clinicians whose interactions are dictated by detailed behavioral protocols that tell them what to do, what to say, and how to say it may be experienced by parents as insincere and as delivering lines from a script rather than empathizing with their grief. Clinicians need to try to appreciate as much as possible, within the restrictions of time and setting, the individualized meanings of loss to parents. After early term losses and pregnancy termination because of fetal anomaly, it is especially important to understand whether the parent is experiencing the loss as the death of a baby or the ending of a pregnancy. It is no help clinically to encourage personification of a fetus when parents have given the clear message that this is not a baby to them. Telling parents the "right" thing to do may deprive them of a crucial aspect of the process that empowers parents after they experience the helplessness associated with perinatal loss—making their own decisions. For example, it is valid to discuss with parents the fact that beginning another pregnancy soon after a perinatal loss may make it more challenging to separate identities of the two babies; however, instructing them to wait at least 6 months is advice that will be neither appreciated nor necessarily followed.

C. Follow-Up Care: A serious deficiency in the management of perinatal loss at most hospitals is the lack of follow-up care. Parents are typically in a state of shock when this sudden, unexpected death occurs. They often are not able to hear completely or understand what they are told in the hospital, and a follow-up appointment within a week is valuable to review what was discussed and answer any questions they may have.

Because a sizable proportion of parents are at risk for continued psychological problems, follow-up appointments over the next year are recommended to provide support, give autopsy results, and make referral for counseling and psychotherapy when appropriate. Unremitting grief, depression, impaired job and interpersonal functioning, psychosomatic symptoms, and increased substance use all warrant mental health consultation. Optimally, clinicians have access to psychotherapists who are familiar with the unique aspects of perinatal loss.

Even when referral is unnecessary, most parents appreciate the concern demonstrated by follow-up appointments. This function is best accomplished in office visits, to underscore the importance of face-to-face meetings, rather than brief phone calls.

D. Use of Medications: With the increased use of the selective serotonin reuptake inhibitors (eg, fluoxetine, sertraline, and paroxetine), which have fewer side effects than older antidepressants, these drugs are being prescribed increasingly for dysthymic disorders and depressive reactions associated with bereavement. If the bereaved is able to bond with an empathic therapist, medications usually are not necessary, because considerable symptomatic relief is achieved over 3–4 months of weekly psychotherapy. In the presence of immobilizing depression, persistent suicidal ideation, or both, antidepressant medication and psychotherapy both may be needed. Patients who require medications often have prior major affective disorder, serious personality disorder, or history of trauma rather than solely a severe reaction to perinatal loss.

Future Directions

A. Coping With Related Losses: Perinatal loss accompanied by infertility presents additional challenges. When patients with these losses present for psychological help, it is difficult to engage them in treatment, and they often leave quickly. The strain of grieving over a perinatal loss is compounded by the additional stress of infertility, with both losses interfering with the achievement of parenthood and reducing self-esteem. Support groups—especially those oriented to couples dealing with both losses—

offer a valuable normalizing environment in which the multiple pains and hardships of reproductive losses may be shared.

Pregnancy termination after fetal anomaly usually results in profound grief, indistinguishable from that following perinatal loss. Yet many physicians do not provide the necessary follow-up and support, mistakenly assuming that emotional reactions will be like the more benign aftermath of most elective abortions. On the basis of a clinical study, Leon (in press) emphasizes that this reproductive loss may be even more difficult to manage than perinatal loss; additional psychological burdens it presents include the challenge of making the decision to terminate the pregnancy, the psychological quandary of whether a pregnancy or a life has been ended, the amplified shame and reluctance to share this loss with others because of the current controversy regarding elective abortion, and the anxiety and guilt in telling (or not telling) one's other children about the nature of the loss. It is especially important for clinicians to provide emotional support and understanding for this often overlooked reproductive loss, making use of pamphlets that normalize intense reactions.

B. Subcultural Differences: In addition to being sensitive to individual differences, it is important for clinicians to understand how patients from different subcultures may respond to perinatal loss. How openly grief is expressed both within and outside the family; religious beliefs about when life begins, the meaning of death, and funeral rites; and the role of indigenous healers in bereavement are a few of the factors that need to be considered; in addition, global differences in language and style of interaction can complicate the clinicians's work with families of a different culture. Being prepared to listen and learn is crucial. Becoming familiar with aspects of a cultural group, particularly views about pregnancy and death, is helpful as long as it does not promote stereotypic expectations.

C. Need for Clinical Studies: A scarcity of qualitative studies of perinatal loss continues to limit a deeper understanding of the dimensions and meanings of this loss. More clinical studies are needed to develop interventions, especially studies that involve fathers and families as well as mothers. Normative nonclinical studies that go into greater depth than the self-reports found in the anecdotal handbook literature while preserving the breadth of that approach are needed to delineate further the unique aspects of perinatal loss.

REFERENCES

Davis DL, Stewart M, Harmon RJ: Postponing pregnancy after perinatal death. J Am Acad Child Adolesc Psychiatry 1989;28:481.

Downey J, McKinney M: The psychiatric status of women presenting for infertility evaluation. Am J Orthopsychiatry 1992;62:196.

Lasker JN, Toedter LJ: Acute vs. chronic grief: The case of pregnancy loss. Am J Orthopsychiatry 1991;61:510.

Lawson LV: Culturally sensitive support for grieving parents. Am J Matern Child Nurs 1990;15:76.

Leon IG: Perinatal loss: A critique of current hospital practices. Clin Pediatr 1992;31:366.

Leon IG: Pregnancy termination after fetal anomaly: Clinical considerations. Infant Ment Health J. [In press.]

Leon IG: The psychoanalytic conceptualization of perinatal loss: A multidimensional model. Am J Psychiatry 1992; 149:1464.

Leon IG: *When a Baby Dies: Psychotherapy for Pregnancy and Newborn Loss.* Yale University Press, 1990.

Minnick MA: *A Time to Decide, A Time to Heal,* 4th ed. Pineapple Press, 1994.

Murray J, Callan VJ: Predicting adjustment to perinatal death. Br J Med Psychol 1988;61:237.

Silver D, Lester E, Campbell BK (editors): Pregnancy. Psychoanal Inquiry 1988;8:135.

Theut SK et al: Resolution of parental bereavement after a perinatal loss. J Am Acad Child Adolesc Psychiatry 1990; 29:521.

Zeanah CH: Adaptation following perinatal loss: A critical review. J Am Acad Child Adolesc Psychiatry 1989; 28:467.

Zeanah CH et al: Do women grieve after terminating pregnancies because of fetal anomalies? A controlled investigation. Obstet Gynecol 1993;82:270.

Appendix A: Roadblock Survey

I. Overt roadblocks
   A. Dysfunctional family issues
      1. Was a parent or primary caretaker an alcoholic or problem drinker?
      2. Did you experience physical, sexual, or emotional abuse as a child?
      3. Did a parent or primary caretaker suffer from emotional illness?
      4. Did you experience parental death or divorce as a child (younger than 12 years)?
      5. Did you feel abandoned by a parent or primary caretaker who was chronically unavailable because of work, illness, or family strife?
      6. Does your current spouse or did a past spouse have a problem with substance abuse (alcohol or drugs) or other compulsive behaviors?
      7. Have you ever had a problem with substance abuse or other compulsive behaviors?
      8. Have you or your children been subject to physical, sexual, or emotional abuse in any of your marriages or relationships?
   B. Binge eating
      1. Do you eat what most people would consider large amounts of food and feel out of control of your eating?
      2. Do you snack constantly throughout the day, even when not really hungry, and feel out of control of your eating?
      3. Do you induce vomiting, use laxatives or water pills, or exercise specifically to lose weight or avoid gaining weight after binge eating?
   C. Moods and energy
      1. Do you have persistent tension, anxiety, irritability, or insomnia?
      2. Do you have persistent sadness, daytime sleepiness, or fatigue?
      3. Do you have trouble making decisions or getting started doing things?

II. Subtle roadblocks
   1. Do you have a stressful or unsatisfying marriage or family life?
   2. Did your family when you were growing up, or does your family now, have any of the following dysfunctional features?
      a. Perfectionism
      b. Rigid rules, life-style, or belief systems
      c. "No talk rule" keeping "family secrets"
      d. Inability to identify or express feelings
      e. Triangulation (a communication pattern using one person as intermediary)
      f. Double binds (all choices given family members are negative ones)
      g. Double messages ("Of course I love you, dear," as Mom tenses up and grits her teeth)
      h. Inability to play, have fun, be spontaneous
      i. High tolerance for inappropriate behavior
      j. Overinvolvement of family members in each other's lives

If you answered yes to any of the preceding questions, "recovery" from roadblock issues may be important for successful management of your weight.

Appendix B: Weight & Management Primer for Primary Care Practitioners

1. Understand the disease
   a. The patient has low self-esteem, often comes from a dysfunctional family, and often has poor interpersonal relationships. Depression, codependency, and personality disorders are common comorbidities.
   b. Personal growth and recovery from a dysfunctional family background may be as important as diet and exercise.
   c. Long-term supportive, nonjudgmental relationships are a key part of recovery.
2. Weight loss is not the basis of your relationship with the patient. Information such as the following should be conveyed: "I am happy to be your physician no matter what your weight. My job is to monitor and treat any complications of obesity such as diabetes, high blood pressure, high cholesterol, or gallbladder disease. I will support any efforts you make to control your weight."
3. Relapses are to be expected.
   a. Try not to show disappointment and frustration when the patient regains some weight. The patient feels as frustrated as you do.
   b. "Starting over" is not failure but is the process by which success is achieved. Encourage reversal of small weight gains when they occur. "Is your maintenance program over? If not, why not go back? Just about everyone in your group will put on some weight at one point or another. The group will be very understanding and will not shame you." "All professional athletes need to go to spring training, every year." "It is how you bounce back that is important."
4. Dispel the belief that "I should be able to do this on my own." Say something like the following: "Every competitor or star performer has a coach." "Research has shown that getting extra support from group or individual counseling improves your chances of success." "Overeaters Anonymous or other twelve-step programs are free and can be effective alone or with other counseling."
5. Strive for persistence, not perfection. Encourage patients not to be so hard on themselves. "You lost 50 pounds and put on just 10 pounds; that's great!" "Your blood pressure and blood sugar are still much improved." "It's okay to have an occasional slip." "We can learn from our mistakes and do a better job next time."
6. Recommend books for the patient to read. Recovery-oriented books can help patients realize that they are not alone and that success is possible. Patients can learn that much of their difficulty in dealing with the world is related to their stressful family of origin and not to some inherent personal flaw.
7. Personal growth and recovery are necessary ingredients. Weight loss by itself is not enough. Weight control, however, can be a catalyst for the patient for improving her whole life if she addresses the multiple factors contributing to the obesity.

Appendix C

One practical approach to adjustment of out of range values:

> For international normalized ratio (INR) Goal 2–3
>
> Tolerate a single low/high 1.5–3.5
> Adjust for 2 in a row or 2/3 out of range

If INR < 2	Increase weekly dose 10–15%
If INR 3–3.5	Decrease weekly dose 5–15%
If INR 3.6–4	Hold warfarin 1 day
	Decrease weekly dose 10–15%
If INR > 4	Hold warfarin 2 days
	Decrease weekly dose 10–15%

Then recheck PT in 1 week

MD, RN, or qualified pharmacist must evaluate in person or by phone for clinical bleeding, drug or diet interactions, and compliance to judge need for clinic visit and "nonalgorithm" adjustment.

From: VMMC Cardiology Anticoagulation Clinic, Edward F. Gibbons MD, Linda Baird, RN.

Warfarin dosing schedule.

Sun	Mon	Tues	Wed	Thurs	Fri	Sat		Weekly Total		Plus 5%	Plus 10%	Plus 15%		Minus 5%	Minus 10%	Minus 15%
2	2	2	2	2	2	2		14		15	15	16		13	13	12
2	3	2	2	2	3	2		16		17	18	18		15	14	14
2.5	2.5	2.5	2.5	2.5	2.5	2.5		17.5		18	19	20		17	16	15
2.5	2.5	2.5	5	2.5	2.5	2.5		20		21	22	23		19	18	17
2.5	5	2.5	2.5	2.5	5	2.5		22.5		24	25	26		21	20	19
2.5	5	2.5	5	2.5	5	2.5		25		26	28	29		24	23	21
5	2.5	5	2.5	5	2.5	5		27.5		29	30	32		26	25	23
5	2.5	5	5	5	2.5	5		30		32	33	35		29	27	26
5	5	5	2.5	5	5	5		32.5		34	36	37		31	29	28
5	5	5	5	5	5	5		35		37	39	40		33	32	30
5	5	5	7.5	5	5	5		37.5		39	41	43		36	34	32
5	7.5	5	5	5	7.5	5		40		42	44	46		38	36	34
5	7.5	5	7.5	5	7.5	5		42.5		45	47	49		40	38	36
7.5	5	7.5	5	7.5	5	7.5		45		47	50	52		43	41	38
7.5	5	7.5	7.5	7.5	5	7.5		47.5		50	52	55		45	43	40
7.5	7.5	7.5	5	7.5	7.5	7.5		50		53	55	58		48	45	43
7.5	7.5	7.5	7.5	7.5	7.5	7.5		52.5		55	58	60		50	47	45
7.5	7.5	7.5	10	7.5	7.5	7.5		55		58	61	63		52	50	47
7.5	10	7.5	7.5	7.5	10	7.5		57.5		60	63	66		55	52	49
7.5	10	7.5	10	7.5	10	7.5		60		63	66	69		57	54	51
10	7.5	10	7.5	10	7.5	10		62.5		66	69	72		59	56	53
10	7.5	10	10	10	7.5	10		65		68	72	75		62	59	55
10	10	10	7.5	10	10	10		67.5		71	74	78		64	61	57
10	10	10	10	10	10	10		70		74	77	81		67	63	60
10	10	10	12.5	10	10	10		72.5		76	80	83		69	65	62
10	12.5	10	10	10	12.5	10		75		79	83	86		71	68	64
10	12.5	10	12.5	10	12.5	10		77.5		81	85	89		74	70	66
12.5	10	12.5	10	12.5	10	12.5		80		84	88	92		76	72	68
12.5	10	12.5	12.5	12.5	10	12.5		82.5		87	91	95		78	74	70
12.5	12.5	12.5	10	12.5	12.5	12.5		85		89	94	98		81	77	72
12.5	12.5	12.5	12.5	12.5	12.5	12.5		87.5		92	96	101		83	79	74
12.5	12.5	12.5	15	12.5	12.5	12.5		90		95	99	104		86	81	77
12.5	15	12.5	12.5	12.5	15	12.5		92.5		97	102	106		88	83	79
12.5	15	12.5	15	12.5	15	12.5		95		100	105	109		90	86	81
15	12.5	15	12.5	15	12.5	15		97.5		102	107	112		93	88	83
15	12.5	15	15	15	12.5	15		100		105	110	115		95	90	85
15	15	15	12.5	15	15	15		102.5		108	113	118		97	92	87
15	15	15	15	15	15	15		105		110	116	121		100	95	89

Daily wrfarin dose (mg)   New weekly warfarin dose (mg)

Appendix D

PRE-PARTICIPATION PHYSICAL EXAMINATION

Name _____ Date _____ Date of Birth _____ Sex _____

Local Address _____ Sport _____

_____ Phone # ( )_____

Home Address _____ Phone # ( )_____

Parent/Guardian _____ Phone # ( )_____

Emergency Contact _____ Phone # ( )_____

Family Doctor _____ Phone # ( )_____

Address _____ Date of Last Exam _____

Health Insurance Company _____ **Policy #** _____

The following questions are to be answered yes or no. Please check the appropriate box. Comment on all "yes" answers.

YES   NO   Comments

Has anyone in your immediate family ever had:

( )   ( )   Diabetes (high blood sugar)? _____

( )   ( )   Sudden death (age less than 50)? _____

( )   ( )   High blood pressure, high cholesterol? _____

( )   ( )   Heart attack (age less than 50)? _____

( )   ( )   Asthma, or sickle cell anemia? _____

( )   ( )   Convulsions (seizures) or epilepsy? _____

Have you ever had or do you now have:

( )   ( )   Chest pain with or after exercise? _____

( )   ( )   Dizziness with or after exercise? _____

( )   ( )   High blood pressure? _____

( )   ( )   Racing of the heart/irregular rhythm? _____

( )   ( )   Wheezing/cough with exercise, or asthma? _____

( )   ( )   Weakness, fatigue, or anemia? _____

( )   ( )   Heart murmur? _____

Have you ever had:

( )   ( )   Loss of consciousness? _____

( )   ( )   Concussion? _____

YES	NO		Comments
( )	( )	Convulsions (seizures) or epilepsy?	_____
( )	( )	Neck injury?	_____
( )	( )	"Stinger", "burner", or "pinched nerve"?	_____

Have you ever:

( )	( )	Been hospitalized for a medical problem?	_____
( )	( )	Had infectious mononucleosis? If yes, + blood test? Y / N	_____
( )	( )	Had heat exhaustion or intolerance?	_____
( )	( )	Been hospitalized or had surgery?	_____
( )	( )	Broken a bone?	_____
( )	( )	Had a muscle injury?	_____
( )	( )	Had a knee injury? R ( ) L ( ) Ligament ( ) Meniscus ( ) Other ( )	
( )	( )	If yes, did you have surgery? Result;	_____
( )	( )	Had a shoulder injury? R ( ) L ( )	_____
( )	( )	If yes, did you have surgery? Result;	_____
( )	( )	Had a back injury?	_____
( )	( )	If yes, did you have surgery? Result;	_____
( )	( )	Had any other joint injuries?	_____
( )	( )	Please check appropriate box(es);	_____
		( ) Hip ( ) Elbow ( ) Wrist ( ) Foot ( ) Other	

Have you had or do you now have:

( )	( )	Hearing loss or perforated eardrum?	_____
( )	( )	Headaches or migraines?	_____
( )	( )	Dental plate or orthotic work?	_____
( )	( )	Impaired vision, wear glasses/contacts?	_____
( )	( )	Hernia?	_____
( )	( )	Loss of function or absence or testicle (males)?	_____

Have you in the past, or do you currently use, or have concerns about:

( )	( )	Cigarettes, chewing tobacco, or marijuana?	_____
( )	( )	Alcohol?	_____
( )	( )	Recreational drugs?	_____
( )	( )	Steroids?	_____
( )	( )	Vitamins or supplements?	_____
( )	( )	Wt loss meds, laxatives, self-induced vomiting?	_____

Do you:

( )	( )	Feel out of control when you are stressed?	_____
( )	( )	Have a history of depression, or feel depressed?	_____
( )	( )	Wear a seat belt at least 90% of the time?	_____
( )	( )	Wear a bicycle/motorcycle helmet?	_____
( )	( )	Understand and regularly perform a self-breast exam or self-testicular exam?	_____
( )	( )	Practice safe sex? (abstinence, condoms)	_____
( )	( )	Have a history of > 2 sexual partners in the last 6 mo.?	_____
( )	( )	Have a history of any sexually transmitted disease?	_____
( )	( )	Have any additional concerns or questions?	_____

What is your present weight? _____

Are you happy with your present weight? _____

  If not, what is your desired weight? _____

In the last 2 days, how many servings of each of the following have you eaten? (circle)

Grains (cereal, bread, rice, pasta)	0 1 2 3 4 >4	Fruits 0 1 2 3 4 >4
Dairy products (mik, yogurt, cheese)	0 1 2 3 4 >4	Red meat 0 1 2 3 4 >4
Beans, nuts, tofu	0 1 2 3 4 >4	Vegetables 0 1 2 3 4 >4
Chicken, Fish	0 1 2 3 4 >4	Eggs 0 1 2 3 4 >4

How many meals do you eat each day? _____   Do you diet regularly? _____

Are there certain foods you do not like? _____

Do you ever feel out of control of your eating patterns? _____

Have you ever tried to control you weight by;   Excessive exercise? _____

    Vomiting? _____   Diet pills? _____   Laxatives _____   Diuretics? _____

Have you ever had an eating disorder? _____

List any current medications: (include vitamins, over the counter medications, supplements, and birth control pills)

_____

_____

List any allergies: (animals, food, pollen, medications)

_____

_____

_____

IMMUNIZATION HISTORY

(1) Tetanus/Diphtheria
_____ Primary series of DPT complete
_____ Tetanus booster (within 10 yrs.)

(2) MMR (Measles, mumps, rubella)
If had MMR vaccine, omit (3) (4) (5)
_____ Dose 1; after 12 mo. and before 5 yr old
_____ Dose 2; 5 yrs. old or after

(3) Measles (Rubeola)
_____ Had disease, confirmed by office record
_____ Has immune titre report, specify date
_____ Dose 1; Between 12 mo. and 5 yrs. old
_____ Dose 2; After 5 yrs.

(4) Rubella
_____ Has report of immune titre, specify date
_____ Vaccine at age 12 mo. or older

(5) Mumps
_____ Had disease confirmed by office record
_____ Vaccine at age 12 mo. or older

(6) Polio
_____ Completed primary vacination series
Type of vaccine; _____ oral
                 _____ inactivated
                 _____ E-IPV
                 _____ Booster

Tuberculosis test;   Date of most recent test and rusult;   PPD _____   CXR _____

- -

I, _____, declare that all of the above information is true to the best of my knowledge.

    (Signature) _____   Date _____

(Signature of parent if < 18 yrs. old) _____   Date _____

PHYSICAL EXAMINATION: (To be completed by physician)

Blood pressure _____   Pulse _____   Height _____   Weight _____

Vision   R 20/ _____   L 20/ _____   corrected Y / N   Pupil size; equal / unequal

Normal	Abnormal		Comments
( )	( )	HEENT	_____
( )	( )	Thyroid	_____
( )	( )	Lymphatics	_____
( )	( )	Cardiac	_____
( )	( )	Lungs	_____
( )	( )	Skin	_____
( )	( )	Abdominal	_____
( )	( )	Genitalia	Hernia? Y / N _____

Normal	Abnormal		Comments
( )	( )	Musculoskeletal:	
( )	( )	Neck	_____
( )	( )	Shoulder	_____
( )	( )	Elbow	_____
( )	( )	Wrist, hand	_____
( )	( )	Back	Scoliosis? Y / N _____
( )	( )	Knee	_____
( )	( )	Ankle, foot	_____
( )	( )	Neurologic	_____

Other: _____

I certify that I have reviewed the history and examined the above athlete, and recommend sports activity:

      Clearance with no limitations _____

      Clearance pending further evaluation or testing _____

      Referral to _____ prior to clearance

      Clearance with limitations _____

      Disqualification from competition _____

Signature of Examining Physician _____ Date _____

Appendix E

INTERCURRENT/FINAL PRE-PARTICIPATION PHYSICAL EXAMINATION

Today's Date _____   Sport; _____

Date of Entrance Physical Exam _____

Master Problem List: Date Identified   Date Resolved

1.

2.

3.

4.

5.

Past Medical History; Since your initial pre-participation physical examination have you had any of the following; (If yes, please explain what, when, and all details.)

Yes	No		Comments
( )	( )	1. Presently taking medication (include over the counter medicine and birth control pills)	_____
( )	( )	2. Allergic to medicine, food, bee stings?	_____
( )	( )	3. Wearing any **new** appliances? (glasses, contacts, braces, dentures, hearing aids)	_____
( )	( )	4. **New** medical problem requiring treatment or medications?	_____
( )	( )	5. Surgical operations or accidents?	_____
( )	( )	6. Injuries related to sports participation?	_____
( )	( )	7. Fainting or dizziness with exercise?	_____
( )	( )	8. Head injury or loss of consciousness?	_____
( )	( )	9. Menstrual dysfunction (females)? Date of last menstrual period _____
( )	( )	10. Nutrition/weight control problem	_____
( )	( )	11. Emotional problem	_____

Review of Systems; Please check if you have developed any new problem in the following areas of your body since your last examination.

_____ Skin	_____ Neck	_____ Genital
_____ Head	_____ Lungs	_____ Heart
_____ Eyes	_____ Mouth/throat	_____ Abdomen
_____ Knees	_____ Shoulders	_____ Hip
_____ Ankle/Foot	_____ Hand/wrist	_____ Back

I would like to meet with the team physician _____
I certify that the above information is correct to the best of my knowledge.
Student athlete signature _____   Date _____
Blood pressure _____   Pulse _____   Ht _____   Wt _____   Visual Acuity L ___/___   R ___/___
Athletic Trainer's signature _____   Date _____

Appendix F

SUPPLEMENTAL HISTORY FOR THE FEMALE ATHLETE

1. At what age did you have your first menstrual cycle? _____
2. How many days does your cycle last? _____ How many days between cycles? _____
3. How many periods have you had in the past 12 months? _____
4. What is the date of your last menstrual cycle? _____
5. Do you ever have cramping with your period? _____
6. If so, do you do anything to lessen your symptoms? _____
7. Have you ever had "irregular" cycles (shorter than 21 days, or with more than 35 days between cycles)? _____
8. Have you ever had heavy bleeding? _____
9. Have you ever stopped having a period? _____
   If so, for how long? (Give details) _____
10. Have you ever had a stress fracture? If so, please list sites, dates, method of diagnosis (X-ray, bone scan) _____
11. Is there any family history of osteoporosis (thinning of the bones)? _____
12. When was your last pelvic exam? _____ Last Breast Exam? _____
13. Have you ever had an abnormal pelvic exam or PAP smear? _____
14. Do you/have you ever taken birth control pills or hormones? _____
15. Has a physician ever told you that you had anemia (low hematocrit or iron)? _____
16. What is you present weight? _____ Present height? _____
17. Are you happy with your present weight? _____ If not, what is your desired weight? _____
18. Does your weight fluctuate? _____ Highest weight _____ Lowest weight _____
19. Do you have trouble maintaining your optimal weight? _____
20. Do you diet regularly? _____
21. Do you ever feel out of control of your eating patterns? _____
22. Have you ever tried to control your weight by; Vomiting? _____ Diet pills? _____
    Laxatives? _____ Diuretics? _____ Excessive exercise? _____
23. Have you ever had an eating disorder? _____
24. Do you take vitamins or supplements? _____

25. In the last 2 days, how many servings of each have you eaten? (circle)

Grains (cereal, bread, rice, pasta)	0 1 2 3 4 >4	Fruits	0 1 2 3 4 >4
Dairy products (mik, yogurt, cheese)	0 1 2 3 4 >4	Red meat	0 1 2 3 4 >4
Beans, nuts, tofu	0 1 2 3 4 >4	Vegetables	0 1 2 3 4 >4
Chicken, Fish	0 1 2 3 4 >4	Eggs	0 1 2 3 4 >4

26. How many meals do you eat each day? _____

27. How much alcohol do you drink at one time? (avg.) _____   Per week (avg)? _____

28. Do you smoke cigarettes? _____   Would you like to see the sports nutritionist? _____

Appendix G

DAILY RATINGS FORM*

Name: _____   Date Starting: ___ ___ / ___ ___ / ___ ___
                                            Date Ending: ___ ___ / ___ ___ / ___ ___

This section is to be completed by the Data Processing Staff:

ID No. __ __ __ __ __ __ __ __ __   Study No. ____ ____   Group No. ____ ____

Reason for collection of ratings: _____

INSTRUCTIONS

There are 21 items listed on the following pages and three blanks where you can add items describing other changes that bother you.

1. Start your ratings on the line with the correct day of the week for the first day's ratings.
2. Rate each item each day for a total of at least 21 items.
3. Make the ratings each evening just before going to sleep.
4. Note those days on which you are menstruating by writing "YES" in the column labeled "Menstruating?".
5. Comment on page 8 if anything has happened that may have affected your physical or psychological behavior for that day (e.g., illness, bad news).
6. The ratings should indicate the degree to which you experienced the feelings or behaviors described in the item on that particular day. Sometimes you may have feelings that are contradictory, such as feeling both sad and happy. If so, rate both the items if both have occurred.
7. The levels of severity for rating each item are given at the top of each page.
8. It is usually a good idea to "post" the ratings where you will see them each evening (e.g., on the closet door, on the door of the medicine cabinet, inside the door of the medicine cabinet, on the night table beside the bed).
9. If you forget to make the ratings on any evening, try to do it as early as possible on the next day or so.

TURN EACH PAGE EACH DAY AND RATE A TOTAL OF AT LEAST 21 ITEMS DAILY.

ADDITIONAL INSTRUCTIONS FOR STUDY.

All information contained on this form and data summarized from it will be kept confidential. Any written or verbal reports will be done in a way which precludes identification of individuals.

*Developed by Jean Endicott, Ph.D., Sybil Schacht, M.S.W., and Uriel Halbreich, M.D. Available from Dr. Endicott, Research Assessment and Training Unit, 722 West 168th Street, New York, N.Y. 10032.

Name: _____ ID No.: _ _ _ _ _ _ _ _ Date: _ _ / _ _ / _ _

Severity Ratings: 1 = Not at all, 2 = Minimal, 3 = Mild, 4 = Moderate, 5 = Severe, 6 = Extreme

Day	Date	Menstru- ating?	Stay at home, avoid social activity	Increased enjoy- ment and efficiency	Less work (job, house, school), impaired	Feel bloated have edema	Comments on page 8	
Mon.	___/___	_____	1 2 3 4 5 6	1 2 3 4 5 6	1 2 3 4 5 6	1 2 3 4 5 6	Yes	No
Tues.	___/___	_____	1 2 3 4 5 6	1 2 3 4 5 6	1 2 3 4 5 6	1 2 3 4 5 6	Yes	No
Wed.	___/___	_____	1 2 3 4 5 6	1 2 3 4 5 6	1 2 3 4 5 6	1 2 3 4 5 6	Yes	No
Thurs.	___/___	_____	1 2 3 4 5 6	1 2 3 4 5 6	1 2 3 4 5 6	1 2 3 4 5 6	Yes	No
Fri.	___/___	_____	1 2 3 4 5 6	1 2 3 4 5 6	1 2 3 4 5 6	1 2 3 4 5 6	Yes	No
Sat.	___/___	_____	1 2 3 4 5 6	1 2 3 4 5 6	1 2 3 4 5 6	1 2 3 4 5 6	Yes	No
Sun.	___/___	_____	1 2 3 4 5 6	1 2 3 4 5 6	1 2 3 4 5 6	1 2 3 4 5 6	Yes	No
Mon.	___/___	_____	1 2 3 4 5 6	1 2 3 4 5 6	1 2 3 4 5 6	1 2 3 4 5 6	Yes	No
Tues.	___/___	_____	1 2 3 4 5 6	1 2 3 4 5 6	1 2 3 4 5 6	1 2 3 4 5 6	Yes	No
Wed.	___/___	_____	1 2 3 4 5 6	1 2 3 4 5 6	1 2 3 4 5 6	1 2 3 4 5 6	Yes	No
Thurs.	___/___	_____	1 2 3 4 5 6	1 2 3 4 5 6	1 2 3 4 5 6	1 2 3 4 5 6	Yes	No
Fri.	___/___	_____	1 2 3 4 5 6	1 2 3 4 5 6	1 2 3 4 5 6	1 2 3 4 5 6	Yes	No
Sat.	___/___	_____	1 2 3 4 5 6	1 2 3 4 5 6	1 2 3 4 5 6	1 2 3 4 5 6	Yes	No
Sun.	___/___	_____	1 2 3 4 5 6	1 2 3 4 5 6	1 2 3 4 5 6	1 2 3 4 5 6	Yes	No
Mon.	___/___	_____	1 2 3 4 5 6	1 2 3 4 5 6	1 2 3 4 5 6	1 2 3 4 5 6	Yes	No
Tues.	___/___	_____	1 2 3 4 5 6	1 2 3 4 5 6	1 2 3 4 5 6	1 2 3 4 5 6	Yes	No
Wed.	___/___	_____	1 2 3 4 5 6	1 2 3 4 5 6	1 2 3 4 5 6	1 2 3 4 5 6	Yes	No
Thurs.	___/___	_____	1 2 3 4 5 6	1 2 3 4 5 6	1 2 3 4 5 6	1 2 3 4 5 6	Yes	No
Fri.	___/___	_____	1 2 3 4 5 6	1 2 3 4 5 6	1 2 3 4 5 6	1 2 3 4 5 6	Yes	No
Sat.	___/___	_____	1 2 3 4 5 6	1 2 3 4 5 6	1 2 3 4 5 6	1 2 3 4 5 6	Yes	No
Sun.	___/___	_____	1 2 3 4 5 6	1 2 3 4 5 6	1 2 3 4 5 6	1 2 3 4 5 6	Yes	No
Mon.	___/___	_____	1 2 3 4 5 6	1 2 3 4 5 6	1 2 3 4 5 6	1 2 3 4 5 6	Yes	No
Tues.	___/___	_____	1 2 3 4 5 6	1 2 3 4 5 6	1 2 3 4 5 6	1 2 3 4 5 6	Yes	No
Wed.	___/___	_____	1 2 3 4 5 6	1 2 3 4 5 6	1 2 3 4 5 6	1 2 3 4 5 6	Yes	No
Thurs.	___/___	_____	1 2 3 4 5 6	1 2 3 4 5 6	1 2 3 4 5 6	1 2 3 4 5 6	Yes	No
Fri.	___/___	_____	1 2 3 4 5 6	1 2 3 4 5 6	1 2 3 4 5 6	1 2 3 4 5 6	Yes	No
Sat.	___/___	_____	1 2 3 4 5 6	1 2 3 4 5 6	1 2 3 4 5 6	1 2 3 4 5 6	Yes	No
Sun.	___/___	_____	1 2 3 4 5 6	1 2 3 4 5 6	1 2 3 4 5 6	1 2 3 4 5 6	Yes	No
Mon.	___/___	_____	1 2 3 4 5 6	1 2 3 4 5 6	1 2 3 4 5 6	1 2 3 4 5 6	Yes	No
Tues.	___/___	_____	1 2 3 4 5 6	1 2 3 4 5 6	1 2 3 4 5 6	1 2 3 4 5 6	Yes	No
Wed.	___/___	_____	1 2 3 4 5 6	1 2 3 4 5 6	1 2 3 4 5 6	1 2 3 4 5 6	Yes	No
Thurs.	___/___	_____	1 2 3 4 5 6	1 2 3 4 5 6	1 2 3 4 5 6	1 2 3 4 5 6	Yes	No
Fri.	___/___	_____	1 2 3 4 5 6	1 2 3 4 5 6	1 2 3 4 5 6	1 2 3 4 5 6	Yes	No
Sat.	___/___	_____	1 2 3 4 5 6	1 2 3 4 5 6	1 2 3 4 5 6	1 2 3 4 5 6	Yes	No
Sun.	___/___	_____	1 2 3 4 5 6	1 2 3 4 5 6	1 2 3 4 5 6	1 2 3 4 5 6	Yes	No
Mon.	___/___	_____	1 2 3 4 5 6	1 2 3 4 5 6	1 2 3 4 5 6	1 2 3 4 5 6	Yes	No
Tues.	___/___	_____	1 2 3 4 5 6	1 2 3 4 5 6	1 2 3 4 5 6	1 2 3 4 5 6	Yes	No
Wed.	___/___	_____	1 2 3 4 5 6	1 2 3 4 5 6	1 2 3 4 5 6	1 2 3 4 5 6	Yes	No
Thurs.	___/___	_____	1 2 3 4 5 6	1 2 3 4 5 6	1 2 3 4 5 6	1 2 3 4 5 6	Yes	No
Fri.	___/___	_____	1 2 3 4 5 6	1 2 3 4 5 6	1 2 3 4 5 6	1 2 3 4 5 6	Yes	No
Sat.	___/___	_____	1 2 3 4 5 6	1 2 3 4 5 6	1 2 3 4 5 6	1 2 3 4 5 6	Yes	No
Sun.	___/___	_____	1 2 3 4 5 6	1 2 3 4 5 6	1 2 3 4 5 6	1 2 3 4 5 6	Yes	No

Name: _____ ID No.: _ _ _ _ _ _ _ _ Date: __ __ / __ __ / __ __

Severity Ratings: 1 = Not at all, 2 = Minimal, 3 = Mild, 4 = Moderate, 5 = Severe, 6 = Extreme

Day	Date	Menstru-ating?	Active, restless	Mood swings	Depressed, sad, low, blue, lonely	Anxious, jittery, nervous	Comments on page 8	
Mon.	___/___	___	1 2 3 4 5 6	1 2 3 4 5 6	1 2 3 4 5 6	1 2 3 4 5 6	Yes	No
Tues.	___/___	___	1 2 3 4 5 6	1 2 3 4 5 6	1 2 3 4 5 6	1 2 3 4 5 6	Yes	No
Wed.	___/___	___	1 2 3 4 5 6	1 2 3 4 5 6	1 2 3 4 5 6	1 2 3 4 5 6	Yes	No
Thurs.	___/___	___	1 2 3 4 5 6	1 2 3 4 5 6	1 2 3 4 5 6	1 2 3 4 5 6	Yes	No
Fri.	___/___	___	1 2 3 4 5 6	1 2 3 4 5 6	1 2 3 4 5 6	1 2 3 4 5 6	Yes	No
Sat.	___/___	___	1 2 3 4 5 6	1 2 3 4 5 6	1 2 3 4 5 6	1 2 3 4 5 6	Yes	No
Sun.	___/___	___	1 2 3 4 5 6	1 2 3 4 5 6	1 2 3 4 5 6	1 2 3 4 5 6	Yes	No
Mon.	___/___	___	1 2 3 4 5 6	1 2 3 4 5 6	1 2 3 4 5 6	1 2 3 4 5 6	Yes	No
Tues.	___/___	___	1 2 3 4 5 6	1 2 3 4 5 6	1 2 3 4 5 6	1 2 3 4 5 6	Yes	No
Wed.	___/___	___	1 2 3 4 5 6	1 2 3 4 5 6	1 2 3 4 5 6	1 2 3 4 5 6	Yes	No
Thurs.	___/___	___	1 2 3 4 5 6	1 2 3 4 5 6	1 2 3 4 5 6	1 2 3 4 5 6	Yes	No
Fri.	___/___	___	1 2 3 4 5 6	1 2 3 4 5 6	1 2 3 4 5 6	1 2 3 4 5 6	Yes	No
Sat.	___/___	___	1 2 3 4 5 6	1 2 3 4 5 6	1 2 3 4 5 6	1 2 3 4 5 6	Yes	No
Sun.	___/___	___	1 2 3 4 5 6	1 2 3 4 5 6	1 2 3 4 5 6	1 2 3 4 5 6	Yes	No
Mon.	___/___	___	1 2 3 4 5 6	1 2 3 4 5 6	1 2 3 4 5 6	1 2 3 4 5 6	Yes	No
Tues.	___/___	___	1 2 3 4 5 6	1 2 3 4 5 6	1 2 3 4 5 6	1 2 3 4 5 6	Yes	No
Wed.	___/___	___	1 2 3 4 5 6	1 2 3 4 5 6	1 2 3 4 5 6	1 2 3 4 5 6	Yes	No
Thurs.	___/___	___	1 2 3 4 5 6	1 2 3 4 5 6	1 2 3 4 5 6	1 2 3 4 5 6	Yes	No
Fri.	___/___	___	1 2 3 4 5 6	1 2 3 4 5 6	1 2 3 4 5 6	1 2 3 4 5 6	Yes	No
Sat.	___/___	___	1 2 3 4 5 6	1 2 3 4 5 6	1 2 3 4 5 6	1 2 3 4 5 6	Yes	No
Sun.	___/___	___	1 2 3 4 5 6	1 2 3 4 5 6	1 2 3 4 5 6	1 2 3 4 5 6	Yes	No
Mon.	___/___	___	1 2 3 4 5 6	1 2 3 4 5 6	1 2 3 4 5 6	1 2 3 4 5 6	Yes	No
Tues.	___/___	___	1 2 3 4 5 6	1 2 3 4 5 6	1 2 3 4 5 6	1 2 3 4 5 6	Yes	No
Wed.	___/___	___	1 2 3 4 5 6	1 2 3 4 5 6	1 2 3 4 5 6	1 2 3 4 5 6	Yes	No
Thurs.	___/___	___	1 2 3 4 5 6	1 2 3 4 5 6	1 2 3 4 5 6	1 2 3 4 5 6	Yes	No
Fri.	___/___	___	1 2 3 4 5 6	1 2 3 4 5 6	1 2 3 4 5 6	1 2 3 4 5 6	Yes	No
Sat.	___/___	___	1 2 3 4 5 6	1 2 3 4 5 6	1 2 3 4 5 6	1 2 3 4 5 6	Yes	No
Sun.	___/___	___	1 2 3 4 5 6	1 2 3 4 5 6	1 2 3 4 5 6	1 2 3 4 5 6	Yes	No
Mon.	___/___	___	1 2 3 4 5 6	1 2 3 4 5 6	1 2 3 4 5 6	1 2 3 4 5 6	Yes	No
Tues.	___/___	___	1 2 3 4 5 6	1 2 3 4 5 6	1 2 3 4 5 6	1 2 3 4 5 6	Yes	No
Wed.	___/___	___	1 2 3 4 5 6	1 2 3 4 5 6	1 2 3 4 5 6	1 2 3 4 5 6	Yes	No
Thurs.	___/___	___	1 2 3 4 5 6	1 2 3 4 5 6	1 2 3 4 5 6	1 2 3 4 5 6	Yes	No
Fri.	___/___	___	1 2 3 4 5 6	1 2 3 4 5 6	1 2 3 4 5 6	1 2 3 4 5 6	Yes	No
Sat.	___/___	___	1 2 3 4 5 6	1 2 3 4 5 6	1 2 3 4 5 6	1 2 3 4 5 6	Yes	No
Sun.	___/___	___	1 2 3 4 5 6	1 2 3 4 5 6	1 2 3 4 5 6	1 2 3 4 5 6	Yes	No
Mon.	___/___	___	1 2 3 4 5 6	1 2 3 4 5 6	1 2 3 4 5 6	1 2 3 4 5 6	Yes	No
Tues.	___/___	___	1 2 3 4 5 6	1 2 3 4 5 6	1 2 3 4 5 6	1 2 3 4 5 6	Yes	No
Wed.	___/___	___	1 2 3 4 5 6	1 2 3 4 5 6	1 2 3 4 5 6	1 2 3 4 5 6	Yes	No
Thurs.	___/___	___	1 2 3 4 5 6	1 2 3 4 5 6	1 2 3 4 5 6	1 2 3 4 5 6	Yes	No
Fri.	___/___	___	1 2 3 4 5 6	1 2 3 4 5 6	1 2 3 4 5 6	1 2 3 4 5 6	Yes	No
Sat.	___/___	___	1 2 3 4 5 6	1 2 3 4 5 6	1 2 3 4 5 6	1 2 3 4 5 6	Yes	No
Sun.	___/___	___	1 2 3 4 5 6	1 2 3 4 5 6	1 2 3 4 5 6	1 2 3 4 5 6	Yes	No

Name: _____ ID No.: _ _ _ _ _ _ _ _ _ Date: _ _ / _ _ / _ _

Severity Ratings: 1 = Not at all, 2 = Minimal, 3 = Mild, 4 = Moderate, 5 = Severe, 6 = Extreme

Day	Date	Menstru- ating?	Irritable, angry, impatient	Appetite up, eat more, crave foods	More sleep, naps, say in bed	Low energy, tired, weak	Comments on page 8	
Mon.	___/___	_____	1 2 3 4 5 6	1 2 3 4 5 6	1 2 3 4 5 6	1 2 3 4 5 6	Yes	No
Tues.	___/___	_____	1 2 3 4 5 6	1 2 3 4 5 6	1 2 3 4 5 6	1 2 3 4 5 6	Yes	No
Wed.	___/___	_____	1 2 3 4 5 6	1 2 3 4 5 6	1 2 3 4 5 6	1 2 3 4 5 6	Yes	No
Thurs.	___/___	_____	1 2 3 4 5 6	1 2 3 4 5 6	1 2 3 4 5 6	1 2 3 4 5 6	Yes	No
Fri.	___/___	_____	1 2 3 4 5 6	1 2 3 4 5 6	1 2 3 4 5 6	1 2 3 4 5 6	Yes	No
Sat.	___/___	_____	1 2 3 4 5 6	1 2 3 4 5 6	1 2 3 4 5 6	1 2 3 4 5 6	Yes	No
Sun.	___/___	_____	1 2 3 4 5 6	1 2 3 4 5 6	1 2 3 4 5 6	1 2 3 4 5 6	Yes	No
Mon.	___/___	_____	1 2 3 4 5 6	1 2 3 4 5 6	1 2 3 4 5 6	1 2 3 4 5 6	Yes	No
Tues.	___/___	_____	1 2 3 4 5 6	1 2 3 4 5 6	1 2 3 4 5 6	1 2 3 4 5 6	Yes	No
Wed.	___/___	_____	1 2 3 4 5 6	1 2 3 4 5 6	1 2 3 4 5 6	1 2 3 4 5 6	Yes	No
Thurs.	___/___	_____	1 2 3 4 5 6	1 2 3 4 5 6	1 2 3 4 5 6	1 2 3 4 5 6	Yes	No
Fri.	___/___	_____	1 2 3 4 5 6	1 2 3 4 5 6	1 2 3 4 5 6	1 2 3 4 5 6	Yes	No
Sat.	___/___	_____	1 2 3 4 5 6	1 2 3 4 5 6	1 2 3 4 5 6	1 2 3 4 5 6	Yes	No
Sun.	___/___	_____	1 2 3 4 5 6	1 2 3 4 5 6	1 2 3 4 5 6	1 2 3 4 5 6	Yes	No
Mon.	___/___	_____	1 2 3 4 5 6	1 2 3 4 5 6	1 2 3 4 5 6	1 2 3 4 5 6	Yes	No
Tues.	___/___	_____	1 2 3 4 5 6	1 2 3 4 5 6	1 2 3 4 5 6	1 2 3 4 5 6	Yes	No
Wed.	___/___	_____	1 2 3 4 5 6	1 2 3 4 5 6	1 2 3 4 5 6	1 2 3 4 5 6	Yes	No
Thurs.	___/___	_____	1 2 3 4 5 6	1 2 3 4 5 6	1 2 3 4 5 6	1 2 3 4 5 6	Yes	No
Fri.	___/___	_____	1 2 3 4 5 6	1 2 3 4 5 6	1 2 3 4 5 6	1 2 3 4 5 6	Yes	No
Sat.	___/___	_____	1 2 3 4 5 6	1 2 3 4 5 6	1 2 3 4 5 6	1 2 3 4 5 6	Yes	No
Sun.	___/___	_____	1 2 3 4 5 6	1 2 3 4 5 6	1 2 3 4 5 6	1 2 3 4 5 6	Yes	No
Mon.	___/___	_____	1 2 3 4 5 6	1 2 3 4 5 6	1 2 3 4 5 6	1 2 3 4 5 6	Yes	No
Tues.	___/___	_____	1 2 3 4 5 6	1 2 3 4 5 6	1 2 3 4 5 6	1 2 3 4 5 6	Yes	No
Wed.	___/___	_____	1 2 3 4 5 6	1 2 3 4 5 6	1 2 3 4 5 6	1 2 3 4 5 6	Yes	No
Thurs.	___/___	_____	1 2 3 4 5 6	1 2 3 4 5 6	1 2 3 4 5 6	1 2 3 4 5 6	Yes	No
Fri.	___/___	_____	1 2 3 4 5 6	1 2 3 4 5 6	1 2 3 4 5 6	1 2 3 4 5 6	Yes	No
Sat.	___/___	_____	1 2 3 4 5 6	1 2 3 4 5 6	1 2 3 4 5 6	1 2 3 4 5 6	Yes	No
Sun.	___/___	_____	1 2 3 4 5 6	1 2 3 4 5 6	1 2 3 4 5 6	1 2 3 4 5 6	Yes	No
Mon.	___/___	_____	1 2 3 4 5 6	1 2 3 4 5 6	1 2 3 4 5 6	1 2 3 4 5 6	Yes	No
Tues.	___/___	_____	1 2 3 4 5 6	1 2 3 4 5 6	1 2 3 4 5 6	1 2 3 4 5 6	Yes	No
Wed.	___/___	_____	1 2 3 4 5 6	1 2 3 4 5 6	1 2 3 4 5 6	1 2 3 4 5 6	Yes	No
Thurs.	___/___	_____	1 2 3 4 5 6	1 2 3 4 5 6	1 2 3 4 5 6	1 2 3 4 5 6	Yes	No
Fri.	___/___	_____	1 2 3 4 5 6	1 2 3 4 5 6	1 2 3 4 5 6	1 2 3 4 5 6	Yes	No
Sat.	___/___	_____	1 2 3 4 5 6	1 2 3 4 5 6	1 2 3 4 5 6	1 2 3 4 5 6	Yes	No
Sun.	___/___	_____	1 2 3 4 5 6	1 2 3 4 5 6	1 2 3 4 5 6	1 2 3 4 5 6	Yes	No
Mon.	___/___	_____	1 2 3 4 5 6	1 2 3 4 5 6	1 2 3 4 5 6	1 2 3 4 5 6	Yes	No
Tues.	___/___	_____	1 2 3 4 5 6	1 2 3 4 5 6	1 2 3 4 5 6	1 2 3 4 5 6	Yes	No
Wed.	___/___	_____	1 2 3 4 5 6	1 2 3 4 5 6	1 2 3 4 5 6	1 2 3 4 5 6	Yes	No
Thurs.	___/___	_____	1 2 3 4 5 6	1 2 3 4 5 6	1 2 3 4 5 6	1 2 3 4 5 6	Yes	No
Fri.	___/___	_____	1 2 3 4 5 6	1 2 3 4 5 6	1 2 3 4 5 6	1 2 3 4 5 6	Yes	No
Sat.	___/___	_____	1 2 3 4 5 6	1 2 3 4 5 6	1 2 3 4 5 6	1 2 3 4 5 6	Yes	No
Sun.	___/___	_____	1 2 3 4 5 6	1 2 3 4 5 6	1 2 3 4 5 6	1 2 3 4 5 6	Yes	No

Name: _____ ID No.: __ __ __ __ __ __ __ __   Date: __ __ / __ __ / __ __

Severity Ratings: 1 = Not at all, 2 = Minimal, 3 = Mild, 4 = Moderate, 5 = Severe, 6 = Extreme

Day	Date	Menstru-ating?	Headaches	Back, joint, or muscle pain	Abdominal pain	Breast pain	Comments on page 8	
Mon.	___/___	___	1 2 3 4 5 6	1 2 3 4 5 6	1 2 3 4 5 6	1 2 3 4 5 6	Yes	No
Tues.	___/___	___	1 2 3 4 5 6	1 2 3 4 5 6	1 2 3 4 5 6	1 2 3 4 5 6	Yes	No
Wed.	___/___	___	1 2 3 4 5 6	1 2 3 4 5 6	1 2 3 4 5 6	1 2 3 4 5 6	Yes	No
Thurs.	___/___	___	1 2 3 4 5 6	1 2 3 4 5 6	1 2 3 4 5 6	1 2 3 4 5 6	Yes	No
Fri.	___/___	___	1 2 3 4 5 6	1 2 3 4 5 6	1 2 3 4 5 6	1 2 3 4 5 6	Yes	No
Sat.	___/___	___	1 2 3 4 5 6	1 2 3 4 5 6	1 2 3 4 5 6	1 2 3 4 5 6	Yes	No
Sun.	___/___	___	1 2 3 4 5 6	1 2 3 4 5 6	1 2 3 4 5 6	1 2 3 4 5 6	Yes	No
Mon.	___/___	___	1 2 3 4 5 6	1 2 3 4 5 6	1 2 3 4 5 6	1 2 3 4 5 6	Yes	No
Tues.	___/___	___	1 2 3 4 5 6	1 2 3 4 5 6	1 2 3 4 5 6	1 2 3 4 5 6	Yes	No
Wed.	___/___	___	1 2 3 4 5 6	1 2 3 4 5 6	1 2 3 4 5 6	1 2 3 4 5 6	Yes	No
Thurs.	___/___	___	1 2 3 4 5 6	1 2 3 4 5 6	1 2 3 4 5 6	1 2 3 4 5 6	Yes	No
Fri.	___/___	___	1 2 3 4 5 6	1 2 3 4 5 6	1 2 3 4 5 6	1 2 3 4 5 6	Yes	No
Sat.	___/___	___	1 2 3 4 5 6	1 2 3 4 5 6	1 2 3 4 5 6	1 2 3 4 5 6	Yes	No
Sun.	___/___	___	1 2 3 4 5 6	1 2 3 4 5 6	1 2 3 4 5 6	1 2 3 4 5 6	Yes	No
Mon.	___/___	___	1 2 3 4 5 6	1 2 3 4 5 6	1 2 3 4 5 6	1 2 3 4 5 6	Yes	No
Tues.	___/___	___	1 2 3 4 5 6	1 2 3 4 5 6	1 2 3 4 5 6	1 2 3 4 5 6	Yes	No
Wed.	___/___	___	1 2 3 4 5 6	1 2 3 4 5 6	1 2 3 4 5 6	1 2 3 4 5 6	Yes	No
Thurs.	___/___	___	1 2 3 4 5 6	1 2 3 4 5 6	1 2 3 4 5 6	1 2 3 4 5 6	Yes	No
Fri.	___/___	___	1 2 3 4 5 6	1 2 3 4 5 6	1 2 3 4 5 6	1 2 3 4 5 6	Yes	No
Sat.	___/___	___	1 2 3 4 5 6	1 2 3 4 5 6	1 2 3 4 5 6	1 2 3 4 5 6	Yes	No
Sun.	___/___	___	1 2 3 4 5 6	1 2 3 4 5 6	1 2 3 4 5 6	1 2 3 4 5 6	Yes	No
Mon.	___/___	___	1 2 3 4 5 6	1 2 3 4 5 6	1 2 3 4 5 6	1 2 3 4 5 6	Yes	No
Tues.	___/___	___	1 2 3 4 5 6	1 2 3 4 5 6	1 2 3 4 5 6	1 2 3 4 5 6	Yes	No
Wed.	___/___	___	1 2 3 4 5 6	1 2 3 4 5 6	1 2 3 4 5 6	1 2 3 4 5 6	Yes	No
Thurs.	___/___	___	1 2 3 4 5 6	1 2 3 4 5 6	1 2 3 4 5 6	1 2 3 4 5 6	Yes	No
Fri.	___/___	___	1 2 3 4 5 6	1 2 3 4 5 6	1 2 3 4 5 6	1 2 3 4 5 6	Yes	No
Sat.	___/___	___	1 2 3 4 5 6	1 2 3 4 5 6	1 2 3 4 5 6	1 2 3 4 5 6	Yes	No
Sun.	___/___	___	1 2 3 4 5 6	1 2 3 4 5 6	1 2 3 4 5 6	1 2 3 4 5 6	Yes	No
Mon.	___/___	___	1 2 3 4 5 6	1 2 3 4 5 6	1 2 3 4 5 6	1 2 3 4 5 6	Yes	No
Tues.	___/___	___	1 2 3 4 5 6	1 2 3 4 5 6	1 2 3 4 5 6	1 2 3 4 5 6	Yes	No
Wed.	___/___	___	1 2 3 4 5 6	1 2 3 4 5 6	1 2 3 4 5 6	1 2 3 4 5 6	Yes	No
Thurs.	___/___	___	1 2 3 4 5 6	1 2 3 4 5 6	1 2 3 4 5 6	1 2 3 4 5 6	Yes	No
Fri.	___/___	___	1 2 3 4 5 6	1 2 3 4 5 6	1 2 3 4 5 6	1 2 3 4 5 6	Yes	No
Sat.	___/___	___	1 2 3 4 5 6	1 2 3 4 5 6	1 2 3 4 5 6	1 2 3 4 5 6	Yes	No
Sun.	___/___	___	1 2 3 4 5 6	1 2 3 4 5 6	1 2 3 4 5 6	1 2 3 4 5 6	Yes	No
Mon.	___/___	___	1 2 3 4 5 6	1 2 3 4 5 6	1 2 3 4 5 6	1 2 3 4 5 6	Yes	No
Tues.	___/___	___	1 2 3 4 5 6	1 2 3 4 5 6	1 2 3 4 5 6	1 2 3 4 5 6	Yes	No
Wed.	___/___	___	1 2 3 4 5 6	1 2 3 4 5 6	1 2 3 4 5 6	1 2 3 4 5 6	Yes	No
Thurs.	___/___	___	1 2 3 4 5 6	1 2 3 4 5 6	1 2 3 4 5 6	1 2 3 4 5 6	Yes	No
Fri.	___/___	___	1 2 3 4 5 6	1 2 3 4 5 6	1 2 3 4 5 6	1 2 3 4 5 6	Yes	No
Sat.	___/___	___	1 2 3 4 5 6	1 2 3 4 5 6	1 2 3 4 5 6	1 2 3 4 5 6	Yes	No
Sun.	___/___	___	1 2 3 4 5 6	1 2 3 4 5 6	1 2 3 4 5 6	1 2 3 4 5 6	Yes	No

Name: _____ ID No.: __ __ __ __ __ __ __ __   Date: __ __ / __ __ / __ __

Severity Ratings: 1 = Not at all, 2 = Minimal, 3 = Mild, 4 = Moderate, 5 = Severe, 6 = Extreme

Day	Date	Menstru-ating?	More sexual interest	Less sexual interest	Drink alcohol, use nonprescribed drugs	Drink coffee, tea, cold drinks	Comments on page 8	
Mon.	___/___	___	1 2 3 4 5 6	1 2 3 4 5 6	1 2 3 4 5 6	1 2 3 4 5 6	Yes	No
Tues.	___/___	___	1 2 3 4 5 6	1 2 3 4 5 6	1 2 3 4 5 6	1 2 3 4 5 6	Yes	No
Wed.	___/___	___	1 2 3 4 5 6	1 2 3 4 5 6	1 2 3 4 5 6	1 2 3 4 5 6	Yes	No
Thurs.	___/___	___	1 2 3 4 5 6	1 2 3 4 5 6	1 2 3 4 5 6	1 2 3 4 5 6	Yes	No
Fri.	___/___	___	1 2 3 4 5 6	1 2 3 4 5 6	1 2 3 4 5 6	1 2 3 4 5 6	Yes	No
Sat.	___/___	___	1 2 3 4 5 6	1 2 3 4 5 6	1 2 3 4 5 6	1 2 3 4 5 6	Yes	No
Sun.	___/___	___	1 2 3 4 5 6	1 2 3 4 5 6	1 2 3 4 5 6	1 2 3 4 5 6	Yes	No
Mon.	___/___	___	1 2 3 4 5 6	1 2 3 4 5 6	1 2 3 4 5 6	1 2 3 4 5 6	Yes	No
Tues.	___/___	___	1 2 3 4 5 6	1 2 3 4 5 6	1 2 3 4 5 6	1 2 3 4 5 6	Yes	No
Wed.	___/___	___	1 2 3 4 5 6	1 2 3 4 5 6	1 2 3 4 5 6	1 2 3 4 5 6	Yes	No
Thurs.	___/___	___	1 2 3 4 5 6	1 2 3 4 5 6	1 2 3 4 5 6	1 2 3 4 5 6	Yes	No
Fri.	___/___	___	1 2 3 4 5 6	1 2 3 4 5 6	1 2 3 4 5 6	1 2 3 4 5 6	Yes	No
Sat.	___/___	___	1 2 3 4 5 6	1 2 3 4 5 6	1 2 3 4 5 6	1 2 3 4 5 6	Yes	No
Sun.	___/___	___	1 2 3 4 5 6	1 2 3 4 5 6	1 2 3 4 5 6	1 2 3 4 5 6	Yes	No
Mon.	___/___	___	1 2 3 4 5 6	1 2 3 4 5 6	1 2 3 4 5 6	1 2 3 4 5 6	Yes	No
Tues.	___/___	___	1 2 3 4 5 6	1 2 3 4 5 6	1 2 3 4 5 6	1 2 3 4 5 6	Yes	No
Wed.	___/___	___	1 2 3 4 5 6	1 2 3 4 5 6	1 2 3 4 5 6	1 2 3 4 5 6	Yes	No
Thurs.	___/___	___	1 2 3 4 5 6	1 2 3 4 5 6	1 2 3 4 5 6	1 2 3 4 5 6	Yes	No
Fri.	___/___	___	1 2 3 4 5 6	1 2 3 4 5 6	1 2 3 4 5 6	1 2 3 4 5 6	Yes	No
Sat.	___/___	___	1 2 3 4 5 6	1 2 3 4 5 6	1 2 3 4 5 6	1 2 3 4 5 6	Yes	No
Sun.	___/___	___	1 2 3 4 5 6	1 2 3 4 5 6	1 2 3 4 5 6	1 2 3 4 5 6	Yes	No
Mon.	___/___	___	1 2 3 4 5 6	1 2 3 4 5 6	1 2 3 4 5 6	1 2 3 4 5 6	Yes	No
Tues.	___/___	___	1 2 3 4 5 6	1 2 3 4 5 6	1 2 3 4 5 6	1 2 3 4 5 6	Yes	No
Wed.	___/___	___	1 2 3 4 5 6	1 2 3 4 5 6	1 2 3 4 5 6	1 2 3 4 5 6	Yes	No
Thurs.	___/___	___	1 2 3 4 5 6	1 2 3 4 5 6	1 2 3 4 5 6	1 2 3 4 5 6	Yes	No
Fri.	___/___	___	1 2 3 4 5 6	1 2 3 4 5 6	1 2 3 4 5 6	1 2 3 4 5 6	Yes	No
Sat.	___/___	___	1 2 3 4 5 6	1 2 3 4 5 6	1 2 3 4 5 6	1 2 3 4 5 6	Yes	No
Sun.	___/___	___	1 2 3 4 5 6	1 2 3 4 5 6	1 2 3 4 5 6	1 2 3 4 5 6	Yes	No
Mon.	___/___	___	1 2 3 4 5 6	1 2 3 4 5 6	1 2 3 4 5 6	1 2 3 4 5 6	Yes	No
Tues.	___/___	___	1 2 3 4 5 6	1 2 3 4 5 6	1 2 3 4 5 6	1 2 3 4 5 6	Yes	No
Wed.	___/___	___	1 2 3 4 5 6	1 2 3 4 5 6	1 2 3 4 5 6	1 2 3 4 5 6	Yes	No
Thurs.	___/___	___	1 2 3 4 5 6	1 2 3 4 5 6	1 2 3 4 5 6	1 2 3 4 5 6	Yes	No
Fri.	___/___	___	1 2 3 4 5 6	1 2 3 4 5 6	1 2 3 4 5 6	1 2 3 4 5 6	Yes	No
Sat.	___/___	___	1 2 3 4 5 6	1 2 3 4 5 6	1 2 3 4 5 6	1 2 3 4 5 6	Yes	No
Sun.	___/___	___	1 2 3 4 5 6	1 2 3 4 5 6	1 2 3 4 5 6	1 2 3 4 5 6	Yes	No
Mon.	___/___	___	1 2 3 4 5 6	1 2 3 4 5 6	1 2 3 4 5 6	1 2 3 4 5 6	Yes	No
Tues.	___/___	___	1 2 3 4 5 6	1 2 3 4 5 6	1 2 3 4 5 6	1 2 3 4 5 6	Yes	No
Wed.	___/___	___	1 2 3 4 5 6	1 2 3 4 5 6	1 2 3 4 5 6	1 2 3 4 5 6	Yes	No
Thurs.	___/___	___	1 2 3 4 5 6	1 2 3 4 5 6	1 2 3 4 5 6	1 2 3 4 5 6	Yes	No
Fri.	___/___	___	1 2 3 4 5 6	1 2 3 4 5 6	1 2 3 4 5 6	1 2 3 4 5 6	Yes	No
Sat.	___/___	___	1 2 3 4 5 6	1 2 3 4 5 6	1 2 3 4 5 6	1 2 3 4 5 6	Yes	No
Sun.	___/___	___	1 2 3 4 5 6	1 2 3 4 5 6	1 2 3 4 5 6	1 2 3 4 5 6	Yes	No

Name: _____   ID No.: _ _ _ _ _ _ _ _   Date: _ _ / _ _ / _ _

Severity Ratings: 1 = Not at all, 2 = Minimal, 3 = Mild, 4 = Moderate, 5 = Severe, 6 = Extreme

Day	Date	Menstru- ating?	Smoke	_____	_____	_____	Comments on page 8	
Mon.	___/___	_____	1 2 3 4 5 6	1 2 3 4 5 6	1 2 3 4 5 6	1 2 3 4 5 6	Yes	No
Tues.	___/___	_____	1 2 3 4 5 6	1 2 3 4 5 6	1 2 3 4 5 6	1 2 3 4 5 6	Yes	No
Wed.	___/___	_____	1 2 3 4 5 6	1 2 3 4 5 6	1 2 3 4 5 6	1 2 3 4 5 6	Yes	No
Thurs.	___/___	_____	1 2 3 4 5 6	1 2 3 4 5 6	1 2 3 4 5 6	1 2 3 4 5 6	Yes	No
Fri.	___/___	_____	1 2 3 4 5 6	1 2 3 4 5 6	1 2 3 4 5 6	1 2 3 4 5 6	Yes	No
Sat.	___/___	_____	1 2 3 4 5 6	1 2 3 4 5 6	1 2 3 4 5 6	1 2 3 4 5 6	Yes	No
Sun.	___/___	_____	1 2 3 4 5 6	1 2 3 4 5 6	1 2 3 4 5 6	1 2 3 4 5 6	Yes	No
Mon.	___/___	_____	1 2 3 4 5 6	1 2 3 4 5 6	1 2 3 4 5 6	1 2 3 4 5 6	Yes	No
Tues.	___/___	_____	1 2 3 4 5 6	1 2 3 4 5 6	1 2 3 4 5 6	1 2 3 4 5 6	Yes	No
Wed.	___/___	_____	1 2 3 4 5 6	1 2 3 4 5 6	1 2 3 4 5 6	1 2 3 4 5 6	Yes	No
Thurs.	___/___	_____	1 2 3 4 5 6	1 2 3 4 5 6	1 2 3 4 5 6	1 2 3 4 5 6	Yes	No
Fri.	___/___	_____	1 2 3 4 5 6	1 2 3 4 5 6	1 2 3 4 5 6	1 2 3 4 5 6	Yes	No
Sat.	___/___	_____	1 2 3 4 5 6	1 2 3 4 5 6	1 2 3 4 5 6	1 2 3 4 5 6	Yes	No
Sun.	___/___	_____	1 2 3 4 5 6	1 2 3 4 5 6	1 2 3 4 5 6	1 2 3 4 5 6	Yes	No
Mon.	___/___	_____	1 2 3 4 5 6	1 2 3 4 5 6	1 2 3 4 5 6	1 2 3 4 5 6	Yes	No
Tues.	___/___	_____	1 2 3 4 5 6	1 2 3 4 5 6	1 2 3 4 5 6	1 2 3 4 5 6	Yes	No
Wed.	___/___	_____	1 2 3 4 5 6	1 2 3 4 5 6	1 2 3 4 5 6	1 2 3 4 5 6	Yes	No
Thurs.	___/___	_____	1 2 3 4 5 6	1 2 3 4 5 6	1 2 3 4 5 6	1 2 3 4 5 6	Yes	No
Fri.	___/___	_____	1 2 3 4 5 6	1 2 3 4 5 6	1 2 3 4 5 6	1 2 3 4 5 6	Yes	No
Sat.	___/___	_____	1 2 3 4 5 6	1 2 3 4 5 6	1 2 3 4 5 6	1 2 3 4 5 6	Yes	No
Sun.	___/___	_____	1 2 3 4 5 6	1 2 3 4 5 6	1 2 3 4 5 6	1 2 3 4 5 6	Yes	No
Mon.	___/___	_____	1 2 3 4 5 6	1 2 3 4 5 6	1 2 3 4 5 6	1 2 3 4 5 6	Yes	No
Tues.	___/___	_____	1 2 3 4 5 6	1 2 3 4 5 6	1 2 3 4 5 6	1 2 3 4 5 6	Yes	No
Wed.	___/___	_____	1 2 3 4 5 6	1 2 3 4 5 6	1 2 3 4 5 6	1 2 3 4 5 6	Yes	No
Thurs.	___/___	_____	1 2 3 4 5 6	1 2 3 4 5 6	1 2 3 4 5 6	1 2 3 4 5 6	Yes	No
Fri.	___/___	_____	1 2 3 4 5 6	1 2 3 4 5 6	1 2 3 4 5 6	1 2 3 4 5 6	Yes	No
Sat.	___/___	_____	1 2 3 4 5 6	1 2 3 4 5 6	1 2 3 4 5 6	1 2 3 4 5 6	Yes	No
Sun.	___/___	_____	1 2 3 4 5 6	1 2 3 4 5 6	1 2 3 4 5 6	1 2 3 4 5 6	Yes	No
Mon.	___/___	_____	1 2 3 4 5 6	1 2 3 4 5 6	1 2 3 4 5 6	1 2 3 4 5 6	Yes	No
Tues.	___/___	_____	1 2 3 4 5 6	1 2 3 4 5 6	1 2 3 4 5 6	1 2 3 4 5 6	Yes	No
Wed.	___/___	_____	1 2 3 4 5 6	1 2 3 4 5 6	1 2 3 4 5 6	1 2 3 4 5 6	Yes	No
Thurs.	___/___	_____	1 2 3 4 5 6	1 2 3 4 5 6	1 2 3 4 5 6	1 2 3 4 5 6	Yes	No
Fri.	___/___	_____	1 2 3 4 5 6	1 2 3 4 5 6	1 2 3 4 5 6	1 2 3 4 5 6	Yes	No
Sat.	___/___	_____	1 2 3 4 5 6	1 2 3 4 5 6	1 2 3 4 5 6	1 2 3 4 5 6	Yes	No
Sun.	___/___	_____	1 2 3 4 5 6	1 2 3 4 5 6	1 2 3 4 5 6	1 2 3 4 5 6	Yes	No
Mon.	___/___	_____	1 2 3 4 5 6	1 2 3 4 5 6	1 2 3 4 5 6	1 2 3 4 5 6	Yes	No
Tues.	___/___	_____	1 2 3 4 5 6	1 2 3 4 5 6	1 2 3 4 5 6	1 2 3 4 5 6	Yes	No
Wed.	___/___	_____	1 2 3 4 5 6	1 2 3 4 5 6	1 2 3 4 5 6	1 2 3 4 5 6	Yes	No
Thurs.	___/___	_____	1 2 3 4 5 6	1 2 3 4 5 6	1 2 3 4 5 6	1 2 3 4 5 6	Yes	No
Fri.	___/___	_____	1 2 3 4 5 6	1 2 3 4 5 6	1 2 3 4 5 6	1 2 3 4 5 6	Yes	No
Sat.	___/___	_____	1 2 3 4 5 6	1 2 3 4 5 6	1 2 3 4 5 6	1 2 3 4 5 6	Yes	No
Sun.	___/___	_____	1 2 3 4 5 6	1 2 3 4 5 6	1 2 3 4 5 6	1 2 3 4 5 6	Yes	No

Name: _____ ID No.: _ _ _ _ _ _ _ _   Date: _ _ / _ _ / _ _

Note if anything happened on the day that may have affected your physical or mental feelings or behaviors. For example, car accident, bad cold, etc. Continue on back if necessary.

Comments:

Mon. ___/___ ___ _____
Tues. ___/___ ___ _____
Wed. ___/___ ___ _____
Thurs. ___/___ ___ _____
Fri. ___/___ ___ _____
Sat. ___/___ ___ _____
Sun. ___/___ ___ _____

Mon. ___/___ ___ _____
Tues. ___/___ ___ _____
Wed. ___/___ ___ _____
Thurs. ___/___ ___ _____
Fri. ___/___ ___ _____
Sat. ___/___ ___ _____
Sun. ___/___ ___ _____

Mon. ___/___ ___ _____
Tues. ___/___ ___ _____
Wed. ___/___ ___ _____
Thurs. ___/___ ___ _____
Fri. ___/___ ___ _____
Sat. ___/___ ___ _____
Sun. ___/___ ___ _____

Mon. ___/___ ___ _____
Tues. ___/___ ___ _____
Wed. ___/___ ___ _____
Thurs. ___/___ ___ _____
Fri. ___/___ ___ _____
Sat. ___/___ ___ _____
Sun. ___/___ ___ _____

Mon. ___/___ ___ _____
Tues. ___/___ ___ _____
Wed. ___/___ ___ _____
Thurs. ___/___ ___ _____
Fri. ___/___ ___ _____
Sat. ___/___ ___ _____
Sun. ___/___ ___ _____

Mon. ___/___ ___ _____
Tues. ___/___ ___ _____
Wed. ___/___ ___ _____
Thurs. ___/___ ___ _____
Fri. ___/___ ___ _____
Sat. ___/___ ___ _____
Sun. ___/___ ___ _____

Appendix H

PREMENSTRUAL ASSESSMENT FORM—PAST CYCLE VERSION
(PAF—PCV)

Uricl, Halbreich, M.D., Jean Endicott, Ph.D., and Sybil Schacht, M.S.W

This version of the PAF is used to describe changes which occurred during the premenstrual period of the past menstrual cycle. It is generally used in studies in which the regular, 3 cycle, PAF has been completed initially and this form is used for subsequent ratings.

Card No.: _____   ID No.: __ __ __ __ __ __ __   Study No.: __ __
         2-2   2-201   22-229

Name: _____   Phone No.: _____

Dates covered by premenstrual period described: From __ __ __ __ __ __   to __ __ __ __ __ __
                                                           23-289   22-24

Were daily ratings made during the cycle which included the premenstrual period described on the form?

Were daily ratings...	1—No	2—Yes	23
Did you take your temperature?	1—No	2—Yes	26
Was there anything unusual about you cycle?	1—No	2—Yes (describe) _____	27

Was the onset of menses: 1—Early   2—Late   3—On time   28

Did you take any medication during the menstrual cycle or during the premenstrual period? 1—No   2—Yes 29

If yes, please list all medications, dosages, and dates taken. If you are taking medication as part of a study and do not know the name, put "study medication," number of pills, and dates taken. List all medications regardless of reason taken, note reason.

Name of Medication	Dosage/number of pills	Dates taken (from–to)	Reason
_____	30–31_____	_____	_____
_____	32–33_____	_____	_____
_____	34–35_____	_____	_____
_____	36–37_____	_____	_____
_____	38–39_____	_____	_____
_____	40–41_____	_____	_____

Did you take a "study medication?"   1—No   2—Yes   42

If yes, do you think you had any side effects?   1—No   2—Yes (describe) _____ 43

_____

_____

_____

Were you physically ill during the cycle?   1—No   2—Yes (describe and give dates) _____ 44

_____

_____

_____

(Please turn the page.) _____

1—Not applicable, not present at all, or no change from usual level, 2—Minimal change,
3—Mild change,   4—Moderate change,   5—Severe change,   6—Extreme change

Usual Level of Change During
Last Premenstrual Period

Changes Present During Premenstrual Period

Item	1	2	3	4	5	6	
Have rapid changes in mood (e.g., laughing, crying, angry, happy, etc.) all within the same day.	1	2	3	4	5	6	215
Have decreased energy or tend to fatigue easily	1	2	3	4	5	6	216
Have decreased ability to coordinate fine movements, poor motor coordination or clumsiness	1	2	3	4	5	6	217
Feel anxious or more anxious	1	2	3	4	5	6	218
Sleep too much or have difficulty getting up in the morning or from naps.	1	2	3	4	5	6	219
Have a feeling of malaise (i.e., general, non-specific bad feeling or vague sense of mental or physical ill-health)	1	2	3	4	5	6	220
Feel jittery or restless	1	2	3	4	5	6	221
Have loss of appetite	1	2	3	4	5	6	222
Have pain, tenderness, enlargement, or swelling of breasts	1	2	3	4	5	6	223
Have headaches or migraines	1	2	3	4	5	6	224
Be more easily distracted (i.e., attention shifts easily and rapidly)	1	2	3	4	5	6	225
Tend to have accidents, fall, cut self, or break things unintentionally	1	2	3	4	5	6	226
Have nausea or vomiting	1	2	3	4	5	6	227
Show physical agitation (e.g., fidgeting, hand wringing, pacing, can't sit still)	1	2	3	4	5	6	228
Have feelings of weakness	1	2	3	4	5	6	229
Feel that you just "can't cope" or are overwhelmed by ordinary demands	1	2	3	4	5	6	230
Feel insecure	1	2	3	4	5	6	231
Have "flare-ups" of allergy, breathing difficulties, stuffy feeling, or watery discharge from the nose	1	2	3	4	5	6	232
Feel depressed	1	2	3	4	5	6	233
Have periods of dizziness, faintness, vertigo (room spinning), ringing in the ears, numbness, tingling of skin, trembling, lightheadedness	1	2	3	4	5	6	234
Tend to "nag" or quarrel over unimportant issues	1	2	3	4	5	6	235
Think of what it would be like to do something to self, like crash the car, wish to go to sleep and not wake up, or have thoughts of death or suicide	1	2	3	4	5	6	236
Feel less desire to talk or move about (it takes an effort to do so)	1	2	3	4	5	6	237
Become more forgetful	1	2	3	4	5	6	238
Feel dissatisfied with personal appearance	1	2	3	4	5	6	239
Tend to have backaches, joint and muscle pains or stiffness	1	2	3	4	5	6	267
Family or friends know "she is in one of her moods today"	1	2	3	4	5	6	268
Feel "at war" on awakening or have complaints or outbursts about old irritants.	1	2	3	4	5	6	269
Act spiteful	1	2	3	4	5	6	270
Feel lonely	1	2	3	4	5	6	271
Urinate less frequently or in lesser amounts	1	2	3	4	5	6	272
Have weight gain	1	2	3	4	5	6	273
Tend to be intolerant or impatient or to lose the ability to respond to or understand the faults, needs or errors of others	1	2	3	4	5	6	274
Tend to be overtalkative	1	2	3	4	5	6	275
Have relatively steady abdominal heaviness, discomfort or pain	1	2	3	4	5	6	276
Have increased sexual activity or interest (fantasy, with self, with others)	1	2	3	4	5	6	277
Have trouble sleeping	1	2	3	4	5	6	278
Check, if wake early in morning and can't get back to sleep							214

Changes Present During Premenstrual Period	Usual Level of Change During Last Premenstrual Period						
Have intermittent pain or cramps in the abdomen _ _ _ _ _ _ _ _ _ _ _ _ _ _ _ _	1	2	3	4	5	6	215
Have a decrease in self-esteem (i.e., don't feel good about self or feel a failure)	1	2	3	4	5	6	216
Tend to blame others for problems (personal, at home, work, school, etc)_ _ _	1	2	3	4	5	6	217
Have increase in activity, organization, efficiency, or involvement socially, at home or work _	1	2	3	4	5	6	218
Tend to brood over unpleasant events _	1	2	3	4	5	6	219
Have skin problems such as acne, pimples, etc _ _ _ _ _ _ _ _ _ _ _ _ _ _	1	2	3	4	5	6	220
Have edema, swelling, puffiness, or "water retention" _ _ _ _ _ _ _ _ _ _ _ _	1	2	3	4	5	6	221
Stay at home more _	1	2	3	4	5	6	222
Have less sexual interest or activity (fantasy, self, others) _ _ _ _ _ _ _ _ _ _	1	2	3	4	5	6	223
Tend to avoid social activities _	1	2	3	4	5	6	224
Feel bloated _	1	2	3	4	5	6	225
Have lowered performance, output, efficiency or ease, in tasks at work, at home, or with hobbies, etc _ _ _ _ _ _ _ _ _ _ _ _ _ _ _ _ _ _	1	2	3	4	5	6	226
Miss time at work because of premenstrual changes _ _ _ _ _ _ _ _ _ _ _ _ _	1	2	3	4	5	6	227
Want to be alone _	1	2	3	4	5	6	228

Subject Index

NOTE: Page numbers in bold face type indicate a major discussion. A *t* following a page number indicates tabular material and an *i* following a page number indicates an illustration. Drugs are listed under their generic names. When a drug trade name is listed, the reader is referred to the generic name.

(more on reverse)

Clinical Science Textbooks

Understanding Health Policy:
A Clinical Approach
Bodenheimer & Grumbach
1995, ISBN 0-8385-3678-6, A3678-8

Clinical Cardiology, 6/e
Cheitlin, Sokolow, & McIlroy
1993, ISBN 0-8385-1093-0, A1093-2

Fluid & Electrolytes
Physiology & Pathophysiology
Cogan
1991, ISBN 0-8385-2546-6, A2546-8

Basic & Clinical Biostatistics, 2/e
Dawson-Saunders & Trapp
1994, ISBN 0-8385-0542-2, A0542-9

Basic Gynecology and Obstetrics
Gant & Cunningham
1993, ISBN 0-8385-9633-9, A9633-7

Review of General Psychiatry, 4/e
Goldman
1995, ISBN 0-8385-8421-7, A8421-8

Principles of Clinical
Electrocardiography, 13/e
Goldschlager & Goldman
1990, ISBN 0-8385-7951-5, A7951-5

Clinical Neurology, 2/e
Greenberg, Aminoff, & Simon
1993, ISBN 0-8385-1311-5, A1311-8

Medical Epidemiology
Greenberg, Daniels, Flanders, Eley, &
Boring
1993, ISBN 0-8385-6206-X, A6206-5

Basic & Clinical Endocrinology, 4/e
Greenspan & Baxter
1994, ISBN 0-8385-0560-0, A0560-1

Occupational Medicine
LaDou
1990, ISBN 0-8385-7207-3, A7207-2

Primary Care of Women
Lemcke, Pattison, Marshall, & Cowley
1995, ISBN 0-8385-9813-7, A9813-5

Clinical Anesthesiology, 2/e
Morgan & Mikhail
1995, ISBN 0-8385-1381-6, A1381-1

Dermatology
Orkin, Maibach, & Dahl
1991, ISBN 0-8385-1288-7, A1288-8

Rudolph's Fundamentals of
Pediatrics
Rudolph & Kamei
1994, ISBN 0-8385-8233-8, A8233-7

Genetics in Clinical Medicine and
Primary Care
Seashore
1995, ISBN 0-8385-3128-8, A3128-4

Smith's General Urology, 14/e
Tanagho & McAninch
1995, ISBN 0-8385-8612-0, A8612-2

Clinical Oncology
Weiss
1993, ISBN 0-8385-1325-5, A1325-8

General Opthalmology, 14/e
Vaughan, Asbury, & Riordan-Eva
1995, ISBN 0-8385-3127-X, A3127-6

CURRENT Clinical References

CURRENT Critical Care Diagnosis &
Treatment, 2/e
Bongard & Sue
1995, ISBN 0-8385-1454-5, A1454-6

CURRENT Diagnosis & Treatment in
Cardiology
Crawford
1995, ISBN 0-8385-1444-8, A1444-7

CURRENT Diagnosis & Treatment in
Vascular Surgery
Dean, Yao, & Brewster
1995, ISBN 0-8385-1351-4, A1351-4

CURRENT Obstetric & Gynecologic
Diagnosis & Treatment, 8/e
DeCherney & Pernoll
1994, ISBN 0-8385-1447-2, A1447-0

CURRENT Pediatric Diagnosis &
Treatment, 12/e
Hay, Groothuis, Hayward, & Levin
1995, ISBN 0-8385-1446-4, A1446-2

CURRENT Emergency Diagnosis &
Treatment, 5/e
Saunders & Ho
1995, ISBN 0-8385-1450-2, A1450-4

CURRENT Diagnosis & Treatment in
Orthopedics
Skinner
1995, ISBN 0-8385-1009-4, A1009-8

CURRENT Medical Diagnosis &
Treatment 1995
Tierney, McPhee, & Papadakis
1995, ISBN 0-8385-1449-9, A1449-6

CURRENT Surgical Diagnosis &
Treatment, 10/e
Way
1994, ISBN 0-8385-1439-1, A1439-7

LANGE Clinical Manuals

Dermatology
Diagnosis and Therapy
Bondi, Jegasothy, & Lazarus
1991, ISBN 0-8385-1274-7, A1274-8

Practical Oncology
Cameron
1994, ISBN 0-8385-1326-3, A1326-6

Office & Bedside Procedures
Chesnutt, Dewar, Locksley, & Tureen
1993, ISBN 0-8385-1095-7, A1095-7

Psychiatry
Diagnosis & Therapy 2/e
Flaherty, Davis, & Janicak
1993, ISBN 0-8385-1267-4, A1267-2

Neonatology
Management, Procedures, On-Call
Problems, Diseases and Drugs, 3/e
Gomella
1994, ISBN 0-8385-1331-X, A1331-6

Practical Gynecology
Jacobs & Gast
1994, ISBN 0-8385-1336-0, A1336-5

Drug Therapy, 2/e
Katzung
1991, ISBN 0-8385-1312-3, A1312-6

Ambulatory Medicine
The Primary Care of Families
Mengel & Schwiebert
1993, ISBN 0-8385-1294-1, A1294-6

Poisoning & Drug Overdose, 2/e
Olson
1994, ISBN 0-8385-1108-2, A1108-8

Internal Medicine
Diagnosis and Therapy, 3/e
Stein
1993, ISBN 0-8385-1112-0, A1112-0

Surgery
Diagnosis & Therapy
Stillman
1989, ISBN 0-8385-1283-6, A1283-9

Medical Perioperative Management
Wolfsthal
1989, ISBN 0-8385-1298-4, A1298-7

LANGE Handbooks

Handbook of Gynecology &
Obstetrics
Brown & Crombleholme
1993, ISBN 0-8385-3608-5, A3608-5

HIV/AIDS Primary Care Handbook
Carmichael, Carmichael, & Fischl
1995, ISBN 0-8385-3557-7, A3557-4

Pocket Guide to Diagnostic Tests
Detmer, McPhee, Nicoll, & Chou
1992, ISBN 0-8385-8020-3, A8020-8

Handbook of Poisoning
Prevention, Diagnosis & Treatment,
12/e
Dreisbach & Robertson
1987, ISBN 0-8385-3643-3, A3643-2

Handbook of Clinical Endocrinology,
2/e
Fitzgerald
1992, ISBN 0-8385-3615-8, A3615-0

Clinician's Pocket Reference, 7/e
Gomella
1993, ISBN 0-8385-1222-4, A1222-7

Surgery on Call, 2/e
Gomella & Lefor
1995, ISBN 0-8385-8746-1, A8746-8

Pocket Guide to Commonly
Prescribed Drugs
Levine
1993, ISBN 0-8385-8023-8, A8023-2

Handbook of Pediatrics, 17/e
Merenstein, Kaplan, & Rosenberg
1994, ISBN 0-8385-3657-3, A3657-2

 Appleton & Lange • 25 Van Zant Street • P.O. Box 5630 • Norwalk, CT • 06856